Osteoarthritis

Second edition

Oxford Medical Publications

Osteoarthritis

Second edition

Edited by

Kenneth D. Brandt

Rheumatology Division, Department of Medicine, and Department of Orthopaedic Surgery
Indiana University School of Medicine
USA

Michael Doherty

Nottingham University Medical School
Nottingham
UK

L. Stefan Lohmander

University Hospital
Lund
Sweden

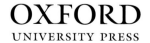

OXFORD
UNIVERSITY PRESS

OXFORD
UNIVERSITY PRESS

Great Clarendon Street, Oxford OX2 6DP

Oxford University Press is a department of the University of Oxford.
It furthers the University's objective of excellence in research, scholarship,
and education by publishing worldwide in

Oxford New York

Auckland Cape Town Dar es Salaam Hong Kong Karachi
Kuala Lumpur Madrid Melbourne Mexico City Nairobi
New Delhi Shanghai Taipei Toronto

With offices in

Argentina Austria Brazil Chile Czech Republic France Greece
Guatemala Hungary Italy Japan South Korea Poland Portugal
Singapore Switzerland Thailand Turkey Ukraine Vietnam

Oxford is a registered trade mark of Oxford University Press
in the UK and in certain other countries

Published in the United States
by Oxford University Press Inc., New York

© Oxford University Press, 2003

British Library Cataloguing in Publication Data

Data available

Library of Congress Cataloging in Publication Data

ISBN 0 19 850967 7 (Hbk.)

10 9 8 7 6 5 4 3 2

Typeset in Minion
by Newgen Imaging Systems (P) Ltd., Chennai, India
Printed in China

Acknowledgements

The efficient and highly competent secretarial support that the editors received from Joanna Ramowski in Nottingham and Viveca Wiklund in Lund is hugely appreciated; without their efforts this book would not have seen the light of day. In Indianapolis, as usual, Deborah Jenkins provided excellent secretarial support. In addition, as was the case when we put together the 1st edition of this book, the initiative, enthusiasm, and dedication to the task shown by Kathie Lane was exemplary. Her professionalism in working with the editors and representatives of the Oxford University Press and, particularly, her help in proofing and editing, make this book much better than it would have been otherwise. Furthermore, without her diplomacy in reeling in chapters that seemed to be in limbo, we could not have met our deadline.

Finally, we are grateful to Pharmacia for their generous support, which helped defray production costs for the 2nd edition and, in particular, permitted the use of colour throughout the book.

Preface

A number of exciting new developments make it highly desirable at this time to summarize the large body of knowledge related to the etiopathogenesis and management of osteoarthritis. For years, many primary care physicians and, indeed, many rheumatologists have considered osteoarthritis to be a boring condition for which they had little to offer patients. Osteoarthritis has been viewed by physicians and surgeons, erroneously, as an inevitable consequence of aging or repetitive usage of a joint and a condition which, once it becomes symptomatic, progresses inexorably. Doctors and allied health professionals have conveyed these misconceptions and oversimplifications to millions of patients. Consider the nihilism, pessimism and futility engendered in those patients by such remarks!

But things are changing—and changing rapidly. Our understanding of mechanisms underlying the breakdown of articular cartilage in osteoarthritis has grown greatly in the past several years—perhaps to an even greater extent than our awareness that osteoarthritis is not a disease simply of cartilage, but of an organ, the diarthrodial joint. Osteoarthritis represents failure of the joint. It may be due in some instances to a primary abnormality in the articular cartilage, but in other cases the initial problem resides in the underlying bone, the synovium, the supporting ligaments or the neuromuscular system.

The above two paragraphs are quotations from the Preface to the 1st edition of *Osteoarthritis*. And how rapidly things continue to change! For example, the 4 year interval between the publication of the 1st edition and the 2nd has witnessed the important development of cyclooxygenase-2 selective inhibitors, such as celecoxib and rofecoxib, which are now used widely in management of osteoarthritis (OA). The new chapter on nonsteroidal anti-inflammatory drugs (NSAIDs) in the 2nd edition discusses this topic in considerable detail. The juxtaposed chapter on economic considerations in pharmacologic management of OA has also been entirely rewritten. Both chapters have new authors.

Another important therapeutic development in the interval between the 1st and 2nd editions is intra-articular hyaluronan therapy. The true efficacy of this treatment with respect to relief of joint pain and modification of structural damage in the OA joint has generated sufficient heat and controversy that an entire chapter is now devoted to this topic. Given that results of sham-controlled clinical trials of joint irrigation are now available, a chapter also on this form of intra-articular therapy is now included.

The 2nd edition differs from the 1st also in a number of other significant respects: The chapters on physical therapy and occupational therapy have been rewritten, with new authorship for both. Chapters have also been added on exercise in management of OA; weight loss and patient adherence. The section of the book dealing with the pathogenesis of OA has been updated considerably, in the light of new knowledge: chapters have been added which discuss protective muscular reflexes; proprioception; the importance of local mechanical factors, such as joint laxity and malalignment; peripheral and central mechanisms relating to the pathogenesis of OA pain; and the possible role of vitamin deficiencies and antioxidants in the pathogenesis of OA. The importance of bone in the pathogenesis of OA is reflected by the fact that three chapters are now devoted to this topic. Whereas discussion of hereditary OA was covered in a single chapter in the 1st edition, three chapters are now devoted to genetic aspects of OA. The chapter on synovial physiology has also been wholly rewritten.

The section of the book dealing with therapy continues to reflect the recognition that optimal management of OA requires a comprehensive program involving both pharmacologic agents and nonmedicinal measures and, in some cases, surgery. It is the belief of the editors that it remains necessary to dispel the widely held notion that medical management is 'conservative' while surgery is 'radical' therapy, whereas the opposite is often true—i.e., withholding surgery from patients with advanced disease while they become increasingly deconditioned is, in fact, the radical approach; in such instances it may be much more conservative to operate. A recent analysis of outcomes of patients undergoing total hip and total knee arthroplasty supports that view.

As indicated in the 1st edition, studies of animal models have shown that the development and progression of OA may be prevented or retarded with pharmacologic or biologic agents. The past few years have witnessed further progress in the development of disease-modifying drugs for osteoarthritis (DMOADs). Clinical trials of such therapy have already been undertaken in humans. A new chapter is devoted to the possible role of nutraceuticals, such as glucosamine and chondroitin sulfate, in modification of structural damage in the OA joint. The outcome measures available for assessment of a DMOAD effect in clinical trials, and limitations thereof, are also discussed.

The numerous changes that have been made in the 2nd edition of *Osteoarthritis* reflect the rapid, broad, exciting progress which has occurred in the past few years. The new topics and changes in authorship, providing expertise in the new areas of discussion, reflect those changes. For the editors, these changes have assured that their work on this book has been both educational and fun.

The primary care physician, clinical rheumatologist, orthopaedic surgeon, allied health professional, basic researcher, those in the pharmaceutical industry who are involved in development of drugs and biologicals for osteoarthritis, and regulatory agency staff should all find this book useful. The high prevalence of OA—which will continue to increase because of the aging of the population—guarantees that health professionals will see a growing number of patients with OA. The need for a timely review of the evidence that drives our current understanding of optimal management of OA and of the basic mechanisms involved in its etiopathogenesis serves as the rationale for the 2nd edition, whose authors continue to represent experts on OA from both sides of the Atlantic.

Kenneth D. Brandt   March 2003
Michael Doherty
L. Stefan Lohmander

Contents

List of Contributors

Abramson, Steven B.; New York University School of Medicine, Hospital for Joint Diseases, New York, NY, USA

Anis, Aslam H.; Centre for Health Evaluation and Outcome Sciences, St. Paul's Hospital, Vancouver, BC, Canada

Ang, Dennis C.; Rheumatology Division, Indiana University School of Medicine Indianapolis, IN, USA

Aspnes, Ann; Department of Psychiatry and Behavioral Sciences, Duke University Medical Center, Durham, NC, USA

Ayral, Xavier; Department of Rheumatology, Cochin Hospital, René Descartes University, Paris, France

Barlow, Julie; The Interdisciplinary Research Centre in Health, Coventry University, Coventry, UK

Bayliss, Michael; Department of Veterinary Basic Sciences, The Royal Veterinary College, London, UK

Bellamy, Nicholas; CONROD, Faculty of Health Sciences, University of Queensland, Queensland, Australia

Bischoff, Heike A.; Department of Medicine, Harvard Medical School, Brigham & Women's Hospital, Boston, MA, USA

Bradley, John D.; Rheumatology Division, Indiana University School of Medicine, and Wishard Memorial Hospital, Indianapolis, IN, USA

Brandt, Kenneth D.; Rheumatology Division, Department of Medicine, and Department of Orthopaedic Surgery, Indiana University School of Medicine, Indianapolis, IN, USA

Buckland-Wright, J. Christopher; University of London, Applied Clinical Anatomy Research Centre, King's College London, School of Biomedical Sciences, London, UK

Buckwalter, Joseph A.; Department of Orthopaedic Surgery, University of Iowa Hospitals, Iowa city, IA, USA

Burr, David B.; Department of Anatomy and Cell Biology, Indiana University School of Medicine, Indianapolis, IN, USA

Caldwell, David S.; Division of Rheumatology and Immunology, Department of Medicine, Duke University Medical Center, Durham, NC, USA

Carr, Alison; Academic Rheumatology, University of Nottingham, Nottingham, UK

Cibere, Jolanda; Arthritis Research Centre of Canada, Vancouver, BC, Canada

Cooper, Cyrus; MRC Environmental Epidemiology Unit, Southampton General Hospital, University of Southampton, Southampton, UK

Dennison, Elaine; MRC Environmental Epidemiology Unit, Southampton General Hospital, University of Southampton, Southampton, UK

Dieppe, Paul MRC Health Services Research Collaboration, University of Bristol, Bristol, UK

DiMicco, Michael A.; Centre for Biomedical Engineering, Massachusetts institute of Technology, and Children's Hospital, Harvard Medical School, Cambridge, MA, USA

Doherty, Michael; Academic Rheumatology, Nottingham City Hospital, Nottingham, UK

Felson, David; Boston University Arthritis Center and the Department of Medicine at Boston City and Boston University Medical Center Hospital, Boston, MA, USA

Flores, Raymond; Department of Medicine, University of Maryland School of Medicine, Baltimore, MD, USA

Ghosh, Peter; Institute of bone and joint research, Royal North Shore Hospital, St Leonards, NSW, Australia

Griffiths, R.J.; Inflammation Biology, Pfizer Global Research and Development, Groton, CT, USA

Grodzinsky, Alan J.; Departments of Electrical and Mechanical Engineering and Biological Engineering Division, Massachusetts Institute of Technology, Cambridge, MA, USA

Hadler, Nortin M.; Department of Medicine, University of North Carolina at Chapel Hill School of Medicine, Chapel Hill, NC, USA

Hart, Deborah J.; Department of Rheumatology, St. Thomas' Hospital, London, UK

Hassett, Geraldine; Department of Rheumatology, St. Thomas' Hospital, London, UK

Heinegard, Dick; Department of Cell and Molecular Biology, University of Lund, Lund, Sweden

Hochberg, Marc; Departments of Medicine and Epidemiology and Preventive Medicine, University of Maryland School of Medicine, Baltimore, MD, USA

Hurley, Michael V.; Rehabilitation Research Unit, Physiotherapy Division, King's College London, London, UK

Hung, Clark T.; Department of Biomedical Engineering, Columbia University, New York, NY, USA

Hunziker, Ernst B.; ITI Research Institute, University of Bern, Switzerland

Ingvarsson, Thorvaldur; Akureyri University Hospital, Akureyri, Iceland

Jones, Adrian; Rheumatology Unit, Nottingham City Hospital, Nottingham, UK

Kashikar-Zuck, Susmita; Department of Psychiatry and Behavioral Sciences, Duke University Medical Center, Durham, NC, USA

Keefe, Francis J.; Department of Psychiatry and Behavioral Sciences, Duke University Medical Center, Durham, NC, USA

Kidd, Bruce; Bone and Joint Research Unit, St. Barts and the Royal London School of Medicine and Dentistry, London, UK

Kim, Young-Jo; Children's Hospital, Harvard Medical School, Boston, MA, USA

Knutson, Kaj; Department of Orthopaedics, University Hospital, Lund, Sweden

Kraus, Virginia Byers; Department of Medicine, Division of Rheumatology, Duke University Medical Center, Durham, NC, USA

Kroenke, Kurt; Regenstrief Institute for Health Care, Indianapolis, IN, USA

Liang, H. Mathew; Department of Medicine, Harvard Medical School, Brigham & Women's Hospital, Boston, MA, USA

Lohmander, L. Stefan; Department of Orthopedics, University Hospital, Lund, Sweden

Lorenzo, Pilar; Department of Cell and Molecular Biology, University of Lund, Lund, Sweden

Lorig, Kate; Stanford University, Palo Alto, CA, USA

Manek, Nisha; Twin Research and Genetic Epidemiology Unit, St. Thomas' Hospital, London, UK

Marra, Carlo A.; Centre for Health Evaluation and Outcome Sciences, St. Paul's Hospital, Vancouver, BC, Canada

Martin, Eden R.; Department of Medicine, Section of Medical Genetics, Duke University Medical Center, Durham, NC, USA

Mazucca, Steven A.; Rheumatology Division, Indiana University School of Medicine, Indianapolis, IN, USA

McAlindon, Timothy E.; Boston University School of Medicine, Boston, MA, USA

Melvin, Jeanne L.; Chronic Pain and Fibromyalgia Management Programs, Cedars-Sinai Medical Center, Los Angeles, CA, USA

Minor, Marian A.; Department of Physical Therapy, School of Health Professions, University of Missouri, Columbia, MO, USA

Mow, Van C.; Department of Biomedical Engineering and New York Orthopaedic Hospital Research Laboratory, Columbia University, New York, NY, USA

Myers, Stephen L.; Eli Lilly and Company, Indianapolis, IN, USA

Muir, Kenneth R.; Department of Public Health Medicine and Epidemiology, Queen's Medical Center, Nottingham, UK

O'Connor, Brian L.; Indiana University School of Medicine, Indianapolis, IN, USA

O'Reilly, Sheila; Rheumatology Unit, Nottingham City Hospital, Nottingham, UK

Peterfy, Charles G.; Synarc, San Francisco, CA, USA

Plaas, Anna H.K.; Biochemistry and Molecular Biology, University of South Florida, and Center for Research in Paediatric Orthopaedics, Shriners Hospital, Tampa, FL, USA

Poole, A. Robin; Joint Diseases Laboratory and Department of Surgery, Shriner's Hospital for Crippled Children, Montreal, Quebec, Canada

Pritzker, Kenneth P.H.; Pathology and Laboratory Medicine, Mount Sinai Hospital, Toronto, Ontario, Canada and University of Toronto, Canada

Reid, David M.; Department of Medicine and Therapeutics, University of Aberdeen, Aberdeen, UK

Rogers, Juliet; Bristol Royal Infirmary, Bristol, UK (deceased)

Roos, Ewa M.; Department of Orthopedics, University Hospital, Lund, Sweden

Rosenthal, Ann K.; Division of Rheumatology, Department of Medicine, Medical College of Wisconsin, and the Zablocki Veterans Administration Medical Center, Milwaukee, WI, USA

Ryan, Lawrence M.; Division of Rheumatology, Department of Medicine, Medical College of Wisconsin, Milwaukee, WI, USA

Sandy, John D.; Department of Pharmacology and Therapeutics, University of South Florida, and Senior Scientist, Center for Research in Skeletal Development and Pediatric Orthopedics, Shriners Hospital, Tampa, FL, USA

Schrier, D.J.; Inflammation Pharmacology, Pfizer Global Research and Development, Ann Arbor, MI, USA

Schauwecker, Donald S.; Department of Radiology, Indiana University School of Medicine, Indianapolis, IN, USA

Sharma, Leena; Division of Rheumatology, Northwestern University Medical School, Chicago, IL, USA

Simkin, Peter A.; Division of Rheumatology, University of Washington, Seattle, WA, USA

Spector, Tim D.; Twin Research and Genetic Epidemiology Unit, St Thomas' Hospital, London, UK

Stefansson, Stefan Einar; deCODE, Reykjavik, Iceland

Tyler, Jenny; Strangeways Research Laboratory, Cambridge, UK

van Beuningen, Henk M.; University Medical Centre Nijmegen, Nijmegen, the Netherlands

van der Kraan, Peter M.; University Medical Centre Nijmegen, Nijmegen, the Netherlands

van den Berg, Wim B.; University Medical Centre Nijmegen, Nijmegen, the Netherlands

Vilensky, Joel A.; Indiana University School of Medicine, Fort Wayne, IN, USA

Walsh, Nicola; Rehabilitation Research Unit, Physiotherapy Division, King's College London, London, UK

Watt, Iain; Directorate of Clinical Radiology, Bristol Royal Infirmary, Bristol, UK

Webber, Jonathan; Clinical Nutrition Unit, Queen's Medical Center, Nottingham, UK

Westacott, C.I.; Department of Pathology and Microbiology, University of Bristol, School of Medical Sciences, University Walk, Bristol, UK

Weinberger, Morris; Department of Health Policy and Administration, University of North Carolina at Chapel Hill, Chapel Hill, NC, USA

Yelin, Edward; Arthritis Research Group, University of California, San Francisco, CA, USA

1 Definition and classification of osteoarthritis

Raymond H. Flores and Marc C. Hochberg

Osteoarthritis (OA), formerly referred to as osteoarthrosis and degenerative joint disease, is the most common form of arthritis.[1,2] Prior to 1986, no standard definition of OA existed; most authors described OA as a disorder of unknown etiology that primarily affects the articular cartilage and subchondral bone in contrast to rheumatoid arthritis, a disorder that primarily affects the synovial membrane. In that year, the Subcommittee on Osteoarthritis of the American College of Rheumatology Diagnostic and Therapeutic Criteria Committee, proposed the following definition of OA: a heterogeneous group of conditions that lead to joint symptoms and signs which are associated with the defective integrity of articular cartilage, in addition to related changes in the underlying bone at the joint margins.[3]

A more comprehensive definition of OA was developed at the 'Workshop on Etiopathogenesis of Osteoarthritis' sponsored by the National Institute of Arthritis, Diabetes, Digestive, and Kidney Diseases, the National Institute on Aging, the American Academy of Orthopedic Surgeons, the National Arthritis Advisory Board, and the Arthritis Foundation.[4] This definition summarized the clinical, pathophysiologic, biochemical, and biomechanical changes that characterize OA:

> Clinically, the disease is characterized by joint pain, tenderness, limitation of movement, crepitus, occasional effusion, and variable degrees of local inflammation, but without systemic effects. Pathologically, the disease is characterized by irregularly distributed loss of cartilage more frequently in areas of increased load, sclerosis of subchondral bone, subchondral cysts, marginal osteophytes, increased metaphyseal blood flow, and variable synovial inflammation. Histologically, the disease is characterized early by fragmentation of the cartilage surface, cloning of chondrocytes, vertical clefts in the cartilage, variable crystal deposition, remodeling, and eventual violation of the tidemark by blood vessels. It is also characterized by evidence of repair, particularly in osteophytes, and later by total loss of cartilage, sclerosis, and focal osteonecrosis of the subchondral bone. Biomechanically, the disease is characterized by alteration of the tensile, compressive, and shear properties and hydraulic permeability of the cartilage, increased water, and excessive swelling. These cartilage changes are accompanied by increased stiffness of the subchondral bone. Biochemically, the disease is characterized by reduction in the proteoglycan concentration, possible alterations in the size and aggregation of proteoglycans, alteration in collagen fibril size and weave, and increased synthesis and degradation of matrix macromolecules.

The current definition was developed in 1994 at a workshop entitled 'New Horizons in Osteoarthritis' sponsored by the American Academy of Orthopedic Surgeons, the National Institute of Arthritis, Musculoskeletal and Skin Diseases, the National Institute on Aging, the Arthritis Foundation, and the Orthopaedic Research and Education Foundation.[5] This definition underscores the concept that OA may not represent a single disease entity:

> Osteoarthritis is a group of overlapping distinct diseases, which may have different etiologies but with similar biologic, morphologic, and clinical outcomes. The disease processes not only affect the articular cartilage, but involve the entire joint, including the subchondral bone, ligaments, capsule, synovial membrane, and periarticular muscles. Ultimately, the articular cartilage degenerates with fibrillation, fissures, ulceration, and full thickness loss of the joint surface. ... OA diseases are a result of both mechanical and biologic events that destabilize the normal coupling of degradation and synthesis of articular cartilage chondrocytes and extracellular matrix, and subchondral bone. Although they may be initiated by multiple factors, including genetic, developmental, metabolic, and traumatic, OA diseases involve all of the tissues of the diarthrodial joint. Ultimately, OA diseases are manifested by morphologic, biochemical, molecular, and biomechanical changes of both cells and matrix which lead to a softening, fibrillation, ulceration, loss of articular cartilage, sclerosis and eburnation of subchondral bone, osteophytes, and subchondral cysts. When clinically evident, OA diseases are characterized by joint pain, tenderness, limitation of movement, crepitus, occasional effusion, and variable degrees of inflammation without systemic effects.

Classification of osteoarthritis

OA, as noted above, is a disorder of diverse etiologies, which affects both the small and large joints, either singly or in combination. Table 1.1 contains a classification schema for OA developed at the 'Workshop on Etiopathogenesis of Osteoarthritis'[4] in which idiopathic OA is divided into two forms: localized or generalized; the latter represents the form of OA described by Kellgren and Moore involving three or more joint groups.[6] Furthermore, generalized OA may occur with or without Heberden's and Bouchard's nodes, that is as either a nodal or non-nodal form.

The classification of OA into idiopathic (primary) and secondary forms was based on the knowledge that OA could result from some recognized causative factors. These factors operate largely through two mechanisms: abnormalities of the biomaterials of the joint, usually the articular cartilage; and abnormalities of the biomechanics of the joint, usually due to the abnormal joint structure, resulting in abnormalities in the distribution of loading forces across the joint. Thus, patients with an underlying disease that appears to have caused their OA are classified as having secondary OA. A detailed discussion of several forms of secondary OA can be found elsewhere.[7] While this classification is helpful for teaching and research purposes, it has obvious deficiencies as some risk factors for idiopathic OA, for example obesity, may be considered, alternatively, as causes of secondary OA (see Chapter 2).

Diagnostic criteria for osteoarthritis

Radiographic criteria

Classically, the diagnosis of OA in epidemiological studies has relied on the characteristic radiographic changes described by Kellgren and Lawrence in 1957[8] and illustrated in the *Atlas of Standard Radiographs*.[9] The cardinal radiographic features of OA include: (1) the formation of osteophytes on the joint margins or in ligamentous attachments, as on the tibial spines;

Table 1.1 Classification of osteoarthritis*

I   Idiopathic

  A   Localized

    1   Hands: e.g. Heberden's and Bouchard's nodes (nodal), erosive interphalangeal arthritis (non-nodal), carpal-1st metacarpal

    2   Feet: e.g. hallux valgus, hallux rigidus, contracted toes (hammer/cock-up toes), talonavicular

    3   Knee: (a) medial compartment; (b) lateral compartment; (c) patello-femoral compartment

    4   Hip: (a) eccentric (superior); (b) concentric (axial, medial); (c) diffuse (coxae senilis)

    5   Spine: (a) apophyseal joints; (b) intervertebral joints (discs); (c) spondylosis (osteophytes); (d) ligamentous (hyperostosis, Forestier's disease, DISH)

    6   Other single sites: e.g. glenohumeral, acromioclavicular, tibiotalar, sacroiliac, temporomandibular

  B   Generalized (GOA) includes three or more areas above (6)

II Secondary

  A   Trauma

    1   Acute

    2   Chronic (occupational, sports)

  B   Congenital or developmental diseases

    1   Localized diseases: e.g. Legg–Calve–Perthes, congenital hip dislocation, slipped epiphysis

    2   Mechanical factors: e.g. unequal lower extremity length, valgus/varus deformity, hypermobility syndromes

    3   Bone dysplasias: e.g. epiphyseal dysplasia, spondyloapophyseal dysplasia, osteonychodystrophy

  C   Metabolic diseases

    1   Ochronosis (alkaptonuria)

    2   Hemochromatosis

    3   Wilson's disease

    4   Gaucher's disease

  D   Endocrine diseases

    1   Acromegaly

    2   Hyperparathyroidism

    3   Diabetes mellitus

    4   Obesity

    5   Hypothyroidism

  E   Calcium deposition diseases

    1   Calcium pyrophosphate dihydrate deposition disease

    2   Apatite arthropathy

  F   Other bone and joint diseases

    1   Localized: e.g. fracture, avascular necrosis, infection, gout

    2   Diffuse: rheumatoid (inflammatory) arthritis, Paget's disease, osteopetrosis, osteochondritis

  G   Neuropathic (Charcot) arthropathy

  H   Endemic disorders

    1   Kashin–Beck

    2   Mseleni

  I   Miscellaneous conditions

    1   Frostbite

    2   Caisson's disease

    3   Hemoglobinopathies

* Reproduced from Ref. 4 with permission.

(2) the periarticular ossicles, chiefly in relation to distal and proximal interphalangeal joints; (3) the narrowing of the joint space associated with sclerosis of subchondral bone; (4) the cystic areas with sclerotic walls situated in the subchondral bone; and (5) the altered shape of the bone ends, particularly the head of the femur. Combinations of these changes considered together led the authors to the development of an ordinal grading scheme for severity of radiographic features of OA: 0 = normal; 1 = doubtful; 2 = minimal; 3 = moderate; and 4 = severe. Different joints are graded using different characteristics. For the small joints of the hands, knees, and hips these differences are summarized in Tables 1.2–1.4 and illustrated in Figs. 1.1–1.5, respectively.

A number of potential limitations of the use of the Kellgren–Lawrence grading scale, as illustrated in the *Atlas on Standard Radiographs*, have been noted.[10–13] Foremost among these is the fact that the radiographs of neither the hips nor knees were taken in the weight-bearing position, limiting the ability of the reader to accurately assess joint-space narrowing as a measure of cartilage loss. In an attempt to address the limitations of a global grading scale, several groups developed radiographic grading schema that focus on the individual radiographic features of OA at specific joint groups; reliable grading scales have been published for the hand,[14] hip,[15,16] knee,[17–20] and for all three of these peripheral joint groups.[21,22] The atlas

Table 1.2 Grades of severity of osteoarthritis in the small joints of the hands*

Distal interphalangeal joints:	
Grade 1	Normal joint except for one minimal osteophyte
Grade 2	Definite osteophytes at two points with minimal subchondral sclerosis and doubtful subchondral cysts, but good joint space and no deformity
Grade 3	Moderate osteophytes, some deformity of bone ends and narrowing of joint space
Grade 4	Large osteophytes and deformity of bone ends with loss of joint space, sclerosis, and cysts
Proximal interphalangeal joints:	
Grade 1	Minimal osteophytosis at one point and possible cyst
Grade 2	Definite osteophytes at two points and possible narrowing of joint space at one point
Grade 3	Moderate osteophytes at many points, deformity of bone ends
Grade 4	Large osteophytes, marked narrowing of joint space, subchondral sclerosis, and slight deformity
First carpometacarpal joint:	
Grade 1	Minimal osteophytosis and possible cyst formation
Grade 2	Definite osteophytes and possible cysts
Grade 3	Moderate osteophytes, narrowing of joint space, and subchondral sclerosis and deformity of bone ends
Grade 4	Large osteophytes, severe sclerosis, and narrowing of joint space

* Modified from Ref. 9. Reproduced from Silman, A.J., Hochberg, M.C. (1993). *Epidemiology of the Rheumatic Diseases.* Oxford: Oxford University Press.

Table 1.3 Grades of severity of osteoarthritis of the knee*

Grade 1	Doubtful narrowing of joint space and possible osteophytic lipping
Grade 2	Definite osteophytes and possible narrowing of joint space
Grade 3	Moderate multiple osteophytes, definite narrowing of joint space and some sclerosis and possible deformity of bone ends
Grade 4	Large osteophytes, marked narrowing of joint space, severe sclerosis, and definite deformity of bone ends

* Taken from Ref. 9. Reproduced from Silman, A.J., Hochberg, M.C. (1993). *Epidemiology of the Rheumatic Diseases.* Oxford: Oxford University Press.

Table 1.4 Grades of severity of osteoarthritis of the hip*

Grade 1	Possible narrowing of joint space medially and possible osteophytes around femoral head
Grade 2	Definite narrowing of joint space inferiorly, definite osteophytes, and slight sclerosis
Grade 3	Marked narrowing of joint space, slight osteophytes, some sclerosis and cyst formation, and deformity of femoral head and acetabulum
Grade 4	Gross loss of joint space with sclerosis and cysts, marked deformity of femoral head and acetabulum, and large osteophytes

* Taken from Ref. 9. Reproduced from Silman, A.J., Hochberg, M.C. (1993). *Epidemiology of the Rheumatic Diseases.* Oxford: Oxford University Press.

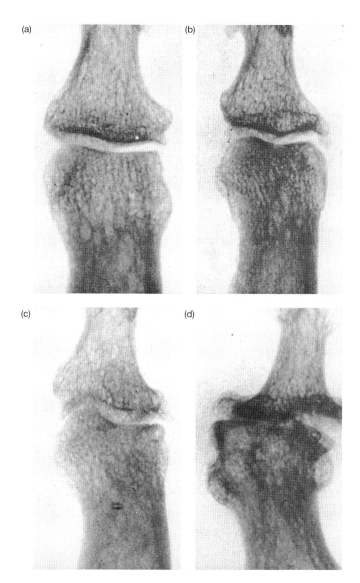

Fig. 1.1 Grades of severity of OA of the distal interphalangeal joints:
(a) Grade 1; (b) Grade 2; (c) Grade 3; (d) Grade 4.

Source: Reproduced from Silman, A.J. and Hochberg, M.C. (1993). *Epidemiology of the Rheumatic Diseases.* Oxford: Oxford University Press.

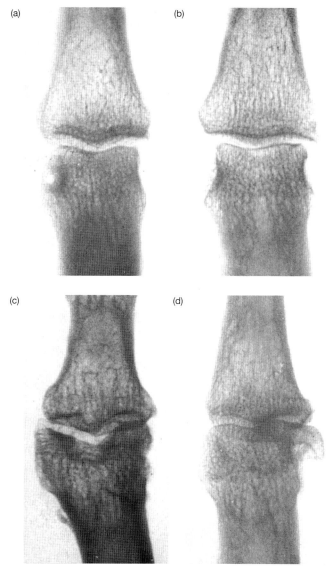

Fig. 1.2 Grades of severity of OA of the proximal interphalangeal joints:
(a) Grade 1; (b) Grade 2; (c) Grade 3; (d) Grade 4.

Source: Reproduced from Silman, A.J. and Hochberg, M.C. (1993). *Epidemiology of the Rheumatic Diseases.* Oxford: Oxford University Press.

published by the Osteoarthritis Research Society International contains 152 black-and-white photos illustrating 39 different radiographic features of OA (Table 1.5).[18] Using this and other published atlases, trained readers have been shown to have excellent intra-reader and very good-to-excellent inter-reader reliability in measuring the presence and severity of OA of the hand, hip, and knee; the results of reliability studies have been reviewed by Lane and Kremer[23] and Sun and colleagues.[24] In a recent study using radiographs from subjects registered in the Australian Twin Registry, inter-rater and intra-rater agreement varied by different anatomic sites and different radiographic features.[25] The authors concluded that a single experienced assessor could reliably classify subjects as having radiographic OA at the hand, hip, and knee; when less experienced assessors were involved, however, independent examinations should be made by at least two persons with either adjudication or a consensus reached on disparate examinations.

The validity of using individual radiographic features and a revised composite grading scale has been demonstrated in several studies. Croft *et al.* examined the association of individual radiographic features of OA of the hip with reported hip pain in 759 men, 60–75 years of age, who had undergone intravenous urograms.[15] The radiographic feature most strongly associated with reported hip pain was joint-space width, at the narrowest point,

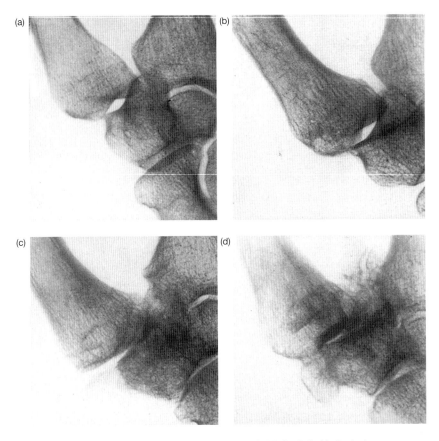

Fig. 1.3 Grades of severity of OA of the first carpometacarpal joint: (a) Grade 1; (b) Grade 2; (c) Grade 3; (d) Grade 4.

Source: Reproduced from Silman, A.J. and Hochberg, M.C. (1993). *Epidemiology of the Rheumatic Diseases*. Oxford: Oxford University Press.

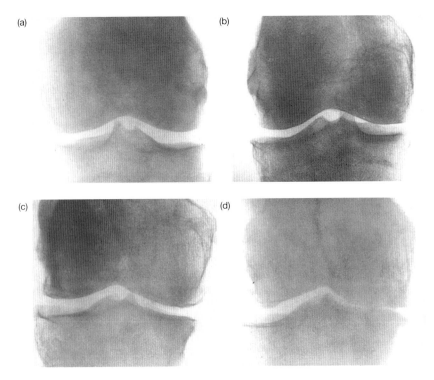

Fig. 1.4 Grades of severity of OA of the knee: (a) Grade 1; (b) Grade 2; (c) Grade 3; (d) Grade 4.

Source: Reproduced from Silman, A.J. and Hochberg, M.C. (1993). *Epidemiology of the Rheumatic Diseases*. Oxford: Oxford University Press.

Table 1.5 Radiographic features of osteoarthritis illustrated in the Atlas of the Osteoarthritis Research Society International*

Joint group and feature	Range of grades
Hand	
Marginal osteophytes	0–3
Joint-space narrowing	0–3
Subchondral sclerosis	0–3
Subchondral erosions	0–3
Malalignment	0–3
Hip	
Marginal osteophytes	0–3
Joint-space narrowing	0–3
Subchondral sclerosis	0–3
Subchondral lucencies	0–3
Femoral buttressing	0–3
Knee (Tibiofemoral joint)	
Marginal osteophytes	0–3
Joint-space narrowing	0–3
Subchondral sclerosis	0–3
Subchondral erosions	0–3
Malalignment	0–3
Attrition	0–3
Tibial spine hypertrophy	0–1
Knee (Patellofemoral joint)	
Marginal osteophytes	0–3
Joint-space narrowing	0–3
Subchondral sclerosis	0–1
Medial subluxation	0–1
Lateral subluxation	0–3

* Modified from Ref. 18.

measured in millimeters; in addition, an overall qualitative grade of 3 or higher (Table 1.6) was strongly associated with reported hip pain. These findings were subsequently confirmed by Scott *et al.* in an analysis of data from women aged 65 and older, who had pelvic radiographs obtained at entry into the 'Study of Osteoporotic Fractures', a longitudinal epidemiologic study of risk factors for osteoporotic fractures.[26] In a more recent study, Ingvarsson and colleagues compared the reliability of measuring minimum joint space with the Kellgren–Lawrence global scale for assessing the prevalence of hip OA using colon radiographs in Iceland.[27] They noted that the measurement of the minimum joint space had better intra-observer and inter-observer reliability than the global grade, although prevalence estimates were similar between the two methods. Based on the validity of the association of individual radiographic features with hip pain, and the greater reliability of scoring individual features, as compared to the global Kellgren–Lawrence score,[15,16,27] future population-based epidemiological studies of OA of the hip should rely on the presence of individual radiographic features and the Croft or modified Croft global scales, rather than on the Kellgren–Lawrence grading scale, for classifying cases of OA of the hip.[28]

Spector *et al.* examined the association of the individual radiographic features of knee OA with reported knee pain in 977 women aged 45–64 years who were participants in the Chingford Study, a longitudinal study

Table 1.6 Croft's overall qualitative grading of hip OA*

Grade	Definition
0	No changes of osteoarthritis
1	Osteophytosis only
2	Joint-space narrowing only
3	Two of osteophytosis, joint-space narrowing, subchondral sclerosis, and cyst formation
4	Three of osteophytosis, joint-space narrowing, subchondral sclerosis, and cyst formation
5	As in grade 4, but with deformity of the femoral head

* Modified from Ref. 13.

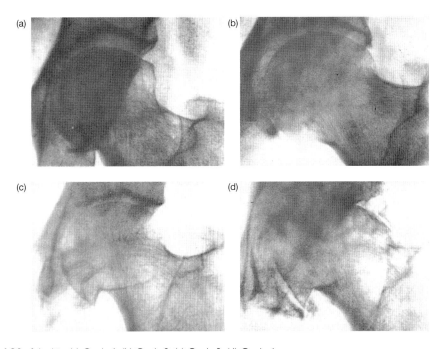

(a)   (b)   (c)   (d)

Fig. 1.5 Grades of severity of OS of the hip: (a) Grade 1; (b) Grade 2; (c) Grade 3; (d) Grade 4.

Source: Reproduced from Silman, A.J. and Hochberg, M.C. (1993). *Epidemiology of the Rheumatic Diseases.* Oxford: Oxford University Press.

of musculoskeletal disease in women recruited from a single general practice in Chingford, East London, England.[29] They noted that, among the individual radiographic features of OA, a definite osteophyte in the medial compartment was most strongly associated with reported knee pain. The odds ratio for the association of grade 1–3 osteophytes with knee pain and the proportion of subjects with grade 1–3 osteophytes who had knee pain were both similar to those for the Kellgren–Lawrence grade 2–4 changes.

In an analysis of data from the Baltimore Longitudinal Study on Aging, Lethbridge-Cejku *et al.* examined the association of individual radiographic features and the global Kellgren–Lawrence grade with reported knee pain among 452 men and 223 women, aged 18 and older.[30] In support of the findings of Spector *et al.*,[29] they found that the strength of the association of definite grade 1–3 osteophytes with current knee pain was similar to that for grade 2 or higher OA, using the Kellgren–Lawrence scale; the odds ratios were 4.4 (95 per cent confidence intervals: 2.6, 7.5) and 4.8 (2.5, 8.5), respectively. This relationship was stronger, and remained consistent, among the more severe grades of OA: grade 2–3 osteophytes were associated with current knee pain with an odds ratio of 17.1 (7.5, 38.7), while a Kellgren–Lawrence grade of 3–4 was associated with current knee pain with an odds ratio of 20.8 (8.6, 50.4). Both these studies provided data derived from the standing, extended knee radiographs of the tibiofemoral joint.

Felson and colleagues examined the association between clinically diagnosed knee OA, defined as frequent knee symptoms plus crepitus on physical examination, with radiographic features present on either anteroposterior weight-bearing or lateral semi-flexed weight-bearing knee radiographs.[31] The radiographic definitions that best identified knees with clinical OA were the presence of a moderate or larger osteophyte, or the presence of moderate or greater joint-space narrowing plus at least one bony feature (cyst, sclerosis, or osteophyte). Adding information from the lateral views of the patellofemoral joint enhanced the ability to more efficiently distinguish clinical knee OA from those without clinical knee OA. This study, however, did not have skyline views of the patellofemoral joint, as illustrated in the atlas published by the Osteoarthritis Research Society International.[22] A study by Lanyon and colleagues, however, did include both an anteroposterior standing and midflexion skyline radiograph of the knee.[32] These authors noted that a case definition based on the presence of a definite osteophyte was more efficient at predicting pain than definitions based on joint-space width. Furthermore, the addition of the patellofemoral joint improved sensitivity for the presence of knee pain. Thus, the use of skyline views of the patellofemoral joint combined with standing views of the tibiofemoral joint is preferable for epidemiological studies. Based on the validity of the association of individual radiographic features with knee pain, future population-based epidemiologic studies of OA of the knee should rely on the use of individual features alone or in combination to classify cases.[33] Protocols for the precise positioning of the tibiofemoral and patellofemoral compartments of the knee joint have been published.[34]

Clinical criteria

As noted above, there are potential limitations to the use of only radiographic criteria for a case definition, especially in clinical research studies of patients with OA. In particular, although a statistical association exists between the radiographic changes of OA and reported pain at both the hip and knee, in the individual patient there is often a poor correlation between the severity of radiographic changes and clinical symptomatology.[35]

At the Third International Symposium on Population Studies of the Rheumatic Diseases in 1966, the Subcommittee on Diagnostic Criteria for Osteoarthrosis recommended that population-based studies should investigate the validity of certain historical, physical, and laboratory findings in predicting the typical radiographic features of OA on a joint-by-joint basis.[36] Such historical features include pain on motion, pain at rest, nocturnal joint pain, and morning stiffness. Features present on physical examination include bony enlargement and expansion, limitation of motion, and crepitus. Laboratory features include the erythrocyte sedimentation rate, tests for rheumatoid factor, serum uric acid concentration, and appropriate analyses of synovial fluid.

In 1981, the Subcommittee on Osteoarthritis of the American College of Rheumatology Diagnostic and Therapeutic Criteria Committee was established to develop clinical criteria for the classification of OA.[37] Over the last decade, the Subcommittee has developed and published sets of classification criteria for OA of the knee,[3] hand,[38] and hip.[39] Altman modified the criteria sets into algorithms, facilitating their use in clinical research and population-based studies.[40] The algorithms for classification of OA of the knee (Table 1.7), hand (Table 1.8), and hip (Table 1.9), were all developed using patients with site-specific joint pain due to other types of arthritis or musculoskeletal diseases as the comparison groups. For OA of the knee, data on 85 historical, physical, laboratory, and radiographic features were collected from 130 patients with symptomatic OA of the knee and 105 control patients with knee pain due to other etiologies; 55 of the controls had rheumatoid arthritis.[3] For OA of the hand, the Subcommittee collected data on 51 historical, physical, laboratory, and radiographic features from 100 patients with symptomatic hand OA and 99 control patients with hand

Table 1.7 Algorithm for classification of osteoarthritis of the knee, Subcommittee on Osteoarthritis, American College of Rheumatology Diagnostic and Therapeutic Criteria Committee*

Clinical

1 Knee pain for most days of prior month

2 Crepitus on active joint motion

3 Morning stiffness <30 minutes in duration

4 Age >38 years

5 Bony enlargement of the knee on examination

Osteoarthritis is present if items 1, 2, 3, 4 or items 1, 2, 5 or items 1 and 5, are present. Sensitivity and specificity are 89 and 88%, respectively.

Clinical, laboratory, and radiographic

1 Knee pain for most days of prior month

2 Osteophytes at joint margins (X-ray spurs)

3 Synovial fluid typical of osteoarthritis (laboratory)

4 Age >40 years

5 Morning stiffness <30 minutes

6 Crepitus on active joint motion

Osteoarthritis is present if items 1 and 2 or items 1, 3, 5, 6 or items 1, 4, 5, 6 are present. Sensitivity and specificity are 94 and 88%, respectively.

* Modified from Refs 3 and 27. Reproduced from Silman, A.J., Hochberg, M.C. (1993). *Epidemiology of the Rheumatic Diseases*. Oxford: Oxford University Press.

Table 1.8 Algorithm for classification of OA of the hand, Subcommittee on Osteoarthritis, American College of Rheumatology Diagnostic and Therapeutic Criteria Committee*

Clinical

1 Hand pain, aching, or stiffness for most days of prior month.

2 Hard tissue enlargement of ≥2 of 10 selected hand joints[†]

3 Fewer than 3 swollen MCP joints.

4 Hard tissue enlargement of 2 or more DIP joints.

5 Deformity of 2 or more of 10 selected hand joints[†]

Osteoarthritis is present if items 1, 2, 3, 4 or items 1, 2, 3, 5 are present. Sensitivity and specificity are 92 and 98%, respectively.

DIP, distal interphalangeal; PIP, proximal interphalangeal; MCP, metacarpophalangeal; CMC, carpo-metacarpal.

* Modified from Refs 25 and 27. Reproduced from Silman, A.J., Hochberg, M.C. (1993). *Epidemiology of the Rheumatic Diseases*. Oxford: Oxford University Press.

† The 10 selected hand joints include bilateral 2nd and 3rd DIP joints, 2nd and 3rd PIP joints, and 1st CMC joints.

Table 1.9 Algorithm for classification of hip OA, Subcommittee on Osteoarthritis, American College of Rheumatology Diagnostic and Therapeutic Criteria Committee*

Clinical, laboratory, and radiographic
1 Hip pain for most days of the prior month
2 Femoral and/or acetabular osteophytes on radiograph
3 Erythrocyte sedimentation rate <20 mm/h
4 Axial joint-space narrowing on radiograph

Osteoarthritis is present if items 1 and 2 or items 1, 3, 4 are present. Sensitivity and specificity are 91 and 89%, respectively.

* Modified from Refs 26 and 27. Reproduced from Silman, A.J., Hochberg, M.C. (1993). *Epidemiology of the Rheumatic Diseases*. Oxford: Oxford University Press.

pain of other etiologies: 74 had rheumatoid arthritis.[38] For OA of the hip, data on 76 historical, physical, laboratory, and radiographic features were collected from 114 patients with symptomatic OA of the hip and 87 control patients with hip pain of other etiologies: 37 had rheumatoid arthritis.[39] At all joint sites, the sensitivity, specificity, and accuracy of these algorithms approached or exceeded 90 per cent. Misclassification bias, therefore, would not likely be a major problem in clinical research studies that employed these criteria.

Because the major inclusion parameter is joint pain on most days of the prior month, these criteria sets identify patients with clinically important OA. This contrasts with the identification of cases of OA based on radiographic features alone, insofar as many, if not most, subjects with radiographic evidence of OA do not report joint pain.[35,41] Therefore, estimates of the prevalence of OA will be lower when based on the American College of Rheumatology criteria as compared to the traditional radiographic criteria. In population-based studies, misclassification, particularly of false-negative cases, may be considerable because of the high proportion of subjects with radiographic evidence of OA who do not have joint pain. For example, in one study of 400 women aged 45–65 years, Hart and colleagues noted that the prevalence of symptomatic knee OA was only 2.3 per cent compared to a prevalence of radiographic knee OA of 17 per cent.[42] In another study of an elderly population in Iceland, Aspelund and colleagues noted that the majority of persons who fulfilled the classification criteria for hand OA lacked symptoms on most days of the prior month; furthermore, symptoms, when present, were episodic in almost one-third of the group.[43] They concluded that the clinical criteria were of limited use in population surveys. Readers need to be aware of the difference between prevalence estimates based on radiographic or clinical criteria for case definitions when reviewing published studies.

McAlindon and Dieppe reviewed both the process and development of the American College of Rheumatology criteria for OA of the knee.[44] They noted several potential limitations, including the lack of age- and gender-matched controls, inclusion of controls with rheumatoid arthritis, use of criterion items that were largely subjective and not validated, and the absence of a definition or test for OA. Their comments were echoed by Balint and Szebenyi.[45] The comments were addressed by Altman *et al.* who noted that the methodology used to construct the criteria adjusted for differences between cases and controls, and that the final items included in the criteria sets could be reliably and objectively measured.[46]

The validity of the criteria for classifying patients with hip OA was examined in a primary care setting.[47] The authors noted an excellent agreement between the use of the classification tree approach and the criteria set including radiographic findings, but poor agreement when only clinical variables were included. They suggested that radiographic information was necessary to apply the criteria for hip OA in clinical practice.

In a more recent study, 85 pairs of twins registered in the Australian Twin Registry were examined as part of a study to determine the reliability of the ACR clinical criteria.[48] Two rheumatologists performed independent clinical assessments blinded to laboratory or radiographic data. While inter-rater agreement varied by different anatomic sites, it was excellent at all sites. The authors concluded that a single experienced assessor could reliably classify subjects as having clinical OA at the hand, hip, and knee.[48]

In summary, OA is a complex disorder that may result from many potential etiologies. Definitions of OA developed at multidisciplinary conferences, with international representation of experts, reflect this complexity. It is difficult, however, to apply these definitions to case definition and diagnosis in the community or clinic setting.

In the community setting, the criteria for case definitions have traditionally relied on the presence of radiographic features of OA, codified using the Kellgren–Lawrence grading schema as illustrated in the *Atlas of Standard Radiographs*. Recently, however, the use of reliable atlases for grading the severity of the individual radiographic features of OA and of modified global scales has received an enthusiastic acceptance among rheumatic disease epidemiologists. In the clinic setting, however, a case definition based on radiographic features alone has limitations. For purposes of clinical research, including therapeutic trials, classification criteria have been developed that use combinations of symptoms, physical findings, laboratory data, and radiographic features, and have high levels of sensitivity and specificity. These classification criteria have been endorsed by the Osteoarthritis Research Society International, for use as inclusion criteria for patients in clinical research studies, including clinical trials.[49,50]

Key points

1. The definition of OA has evolved over the past two decades and now recognizes OA as a syndrome with many complex etiologies rather than as a single disease entity.

2. In epidemiological studies, radiographic criteria remain the basis for classifying subjects as having OA.

3. Clinical criteria identify persons with symptomatic disease and should be used for the entry of subjects into clinical trials.

References

(An asterisk denotes recommended reading.)

1. **Scott, J.C., Lethbridge-Cejku, M., and Hochberg, M.C.** (1999). Epidemiology and economic consequences of osteoarthritis: the American viewpoint. In: J-Y. Reginster, J-P. Pelletier, J. Martel-Pelletier, and Y. Henroitin (eds). *Osteoarthritis: Clinical and Experimental Aspects*. Berlin: Springer, pp. 20–38.

2. **Scott, J.C. and Hochberg, M.C.** (1998). Arthritis and other musculoskeletal diseases. In: R.C. Brownson, P.L. Remington, and J.R. Davis (eds). *Chronic Disease Epidemiology and Control, 2nd edition*. Washington, DC: American Public Health Association, pp. 465–89.

3. *Altman, R., Asch, E., Bloch, D., Bole, G., Borenstein, D., Brandt, K., *et al.* (1986). Development of criteria for the classification and reporting of osteoarthritis: classification of osteoarthritis of the knee. *Arthritis Rheum* 29:1039–49.

   The American College of Rheumatology classification schema for OA as well as the preliminary criteria for classification of OA of the knee are provided in this article.

4. **Brandt, K.D., Mankin, H.J., and Shulman, L.E.** (1986). Workshop on etiopathogenesis of osteoarthritis. *J Rheumatol* 13:1126–60.

5. **Keuttner, K. and Goldberg, V.M.** (ed.) (1995). *Osteoarthritic Disorders*. Rosemont: American Academy of Orthopedic Surgeons, pp. xxi–v.

6. **Kellgren, J.H. and Moore, R.** (1952). Generalised osteoarthritis and Heberden's nodes. *Br Med J* 1:181–7.

7. **Schumacher, H.R. Jr.** (2001). Secondary osteoarthritis. In: R.W. Moskowitz, D.S. Howell, R.D. Altman, J.A. Buckwalter, and V.M. Goldberg (eds). *Osteoarthritis: Diagnosis and Medical/Surgical Management, 3rd edition*. Philadelphia: WB Saunders, pp. 327–58.

8. *Kellgren, J.H. and Lawrence, J.S.* (1957). Radiologic assessment of osteoarthrosis. *Ann Rheum Dis* 16:494–501.

This landmark paper presents the radiographic features of OA for each of the most common sites affected.

9. The Department of Rheumatology and Medical Illustration, University of Manchester (1973). *The Epidemiology of Chronic Rheumatism, Vol. 2, Atlas of Standard Radiographs of Arthritis*. Philadelphia: FA Davis, pp. 1–15.

10. **Spector, T.D. and Cooper, C.** (1993). Radiographic assessment of osteoarthritis in population studies: whither Kellgren and Lawrence? *Osteoarthritis Cart* **1**:203–6.

11. **Spector, T.D. and Hochberg, M.C.** (1994). Methodological problems in the epidemiological study of osteoarthritis. *Ann Rheum Dis* **53**:143–6.

12. **Hart, D.J. and Spector, T.D.** (1995). Radiographic criteria for epidemiologic studies of osteoarthritis. *J Rheumatol* **22**(Suppl 43):46–8.

13. **Hart, D.J. and Spector, T.D.** (1995). The classification and assessment of osteoarthritis. *Bailliéres Clin Rheumatol* **9**:407–32.

14. **Kallman, D.A., Wigley, F.M., Scott, W.W. Jr., Hochberg, M.C., and Tobin, J.D.** (1989). New radiographic grading scales for osteoarthritis of the hand. *Arthritis Rheum* **32**:1548–91.

15. **Croft, P., Cooper, C., Wickham, C., and Coggon, D.** (1990). Defining osteoarthritis of the hip for epidemiologic studies. *Am J Epidemiol* **132**:514–22.

16. **Lane, N.E., Nevitt, M.C., Genant, H.K., Hochberg, M.C.** (1993). Reliability of new indices of radiographic osteoarthritis of the hand and hip and lumbar disc degeneration. *J Rheumatol* **20**:1911–8.

17. **Spector, T.D., Cooper, C., Cushnaghan, J., Hart, D.J., and Dieppe, P.A.** (1992). *A Radiographic Atlas of Knee Osteoarthritis*. London: Springer.

18. **Scott, W.W. Jr., Lethbridge-Cejku, M., Reichle, R., Wigley, F.M., Tobin, J.D., and Hochberg, M.C.** (1993). Reliability of grading scales for individual radiographic features of osteoarthritis of the knee: the Baltimore Longitudinal Study of Aging atlas of knee osteoarthritis. *Invest Radiol* **28**:497–501.

19. **Cooke, T.D.V., Kelly, B.P., Harrison, L., Mohamed, G., and Khan, B.** (1999). Radiographic grading for knee osteoarthritis: a revised scheme that relates to alignment and deformity. *J Rheumatol* **26**:641–4.

20. **Nagaosa, Y., Mateus, M., Hassan, B., Lanyon, P., and Doherty, M.** (2000). Development of a logically devised line drawing atlas for grading of knee osteoarthritis. *Ann Rheum Dis* **59**:587–95.

21. **Burnett, S., Hart, D.J., Cooper, C., and Spector, T.D.** (1994). *A Radiographic Atlas of Osteoarthritis*. London: Springer.

22. *Altman, R.D., Hochberg, M.C., Murphy, W.A. Jr., Wolfe, F., and Lequesne, M.** (1995). Atlas of individual radiographic features in osteoarthritis. *Osteoarthritis Cart* **3**(Suppl. A):3–70.

The photographs reproduced in this paper are the standards developed by the Osteoarthritis Research Society International (OARSI) for grading the individual radiographic features of OA at the most common sites affected.

23. **Lane, N.E. and Kremer, L.B.** (1995). Radiographic indices for osteoarthritis. *Rheum Dis Clin North Am* **21**:379–94.

24. **Sun, Y., Gunther, K.P., and Brenner, H.** (1997). Reliability of radiographic grading of osteoarthritis of the hip and knee. *Scand J Rheumatol* **36**:155–65.

25. **Bellamy, N., Tesar, P., Walker, D., Klestov, A., Muirden, K., Kuhnert P,** *et al.* (1999). Perceptual variation in grading hand, hip and knee radiographs: observations based on an Australian twin registry study of osteoarthritis. *Ann Rheum Dis* **58**:766–9.

26. **Scott, J.C., Nevitt, M.C., Lane, N.E., Genant, H.K., and Hochberg, M.C.** (1992). Association of individual radiographic features of hip osteoarthritis with pain. *Arthritis Rheum* **35**(Suppl. 9):S81.

27. **Ingvarsson, T., Hagglund, G., Lindberg, H., Lohmander, L.S.** (2000). Assessment of primary hip osteoarthritis: comparison of radiographic methods using colon radiographs. *Ann Rheum Dis* **59**:650–3.

28. **Nevitt, M.C.** (1996). Definition of hip osteoarthritis for epidemiological studies. *Ann Rheum Dis* **55**:652–5.

29. **Spector, T.D., Hart, D.J., Byrne, J., Harris, P.A., Dacre, J.E., and Doyle, D.V.** (1993). Defining the presence of osteoarthritis of the knee in epidemiologic studies. *Ann Rheum Dis* **52**:790–4.

30. **Lethbridge-Cejku, M., Scott, W.W. Jr, Reichle, R., Ettinger, W.H., Zonderman, A., Costa, P.,** *et al.* (1995). Association of radiographic features of osteoarthritis of the knee with knee pain: Data from the Baltimore Longitudinal Study of Aging. *Arthritis Care Res* **9**:182–8.

31. **Felson, D.T., McAlindon, T.E., Anderson, J.J., Naimark, A., Weissman, B.W., Aliabadi, P.,** *et al.* (1997). Defining radiographic osteoarthritis for the whole knee. *Osteoarthritis Cart* **5**:241–50.

32. **Lanyon, P., O'Reilly, S., Jones, A., and Doherty, M.** (1998). Radiographic assessment of symptomatic knee osteoarthritis in the community: definitions and normal joint space. *Ann Rheum Dis* **57**:595–601.

33. **Jacobson LT.** (1996). Definitions of osteoarthritis in the knee and hand. *Ann Rheum Dis* **55**:656–8.

34. *Buckland-Wright, C.** (1995). Protocols for precise radio-anatomical positioning of the tibiofemoral and patellofemoral compartments of the knee. *Osteoarthritis Cart* **3**(Suppl A):71–80.

This article provides standardized protocols for positioning patients to obtain optimal radiographic views for determining the presence and progression of osteoarthritis.

35. **Creamer, P. and Hochberg, M.C.** (1997). Why does osteoarthritis of the knee hurt—sometimes? *Br J Rheumatol* **37**:726–8.

36. **Bennett, P.H. and Wood, P.H.N.** (ed.) (1968). *Population Studies of the Rheumatic Diseases. International Congress Series No. 148*. Excerpta Medica Foundation: Amsterdam, pp. 417–19.

37. **Altman, R.D., Meenan, R.F., Hochberg, M.C., Bole, G.G. Jr, Brandt, K., Cooke, T.D.V.,** *et al.* (1983). An approach to developing criteria for the clinical diagnosis and classification of osteoarthritis: a status report of the American Rheumatism Association Diagnostic Subcommittee on Osteoarthritis. *J Rheumatol* **10**:180–3.

38. **Altman, R., Alarcon, G., Appelrough, D., Bloch, D., Borenstein, D., Brandt, K.,** *et al.* (1990). The American College of Rheumatology criteria for the classification and reporting of osteoarthritis of the hand. *Arthritis Rheum* **33**:1601–10.

39. **Altman R, Alarcon G, Appelrough D, Bloch D, Borenstein D, Brandt K,** *et al.* (1991). The American College of Rheumatology criteria for the classification and reporting of osteoarthritis of the hip. *Arthritis Rheum* **34**: 505–14.

40. **Altman, R.** (1991). Classification of disease: osteoarthritis. *Sem Arthritis Rheum* **20**(6,Suppl 2):40–7.

41. **Lawrence, J.S., Bremner, J.M., and Bier, F.** (1966). Osteoarthritis: prevalence in the population and relationship between symptoms and X-ray changes. *Ann Rheum Dis* **25**:1–25.

42. **Hart, D.J., Leedham-Green, M., and Spector, T.D.** (1991). The prevalence of knee osteoarthritis in the general population using different clinical criteria: the Chingford Study. *Br J Rheumatol* **30**(Suppl. 2):72.

43. **Alpelund, G., Gunnarsdottir, S., Jonsson, P., and Jonsson, H.** (1996). Hand osteoarthritis in the elderly: application of clinical criteria. *Scand J Rheumatol* **25**:34–6.

44. **McAlindon, T. and Dieppe, P.** (1989). Osteoarthritis: definitions and criteria. *Ann Rheum Dis* **48**:531–2.

45. **Balint, G. and Szebenyi, B.** (1996). Diagnosis of osteoarthritis: guidelines and current pitfalls. *Drugs* **52**(Suppl. 3):1–13.

46. **Altman, R.D., Bloch, D.A., Brandt, K.D., Cooke, D.V., Greenwald, R.A., Hochberg, M.C.,** *et al.* (1990). Osteoarthritis: definitions and criteria. *Ann Rheum Dis* **49**:201.

47. **Bierma-Zeinstra, S., Bohnen, A., Ginai, A., Prins, A., and Verhaar, J.** (1999). Validity of American College of Rheumatology criteria for diagnosing hip osteoarthritis in primary care research. *J Rheumatol* **26**:1129–33.

48. **Bellamy, N., Klestov, A., Muriden, K., Kuhnert, P., Do, K.A., O'Gorman, L., and Martin, N.** (1999). Perceptual variation in categorizing individuals according to American College of Rheumatology classification criteria for hand, knee, and hip osteoarthritis (OA): observations based on an Australian Twin Registry study of OA. *J Rheumatol* **26**:2654–8.

49. **Altman, R., Brandt, K., Hochberg, M., and Moskowitz, R.** (for the Task Force) (1996). Design and conduct of clinical trials in patients with osteoarthritis: recommendations from a task force of the Osteoarthritis Research Society. *Osteoarthritis Cart* **4**:217–43.

This article provides the OARSI guidelines for designing and conducting trials in patients with osteoarthritis of the hip or knee. A companion article on guidelines for designing and conducting trials in patients with osteoarthritis of the hand is in preparation and will be published in Osteoarthritis Cart in 2002.

50. **Altman, R. and Maheu, E.** (for the Task Force) (2002). Design and conduct of clinical trials in patients with osteoarthritis of the hand: recommendations from a task force of the Osteoarthritis Research Society. *Osteoarthritis Cart* **10**:in press.

2 Epidemiology of osteoarthritis

David T. Felson

Impact of OA

Osteoarthritis is the most common form of arthritis. Its high prevalence, especially in the elderly, and the frequency of OA-related physical disability make OA one of the leading causes of disability in the elderly, especially with respect to weight-bearing functional tasks.[1] According to a report on the prevalence of arthritis: 'By 2020 the estimated number of persons with arthritis is projected to increase by 57 per cent and activity limitations associated with arthritis by 66 per cent'. These projected increases are largely attributable to the high prevalence of OA among older persons and the increasing average age of the US population.[2]

Epidemiology is the study of disease in populations and its association with characteristics of people and their environments. Epidemiological studies document the burden of disease in society and evaluate risk factors for disease that, if modified, might lead to disease prevention and a lessening of the burden of disability associated with disease. Identifying modifiable risk factors for OA is the first step to prevent this disease and lower its formidable burden in our society.

Prevalence and incidence of OA

Osteoarthritis is an extremely common joint disorder in all populations. It often affects certain joints, yet spares others. For example, in the hands, the distal interphalangeal (DIP), proximal interphalangeal (PIP) joints, and the carpometacarpal (CMC) joint of the thumb are frequently involved. Other joints commonly affected include the cervical spine, lumbosacral spine, hip, knee, and first metatarsophalangeal (MTP) joint. The ankle, wrist, elbow, and shoulder are usually spared. Our joints were designed and shaped, in an evolutionary sense, when humans were brachiating apes. Only later did humans develop a pincer grip capability[3] and full weight-bearing on their legs. These evolutionary differences in joint function and, possibly, differences in the composition of articular cartilage among the different joints, predispose some joints to cartilage breakdown, leading to OA.

Osteoarthritis can be defined in many ways. On the one hand, there is structural change in a joint often assessed by radiograph. Radiographic changes of OA include osteophytes and joint-space narrowing, the latter reflecting cartilage loss. Many persons with radiographic OA do not have joint symptoms. Secondly, one can assess the occurrence of joint symptoms. While this is an appealing definition from a clinical and public health standpoint, many with joint symptoms do not have radiographic changes of disease and may not have OA. Prevalence estimates across studies vary because of the inconsistent definitions of symptoms and radiographic change. The only exception to this is the Kellgren and Lawrence scale, which has been widely used to evaluate the prevalence of radiographic OA in most joints.

Radiographic disease is highly prevalent with radiographic hand OA occurring in approximately 32.5 per cent of adults aged 30 and over.[4] The prevalence of radiographic knee and hip OA has been best studied in the population surveys of elders. The Framingham Study suggests that radiographic knee OA occurs in 33 per cent of people aged 63 and over, and studies from the United States of America and Europe suggest that radiographic hip OA occurs in roughly 3–4 per cent of elders.[5]

Symptomatic OA is generally defined as frequent joint pain plus radiographic change; its prevalence in the knee has ranged in different studies from 1.6–9.4 per cent of adults and in 10–15 per cent of elders. Symptomatic hip OA occurs in anywhere from 0.7–4.4 per cent of adults, and, using British data from the 1960s, symptomatic hand OA occurs in about 2.6 per cent of adults.

The prevalence of knee pain and OA by radiograph represents a good example of how the prevalence of OA differs depending on how the disease is defined. Approximately 25 per cent of adults aged 55 and over experience knee pain for a prolonged period every year (lasting at least a month). Of these, roughly half have evidence of radiographic OA[6] (see Fig. 2.1). Even though they have frequent knee pain, many of these persons do not necessarily experience limited function from this pain, so that when one addresses the prevalence of knee pain with limitation, it is roughly half the previous prevalence. Severely disabling knee pain is relatively uncommon. A similar relationship between disabling joint pain and radiographic change exists for most regions of the body affected by OA.

The prevalence of OA in all joints is strikingly correlated with age. Regardless of how OA is defined, it is uncommon in adults aged under 40 and extremely prevalent in those aged above 60. Radiographic hand OA, for example, was present in only about 5 per cent of adults aged under 35, but was seen in over 70 per cent of those who were aged 65 or older.[7]

Osteoarthritis has a higher prevalence, and more often exhibits a generalized distribution, in women than in men. Before the age of 50, men have a higher prevalence than women, but after the age of 50 women have a higher prevalence, and this sex difference in prevalence further increases with age.[8,9] These gender and age-related prevalence patterns are consistent with a role of post-menopausal hormone deficiency in increasing the risk of OA.

Cross-national and cross-racial studies often produce insights about disease etiology. With respect to OA, black women have been reported to have higher rates of knee OA than white women[10] even after adjustment for age and weight. The results in black men have been inconsistent. However, studies suggest very low rates of hip OA among the black populations in Jamaica, South Africa, Nigeria, and Liberia (1–4 per cent for radiographic OA), in comparison with European populations (7–25 per cent). In Blackfeet and Pima Native Americans, the rates of hip OA are intermediate between those for blacks and whites,[11] even though the Pimas weigh more, on average, than Caucasians.

The rates of hip OA are much lower in Asians than in Caucasians. The rate of hip arthroplasty for OA in people of Asian extraction is lower than that in Caucasians in the United States of America.[12] Using standard methods across population-based groups, Nevitt *et al.*[13] report that symptomatic and radiographic hip OA are far less prevalent in Chinese than in Caucasians from the United States of America. The low rate of hip OA in Asians is not matched by a low rate of knee OA, as Zhang *et al.*[14] using standardized methods across populations, found that knee OA prevalence was actually more prevalent in Chinese than in Caucasian women and equally

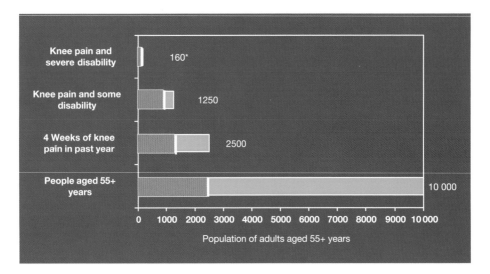

Fig. 2.1 Prevalence of knee pain and osteoarthritis in persons aged 55 and over. *The proportion with radiographic evidence in this category is not known, though it seems likely to be high. The shading represents the proportion in each category with radiographic evidence of knee osteoarthritis.

Source: Taken from Peat et al.[6]

prevalent among men. Although it was initially felt that these racial differences in hip OA prevalence might be attributed to an absence of developmental hip abnormalities in Asians, studies of the Chinese in Hong Kong[15,16] fail to confirm a lower prevalence of developmental hip abnormalities. Thus, the explanation for these racial differences in prevalence is unclear.

Generalized OA involves hand joints, including the DIP, PIP, and the first CMC joints; cervical spine; lumbosacral spine and knees; and may include the hips. There are two types of generalized OA: nodal OA (Heberden's nodes) and non-nodal OA.[17] There is little question that this entity exists; OA in one joint is associated with the presence of OA in other joints, even after adjusting for age and sex. Generalized OA is most common in older women and may be inherited in a polygenic pattern.[18]

Because the risk of mortality may be increased in those with OA[19,20] prevalence estimates may give erroneous estimates of actual disease incidence, that is the new occurrence of disease. A large-scale study from a Massachusetts health maintenance organization[21] reported that the age- and sex-standardized incidence rate for symptomatic hand OA was 100 per 100 000 person years. For hip OA the rate was 88 per 100 000 person years and for knee OA 240 per 100 000 person years. The incidence of hand, knee, and hip OA all increased with age (Fig. 2.2) and for each joint was higher in women than in men after the age of 50. At the age of 70–89, the knee OA rates among women reached a maximum incidence of 1 per cent per year. Interestingly, a leveling off or decline in the incidence of symptomatic OA occurred in both sexes around the age of 80. In studies in which serial knee radiographs were obtained,[22] rates of incident symptomatic OA in women were 1 per cent per year. Radiographic OA of the knee (often asymptomatic) was more frequent with an incidence of 2 per cent per year in women.[23]

The descriptive epidemiology of OA

♦ The most common form of arthritis

♦ Occurs most frequently in knees, hands (DIPs, PIPs, MCPs, thumb base), hips, back, neck and spares wrists, ankles

♦ Incidence and prevalence higher in women than in men, especially after the age of 50

♦ Many have joint symptoms without X-ray change and vice versa

♦ Emerging information on racial differences in occurrence may provide etiologic clues to disease

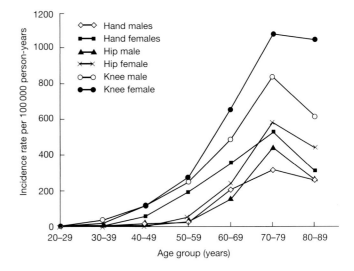

Fig. 2.2 Incidence of OA of the hand, hip, and knee, in members of the Fallon Community Health Plan, 1991–2, by age and sex.

Source: Taken from Oliveria et al.[21]

Risk factors for OA

Individual joints become especially susceptible to OA when local factors in the joint combine with systemic vulnerability. Such local factors might include joint deformity or malalignment, but by far the most common local factor we recognize is previous major injury to a joint, which has left the joint vulnerable. Local factors may be powerful determinants of OA by themselves such that a joint may be sufficiently deformed or affected by a major injury as to inevitably lead to OA. But more commonly, this injury acts on a joint within a person whose own systemic vulnerability to OA varies depending on their age and other factors. Thus, in many cases there is interplay of systemic and local vulnerability factors.

Within that local and systemic environment, a variety of loading-related factors exert influence over whether a joint develops OA. The primary factors are obesity and particular physical activities, which we shall call extrinsic factors (see Fig. 2.3). Thus, a person who participates in activities

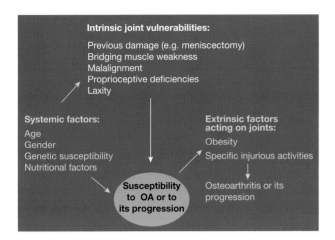

Fig. 2.3 Risk factors and how they interact to cause OA.

that repeatedly injure joints is more likely to develop OA in that joint if they have either local or systemic vulnerabilities. Genetic susceptibilities may be a prime example of the mechanism by which OA occurs in this fashion. Persons who have known mutations predisposing to OA do not get OA in all joints; rather in isolated joints, presumably those in which there is either some local vulnerability or extrinsic injury produces OA. The sections below detail the evidence for the contribution for specific systemic, local, and extrinsic factors and their relation to the development of OA.

Systemic risk factors

The most potent systemic vulnerabilities are increasing age and female gender. While getting older does not cause OA per se, disease incidence and prevalence increase dramatically with age. Further, given this interaction of systemic vulnerabilities and either local or extrinsic factors, it is not surprising that those who sustain major knee injuries after the age of 30 are at a much higher risk of rapidly developing OA[48] than persons under the age of 30 who sustain similar injuries.

Also, as noted above, racial factors provide another systemic vulnerability with those of Asian extraction having very low rates of hip OA. Other racial differences in disease occurrence are yet to be identified.

Heritability and genetics. Like many other chronic diseases of onset in middle and later years, a large proportion of the occurrence of OA is due, in part, to inheritance. The proportion of OA cases attributable to inheritance varies according to the joint. For example, the proportion of hand and hip OA due, in part, to inheritance is over 50 per cent, yet the proportion of knee OA ranges from 10–30 per cent.[24,25] Also, heritability of disease is higher in early onset of disease than it is among those who have onset of disease later in life. The details of the heritability of OA and identified genetic factors that may predispose to disease are discussed in later chapters.

Bone density and OA. Persons with osteoporosis exhibit a lower than expected rate of OA.[26] Further, bone density is greater in patients with OA than in age-matched controls, even at sites distant from the OA joint.[27,28] Some, but not all, of the increase in bone mass may be explained by the association of OA with obesity, which protects against osteoporosis. Also, osteophyte formation, not cartilage loss, may be linked to high bone mass,[29] and a circulating bone growth factor may enhance the growth of osteophytes and enthesophytes, extra bone formation at the sites of ligament and tendon insertions.[30] The relation of that circulating or local factor and systemic bone mineral density is unknown.

Emerging longitudinal studies are beginning to suggest a complex relationship between bone density and OA. In one study,[31] while women with incident hand OA had higher bone density than women without it, bone turnover assessed by osteocalcin levels was actually lower in those with incident OA. In the Framingham Study where subjects were followed longitudinally to evaluate a change in OA, high bone density increased the risk of

developing new radiographic knee OA, but, paradoxically, those with OA who had high bone mineral density had a much lower risk of disease progression by radiograph (joint space loss) than those with low bone density.[32]

Estrogen deficiency in women. In addition to the high incidence of OA in women after the age of 50—the approximate age of menopause—some women develop 'menopausal arthritis' (rapidly progressive hand OA) at the time of menopause.[33] These gender and age-related prevalence patterns are consistent with a role for post-menopausal hormone deficiency in increasing the risk of OA. In coronary artery disease, gout, and osteoporosis—diseases for which the risk in women rises dramatically after menopause as it does in OA—estrogen loss has been strongly implicated as a risk factor.

Most, but not all, epidemiologic studies[34–36] provide evidence that estrogen replacement therapy (ERT) is associated with a reduction in the risk of knee and hip OA. For example, both the Study of Osteoporotic Fractures (SOF)[28] and the Framingham Study[35] have reported a lower prevalence of OA among those reporting long-term use of ERT, than among non-users or among women who used ERT for shorter periods (OR for more than 10 years of ERT use, for both SOF and the Framingham Study = 0.6). In both studies the inverse association was stronger when analysis was restricted to more severe OA or to bilateral radiographic OA. Follow-up of the Framingham[37] and Chingford Study[38] subjects suggested that women in ERT were less likely than those not on ERT to have incident or progressive OA. Further, ERT users may have more cartilage in their knees than non-users.[39] Clinical OA, however, may not be less prevalent among ERT users,[40] possibly because ERT users see doctors more often and are therefore more likely to get their OA diagnosed, a form of detection bias. Lastly, while ERT may prevent structural changes of OA such as cartilage loss, clinical trial evidence suggests it does not have a measurable effect on knee symptoms.[41]

Nutritional factors. Vitamin C or ascorbic acid has a multitude of functions within cartilage. Among others, it protects against damage by reactive oxygen species and it serves as a cofactor for enzymes contributing to type II collagen synthesis. In a longitudinal study based in Framingham, low vitamin C intake was associated with accelerated radiographic progression of OA in those with prevalent disease at baseline. It was unassociated with incident disease.

Using the same study subjects, a similar protective effect on disease progression of high levels and intakes of vitamin D was seen.[42] The rationale behind vitamin D is on the surface more farfetched, although chondrocytes at the basal level of cartilage redevelop vitamin D receptors in OA, and vitamin D sufficiency is necessary for active bone turnover, which may be critical in OA. The vitamin D results have been reexamined in a longitudinal hip study and similar results have been reported.[43]

Local risk factors: intrinsic (in local joint environment)

Congenital and developmental deformities and hip OA. Three uncommon developmental abnormalities, congenital dislocation, Legg-Perthes disease, and slipped femoral capital epiphysis, lead invariably to hip OA in later life. Milder developmental abnormalities, including sub-clinical variants of these developmental diseases may also presage hip OA. Circumstantial evidence for this link includes the unusual predominance of hip OA in men,[44] the striking racial disparities in the prevalence of hip OA, and the weak association with hip OA of such traditional risk factors as obesity, suggesting the importance of other risk factors. Acetabular dysplasia, a mild variant of congenital dislocation in which the acetabulum is shallow, increases the risk of incident hip OA in women and may account for a substantial proportion of hip OA in women, although probably not in men.[45,46]

Major joint injury. With a major joint injury, a person can sustain permanent damage of many of the structures within a joint. This damage alters the biomechanics of the joint, increases stress across particular areas of the joint and often dramatically increases the risk of OA. Joint cartilage and other joint structures are often damaged by sudden injuries such as fractures or ligamentous tears. Acute major knee injuries including cruciate ligament and meniscal tears are common causes of knee OA especially among men.[47,48] Such injuries are prevalent[49] in young women athletes and increase their risk of developing OA at a young age. Epidemiologic studies have documented that those with a history of major knee injury are a high risk of later, usually ipsilateral, knee OA. In the Framingham study,[50] men with a history of major knee injuries had a relative risk of 3.5 for subsequent knee OA; for women the relative risk was 2.2 (both $p < 0.05$). At sites in which the disease is generally uncommon, for example, the ankle and shoulder joints, major joint injury may account for a large proportion of all cases of OA.

There is clearly interplay between systemic and local injury factors. For example, those sustaining major knee injuries of their knees develop OA in the knees rapidly if they are older but are less likely to develop OA with such rapidity if they are younger.[51] Either partial or complete meniscus removal, done when the meniscus is injured increases local stresses and laxity within the knee[52] and is itself a prominent cause of OA.[53] Hip injuries may also cause OA there, but longitudinal studies evaluating this issue are lacking.

Other local risk factors. Those with joint deformities from fractures, osteonecrosis, or other reasons are at high risk for OA also because of the biomechanical modifications that occur with joint deformity. This constitutes one of the reasons why those with destructive inflammatory arthritis are at a high risk for getting secondary OA. Lastly, malalignment especially in the knees has recently been linked to rapid disease progression for those who already have knee OA.[54] By altering loading across joints, malalignment may contribute to OA incidence in the knees and other joints.

Extrinsic risk factors (factors acting on the joint)

Obesity. Population-based studies consistently show that overweight persons are at higher risk of knee OA than non-overweight controls. Estimates of risk vary from population to population and depend, to some degree, on the criteria for overweight and the definition of OA. In NHANES I, which was conducted throughout the United States of America from 1971–5,[55] the risk of radiographic OA in obese women (body mass index, BMI, greater than 30 but less than 35) was almost four times that in women whose BMI was lower than 25. For men in the same overweight category the risk was 4.8 times greater than that for men of normal weight. Three to six times body weight is exerted across the knee during single leg stance in walking;[56] therefore, any increase in weight may be multiplied by this factor to reveal the excess force across the knee of an overweight person during walking. In addition to increasing the risk of tibiofemoral OA, obesity augments the risk of disease in the patellofemoral joint. Not only does obesity occur with knee OA more than expected, it actually[57,58] *precedes* the development of knee OA, suggesting it causes disease, probably through excess loading. The relation of obesity to hip OA is weaker than with knee OA, a difference that is possibly due to the different multiplier effects of body weight across the two joint sites or differences in distribution of load across the hip and knee during weight-bearing.[59]

Weight could act to cause OA via two mechanisms: first, and most logically, because it increases the amount of load across a joint, obesity could induce cartilage breakdown simply on the basis of excess load. This could account for the apparent causal relationship between weight and knee and hip OA. Indeed, the association of obesity and knee OA is so strong that it is not likely to be explained by confounding factors. Surprisingly, people who are overweight may be at slightly higher risk of hand OA.[60] The load theory does not explain the relationship between overweight and hand OA, which suggests the involvement of a systemic factor. Following this line of reasoning, it has been speculated that a circulating factor that acts to accelerate cartilage breakdown may be present in overweight persons, serving as a second mechanism leading to OA.

In addition, bone mineral density is increased in overweight persons and this (or the absence of osteoporosis) may be a risk factor for OA.[61] Additional evidence in favor of a systemic factor is the possibility that the relationship between overweight and OA is stronger in women than in men.[62]

Does losing weight lower the risk of OA? For the Framingham women whose baseline BMI values were greater than 25, that is, greater than the median, weight loss significantly lowered the rate of incident symptomatic knee OA.[63] The adjusted odds ratio per two units of BMI (approximately 5 kg for a woman of normal height) was 0.41, a reduction of more than 50 per cent in the risk of developing knee OA. Weight gain was associated with a slightly increased rate of subsequent knee OA (odds ratio 1.28 for a two-unit weight gain). For women whose baseline weight was lower than the median, neither weight gain nor weight loss significantly affected their risk of later disease.

Substantial weight loss (dropping from obese to overweight, or from overweight to normal weight range) would prevent about 21 per cent of knee OA in men; in women (in whom the association of obesity and knee OA is stronger), 33 per cent of knee OA would be prevented.[64] For women, weight accounts for more OA than any other known factor; for men, overweight is second to knee injury as a preventable cause of knee OA.

Not only does being overweight increase the risk for OA, but for those with established knee OA it increases the odds of disease progression.[65–67] Furthermore, those with OA in one knee are at higher risk of developing OA in the other knee if they are overweight.[68] The effect of obesity on OA progression in joints other than the knee has not been studied.

In those who already have OA, weight change is likely to affect symptoms. McGoey *et al.*[69] studied morbidly obese women at the time of their gastric stapling operation and one year later, at which time their mean weight loss was approximately 45 kg. The proportion with knee symptoms dropped from 57 to 14 per cent during this interval and the prevalence of other regional symptoms, for example, hip pain and back pain, fell commensurately. Unfortunately, the authors did not definitively ascertain whether these subjects had OA.

In another study, 30 obese women (48.7 per cent above ideal weight) with knee or hip OA were randomized to phentermine, an appetite suppressant, or placebo, with all subjects instructed to eat a low-energy diet.[70] Six months later, among 22 patients who remained in the trial, those taking phentermine had lost 6.3 kg and those in the placebo group 4.5 kg ($p = NS$). The amount of weight loss correlated significantly with improvement in a clinical score, which combined symptoms and physical findings. For knee OA, the correlation between weight loss and improvement was especially strong ($r = 0.66$, $p < 0.01$).

Muscle weakness. It has long been recognized that persons with knee OA have weaker quadriceps than those without the disease.[71,72] In a longitudinal follow-up study, women with incident knee OA were weaker at baseline than women who did not develop knee OA.[73] The same was not necessarily true for men, but the numbers were small. Quadriceps contraction may decelerate impulse loading during gait and therefore protect the knee from damage.[74] Since muscle contraction across a joint may be the main source of joint loading, strength may not protect all joints from getting OA. Increased grip strength has been found to be associated with high rates of OA in proximal hand joints like the MCP and base of the thumb, suggesting that increased loading on the basis of powerful muscle contraction can actually damage joints.[75]

Repeated use of joint. There are two types of activities that involve the repeated use of a joint and have been the focus of epidemiologic studies, occupational and athletic activities.

Occupational activities and OA. Farmers are at high risk for hip OA. Among farmers, standing, bending, walking long distances over rough ground, lifting, moving heavy objects, and tractor driving all appear to pose high risks for hip OA, while climbing was not implicated as a risk factor.[76]

Also, jackhammer operators have a high rate of OA in the upper extremity joints that are otherwise rarely affected by disease. Jackhammers impart high impulse loads across joints that are not designed to sustain them. Vibratory tools may subvert the effectiveness of joint shock absorbers, such as muscles, leading to the transmission of excess stress across the joint and leading to joint injury.

Miners have high rates of OA in the knees and spine,[77] while shipyard and dockyard workers have a higher prevalence of OA in the knees and fingers than office workers. Cotton mill workers may have high rates of hand OA compared to controls.[78]

While there are jobs that clearly predispose to OA through joint overuse, there are stereotyped activities that themselves cause OA. Women whose jobs require a fine pincer grip (increasing the stress across DIP joints) in a Virginia textile mill had significantly more DIP joint OA than women whose jobs required repeated power grip, a motion that does not stress the DIP joints.[79] Workers whose jobs required regular knee bending and lifting or carrying heavy loads[80–83] had a higher rate of knee OA than workers whose jobs did not entail these activities.

With respect to the prevention of OA, occupational activities may be extremely important. In a study of older male workers, the proportion of OA potentially attributable to occupational knee bending was higher (32 per cent) than that attributable to obesity (24 per cent).[84] If specific job-related tasks, which increase the risk of OA, were changed or avoided many cases of OA would be prevented. Unfortunately, occupation-related OA is not an easy target for disease prevention. Jobs contain complex ergonomic activities and isolating the injurious ones may be difficult. Also, workers often change jobs or rotate to other tasks. Elimination of all jobs involving substantial physical labor is not realistic, but minor alterations in ergonomic activities might lower job-related OA risk if specific tasks are shown as being linked to a high rate of OA.

Leisure time physical activities and OA. With exercise already assuming a major role in OA treatment, it appears paradoxical to consider the idea that exercise *per se* may actually cause OA. But the evidence suggests that certain types of exercise may indeed do so. The association of running with OA is of special interest (see Table 2.1). Most studies evaluating recreational running have not shown that runners have an increased risk of knee OA, although studies of hip OA have not been consistent. What has emerged, however, is an intriguing relation between elite running[85] and OA of both the knee and hip. Professional runners and those on Olympic teams followed over time have substantially higher rates of OA in weight-bearing joints than age-matched controls. Studies of recreational runners have two important methodological limitations: first, they often miss persons who stop running because they develop knee or hip pain because of early disease and secondly, they often fail to have information on and adjust for a history of major knee injury. One study suggests that runners who get OA are those with the history of major knee injury.[86]

Like occupational activities, OA in athletes seems to occur in especially over-used joints so that weight lifters who squat and then lift heavy weights have a high risk of patellofemoral OA, whereas soccer players have a higher risk of tibiofemoral knee OA.[87]

Given the widespread prescription to adopt a healthier more exercise-filled lifestyle, large-scale longitudinal epidemiologic studies of the consequences of exercise on OA contain cautionary notes. In a large-scale study of women followed for hip OA, those with increased levels of physical activity either as a teenager or at age 50 were at a higher risk of developing symptomatic OA later in life[88] than women who were sedentary. In a prospective follow-up of elders in Framingham, those who reported heavy physical activity were at a three-fold increased risk of developing both radiographic and symptomatic knee OA at follow-up compared to those who were inactive. Not all literature is consistent on this matter, however.[89] Since physical activity in general has so many salutatory effects, identifying the particular activities that pose risks of long-term joint damage (such as those listed above) is preferred to stigmatizing physical activity because it might, in some cases, be risky. Because of the systemic vulnerability to OA among those who are aged, this group may be at a high risk of OA when they become physically active later in life.[90]

Risk factors for symptoms

Only approximately half of those with radiographic OA have frequent joint symptoms. From a clinical and public health perspective, understanding the etiology of joint symptoms is critical. In a recent MRI-based study in which those with knee symptoms were compared to others of a comparable age and radiographic disease, MRI features that distinguished those with knee symptoms from those without were bone marrow edema lesions, synovial thickening, and effusions.[91] Large bone marrow edema lesions were present almost exclusively in those with knee pain and were absent in those without it, even if they had radiographic disease. Symptom severity was strongly correlated with an MRI finding of synovitis.[92] Findings from this study suggest that synovial inflammation and its product, joint effusion, and bone marrow lesions might be uniquely correlated with the development of knee pain.

Table 2.1 Controlled studies on running and OA

Author (year)	Joint	No. of subjects	Time elapsed since running (years)	OA in runners compared to controls
Sohn and Micheli (1985)	Knee	504	25	No increase in knee complaints over controls (swimmers)
Lane et al. (1993)	Knee	33	5	No increase in OA
Panush (1994)	Knee	12	8	No increase in OA
Harris et al. (1995)	Knee	73	0–40	Increase in osteophytes in runners
Kujala et al. (1995)*	Knee	28	35	Non-significant increase (OR = 4.8) of knee OA in runners vs. shooters
Spector et al. (1996)*	Knee	73	0–40	Increase in osteophytes in runners
Puranen (1975)*	Hip	60	20	No increase in OA
Marti et al. (1989)*	Hip	27	15	Runners had more OA than controls
Vingard et al. (1993)*	Hip, Knee	233	20–50	Runners had more OA (RR = 2.1, p = NS)
Kujala et al. (1994)	Hip, and Ankle	100	30	Runners had more hospitalization for knee and hip OA (RR = 1.8; 95% CI 0.9–3.6)
Cheng et al. (2000)	Hip and Knee	16	0–25	Male but not female runners (> 20 miles/week) had more OA than non-runners (OR = 1.6; 95% CI 1.1–2.3)

* Studies of elite runners.

Table 2.2 Do biomechanical factors affect the knee differently at different stages of OA?

	Odds ratio for	
	Incident (new) disease	Progressive disease
High BMI*	9.1	2.6
Previous knee injury*	4.8	1.2
Regular sports*	3.2	0.7
High bone density†	2.3	0.1

* Taken from Cooper et al., 2000.[94]

† Taken from Zhang et al., 2000.[33]

Risk factors for incidence vs. progression

Many of the risk factors discussed above may operate differently on joints at different stages of disease. Studies have suggested, for example, that vitamin D deficiency may accelerate the risk of OA progression but does not appear to affect the risk of incident disease. Vitamin C deficiency may have similar effects.[89] As noted above, bone density may actually have opposite effects at different disease stages with high bone density increasing the risk of incident disease yet delaying progression. Some factors such as obesity, previous knee injury, and regular sports prescriptions, have been strongly linked to incidence yet in the same populations appear unrelated to the risk of progression[90] (see Table 2.2).

It would be unusual if risk factors varied at different stages of the disease, but when disease is present the joint becomes more vulnerable and one might expect risk factors to act in a more potent fashion, although the data do not necessarily suggest they do. Other explanations for the differences reported between risk factors for incidence and progression include: the numbers are small in each of these studies and differences reported may not reflect real ones; risk factors for incidence are really risk factors for osteophytes and those for progression are risk factors for joint space or cartilage loss; and lastly that risk factors really do differ at different stages of the disease perhaps because of the different metabolic or restorative powers of the joint.

References

(An asterisk denotes recommended reading.)

1. Guccione, A.A., Felson, D.T., Anderson, J.J., et al. (1994). The effects of specific medical conditions on the functional limitations of elders in the Framingham Study. Am J Public Health 84:351–8.

2. US Department of Health and Human Services (1995). CDC: Prevalence and impact of arthritis among women—United States, 1989–1991. MMWR 44:329–34.

3. Hutton, C.W. (1987). Hypothesis. Generalised osteoarthritis: an evolutionary problem? Lancet 1:1463–5.

4. Lawrence, R.C., Helmick, C.G., Arnett, F.C., et al. (1998). Estimates of the prevalence of arthritis and selected musculoskeletal disorders in the United States. Arthritis Rheum 41:778–99.

5. Nevitt, M.C., Lane, N.C., Scott, J.C., et al. (1995). Radiographic osteoarthritis of the hip and bone mineral density. Arthritis Rheum 38:907–16.

6. *Peat, G., McCarney, R., and Croft, P. (2001). Knee pain and osteoarthritis in older adults: a review of community burden and current use of primary health care. Ann Rheum Dis 60:91–7.

   This article provides a clear explanation and supporting data on the prevalence of knee pain and OA in the community and how these vary depending on the definition.

7. Engel, A. (1968). Osteoarthritis and body measurements. Rockville MD: National Center for Health Statistics, Series 11, no. 29, PHS publication no. 1999.

8. Felson, D.T., Naimark, A., Anderson, J., Kazis, L., Castelli, W., and Meenan, R.F. (1987). The prevalence of knee osteoarthritis in the elderly. Arthritis Rheum 30(8):914–18.

9. Van Saase, J.L.C.M., Van Romunde, L.K.J., Cats, A., Vandenbroucke, J.P., and Valkenburg, H.A. (1989). Epidemiology of osteoarthritis: Zoetermeer survey. Comparison of radiological osteoarthritis in a Dutch population with that in 10 other populations. Ann Rheum Dis 48:271–80.

10. Anderson, J. and Felson, D.T. (1988). Factors associated with osteoarthritis of the knee in the First National Health and Nutrition Examination Survey (NHANES I). Am J Epidemiol 128:179–89.

11. Lawrence, J.S. and Sebo, M. (1980). 'The geography of osteoarthritis'. In The Aetiopathogenesis of Osteoarthritis, Baltimore: University Park Press, pp. 155–83.

12. Hoaglund, F.T., Oishi, C.S., and Gialamas, G.G. (1995). Extreme variations in racial rates of total hip arthroplasty for primary coxarthrosis: A population-based study in San Francisco. Ann Rheum Dis 54:107–10.

13. Nevitt, M., Xu, L., Zhang, Y., et al. (2000). Chinese in Beijing have a very low prevalence of hip OA compared to U.S. Caucasians. Arthritis Rheum 43:S171.

14. Zhang, Y., Xu, L., Nevitt, M.C., et al. (2001). Comparison of the prevalence of knee osteoarthritis between the elderly Chinese population in Beijing and Whites in the U.S.: The Beijing Osteoarthritis Study. Arthritis Rheum 44:2065–71.

15. Hoaglund, F.T., Yau, A.C.M.C., and Wong, W.I. (1973). Osteoarthritis of the hip and other joints in Southern Chinese in Hong Kong. J Bone Joint Surg 55(A):545–57.

16. Lau, E. and Lin, F. (1994). Low prevalence of osteoarthritis of the hip in Chinese men. Arthritis Rheum 37(Suppl.):S239.

17. Kellgren, J.H. and Moore, R. (1952). Generalized osteoarthritis and Heberden's nodes. Br Med J 1:181–7.

18. Lawrence, J.S. (1977). Osteoarthrosis. In J.S. Lawrence (ed.). Rheumatism in Populations. London: Heinemann.

19. Cerhan, J.R., Wallace, R.B., El-Khoury, G.Y., Moore, T.E., and Long, C.R. (1995). Decreased survival with increasing prevalence of full-body, radiographically defined osteoarthritis in women. Am J Epidemiol 141:225–34.

20. Monson, R.R. and Hall, A.P. (1976). Mortality among arthritics. J Chronic Dis 29:359–467.

21. Oliveria, S.A., Felson, D.T., Reed, J.I., Cirillo, P.A., and Walker, A.M. (1995). Incidence of symptomatic hand, hip, and knee osteoarthritis among patients in a health maintenance organization. Arthritis Rheum 38:1134–41.

22. Felson, D.T., Zhang, Y., Hannan, M.T., et al. (1995). The Incidence and natural history of knee osteoarthritis in the elderly: The Framingham Osteoarthritis Study. Arthritis Rheum 38:1500–5.

23. Hart, D.J., Doyle, D.V., and Spector, T. (1999). Incidence and risk factors for radiographic knee osteoarthritis in middle-aged women. Arthritis Rheum 42:17–24.

24. Demissie, S., Cupples, L.A., Myers, R., Aliabadi, P., Levy, D., and Felson, D.T. (2002). Genome scan for quantity of hand osteoarthritis: the Framingham study. Arthritis Rheum 46:946–52.

25. *Spector, T.D., Cicuttini, F., Baker, J., Loughlin, J., and Hart, D. (1996). Genetic influences on osteoarthritis in women: a twin study. Br Med J 312:940–4.

   In data from a large twin study, these investigators reported that radiographic OA was highly heritable, especially OA in the hand joints.

26. Hart, D.J., Mootoosamy, I., Doyle, D.V., and Spector, T.D. (1994). The relationship between osteoarthritis and osteoporosis in the general population: the Chingford Study. Ann Rheum Dis 53:158–62.

27. Gevers, G., Dequeker, J., Martens, M., et al. (1989). Biomechanical characteristics of iliac crest bone in elderly women according to osteoarthritis grade at the hand joints. J Rheumatol 16:660–3.

28. Dequeker, J., Boonen, N., Aerssens, J., Westhovens, R. (1996). Inverse relationship osteoarthritis–osteoporosis: what is the evidence? What are the consequences? (Editorial). Br J Rheumatol 35:813–20.

29. Hannan, M.T., Anderson, J.J., Zhang, Y., Levy, D., and Felson, D.T. (1993). Bone mineral density and knee osteoarthritis in elderly men and women. *Arthritis Rheum* **36**:1671–80.

30. Rogers, J., Shepstone, L., Dieppe, P. (1997). Bone formers: osteophyte and enthesophyte formation are positively associated. *Ann Rheum Dis* **56**:85–90.

31. Sowers, M., Lachance, L., Jamadar, D., *et al.* (1999). The associations of bone mineral density and bone turnover markers with osteoarthritis of the hand and knee in pre- and perimenopausal women. *Arthritis Rheum* **42**:483–9.

32. Zhang, Y., Hannan, M.T., Chaisson, C.E., *et al.* (2000). Bone mineral density and risk of incident and progressive radiographic knee osteoarthritis in women: the Framingham study. *J Rheumatol* **27**:1032–7.

33. Kellgren, J.H. and Moore, R. (1952). Generalized osteoarthritis and Heberden's nodes. *Br Med J* **1**:181–7.

34. Nevitt, M.C., Cummings, S.R., Lane, N.E., Genant, H.K., and Pressman, A.R. (1994). Current use of oral estrogen is associated with a decreased prevalence of radiographic hip OA in elderly white women. *Arthritis Rheum* **37**(Suppl.):S212.

35. Hannan, M.T., Felson, D.T., Anderson, J.J., Naimark, A., and Kannel, W.B. (1990). Estrogen use and radiographic osteoarthritis of the knee in women. *Arthritis Rheum* **33**:525–32.

36. Wolfe, F., Altman, R., Hochberg, M., Lane, N., Luggan, M., and Sharp, J. (1994). Postmenopausal estrogen therapy is associated with improved radiographic scores in OA and RA. *Arthritis Rheum* **37**(Suppl.):S231.

37. Zhang, Y, McAlindon, T.E., Hannan, M.T., *et al.* (1998). Estrogen replacement therapy and worsening of radiographic knee osteoarthritis. *Arthritis Rheum* **41**:1867–73.

38. Hart, D.J., Doyle, D.V., and Spector, T.D. (1999). Incidence and risk factors for radiographic knee osteoarthritis in middle-aged women: the Chingford Study. *Arthritis Rheum* **42**:17–24.

39. Wluka, A.E., Davis, S.R., Bailey, M., Stuckey, S.L., and Cicuttini, F.M. (2001). Users of oestrogen replacement therapy have more knee cartilage than non-users. *Ann Rheum Dis* **60**:332–6.

40. Sandmark, H., Hogstedt, C., Lewold, S., and Vingard, E. (1999). Osteoarthrosis of the knee in men and women in association with overweight, smoking, and hormone therapy. *Ann Rheum Dis* **58**:151–5.

41. Nevitt, M.C., Felson, D.T., Williams, E.N., and Grady, D. (for the Heart and Estrogen/Progestin Replacement Study Research Group) (2001). The effect of estrogen plus progestin on knee symptoms and related disability in postmenopausal women. *Arthritis Rheum* **44**:811–8.

42. *McAlindon, T.E., Felson, D.T., Zhang, Y., *et al.* (1996). Relation of dietary intake and serum levels of Vitamin D to progression of osteoarthritis of the knee among participants in the Framingham Study. *Ann Intern Med* **125**:353–9.

   A longitudinal study suggesting that low 25-OH vitamin D levels increase the risk of progressive radiographic knee OA.

43. Lane, N.E., Gore, L.R., Cummings, S.R., *et al.* (1999). Serum vitamin D levels and incident changes of radiographic hip osteoarthritis. *Arthritis Rheum* **42**:854–60.

44. Kellgren, J.H. (1961). Osteoarthritis in patients and populations. *Br Med J* **243**:1–6.

45. Solomon, L. (1976). Patterns of osteoarthritis of the hip. *J Bone Joint Surg* **58**(B):176–83.

46. Lane, N.E., Lin, P., Christiansen, L., *et al.* (2000). Association of mild acetabular dysplasia with an increased risk of incident hip osteoarthritis in elderly white women. *Arthritis Rheum* **43**:400–4.

47. Jacobsen, K. (1977). Osteoarthrosis following insufficiency of the cruciate ligaments in man. *Acta Orthop Scand* **48**:520–6.

48. Roos, H.P., Lauren, M., Adalberth, T., Roos, E.M., Jonsson, K., and Lohmander, L.S. (1998). Knee osteoarthritis after meniscectomy. *Arthritis Rheum* **41**:687–93.

49. Roos, H.P., Ostenberg, A. (2000). A prospective study of female soccer players with anterior cruciate ligament tear. Radiographic findings and symptoms 12 years after injury. *Arthritis Rheum* **43**:913.

50. Felson, D.T. (1990). The epidemiology of knee osteoarthritis: results from the Framingham osteoarthritis study. *Sem Arthritis Rheum* **20**: 42–50.

51. *Roos, H.P., Adalberth, T., Dahlberg, L., Lohmander, L.S. (1995). Osteoarthritis of the knee after injury to the anterior cruciate ligament or meniscus: the influence of time and age. *Osteoarthritis Cart* **3**:261–7.

   An important article suggesting that knee injury causes accelerated development of OA if it occurs after age 30.

52. Walker, P.S., Erkman, M.J. (1975). The role of the menisci in force transmission across the knee. *Clin Orthop Rel Res* **109**:184–192.

53. Englund, M., Roos, E.M., Roos, H.P., Lohmander, L.S. (2001). Patient-relevant outcomes fourteen years after meniscectomy: influence of types of meniscal tear and size of resection. *Rheumatology* **40**:631–639.

54. Sharma, L., Song, J., Felson, D.T., Cahue, S., Shamiyeh, E., Dunlop, D.D. (2001). The role of knee alignment in disease progression and functional decline in knee osteoarthritis. *JAMA* **286**:188–195.

55. Anderson, J. and Felson, D.T. (1988). Factors associated with osteoarthritis of the knee in the First National Health and Nutrition Examination Survey (NHANES I). *Am J Epidemiol* **128**:179–89.

56. Maquet, P. (1976). *Biomechanics of the Knee*. Springer-Verlag, New York.

57. Felson, D.T., Anderson, J.J., Naimark, A., Walker, A.M. and Meenan, R.F. (1988). Obesity and knee osteoarthritis. *Ann Intern Med* **109**:18–24.

58. Schouten, J. (1991). A 12-year follow-up study of osteoarthritis of the knee in the general population, Thesis, Erasmus University, pp. 149–64.

59. Heliovaara, M., Mkel, M., and Impivaara, O., *et al.* (1993). Association of overweight, trauma and workload with coxarthrosis: a health survey of 7,217 persons. *Acta Orthop Scand* **64**:513–18.

60. Carman, W.J., Sowers, M.F., Hawthorne, V.M., and Weissfeld, L.A. (1994). Obesity as a risk factor for osteoarthritis of the hand and wrist: a prospective study. *Am J Epidemiol* **39**:119–29.

61. Hannan, M.T., Anderson, J.J., Zhang, Y., Levy, D., and Felson, D.T. (1993). Bone mineral density and knee osteoarthritis in elderly men and women: the Framingham Study. *Arthritis Rheum* **36**:1671–80.

62. *Felson, D.T., Zhang, Y., Anthony, J.M., Naimark, A., and Anderson, J.J. (1992). Weight loss reduces the risk for symptomatic knee osteoarthritis in women. *Ann Intern Med* **116**:535–9.

   Longitudinal study of women suggesting that weight 12 years prior to onset of symptomatic OA increases risk, and that modest weight loss (approximately 12 lbs) can dramatically lower the risk of developing disease, especially among those who are overweight at baseline.

63. Schouten, J.S.A.G., van den Ouweland, and Valkenburg, H.A. (1992). A 12-year follow-up study in the general population on prognostic factors of cartilage loss in osteoarthritis of the knee. *Ann Rheum Dis* **51**:932–7.

64. *Felson, D.T. and Zhang, Y.Q. (1998). An update on the epidemiology of knee and hip osteoarthritis with a view to prevention. *Arthritis Rheum* **41**:1343–55.

   A comprehensive recent review of disease epidemiology including data on prevalence of disease in knee and hip and a critical review of current thinking about risk factors.

65. Schouten, J.S.A.G., van den Ouweland, and Valkenburg, H.A. (1992). A 12-year follow-up study in the general population on prognostic factors of cartilage loss in osteoarthritis of the knee. *Ann Rheum Dis* **51**:932–7.

66. Dougados, M., Gueguen, A., Nguyen, M., *et al.* (1992). Longitudinal radiologic evaluation of osteoarthritis of the knee. *J Rheumatol* **19**:378–83.

67. Altman, R.D., Fried, J.F., Bloch, D.A., *et al.* (1987). Radiographic assessment of progression in osteoarthritis. *Arthritis Rheum* **30**:1214–25.

68. Spector, T.D., Hart, D.J., and Doyle, D.V. (1994). Incidence and progression of osteoarthritis in women with unilateral knee disease in the general population: the effect of obesity. *Ann Rheum Dis* **53**:565–8.

69. McGoey, B.V., Deitel, M., Saplys, R.J.F., and Kliman, M.E. (1990). Effect of weight loss on musculoskeletal pain in the morbidly obese. *J Bone Joint Surg* **72**(B):322–3.

70. Williams, R.A. and Foulsham, B.M. (1981). Weight reduction in osteoarthritis using phentermine. *The Practitioner* **225**:231–2.

71. Slemenda, C., Brandt, K.D., Heilman, *et al.* (1997). Quadriceps weakness and osteoarthritis of the knee. *Ann Intern Med* **127**:97–104.

72. Madsen, O.R., Bliddal, H., Egsmose, C., and Sylvest, J. (1995). Isometric and isokinetic quadriceps strength in gonarthrosis; inter-relations between quadriceps strength, walking ability, radiology, subchondral bone density and pain. *Clin Rheumatol* **14**:308–14.

73. *Slemenda, C., Heilman, D.K., Brandt, K.D., *et al.* (1998). Reduced quadri-ceps strength relative to body weight. A risk factor for knee osteoarthritis in women? *Arthritis Rheum* **41**:1951–9.

Compared to women who did not get OA, those who developed incident radiographic OA had weaker quadriceps 3 years earlier. No association of quadriceps weakness with incident OA was found in men.

74. Jefferson, R.J., Collins, J.J., Whittle, M.W., Radin, E.L., and O'Connor, J.J. (1990). The role of the quadriceps in controlling impulsive forces around heel strike. *Proc Instn Mech Engrs* **204**:21–8.

75. Chaisson, C.E., Zhang, Y., Sharma, L., Kannel, W., Felson, D.T. (1999). Grip strength and the risk of developing radiographic hand osteoarthritis: results from the Framingham study. *Arthritis Rheum* **42**:33–8.

76. Croft, P., Coggon, D., Cruddas, M., and Cooper, C. (1992). Osteoarthritis of the hip: an occupational disease in farmers. *Br Med J* **304**:1269–72.

77. Kellgren, J.H. and Lawrence, J.S. (1952). Rheumatism in miners. II: X-ray study. *Br J Ind Med* **9**:197–207.

78. Lawrence, J.S. (1961). Rheumatism in cotton operatives. *Br J Ind Med* **18**:270–6.

79. Hadler, N.M., Gillings, D.B., Imbus, R. *et al.* (1978). Hand structure and function in an industrial setting. *Arthritis Rheum* **21**:210–20.

80. Anderson, J. and Felson, D.T. (1988). Factors associated with osteoarthritis of the knee in the First National Health and Nutrition Examination Survey (NHANES I). *Am J Epidemiol* **128**:179–89.

81. Kujala, U.M., Kettunen, J., Paananen, H., *et al.* (1995). Knee osteoarthritis in former runners, soccer players, weight lifters and shooters. *Arthritis Rheum* **38**:539–46.

82. Felson, D.T., Hannan, M.T., Naimark, A., *et al.* (1991). Occupational phys-ical demands, knee bending, and knee osteoarthritis: results from the Framingham Study. *J Rheumatol* **18**:1587–92.

83. Cooper, C., McAlindon, T., Coggon, D., Egger, P., and Dieppe, P. (1994). Occupational activity and osteoarthritis of the knee. *Ann Rheum Dis* **53**:90–3.

84. Anderson, J., and Felson, D.T. (1988). Factors associated with osteoarthritis of the knee in the First National Health and Nutrition Examination Survey (NHANES I). *Am J Epidemiol* **128**:179–89.

85. Spector, T.D., Harris, P.A., Hart, D.J., *et al.* (1996). Risk of osteoarthritis asso-ciated with long-term weight-bearing sports. *Arthritis Rheum* **39**:988–95.

86. McDermott, M. and Freyne, P. (1983). Osteoarthrosis in runners with knee pain. *Br J Sports Med* **17**:84–7.

87. Kujala, U.M., Kettunen, J., Paananen, H., *et al.* (1995). Knee osteoarthritis in former runners, soccer players, weight lifters, and shooters. *Arthritis Rheum* **38**:539–46.

88. Lane, N.E., Hochberg, M.C., Pressman, A., Scott, J.C., and Nevitt, M.C. (1999). Recreational physical activity and the risk of osteoarthritis of the hip in elderly women. *J Rheumatol* **26**:849–540.

89. Manninen, P., Riihimaki, H., Heliovaara, M., Suomalainen, O. (2001). Physical exercise and risk of severe knee osteoarthritis requiring arthro-plasty. *Rheumatology* **40**:432–7.

90. McAlindon, T.E., Wilson, W.F., Aliabadi, P., Weissman, B., Felson, D.T. (1999). Level of physical activity and the risk of radiographic and sympto-matic knee osteoarthritis in the elderly: the Framingham study. *Am J Med* **106**:151–7.

91. Felson, D.T., Chaisson, C.E., Hill, C.L., *et al.* (2001). The association of bone marrow lesions with pain in knee osteoarthritis. *Ann Intern Med* **134**:541–9.

92. *Hill, C.L., Gale, D.G., Chaisson, C.E., *et al.* (2001) Knee effusions, popliteal cysts and synovial thickening: association with knee pain in those with and without osteoarthritis. *J Rheumatol* **28**:1330–7.

Compared to persons without knee pain, those with knee pain more often had synovitis and effusions on their knee MRI's. Prior reference (Felson et al.) suggested that also those with knee pain more often had bone marrow edema lesions. These two studies provide evidence that bone marrow edema, synovitis, and effusions are the structural findings correlated with knee pain in OA.

93. Oliveria, S.A., Felson, D.T., Reed, J.I., Cirillo, P.A., and Walker, A.M. (1995). Incidence of symptomatic hand, hip, and knee osteoarthritis among patients in a health maintenance organization. *Arthritis Rheum* **38**:1134–41.

94. Cooper, C., McAlindon, T.E., Goggon, D., Egger, P., and Dieppe, P. (1994). Occupational activity and osteoarthritis of the knee. *Ann Rheum Dis* **53**:90–3.

3 The economics of osteoarthritis

Edward Yelin

Demographers and economists traditionally divide chronic diseases into two groups: those of high prevalence and low-average impact, for example, chronic sinusitis; and those of low prevalence and high-average impact, for example, systemic lupus erythematosus.[1] OA sits astride these two major classifications: it is clearly a high prevalence condition, but it must also be classified as one with at least a moderate, if not a high level of impact. More importantly, because OA is associated with age,[2] the aging of the population puts a higher proportion of the total population at risk for OA. Moreover, the aging of the population puts a higher proportion of persons with OA in the age groups in which the severity of the disease is greatest. This combination of high and growing prevalence, and moderate to severe impact, makes OA an important condition in health policy concerns.

Interestingly, the condition has received relatively scant attention in the cost-of-illness literature. Instead, health services researchers from the rheumatology community have focussed on the cost of rheumatoid arthritis (RA) in clinical samples, probably because it is a more prominent condition in the practices of rheumatologists.[3–9] On the other hand, in their own studies, demographers and economists tend to focus on the more encompassing rubrics of musculoskeletal disease or all forms of arthritis, probably because the data sets they analyse do not include discrete diagnoses, such as OA. However, persons with OA constitute a large fraction of all persons with musculoskeletal conditions and, therefore, of the costs of these diseases.

This chapter reviews the studies of the economic impact of musculoskeletal disease and all forms of arthritis, in general, conducted on random samples of the population; summarizes the small literature on the cost of OA, in particular, based on clinical samples, including those conducted in managed care environments in the United States of America; compares results from clinical studies of OA and RA; and then uses the 1979–81 National Health Interview Survey to make preliminary estimates of the absolute national cost of arthritis and of the increment in costs experienced by persons with arthritis compared to those of similar age, sex, and race without arthritis. The pharmacoeconomics of treatment of OA are discussed specifically in Chapter 8.

Cost-of-illness studies

The costs of illness are divided into two distinct spheres, those due to direct expenditures for medical care services and those due to the indirect impact of illness on function, principally measured by lost wages due to reduced work effort or total cessation of work activities.[10–13]

National studies of the cost of musculoskeletal diseases

Five studies of the cost of musculoskeletal diseases in the United States of America have been published, the two most recent of which presented the costs of arthritis separately. In addition, studies of the economic impact of musculoskeletal disease in Canada, Australia, France, and the United Kingdom have recently been completed. Table 3.1 summarizes the results of these studies. In the first systematic study of the cost of illness, Rice[10] reported that in the United States of America in 1963, musculoskeletal conditions accounted for $4 billion in total costs, half of which was attributed to the direct costs of medical care and the other half to wage losses and the imputed value of homemaker losses. This sum was equivalent to 0.7 per cent of the gross national product (GNP).

The relative magnitude of the total costs of musculoskeletal disease in the United States of America remained fairly stable through 1980, though the proportion due to medical care and wage losses changed substantially.[14,15] In the 1960s, real wages were rising rapidly, while medical care inflation had not yet become a significant problem. Accordingly, the proportion of total costs due to lost wages rose between the 1963 and 1972 studies. In contrast, after the oil shock of the early 1970s, real wages stagnated while medical care prices rose quickly. By 1980, direct costs of musculoskeletal disease accounted for more than 60 per cent of the total costs of this group of illnesses. However, by 1988, total costs had increased to $124 billion, with more than half associated with indirect costs.[16]

The most recent national study of the costs of musculoskeletal conditions concerned 1995.[17] In that year, the total costs of these illnesses amounted to $215 billion, or about 2.9 per cent of the GNP. Less than half of the total was due to direct costs of medical care; the balance was due to wage losses. In the same study, the cost of arthritis alone was estimated to be $83 billion, with about three-quarters of that total due to lost wages.

These studies of the national economic impact of musculoskeletal conditions in the United States of America suggest a large increase in costs occurred between 1980 and 1988, differences among the studies in methods notwithstanding.[18]

The relative magnitude of the costs of musculoskeletal conditions in Canada, Australia, and the United Kingdom would appear to be similar to that in the United States of America.[19–22] For example, in 1986 the total costs of musculoskeletal conditions in Canada was approximately 1.7 per cent of the GNP, or about half-way between the estimates for the United States of America for 1988 of the costs of all forms of arthritis alone and all forms of musculoskeletal disease. In addition to the studies of all forms of musculoskeletal conditions in various nations, a study has been published concerning the costs of OA, in particular, in France; total costs of OA were approximately 6 billion francs per year.[22]

Costs of osteoarthritis from studies using clinical samples

Only four studies of the costs of osteoarthritis have been derived from clinical samples and in only one of these was indirect cost due to lost wages assessed. Table 3.2 summarizes the result of these studies, expressing all costs in 1999 terms. The study by Liang et al.[25] derives from a random sample of those who had ever attended a tertiary care facility. They reported that physician visits accounted for only a small portion of direct costs of medical care; the majority of direct costs were due to a handful of hospital admissions and

Table 3.1 Cost of musculoskeletal diseases in the current US, Canadian, and Australian dollars, French francs, and British pounds and as a % of Gross National Product (GNP)

Year	Direct ($ billion)	Indirect ($ billion)	Total ($ billion)	% of GNP		
All Musculoskeletal conditions-US						
1963	2	2	4	0.7		
1972	4	5	9	0.7		
1980	13	8	21	0.8		
1988	60	64	124	2.5		
1995	89	126	215	2.9		
All Forms of Arthritis-US						
1988	13	42	55	1.2		
1995	22	61	83	1.1		
Country	**Year**	**Currency**	**Direct**	**Indirect**	**Total**	**% of GNP**
All Forms of Musculoskeletal Condtions: Non-US						
Canada	1986	dollars-billions	2	6	8	1.7
Australia	1994	dollars-billions	1	4	5	1.3
United Kingdom	1986	pounds-billions	1	3	4	1.1
Osteoarthritis: Non-US						
France	1991	francs-billions	4	2	6	n/a

Source: US, Refs 10, 14–17; Canada, Ref. 19; Australia, Ref. 20; United Kingdom, Ref. 21; France, Ref. 22. Adopted from Ref. 23.

Table 3.2 Costs of osteoarthritis, in 1999 dollars, from four studies using clinical samples

Study	Year	Direct costs				Indirect Costs	Total Costs
		Physician	Hospital	Other	Total		
Liang *et al.*	1984	183	628	958	1769	12 032	13 801
Holman *et al.*	1988	1294	846		2157		
Gabriel *et al.*	1995				2427		
Lanes *et al.*	1997	135	280	196	611		

Notes: All costs have been expressed in 1999 terms by inflating study year costs by the change in the Consumer Price Index (24, p. 487). In the study by Liang et al.,[25] indirect costs were estimated jointly for persons with OA and RA; this amount was applied here for the persons with OA. In the study by Holman et al.,[26] neither 'other' costs nor indirect costs were reported. The study by Gabriel et al.[27] reported the frequency of changes in employment, but not the associated indirect costs. Lanes et al.[28] reported costs incurred by a member of a health maintenance organization.

to the category 'other', which include prescription and non-prescription drugs and medical devices. Indirect costs of OA dwarfed medical costs, averaging $12 032 in 1999 terms among all persons with OA.

The study by Holman et al.[26] was limited to costs of physician visits and hospital admissions. It was conducted in Northern California and included respondents receiving care in the fee-for-service sector, in a pre-paid group practice, and in an experimental center designed to lower utilization rates. The authors reported that the magnitude of the costs of hospitalization in their study was similar to that in the study by Liang et al., but they also reported much higher costs due to physician visits, and overall direct medical care costs more than 20 per cent higher, even though the costs of drugs and devices were not estimated. Interestingly, costs were lower in the experimental setting than in the pre-paid group practice, and lower in the pre-paid group practice than under fee-for-service. This suggests that medical care costs of OA can be reduced through both financial incentives to providers and patients and through non-monetary incentives in a practice designed to reduce utilization through more interactive relationships between patients and physicians.

Gabriel et al.[27] assembled a database of all persons with a diagnosis of OA among residents of Olmstead County, Minnesota. This sample approximates a true population-based study, with the caveat that those who have OA but have not received a diagnosis would not appear in the database. In this study, the authors did not report direct medical costs by category. Moreover, they accounted only for costs that generated medical bills. Nonetheless, their estimate of overall annual direct medical care costs for OA—$2427 per person in 1999 terms—exceeds the estimates from the two previous studies. Although Gabriel et al. did not estimate the wage losses associated with OA, they noted that about 11 per cent of persons with OA reduced their hours of work, 9 per cent reported being unable to get a job, and 14 per cent retired early due to this condition.

In another study using a clinical sample, Lanes et al.[28] analysed costs among members of a single health maintenance organization, and found costs to be considerably lower than other studies (direct costs totalled only $611 in 1999 terms), perhaps indicating lower costs in that form of managed-care organization than in other systems of care.

Comparison of the costs of OA and RA

Table 3.3 compares the per-case costs of OA and RA by averaging values from each of the studies using clinical samples (two values are provided for

Table 3.3 Costs, in 1999 dollars, of rheumatoid arthritis and osteoarthritis from average of clinical studies

Study	Physician	Hospital	Other	Total Direct Costs	Indirect Costs	Total
OA-including Lanes et al.	537	585	577	1699	12032	13731
OA-excluding Lanes et al.	738	737	958	2433	12032	14465
RA	1082	3361	1397	5840	18907	24747

Notes: All costs have been expressed in 1999 terms by inflating study year costs by the change in the Consumer Price Index (32, p. 487). The first estimate of the costs of OA was obtained by averaging the four studies summarized in Table 3.2, or, where only one study provided as estimate, using that one value. The second estimate of the costs of OA excludes the value from the study of Lanes et al.[28] because the latter study is an outlier among the four studies. The costs of RA were estimated in a fashion similar to that for the OA estimates, using the studies of Meenan et al.[3] and Lubeck et al.[4]

OA, including and excluding the study by Lanes et al. because the costs in that study appear to be systematically lower than those in the other three studies). Not surprisingly, the per-case costs of RA exceed the costs of OA in every category, with the costs of hospital admissions accounting for the largest relative difference. Overall, the per-case cost of RA is more than 1.7 times as great as the per-case cost of OA, even if the results of Lanes et al. are excluded. Nevertheless, because the prevalence of OA is so great, OA has a far greater overall impact on the economy than RA. Assuming a liberal estimate of the prevalence of RA of 1.0 per cent of the total population, a conservative estimate of the prevalence of OA of 4.2 per cent of males and 9.0 per cent of females 20 years of age or over;[2] estimates of the per-case cost of OA, including those from Lanes et al.; and the US population in 1999,[24] there are 2.73 million persons with RA and 13.03 million with OA in the nation. Accordingly, the total costs of OA, at $178.9 billion, are about 2.65 times as large as the total costs of RA, at $67.5 billion. Even using the highest published estimates for the prevalence of RA—2 per cent,[2] the national cost of OA would still exceed the national cost of RA by about 50 per cent. It should be noted that the combined cost of OA and RA— about $246 billion—is far larger than the most recent estimate of the cost of all forms of arthritis from a US national study in 1995,[18] $83 billion, or about $91 billion in 1999 terms (Table 3.1). The higher estimate from the clinical samples may be due to the greater severity of the disease among persons sampled in clinical environments. Alternatively, the difference may be due to the greater level of detail in the enumeration of costs in the clinical studies.

National community-based estimates of the impact of arthritis

In studies using clinical samples, researchers are able to customize data collection to ensure relatively complete enumeration of the impacts of illness. However, the sample of persons with the illness is biased, either because those who receive a diagnosis may have inherently better access to care, or because they may have more severe illness than those who do not.

In part, to avoid the bias from sampling in clinical environments, the federal government in the United States of America instituted an annual community-based survey of the health of the population—the National Health Interview (HIS).[29] In the HIS, individuals self-report their symptoms and, unless a physician has told the individual a specific diagnosis associated with the symptoms, a general diagnostic code, such as arthritis, is given. The analysis reported below provides estimates of the impact of all forms of self-reported arthritis for the years 1989–91 (using three years reduces the sampling variability associated with any one year's data). OA accounts for most of the subjects in this diagnostic classification.[30]

Over the period 1989–91, an average of 30.8 million individuals reported symptoms consistent with arthritis, providing an overall prevalence rate of 12.3 per cent, that is, roughly twice the rate that has been estimated from epidemiological studies of OA based on physician examination.[2] Table 3.4 summarizes the average and total health care utilization of these individuals self-reporting arthritis. Overall, they made a mean of 7.34 visits to physicians in the year prior to the interview, or 226.3 million visits overall. In addition, they experienced an average of 0.22 hospital admissions per person, amounting to 6.9 million admissions in the nation as a whole.

Table 3.4 Per capita and total utilization of persons reporting arthritis, US, 1989–91

Type of utilization	Mean	Total (millions)
Visits to physicians	7.34	226.3
Hospital admissions	0.22	6.9
Hospital days	1.58	48.8
Length of admissions (in days)	7.07	

Source and note: Author's analysis of 1989–91 National Health Interview Surveys. Estimates based on averaging across the three surveys.

These hospital admissions totaled 48.8 million days; the average length of stay was 7.07 days per admission.

Table 3.5 provides estimates of the economic impact of this medical care utilization and of the wage losses associated with arthritis. These estimates were made by multiplying the number of units of physician visits used by $90 (the approximate average of the costs of a physician visit in the nation in 1999), and the number of hospital admissions by $8220 (the average cost of all hospital stays in the United States of America in that year). Using these unit prices, all persons self-reporting arthritis incurred $2.0 billion in costs due to physician visits and $56.7 billion in costs due to hospital admissions in the years 1989–91. Because many of the hospital admissions for arthritis include surgical procedures, including total joint replacement surgery, and surgical admissions are more expensive than this average, the 'true' cost of the admissions probably exceeds the $56.7 billion estimate. Even without adjusting the unit price of hospital admissions to take surgery into account, the annual cost of medical care for arthritis is at least $58.7 billion. Including the costs of drugs and devices, which are not enumerated in the HIS, would substantially increase this total.

In addition, 14.1 per cent fewer of those with arthritis are in the labor force than persons without arthritis. Thus, 2.34 million persons with arthritis were not working who would have been working if they had the same labor force participation rates as persons without arthritis. If a unit price for wage losses, based on average earnings among all US workers in 1999, is applied, the indirect costs of arthritis total at least $66.8 billion. This figure omits all losses due to reduction in hours worked or the lesser degree of career advancement experienced by persons with arthritis in comparison with those without arthritis.

Even though the estimate of the direct costs omits common expenses for arthritis, and the estimate of indirect costs omits partial work disability, the estimate of the total cost of arthritis—$125.5 billion—represents 1.4 per cent of the gross domestic product for the United States of America for the year 1999.[24]

Table 3.5 provides estimates of the total costs incurred by persons with arthritis. Table 3.6, in contrast, shows the increment in costs experienced by persons with arthritis relative to the remainder of the population and assuming persons with arthritis have the same age, race, and sex distribution as those without arthritis. Persons with arthritis make slightly less than one more visit per physician year than similar persons without arthritis.

Table 3.5 Estimates of the absolute national costs of arthritis in 1999, US, 1989–91

Direct costs							
Physician visits			**Hospital admissions**			**Total**	
Number	**Unit price**	**Total**	**Number**	**Unit price***	**Total**		
226.3 mil	$90	$2.0 bil	6.9 mil	$8220	$56.7 bil	$58.7 bil	
Indirect costs							
Number leaving work†	**Unit price‡**	**Total**		**Total costs**			
2.34 mil	$28,548	$66.8 bil		$125.5 bil			

Source and notes: Author's analysis of 1989–91 National Health Interview Surveys.

* Unit price of hospital admission based on average cost of patient stay in US short-term hospitals in 1992 (33, p. 127), with the value inflated to 1999 terms using the Medical Care Component of the Consumer Price Index (24, p. 487).

† Number of persons who left work based on difference in age, sex, and race matched labor force participation rates of persons without arthritis and actual labor force participation rate of persons with arthritis (14.1%).

‡ Unit price of cessation of work based on the US median weekly wage times 52 weeks (24, p. 437).

Table 3.6 Estimates of the incremental national costs of arthritis in 1994, US, 1989–91

Direct costs							
Physician visits			**Hospital admissions**			**Total**	
Incremental#	**Unit price**	**Total**	**Incremental***	**Unit price#**	**Total**		
0.98 mil	$90	$0.1 bil	0.06 mil	$8220	$0.5 bil	$0.6 bil	
Indirect costs							
Incremental#	**Leaving work†**	**Unit price‡**	**Total**	**Total costs**			
1.00 mil		$28,548	$28.6 bil	$29.2 bil			

Source and notes: Author's analysis of 1989–91 National Health Interview Surveys.

* Incremental number of physician visits and hospital admissions per person based on regressions estimating the utilization among persons with OA assuming the age, sex, and race distribution in the remainder of the population.

Unit price of hospital admission based on average cost of patient stay in US short-term hospitals in 1992 (31, p. 127), with this value inflated to 1999 terms using the Medical Care Component of the Consumer Price Index (24, p. 487).

† Number of persons who left work based on difference in labor force participation of persons without arthritis, and the estimated labor force participation rate of persons with arthritis and the same distribution of age, sex, and race as persons without arthritis (6.0%).

‡ Unit price of cessation of work based on the US median weekly wage times 52 weeks (24, p. 437).

Accordingly, the incremental costs of their physician visits are relatively small—$0.1 billion. The incremental cost of their hospitalizations is much larger: based on an excess of 0.06 admissions per capita and a unit cost of $8220 per admission, the increment in the costs of the hospital admissions of persons with arthritis is $0.5 billion. Thus, of the total incremental medical care costs of $0.6 billion incurred by persons with arthritis, more than 80 per cent is due to excess hospital admissions.

However, the incremental costs of wage losses dwarf even those due to hospitalization. In the period 1989–91, an extra 1.0 million persons with arthritis were out of work, relative to the expected labor force participation rate of persons with the same age, sex, and race characteristics but without arthritis. After multiplying this number by the average wages of US workers, the increment in wage losses totals $28.6 billion. All told, the increment in wage losses of persons with arthritis relative to those without is far larger than the increment in direct medical care costs.

Policymakers concerned about the medical care costs of arthritis would do well to focus on reducing hospital admissions, since excess admissions are responsible for the bulk of the increment in medical care costs. Although one cannot easily attribute surgical procedures to particular conditions in the HIS, we know from other sources of data that surgical admissions

account for a large proportion of the increment in costs attributable to hospitalization.[32] To an even greater extent, policymakers would do well to emphasize the impact of arthritis on work, since wage losses account for almost two-thirds of the incremental cost of arthritis.

Summary and conclusions

In contrast to RA, the cost of OA has been the subject of few studies. From these studies, the annual cost of OA would appear to be in the range of from $13 000–15 000 per case, with most of the costs due to lost wages. Though its per-case cost is lower than that of RA, because of the much greater prevalence of OA, the overall economic impact of OA is much greater. However, it is very difficult to provide a good estimate of the exact magnitude of the economic cost of OA for the nation. In self-report studies, such as the HIS, the prevalence of OA is under-reported; most OA is classified under the more encompassing rubric of 'all forms of arthritis'. Indeed, a diagnosis of OA occurs relatively infrequently in the clinical environment, because physicians often do not differentiate among musculoskeletal complaints in their treatment plans. As shown above, it can be estimated that the economic impact of this more encompassing rubric is $125.5 billion, and that people with arthritis incur incremental costs of about $29.2 billion, mostly due to lost wages. The estimates of the per-case cost and of the national impact must both be viewed as preliminary, however, in the former case because the clinical studies are few and not as systematic as studies of the cost of RA and in the latter case because of the lack of differentiation of OA from other forms of musculoskeletal disease in the relevant databases.

However, to a certain extent these shortcomings in the literature reflect a shortcoming of concern about OA itself. Even these preliminary findings should indicate to policymakers that the combination of high prevalence, and moderate to high impact, combine to make OA a costly illness. It is time to conduct more systematic studies on the economic impact of OA, so that we can plan adequately for the pandemic of OA we face with the aging of the population.

Key points

1. Musculoskeletal conditions account for as much as 1.1–2.9 per cent of the GNP of nations with advanced economies, including the direct costs associated with medical care and the indirect costs due to lost function and work disability.

2. All forms of arthritis account for as much as 1.2 per cent of the GDP of the United States of America.

3. The direct cost of OA averages between $1699 and 2433, while indirect costs are $12 032, in 1999 terms.

4. Even though the per-case cost of RA is higher than that of OA because of the much higher prevalence of OA, the total costs of OA—$178.9 billion in 1999 terms—exceed those of RA by at least 50 per cent.

5. Most of the increment in costs of arthritis beyond that expected of persons of similar age and gender is due to work loss, not to expenditures for medical care.

References

(An asterisk denotes recommended reading.)

1. *Verbrugge, L. and Patrick, D. (1995). Seven chronic conditions: their impact on US adults' activity levels and use of medical services. *Am J Public Health* **85**:173–82.
   This article shows the differential impact of various chronic conditions on disability and access to medical care. It demonstrates that arthritis is among the leading causes of disability, starting in middle age, but is not among the leading reasons for physician visits or hospital admissions in any age group.

2. Silman, A. and Hochberg, M. (1993). In *Epidemiology of the rheumatic diseases*. Oxford: Oxford University Press, pp. 257–88.

3. Meenan, R., Yelin, E., Henke, C., Curtis, D., and Epstein, W. (1978). The costs of rheumatoid arthritis. *Arthritis Rheum* **21**:827–33.

4. Lubeck, D., Spitz, P., Fries, J., Wolfe, F., Mitchell, D., and Roth, S. (1986). A multicenter study of annual health services utilization and costs in rheumatoid arthritis. *Arthritis Rheum* **29**:488–93.

5. Thompson, M., Read, J., and Liang, M. (1984). Feasibility of willingness-to-pay measurements in chronic arthritis. *Med Decis Making* **4**:195–212.

6. Stone, C. (1984). The lifetime costs of rheumatoid arthritis. *J Rheumatol* **11**:819–27.

7. Pugner, K., Scott, D., Holmes, J., and Hieke, K. (2000). The costs of rheumatoid arthritis: an international long-term view. *Sem Arthritis Rheum* **29**:305–20.

8. Albers, J., Kuper, H., van Riel, P., Prevoo, M., Van't Hof, M., van Gestel, A., and Severens, J. (1999). Socio-economic consequences of rheumatoid arthritis in the first years of the disease. *Rheumatology* **38**:423–30.

9. Merkesdal, S., Ruof, J., Schoofski, O., Bernitt, K., Zeidler, H., and Mau, W. (2001). Indirect costs in early rheumatoid arthritis. *Arthritis Rheum* **44**:528–34.

10. Rice, D. (1966). Estimating the cost of illness. *Health Econ Ser*, No. 6, National Center for Health Statistics.

11. Walker, K. and Gauger, W. (1970, revised 1980). The dollar value of household work. In *Information Bulletin*, No. 60. Ithaca, New York: New York State College of Human Ecology.

12. Lubeck, D. and Yelin, E. (1988). A question of value: measuring the impact of chronic disease. *Milbank Quart* **66**:445–64.

13. Reisine, S., Goodenow, C., and Grady, K. (1987). The impact of rheumatoid arthritis on the Homemaker. *Soc Sci Med* **25**:89–95.

14. Cooper, B. and Rice, D. (1976). The economic cost of illness revisited. *Soc Sec Bull* **39**:21–35.

15. Rice, D., Hodgson, T., and Kopstein, A. (1985). The economic costs of illness: a replication and update. *Health Care Finance Rev* **7**:61–80.

16. *Rice, D. (1992). Cost of musculoskeletal conditions. In A. Pramer, S. Furner, and D. Rice (eds.) *Musculoskeletal Conditions in the US*. Chicago: American Academy of Orthopedics, pp. 143–70.
   This article documents the high toll that all forms of musculoskeletal disease, but especially arthritis, played in the national economy in the early 1990s. Using methods from prior studies, the author shows that the impact of these conditions has grown dramatically because of the aging of the population.

17. Rice, D. (1999). Cost of musculoskeletal conditions. In A. Pramer, S. Furner, and D. Rice (eds.) *Musculoskeletal conditions in the US* (2nd ed.), Chigaco: American Academy of Orthopedics, pp. 141–62.

18. *Yelin, E. and Callahan, L. (1995). The economic cost and social and psychological impact of musculoskeletal conditions. *Arthritis Rheum* **38**:1351–62.
   This article, written by members of the National Arthritis Data Task Force, is a comprehensive review of the literature on the economic costs and psychological impact of musculoskeletal conditions. It can be used to access the key articles in the cost of arthritis literature.

19. Badley, E. (1995). The economic burden of musculoskeletal disorders in Canada is similar to that for cancer, and may be higher. *J Rheumatol* **22**:204–6.

20. Arthritis Foundation of Australia. (1994). In *Industry Commission Report. Cost of Arthritis to the Australian Community*, pp. 14–22.

21. Freedman, D. (1989). *Arthritis: the painful challenge*, Searle Social Research Fellowship Report.

22. Levy, E., Ferme, A., Perocheau, D., and Bono, I. (1993). Les couts socio-economiques de l'arthrose en France. *Rev Rheum* **60**:63s–67s.

23. March, L. and Bachmeier, C. (1997). Economics of osteoarthritis: a global perspective. *Bailliere's Clin Rheum* **11**:817–34.

24. USGPO. (2000). *Statistical Abstract of the US, 2000*, p. 13, 127, 437, 487.

25. Liang, M., Larson, M., Thompson, M., Eaton, H., McNamera, E., and Katz, R., et al. (1984). Costs and outcomes in rheumatoid and osteoarthritis. *Arthritis Rheum* **27**:522–9.

26. Holman, H., Lubeck, D., Dutton, D., and Brown, B. (1988). Improving health service performance by modifying medical practices. *Trans Assoc Am Phys* **101**:173–9.

27. *Gabriel, S., Crowson, C., and O'Fallon, W. (1995). Costs of osteoarthritis: estimates from a geographically defined population. *J Rheumatol* **22**(Suppl. 43):23–5.
   This article is unique among studies of the costs of arthritis because of the combination of the community-based sampling frame and certainty of diagnosis provided by a database of all medical care encounters in the area surrounding Rochester, Minnesota.

28. *Lanes, S., Lanza, L., Randensky, P., Yood, R., Meenan, R., Walker, A., and Dreyer, N. (1997). Resource utilization and cost of care for rheumatoid arthritis and osteoarthritis in a managed care setting. *Arthritis Rheum* **40**:1475–81.
   This article provided the first indication of the extent of the medical care utilization and economic costs for RA in a closed-system sample, that is, in a managed care organization.

29. Kovar, M. and Poe, G. (1985). National Health Interview Survey design, 1973–84 and procedures, 1975–83. *Vital Health Stat* **18** (Series 1):1–130.

30. LaPlante, M. (1988). *Data on disability from the National Health Interview Survey*, National Institute on Disability and Rehabilitation Research, Washington, DC.

31. USGPO (1994). *Statistical Abstract of the US, 1994*, p. 127.

32. Felts, W. and Yelin, E. (1989). The economic impact of the rheumatic diseases in the United States. *J Rheumatol* **16**:867–84.

4

Genetic aspects of osteoarthritis

4.1 Evidence for the inheritance of osteoarthritis

Nisha J. Manek and Tim D. Spector

Genetic studies are under way for many complex traits, spurred by the improvement in genetic tools and resources during the past decade. The mechanism by which DNA sequence variations or alleles in genes contribute to differences within the human population with respect to the occurrence of OA is unknown.

Epidemiological studies have provided evidence to support the long-standing clinical perspective that environmental factors predominate in the etiology of OA. Important risk factors affecting disease status include age, occupation, body mass index, trauma, and joint deformity.[1] Conversely, genetic liability is traditionally seen to predominate in only a small minority of the OA population. Families that transmit OA as a simple Mendelian genetic trait have been described but are rare. Partitioning OA into these two conceptual groups, that is, strongly genetic or strongly environmental, neglects the majority of the population in which the interplay between genes and environment in the occurrence of 'common' OA remains significant.

To study sources of individual differences (i.e., the variance) in a phenotype such as OA, genetically related subjects are required and methods of assessing genetic influence in common OA include estimations of relative risk such as sibling recurrence risk (λ_s). This is an estimate of familiality or the risk of disease in first-degree relatives of the patients affected with OA (see practice point 1) and depends on the choice of controls and prevalence in the general population. Estimation of genetic relative risk in family studies, however, does not provide information about the number of genes that contribute to this risk or the strength of each gene's contribution.

A second method of assessing the genetic influence in OA is the total heritability (h^2) estimate. This is usually defined as the proportion of population variance explained by genetic factors.[2] It can be calculated by comparing the liability to OA in first-degree relatives to that in more distant relatives, spouses, or unrelated individuals. Twins are a useful group matched for upbringing and age, where identical or monozygotic (MZ) twins share 100 per cent of their genes and non-identical or dizygotic (DZ) twins share 50 per cent of their genes. It is assumed that both twins have roughly the same family environment, and that therefore any greater similarity between the MZ and DZ twins is due to genetic influences.[3] As well as estimating traditional heritability without many of the problems of family studies, comparison of the covariance (or correlation) in OA between the MZ and DZ twins allows separation of the observed phenotypic variance into additive and dominant genetic components and into common and unique environmental components. This is reviewed in detail elsewhere.[4]

This chapter reviews evidence of the extent of genetic variation in both common and rare forms of OA.

Family studies: establishing familial risk of OA

As early as 60 years ago, in 1941, Stecher[5] observed the familial nature of idiopathic Heberden's nodes, which he concluded was explained best by hereditary factors. Other earlier clinical studies by Kellgren and associates[6] and Lawrence and Moore[7] on generalized OA and other OA subtypes, suggested that specific forms of common OA cluster within families. A retrospective radiographic analysis of hip OA by Lindberg provided further support for this observation.[8] In this study, siblings of patients who had undergone hip replacement were noted to have twice the incidence of hip OA than that of age- and sex-matched control subjects. Chitnavis *et al.*[9] have estimated the relative risks of advanced, symptomatic OA of the hip and knee in siblings of probands having total joint replacement for OA. Spouse-based controls were used to correct for environmental influences. A sibling relative risk of 1.9 for total hip replacement and 4.8 for total knee replacement was calculated. The overall combined relative risk for joint replacement was 2.3. A sibling study by Lanyon and colleagues[10] showed that siblings of patients with hip OA of sufficient severity to warrant total hip replacement have a high risk of radiographic hip OA. Each study, despite using different approaches, demonstrates that relatives of affected individuals have higher rates of OA than the general population. Table 4.1 summarizes these trials. Clustering of OA within families is suggestive of a genetic contribution to common OA, but they do not provide conclusive evidence. Clearly, familial aggregation of disease might also be explained by non-genetic factors owing to siblings sharing important environmental influences. Therefore, an alternative explanation for familial aggregation of disease is that members within a family and members within a racial group share similar environmental influences.

Twin pair studies: heritability estimates for OA

The publication in 1996 of the first large-scale OA twin study by Spector *et al.*[11] gave compelling support that the familial clustering was due to a major genetic contribution to common OA. Using a cohort of 130 MZ and 120 DZ female twin pairs in the age group 48–70 years, a higher intra-class correlation among MZ twins compared with DZ twins was observed for several clinical and radiographic features of OA. Significant differences in OA concordance between the MZ and DZ twin pairs remained after control of environmental contributors such as weight, smoking, and oestrogen replacement. The study revealed an h^2 between 39–65 per cent, with a concordance rate in the MZ twin pairs of 0.64 compared with 0.38 in the DZ pairs. Incomplete concordance in the MZ twin pairs clearly demonstrated an environmental component to disease expression. A twin study focusing on radiographic hip OA in female twins was carried out by the same group.[12] An h^2 of approximately 50 per cent was determined for disease defined by joint-space narrowing at the hip joint. A questionnaire based twin study from Finland included both male (577 MZ and 1180 DZ) and female (836 MZ and 1502 DZ) twin pairs.[13] Recalled OA at any joint was used as the criterion for disease and an h^2 of 44 per cent was obtained for women. Interestingly, this Finnish study detected no genetic component to male disease, with a concordance of 0.34 in MZ male twin pairs and 0.38 in

Table 4.1 Family studies of OA with relative risk estimations

Study	Proband	Relatives	Controls	Relative risk
Stecher[5]	Women with idiopathic Heberden's nodes	Sisters mothers	Women in the population	3-fold for sisters 2-fold for mothers
Kellgren et al.[6]	Men and women with primary generalized OA	Siblings	Age- and sex-matched controls	2-fold for siblings
Lindberg[8]	Men and women with hip OA	Siblings	Age- and sex-matched controls from the same hospital	2-fold for siblings
Chitnavis et al.[9]	Men and women with hip and knee arthroplasty	Siblings	Spouses	2-fold for siblings
Lanyon et al.[10]	Men and women with severe hip OA	Siblings	Age- and sex-matched controls	7-fold for siblings

Table 4.2 Heritability (h^2) of OA

Author	Study group	Controls	h^2
Twin studies			
Spector et al.[11]	130 female MZ twin pairs	120 female DZ twin pairs	0.39 for knee OA 0.65 for hand OA
MacGregor et al.[12]	135 female MZ twin pairs Hip radiographic OA	277 female DZ twin pairs Hip radiographic OA	0.64 for hip JSN 0.58 for OA overall (radiographic)
Kaprio et al.[13]	577 male MZ twin pairs 836 female MZ twin pairs	1180 male DZ pairs 1502 female DZ pairs	0.44 for OA, any site in female twin pairs only. No evidence of h^2 in male twin pairs
Population studies			
Felson et al.[16]	337 nuclear families from the Framingham Heart Study ascertained independently of OA status	Spouses	0.42 for generalized OA
Bijkerk et al.[14]	118 Probands with multiple affected joint sites and 257 of their siblings	1587 indivduals randomly selected from the Rotterdam study of aging	0.75 for disk degeneration 0.56 for hand OA
Hirsch et al.[15]	167 families in the Baltimore Longitudinal Study of Aging	Regression analysis of OA presence, absence and severity in sibs and offspring	Increased correlation identified for hand and polyarticular OA: $r = 0.33 - 0.81$, no direct h^2 estimate
Chitnavis et al.[9]	402 probands with TKR or THR for idiopathic OA	Prevalence of TKR and THR for idiopathic OA in 1171 siblings and 376 spouses	0.27 for THR 0.31 for THR or TKR [all relatives included]

MZ, monozygotic (identical) twins; DZ, dizygotic (non-identical) twins; TKR, total knee replacement; THR, total hip replacement; JSN, joint-space narrowing.

DZ male twin pairs. This result suggests the possibility that genes play a more significant role in the development of OA in females.

Population studies: heritability estimates

Other population-based studies also support a genetic contribution to common OA risk (see Table 4.2). Bijkerk and co-workers[14] compared the joint specific frequency of OA between the probands and their siblings enrolled in the Rotterdam study and noted a high level of familial correlation for hand OA (h^2 of 0.56), but no correlation for hip or knee OA. The h^2 for a score that summed the number of joints affected in the knees, hips, hands, and spine was 0.78. Hirsch et al.[15] studied the familial aggregation of OA by determining siblings' correlations for the disease in a cohort of patients collected by the Baltimore Longitudinal Study on Ageing. Increased correlation for hand and polyarticular OA demonstrated clear familial aggregation of OA.

To understand the mechanism by which OA genetic susceptibility is transmitted, Felson *et al.*[16] conducted a segregation analysis of 337 nuclear families and their adult offspring from the Framingham study. Parent–offspring and sibling–sibling correlation were determined for primary OA of hand and knee radiographs and were in the range 0.115–0.306. In segregation analyses, the best-fitting models were mixed models with a Mendelian mode of inheritance and a residual multi-factorial component representing either polygenic or environmental factors. The Mendelian recessive model provided the best fit, although in a subsequent reanalysis Spector *et al.* found that other non-Mendelian models also fitted the data equally.[17]

Hereditary disorders causing premature OA

Osteochondrodysplasias, the developmental defects affecting cartilage and bone, comprise a large and heterogeneous group of disorders. These heritable disorders predispose to OA by affecting joint shape, mobility, and matrix composition. To date the genetic bases for only a few of the over 150 types have been identified.[18] An online history of skeletal dysplasias and their responsible genes can be found at www.csmc.edu/genetics/skeldys.

The majority of these Mendelian genetic disorders can be diagnosed before the onset of adult OA symptoms on the basis of clinical and radiological examinations during childhood and young adulthood (see practice point 2). A proper diagnosis is of practical importance with respect to genetic and occupational counselling. The skeletal dysplasias are discussed more fully in the chapter on specific gene defects associated with OA (see Chapter 4.2). However, even in aggregate, the percentage of common OA due to well-characterized genetic syndromes will be low (<1 per cent) among the osteoarthritic population. The study of heritable arthropathies not only illustrates the significant progress that has been made in the understanding of the genetics of these diseases, but also highlights some important observations that are pertinent in considering the genetic variation associated with common OA. These include:

1. Locus heterogeneity whereby similar clinical phenotypes can result from mutations in different genes. An example is multiple epiphyseal dysplasia (MED) (see practice point 3).

2. Different mutations within the same gene can cause different phenotypes. For example, different mutations in the COL2A1 gene are associated with the Stickler syndrome, neonatal achondrogenesis II/hypochondrogenesis, Kniest dysplasia as well as SED.

3. Different mutations within the same gene can cause identical phenotypes. For example, at least 20 different mutations within the COL2A1 gene on chromosome 12 have been associated with the Stickler syndrome.[19,20]

Identifying disease genes in heritable OA

Linkage analysis. The first step for establishing the involvement of a candidate gene in heritable OA is the performance of genetic linkage analyses of large kindred populations. Linkage analysis has been utilized widely for linkage studies of type II collagen gene COL2A1 mutations to heritable cartilage diseases. The OA in these pedigrees is best described as secondary and related to chondrodysplasia and not the common primary form.

Linkage analysis, in simple Mendelian disorders, tests for the co-segregation of two polymorphic loci. A statistical calculation termed the LOD score is a measure of the likelihood that a known normal allele and the mutant allele in question for a disease syndrome co-segregate in a family because they are physically close on the same chromosome versus the two genes being on different chromosomes and travelling together by chance alone. For simple Mendelian genetic diseases, a LOD score above 3.0 is considered strong statistical evidence of linkage. For complex genetic diseases or traits dependent on the number of markers used and information content, higher LOD scores are required for strong statistical evidence of linkage. Lander and Kruglyak have reviewed the linkage analysis for complex traits in an excellent review.[21]

Candidate gene linkage studies. Linkage analysis of affected sibling pairs gives a robust analysis especially in addressing uncertainties such as possible environmental con-founders in expression of phenotypes or uncertain inheritance patterns. Few studies have focused on families where OA is the only and primary disease process without any chondrodysplasia. The other major limitation to the studies has been the small numbers of sibling pairs, many with less than 80 pairs[22–29] (See Table 4.3). Genetic studies have shown a positive linkage to COL2A1 in two Finnish families having familial OA with classic clinical and radiographic findings.[23,30] Mutation analysis of the COL2A1 gene in 45 unrelated patients with familial OA found only a single putative COL2A1 mutation.[31] This result suggests that among patients with common OA, the incidence of COL2A1 mutations is low, probably even below 2 per cent. Loughlin and co-workers[25] have investigated candidate genes as susceptibility

Table 4.3 Candidate gene studies in OA

Gene	Number	Association result*	Author(s)
COL2A1	$n = 86$	+	Hull and Pope, 1989
COL2A1	$n = 91$	NS	Vikkula, 1993
COL2A1	$n = 21$ pairs	NS	Priestly, 1991
COL2A1	$n = 38$ pairs	NS	Loughlin, 1994
CRTL1	$n = 38$ pairs	NS	Loughlin, 1994
CRTM	$n = 38$ pairs	NS	Loughlin, 1994
CRTM	$n = 261$	+	Muelenbelt, 1997
2q	$n = 99$ pairs	+	Wright, 1996
VDR	$n = 351$	+	Keen, 1997
VDR	$n = 846$	+	Uitterlinden, 1997

*NS: not significant.

loci in affected sibling pairs. They tested for linkage of the COL2A1 locus in 48 sibling pairs with generalized OA (primary OA in 3 joint groups) but found no evidence of linkage. Two other genes encoding secreted proteins in cartilage link protein (CRTL1) and cartilage matrix protein (CRTM) were also evaluated for linkage, but neither gene could be substantially associated with OA risk. However, the sample size was too small and lacked power. Mustafa *et al.*[32] examined a number of candidates using a cohort of 481 affected sibling pairs ascertained by joint replacement surgery for OA (hip, knee, or hip and knee). Suggestive linkage was obtained to the COL9A1 gene in female affected pairs who were concordant for hip OA, with a LOD score of 2.3.

Meulenbelt *et al.*[33] reported a large Dutch family that has primary OA of the knees, hands, and the spine, in four generations with disease onset in the third and fifth decades. The transmittance of OA in this family appears to be autosomal dominant and ten candidate genes were excluded as the mutant locus, including several that encode structural proteins of the cartilage extra-cellular matrix. A genome-wide scan has now linked the OA in this family to micro-satellite markers on chromosome 2q.[34] Roby *et al.*[35] also excluded several candidate genes in a South African family of Dutch origin in which severe early-onset hip OA segregates as an autosomal dominant trait. The group subsequently mapped the disease to chromosome 4q35 (LOD score of 5.7).

Genome-wide linkage studies. Scans with the use of affected sibling pairs or other affected relative pairs is a powerful approach especially if the genetic variants under study have a high relative risk for predisposition to OA. Siblings and other relatives who are concordant for OA because of genetic predisposition will inherit their OA-predisposing alleles in common more than would be expected by chance alone. On the other hand, siblings who are discordant for OA would be expected to inherit an OA predisposing allele in common less than would be expected by chance alone. Chapman and colleagues[36] performed a two-stage genome-wide scan of 481 affected sibling pairs who were concordant for having undergone joint replacement surgery for primary OA. Analyses of their data suggested a potential OA susceptibility region on chromosome 11q13 in the females with hip OA of the sibling pairs. Subsequent stratification of this cohort based on gender and site of involvement suggested other potential disease-predisposing genes on chromosomes 4, 6, and 16.[37] In a smaller cohort of 27 Finnish families with hand OA, Leppavuori *et al.*[38] performed a genome-wide scan using 302 micro-satellites. Eight regions supported linkage with LOD scores >1.0 on chromosomes 2q, 4q, 7p, 8q, 9p, 9q, 10p, and 12q. The X centromeric region also supported the linkage but at a lower level of significance. In the second stage, additional markers and family members were genotyped in these chromosomal regions and supported linkage to chromosome 2q. Wright *et al.*[27] genotyped 12 micro-satellite markers in 44 generalized nodal families in Nottingham, UK. Three of the twelve markers demonstrated linkage to chromosome 2q. However, the regions of chromosome 2, predicted to contain nodal OA susceptibility genes by

Leppavuori and Wright, do not overlap suggesting that this chromosome may contain more than one OA susceptibility gene.

Overall linkage analysis of affected sibling pairs has so far identified regions of suggestive linkage on chromosomes 2q, 4q, 6, 7p, 11q, 16, and Xcen. Of these, chromosome 2q looks promising as it gave positive results in genome screens performed in Oxford, Finland, and Nottingham as well as being linked in the Dutch pedigree.

Association analysis. Another contemporary approach for evaluating candidate genes as risk factors for common OA has employed allelic association studies using case-control cohorts. Several OA association analyses have been carried out[22–24,26,28,29,39–54] (Table 4.4). Two main underlying assumptions are pertinent in this approach. One is that OA risk in apparently unrelated affected individuals is actually due to their inheriting the same OA-predisposing allele from a distant common ancestor. The second assumption is the prediction of the allele being disease causing. A number of different genes have been studied by tests of allelic association in the osteoarthritic population. These include the COL2A1 gene, CRTLI and CRTM proteins, vitamin D receptor, oestrogen receptor, insulin-like growth factor 1, transforming growth factor β-1 (TGF-β1), and aggrecan.

The first COL2A1 study reported the association of an intragenic dimorphism with radiographic OA in a British cohort.[22] Meulenbelt *et al.*[43]

investigated whether radiographic OA (ROA) is associated with specific haplotypes of the COL2A1 gene in a large population-based study. The VNTR allele and the *Hind*III polymorphism showed significant association for ROA.

The vitamin D receptor (VDR) has received considerable attention in OA. It is a gene implicated in regulating bone mass and density. Keen *et al.*[28] compared the allele frequencies and genotypes of an intragenic TaqI dimorphism between females with primary radiographic knee OA and female controls. An allele of the Taq1 dimorphism was associated with knee OA and particularly with osteophytes. Furthermore, the TaqI allele was the haplotype associated with ROA at the knee joint in a study from Rotterdam.[29] The COL2A1 and VDR genes are physically close on chromosome 12q and one could surmise that an association to COL2A1 may in fact be to the VDR gene and vice versa. Both genes alternatively, could harbour susceptibility to OA. Uitterlinden looked at this possibility[55] by typing their subjects for the COL2A1. They have found that both genes appear to encode susceptibility for knee OA, with COL2A1 associated with joint-space narrowing and VDR associated with osteophytes.

A number of other different genes have been studied by tests of allelic association including CRTLI and CRTM proteins,[26] estrogen receptor,[49] insulin-like growth factor 1,[50] aggrecan[47] without firm conclusions or

Table 4.4 Primary OA association studies

Locus	Site of OA	Results	Author
COL1A1	Female hip OA	No association	Aerssens, 1998
	Hip or knee (both sexes)	Association	Loughlin, 2000
COL2A1	Female (more than one joint)	Association	Hull & Pope, 1989
	PGOA/chondrodysplasia	Association	Knowlton, 1990
	Nodal GOA	No association	Priestley, 1991
	Hand or generalized OA	No association	Vikkula, 1993
	Generalized OA both sexes	Association	Loughlin, 1995
	Female hip	No association	Aerssens, 1998
	Generalized OA both sexes	Association	Meulenbelt, 1999
	Knee OA (JSN)	Association	Uitterlinden, 2000
COL9A1	Knees, hips, hands or spine (female)	Association	van Duijn, 1998
COL11A2	Knees, hips, hands or spine	No association	van Duijn, 1998
	Hand OA,	Association	Leppavuori, 2000
CRTM	Hip or knee	Association (male)	Meulenbelt, 1997
	Hip or knee	No Association	Loughlin, 2000
CRTL1	Hip or knee	No association	Meulenbelt, 1997
Aggrecan	Male hand or knee	Association (hand)	Horton, 1998
	Female spine	Association	Kawaguchi, 1999
ER	Generalized OA	Association	Ushiyama, 1998
IGF-1	Hand, hip, knee, or spine	Association	Meulenbelt, 1998
TGF-β1	Female spine (osteophytes)	Association	Yamada, 2000
VDR	Female knee	Association	Keen, 1997
	Knee OA (osteophytes)	Association	Uitterlinden, 1997
	Female hip OA	No association	Aerssens, 1998
	Spine	Association	Jones, 1998
	Male spine	Association	Videman, 1998
	Hand, hip or knee	No association	Huang, 2000
	Hip or knee	No association	Loughlin, 2000
	Knee OA (osteophytes)	Association	Uitterlinden, 2000

CRTM, matrillin 1; CRTL, cartilage link protein; VDR, vitamin D receptor; ER, estrogen receptor; IGF-1, insulin-like growth factor-1; TGF-β1, transforming growth factor β1.

confirmation. A Japanese group has found TGF-β1 to be related to disc degeneration.[51] Lumbar disc degeneration has also been associated with collagen 9 mutations in the Finnish population[56] but its relationship to OA at other sites is unclear. Of the collagen genes, association studies have looked at COL1A1,[39,40] COL2A1,[39,42,57] COL9A1,[45] COL11A2.[45,46] Only COL9A1 and COL11A2 candidate genes reside on a chromosome, chromosome 6, which has some evidence for linkage in the genome-wide scans.

Allelic association studies are challenging to perform, as there may exist a number of different genetic loci that independently contribute to the risk of OA. Also there are the difficulties encountered in selection/stratification bias and ethnic or phenotypic differences, for instance comparing hip OA with knee OA, or comparing ROA with end-stage OA. To overcome these problems, a large number (thousands or tens of thousands) of patients and control subjects could be required to identify an individual locus because it confers a risk in only a subset or small percentage of the osteoarthritic population.

Defining the OA phenotype

OA is now recognized as a heterogeneous group of conditions with a wide variety of different pathological processes leading to a common outcome of joint destruction and disability. Linkage studies focusing on the end result of OA, by examining the genetics of severe disease or joint replacement as a categorical variable is a crude and underpowered approach to the problem. Even using global scores from joint radiographs may be too insensitive. A more useful understanding of the physiology and genetic mechanisms of the complex disease may be obtained by studying intermediate phenotypes individually or in combination. These are obtained by dividing OA into its constituent parts; for example, bone turnover, subchondral bone sclerosis, osteophyte formation, cartilage turnover and breakdown, cartilage swelling, hydration, and volume. These intermediate phenotypes may operate independently or together in clusters determined by pleiotropic genes. A number of linkage simulations have suggested that the poor power of linkage studies can be enhanced upto three-fold by combining the correct number of correlated phenotypes in analysis. The exact optimum number and degree of correlation remains to be determined in practice. A common thread among reported family studies has been that the genetic influences on OA appear to be strongest for generalized OA, suggesting some common susceptibility genes. The definition of 'generalized OA', however, has no consensus by clinicians and epidemiologists and in general has weighted heavily toward hand OA in the clinical studies.[11,16] Furthermore, the prevalence of disease at any given joint site increases steeply with age, and it is not clear that clustering between sites is greater than would be expected from the effects of age. There is a tendency towards polyarticular OA among women aged 45–64 years,[58] but there is no single threshold number of joint sites that can be used to define generalized OA.

Conclusions

Twin pair, sibling risk, and segregation studies have demonstrated that primary OA is a complex genetic disease. Linkage analysis of affected sibling pairs and rare pedigrees in which OA segregates as a Mendelian trait has revealed chromosomes 2, 4, and 16 as positive in more than one genome-wide scan. Analysis of several known candidate genes has revealed evidence for COL2A1 and VDR genes. Tremendous effort and expense have already been committed to finding genes that confer risk for both rare and common forms of OA, and future efforts to identify OA genes will involve intense investigations of those chromosomes highlighted by linkage studies. The genetic study of OA is certain to lead to new therapeutic approaches for preventing and treating OA, as there undoubtedly will be a better understanding of joint development and homeostasis.

Practice point 1: methods of genetic assessment in OA

Relative risk to siblings (λ_S)

Risk estimates based on the presence of OA in siblings of patients with OA and matched controls is obtained by:

$$(\lambda_s) = \frac{\text{per cent siblings with idiopathic OA}}{\text{per cent controls with idiopathic OA}}$$

- Controls in sibling and relative studies ideally resemble siblings with respect to environmental risk factors but differ from them in regard to possible genetic determinants
- Controls should also be representative of the general population in terms of their susceptibility to disease

h^2 estimation

- A measure of the proportion of total variance of disease in a population that is due to genetic influences
- Genetic components include *additive* genetic effects (the effect of individual alleles on the trait) and *non-additive* genetic effects secondary to genetic dominance (the effect due to non-linear interaction between alleles at a single locus)

Twin pair studies

- In the classic twin method, the difference between intra-class correlations for MZ twins and those for DZ twins is doubled to provide a crude estimate of heritability with the remaining population variance attributed to environmental factors

$$h^2 = 2(r_{MZ} - r_{DZ})$$

Practice point 2: features of simple Mendelian disorders

- Onset of symptoms at childhood or teenage years
- Multiple joints affected
- Unusual joint distribution such as elbow and ankle
- Other first degree relatives and family (siblings, offspring, parents) have similar findings
- Radiographic evidence of skeletal disease at sites other than the symptomatic joint, such as the spine
- There may be a disproportionate short stature or altered body habitus
- A proper diagnosis is of practical importance with respect to genetic and occupational counselling

Practice point 3

- Careful subdivision of OA phenotypes reduces the possibility that locus heterogeneity will confound the search for common genetic variants that contribute to common OA.
- Any genetic mutation associated with a Mendelian disorder that has OA as a component feature is capable of causing OA in isolation given the right mutation
- Persons with the same subtype of OA cannot be assumed to have the same predisposing genetic variant; the genetic change within the gene may have arisen independently among the affected individuals

References

(An asterisk denotes recommended reading.)

1. Cooper, C., McAlindon, T., Snow, S., *et al.* (1994). Mechanical and constitutional risk factors for symptomatic knee osteoarthritis: differences between medial tibiofemoral and patellofemoral disease. *J Rheumatol* **21**(2):307–13.

2. Reich, T., James, J.W., and Morris, C.A. (1972). The use of multiple thresholds in determining the mode of transmission of semi-continuous traits. *Ann Hum Genet* **36**(2):163–84.

3. Spector, T.D., Snieder, H., and MacGregor, A.J. (2000). Advances in twin and sib-pair analysis (1st ed.). Oxford: Oxford University Press.

4. *MacGregor, A.J., Spector, T.D. (1999). Twins and the genetic architecture of osteoarthritis. *Rheumatology* **38**(7):583–8.
   A good review of the use of twin pairs in genetic studies with emphasis on OA.

5. Stecher, R.M. (1941). Heberden's nodes. Hereditary in hypertrophic arthritis of finger joints. *Am J Med Sci* **201**:801–9.

6. Kellgren, J.H., Lawrence, J.S., and Bier, F. (1963). Genetic factors in generalized osteoarthrosis. *Ann Rheum Dis* **22**:237–55.

7. Lawrence, J.S. and Moore, J. (1952). Generalized osteoarthritis and Heberden's nodes. *Br Med J* **1**:181–7.

8. Lindberg, H. (1986). Prevalence of primary coxarthrosis in siblings of patients with primary coxarthrosis. *Clin Orthop* **203**:273–5.

9. Chitnavis, J., Sinsheimer, J.S., Clipsham, K., *et al.* (1997). Genetic influences in end-stage osteoarthritis. Sibling risks of hip and knee replacement for idiopathic osteoarthritis. *J Bone Joint Surg Br* **79**(4):660–4.

10. Lanyon, P., Muir, K., Doherty, S., and Doherty, M. (2000). Assessment of a genetic contribution to osteoarthritis of the hip: sibling study. *Br Med J* **321**:1179–83.

11. Spector, T.D., Cicuttini, F., Baker, J., Loughlin, J., and Hart, D. (1996). Genetic influences on osteoarthritis in women: a twin study. *Br Med J* **312**:940–3.

12. MacGregor, A.J., Antoniades, L., Matson, M., Andrew, T., and Spector, T.D. (2000). The genetic contribution to radiographic hip osteoarthritis in women: results of a classic twin study. *Arthritis Rheum* **43**(11):2410–16.

13. Kaprio, J., Kujala, U.M., Peltonen, L., and Koskenvuo, M. (1996). Genetic liability to osteoarthritis may be greater in women than men. *Br Med J* **313**:232.

14. Bijkerk, C., Houwing-Duistermaat, J.J., Valkenburg, H.A., *et al.* (1999). Heritabilities of radiologic osteoarthritis in peripheral joints and of disc degeneration of the spine. *Arthritis Rheum* **42**(8):1729–35.

15. Hirsch, R., Lethbridge-Cejku, M., Hanson, R., *et al.* (1998). Familial aggregation of osteoarthritis: data from the Baltimore Longitudinal Study on Aging. *Arthritis Rheum* **41**(7):1227–32.

16. Felson, D.T., Couropmitree, N.N., Chaisson, C.E., *et al.* (1998). Evidence for a Mendelian gene in a segregation analysis of generalized radiographic osteoarthritis: the Framingham Study. *Arthritis Rheum* **41**(6):1064–71.

17. Spector, T.D., Snieder, H., and Keen, R. (1999). Interpreting the results of a segregation analysis of generalized radiographic osteoarthritis: comment on the article by Felson *et al.* *Arthritis Rheum* **42**(5):1068–70.

18. International nomenclature and classification of the osteochondrodysplasias (1997). (International Working Group on Constitutional Diseases of Bone 1998.) *Am J Med Genet* **79**(5):376–82.

19. Annunen, S., Korkko, J., Czarny, M., *et al.* (1999). Splicing mutations of 54-bp exons in the COL11A1 gene cause the Marshall syndrome, but other mutations cause overlapping Marshall/Stickler phenotypes. *Am J Hum Genet* **65**(4):974–83.

20. Snead, M.P. and Yates, J.R. (1999). Clinical and molecular genetics of Stickler syndrome. *J Med Genet* **36**(5):353–9.

21. Lander, E. and Kruglyak, L. (1995). Genetic dissection of complex traits: guidelines for interpreting and reporting linkage results. *Nat Genet* **11**(3):241–7.

22. Hull, R. and Pope, F.M. (1989). Osteoarthritis and cartilage collagen genes. *Lancet* **1**(8650):1337–8.

23. Vikkula, M., Palotie, A., and Ritvaniemi, P., *et al.* (1993). Early-onset osteoarthritis linked to the type II procollagen gene. Detailed clinical phenotype and further analyses of the gene. *Arthritis Rheum* **36**(3):401–9.

24. Priestley, L., Fergusson, C., Ogilvie, D., *et al.* (1991). A limited association of generalized osteoarthritis with alleles at the type II collagen locus: COL2A1. *Br J Rheumatol* **30**(4):272–5.

25. Loughlin, J., Irven, C., Fergusson, C., and Sykes B. (1994). Sibling pair analysis shows no linkage of generalized osteoarthritis to the loci encoding type II collagen, cartilage link protein or cartilage matrix protein. *Br J Rheumatol* **33**(12):1103–6.

26. Meulenbelt, I., Bijkerk, C., De Wildt, S.C., *et al.* (1997). Investigation of the association of the CRTM and CRTL1 genes with radiographically evident osteoarthritis in subjects from the Rotterdam study [see comments]. *Arthritis Rheum* **40**(10):1760–5.

27. Wright, G.D., Hughes, A.E., Regan, M., and Doherty, M. (1996). Association of two loci on chromosome 2q with nodal osteoarthritis. *Ann Rheum Dis* **55**(5):317–9.

28. Keen, R.W., Hart, D.J., Lanchbury, J.S., and Spector, T.D. (1997). Association of early osteoarthritis of the knee with a Taq I polymorphism of the vitamin D receptor gene. *Arthritis Rheum* **40**(8):1444–9.

29. Uitterlinden, A.G., Burger, H., Huang, Q., *et al.* (1997). Vitamin D receptor genotype is associated with radiographic osteoarthritis at the knee. *J Clin Invest* **100**(2):259–63.

30. Palotie, A., Vaisanen, P., Ott, J., *et al.* (1989). Predisposition to familial osteoarthrosis linked to type II collagen gene. *Lancet* **1**(8644):924–7.

31. Ritvaniemi, P., Korkko, J., Bonaventure, J., *et al.* (1995). Identification of COL2A1 gene mutations in patients with chondrodysplasias and familial osteoarthritis. *Arthritis Rheum* **38**(7):999–1004.

32. Mustafa, Z., Chapman, K., Irven, C., *et al.* (2000). Linkage analysis of candidate genes as susceptibility loci for osteoarthritis-suggestive linkage of COL9A1 to female hip osteoarthritis. *Rheumatology* **39**(3):299–306.

33. Meulenbelt, I., Bijkerk, C., Breedveld, F.C., and Slagboom, P.E. (1997). Genetic linkage analysis of 14 candidate gene loci in a family with autosomal dominant osteoarthritis without dysplasia. *J Med Genet* **34**(12):1024–7.

34. Loughlin, J. (2001). Genetic epidemiology of primary osteoarthritis. *Curr Opin Rheumatol* **13**(2):111–16.

35. Roby, P., Eyre, S., Worthington, J., *et al.* (1999). Autosomal dominant (Beukes) premature degenerative osteoarthropathy of the hip joint maps to an 11-cM region on chromosome 4q35. *Am J Hum Genet* **64**(3):904–8.

36. *Chapman, K., Mustafa, Z., Irven, C., *et al.* (1999). Osteoarthritis-susceptibility locus on chromosome 11q, detected by linkage. *Am J Hum Genet* **65**(1):167–74.
   The first published genome scan for OA susceptibility locus.

37. *Loughlin, J., Mustafa, Z., Irven, C., *et al.* (1999). Stratification analysis of an osteoarthritis genome screen-suggestive linkage to chromosomes 4, 6, and 16. *Am J Hum Genet* **65**(6):1795–8.
   Additional loci detected by stratification of a genome scan.

38. Leppavuori, J., Kujala, U., Kinnunen, J., *et al.* (1999). Genome scan for predisposing loci for distal interphalangeal joint osteoarthritis: evidence for a locus on 2q. *Am J Hum Genet* **65**(4):1060–7.

39. Aerssens, J., Dequeker, J., Peeters, J., Breemans, S., and Boonen, S. (1998). Lack of association between osteoarthritis of the hip and gene polymorphisms of VDR, COL1A1, and COL2A1 in postmenopausal women. *Arthritis Rheum* **41**(11):1946–50.

40. Loughlin, J., Sinsheimer, J.S., Mustafa, Z., *et al.* (2000). Association analysis of the vitamin D receptor gene, the type I collagen gene COL1A1, and the estrogen receptor gene in idiopathic osteoarthritis. *J Rheumatol* **27**(3):779–84.

41. Knowlton, R.G., Katzenstein, P.L., Moskowitz, R.W., *et al.* (1990). Genetic linkage of a polymorphism in the type II procollagen gene (COL2A1) to primary osteoarthritis associated with mild chondrodysplasia. *N Engl J Med* **322**(8):526–30.

42. Loughlin, J., Irven, C., Athanasou, N., Carr, A., and Sykes, B. (1995). Differential allelic expression of the type II collagen gene (COL2A1) in osteoarthritic cartilage. *Am J Hum Genet* **56**(5):1186–93.

43. Meulenbelt, I., Bijkerk, C., De Wildt, S.C., *et al.* (1999). Haplotype analysis of three polymorphisms of the COL2A1 gene and associations with generalized radiological osteoarthritis. *Ann Hum Genet* **63**(Pt 5):393–400.

44. *Uitterlinden, A.G., Burger, H., van Duijn, C.M., *et al.* (2000). Adjacent genes, for COL2A1 and the vitamin D receptor, are associated with separate features of radiographic osteoarthritis of the knee. *Arthritis Rheum* **43**(7):1456–64.
   Determines possible linkage disequilibrium between VDR and COL2A1 genes.

45. van Duijn, C.M., Bijkerk, C., Houwing-Duistermaat, J.J., *et al.* (1998). A population based study of the genetics of osteoarthritis [abstract]. *Am J Hum Genet* **63**(Suppl.):1282.

46. Leppavuori, J.K., Pastinen, T., Kujala, U. *et al.* (2000). Array-based candidate gene analysis identify COL11A2 on 6p21.3 as predisposing locus for distal interphalangeal joint osteoarthritis [abstract]. *Am J Hum Genet* **67**(Suppl.):125.

47. Horton, W.E. Jr, Lethbridge-Cejku, M., Hochberg, M.C., *et al.* (1998). An association between an aggrecan polymorphic allele and bilateral hand osteoarthritis in elderly white men: data from the Baltimore Longitudinal Study of Aging (BLSA). *Osteoarthritis Cart* **6**(4):245–51.

48. Kawaguchi, Y., Osada, R., Kanamori, M., *et al.* (1999). Association between an aggrecan gene polymorphism and lumbar disc degeneration. *Spine* **24**(23):2456–60.

49. Ushiyama, T., Ueyama, H., Inoue, K., Nishioka, J., Ohkubo, I., and Hukuda, S. (1998). Estrogen receptor gene polymorphism and generalized osteoarthritis. *J Rheumatol* **25**(1):134–7.

50. Meulenbelt, I., Bijkerk, C., Miedema, H.S., *et al.* (1998). A genetic association study of the IGF-1 gene and radiological osteoarthritis in a population-based cohort study (the Rotterdam Study). *Ann Rheum Dis* **57**(6):371–4.

51. Yamada, Y., Okuizumi, H., Miyauchi, A., Takagi, Y., Ikeda, K., Harada, A. (2000). Association of transforming growth factor beta1 genotype with spinal osteophytosis in Japanese women. *Arthritis Rheum* **43** (2):452–60.

52. Jones, G., White, C., Sambrook, P., Eisman, J. (1998). Allelic variation in the vitamin D receptor, lifestyle factors and lumbar spinal degenerative disease. *Ann Rheum Dis* **57**(2):94–9.

53. Videman, T., Leppavuori, J., Kaprio, J., *et al.* (1998). Intragenic polymorphisms of the vitamin D receptor gene associated with intervertebral disc degeneration. *Spine* **23**(23):2477–85.

54. Huang, J., Ushiyama, T., Inoue, K., Kawasaki, T., and Hukuda, S. (2000). Vitamin D receptor gene polymorphisms and osteoarthritis of the hand, hip, and knee: a case-control study in Japan. *Rheumatology* **39**(1):79–84.

55. Uitterlinden, A.G., Burger, H., van Duijn, C.M., *et al.* (2000). Adjacent genes, for COL2A1 and the vitamin D receptor, are associated with separate features of radiographic osteoarthritis of the knee. *Arthritis Rheum* **43**(7):1456–64.

56. Paassilta, P., Lohiniva, J., Goring, H.H., *et al.* (2001). Identification of a novel common genetic risk factor for lumbar disk disease. *JAMA* **285**(14):1843–9.

57. Vikkula, M., Nissila, M., Hirvensalo, E., *et al.* (1993). Multiallelic polymorphism of the cartilage collagen gene: no association with osteoarthrosis. *Ann Rheum Dis* **52**(10):762–4.

58. Cooper, C., Egger, P., Coggon, D., *et al.* (1996). Generalized osteoarthritis in women: pattern of joint involvement and approaches to definition for epidemiological studies. *J Rheumatol* **23**(11):1938–42.

4.2 Specific gene defects associated with osteoarthritis

Thorvaldur Ingvarsson and Stefan Einar Stefansson

The recent publication of a first draft of the human genomic sequence will facilitate the search for OA genes but the obstacles remain significant. For example, the identification of positional candidates still depends on uncovering evidence of linkage between a chromosomal region and an OA phenotype. Once a chromosomal region has been found to link to OA it will be necessary to find a gene in the linked region and for this it will in many cases be necessary to narrow the region down, by applying additional marker sets, to a more manageable size for DNA sequencing or other mutation detection techniques. However, it is not sufficient merely to show an association between a variant in a candidate gene and a phenotype, since such an association may merely reflect linkage disequilibrium. The variant, such as a missense mutation, must also be shown to alter the biological function of a protein in animal models or a tissue such as cartilage that relates to OA. For putative mutations in regulatory regions this chain of evidence becomes even more crucial. Current developments in molecular biology such as micro-array chips now allow the simultaneous large-scale identification of thousands of genes with differential expression in disease. This will enhance our ability to identify candidate molecules and processes that are relevant to OA pathology.

Multiple pathogenetic mechanisms are implicated in the development of OA. Continued studies of the kind outlined here will clarify the complex genetic background of OA and identify genetic variation associated with the disease. In addition to improving our understanding of the pathogenesis of OA and identifying new molecular targets for treatment, this knowledge will also allow a better insight into the interactions between the genetic background and the environmental factors that initiate and drive OA.

Is OA subject to major gene effects?

Given that genetic factors may play a major role in the etiology of OA, the question arises whether these influences are exerted by one or a few 'major genes' each with a relatively large effect, such as the COL2A1 gene, or by a large number of 'polygenes', each with a relatively minor effect. Presumably, in the monogenic form of OA the genes would be easier to identify and could have greater relevance to public health. Complex segregation analysis can be used to study the mode of inheritance of a trait and in particular to infer whether the distribution of the trait within pedigrees is compatible with the action of a major gene. This was done by Felson and co-workers in 1998,[1] concluding that in generalized OA (in this study hand and knee OA) there was evidence to support a significant genetic contribution, with evidence for a major recessive gene and a multi-factorial component, representing either polygenic or environmental factors. However, the evidence is not yet conclusive that 'common OA' is influenced by major genes.[2] On the contrary, several susceptible loci for OA have been suggested and each of them is thought to include a possible gene for OA. This could support the notion that the inherited OA is a polygenic disease.

The study of candidate genes for OA by association analysis

A candidate gene is defined as a gene whose protein product, based on its biological activity, can plausibly be assumed to influence the disease (phenotype) under consideration. The candidate gene can be directly screened for mutations in the affected family or individuals. The main problem with this approach is that the number of these proteins is already large, and as more is learned about cartilage and bone biology the list of potential candidate genes keeps growing. The chances of a 'lucky hit' would seem to be remote. Indeed studies of candidate genes have been disappointing, with the exception of some of the chondrodysplasia families.

Most of the association analyses for OA, which have targeted candidate genes, have tended to be genes encoding structural proteins of the extracellular matrix of cartilage and bone or genes implicated in the regulation of bone density.

Some examples of known mutations in candidate genes follow (see Table 4.5 for more information).

COL2A1

A large number of mutations (over 100) have been reported in the COL2A1 gene on chromosome 12, which codes for II collagen.[3] The clinical phenotypes have ranged widely in severity from the achondrogenesis type II and hypochondrogenesis at the severe end of the spectrum to very mild spondyloepiphyseal dysplasia (SED) with precocious OA, often called late onset SED. Further phenotypes have included early onset premature generalized OA (PGOA),[4,5] families with crystal deposition disease phenotypes of intermediate severity,[6] SED-congenita, and Kniest dysplasia. Mutations have also been described in Stickler dysplasia, in which skeletal phenotype is typical with OA rather than short stature, including eye and inner ear abnormalities. See Table 4.5 and Refs 2 and 13 for further details.

COL11A2

Mutations have been described in the COL11A2 gene, which encode the alpha-2 chain of type XI collagen[3,7] in families with Stickler syndromes presenting mild SED, premature OA and sensorineural hearing loss, but lacking the eye involvement.

COL9A1

Several mutations have been found in the gene for type IX collagen,[7] all associated with Schmid metaphyseal chondrodysplasia, which is a relatively mild chondrodysplasia.

Table 4.5 Examples of known genes associated with OA mutations, their chromosomal location and the respective protein

Gene/locus	Chromosome	Gene product function	Clinical phenotype	Known mutations	Reference	Protein
COL11A1	1p21	Extracellular matrix protein	Knee, hip, hand	No	3,7	Alpha-1-chain type XI collagen
COL11A2	6p21.3	Extracellular matrix protein	Stickler dysplasia-SED late onset, knee, hip, hand	Yes	3	Alpha-2-chain type XI collagen
COL2A1	12q13-q14	Extracellular matrix protein	Achondrogenesis Hypochondrogenesis SED congenita SED late onset Kniest dysplasia Stickler dysplasia	Yes hundreds	2	Alpha-1-chain type II collagen
COL9A1	6q12-q13	Extracellular matrix protein	Knee, hip, hand	Yes	4	Alpha-1-chain type IX collagen
COL9A2	1p32	Extracellular matrix protein	Multiple epiphyseal dysplasia	Yes	3	Alpha-2-chain type IX collagen
COL10A1	6p	Extracellular matrix protein hypertrophic cartilage	Schmid metaphyseal chondrodysplasia	Yes several	3	Alpha-1-chain type X collagen
COMP	19p13.1	Extracellular matrix protein	Multiple epiphyseal dysplasia (Fairbanks) Pseudoachondroplasia	Yes many	3	cartilage oligomeric matrix protein
FGFR3	4p16.3	Tyrosine kinase transmembrane receptor for FGFs	Thanotophoric dysplasia Achondrodysplasia Hypochondrodysplasia	Yes many	3,65–66	
PTHrPR	11p15.3	G-protein transmembrane receptor for PTH and PTHrP	Jansen metaphyseal chondrodysplasia	Yes	3	G-protein
CRTL1	5q13-14.1	Cartilage link protein	Hip or knee		53	Cartilage link protein
DTDST	5q31-q34	Transmembrane sulfate transporter	Achondrogenesis type IB Atelosteogenesis type II Diastrophic dysplasia	Yes several	3	diastrophic dysplasia sulfate transporter
VDR	12q13-q14	Vitamin D-receptor	Hip, knee, hand, spine	Unknown loci	9,10,54–56	

COL9A2

Mutations have been found in the type IX collagen in a multiple epiphyseal dysplasia (MED) family (EDM2) on chromosome 1.[41] Type I collagen is a quantitatively minor cartilage collagen thought to participate in the regulation of collagen fibril assembly in cartilage matrix.

FGFR3

Mutations in the gene for fibroblast growth factor receptor 3 are known in achondroplasia and hypochondroplasia.[66,67] The gene is located on chromosome 4.

COMP

Cartilage oligomeric matrix protein (COMP) is a member of the thrombospondin protein family. It is found in the extracellular matrix of cartilage and to a lesser extent in other connective tissues. The function of COMP is not well-defined.[3] Mutations have been described in the COMP gene located on chromosome 19 in pseudoachondroplasia and MED. It is postulated that pseudoachondroplasia and some forms of MED could share common pathogenetic features.

DTDST

The gene DTDST (diastrophic dysplasia sulfate transporter) is located on chromosome 5q and is responsible for chondrodiastrophic dysplasia. Several mutations are known.[7]

MATN3 (Matrilin-3)

The gene MATN3 (matrilin-3) is located on chromosome 2p and mutations have been described associated with MED.[8]

VDR

A VDR haplotype was shown to be associated with higher risk for knee OA in both women and men.[9] The authors concluded that the two- to three-fold risk increase associated with this haplotype was due to increased osteophytosis rather than joint-space narrowing, suggesting that radiological changes indicative of cartilage degeneration were not associated with this haplotype. In further support of an association of the VDR with OA, a British survey showed that women with a specific VDR haplotype had a three-fold increase of knee OA.[10]

It is interesting to note, however, that the VDR gene locus is located in close proximity (within 100 000 base pairs) of the type II collagen gene (COL2A1) on chromosome 12q. Accordingly, it was speculated that the VDR is not the causative locus, but that it may be in linkage disequilibrium with a neighboring disease-causing gene.[11]

Adding further complexity, a recent study suggested that the COL2A1 and the VDR genes are associated with separate features of ROA of the knee. The investigators concluded that both genes are involved in knee OA, but with separate features of radiographic knee OA: the COL2A1 phenotype is associated with joint-space narrowing, while the VDR phenotype is associated with osteophytes.[12]

Association and linkage studies

Before investing major resources in the detailed study of a potential candidate gene, a strong prior hypothesis implicating the proposed candidate gene is needed, rather than just a general sense based on its biology. Such information can be gained in association studies, which can be done on both related and unrelated individuals. In this case one or several markers are selected for study, which are located within or adjacent to the candidate gene and the association of these and other markers with the phenotype is investigated. Population stratification with the existence of more than one ancestral source of population gene pool represents a major limitation of this study design. If, as likely, the various ancestral sources differ both in their susceptibility to various diseases and in the frequency of various genetic markers, false associations may be observed between genetic markers and phenotypes. It is likely that population stratification is at least partly responsible for some of the associations between candidate gene polymorphisms and diseases that have later proven to be nonreplicable. Examples of loci that are associated with OA are shown in Table 4.6 and candidate gene polymorphisms associated with OA in Table 4.7.

Inherited specific forms of OA and mutations associated with OA in rare Mendelian families

During the last decade several groups have reported linkage analysis of candidate genes to OA in families in which the disease was transmitted as a dominant trait, often with incomplete penetrance. It soon became apparent, that affected individuals in these families had mild osteochondrodysplasias or other rare diseases that can predispose to OA and that the OA in these families is best described as secondary and not the common primary OA. Recently, a number of groups have described families with early onset OA in the absence of chondrodysplasia.[13]

This gave evidence for the existence of a genetic predisposition to OA, for example by a number of rare subtypes of OA including familial calcium pyrophosphate deposition disease, Stickler syndrome, and some chondrodysplasias that have a genetic basis.[14] The spectrum of these particular hereditary forms of OA is quite varied encompassing mild disorders, which do not become clinically apparent until late adult life, to very severe forms that manifest during childhood. Many of these disorders have been classified as secondary OA.[15] They all have the common characteristic of being associated with mutations in genes encoding macromolecules predominantly expressed in cartilage. Genes that may be involved in these diseases include those encoding cartilage-specific collagens (types II, IX, X, and XI), proteoglycan core protein and link proteins, noncollagenous components of the cartilage matrix, growth factors involved in cartilage differentiation or in the regulation of chondrocyte proliferation and specific gene expression, and genes encoding enzymes involved in various cartilage-specific metabolic pathways. Thus, these disorders may be seen to represent a distinct subgroup of OA that can be separated from secondary OA.[14]

After the initial descriptions of genetic linkage between the phenotype of precocious OA and the type II procollagen gene COL2A1 on chromosome 12,[16] a large number of mutations in the genes encoding structural and functional components of cartilage have been identified in various hereditary diseases affecting this tissue.[17–19] Progress on the elucidation of gene mutations in hereditary OA has been most substantial for COL2A1, the gene encoding for type II collagen, the most abundant collagen in articular cartilage. Accordingly, the term 'type II collagenopathies' has been used to describe hereditary cartilage diseases in which their primary defect is mutation in COL2A1.[20] Over 100 mutations are known in the COL2A1

Table 4.6 Quantitative trait loci (QTL) associated with osteoarthritis

Chromosome	Joint(s) affected	Phenotype	Reference
8q	GOA	Early-onset OA-CPDD (1 family)	27
2q23-35	Hand	Nodal OA	47
11q	Hip, knee	Female	45
2q	Hip, knee	OA of the hip	2
4q	Hip, knee	Female OA of the hip	2
6p/6q	Hip	OA of the hip	2
11q	Hip	Female OA	2
16p/16q	Hip	Female OA of the hip	2
2q12-13	Hand	Dip OA	48
4q26-27	Hand	Dip OA	48
7p15-21	Hand	Dip OA	48
X-cen	Hand	Dip OA	48
4q35	Hip	Premature degenerative OA of the hip	49
6q12-13	Hip, knee	Female OA of the hip	50
6p21.3	Hip	Female OA of the hip	50
2q31	Hip, knee	Familial OA of the hip	46
16q	Hip	Familial OA of the hip	51

CPDD, calcium pyrophosphate deposition disease; GOA, generalized osteoarthritis; OA, osteoarthritis.

Table 4.7 Candidate gene polymorphisms associated with osteoarthritis

Genetic polymorphism	Phenotype	Association found?	Reference
VDR	Female knee OA	Yes	10
	Knee OA (osteophytes)	Yes	9
	Female OA (hip replacements)	No	54
	Hand, hip, knee OA	No	55
	Idiopathic OA	No	56
COL2A1	GOA/chondrodysplasia	Yes	57
	Nodal GOA	No	58
	GOA, finger joints	No	43
	GOA	Yes	59
	Female OA (hip replacement)	No	54
	GOA	Yes	60
	Knee OA	Yes	12
COL1A1	Female OA (hip replacement)	No	54
	Idiopathic female OA	Yes	56
ER alfa	GOA	Yes	61
	Idiopathic OA	No	56
TGFB1	Spine OA (osteophytes)	Yes	62
IGF-I	GOA	Yes	63
Aggrecan proteoglycan	Male bilateral hand OA	Yes	64

OA, osteoarthritis; COL, collagen; ER, estrogen receptor; GOA, generalized osteoarthritis; IGF, insulin-like growth factor; TGF, transforming growth factor; JS, joint space.

gene associated with different forms of hereditary cartilage aberrations and OA. These mutations are of considerable scientific interest, but there is yet little evidence that common forms of OA are due to mutations in type II collagen, as a fact even the opposite.[21]

Genome-wide scanning for linkage to OA phenotypes

With the increasing availability of large numbers of highly informative genetic markers, particularly micro-satellite markers that now span the entire genome, the strategy of whole-genome scanning for linkage to phenotypes of interest has become feasible.

Primary generalized OA (PGOA)

PGOA is thought to be the most common form of inherited OA. It is characterized by the familial trait of hand OA (Heberden's and Bouchard's nodes) and premature alterations in multiple joints.[22] Typically, the clinical and radiological features have a precocious onset and an accelerated progression. Generally, the loss of articular cartilage is concentric in the knees and hips. The radiographic appearance is indistinguishable from that of nonhereditary OA, except for the premature occurrence, increased severity, and rapid progression.[14] In the hand the DIP, PIP, and CMC I joints are involved. The hip is affected in early adult life.

Mutations in COL2A1 genes have been identified in affected members of several families with generalized OA with premature onset and rapid progression. However, all these families also display evidence of mild SED.[14] Conversely, however, a recent study analysing COL2A1 for mutations in 47 families with early onset generalized OA without SED, identified a possible COL2A1 mutation in only one of the cases. Further screenings of families with generalized OA showed that only some two per cent of them had a mutation in the COL2A1 gene, suggesting that only a small proportion of OA can be explained by this genetic variation.[23] Other reports suggest that COL2A1 is not the disease locus in families with premature generalized OA, without evidence of SED.[6]

A genetic predisposition in primary generalized OA has also been suggested to be associated with HLA-A1B8 and HLA-B8 haplotypes[24] and with alfa-1-antitrypsin isoform patterns, while other studies have failed to confirm this association.[25]

Familial calcium pyrophosphate deposition

This condition is also known as familial chondrocalcinosis. Following an initial description of the disease in five Czech families,[26] multiple ethnic series have been reported.[14] The condition appears to be inherited in an autosomal dominant manner with precocious onset and severe clinical expression. Radiographs show chondrocalcinosis most frequently in the knees, symphysis pubis, and the wrist. These changes may precede OA changes in the joint. No linkage to the COL2A1 gene on chromosome 12 has been proven, but susceptibility loci have been described on chromosome 5 and 8.[27–29]

A role for the ank gene in controlling tissue calcification in mice has been described.[30] Ongoing investigations explore the role of the ank gene in human OA.[28,29]

Familial hydroxyapatite deposition disease

Another form of inherited crystal deposition disease is due to the deposition of hydroxyapatite crystals in articular cartilage. The mode of inheritance is that of an autosomal dominant pattern with full penetrance. This disorder results in periarticular disease in the form of tendinitis or bursitis and less frequently, true articular disease. The most common locations are the shoulders, wrist, and hips. A recent study of a family from Argentina with this condition and mild SED excluded several candidate genes including type II and X collagen.[31]

Chondrodysplasias

These disorders represent a group of clinically heterogeneous hereditary disorders, characterized by abnormalities in the growth and development of articular and growth plate cartilages. The classifications are based on clinical and radiographic features of the affected individuals. In the future, it will be possible to classify those disorders by the nature of the genetic defects, as the gene mutations responsible for these diseases are identified. Several of them are associated with the development of premature OA. Linkage to COL2A1 has been demonstrated in some cases and excluded in others.[14] These disorders include SED, Stickler syndrome, Kniest dysplasia, MED, and metaphyseal chondrodysplasias.

Spondyloepiphyseal dysplasias

SED is a heterogeneous group of autosomal dominant disorders characterized by abnormal development of the axial skeleton and severe alterations of the epiphysis of long bones, often resulting in dwarfism with a marked shortening of the trunk and to a lesser extent of the extremities.[14] The phenotype of SED is quite varied, ranging from severe forms that are clinically apparent at birth to milder forms, which manifest in childhood or early adolescence. In the late onset form, early degenerative changes are seen in multiple joints, often as generalized OA. Hip OA may develop in adolescence, worsening in early adulthood. There may be mild epiphyseal abnormality in the peripheral joints, for example in the metacarpal phalangeal joints. The most constant features in peripheral joints are the flattening of the articular surfaces of the ankles and knees and shallowness of femoral inter-condylar notches. In adult classic cases, platyspondyly may be severe, accompanied by severe coxa vara and small and irregular femoral epiphyses. In milder cases the features of SED are not clinically obvious and many patients initially present with severe OA affecting multiple joints.[14] Many different mutations have been described in families with SED. Several supposedly unrelated families have demonstrated coinheritance of primary generalized OA with mild SED with specific alleles of the gene for type II procollagen on chromosome 12.[32–34] This allele has now been cloned and found to contain a single base mutation at position 519 of the alpha-1(II) chain.[33] It was speculated that three of the known families with OA and mild SED and which share this COL2A1 gene defect might be related through an early founder.[34] In SED tarda a different mutation was recently described on chromosome Xp22.[35]

Stickler syndrome

This is a form of inherited OA characterized by ocular involvement associated with severe premature OA. Patients have myopia, hearing loss, and epiphyseal dysplasia and even mandibular dysplasia. Linkage analysis of several Stickler's syndrome kindreds has demonstrated that this disease is linked to COL2A1 in some 25–50 per cent of the families and mutations have been shown.[36] Linkage to collagen XI on chromosome 6 and a mutation in the gene encoding the alpha-2 XI collagen chain was demonstrated in one family.[37]

Kniest dysplasia

Kniest dysplasia is a disorder characterized by an autosomal dominant pattern of inheritance displaying shortening of the trunk and limbs, flattening of the face, and severe joint abnormalities. The majority of affected individuals develop severe premature OA, most prominent in the hips and knee. Mutations in COL2A1 have been identified in Kniest dysplasia.[14]

Multiple epiphyseal dysplasia

MED is a heterogeneous disorder characterized by alterations in epiphyseal growth that cause irregularity and fragmentation of the epiphyses of multiple long bones. Spinal alteration is absent or slight. The condition results in premature OA of both weight-bearing and nonweight-bearing joints, often in childhood or early adulthood. Early studies of MED failed to identify an association with the genes for collagen types II and VI, chondroitin sulfate, proteoglycan core protein, and cartilage link protein. Subsequent studies identified mutations in the gene encoding COMP,[38,39] in the COL9A2 gene,[40,41] and lately in the MATN3 gene on chromosome 2.[8] It is likely that additional and different loci will be identified, since other families with this phenotype have been shown to lack genetic linkage with either COMP or COL9A2.[42]

It has even been shown that mutations in MED can in some cases be joint specific. The type of MED with predominant involvement of the capital femoral epiphyses can have mutations in the COMP gene,[43] and those patients with predominant involvement of knees with relative hip sparing can have COL9A2 or COL9A3 mutations.[43] This suggests that mutations can be joint specific with regard to phenotypic expression. However, we do not as yet know if there are corresponding differences in the developmental or spatial expression patterns of these genes between different joints. Table 4.7 lists examples of known genes and mutations associated with OA.

Metaphyseal chondrodysplasias

More than 150 different types of metaphyseal chondrodysplasias are known. The clinical features of affected individuals include short stature with short limbs, bowed legs, and a waddling gait. Mutations have been shown in the COL2A1 gene.[14]

Model free linkage analysis of affected sibling pairs by genome-wide scanning for chromosomal loci associated with OA

The rarity of families in which primary OA segregates as a Mendelian trait, combined with the potential of osteochondro dysplasias in these families, has promoted the use of affected sibling pairs.

As summarized in Table 4.5, a number of candidate genes have been proposed to be associated with OA, but the results from studies published so far are somewhat conflicting. This may be a reflection of the complexity of the disease and/or be related to the limited power of some of these studies. The pathophysiology of OA is complex and the a priori choice of candidate genes is increasingly difficult and prone to bias. Association studies may provide support for the role of specific candidate genes in an inherited disease, but population heterogeneity provides a limitation to this study design.

Systematic genome-wide scan for linkage of markers to phenotypes of interest, using large numbers of randomly distributed anonymous polymorphic micro-satellite markers together with DNA samples from large families or large numbers of sibling pairs with OA may be used to identify yet other, unknown, predisposing chromosomal loci for OA. However, depending on the density and location of micro-satellite markers used in the genome-wide scan, the chromosomal region implicated may sometimes contain a large number of genes. Often, 300–900 micro-satellite markers are used. The LOD score is used as a measure of support for linkage versus absence of linkage,[44] where a LOD score above 2.0 is sometimes referred to as 'suggestive', and a LOD score above 3.0 as 'significant' linkage. These are, however, arbitrary LOD score cut-off levels and may need to be changed depending on the particular experimental design and statistical analysis performed.

Genome-wide scans are often followed by further scans of the chromosomal region of interest with higher density marker panels, to narrow down the chromosomal region (and number of genes) associating with the phenotype of interest. However, assuming that a gene can eventually be identified through this search strategy, the challenge remains to identify sequence variants that influence the function of the protein and result in the phenotype.

In a study using 481 families with at least two siblings each of whom had undergone one or more of total hip replacement or total knee replacement,

or both, for primary OA, Heberden's nodes were noted in 38.5 per cent of the affected individuals. Using a genome-wide scan, a locus associating with OA in women was identified on chromosome 11q with a LOD score between 2 and 3. The authors suggested that a female-specific susceptibility gene for primary OA was present on chromosome 11q.[45] Further reports on genome-wide scans have indicated the existence of multiple susceptibility loci for OA by stratifying the same material by gender and joint. Thus, linkage to loci on chromosomes 2, 4, 6, and 16 was proposed.[2,46]

Chromosome 2

A suggestion of linkage was based on a LOD score of 1.22 that increased to 2.19 in hip patients, and it was stated that this suggestive linkage was greater for male hip patients. The proposed region 2q31 is at a similar location described in nodal OA[47] and near a locus, which was described for DIP OA.[48] It appears possible that chromosome 2q contains at least one susceptibility locus for OA.

Chromosome 4

The suggestion of linkage was based on a LOD score of 3.9 and centered on the chromosomal region 4q12-21.2, based on female sibling pairs with hip OA.[49] A separate study of a Dutch family with hip OA proposed linkage to a region of chromosome 4 more than 50 cM distal from the locus at 4q12-21.2. These authors concluded that it was unlikely that the two linkages had detected the same locus.[2]

Chromosome 6

Linkage for hip OA was based on an LOD score of 2.9 and centered on a strong candidate gene for OA, COL9A1 at 6q12-13.[2] This locus was further confirmed in an additional report by the same group, suggesting that the COL9A1 gene was associated with susceptibility for hip OA in females.[50]

Chromosome 16

Linkage showed an LOD score of 2.1, but no candidate genes for OA were associated with this locus. Again, the material was stratified for hip OA in women. The authors concluded that their analysis highlighted the potential utility of genome-wide screens, and that stratification of the material revealed additional chromosomal regions that may harbor susceptibility loci for OA in this British population.[2]

A genome-wide scan was done on a large Icelandic family with mainly hip OA, which showed linkage with a LOD score of 2.58 on chromosome 16 at a similar location as in the Loughlin study.[51] This is the first independent description of the same susceptibility locus in two different populations. However, this raises the possibility that they have the same founder. In this context, it is interesting to note that the Icelandic population gene pool has a significant component that appears to originate from Orkney, the Western Isles, and the Isle of Skye (British Isles).[52]

Conclusions

Some conclusions may be drawn from the currently known mutations in diseases associated with OA.

First, no mutation is known today in the 'common' primary form of OA, and most of the mutations are associated with relatively rare syndromes or diseases with what could be classified as secondary OA.

Second, most of the known mutations occur in collagen genes and it is worth noting that mutations in, for example, COL2A1 genes can have clinical phenotypes ranging from mild SED with premature OA of the hips to severe crippling disease from childhood.

Third, the number of newly discovered chondrodysplasia loci is decreasing, but the number of 'the garden-variety OA' loci is increasing.

Fourth, chromosomes 2, 4, and 16 were identified in multiple genome scans and are therefore the most likely to encode susceptibility.

Fifth, ongoing studies will eventually lead to classifications of the 'common OA' based on the causative gene defect, rather than on their variable clinical and radiographic phenotype. Hopefully, these studies will lead to the development of tests that will permit diagnosis of molecular defects, which can lead to therapy.

Key points

1. When should we think of inherited OA?
   a. When there is a rich family history.
   b. An unusually young patient with precocious OA in one or several joints is brought to your attention, and no other secondary cause of OA is known.
2. OA mutations known today are all associated with relatively rare syndromes that have OA as a major component. However, in recent years many loci have been found associated with the 'common OA phenotype'.
3. Several independent genome-wide scans have identified susceptibility associated with chromosomes 2, 4, and 16. Therefore, these chromosomes are most likely to harbor OA susceptibility genes.

Summary

Osteoarthritis (OA) is a heterogeneous and multi-factorial disease with many pathogenetic mechanisms implicated in its development and progression. Although OA is frequently a manifestation of certain metabolic, mechanical, or inflammatory events, several distinct forms of OA are inherited as dominantly acquired Mendelian traits, and evidence is piling up showing that inheritance and possible mutations in genes associated with OA can play a major role in the common form of OA in many joints. By the introduction of new biological methods for finding gene defects the search for possible gene defects have taken mainly three forms:[1] the parametric linkage analysis of rare families in which OA segregates as a Mendelian trait;[2] the model free linkage analysis of affected sibling pairs, and[3] the association analysis of known candidate genes.

Today, mutations known to be associated with OA all occur in relatively rare syndromes or diseases, which have OA as a major component. In recent years many loci have been found associated with the 'common OA phenotype'. Chromosome 2, 4, and 16 were identified in multiple genome scans and are therefore the most likely to encode susceptibility. Association analysis of candidate genes suggests that the syntenic genes for type II collagen and the vitamin D-receptor (12q12-q13.1) may also encode for OA susceptibility. The ongoing studies will eventually lead to classifications of the 'common OA' based on the exact causative gene defects, rather than on their variable clinical and radiographic phenotype. Hopefully, these studies will lead to the development of tests that permit diagnosis of molecular defects, which can lead to therapy of OA.

References

(An asterisk denotes recommended reading.)

1. Felson, D.T., Couropmitree, N.N., Chaisson, C.E., *et al.* (1998). Evidence for a Mendelian gene in a segregation analysis of generalized radiographic osteoarthritis. The Framingham Study. *Arthritis Rheum* **41**:1064–71.
2. *Loughlin, J., Moustafa, Z., Irven, C., *et al.* (1999). Stratification analysis of an osteoarthritis genome screen-suggestive linkage to chromosomes 4, 6, and 16. *Am J Hum Genet* **65**:1795–8.
   A genome scan for OA susceptibility loci.
3. Vikkula, M., Mariman, E., Lui, V., *et al.* (1995). Autosomal dominant and recessive osteochondro dysplasias associated with the COL11A2 locus. *Cell* **80**:431–7.
4. Vikkula, M., Nfissila, M., Hirvensala, E., *et al.* (1993). Multiallelic polymorphism of the cartilage gene: no association with osteoarthritis. *Ann Rheum Dis* **52**:762–4.
5. Ritvaniemi, P., Korkko, J., Bonaventure, J., Vikkula, M., Hyland, J., and Paasilta, P. (1995). Identification of COL2A1 mutations in patients with chondrodysplasias and familial osteoarthritis. *Arthritis Rheum* **38**: 999–1004.
6. *Loughlin, J., Irven, C., Fergusson, C., and Sykes, B. (1994). Sibling pair analysis shown no linkage of generalized osteoarthritis to the loci encoding type II collagen link protein or cartilage matrix protein. *Br J Rheumatol* **33**:1103–6.
   An example of sibling pair analysis.
7. Horton, A.W. (1996). Molecular genetic basis of the human chondrodysplasias. *Endocrin Met Clin North Am* **25**:683–97.
8. Chapmann, L.K., Mortier, R.G., Chapmann, K., *et al.* (2001). Mutation in the region encoding the von Willebrand factor A domain of matrilin-3 are associated with multiple epiphyseal dysplasia. *Nat Genet* **28**(August): 393–6.
9. Uitterlinden, A.G., Burger, H., Huang, Q., *et al.* (1997). Vitamin D receptor genotype is associated with radiographic osteoarthritis at the knee. *J Clin Invest* **100**:259–63.
10. Keen, R.W., Hart, D.J., Lanchbury, J.S., and Spector, T.D. (1997). Association of early osteoarthritis of the knee with a Taq I polymorphism of the vitamin D receptor gene. *Arthritis Rheum* **40**:1444–9.
11. Holderbaum, D., Haqqi, T.M., and Moskowitz (1999). Genetics and osteoarthritis. *Arthritis Rheum* **42**:397–405.
12. Uitterlinden, A.G., Burger, H., van Duijn, C.M., *et al.* (2000). Adjacent genes, for COL2A1 and vitamin D receptor, are associated with separate features of radiographic osteoarthritis of the knee. *Arthritis Rheum* **43**:1456–64.
13. *Loughlin, J. (2001). Genetic epidemiology of primary osteoarthritis. *Curr Opin Rheumatol* **13**:111–6.
    A good review of OA genetic studies to date.
14. Jimenez, S.A., Williams, C.J., and Karasick, D. (1998). Hereditary osteoarthritis. In K.D. Brandt, M. Doherty, and L.S. Lohmander (eds), *Osteoarthritis.* Oxford: Oxford University Press, pp. 31–49.
15. Schumacher Jr., H.R. (1972). Secondary osteoarthritis. In R.W. Moskowitz, D.S. Howell, V.M. Goldberg, and H.J. Mankin (eds), *Osteoarthritis: Diagnosis and Medical/Surgical Management.* Philadelphia: WB Saunders Philadelphia 1972:367–98.
16. Palotie, A., Väisänen, P., Ott, J., *et al.* (1989). Predisposition to familial osteoarthrosis linked to type II collagen gene. *Lancet* **29**(April):924–7.
17. Ala-Kokko, L, Baldwin, C.T., Moskowitz, R.W., and Prockop, D.J. (1990). A single base mutation in the type II procollagen gene (COL2AI) as cause of primary osteoarthritis associated with mild chondrodysplasia. *Proc Nat Acad Sci USA* **87**:6565–8.
18. Williams, C.J. and Jimenez, S.A. (1993). Heredity, genes and osteoarthritis. *Rheum Dis Clin North Am* **19**:523–43.
19. Vikkula, M., Metsaranta, M., and Ala-Kokko, L. (1994). Type II collagen mutation in rare and common cartilage diseases. *Ann Med* **26**:107–14.
20. Spranger, J., Winterpacht, A., and Zabel, B. (1994). The type II collagenopathies: a spectrum of chondrodysplasias. *Eur J Pediatr* **153**:56–65.
21. Loughlin, J., Irven, C., Athanasou, N., Carr, A., and Sykes, B. (1995). Differential allelic expression of the type II collagen gene (COL2A1) in osteoarthritic cartilage. *Am J Hum Genet* **56**:1186–93.
22. Kellgren, J.H., Lawrence, J.S., and Bier, F. (1963). Genetics factors in generalised osteoarthritis. *Ann Rheum Dis* **22**:237–55.
23. Ritvaniemi, P., Korkko, J., Bonaventure, J., *et al.* (1995). Identification of COL2a1 gene mutations in patients with chondrodysplasias and familial osteoarthritis. *Arthritis Rheum* **38**:999–1004.
24. Pattrick, M., Manhire, A., Ward, M., Doherty, M. (1989). HLA-B antigens and alpha-antitrypsin phenotypes in nodal and generalized osteoarthritis and erosive osteoarthritis. *Ann Rheum Dis* **48**:470–5.
25. Cicuttini, F.M. and Spector, T.D. (1996). Genetics of osteoarthritis. *Ann Rheum Dis* **55**:665–7.
26. Zitnan, D. and Sitaj, S. (1963). Chondrocalcinosis articularis. Section I: Clinical and radiological study. *Ann Rheum Dis* **22**:142–69.

27. Baldwin, C.T., Farrar, L.A., Dharmavaram, R., Adair, R., Jimenez, S.A., Anderson, L. (1995). Linkage of early onset osteoarthritis and chondrocalcinosis to human chromosome 8q. *Am J Hum Genet* **56**:692–7.

28. Hughes, A.E., McGibbon, D., Woodward, E., Dixey, J., and Doherty, M. (1995). Localisation of a gene for chondrocalcinosis to chromosome 5p. *Hum Mol Genet* **4**:1225–8.

29. Rojas, K., Serrano de la Pena, L., Gallardo, T., *et al.* (1999). Physical map and characterization of transcripts in the candidate interval for familial chondrocalcinosis at chromosome 5p15.1. *Genomics* **62**:177–83.

30. Ho, A.M., Johnson, M.D., Kingsley, D.M. (2000). Role of the mouse ank gene in control of tissue calcification and arthritis. *Science* **289**:265–70.

31. Marcos, J.C., Arturi, A.S., Babini, C., Jimenez, S.A., Knowlton, R., and Reginato, A.J. (1995). Familial hydroxyapatite chondrocalcinosis with spondyloepiphyseal dysplasia: clinical course and absence of genetic linkage to type II procollagen gene. *J Clin Rheumatol* **1**:171–8.

32. Bleasel, J.F., Bisagnifaure, A., Holderbaum, D., *et al.* (1995). Type II procollagen gene (COL2A1) mutation in exon 11 associated with spondyloepiphyseal dysplasia; tall stature and precocious osteoarthritis. *J Rheumatol* **22**:255–61.

33. Bleasel, J.F., Holderbaum, D., Mallock, V., Haqqi, T.M., Williams, H.J., Moskowitz, R.W. (1996). Hereditary osteoarthritis with mild spondyloepiphyseal dysplasia—are there 'hot spots' on COL2A1? *J Rheumatol* **23**:1594–8.

34. Bleasel, J.F., Holderbaum, D., Brancolini, V., *et al.* (1998). Five families with arginine 519-cysteine mutation in COL2A1: evidence for three distinct founders. *Hum Mutat* **12**:172–6.

35. Gedeon, A.K., Colley, A., Jamieson, R., *et al.* (1999). Identification of the gene (SEDL) causing X-linked spondyloepiphyseal dysplasia tarda. *Nat Genet* **4**:400–4.

36. Francomano, C.A., Liberfarb, R.M., Hirose, T., *et al.* (1987). The Stickler syndrome: Evidence for the close linkage to the structural gene for type II collagen. *Genomics* **1**:293–6.

37. Brunner, H.G., van Beersum, S.E., Warman, M.L., Olsen, B.R., Ropers, H.H., and Mariman, E.C. (1994). A Stickler syndrome gene is linked to chromosome 6 near the COL11A2 gene. *Hum Mol Genet* **3**:1561–4.

38. Briggs, M.D., Hoffman, S.M.G., King, L.M., *et al.* (1995). Pseudoachondroplasia and multiple epiphyseal dysplasia due to mutations in the cartilage oligomeric matrix protein gene. *Nat Genet* **10**:330–6.

39. Hecht, J.T., Nelson, L.D., Crowder, E., Wang, Y., Elder, F.F.B., and Harrison, W.R. (1995). Mutation in exon 17B of cartilage oligomeric matrix protein(COMP) cause pseudochondroaplasia. *Nat Genet* **10**:325–9.

40. Briggs, M.D., Choi, H.C., Warman, M.L., Loughlin, J.A., Wordsworth, P., and Sykes, B.C. (1994). Genetic mapping of a locus for multiple epiphyseal dysplasia (EDM2) to a region of chromosome 1 containing a type IX collagen gene. *Am J Hum Genet* **55**:678–84.

41. Muragaki, Y., Mariman, E.C.M., van Beersum, S.E.C., Perälä, M., van Mourik, J.B.A., and Warman, M.L. (1996). A mutation in the gene encoding the alfa2 chain of the fibril associated collagen IX, COL9A2, causes multiple epiphyseal dysplasia (EDM2). *Nat Genet* **12**:103–5.

42. Deere, M., Blanton, S.H., Scott, C.I., Langer, L.O., Pauli, R.M., Hecht, J.T. (1995). Genetic heterogeneity in multiple epiphyseal dysplasia. *Am J Hum Genet* **56**:698–704.

43. Unger, L.S., Briggs, M.D., Holden, P., *et al.* (2001). Multiple epiphyseal dysplasia:radiographic abnormalities correlated with genotype. *Pediatr Radiol* **31**:10–18.

44. Lander, E., and Kruglyak, L. (1995). Genetic dissection of complex traits: guidelines for interpreting and reporting linkage results. *Nat Genet* **11**:241–7.

45. Chapman, K., Moustafa, Z., Irven, C., *et al.* (1999). Osteoarthritis-susceptibility locus on chromosome 11q, detected by linkage. *Am J Hum Genet* **65**:167–74.

46. Loughlin, J., Moustafa, Z., Smith, A., *et al.* (2000). Linkage analysis of chromosome 2q in osteoarthritis. *Rheumatology* **39**:377–81.

47. Wright, G.D., Hughes, A.E., Regan, M., Doherty, M. (1996). Association of two loci on chromosome 2q with nodal osteoarthritis. *Ann Rheum Dis* **55**:317–319.

48. Leppavouri, J., Kujala, U., Kinnunen, J., *et al.* (1999). Genome scan for predisposing loci for distal interfalangeal joint osteoarthritis: evidence for a locus on 2q. *Am J Hum Genet* **65**:1060–7.

49. Roby, P., Eyre, S., Worthington, J., *et al.* (1999). Autosomal dominant (Beukes) premature degenerative osteoarthropathy of the hip joint maps to an 11-cM region on chromosome 4q35. *Am J Hum Genet* **64**:904–8.

50. Mustafa, Z., Chapman, K., Irven, C., *et al.* (2000). Linkage analysis of candidate genes as susceptibility loci for osteoarthritis-suggestive linkage of COL9A1 to female hip osteoarthritis. *Rheumatology* **39**:299–306.

51. *Ingvarsson, Th., Stefánsson, E.S., Gulcher, J.R., *et al.* (2001). A large Icelandic family with early osteoarthritis of the hip associated with a susceptibility loci on chromosome 16. *Arthritis Rheum* **44**:2548–55.
    This is the first independent description of the same susceptibility locus in two different populations.

52. Helgason, A., Sigurdardóttir, S., Gulcher, J.R., Ward, R., and Stefánsson, K. (2000). mtDNA and the origin of the Icelanders: deciphering signals of recent population history. *Am J Hum Genet* **66**:999–1116.

53. Meulenbelt, I., Biijerk, C., de Wildt, S.C.M., *et al.* (1997). Investigation of the assocation of the CRTM and CRTL1 genes with radiologically evident osteoarthritis in subjects from the Rotterdam study. *Arthritis Rheum* **40**:1760–5.

54. Aerssens, J., Dequeker, J., Peeters, J., Breemans, S., and Boonen, S. (1998). Lack of association between osteoarthritis of the hip and gene polymorphisms of VDR, COL1A1, and COL2A1 in post-menopausal women. *Arthritis Rheum* **41**:1946–50.

55. Huang, J., Hushiyama, T., Inoue, K., Kawasaki, T., and Hukuda, S. (2000). Vitamin D receptor gene polymorphisms and osteoarthritis of the hand, hip and knee: a case-control study in Japan. *Rheumatoloy* **39**:79–84.

56. Loughlin, J., Sinsheimer, J.S., Mustafa, Z., *et al.* (2000). Association of the vitamin D receptor gene, the type I collagen gene COL1A1, and the estrogen receptor gene in idiopathic osteoarthritis. *J Rheumatol* **27**:779–84.

57. Knowlton, R.G., Katzenstein, P.L., Moskowitz, R.W., *et al.* (1990). Genetic linkage of a polymorphism in the type II procollagen gene (COL2A1) to primary osteoarthritis associated with mild chondrodysplasia. *N Engl J Med* **22**:526–30.

58. Priestley, L., Fergusson, C., Ogilvie, D., *et al.* (1991). A limited association of generalized osteoarthritis with alleles at the type II collagen locus: COL2A1. *Br J Rheumatol* **30**:272–5.

59. Loughlin, J., Irven, C., Athanasou, N., Carr, A., and Sykes, B. (1995). Differential allelic expression of the type II collagen gene (COL2A1) in osteoarthritic cartilage. *Am J Hum Genet* **56**:1186–93.

60. Meulenbelt, I., Biykerk, C., de Wildt, S.C., *et al.* (1999). Haplotype analysis of three polymorphisms of the COL2A1 gene and association with generalized radiological osteoarthritis. *Ann Hum Genet* **63**:393–400.

61. Ushiyama, T., Ueyama, H., Inoue, K., Nisshioka, J., Onkubo, I., and Hukuda, S. (1998). Estrogen receptor gene polymorphism and generalized osteoarthritis. *J Rheumatol* **25**:134–7.

62. Yamada, Y., Okuizumi, H., Miyauchi, A., Takagi, Y., Ikeda, K., and Harada, A. (2000). Association of transforming growth factor beta 1 genotype with spinal osteophytosis in Japanese women. *Arthritis Rheum* **43**:452–60.

63. Meulenbelt, I., Bijkerk, C., Miedema, H.S., *et al.* (1998). A genetic association study of the IGF-I gene and radiological osteoarthritis in a population-based cohort study (the Rotterdam study). *Ann Rheum Dis* **57**:371–4.

64. Horton Jr., W.E., Lethbridge-Cejku, M., Hochberg, M.C., *et al.* (1998). An association between an aggrecan polymorphic allele and bilateral hand osteoarthritis in elderly white men: data from the Baltimore Longitudinal Study of Aging (BLSA). *Osteoarthritis Cart* **6**:245–51.

65. Shiang, R., Thompson, L.M., Zhu, Y.Z., *et al.* (1994). Mutations in the transmembrane domain of FGFR3 cause the most common genetic form of dwarfism, achondroplasia. *Cell* **78**:335–42.

66. Bellus, G.A., McIntosh, I., Smith, E.A., *et al.* (1995). A recurrent mutation in the tyrosine kinase domain of fibroblast growth factor receptor 3 causes hypochondroplasia. *Nat Genet* **10**:357–9.

4.3 Laboratory approaches to the identification of genetic association in osteoarthritis

Virginia B. Kraus and Eden R. Martin

Osteoarthritis is a common multifactorial disease with a strong genetic component. Considered from a genetic standpoint, it is a complex disorder resulting from the combined effects of genes at two or more locations in the genome, or interplay of variant genes and environmental exposures or events. Complex disorders differ from the Mendelian inherited disorders, which occur as a result of a single variant gene. To date, studies have demonstrated that OA is only rarely transmitted as a Mendelian trait. Methods of genetic analysis are currently available and rapidly evolving[1] to elucidate the genetic etiologies of even complex disorders like OA. What seems a daunting task is made more manageable by considering the fact that identifying even one causal gene in a complex disorder has the potential to 'tag' a member of a key disease pathway wherein may reside many of the genetic etiologies.[2] The common laboratory approaches to the identification of OA susceptibility genes are described below.

Genetic mapping

The process of identifying genetic causality or susceptibility involves genetic mapping. Genetic mapping is a multistep process involving three fundamental elements: defining and collecting the data set, genotyping markers, and performing the statistical analysis. The steps involved in this process are summarized in Fig. 4.1.

Defining and collecting the data set

The success of any form of genetic analysis is critically dependent on clearly, and as unequivocally as possible, defining the disease phenotype. The phenotype is the expression of the genotype, modified by the environment, manifested as functional or structural characteristics of an individual, such as the appearance, physical features, or physiology. In the case of OA, the sites and severity of joint involvement define the phenotype. Genetic mapping could be thought of as phenotype mapping because the genotype, the group of alleles (DNA sequences) that an individual carries, is identified as being related to a specific phenotype.

Qualitative or quantitative traits or a combination of the two can define the phenotype. Qualitative traits are discontinuous and scored by their presence or absence. Family members in genetic studies are classified as affected, unaffected, or unknown based upon the phenotype definition. The presence or absence of radiographic joint disease is an example of a qualitative trait for OA studies. A qualitative trait implies a threshold value or combination of factors that distinguishes the norm from the disease state. The level at which the threshold is set defines the study phenotype and may be somewhat arbitrary in the absence of abundant epidemiological data concerning the trait. For most OA studies, a Kellgren–Lawrence grade of 2 or greater is accepted as defining a threshold of disease that is widely accepted as representative of OA. However, variations in organisms are usually quantitative not qualitative.[3] Quantitative traits are continuously distributed measurements of disease that encompass a range of values. For instance, the severity grade of OA based upon the Kellgren–Lawrence grading scheme in the range 0–4 is a quantitative trait of OA. The Kellgren–Lawrence scores from multiple joint sites can also be combined into a sum score to represent a quantitative trait of disease burden.[4] Quantitative traits might also include serum biomarker measures representative of cartilage matrix metabolism. The potential for cartilage biomarkers to serve as quantitative traits of OA was illustrated in a study performed in families with known collagen II mutations.[5] Serum levels of cartilage oligomeric protein and keratan sulphate were elevated in mutation-positive individuals and individuals with OA regardless of mutation status, illustrating the potential for cartilage biomarkers to function as quantitative traits in genetic analyses. The increased serum levels of these two biochemical markers in mutation-positive individuals who had not yet developed radiographic evidence of disease, further illustrates the potential for biomarkers to provide a more precise method of differentiating truly unaffected cases from apparently unaffected cases that have not yet developed radiographic signs of disease. The use of any quantitative traits for defining phenotype is subject to refinement as knowledge of the disease is advanced. Therefore, these types of methodologies are expected to improve in the coming years as the understanding of OA progresses.

To make the effect of genes more easily detectable, the sampled population may be restricted to extremes of the phenotype, such as those with very young onset or with unusual presentations or more widespread or severe disease. One approach taken in OA research has been to evaluate the families of individuals who have undergone a total joint replacement.[6,7] Although total joint replacement is not a perfect surrogate for disease severity, this approach has led to successful linkage of disease phenotype to regions of interest within the genome. Still others have adopted the approach of ascertaining generalized OA manifesting at multiple joint sites on the hypothesis that this may represent a more severe form of the disease (for instance the ongoing Genetics of Generalized OA or GOGO Consortium study [unpublished] and Refs 8 and 9). To reduce the effect of known environmental confounders, the sample might be restricted to a genetically homogeneous population such as has been done in OA studies in Iceland[2] and Finland.[10] However, the more restrictions placed upon the sampled population, the greater the risk incurred of limiting inferences about the genetic basis for the disease in the general population.

Phenotype is also subject to heterogeneity for many reasons (Table 4.8). Phenotype is influenced by penetrance and expressivity. Penetrance is the

Table 4.8 Types of heterogeneity contributing to phenotypic variation

- ◆ Clinical
    - ■ Affected individuals vary in clinical expression
- ◆ Genetic
    - ■ Locus: Different genes lead to same disease
    - ■ Allelic: Different alleles of same gene lead to same/different disease

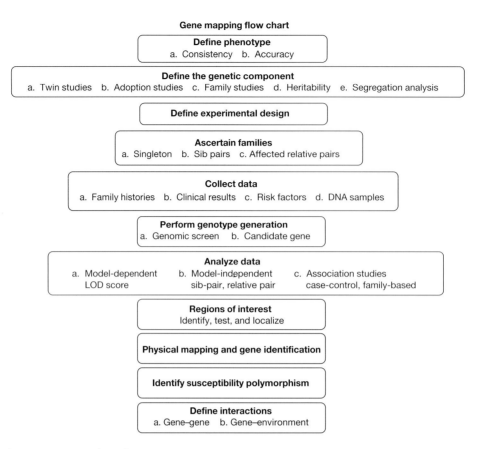

Fig. 4.1 The steps involved in genetic mapping of complex traits.

Source: Adapted from Haines and Pericak-Vance 1998,[40] and used with the kind permission of the authors.

proportion of individuals with a risk genotype that expresses the disease phenotype and expressivity is the severity of the phenotype. OA is an example of a disease with an age-dependent penetrance generally appearing after the fourth decade of life and progressing over time.[11] OA is also known for its gender-influenced expression with women more often manifesting generalized joint disease than men.[12] Well-chosen phenotypes or disease subtypes based upon epidemiological data can identify more homogeneous families for analysis and add to the ultimate success of genetic mapping.

The genetic analysis requires a sample for DNA isolation from each subject. DNA can be isolated from blood or tissue. In humans, lymphocytes from blood provide the source of DNA as opposed to mature red blood cells, which are devoid of nuclei and thus devoid of DNA. In general, a total of 30 ml of blood provides adequate amounts of DNA for a genetic screen (extracted from 10 ml) leaving some additional blood that can be stored as a back up. At room temperature, DNA is most stable when EDTA or acid dextrose is used as the anticoagulant.[13] DNA can be extracted from fresh or frozen isolated lymphocytes or whole blood. Samples for DNA extraction can be held at 4 °C for up to several days, however, if longer lag times are anticipated, the samples should be stored at −80 °C as soon after collection as possible.[13] Squamous cells from the buccal mucosa are a readily accessible source of DNA and provide an alternative means of acquiring a DNA sample when it is not possible to obtain blood. In addition, tissue, fixed or fresh, from any organ can also serve as a source of DNA. Inexhaustible supplies of DNA from specific individuals are made possible by immortalizing their lymphocytes *in vitro* with Epstein Barr virus.[14] It is generally recommended that cards containing spots of dried blood be prepared for each individual at the time of blood sampling to provide a cross check of sample

identity in case of any mix up in the future. Attention must also be given to careful sample labelling, as the genetic analysis will be substantially weakened if significant numbers of DNA samples are mislabelled.[15]

Genotyping markers

Gene discovery in humans advanced dramatically with the discovery in 1980 that variations in human DNA could be assayed directly and used as genetic markers.[16] The process of characterizing markers in the genome to genetically map a trait is genotyping. By the time samples make it to the genotyping stage, they have usually been through a long journey. The particular choice of marker type to evaluate is dependent upon the accuracy, rapidity, and expense involved in the genotyping assay. In genetic mapping, usually the DNA markers themselves are not functionally important; rather they serve to correlate mutant phenotypes with specific molecular regions within the genome and thus provide convenient reference points, which enable disruptions of specific regions to be identified. Progress in the human genome project has enhanced the ability to detect DNA sequence variants, thus expanding the catalogue of useful markers.

Markers that are useful for genetic analysis are of several types (Table 4.9). Simple-sequence length polymorphisms (SSLPs) are short segments of DNA repeated in tandem.[3] By definition, to be classified as a polymorphism, a variant must be present in 1 per cent or more of the population.[17] Short tandem repeats can be further separated into micro-satellite markers and mini-satellite markers. Micro-satellite markers (also called simple sequence repeats/SSRs or short tandem repeat polymorphisms/STRPs) consist of repeating units of one, two, three, or four nucleotides. The most common type consists of repeats of CA and its complement GT. About 10 000 human micro-satellites have been identified and mapped in the human genome. Informative micro-satellites, those useful for genetic analyses, have been observed to occur on average every 20 000 base-pairs in the human genome.[15] Mini-satellite markers consist of repeats of more complex units of DNA with variation in the number of tandem repeats (VNTRs), usually in the range of 14–100 base-pairs in length.[18] SSLPs have proven very useful in genetic studies due to the large variation in alleles made possible by the association of differing DNA sequences, unit lengths, and repeat numbers. Moreover, they tend to show high levels of heterozygosity, meaning

Table 4.9 Types of markers useful for genetic analysis

Simple-Sequence Length Polymorphisms (SSLPs)

◆ Microsatellites
- Multiply repeated short sequence elements of DNA
  - Mononucleotides (repeats of 1-base pair units)
  - Dinucleotides (repeats of 2-base pair units)
  - Trinucleotides (repeats of 3-base pair units)
  - Tetranucleotides (repeats of 4-base pair units)
◆ Minisatellites
- Multiply repeated longer, more complex units of DNA
  - Variable number tandem repeats (VNTRs)

Single Nucleotide Polymorphisms (SNPs)

- Point mutations in DNA
  - Type I   mutation in coding region leading to non-conservative change in protein sequence
  - Type II   mutation in coding region leading to conservative change in protein sequence
  - Type III mutation in coding region leading to no change in protein sequence
  - Type IV   mutation in non-coding 5′ untranslated region
  - Type V   mutation in non-coding 3′ untranslated region
  - Type VI   mutation in other non-coding regions

Restriction fragment length polymorphisms (RFLPs)

- Create or destroy a restriction site in DNA

Table 4.10 Useful Internet addresses

◆ Online Mendelian inheritance in man (OMIM)
- USA: http://www.ncbi.nlm.nih.gov/Omim/
- UK: http://www.hgmp.mrc.ac.uk/omim/
◆ Genome browser
- http://www.ensembl.org/
◆ SNP database (dbSNP)
- http://www.ncbi.nlm.nih.gov/SNP/
◆ Genetic analysis software
- http://linkage.rockefeller.edu/soft/
◆ NIH sponsored mammalian genotyping services
- http://research.marshfieldclinic.org/genetics/
- http://www.cidr.jhmi.edu

that a large number of different alleles tend to be found fairly commonly in the population. Information on several thousand micro-satellite markers is electronically accessible to investigators through genome databases (see Table 4.10 for useful Internet addresses).[18]

Another major class of markers useful for genetic analyses is the single nucleotide polymorphisms (SNPs). SNPs are single base-pair sites within the genome at which more than one of the four possible base pairs is commonly found in the population.[3] SNPs occur on average every 1000 base pairs (some estimate even closer) and are the most common type of sequence change in the genome, outweighing insertions, deletions, and copy-number variations in nucleotide repeat motifs.[19] SNPs have been categorized into six types based upon location relative to a gene and ability to result in an amino acid substitution within a protein[20] (Table 4.9). SNPs within a region of a gene coding for protein are termed Types I–III or cSNPs (coding SNPs). It has been estimated that the genome contains between 30 000 and 100 000 human genes[2,21,22] with approximately 4 cSNPs per gene.[23] SNPs in non-coding regions are designated Types IV–VI with an estimated 440 000 in untranslated portions of genes and more than 1 million in other non-coding regions of DNA. Restriction fragment length polymorphisms or RFLPs can be SNPs or small deletions, insertions, or changes affecting a few bases that create or destroy a restriction site in DNA (sites recognized by bacterial enzymes that cut DNA at specific base sequences in the genome). These were the first DNA markers to be generally used in genomic characterization.[16]

To reduce costs a two-stage strategy is often adopted for a genetic screen, the process of genotyping markers. The whole genome of the first sample set is genotyped, while the regions of interest showing potential linkage to the disease phenotype, are genotyped in the second sample set. The most common approach currently involves genotyping a dense set of uniformly spaced micro-satellite markers to systematically screen the genome. On average, 350–400 markers 10 centiMorgan apart (estimated to be approximately equivalent to 10 million base-pairs apart) are mapped in a primary genome screen.[3] SNP analyses promise to accelerate the mapping of complex traits in the future by allowing for a much denser screen, but currently SNP mapping at such density is too costly (estimated, at a minimum, to require mapping one SNP every 30 kb for a total of 100 000 SNPs for a full genome scan). Approximately three- to four-fold more SNPs must be analysed than micro-satellites for the same information content, thus, their most immediate use is in fine mapping once locations of interest in the genome are identified. There exists a relative deficiency of types I and IV SNPs in the genome, relative to the other types, suggesting the influence of selection pressure on SNPs in these regions.[20] It has been hypothesized that the mapping of types I and IV SNPs in coding and promoter regions is more likely to identify DNA regions with functional significance, which influence phenotypic traits, than the mapping of random SNPs.[20] This approach would theoretically reduce the total number of SNPs required in a screen and therefore reduce the expense of genotyping.

Numerous methods of genotyping have emerged. Technology is advancing rapidly in this area, therefore, we list below only a few of the major techniques currently utilized including RFLPs, mini-satellite, micro-satellite and SNP detection methods. RFLPs are detected by Southern blotting that entails digesting genomic DNA with a particular restriction enzyme and evaluating the fragment sizes yielded upon hybridization of a radiolabelled probe to a region of interest. The frequency of occurrence of RFLPs is dependent on the length of the sequence recognized by the restriction enzyme. For instance, a restriction enzyme that recognizes six-base sequences will cleave a DNA molecule approximately once every $4^6 = 4096$ base-pairs, based upon the probability that a specific base (of which there are four) will be found at each of the six positions.[3] Thus, a panel of 8 enzymes (each recognizing six-base sequences) will sample every $4096/8 = 500$ base-pairs for polymorphisms. A panel of 8 enzymes that recognize four-base sequences can sample about once every 32 base-pairs along the DNA molecule. Insertions and deletions of DNA that can also cause restriction fragment lengths to vary can confound this method. This method has the disadvantages of requiring specific cloned probes for each marker locus and the availability of relatively large

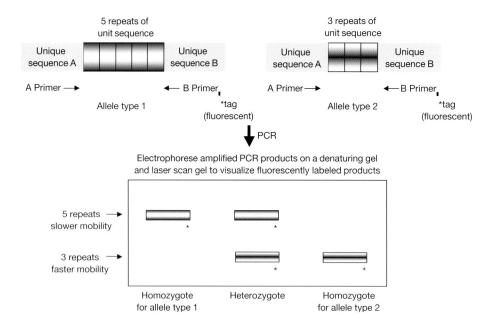

Fig. 4.2 Methodology of genotyping microsatellite markers.

amounts of DNA. Mini-satellite analysis requires only one probe that detects the core sequence of the repetitive element at loci anywhere in the genome.

There are numerous ways to detect micro-satellites. The most amenable to automation and therefore typically employed for high throughput genotyping relies upon PCR with fluorescent-labelled primers (Fig. 4.2). A primer pair for each marker locus is required. The variable number of repeats in the micro-satellite produces PCR fragments of different sizes. The PCR fragments are separated on denaturing acrylamide gels or in capillary tubes and detected by a laser scanner. This method requires only small amounts of DNA. Several sets of PCR primers, each labelled with a distinct fluorescent dye, can be mixed in a single tube if the amplified fragments from each primer set can be sufficiently separated by size from one another, thus further increasing the genotyping output and reducing the cost.

Precise gene localization is most often achieved by candidate gene analysis. The advent of SNP maps facilitated by the SNP Consortium has led to the recent proposal to achieve fine localization via high-density SNP mapping in regions of interest.[24] Many methods exist for detection of SNPs including PCR and DNA chip based methods among others.[15,24,25] To date no one technique has achieved dominance.

Good study design includes running the samples and scoring the marker results without pedigree or disease affection status and the inclusion of blinded duplicate samples. There is an absolute need for a replicate sample especially as complexity of a trait increases. To ultimately establish that a mutation in a particular gene is causative of a disease phenotype, it is necessary to have a physical map of the DNA in the region of interest, a transcript map of the region of interest identifying intron-exon boundaries, and a population survey of the purported mutation to determine that it is not a naturally occurring, inconsequential substitution in the normal population.[26] Fortunately, the human genome project is providing the molecular tools to facilitate this process.

Statistical methods

Statistical methods for identifying genes involved in human disease fall largely into two classes: linkage methods and association methods. Linkage methods use family data and look for the cosegregation of genetic markers and disease. Identification of linkage suggests that the marker and disease loci are physically close together, thus linkage analysis can help to identify regions in the genome containing genetic loci influencing disease. Association methods use either samples of unrelated individuals or family data. These methods attempt to identify specific alleles of genetic markers that are correlated with disease status. Association methods are often used to try to refine the position of disease loci in a previously identified region of linkage or in candidate gene studies.

Linkage methods

Recombination fraction. An individual receives two sets of chromosomes, one set from his/her mother and one set from his/her father. Consider two loci in the genome, 'A' and 'B'. When the individual forms gametes during meiosis, there are four types of gametes that can be formed with respect to the alleles at the two loci (see Fig. 4.3). Two of these gametes are *parental*, one containing the two maternal alleles and the other containing the two paternal alleles. The other two gametes are *recombinant*, each containing one maternal and one paternal allele. If the two loci are *unlinked*, then the four types of gametes are formed with equal frequency. This independent segregation is what is expected if, for example, the two loci are on different chromosomes. If the two loci are *linked*, then recombinant gametes are expected to form less frequently than parental gametes because the parental alleles tend to cosegregate.

Linkage is generally measured by the recombination fraction (typically denoted by θ). The recombination fraction between two loci is the proportion of recombinant gametes. The recombination fraction ranges between 0, if there is linkage (with no recombination), and 0.5, if the loci are unlinked. Tests for linkage test the null hypothesis that $\theta = 0.5$, and a significant result indicates that there is linkage between the loci. Linkage is important, because, in general, the more tightly linked two loci are, the closer together they are physically. So linkage between a marker and disease locus suggests that the marker is close to the unknown disease locus. However, the relationship between linkage and physical distance is quite variable and differs among different regions of the genome and even between the sexes.[27]

Lod score. Tests for linkage are often based on the lod score. First introduced by Morton in 1955,[28] the lod score is the log of the odds of linkage between

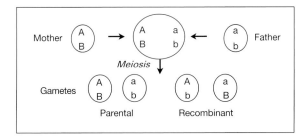

Fig. 4.3 Segregation of alleles at meiosis.

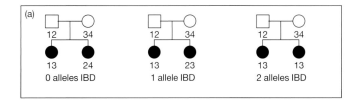

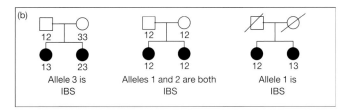

Fig. 4.4 (a) Identity by descent (IBD) among siblings; (b) identity by state (IBS) among siblings.

two loci. A lod score is a measure of the evidence for linkage between two loci in family data. The lod score for $\theta = x$ is:

$$z(x) = \log_{10}\left(\frac{L(\text{family data} \mid \theta = x)}{L(\text{family data} \mid \theta = 0.5)}\right),$$

where $L(\text{family data} \mid \theta = x)$ is the likelihood of the family data (i.e., the probability of observing the family with the specified relationships, affection status, and marker genotype data) if the true recombination fraction is x and $L(\text{family data} \mid \theta = 0.5)$ is the likelihood of the family data when there is no linkage. Statistical tests are usually based on the maximum lod score over all possible values of x. The value of x for which this maximum is obtained is the maximum likelihood estimate of θ. If the maximum occurs at $\theta = 0.5$, then the lod score is 0, indicating no evidence of linkage. If the maximum occurs at $\theta < 0.5$, then the lod score is positive. Lod scores are additive over families, therefore the evidence of linkage increases as more linked families are considered.

Parametric linkage analysis. In linkage analysis to identify genes involved in human genetic disease, the underlying disease locus genotype is typically unknown. However, if there is information about the relationship between the disease locus genotype and phenotype, that is the disease model, then probabilities can be placed on possible genotypes given the phenotype information. Linkage analysis methods that require specification of the disease model are referred to as *parametric linkage* methods. The disease model is usually specified in terms of genotype-specific penetrances: the probability that an individual with a specific genotype is affected with the disease. For example, for a simple recessive disorder, individuals with two copies of the disease allele have probability 1 of being affected, while individuals with other genotypes have probability 0 of being affected. Having this information, along with disease allele frequencies allows us to assign disease locus genotypes with certain probabilities based on the known phenotype information. For the recessive disease example, all affected individuals carry two copies of the disease allele with certainty, while unaffected individuals carry either one or no copies of the disease allele, depending on allele frequencies and the genotypes of their relatives. With this information, the lod score for any family can be computed by considering all possible genotype configurations based on the known phenotype information.

For complex diseases, with many genes and other factors contributing to disease risk, the disease model may not be straightforward, however, parametric linkage analysis may still be used with some success. Often a range of models is considered, with the maximum lod score over models taken to be the best evidence of linkage. Alternatively, non-parametric methods can be used.

Non-parametric linkage analysis. Non-parametric linkage methods do not require specification of the disease model. These methods test for linkage by looking for the increased sharing of alleles among affected relatives, often affected sibling pairs. These are based on the principle that affected relatives should share more alleles *identical by descent* (IBD) than expected by chance at loci linked to the disease locus. Two alleles are IBD if they are descendants of the same parental chromosomes. Figure 4.4 shows an example of siblings who share 0, 1, and 2 alleles IBD. At loci unlinked to the

disease locus, full siblings are expected to share 0, 1, or 2 alleles with probabilities 0.25, 0.5, and 0.25, respectively. So, on average, they are expected to share 1 allele IBD at unlinked loci.

In some cases, it may not be possible to determine whether alleles are IBD. They may be *identical by state* (IBS), that is, be the same allele type, but it may be impossible to tell if they come from copies of the same chromosome. This can occur if the parents are not fully informative (i.e., not different heterozygotes) or if parents' genotypes are unknown. Missing parental data is often a problem for late onset diseases such as OA. Figure 4.4 also shows examples of families in which alleles are IBS, but IBD status is unknown. Identity by state can function as a surrogate for IBD information, allowing one to obtain an estimate of the IBD allele sharing among relatives and thus assess the degree of linkage.

The methods described above focus on identifying linkage with a binary trait, for example, affected or unaffected (for a thorough treatment of parametric and non-parametric linkage methods, see Ott[27]) however there are methods that allow one to test for linkage to quantitative trait loci (QTL) as well. These methods are typically based on a variance components model, and the tests assess whether the additive genetic variance attributed to an unobserved QTL equals zero. The lod score that is equivalent to the classical lod score of linkage analysis can be obtained through a likelihood ratio test. Among many developments of QTL mapping methods, the SOLAR program[29] was developed to perform linkage analysis for quantitative traits based on the variance component method.

Association methods

Measures of association. An alternative to using linkage methods is to use association-based methods. These methods look for a correlation between genotype and phenotype, for example, affection status. An association between genotype and phenotype can occur if the genotype directly influences the disease phenotype by disrupting the function of important proteins. Alternatively, phenotype–genotype correlations may occur if the marker is in linkage disequilibrium with another polymorphism, which influences disease phenotype. *Linkage disequilibrium* refers to the association between alleles at different loci.[30] If there is linkage disequilibrium, then the genotypes at two loci are not independent and this can lead to association between a marker genotype and phenotype, even if the marker is not directly responsible for the disease.

There are several measures of association that are commonly used in epidemiological and genetic studies.[31] Table 4.11 shows how to calculate some common measures of association. The *relative risk* measures the increase in risk of disease among carriers of the risk allele relative to non-carriers.

Table 4.11 Common measures of association

Sample observations

	Carries risk allele	Does not carry risk allele
Affected	a	b
Unaffected	c	d

$(a + b)/(a + b + c + d)$ = disease frequency
$(a + c)/(a + b + c + d)$ = carrier frequency

Measures

Relative Risk	$\dfrac{a/(a + c)}{b/(b + d)}$
Odds Ratio	$\dfrac{ad}{bc}$
Attributable Risk	$\dfrac{a}{a + c} - \dfrac{b}{b + d}$

The relative risk can be estimated only in a random sample. If the sample has been ascertained based on affection status, then the *odds ratio* provides an approximation for the relative risk for diseases with low prevalence. The odds ratio measures the increase in the odds of being a carrier of the risk allele among individuals with disease, relative to the odds of being a carrier of the risk allele among individuals without the disease. A third measure is the *attributable risk*, which is based on the difference between the risk of disease among carriers and the risk among non-carriers.

Case-control tests of association. For common traits, it is possible to test for association in a random sample of individuals from the population. However, for less common traits, such as many genetic diseases, it may be difficult to get sufficient numbers of diseased individuals in a random sample. For this reason, samples are often collected targeting affected individuals (the cases) specifically and then collecting a separate set of unaffected controls for comparison. This design is referred to as a case-control design. To test for association between the marker and disease, allele or genotype frequencies are compared between the case and control samples. A standard chi-square test is often used to assess significant differences between the two populations. Alternatively, a test can be based on the odds ratio, declaring significant association if it's associated confidence interval does not include 1.

A difficulty with case-control tests is that they can be biased if cases and controls are not appropriately matched for factors that may lead to allele frequency differences unrelated to genetic associations. For example, if cases come from one population and controls from another, then we may detect allele frequency differences that merely represent population differences rather than indicating that the marker is associated with disease. This is a particular concern in stratified populations in which the population is subdivided into different strata and disease prevalence and allele frequencies differ between the strata. To overcome these concerns, several family-based tests of association have been proposed.

Family-based tests of association. Family-based tests of association use within-family controls, thus assuring that cases and controls are well-matched for ethnicity. Early family-based tests of association use *family triads*, an affected individual and both parents. Examples of tests for association in triads include the haplotype relative risk (HRR),[32] the haplotype-based haplotype relative risk (HHRR)[33] and the transmission/disequilibrium test (TDT).[34] These tests are based on the observation that, for any triad, there is a pair of alleles that is transmitted from parents to the affected offspring and a pair of alleles that is not transmitted. The transmitted pair of alleles is the case genotype and the non-transmitted pair of alleles functions as a well-matched 'control' genotype. If a particular allele occurs more often in the transmitted pair of alleles than in the non-transmitted pair, then that allele is associated with the disease.

For late-onset diseases, such as OA, it may be difficult to obtain parental genotype data. In this case several tests have been proposed that use unaffected siblings as controls. Examples of these tests include the Sib-TDT[35]

and the sibship disequilibrium test (SDT).[36] These tests compare the genotypes of affected siblings to the genotypes of their unaffected siblings and properly account for the inherent correlation between siblings' genotypes. Like the association tests in family triads, the sibling-based tests assure that cases and controls are well-matched for ethnicity, thus remain valid even in stratified populations. However, these methods may be less powerful than methods that use family triads if there is misclassification of the disease status of the unaffected siblings. The concern is that we have no guarantee that unaffected siblings will remain unaffected, thus statistical power may be compromised. The same concern holds for case-control tests in unrelated individuals, but is magnified in family-based tests since unaffected siblings have an increased chance of carrying the risk allele. One way to decrease potential misclassification is to use older unaffecteds, for example, those older than the age-of-onset of disease in their affected sibling(s). Alternatively, some methods make inference about missing parental genotypes based on the genotypes of offspring, but do not directly use the phenotype information from unaffecteds. These methods avoid concerns regarding misdiagnosis of unaffecteds, but are not robust to population stratification due to assumptions needed to make inference about parental genotypes.

Traditionally family-based tests for association have been proposed for binary traits, however there are several variations that can be applied when the trait is a quantitative variable instead. Like the methods above, these methods test for correlation between the trait and marker genotype and can use data from either family triads or sibships.

Examples in OA. Many of the analyses described above have been used in the search for genes contributing to OA. Parametric linkage analysis has been used in the study of functional candidate genes and in genome screens to identify regions of linkage in large families showing autosomal dominant inheritance for early-onset forms of OA.[36] However families showing clear Mendelian inheritance of OA are rare, therefore larger linkage studies have focused on smaller affected sib-pair families with the more common form of late-onset OA. Several studies have looked for linkage to candidate gene polymorphisms or conducted genome screens using non-parametric linkage methods (see Loughlin 2001 for a review[39]). Several distinct regions have been identified as being linked to OA, however, the only chromosome that has been identified consistently is chromosome 2q. Often stratification by gender or site of OA increased the evidence of linkage, which highlights the importance of considering potentially more homogeneous subsets when testing for genetic linkage. Association methods in unrelated cases and controls have also been used to test candidate genes, which based on function, could be involved in the development and progression of OA. The list of candidate genes tested is long and includes genes which code for structural proteins, such as the collagen genes, and those involved in regulating bone mass and density. Loughlin gives a thorough review of candidate genes that have been tested.[39] The most consistent evidence for association has been with the COL2A1 and VDR genes, which have been tested in several studies; however, even these genes have yielded a mix of positive and negative reports of association. Possible reasons for the inconsistent results in the association studies include phenotypic differences between the studies, population or ethnic differences in the samples, and small sample size leading to low statistical power to detect associations. Additionally, all of the association tests to date have been applied in case-control samples rather than family samples, thus false–positive results due to population stratification cannot be ruled out.

Conclusions

With the advent of genetic maps and advances in molecular biology, the genetic dissection of complex diseases like OA has become possible. To ultimately find the disease susceptibility genes for OA will likely require large sample sets. The concept of multicenter genetic studies in well-characterized populations, as a means of generating large samples of family data using standardized protocols, is ongoing in OA. Even though evidence for a genetic effect from any single study may be moderate, constructive synergism of various sites working with different populations is most likely to achieve our common goal of attaining a better molecular and genetic understanding of OA for the purpose of ameliorating the effects of this disabling disease.

Key points

1. OA is a complex disease with a strong genetic basis due to the influence of multiple genes and environment.

2. The success of genetic analysis is critically dependent upon clearly defining a disease phenotype.

3. Genotyping is the process of characterizing markers in the genome to genetically map a disease phenotype.

4. The two major classes of statistical methods for gene identification are linkage and association methods.

5. Parametric linkage analysis requires knowledge of the nature of inheritance of a disease gene (recessive, dominant, etc.), while non-parametric methods do not.

References

(An asterisk denotes recommended reading.)

1. *Lander, E. and Schork, N. (1994). Genetic dissection of complex traits. *Science* **265**:2037–48.
   A classic description of genetic methodologies and approaches used for complex diseases.

2. Gulcher, J., Kong, A., and Stefansson, K. (2001). The genealogic approach to human genetics of disease. *Cancer J* **7**(1):61–8.

3. Griffiths, A., Miller, J., Suzuki, D., Lewontin, R., and Gelbart, W. (2000). An Introduction to Genetic Analysis (7th ed.). New York: WH Freeman, p. 860.

4. Hirsch, R., Lethbridge-Cejku, M., Hanson, R., *et al.* (1998). Familial aggregation of OA: data from the Baltimore Longitudinal Study on Aging. *Arthritis Rheum* **41**(7):1227–32.

5. Bleasel, J., Poole, A., Heinegard, D., *et al.* (1999). Changes in serum cartilage marker levels indicate altered cartilage metabolism in families with the OA-related type II collagen gene COL2A1 mutation. *Arthritis Rheum* **42**(1):39–45.

6. Ingvarsson, T., Stefansson, S.E., Hallgrimsdottir, I.B., *et al.* (2000). The inheritance of hip OA in Iceland. *Arthritis Rheum* **43**(12):2785–92.

7. Loughlin, J., Mustafa, Z., Smith, A., *et al.* (2000). Linkage analysis of chromosome 2q in OA. *Rheumatology* **39**(4):377–81.

8. Priestley, L., Fergusson, C., Ogilvie, D., *et al.* (1991). A limited association of generalized OA with alleles at the type II collagen locus: COL2A1. *Br J Rheumatol* **30**:272–5.

9. Loughlin, J., Irven, C., Fergusson, C., and Sykes, B. (1994). Sibling pair analysis shows no linkage of generalized OA to the loci encoding type II collagen, cartilage link protein or cartilage matrix protein. *Br J Rheumatol* **33**(12):1103–6.

10. Leppavuori, J., Kujala, U., Kinnunen, J., *et al.* (1999). Genome scan for predisposing loci for distal interphalangeal joint OA: evidence for a locus on 2q. *Am J Hum Genet* **65**(4):1060–7.

11. Dieppe, P., Cushnaghan, J., Tucker, M., Browning, S., and Shepstone, L. (2000). The Bristol 'OA500 study': progression and impact of the disease after 8 years. *Osteoarthritis Cart* **8**(2):63–8.

12. Felson, D. (1995). The epidemiology of OA: prevalence and risk factors. In K. Kuettner and V. Goldberg (eds), *Osteoarthritic Disorders*. Rosemont: American Academy of Orthopaedic Surgeons, pp. 13–24.

13. Vance, J. (1998). The collection of biological samples for DNA analysis. In J. Hanes, and M. Pericak-Vance (eds), *Approaches to Gene Mapping in Complex Human Diseases*. New York: Wiley-Liss, pp. 201–11.

14. Glade, P.R., Beratis, N.G. (1976). Long-term lymphoid cell lines in the study of human genetics. *Prog Medic Genet* **1**:1–48.

15. Weber, J., and Broman, K. (2001). Genotyping for human whole-genome scans: past, present, and future. In D. Rao and M. Province (eds), *Genetic Dissection of Complex Traits*. New York: Academic Press, pp. 77–95.

16. Botstein, D., White, R., Skolnick, M., and Davis, R. (1980). Construction of a genetic linkage map in man using restriction fragment length polymorphisms. *Am J Hum Genet* **32**:314–31.

17. Gelehrter, T., Collins, F., and Ginsburg, D. (1998). *Principles of Medical Genetics* (2nd ed.). Baltimore: Williams Wilkins, p. 410.

18. Vance, J. and Othmane, K. (1998). Methods of genotyping. In J. Hanes and M. Pericak-Vance (eds), *Approaches to Gene Mapping in Complex Human Diseases*. New York: Wiley-Liss, pp. 213–28.

19. Haluska, M., Fan, J-B., and Bentley, K., *et al.* (1999). Patterns of single-nucleotide polymorphisms in candidate genes for blood-pressure homeostasis. *Nat Genet* **22**(July):239–47.

20. Risch, N.J. (2000). Searching for genetic determinants in the new millennium. *Nature* **405**(6788):847–56.

21. Claverie, J-M. (2001). What if there are only 30,000 human genes? *Science* **291**:1255–7.

22. Pennisi, E. (2001). The human genome: news. *Science* **291**:1177–80.

23. Cargill, M., Altshuler, D., Ireland, J., *et al.* (1999). Characterization of single-nucleotide polymorphisms in coding regions of human genes. *Nat Genet* **22**(July):231–8.

24. Carlson, C.S., Newman, T.L., and Nickerson, D.A. (2001). SNPing in the human genome. *Curr Opin Chem Biol* **5**(1):78–85.

25. Kristensen, V., Kelefiotis, D., Kristensen, T., and Borresen-Dale, L. (2001). High-throughput methods for detection of genetic variation. *BioTechniques* **30**(February):318–32.

26. Marchuk, D. (1998). Laboratory Approaches Toward Gene Identification. In J. Hanes, M. Pericak-Vance (eds), *Approaches to Gene Mapping in Complex Human Diseases*. New York: Wiley-Liss, pp. 351–78.

27. *Ott, J. (1999). *Analysis of Human Genetic Linkage* (3rd ed.). Baltimore, MD: The Johns Hopkins University Press.
    A description of statistical methods of genetic linkage analysis in human families.

28. Morton, N. (1955). Sequential tests for the detection of linkage. *Am J Hum Gen* **7**:277–318.

29. Almasy, L. and Blangero, J. (1998). Multipoint quantitative-trait linkage analysis in general pedigrees. *Am J Hum Gen* **62**:1198–211.

30. *Weir, B. (1996). *Genetic Analysis II*. Sunderland, MA: Sinaur.
    A text highlighting concepts from population genetics and disease-gene mapping with a statistical emphasis.

31. *Khoury, M., Beaty, T., and Cohen, B. (1993). *Fundamentals of Genetic Epidemiology*. New York: Oxford University Press.
    A survey of epidemiologic methods specific to analysis of genetic data.

32. Falk, C. and Rubinstein, P. (1987). Haplotype relative risks: an easy reliable way to construct a proper control sample for risk calculations. *Ann Hum Genet* **51**:227–33.

33. Terwilliger, J. and Ott, J. (1992). A haplotype-based 'haplotype relative risk' approach to detecting allelic associations. *Hum Hered* **42**:337–46.

34. Spielman, R., McGinnis, R., and Ewens, W. (1993). Transmission test for linkage disequilibrium: The insulin gene region and insulin-dependent diabetes mellitus (IDDM). *Am J Hum Gen* **52**:506–16.

35. Spielman, R. and Ewens, W. (1998). A sibship test for linkage in the presence of association: The sib transmission/disequilibrium test. *Am J Hum Gen* **62**:450–8.

36. Horvath, S. and Laird, N. (1998). A discordant-sibship test for disequilibrium and linkage: no need for parental data. *Am J Hum Gen* **63**:1886–97.

37. Meulenbelt, I., Bijkerk, C., Breedveld, F.C., and Slagboom, P.E. (1997). Genetic linkage analysis of 14 candidate gene loci in a family with autosomal dominant OA without dysplasia. *J Med Genet* **34**(12):1024–7.

38. Roby, P., Eyre, S., Worthington, J., *et al.* (1999). Autosomal dominant (Beukes) premature degenerative osteoarthropathy of the hip joint maps to an 11-cM region on chromosome 4q35. *Am J Hum Genet* **64**(3):904–8.

39. *Loughlin, J. (2001). Genetic epidemiology of primary OA. *Curr Opin Rheumatol* **13**(2):111–6.
    A succinct review of OA genetic studies to date.

40. *Haines, J. and Pericak-Vance, M. (1998). Overview of mapping common and genetically complex human disease genes. In J. Haines and M. Pericak-Vance (eds), *Approaches to Gene Mapping in Complex Human Diseases*. New York: Wiley-Liss, pp. 1–16.
    A practical guide to medical genetics.

5 Pathology of osteoarthritis

Kenneth P.H. Pritzker

Given the challenge of understanding the pathology of OA, this chapter discusses first the natural history and general pathologic features of the disease, distinguishing OA from pure mechanical effects ('wear and tear') and from aging. Second, the salient histopathologic features of OA are described, with particular reference to pathogenesis and progression. Third, the pathologic characteristics of selected OA subsets and forms of degenerative arthritis that simulate some OA clinical features are discussed. The predilection or sparing of certain joints is considered, emphasizing features of OA peculiar to these joints.

A firm knowledge of the pathology is critically important for accurate clinical diagnosis and therapy of OA. While substantial progress has been made in recent years, many aspects that relate the descriptive pathology to the underlying biologic mechanisms remain elusive. Why has OA pathology been so difficult to characterize specifically? The short answer has four parts:

1. *Clinically, 'OA' means different things to different investigators.* The clinical definition of OA continues to evolve.[1] The widest definition embraces not only primary degenerative joint diseases, but also degenerative changes subsequent to joint inflammation.

2. *Definitions of the histopathologic features of OA have been imprecise.* Imprecision in defining OA histopathologic features can be ascribed, in part, to a lack of understanding of the natural history and, in part, to a lack of precision regarding histologic terminology. Recently, through the efforts of the OA Research Society International (OARSI) Working Group on Osteoarthritis Histopathology, a standard grading system for the pathology of OA has been proposed.[2] Throughout this chapter, we will endeavor to describe histologic features according to this emerging terminology. Accordingly, some terms differ from those employed in the corresponding chapter on OA Pathology that appeared in the first edition of this book.[3]

3. *'Early' changes are studied in late disease.* Few opportunities are available to study 'early OA' with histopathologic/biochemical techniques. Typically, early OA has been studied using tissues from less involved articular surfaces of patients undergoing joint replacement for advanced OA. Most OA animal models are single injury and repair models,[4] whereas cumulative, repetitive episodes of injury and repair are key features of human OA. Studies of the early changes in natural animal models of OA, such as non-human primates that develop spontaneous OA,[5] demonstrate that OA is a systemic joint disease that expresses itself in midlife, that disease activity becomes attenuated in old age, and that OA can be distinguished from the changes of aging.

4. *Human OA is often modified by medical treatment prior to assessment of the pathology.* The various medical treatments that are often employed before an opportunity for pathologic examination arises present a major challenge to precise clinical–pathologic correlation in OA.

Osteoarthritis: natural history and general pathology

OA can be considered as a group of joint diseases characterized by repetitive response to injury with subsequent regenerative, reparative, and degenerative structural changes in all tissues of the joint, including the articular cartilage, bone, synovium, capsule, and periarticular soft tissues.[4] Common to this group of diseases are non-reversible architectural and compositional tissue changes that *progress* toward the functional failure of the joint. As defined above, OA is characterized by ineffective reparative response to joint injury. This implies that OA is distinct from joint injury that results in complete tissue restitution and from changes that result from pure mechanical injury, primary synovial inflammation, or aging. As well, OA with its prominent regenerative and reparative activity contrasts with 'pure' degenerative arthritis, which is characterized by matrix degradation product accumulation and cell death. Table 5.1 illustrates selected differences among the features of OA, aging, material failure of joint tissues, and inflammatory arthritis.

'Pure' OA is seldom seen in human tissues. OA is found in aged joints. Features of the material failure of joint tissue can be seen in both OA and aging. Although mechanical trauma with material failure may lead to a reaction that proceeds to OA, OA is not merely joint aging or failure of the biomaterials of the joint. On the other hand, OA disease activity may be attenuated in the joints of aged individuals.

Mechanical trauma and OA

Formerly, OA was thought to be a disease of 'wear and tear,' in which mechanical forces physically degraded joint tissues, independent of a biologic response. Direct physical effects on joint tissues can be defined and include cartilage fibrillation, abrasion, and crack propagation (vertical fissures or clefts, horizontal splits). Although these mechanical injury effects can be seen in OA, most of the pathologic features of OA are a result of an inadequate and inappropriate *response* to injury of the affected tissues.

Aging and OA

OA is neither a disease of aging nor an inevitable consequence of aging of the joint.[6] Age changes within joint tissues are characterized by a yellow colour[7] and increased autofluorescence, related to accumulation of lipid pigment and advanced glycation endproducts, such as pentosidine.[8] Other age changes include soft tissue atrophy,[9] calcified cartilage atrophy, and focal amyloid deposition.[10] Where tissue diffusion is limited, as in articular cartilage, glycation endproducts, lipid pigment, and amyloid tend to accumulate in increased concentrations. Functionally, this results in decreased responsiveness of chondrocytes to IGF-1[11] and a decreased capacity for cell division and proteoglycan synthesis.[12] These effects account for the attenuation of regenerative and reparative responses when OA occurs with aging.

Table 5.1 OA: comparative histopathologic features

Feature	Reversible injury	OA	Inflammatory arthritis	Aging	Mechanical (loading to failure)
Cartilage mass	Hypertrophy	Hypertrophy, erosion	Resorption, atrophy	No change	No change
Cartilage topographic distribution	Focal	Focal, heterogenous	Joint margins and superficial zone most affected	General, all layers	Focal: at site of forces
Cartilage water	Edema	Edema	Dehydration	Dehydration	No change
Cartilage collagen	Reversible deformation	Pericellular degradation, interterritorial matrix degradation	Degradation maximal at joint margin and superficial zone	↑ Advanced glycation endproducts	Fiber fracture
Cartilage proteoglycan	PG depletion, reversible	PG depletion, not reversible	PG depletion not reversible	↓ PG synthesis	No change
Cartilage matrix degeneration products	Resorption	Accumulative, collagen, PG, etc.	Accumulative, collagen	Accumulative ■ Oxidation ■ Glycation ■ Amyloid	No change
Cell activity	↑ Cell activity, reversible	↑ Cell activity ↑ Cell proliferation	↑ Synovial cell activity ↓ Chondrocyte activity	↓ Chondrocyte activity	Chondrocyte death
Synovium	Mild focal superficial inflammation	Mild, focal superficial inflammation	Intense, general inflammation	Atrophy	Hemorrhage
Bone	No change	Subchondral remodeling	Subchondral resorption	Osteopenia	Microfracture

Histologic features characteristic of joint tissues

Four features characterize each joint tissue: stable cell populations; a high ratio of extracellular matrix to cells; a paucity or absence of blood vessels; and frequent, variable, mechanical stresses. First, each major joint tissue (cartilage, fibrocartilage, bone) is characterized by stable cell populations, such as chondrocytes or osteocytes, which are normally phenotypically monomorphic. With appropriate stimuli, these cell populations replicate and, through enzyme activity, remodel the composition of the surrounding extracellular matrix. These focal changes result in functionally differentiated cells and heterogeneous extracellular matrix domains.

Second, joint function reflects architectural and compositional properties of the extracellular matrix. The matrix is organized into domains, containing local volumes with similar composition. Matrix domains are characterized by the well-defined organization of solid fibers (principally collagen), amorphous solute (proteoglycans, non-collagenous proteins), and aqueous solvent containing ions, such as Ca^{++} and Mg^{++}. This matrix is produced and actively regulated by the cells, each of which regulates a matrix environment 10–30 times its own volume. The composition of the matrix lying furthest from the cell is less closely regulated than the matrix closer to the cell. Particularly in cartilage, this means that matrix degradation products at a distance from the cells are cleared slowly and may accumulate.

Third, articular cartilage is avascular. Other key joint tissues, such as the joint capsule and ligaments, are only poorly vascularized. With the exception of the synovium and bone marrow (which play minor roles in early OA), the reaction to injury (inflammatory response) is devoid of vascular congestion and exudation. In avascular tissues, such as cartilage, the reaction to injury has a defined sequence, involving extracellular edema, matrix degradation by enzymes secreted by endogenous cells, and cell death. This is followed by the resorption of the extracellular matrix, with the accumulation of cell debris and matrix degradation products. Subsequently, repair and regeneration occur, with cell replication and restoration of the organization of the extracellular matrix by the endogenous cells. Within each local tissue domain, the reaction to injury follows the same sequence for each injury episode. The intensity and extent of the reaction is shaped by preceding reactions and depends on the severity of the stimulus and the local composition of the matrix.

Fourth, as load-bearing tissues, joints are subject to repetitive stresses. From time to time, these stresses exceed the capacity of the tissues to effect complete restitution after injury. OA is a group of diseases that may result from the excessive loading of previously normal structures or, alternatively, from normal forces acting on structures that have been altered by systemic disease or previous incomplete repair.

Initially, the reaction to injury is concentrated in load-bearing avascular tissue, such as cartilage. Vascular reaction in OA is seen only adjacent to the site of primary injury, mainly in synovium, capsule, ligaments, and subchondral marrow. Furthermore, this vascular and inflammatory reaction is subdued in comparison with that in inflammatory arthritis.

General pathology

Edema and other features of early or mild non-progressive joint injury are common features of OA activity.[13] It is presumed that injury to a joint in which OA already exists, will invariably lead to a response with inadequate or inappropriate repair, thereby furthering the progression of OA.

OA occurs under three general pathologic conditions: first, OA can develop as a polyarticular disease, with the reaction of joint tissues to (as yet unknown) growth stimuli, mediated by insulin-like growth factor-1 (IGF-1)[11] and/or transforming growth factor-β (TGF-β).[14] Second, OA can develop as a result of other local or systemic disease. Mechanical injury is an example of a common local stimulus; acromegaly is an example of systemic disease. Third, OA can supervene on inflammatory arthritis of various etiologies. Post-inflammatory OA is distinct from other types of OA because inflammation inhibits regenerative and reparative changes in connective tissues.[14] In addition, the pain associated with inflammation inhibits mobility and excessive joint loading. Only after the inflammatory process becomes quiescent, can OA that is secondary to inflammation proceed.

Within each joint, the specific architectural structure has been pre-adapted to mechanical forces.[15] Furthermore, both collagen and chondrocytes have considerable capacity for reversible deformation under load. The normal response to injury results in connective tissue restitution without structural or functional change. OA begins with an inappropriate (exaggerated or inadequate) response to injury that results in non-reversible changes in tissue composition and loss of functional capacity.

Although many morphologic features of primary OA are present also in secondary OA, the following discussion focuses on the reactions of joint tissues in primary OA. The structural changes in earlier and active phases of OA, rather than the end-stage disease, will be emphasized.

The tissue morphology in OA reflects both the current disease activity and the progression of damage that has occurred within the joint over the interval between disease onset and time of sampling.[4,5,16] As joint tissues are affected by common, pathogenetic mechanisms at each stage, the various tissues within the OA joint will show common morphologic features adapted to the histology peculiar to each tissue. Moreover, because systemic factors may drive morphologic changes, similar morphologic features may be seen in different OA joints at the same stage of disease. Load-bearing areas exhibit predominantly degenerative changes, such as condensation of collagen, whereas evidence of regeneration, such as hypertrophy and increased proteoglycan production, is more prominent in adjacent, less heavily loaded areas.[17] As OA progresses, the heterogeneity of the extracellular matrix within the joint increases. This progressive increase in a maladaptive matrix composition further destabilizes the functional integrity of the articular tissue.

OA injury is focused initially, and most intensely, on those joint structures that are subjected to maximal mechanical load. The reaction to injury, although similar in sequence, varies topographically in amplitude and duration from joint to joint and from matrix domain to domain within each joint. Reaction to injury is characterized by edema, followed by destruction and resorption of tissues with the subsequent proliferative regeneration of endogenous cells. This results in hyperplasia, particularly of the chondrocytes in the articular cartilage, and remodeling of the extracellular matrix. This remodeling process results in hypertrophy and architectural distortion of the joint.

Histopathologic features of various tissues of the OA joint

OA involves pathologic changes in all articular and periarticular tissues. In some subsets of OA (e.g., due to ligament laxity) changes in periarticular tissues may precede those in cartilage and bone; in others, pathologic changes are focused first on the areas of the articular cartilage and subchondral bone subject to maximal mechanical stress. The reactions peculiar to each involved joint tissue are described below and summarized in Table 5.2.

Articular cartilage

Articular cartilage pathology in OA is complex. Because disease activity and stage may vary topographically, a brief understanding of normal cartilage structure and function is required prior to discussion of the pathology specific to OA.[18,19]

The articular surfaces of synovial joints are lined by hyaline cartilage. This cartilage consists of a firm, isotropic matrix containing, as major components, type II collagen fibers, aggrecan-type proteoglycans, ions, and water. Important minor components include specialized, structural, non-collagenous proteins and glycoproteins[20] (see chapter 7.2.1.1). Normal, mature articular cartilage is a white, firm, homogenous material that, on conventional histology, appears as an amorphous, extracellular substance interspersed with ovoid chondrocytes. Domains of the extracellular matrix are organized in layers parallel to the joint surface, extending from the joint space to the subchondral bone. In the uncalcified cartilage, the superficial, middle and deep zones vary in thickness, depending on the modality used for visualization. For example, magnetic resonance imaging (MRI) demonstrates a thicker superficial zone, seen histologically.

The superficial zone is relatively rich in collagen fibers organized parallel to the surface in a meshwork containing elongated, flattened chondrocytes.[21] The middle and deep zones consist of a matrix containing vertically aligned collagen fibers that separate chondrons, that is, structures that contain vertically aligned ovoid chondrocytes and pericellular matrix bounded by a discrete collagenous capsule.[21,22] Below the deep zone of the hyaline cartilage lies a layer of calcified cartilage, in which the chondrocytes are

Table 5.2 Pathologic features of OA

Tissue	Activity	Progression	
		Early	Advanced
Cartilage	• Matrix edema	• Fibrillation, superficial zone	• Fissures (clefts), midzone
	• Proteoglycan depletion	• Perichondronal collagen condensation	• Matrix delamination
	• Chondrocyte apoptosis, necrosis	• Chondrocyte proliferation	• Matrix erosion
	• Perichondrocyte proteoglycan		• Matrix fibrosis
	• Chondrocyte hypertrophy with intracellular proteoglycans		• Reparative fibrocartilage
	• Tidemark: active calcification	• Tidemark advancement	• Articular plate disruption
Bone	• Osteoblast/osteoclast activity	• Subchondral thickening	• Eburnated bone surface
	• Decreased mineralization, subchondral plate	• Capillary penetration through the subchondral plate	• Articular plate fractures
			• Corrugated bone surface
			• Osteonecrosis
			• Osteophyte formation
			• Subchondral marrow fibrosis
			• Subchondral cyst formation
Synovium	• Edema	• Lining cell hyperplasia	• Subintimal and perivascular fibrosis
	• Vascular congestion	• Increased collagen at surface	• Fragments of necrotic cartilage and bone
	• Infiltration by occasional lymphocytes and plasma cells	• Focal lymphoid follicles	

embedded in a matrix composed predominantly of calcium apatite crystals.[23] The 'tidemark' is a thin, distinct boundary layer of enhanced calcification lying between the uncalcified and calcified cartilage matrix. The calcified cartilage serves as an intermediate tissue between the hyaline cartilage and bone, whose properties alleviate shear stresses on the bony subchondral plate. Undulation of the tidemark, which develops in OA, serves to further attenuate the shear stresses by converting them to tensile and compressive stresses.

In all the zones of the uncalcified cartilage, water is the dominant matrix component. Water volume and distribution are closely regulated by the arrangement and concentration of the proteoglycan components that, in turn, are regulated by the chondrocytes. The first morphologically recognizable change in OA is edema of the superficial and middle zones of the extracellular matrix.[13,24] Edema expands the cartilage matrix, stretching and thinning the fibrous meshwork of the superficial zone.[21] As a result, the cartilage becomes softer and, therefore, more susceptible to mechanical injury. In conditions such as chondromalacia patella, matrix edema is the dominant feature[25] and can be sufficiently prominent so as to appear as a mucinous cyst within the cartilage. Cartilage edema results from the degradation of matrix proteoglycans, facilitated by the secretion of enzymes from adjacent chondrocytes. This degradation results in the depletion of matrix proteoglycans, decreasing the capacity of the matrix to bind or exclude water (see chapter 7.2.1.4).

If the adjacent chondrocytes survive, the above changes are fully reversible. In the presence of a hyperhydrated extracellular matrix, adjacent chondrocytes produce proteoglycans in excess, a cycle that permits the cartilage to absorb more water and to undergo hypertrophy. The action of physical forces on the softened cartilage and thinned superficial layer can result in matrix fibrillation (cracks in the superficial matrix layer) and matrix fragment delamination,[26] features that are traditionally considered to be typical pathologic characteristics of OA (Figs 5.1 and 5.2). Fibrillation begins almost parallel to the articular surface, reflecting the distribution of shear forces on the superficial collagen fibers. It is not known whether the superficial zone fibrillation is reversible. However, fibrillation itself appears to be non-progressive[12] and may not be associated with the loss of cartilage thickness or other progressive features of OA. Chondrocyte apoptosis (endogenously controlled selective chondrocyte death) in early OA occurs initially in the superficial zone, at the base of the fibrillation.[27] In contrast to necrosis, apoptosis appears to result not from direct mechanical trauma, but from chemical signals derived from matrix degradation products or from adjacent cells.

The plausible sequence for the initial progression of OA in cartilage is as follows: excess mechanical stress induces edema, with stretching and thinning of the superficial layer. Cartilage edema makes the perichondral collagen fibers more susceptible to deformation damage, resulting in increased apoptosis and necrosis of the vulnerable chondrocytes.[28] The resulting decrease in the chondrocyte population decreases the capacity of the tissue to secrete and maintain matrix proteoglycans, initiating a cycle that accelerates the susceptibility to injury. Progressive injury involves vertical crack propagation downward through the cartilage parallel to the radial collagen fibers, creating fissures (clefts). The cycle of reversible proteoglycan depletion, proteoglycan repletion, chondrocyte death, and irreversible proteoglycan depletion is repeated in the cartilage adjacent to the fissures.[29] With further progression, apoptosis is seen within the clustered chondrons.

Within the middle and deep zones of the hyaline cartilage, features of OA progression include chondron enlargement, chondrocyte proliferation (hyperplasia), chondrocyte hypertrophy, and chondrocyte activation. These regenerative features are similar to those seen in the hypertrophic zone of growth plate cartilage.

Triggered by cell and matrix degradation products initially released by mechanical forces, chondrocyte activation appears mediated by TGF-β and other cytokines elaborated by the chondrocytes and, to a lesser extent, by the synovial lining cells.[30,31] Chondrocyte up-regulation produces matrix-degrading proteinases, including metalloproteinases, aggrecanases, plasminogen activators and cathepsins,[31] as well as reactive oxygen species.[32]

As long as matrix degradation is limited to proteoglycan depletion, the cartilage lesion in OA is reversible.[33] In contrast, disruption of the superficial zone of the collagen network is a feature of disease progression. A further indicator of OA progression is perichondral collagen resorption, which occurs in both the superficial and middle zones[21] and decreases the mechanical integrity of the matrix, facilitating the enlargement of the chondron. The affected chondrocytes then become less resistant to mechanical stresses,[22] further amplifying the cycle of chondrocyte apoptosis and necrosis. This rapidly decreases the capacity of the adjacent matrix to maintain its proteoglycan composition. Extension of type II collagen fiber degradation to the midzone of the matrix, first seen in fibers that are oriented parallel to the surface,[21] disrupts the architecture of the cartilage and leads to further tissue breakdown. With extensive collagen disruption, condensation of collagen fibers around chondrons, cartilage delamination, and matrix erosion occur. Again, adjacent to these degenerative changes, reparative features are seen. MRI has confirmed the progressive heterogeneity of the cartilage matrix with OA progression.[16,17] Delaminated fragments of articular cartilage can persist as loose bodies within the joint space, where they can become in vivo cartilage explants that enlarge by chondrocyte proliferation and elaboration of concentric layers of the cartilaginous matrix.[34]

In the depths of the cartilage, the tidemark separating the calcified from the uncalcified zones may be duplicated or reduplicated as the calcified zone expands. Experimentally, advance of the calcified cartilage and tidemark duplication reflect the mechanical unloading of the affected area.[35] Focal active calcification of the tidemark is a further indicator of OA activity;[23] more diffuse calcification within the zone of calcified cartilage is a precursor to capillary invasion and subsequent remodeling of the subchondral bone, which are features of OA progression.[23] In contrast, resorption of subchondral bone and vascular invasion of the calcified layer are promoted by immobilization.[35] Capillaries invasion contributes to the increased remodeling of the cartilage by providing a direct route for the diffusion of systemic hormones and paracrine factors into the deepest layers of the cartilage (see Chapters 7.2.2.1 and 7.2.2.2).

The penetration of blood vessels through the subchondral bone and calcified cartilage provides sites for microfractures extending into the cartilage.[36] Fibroblast ingrowth occurs at these sites. These cells undergo cartilaginous metaplasia and elaborate a fibrous matrix containing type I collagen. Fibrocartilage is elaborated also in and above microfractures within the bony plate that comprises the articular surface at sites that have been denuded of cartilage. In comparison to hyaline cartilage, which contains isotropically oriented type II collagen, the reparative fibrocartilage contains less highly hydrated type I collagen[37] that is usually organized with thicker fibers that are oriented perpendicular to the surface. Although fibrocartilage provides a less adequate articular covering than normal hyaline cartilage, it can provide a functionally acceptable articular surface in the OA joint. Indeed, with joint motion, fibrocartilage can assume many of the characteristics of hyaline cartilage.[38]

Fibrocartilage (meniscus)

The knee, wrist and temporomandibular joints contain menisci composed of fibrochondrocytes embedded in a matrix containing circumferentially oriented type I collagen fibers.[39] Except at the margins, these structures are avascular. Loading injury may produce a vertical disruption of the collagen fiber bundles, with fissure formation and tears that are parallel to the fiber alignment. Loose bodies with fibrocartilage nidus may form. Menisci with tears and other traumatic degeneration can persist without degenerative changes in the OA adjacent cartilage. The response to injury in meniscus consists of focal fibrochondrocyte proliferation adjacent to the fissures, followed by the elaboration of proteoglycans and synthesis of types I and III collagen fibers.[40]

When the reparative process is arrested at the stage of proteoglycan production, cysts can develop.[40] Menisci are usually resistant to vascularization, but with advanced OA, vascularization occurs at the meniscal margins. Typically, the hyaline cartilage subjacent to the meniscus is protected from OA changes until meniscal damage is advanced.

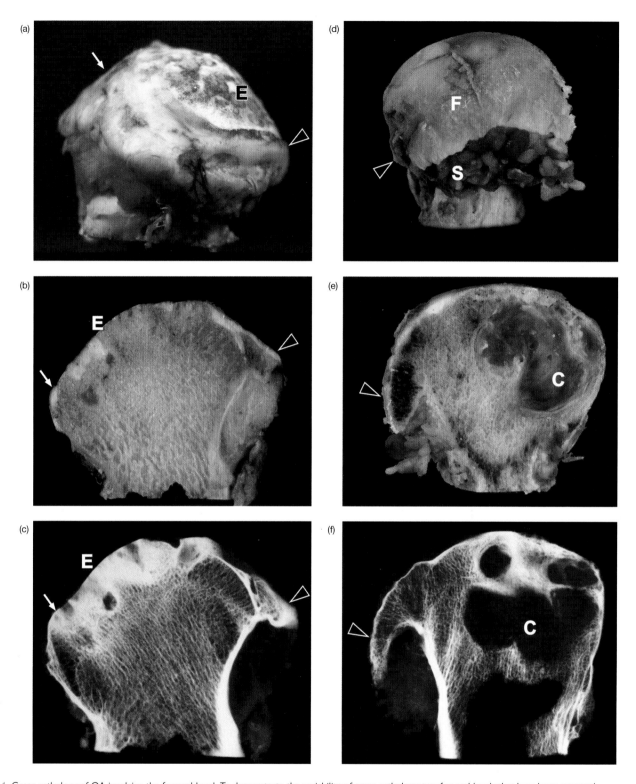

Fig. 5.1 Gross pathology of OA involving the femoral head. To demonstrate the variability of gross pathology, two femoral heads that have been removed surgically because of OA are illustrated. Both specimens show extensive remodeling. The femoral head is shown in a, b, and c with extensive eburnation of the surface and articular plate bone sclerosis: 1a, surface; 1b, cut surface; 1c, specimen X-ray of 1b. Prominent features of OA include: cartilage erosion, ➔; bone eburnation, E; osteophyte formation, ➤. The femoral head with a relative preservation of cartilage, extreme subchondral bone cyst formation, and extreme osteophyte formation is shown in d, e, and f: d, surface; e, cut surface; f, specimen X-ray of e. Prominent OA features include: cartilage fibrillation, F; synovial hypertrophy, S; osteophyte formation, ➤; cyst formation, C.

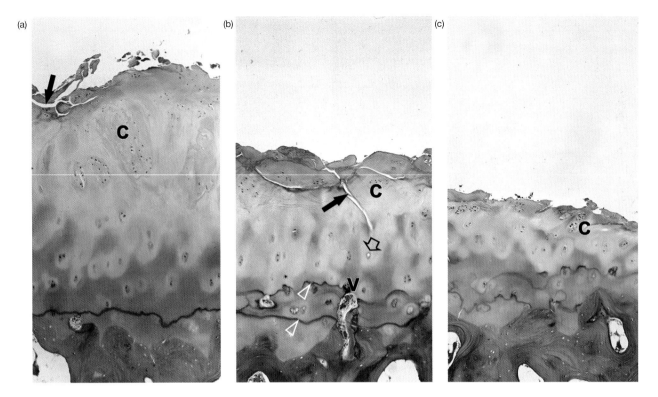

Fig. 5.2 Microscopic pathology of OA articular cartilage. The photomicrographs are taken from different areas of the same specimen: a, early OA; horizontal fibrillation, ➜; chondrocyte clusters, C. b, moderate OA, vertical fissure, ➜; chondrocyte death, ⇨; tidemark undulation and duplication, ➤; vascular penetration into cartilage, V; chondrocyte clusters, C. c, advanced OA, with cartilage erosion; cartilage matrix disorganization; and chondrocyte clusters, C. Hematoxylin and eosin stain, magnification ×40.

Bone

Stimulated by factors such as IGF-1, the subchondral bone in OA reacts to injury in a manner similar to articular cartilage.[41,42] Initially, activation of the osteoclast-osteoblast system results in bone resorption and incremental bone formation that is preferentially restricted to the subchondral plate. Subjacent to the areas of greatest stress, bone formation results in the thickening of the subchondral plate prior to cartilage ulceration (Fig. 5.3). However, the remodeled bone matrix is more hydrated and less dense than bone more distant from the joint surface.[41] Although this subchondral bone is less dense than normal, the overall increase in bone volume renders the articular plate stiffer than normal.[42] Later in the OA process, with extensive erosion or denudation of the cartilage surface, trabecular microfractures may also contribute to the stiffening of subchondral bone (see Chapter 7.2.2.1). With bone resorption, the capillaries penetrate through subchondral bone into the calcified articular cartilage. This can be accompanied by articular cartilage microfracture and resorption of cartilage adjacent to the advancing blood vessel.

Where the cartilage has been eroded completely, the bone surface becomes smooth and shining (burnished, eburnated). Eburnated bone can be observed even when the apposing articular surface is hyaline cartilage. The eburnated bone surface is maintained by subsurface osteocytes within the matrix in a manner analogous to, but less efficient than, that of chondrocytes in the superficial zone of the cartilage. With further progression, the osseous articular surface becomes corrugated with ridges and grooves that are aligned parallel to the plane of joint motion. When bone articulates against bone, both surfaces may exhibit complementary ridges and grooves.[43]

Remodeling of the subchondral plate in OA alters joint loading and results in adaptation by the subjacent bone. With increased stress, this can result in osteosclerosis; with decreased stress, bone resorption leads to

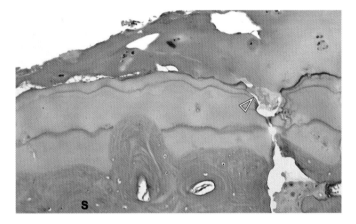

Fig. 5.3 The articular plate in advanced OA. The cartilage is eroded. The tidemark shows undulation and duplication. The subchondral bone, S, is thickened and a fracture through the subchondral bone and calcified cartilage is present, ➜. Hematoxylin and eosin stain, magnification ×100.

osteoporosis. Osteophytes are commonly observed at the margins of OA joints and, occasionally, more centrally, replacing the articular cartilage. It is not known whether osteophytes form in response to altered mechanical stress or as a result of an altered metabolic environment (Fig. 5.4).

Extensive remodeling involves the disruption of the articular plate by microfractures. Bone necrosis with extensive resorption, repair, and apposition of new bone on the subchondral trabecular bone is seen below the articular surface. Scintigraphy may reveal a generalized subarticular zone of

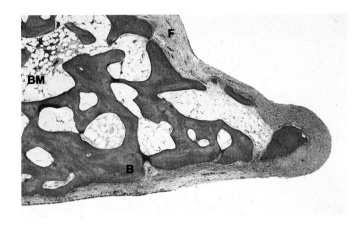

Fig. 5.4 An osteophyte at the articular margin: fibrocartilage, F; bone, B; hematopoietic bone marrow, BM. Hematoxylin and eosin stain, magnification ×2.5.

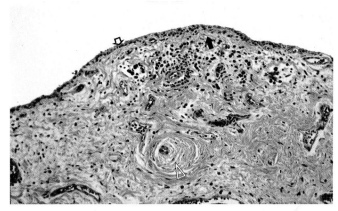

Fig. 5.5 OA synovium: synovial lining cells, ⇨; subintimal fibrosis, ➤; perivascular fibrosis, ➡; infiltrate of plasma cells and lymphocytes, P. Hematoxylin and eosin stain, magnification ×20.

increased uptake. These findings correlate with pain upon joint loading and, as expected, with the progression of OA.[44]

Bone cysts develop beneath the joint surfaces that have been remodeled so that the underlying tissue is subject to less stress than suggested by its anatomic position.[45] Although bone cysts are often called 'geodes',[45] this term is a misnomer because, unlike the geologic structures of the same name, OA cysts do not contain crystals. Bone cysts in OA arise from microfractures through the joint surface into the subjacent osteoporotic domains.

Synovium and synovial fluid

In humans, the synovium consists of a single, discontinuous, intimal layer comprised of macrophages (type A cells) and fibroblasts (type B cells), embedded in connective tissue containing thin collagen fibrils aligned parallel to the synovial surface. No diffusion barrier exists between the synovial space and the adjacent connective tissue.[46]

The early phases of OA are characterized by edema within the synovium. As the edema fluid is resorbed, the matrix proteoglycan content increases. Microvascular congestion and a slight inflammatory reaction are observed. With the progression of OA, the synovial lining becomes more continuous as the intimal cells proliferate and as macrophages migrate into the tissue.[46] Cytokines elaborated by injured chondrocytes appear to be the stimulus for synovial cell proliferation. In repetitive joint injury, the synovial lining cells secrete proteolytic enzymes and hyaluronan. In OA effusions, proteolytic enzymes secreted by the synovium act principally to digest cartilage matrix that has been sheared mechanically from the joint surface. Hyaluronan dampens the intensity of inflammation in the synovial space; facilitates the insudation of water, expanding the volume of synovial effusion; and facilitates the retention of macrophages within the joint. OA synovial effusions are transudates, characterized by high viscosity, a low albumin concentration, and a low cell count (<2000 cells/mm^3), most of which are mononuclear cells.

In established OA, the synovial inflammatory changes do not correlate with the extent or severity of the cartilage lesions.[47] These inflammatory reactions include synovial lining cell hyperplasia, with slight and focal synovial villus formation. Within the synovium, capillary vascular congestion, scattered lymphocytic infiltration, and occasional perivascular lymphoid aggregates are observed. Synovial inflammatory cell infiltrates in OA are a function of the disease activity, rather than disease duration.

In the subintimal synovium, the inflammatory reaction is focal and not as intense as that seen in rheumatoid arthritis (RA). In contrast to RA, however, in the OA synovial lining, the cell activity is insufficient to erode the articular cartilage at the joint margin or to disrupt the cartilage surface. In established OA, focal perivascular lymphoid follicles containing T lymphocytes, B lymphocytes and macrophages may be seen. In contrast to inflammatory arthritis, OA synovium shows relatively few neutrophils and relatively few plasma cells, and a lower level of immunoglobulin synthesis.[46] In advanced OA, circumferential perivascular fibrosis, a hallmark of previous perivascular inflammation, and lamellar collagen fiber deposition are seen in the subintimal synovium (Fig. 5.5).

With the erosion of the cartilage and exposure of a bony articular surface, the cartilage matrix fragments and necrotic bone become incorporated into the synovial membrane, particularly in the synovial recesses of the joint, where they may be surrounded by macrophages, including foreign body giant cells. When this material is abundant, a rapidly destructive arthritis with a neurogenic component must be considered.

Capsule, intra-articular ligaments, bursae

In the joint capsule and intra-articular ligaments, highly oriented type I collagen fiber bundles are arranged between elongated fibrocytes. In the capsule, the reaction to injury in OA is similar to that in synovium. It is characterized by edema and increases in the synthesis of proteoglycans and of collagen fibers that are oriented parallel to the plane of the synovial intima and deposited in a perivascular pattern. Vascular dilatation and congestion may be prominent. In both the capsule and synovial membrane, perineurial and endoneurial fibrosis are common and may be morphologic transducers of the chronic joint pain of OA.[48]

Persistence of a synovial effusion may expand the joint space and distort the architecture of the capsule. The ensuing fibrous reaction alters the capsule physiology making the joint space less compliant and creating a relative barrier to fluid diffusion. Enlargement of the synovial space and persistence of a joint effusion may result in the expansion of bursal structures communicating with the joint space. In advanced OA, these structures participate in the mild chronic synovitis.[47] Movement of the soft tissues over osteophytes can create additional bursae that may communicate with the joint space and participate in the synovial reaction.

Collagenase and other proteolytic enzymes are elaborated by the synovial lining cells and inflammatory cells ingesting fragments of cartilage and bone. This can induce edema and proliferative responses in the ligament and capsule in close proximity to synovium. Laxity of the capsule and ligaments develops as a result of repeated cycles of edema, pain, disuse, and inadequate fibrous repair, and renders the intra-articular ligaments more susceptible to mechanical injury which, in turn, alters the contact areas of the articular cartilage surfaces subjected to impact loading, further facilitating injury.

Extra-articular connective tissues and muscle

OA joints can be either relatively stiff or lax. In joints in which movement is limited by pain, the range of motion may ultimately become restricted by fibrosis of the joint capsule, tendons, and fascia. Joint laxity develops partly by the adaptation of these structures to repeated effusions and leads to mechanical instability. Unstable joints are subject to increased stresses on normally, relatively unloaded, articular surfaces, provoking additional joint injury (see Chapter 7.2.2.1). Pain in OA characteristically does not occur at the onset of loading, but after sustained loading activity, suggesting edema of entheses and other confined soft tissue sites as the basis for the pain.

The cycle of pain on movement, accompanied by connective tissue edema, leads to muscle dysfunction, with disuse atrophy, reflex inhibition of muscle contraction, and impaired proprioception (see Chapter 7.2.4.3). These effects are seen particularly in the knee and hip, where muscle plays a prominent role in stabilizing the joint and controlling the impact loading.[49]

OA: different features in different joints

While OA involves all of the tissues within a joint, many questions remain about the topographic distribution of OA lesions. Why does OA spare some joints? Why are some joints affected more than others? Can clinical subsets of OA be defined?

Joint sparing and involvement in OA

As the articular cartilage and bone are pre-adapted for normal joint loading, and because joint tissues are presumably all subject to common endocrine and metabolic stimuli, it is plausible that some joints are spared from developing OA by being protected from excessive impulse loading and compressive or shear stresses. For example, the ankle joint is much less likely to develop OA than the knee. Features that may serve to spare the ankle are those that promote mechanical stability and resist freedom of movement, including greater reliance on ligaments than upon muscle contraction for stability and a smaller surface area of synovium, in comparison with the knee.

Different histopathologic features in different OA joints

The varying prominence of OA changes in cartilage, bone, and synovium in different joints, clearly relates to the relative volumes of these tissues within the joint and the biomechanics specific to each joint. For example, in the knee, the relatively large area of synovium facilitates the development of joint effusions. Metacarpophalangeal and interphalangeal joints, in which the subchondral bone and cortical bone subjacent to the subchondral plate are predominant components, will exhibit more bone remodeling than the knee or hip, in which the ratio of cartilage to bone is high. In hand OA, advancement of the zone of calcified cartilage and osteophytosis have been shown to precede joint-space narrowing on the radiograph.[50] As these changes occur, remodeling of subchondral bone may predominate. In joints in which the muscle is required for joint stability, such as the knee, irregular, excessive impact loading results in prominent vertical fissures or horizontal splits in the cartilage. In patients in whom the articular cartilage and subchondral bone are subject to excessive systemic endocrine stimuli, deformation and remodeling will be seen concurrently in multiple joints.

OA subsets

Given our lack of understanding of the etiology and pathogenesis of OA, clinical subsets of OA are defined by the frequency and topographic distribution of changes in various joints.[51] Although OA restricted to the hip appears to be distinct, OA commonly affects both the large (knees) and small joints (hands).[51] As OA progresses, more joints become clinically involved. Knowledge of the comparative pathology in various OA subsets is extremely limited. For example, it is not known whether the pathologic features of OA restricted to the hip are comparable to those in patients who have concurrent hip and knee OA. If differences exist, are they related merely to the effect of knee OA on hip pathology? Are there features, for example, subchondral bone remodeling, that are common to both sites in early OA? If so, what mechanisms are common to the pathogenesis of these features?

Degenerative arthritis with features similar to those of OA

For practical purposes, degenerative arthritis can be defined as arthritis in which the accumulation of matrix products and cell death predominate, and hyperplastic, regenerative tissue responses are muted. A discussion of joint pathology in the various forms of secondary OA is beyond the scope of this chapter. Rather, we will focus on three pathologic conditions that arise frequently in the differential diagnosis of primary idiopathic OA: crystal deposition, osteonecrosis, and rapidly destructive arthropathy, in all of which the pathological changes are chiefly degenerative, with no, or very limited, evidence of regeneration or repair. It is this lack of repair activity that differentiates degenerative arthritis from OA: in both primary OA and secondary OA (i.e., OA developing subsequent to another rheumatic disease, such as RA or septic arthritis) features of regeneration and repair, as well as features of degeneration, are apparent.

Crystals and OA

The relationship of crystal deposition to OA is controversial[52] (see Chapter 7.2.1.6). In gout, in which monosodium urate crystals are deposited on the cartilage surfaces, OA changes proceed either coincidentally or secondarily, as a consequence of repeated episodes of acute gout. In pseudogout or calcium pyrophosphate dihydrate (CPPD) crystal arthropathy, crystals form within the matrix of the hyaline cartilage and fibrocartilage.[53] CPPD crystals can deposit in cartilage in which the key metabolic features of active OA are absent.[54] The presence of crystals within the joint space can incite acute inflammation, with consequent damage to joint structures. Unlike RA, however, crystal-associated inflammation is rarely persistent.

OA and CPPD crystal arthropathy are both common. Therefore, when OA and CPPD crystal arthropathy exist concurrently, OA may have preceded crystal deposition or, as in gout, OA may have arisen as a consequence of matrix damage caused by crystal deposition. It is also possible that crystal deposition and changes of OA may be present in different tissues within the same joint; CPPD deposition is more common in the menisci than in the articular cartilage of patients with OA.

The role of calcium apatite crystals in OA is also in dispute.[55] Apatite crystals, derived from necrotic bone, may be present in the synovial fluid from patients with OA. Crystal deposition within the synovium or cartilage may alter tissue biomechanics and stimulate joint remodeling.

Osteonecrosis and OA

The role of osteonecrosis in the development of OA is also controversial.[56,57] In osteonecrosis due to the disruption of the blood supply to the subchondral bone, the articular cartilage remains intact above a zone of necrotic bone and marrow. Repair begins at the interface between the necrotic and viable bones and proceeds with progressive new bone formation and ingrowth of blood vessels toward the surface. When resorption of bone reaches the subchondral plate, the plate fails, disrupting the articular surface and distorting the joint architecture. The histologic features of primary osteonecrosis with secondary degenerative arthritis can be readily distinguished from those of primary OA with osteonecrosis. In primary osteonecrosis, the articular cartilage shows little or no regenerative features, and the necrotic zone extends as a wedge or cone deep into bone. In primary OA, the articular cartilage shows chondrocyte replication and matrix edema; the osteonecrosis is restricted to the superficial bone, immediately under areas of previous cartilage erosion.

Patients with established OA tend to exhibit lipid abnormalities and hypercoagualability.[57] In advanced primary OA, osteonecrosis can involve the eburnated surface and subjacent bone.[58] This lesion is associated with venous thrombosis, thought to be mediated by the hypercoaguability, hyperfibrinolysis and up-regulation of the plasminogen activator system in osteoclasts and synovial cells.[57] Microthrombi in the capillaries of the subchondral bone may contribute to local ischemia and, consequently, to fracture and focal necrosis of subchondral bone. In comparison with primary osteonecrosis, osteonecrosis seen in the late stages of OA is more limited in extent.[58]

Although population studies show discordance between OA and osteoporosis, degenerative arthritis can supervene on osteoporosis. In the knee, this is recognized as spontaneous osteonecrosis and results from microfractures through osteoporotic bone subjacent to the subchondral plate.[59] In these cases, a sharply circumscribed defect is seen in the articular cartilage and subjacent bone. Failure of repair can lead to degenerative arthritis, which is often more severe in the apposing articular surface.[59] A similar condition in the femoral head was recently characterized as subchondral insufficiency fracture.[60] Like the spontaneous osteonecrosis of the knee, the clinical onset tends to be sudden, without a pre-existing history of arthritis. This condition usually remains stable or is only slowly progressive. Osteonecrosis secondary to fracture of the subchondral plate can be identified by MRI.[61]

Rapidly destructive arthropathy

This rare condition predominantly affects the femoral head and is characterized by very rapid progression, with an interval of only months between onset and extensive joint destruction. Without known preconditions, such as a neuropathic joint, this disease can simulate OA in its initial clinical presentation.[62] Histologically, it is characterized by extensive subchondral bone resorption, far in excess of normal remodeling. This leads to the collapse of the subchondral plate, with secondary necrosis. The stimulus for the resorption of subchondral bone is not known. Hyperparathyroidism has not been implicated.

Conclusion: the future of OA pathology

The study of OA pathology is emerging from the static terrain of morphologic description into a dynamic universe in which histologic lesions are linked to experimentally demonstrated pathophysiology. Increasingly, OA can be confidently separated from other disease processes leading to degenerative arthritis. With the standardization of grading and staging, pathologic examination can be employed to evaluate past treatment or to guide future therapy. As disease-modifying drugs for OA (DMOADs) become available, it will be highly desirable to define structural biomarkers that reflect OA activity and progression and can be quantitated against the potential therapeutic benefit. Development of such markers awaits the development of cost-effective and less invasive methods of sampling joint tissues, more precise understanding of the changes in cartilage, bone and synovial cell populations in OA, and better knowledge of how the composition of the extracellular matrix of articular cartilage, in particular, evolves with disease progression.

Key points

1. OA pathology affects all tissues of the diarthrodial joint, not only the cartilage and bone.

2. OA pathology results from the repeated failure of the tissues to respond adequately to injury.

3. OA pathology is affected by systemic factors, for example, the endocrine status of the patient, as well as by local factors, for example, joint laxity.

4. OA pathology can be grouped into features of OA activity (evidence of the response to injury) and features of OA progression (the residual state of the tissue after the failure of adequate repair and regeneration).

5. Pathologic features that are occasionally associated with OA, such as crystal deposition, should be distinguished from OA-specific pathology.

Acknowledgements

We thank Ms. Theresa Pirogowicz for preparation of the manuscript and Mr. Ken Meats, Image Centre, Mount Sinai Hospital, for assisting in the preparation of the figures.

References

(An asterisk denotes recommended reading.)

1. Hochberg, M.C. (1996). Editorial: Development and progression of osteoarthritis. *J Rheumatol* **23**:1497–9.

2. Pritzker, K.P.H., Ostergaard, K., and Salter, D.M. (2000). Towards standardization of osteoarthritis histopathology: terminology, topology and technology. *Osteoarthritis Cart* **8**(Suppl B):IP010.

3. Pritzker, K.P.H. (1998). Pathology of osteoarthritis. In Brandt, K.D., Doherty, M., and Lohmander, L.S. (eds), *Osteoarthritis*. Oxford: Oxford University Press, pp. 50–61.

4. Pritzker, K.P.H. (1994). Animal models for osteoarthritis: processes, problems and prospects. *Ann Rheum Dis* **53**:406–20.

5. Pritzker, K.P.H. (1992). Cartilage histopathology in human and rhesus macaque osteoarthritis. In K.E. Kuettner (ed.), *Articular Cartilage and Osteoarthritis*. New York: Raven Press, pp. 473–85.

6. Kiss, I., Morocz, I., and Herczeg, L. (1984). Localization and frequency of degenerative changes in the knee joint: evaluation of 200 necropsies. *Acta Morphol Hung* **32**:155–63.

7. Van Der Korst, J.K., Sokoloff, L., and Miller, E.J. (1968). Senescent pigmentation of cartilage and degenerative joint disease. *Arch Pathol* **86**:40–7.

8. DeGroot, J., Verzijl, N., Bank, R.A., Lafeber, F.P., Bijlsma, J.W., and Tekoppele, J.M. (1999). Age-related decrease in proteoglycan synthesis of human articular chondrocytes: the role of nonenzymatic glycation. *Arth Rheum* **42**:1003–9.

9. Goffin, Y. and De Doncker, E. (1980). Alterations histologique et histochimique de la capsule articulaire dans l'arthrose et chez les sujets seniles. *Rev Rhum* **47**(1):15–20.

10. Egan, M.S., Goldenberg, D.L., Cohen, A.S., and Segal, D. (1982). The association of amyloid deposits and osteoarthritis. *Arthritis Rheum* **25**:204–8.

11. Loeser, R.F., Shanker, G., Carlson, C.S., Gardin, J.F., Shelton, B.J., and Sonntag, W.E. (2000). Reduction in the chondrocyte response to insulin-like growth factor 1 in aging and osteoarthritis: studies in a non-human primate model of naturally occurring disease. *Arthritis Rheum* **43**:2110–20.

12. van Valburg, A.A., Wenting, M.J.G., Beekman, B., Te Koppele, J.M., Lafeber, F.P.J.G., and Bijlsma, J.W.J. (1997). Degenerated human articular cartilage at autopsy represents preclinical osteoarthritic cartilage: comparison with clinically defined osteoarthritic cartilage. *J Rheumatol* **24**:358–64.

13. Boegard, T.L., Rudling, O., Petersson, I.F., and Jonsson, K. (2001). Magnetic resonance imaging of the knee in chronic knee pain. A 2-year follow-up. *Osteoarthritis Cart* **9**:473–80.

14. *Goldring, M.B. (2001). The role of the chondrocyte in osteoarthritis. *Arthritis Rheum* **43**:1916–6.
    This article describes the functional activities of chondrocytes, with emphasis on the role of cytokines and paracrine factors.

15. Eckstein, F., Reiser, M., Englmeier, K.H., and Putz, R. (2001). *In vivo* morphometry and functional analysis of human articular cartilage with quantitative magnetic resonance imaging–from image to data, from data to theory. *Anat Embryol* **203**:147–73.

16. Gahunia, H.K., Babyn, P., Lemaire, C., Kessler, M.J., and Pritzker, K.P.H. (1995). Osteoarthritis staging: comparison between magnetic resonance imaging, gross pathology and histopathology in the rhesus macaque. *Osteoarthritis Cart* **3**:169–80.

17. Gahunia, H.K., Lemaire, C., Babyn, P.S., Cross, A.R., Kessler, M.J., and Pritzker, K.P.H. (1995). Osteoarthritis in rhesus macaque knee

joint: quantitative magnetic resonance imaging tissue characterization of articular cartilage. *J Rheumatol* **22**:1747–56.

18. *Gardner, D.L. (1992). *Pathological Basis of the Connective Tissue Diseases*. Philadelphia: Lea & Febiger, pp. 842–943.
    This is a detailed outline of the histologic structure of cartilage.

19. *Ostergaard, K. and Salter, D.M. (1998). Immunohistochemistry in the study of normal and osteoarthritic articular cartilage. *Prog Histochemistry Cytochemistry* **33**:93–168.
    This article provides a comprehensive review of the histochemical characterization of cartilage matrix components in OA.

20. Neame, P.J., Tapp, H., and Azizan, A. (1999). Noncollagenous, nonproteoglycan macromolecules of cartilage. *Cell Mol Life Sci* **55**:1327–40.

21. Hwang, W.S., Li, B., Jin, L.H., Ngo, K., Schachar, N.S., and Hughes, G.N.F. (1992). Collagen fibril structure of normal aging, and osteoarthritic cartilage. *J Pathol* **167**:425–33.

22. Poole, C.A. (1997). Articular cartilage chondrons: form, function and failure. *J Anat* **191**:1–13.

23. Revell, P.A., Pirie, C., Amir, G., Rashad, S., and Walker, F. (1990). Metabolic activity in the calcified zone of cartilage: observations on tetracycline labeled articular cartilage in human osteoarthritic hips. *Rheumatol Int* **10**:143–7.

24. *Gardner, D.L., Salter, D.M., and Oates, K. (1997). Advances in the microscopy of osteoarthritis. *Microscopy Res Tech* **37**:245–70.
    This is an extended review of the application of microscopic techniques to the study of OA.

25. Ohno, O., Naito, J., Iguchi, T., Ishikawa, H., Hirohata, K., and Cooke, T.D.V. (1988). An electron microscopic study of early pathology in chondromalcia of the patella. *J Bone Joint Surg* **70**(A):883–99.

26. Bartel, D.L., Bicknell, V.L., Ithaca, M.S., and Wright, T.M. (1986). The effect of conformity. Thickness and material on stresses in ultra-high molecular weight components for total joint replacement. *J Bone Joint Surg* **68**(A):1041–51.

27. Blanco, F.J., Guitian, R., Vazquez-Martul, E., de Toro, F.J., and Galdo, F. (1998). Osteoarthritis chondrocytes die by apoptosis. A possible pathway for osteoarthritis pathology. *Arthritis Rheum* **41**:284–9.

28. Hashimoto, S., Ochs, R.L., Komiya, S., and Lotz, M. (1998). Linkage of chondrocyte apoptosis and cartilage degradation in human osteoarthritis. *Arthritis Rheum* **41**:1632–8.

29. Kim, H.A., Lee, Y.J., Seong, S.C., Choe, K.W., and Song, Y.W. (2000). Apoptotic chondrocyte death in human osteoarthritis. *J Rheumatol* **27**:455–62.

30. Von den Hoff, H.W., de Koning, M.H.M.T, van Kampen, G.P.J., and van der Korst, J. (1994). Transforming growth factor-B stimulates retinoic acid-induced proteoglycan depletion in intact articular cartilage. *Arch Biochem Biophys* **313**:241–7.

31. Goldring, M.B. (1999). The role of cytokines as inflammatory mediators in osteoarthritis: lessons from animal models. *Connect Tissue Res* **40**:1–11.

32. Flugge, L.A., Miller-Deist, L.A., and Petillo, P.A. (1999). Towards a molecular understanding of arthritis. *Chem Biol* **6**:R157–R166.

33. Paul, P.K., O'Byrne, E., Blancuzzi, V., Wilson, D., Gunson, D., Douglas, F.L., Wang, J.Z., and Mezrich, R.S. (1991). Magnetic resonance imaging reflects cartilage proteoglycan degradation in the rabbit knee. *Skeletal Radiol* **20**:31–6.

34. Barrie, H.J. (1978). Intra-articular loose bodies regarded as organ cultures *in vivo*. *J Pathol* **125**:163–9.

35. O'Connor, K.M. (1997). Unweighting accelerates tidemark advancement in articular cartilage at the knee joint of rats. *J Bone Miner Res* **12**:580–9.

36. Sokoloff, L. (1993). Microcracks in the calcified layer of articular cartilage. *Arch Pathol Lab Med* **117**:191–5.

37. Grynpas, M.D., Eyre, D.R., and Kirschner, D.A. (1980). Collagen type II differs from type I in native molecular packing. *Biochim Biophys Acta* **626**:346–55.

38. Kim, H.K., Moran, M.E., and Salter, R.W. (1991). The potential for regeneration of articular cartilage in defects created by chondral shaving and subchondral abrasion. *J Bone Joint Surg* **73**(A):1301–15.

39. Messner, K. and Gao, J. (1998). The menisci of the knee joint. Anatomical and functional characteristics, and a rationale for clinical treatment. *J Anat* **193**:161–78.

40. Ferrer-Roca, O. and Vilalta, C. (1980). Lesions of the meniscus. Part II: Horizontal cleavages and lateral cysts. *Clin Orth Rel Res* **146**:301–7.

41. Grynpas, M.D., Alpert, I., Katz, I., Lieberman, I., and Pritzker, K.P.H. (1991). Subchondral bone in osteoarthritis. *Calcif Tissue Int* **49**:20–6.

42. Burr, D.B. and Schaffler, M.B. (1997). The involvement of subchondral mineralized tissues in osteoarthritis: quantitative microscopic evidence. *Microscopy Res Tech* **37**:343–57.

43. Rogers, J.M. and Dieppe, P.A. (1993). Ridges and grooves on the bony surfaces of osteoarthritic joints. *Osteoarthritis Cart* **1**:167–70.

44. McCrae, F., Shouls, J., Dieppe, P., and Watt, I. (1992). Scintigraphic assessment of osteoarthritis of the knee joint. *Ann Rheum Dis* **51**:938–42.

45. Bullough, P.G. and Bansal, M. (1988). The differential diagnosis of geodes. *Radiol Clinics NA* **26**:1165–84.

46. Revell, P.A., Mayston, V., Lalor, P., and Mapp, P. (1988). The synovial membrane in osteoarthritis: a histological study including the characterisation of the cellular infiltrate present in inflammatory osteoarthritis using monoclonal antibodies. *Ann Rheum Dis* **47**:300–7.

47. Myers, S.L., Brandt, K.D., Ehlich, J.W., Braunstein, E.M., Shelbourne, K.D., Heck, D.A., and Kalasinski, L.A. (1990). Synovial inflammation in patients with early osteoarthritis of the knee. *J Rheumatol* **17**:1662–9.

48. Rabinowicz, T. and Jacqueline, F. (1990). Pathology of the capsular and synovial hip nerves in chronic hip diseases. *Path Res Pract* **186**:283–92.

49. Hurley, M.V. (1999). The role of muscle weakness in the pathogenesis of osteoarthritis. *Rheum Dis Clin NA* **25**:283–98, vi.

50. Patel, N., Buckland-Wright, C. (1999). Advancement in the zone of calcified cartilage in osteoarthritic hands of patients detected by high definition macroradiography. *Osteoarthritis Cart* **7**:520–5.

51. Felson, D.T. and Zhang, Y. (1998). Review: An update on the epidemiology of knee and hip osteoarthritis with a view to prevention. *Arthritis Rheum* **41**:1343–55.

52. Dieppe, P. and Watt, I. (1985). Crystal deposition in osteoarthritis: an opportunistic event? *Clin Rheum Dis* **11**:367–92.

53. Pritzker, K.P.H., Cheng, P-T., and Renlund, R.C. (1988). Calcium pyrophosphate crystal deposition in hyaline cartilage: ultrastructural analysis and implications for pathogenesis. *J Rheumat* **15**:828–35.

54. Cheng, P-T. and Pritzker, K.P.H. (1983). Pyrophosphate, phosphate ion interaction: effects on calcium pyrophosphate and calcium hydroxyapatite crystal formation in aqueous solutions. *J Rheumat* **10**:769–77.

55. Dieppe, P.A. (1991). Inflammation in osteoarthritis and the role of microcrystals. *Arthritis Rheum* **11**:121–2.

56. Pritzker, K.P.H. (1993). Intra-osseous thrombosis in osteoarthritis: association or causation? *Osteoarthritis Cart* **1**:207–8.

57. Cheras, P.A., Whitaker, A.N., Blackwell, E.A., Sinton, T.J., Chapman, M.D., and Peacock, K.A. (1997). Hypercoagulability and hypofibrinolysis in primary osteoarthritis. *Clin Orth Rel Res* **334**:57–67.

58. Yamamoto, T., Yamaguchi, T., Lee, K.B., and Bullough, P.G. (2000). A clinicopathologic study of osteonecrosis in the osteoarthritic hip. *Osteoarthritis Cart* **8**:303–8.

59. Houpt, J.B., Pritzker, K.P.H, Alpert, B., Greyson, M.D., and Gross, A.E. (1983). Osteonecrosis of the knee—a review. *Sem Arthritis Rheum* **13**:212–27.

60. Yamamoto, T., Bullough, P.G. (1999). Subchondral insufficiency fracture of the femoral head: a differential diagnosis in acute onset of coxarthrosis in the elderly. *Arthritis Rheum* **42**:2719–23.

61. Plenk Jr., H., Gstettner, M., Grossschmidt, K., Breitenseher, M., Urban, M., and Hofmann, S. (2001). Magnetic resonance imaging and histology of repair in femoral head osteonecrosis. *Clin Orthop* **386**:42–53.

62. Mitrovic, D.R. and Riera, H. (1992). Synovial, articular cartilage and bone changes in rapidly destructive arthropathy (osteoarthritis) of the hip. *Rheumatol Int* **12**:17–22.

6 Paleopathology of osteoarthritis

Juliet Rogers and Paul Dieppe

Paleopathology is a term first used by Schufeldt[1] and subsequently popularised by Sir Marc Armand Ruffer[2] at the beginning of the twentieth century as 'the study of disease in the past'. Ruffer was a pathologist in Cairo whose interest was aroused by the study of the extensive collection of mummies and other human remains, which were being discovered with great frequency at this period. Paleopathological evidence is, of course, not restricted to the study of mummified human remains although, because of soft tissue preservation, they are ideal. Paintings, drawings, sculpture, literature, and early medical texts can all be used as evidence for the presence and identification of early disease. The most widespread, common, and direct type of evidence however, particularly for disorders that affect the skeleton, is that derived from the study of human skeletal remains from archaeological sites. Apart from the interest in the occurrence of particular diseases at different time periods, paleopathology can provide invaluable evidence for the frequency, distribution, and variation of expression of individual pathologies through time.[3]

From the earliest organized studies of human skeletal remains, it has been evident that joint disease is the most frequent type of postcranial pathology to be seen. Despite diagnostic confusion and variation in terminology, what is now recognized as OA is, by far, the most common form of these joint diseases: it is reported in hominid fossils,[4] from Neolithic sites,[5] and from Egyptian mummies.[6] The presence of OA is ubiquitous in all the other skeletal sites from earliest times to the postmedieval period,[7] in the UK, Europe,[8] the United States of America,[9] and other areas of the world.[10]

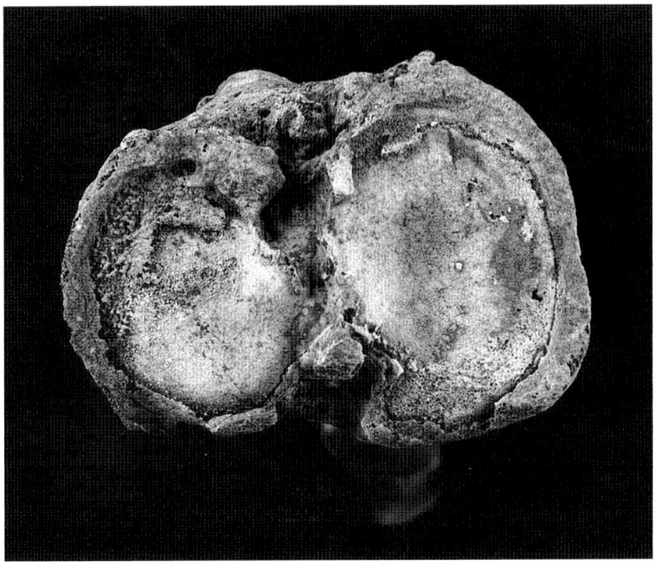

Recognition of OA

OA is customarily recognized in skeletal material by a combination of morphological changes. As in other paleopathological conditions these are generally very easy to see, although postmortem damage may mask some changes. The advantage of skeletal material over clinical observation is the opportunity for direct viewing of every joint in the body from every angle. This allows the recording of OA in unreported or underreported situations and of skeletal changes that are not apparent clinically or radiographically. Conversely, there is the disadvantage that all joints may not be present in every skeleton, thus reducing the quantity and completeness of information for analysis.

The most frequent change is the presence of a rim of osteophyte at the margin of the joint surfaces. Osteophytes are also frequently observed along the upper or lower margins of the vertebral bodies. Around the articular margins, the osteophyte may take the form of a thin sharp rim, a flat ribbon, or a large florid and irregular fringe of bone (Fig. 6.1). They may circle the entire joint margin or only a part. The joint surface itself may exhibit several different abnormalities, either alone or in combination. There may be small areas of new bone formation, one to two centimetres in diameter, in the form of 'buttons' or 'pancakes' of osteophyte on the articular surface itself (Fig. 6.2). Frequently there are areas of pitting, with the openings occasionally visibly connecting with subchondral cysts (Fig. 6.3). The pits can also be very small in diameter and they may be widely spaced or crowded together. The alteration of the shape or contour of the affected bones may

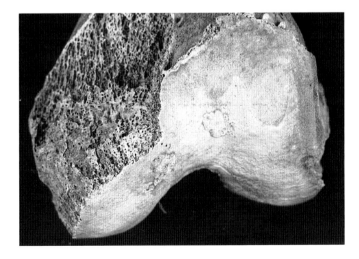

Fig. 6.1 The tibial plateau of a knee joint with prolific osteophyte around the entire joint margin.

Fig. 6.2 The anterior surface of a distal femoral condyle. There is extensive postmortem damage to the medial condyle but it is still possible to see surface osteophyte both on the medial condyle and the patello-femoral joint.

also be seen and can now be measured.[11] The most striking abnormalities, however, are the clearly delineated areas of eburnation or polishing of the joint surface (Fig. 6.4). On some joints the eburnated areas are grooved or scored[12] (Fig. 6.5). This polishing is, presumably caused by the total

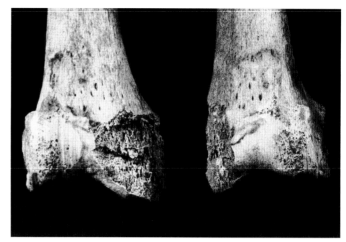

Fig. 6.5 Patello-femoral joints in medieval knees, from the site at Barton-on-Humber. Despite postmortem damage, the grooves can clearly be seen on the eburnated lateral facet of the PF joint.

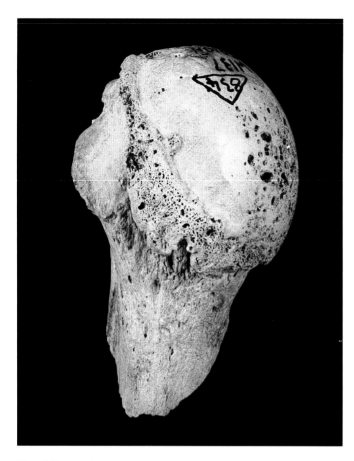

Fig. 6.3 Humeral head with marginal osteophyte, eburnation and, pitting of the articular surface. In this example the pits are restricted to the eburnated area.

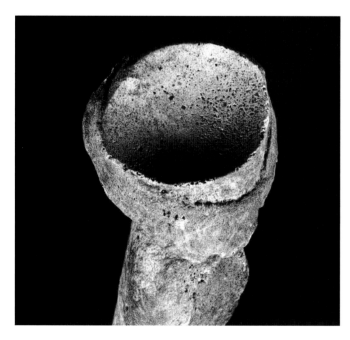

Fig. 6.4 Proximal radial joint with marked bony contour change and eburnation.

degradation of the cartilage, and the friction of the two opposing bone surfaces rubbing together. It is an unequivocal marker of the presence of OA.

Disease definition and assessment

There are, then, several different morphological changes that may be indicative of OA. The relationship between them is often assumed to be linear, as in the radiological stages developed by Kellgren and Lawrence.[13] In this model, osteophyte on its own is scored as being the mildest and earliest sign of OA, developing to the most severe and latest stage marked by the presence of eburnation with grooves. However, osteophytes are an extremely common phenomenon and there is clinical evidence to suggest that they may be a marker of activity or age, rather than OA.[14] Particularly in skeletal material they are easily seen by the direct observation of joints. If, therefore, a positive score for OA is recorded whenever osteophyte is present on its own, OA will be reported with an unexpectedly and erroneously high frequency in many joints. In many reports considering OA in skeletal populations it is not always clear which diagnostic criteria have been used to score OA as present or absent. Furthermore, a study on the interobserver variation in coding OA in skeletal material[15] found that frequently there was incomplete agreement as to whether particular pathological changes were present, and only half the observers agreed on the severity of the changes. It is the case that many different scoring systems can and have been used.[16] These often bear no relationship to the clinical scoring systems, which can add to the confusion and may impair the comparison of skeletal data both between archaeological populations and with clinical data.

Examination of the relationship between visual, radiographic, and pathological changes can be used to help standardize the diagnostic criteria for OA in a paleopathological context. Inspection of a series of cadaveric knees with OA, demonstrates that the region of cartilage degradation has a sharply delineated margin enclosing an area of eburnation. Because of this good correlation between eburnation and cartilage degradation, the presence of eburnation is taken as a pathognomic sign of the presence of OA. Osteophyte is more problematic, as outlined above. The relationship of pitting and bony contour change to the soft tissue pathology and how this relates in dry bone to the X-ray changes is also unclear. So again it is seen that the presence of osteophytes, pitting, or contour change on their own should not be used as a marker for OA. Only if two of the group (pitting of joint surface, osteophyte, bony contour change) are present together[17] should OA be considered as present.

There are, of course, many other bony changes that can be recognized in joints, such as erosion, periosteal reactions, and fractures. Some of these,

(a)

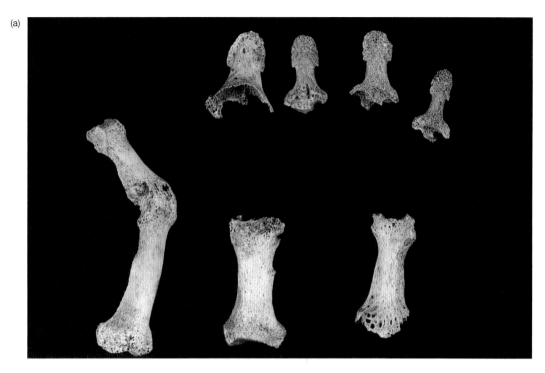

(b)

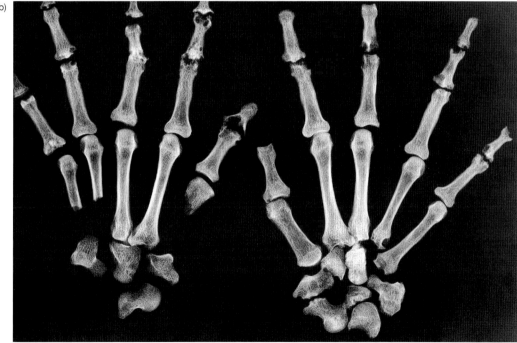

Fig. 6.6 (a) Selected medial and distal phalanges of a skeleton, showing areas of erosion and fusion of one proximal and medial phalanx. (b) X-ray of hand bones from the same skeleton: a possible diagnosis of erosive OA was made for this specimen.

such as erosions, may be due to other forms of arthropathy, which may give rise to secondary OA change. A diagnosis of erosive OA (EOA) has only been suggested in one skeleton, a female recovered from a site in London.[18] The distribution of the erosions on the articular surfaces of the interphalangeal joints and in the carpal bones, with proliferative new bone around the joint margins, is characteristic of EOA (Fig. 6.6). The radiological appearance confirmed the main involvement of the proximal and distal interphalangeal joints. The predominant abnormality was ill-defined bone destruction at the articular surfaces, producing in some fingers a 'gull wing' abnormality and one proximal interphalangeal joint was ankylosed.

The prevalence of OA

The aim of most research on the occurrence of OA in the past is to compare the frequency, distribution or characteristics between various ancient populations and how and why they might differ from those seen now. For this one needs agreed and comparable data and recent work has begun to address this problem.[19,20,16] Even with agreed operational definitions for OA in paleopathological material, as discussed above, there are still problems. In order that data collected from ancient skeletal populations can be compared to modern information, it must be comparable. Clinical data are frequently obtained on the basis of radiographic assessments.[13,21] The visual inspection of skeletal material enables morphological alterations to be observed very easily, but it is not always clear that the visual and radiographic assessments of an osteoarthritic joint are comparable. A study by Rogers et al.[22] demonstrated a frequency of OA in a series of 24 skeletal knees ranging from 21 per cent by visual assessment to 8 per cent in the same knees radiologically assessed (Table 6.1). There is also considerable variation between authors in the way that individual joints are classified. The shoulder joint, for instance, may be defined as the glenohumeral joint or as the glenohumeral joint and acromioclavicular joint.[7,9] Clearly, differences in the definition of what constitutes a particular joint can also produce widely varying values. The knee is another joint that can suffer from confusion over definition between different researchers, some collecting data on the joint as a whole and others recording compartmental changes as separate joints.

A further major problem arises from the paucity of data available on skeletons collected for examination, and the absence of information about the extent to which they are representative of the population from which they come. For example, some burial sites may have a high concentration of clergy, or of some other unrepresentative section of society. It is also difficult to age skeletons accurately, the methods[20] used by biological anthropologists are generally imprecise, only allowing for ageing within a decade after skeletal maturation has been achieved, and with no differentiation after the age of 50, in most cases. For all of these reasons we cannot make accurate comparisons of the prevalence of OA in the modern and ancient population.

Despite this, much interesting and valuable information on the overall prevalence of OA in different populations has been obtained.

Most authors reporting on many different skeletal groups from a wide and varying time span agree that OA is the most commonly reported pathological change and the most frequently occurring joint disease.[23] In a group of Roman British skeletons from Cirencester, for example, Wells[24] reported that 44.8 per cent of the adult population had OA somewhere in the skeleton. When these figures were examined by sex, 51.5 per cent of males and 32.9 per cent of females were affected. In a medieval site in York,[25] at Fishergate, 46.9 per cent of adults had OA in at least one joint— 48 per cent of males and 43.8 per cent of females. Rogers[26] found that only 15 per cent of adult Roman British skeletons had OA—but there were only 15 Roman British skeletons recovered from the site (St Oswald's Priory, Gloucestershire). Larger numbers were recovered for the periods dating, respectively, 900–1120, 1120–1230, and 1600–1850. For the first of these periods, 22 per cent of adults were reported as having OA—28.5 per cent of males and 26.6 per cent of females. The second, later medieval period had 24 per cent of adults with OA—37.5 per cent of males and 25 per cent of females; and, in the postmedieval period dating 1600–1850, the frequency of OA in all adults was 34 per cent—33.3 per cent of males and 39.4 per cent of females. Another site that yielded contemporary skeletal material to support the findings of the last phase of St Oswalds Priory was Christ Church,

Spitalfields, in London. Three hundred and eighty-seven named skeletons were recovered from among a larger assemblage from the crypt of this church. Waldron[27] reported a prevalence of 30.9 per cent of adults with OA, with 34.5 per cent of males and 24.3 per cent of females showing signs of OA change.

Site-specific prevalence

Many reports do not present an overall prevalence of OA for their skeletons but concentrate on the frequency of occurrence at particular joints. The majority of authors agree that OA most commonly affects the spinal facet joints. The prominence of spinal OA is a reasonably constant finding. When more detailed analysis of the peak level of affected vertebrae is undertaken there is also uniformity. Waldron[27] reports that the Spitalfields skeletons have a peak occurrence at Cervical 4/5, Thoracic 4/5, and Lumbar 5. Jurmain and Kilgore[28] find an almost identical picture in a medieval Nubian sample. Merbs,[29] in a detailed and extensive study of Innuit skeletons, found a very similar distribution with peaks of OA frequency at Cervical 2/4, Thoracic 4/5, and Lumbar 5. As well as facet joint involvement of the cervical spine, OA of the odontoid component of atlanto axial joints is also frequently observed (Fig. 6.7).

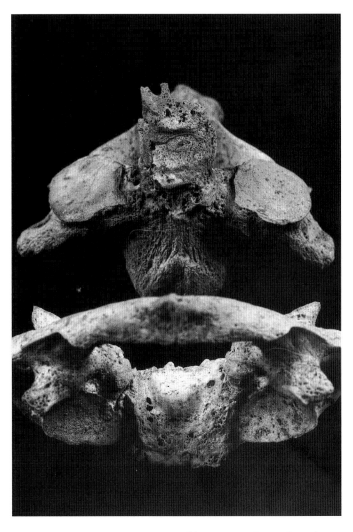

Fig. 6.7 OA of the odontoid articulation of first and second cervical vertebra, with osteophyte and eburnation.

Table 6.1 Frequency of OA in a series of 24 skeletal knees[21]

Normal	Visual appearance		Radiological appearance
	Osteophyte only	OA (eburnation)	OA
8 knees	11 knees	5 knees	2 knees
(33.3%)	(41%)	(21%)	(8%)

Table 6.2 OA of different joints in various skeletal populations

Archeological site	Joints (% skeletons affected)						
	Spine	Shoulder	Elbow	Wrist	Hip	Knee	Ankle
SE USA[8]	—	35.0	40.0	15.0	3.0	27.0	8.0
Fishergate, York[24]	—	12.5	17.0	15.0	18.2	15.2	4.0
Dordrecht, Holland[7]	36.8	14.3	5.6	—	12.0	5.2	—
Trowbridge, Wilts.[27]	—	2.9	1.9	1.4	3.4	1.4	0.4
Castledyke, N. Lincs.[37]	—	7.6	1.8	5.2	2.3	3.8	0.0
England							
premedieval	31.9	31.9	2.1	8.5	12.8	2.1	0.0
medieval	31.7	33.5	2.1	3.6	5.7	5.0	0.0
postmedieval	24.0	27.7	2.6	1.9	2.9	4.4	0.0
St Oswald's Priory, Glos.[25]							
early medieval	18.6	0.0	0.9	5.7	1.9	0.0	0.0
medieval	22.5	0.9	0.0	2.7	4.6	0.9	0.0
post medieval	25.9	0.0	4.6	8.0	3.4	5.7	0.0

The frequency of OA at peripheral joints varies more widely between populations, with Jurmain and Kilgore,[28] for instance, stating that the shoulder and hip are less involved than the knee or elbow, whereas Waldron[7] found the converse. Table 6.2 displays the frequency of OA at different joint sites reported by seven authors for seven different skeletal assemblages. It will be seen that there is a wide variation, some of which can be explained by the inclusion of the acromioclavicular joint within the scoring of the shoulder (Waldron[7] and Bridges[9]). Other variations are likely to be due to the inclusion of too wide a range of bony change within the definition of OA.[8,25,9] The variations seen from the skeletons from the other sites are likely to be real, as the data was collected using the same operational definition of OA.

It can be seen from Table 6.2 that the ankle is very rarely involved in OA, which is similar to the pattern seen today.[30] Other differences are apparent, however, and the findings reported for knee and elbow joint OA raise particularly interesting issues. Rogers and Dieppe[31] reported that in the earlier historical period, hip OA was more frequent than knee OA, but that this ratio changed in the postmedieval period with knee OA becoming more frequent than hip OA. This differs from the pattern most frequently seen in archaeological skeletons in the United States of America,[9,28] where hip OA is less common than knee OA. Not many skeletal reports have covered the precise distribution of knee OA into its component subjoints of patellofemoral and tibiofemoral compartments. In the same study of over 785 skeletons,[31] despite the changing frequency of knee OA, the majority of affected compartments were patellofemoral. This finding has been confirmed by Waldron,[7] but again skeletal populations from the United States of America seem to differ. Merbs[29] reported that the lateral compartment was more frequently involved than the other compartments. In some US populations the medial and patellofemoral compartments are equally involved. One of the most important risk factors for tibiofemoral knee OA is obesity, so it is possible that the relative infrequency of tibiofemoral knee OA in old European populations is explained by a lower prevalence of severe obesity in the past. The elbow joint is interesting for different reasons. It has been found, in several different populations, that skeletal evidence of OA is extremely common in the elbow joint. However, it is rarely reported in contemporary clinical descriptions of OA.[32] This raises the intriguing possibility that elbow OA is relatively asymptomatic, which would result in us not looking for it and therefore not finding it, in the modern clinical setting. Further investigation is needed to find the true prevalence of different joint involvement in different groups and their implications.

Generalized OA and generalized bone formation

The examination of skeletons affords us a unique opportunity to investigate the association of OA between different joints, and thus that of the existence and patterns of 'generalized' forms of OA, and to look for associations between OA and other skeletal changes. However, this has not been possible for most investigators because the requirements include relatively large numbers of skeletons with most joints preserved, in addition to sophisticated statistical analyses. The authors have recently been able to do such work, in conjunction with statistician Lee Shepstone, using a group of 563 well-preserved skeletons from Barton-on-Humber in the United Kingdom. We have obtained good evidence for the existence of at least two forms of generalized OA (i.e., clusters of joints with OA at a much higher association between them than would be expected by chance).[33] We have also found that osteophyte formation as well as eburnation have a higher than expected association with the ossification of entheses, resulting in the concept of a subsection of bone formers in the population (i.e., people whose skeletons react to insult with more bone formation than is generally the case).[34]

The interpretation of OA in osteoarcheology

In most osteoarcheological and paleopathological investigations a special interest is taken in the precise pattern and distribution of OA in different populations. This is because the perception is that OA results from biomechanical stress and that, thus, the pattern of involvement is an imprint of the activity or occupations of the early populations under investigation. A quotation by Calvin Wells[24] perhaps best exemplifies this approach: '*It is the most useful of all diseases for reconstructing the lifestyle of early populations. Its anatomical localisation reflects very closely their occupation and activities…*'.

This concept has helped the widespread dissemination of a preconceived idea of OA as only being caused by activities and occupation. For instance, in a report[35] on the examination of over a thousand skeletons from the Romano–British site at Poundbury, the discussion of OA and other joint disease is placed in a chapter entitled 'Lifestyle and occupation'.

But this approach has also led to some extremely thorough and detailed examinations of the patterns and distributions of the series of bony changes seen in OA. Some of the variations of distribution are, in fact, very likely to be influenced by biomechanical and activity related changes. However, this somewhat simplistic approach of equating a particular pattern with a particular activity is now being questioned.[36] It is very difficult, if not impossible, to test the connection between activity and OA pattern and distribution in an archaeological sample. This is because it is not usually known how representative of the whole historic population the excavated skeletons are. Furthermore, there is rarely, if ever, documentation to link skeletons with particular activities.

The excavation of the 387 named skeletons from Christ Church, Spitalfields, provided a unique opportunity to investigate this further, as there was evidence for the occupation actually followed by these populations. Many of them had been weavers. Waldron and Cox,[37] in a case control study, found no relationship between occupation and OA of the hands or any other joint site.

Comparative animal data

Investigation of the variance of distribution between human populations and primate skeletons is also proving to be a useful area of investigation, providing more insight into the potential contribution of mechanical factors in the pathogenesis of OA at particular joint sites. Jurmain and Kilgore[28] and Lim et al.[38] have shown that there is a similar distribution of OA of the interphalangeal joints between an age-matched group of macaque and human skeletons, but that there was a much lower frequency of thumb-base OA in the macaque group. Investigation of knee OA in the same group of subjects also showed differences, with the humans having a high prevalence of patellofemoral OA. The converse is true of the macaques.[39]

Conclusion

It is clear from the brief discussion of the paleopathology of OA that there are many limitations both in the material and in the methodology and interpretation of findings. Nevertheless, it is also clear that the investigation of the nature and epidemiology of a disease such as OA in earlier populations can provide a valuable type of information to enhance and complement the current research into OA.[29,40] Furthermore, the access to skeletal material provides a unique resource for the investigation of specific questions such as the relationship between the visual, radiological, and pathological appearance of particular pathological changes. Skeletal material can also provide a source of information about the relationship of changes[34,41] throughout the entire skeleton, rather than being restricted to a few symptomatic joints, thus enhancing the possibility of learning something about a systemic bony response.

References

(An asterisk denotes recommended reading.)

1. Schufeldt, R.W. (1893). Notes on paleopathology. *Pop Sci Monthly* **42**:679–84.

2. *Ruffer, M.A. (1913). Studies in palaeopathology in Egypt. *J Pathol Bacteriol* **18**:149–62.

    This is the first significant publication on the use of ancient human remains as a means of exploring disease. Ruffer used mummies as they were more readily available to him than skeletons, which are now the main source of material.

3. Rogers, J. and Dieppe, P. (1990). Skeletal Palaeopathology of the rheumatic diseases. Where are we now? *Ann Rheum Dis* **49**:885–6.

4. Strauss, W.L. and Cave, A.J. (1957). Pathology and posture of Neanderthal man. *Quart Rev Biol* **32**:348–63.

5. Rogers, J.M. (1990). The skeletal remains. In A. Saville (ed.), *Hazelton Long Barrow*. London: English Heritage, pp. 182–97.

6. Ruffer, M.A. (1918). Arthritis deformans and spondylitis in ancient Egypt. *J Pathol Bacteriol* **22**:152–96.

7. Waldron, T. (1995). Changes in the distribution of OA over historical time. *Int J Osteoarchaeol* **5**:385–9.

8. Maat, G., Mastwijk, R.W., and van der Velde, E.A. (1995). Skeletal distribution of degenerative changes in vertebral osteophytosis, vertebral OA and DISH. *Int J Osteoarchaeol* **5**(3):289–98.

9. Bridges, P. (1991). Degenerative joint disease in hunter gatherers and agriculturalists from the South Eastern United States. *Am J Phys Anthropol* **85**:379–91.

10. Kricum, M.E. (1994). Paleoradiology of the prehistoric Australian aboriginies. *Am J Roentgenol* **163**:241–7.

11. Shepstone, L., Rogers, J., Kirwan, J., and Silverman, B. (1999). The shape of the distal femur: A palaeopathological comparison of eburnated and non-eburnated femora. *Ann Rheum Dis* **58**:72–8.

12. Rogers, J. and Dieppe, P. (1993). Ridges and grooves on the bony surfaces of osteoarthritic joints. *Osteoarthritis Cart* **1**:167–70.

13. Kellgren, J.H. and Lawrence, J.S. (1957). Radiological assessment of OA. *Ann Rheum Dis* **16**:494–501.

14. Hernborg, J. and Nilsson, B.E. (1973). The relationship between osteophytes in the knee joint, OA and ageing. *Acta Orthop Scand* **44**:69.

15. Waldron, T. and Rogers, J. (1991). Inter-observer variation in coding OA in human skeletal remains. *Int J Osteoarchaeol* **1**:49–56.

16. Bridges, P. (1993). The effect of variation in methodology on the outcome of osteoarthritic studies. *Int J Osteoarchaeol* **3**:289–95.

17. *Rogers, J. and Waldron, T. (1995). *A Field Guide to Joint Disease in Archaeology*. London: Wiley, pp. 32–46.

    *This excellent book is the current definitive guide to the examination and interpretation of findings on old skeletons. If you want a more readily available journal article, and to confine your attention to arthropathies, then the related reference (J Archaeol Sci **16**:611–25; 1987) is an alternative, but the book is a fascinating read and highly recommended.*

18. Rogers, J., Waldron, T., and Watt, I. (1991). Erosive osteoarthritis in a mediaeval skeleton. *Int J Osteoarchaeol* **1**:151–3.

19. Rogers, J., Waldron, T., Dieppe, P., and Watt, I. (1987). Arthropathies in palaeopathology: the basis of classification according to most probable cause. *J Archaeol Sci* **16**:611–25.

20. Buikstra, J.E. and Ubelaker, D.H. (1994). Standards for data collection from human skeletal remains. *Arkansas Arch Survey Research Series*, No. 44.

21. van Saase, J., van Romande, I.K., Cars, A., Vandenbrouke, J., and Valkenberg, H. (1989). Epidemiology of OA: the Zoctermeer survey. Comparison of radiological arthritis in a Dutch population with that in 10 other populations. *Ann Rheum Dis* **48**:271–80.

22. Rogers, J., Watt, I., and Dieppe, P. (1990). Comparison of visual and radiographic detection of bony changes at the knee joint. *Br Med J* **300**:367–8.

23. Ortner, D.J. and Putschar, W. (1985). Identification of pathological conditions in human skeletal remains. *Smithsonian Contributions to Anthropology*, No. 28, p. 419.

24. Wells, C. (1982). *The Human Burials In Romano-British Cemeteries at Cirencester* (A. McWhirr, L. Viner, and C. Wells (eds)). Cirencester Excavation Committee, p. 152.

25. Stroud, G. (1993). *The Human Bones In Cemeteries of St Andrew Fishergate* (G. Stroud and R. L. Kemp (eds)). York Archaeological Trust.

26. Rogers, J. (forthcoming). *The Human Skeletons In St Oswalds Priory* (Caroline Heighway (ed.)). CBA research report. Council for British Archaeology.

27. *Waldron, T. (1991). Prevalence and distribution of OA in a population from Georgian and early Victorian London. *Ann Rheum Dis* **50**:301–7.

    A large, well-conducted study of osteoarthritis in skeletons. This collection is unique, because complete information on age at death and occupation are available, allowing much more informative comparisons with contemporary data to be made. (see also Waldren and Cox, Brit J Ind Med 46:420–2; 1989).

28. Jurmain, R.D. and Kilgore, L. (1995). Skeletal evidence of osteoarthritis, a palaeopathological perspective. *Ann Rheum Dis* **54**:443–50.

29. Merbs, C.F. (1983). *Patterns of Activity-Induced Pathology in a Canadian Innit Population*. Ottawa: National Museums of Canada, p. 92.

30. **Huch, K., Kuettner, K.E., and Dieppe, P.** (1997). Osteoarthritis in ankle and knee joints. *Sem Arthritis Rheum* **26**:667–74.

31. **Rogers, J. and Dieppe, P.** (1994). Is tibio-femoral osteoarthritis in the knee joint a new disease? *Ann Rheum Dis* **53**:612–13.

32. **Cushingham, J. and Dieppe, P.** (1991). Study of 500 patients with limb joint osteoarthritis. I. Analysis by age, sex, and distribution of symptomatic joint sites. *Ann Rheum Dis* **50**:8–13.

33. **Shepstone, L., Dieppe, P., Rogers, J.** Osteoarthritis – a system disorder of bone. Submitted for publication.

34. *****Rogers, J., Shepstone, L., and Dieppe, P.** (1997). Bone formers: Osteophyte and enthesophyte formation are positively associated. *Ann Rheum Dis* **56**:85–90.

    This paper reports an association between the formation of enthesophytes and osteophytes, the data being derived from a large collection of skeletons from Barton-on-Humbar in the United Kingdom. It suggests that there the generalized tendency for the skeleton to produce bone in response to stress is more pronounced in some individuals ('bone formers') than others, and that this goes someway to explaining the heterogeneity of the OA phenotype.

35. **Molleson, T.** (1993). The human remains in *Poundbury, vol. 2*, monograph series, no. 11, Dorset Natural History and Archaeological Society.

36. **Jurmain, R.D.** (1991). Degenerative changes in peripheral joints as indicators of mechanical stress: opportunities and limitations. *Int J Osteoarchaeol* **3,4**:247–52.

37. **Waldron, H.A. and Cox, M.** (1989). Occupational arthropathy evidence from the past. *Brit J Ind Med* **46**:420–2.

38. *****Lim, K., Rogers, J., Shepstone, L., and Dieppe, P.** (1995). The evolutionary origins of OA: a comparative skeletal study of hand disease in two primates. *J Rheumatol* **22**(11):2132–4.

    This evolutionary hypothesis of OA was first proposed by Charles Hutton in 1987. This paper describes one of the few studies that has tested and extended the hypothesis, using skeletal material from a variety of different primates and relating the distribution of OA to their morphology and joint usage. An example of a paleopathological study that provides data of relevance to the pathogenesis of OA.

39. **Rogers, J., Lim, K., Shepstone, L., and Turnquist, J.** (1996). Distribution of knee OA in human and macaque skeletons. *Am J Phys Anthropol* **22**(Suppl.):202.

40. **Dieppe, P.A. and Rogers, J.** (1985). Two dimensional epidemiology. *Brit J Rheumatol* **24**:310–12.

41. **Boyleston, A., Wiggins, R., and Roberts, C.** (forthcoming). *The human skeletons in the Anglo-Saxon cemetery at Castledyke South, Barton on Humber* (ed. G. Drinkall and M. Foreman).

Acknowledgement

Tragically, Juliet Rogers died in November 2001 during the production of this Second Edition of Osteoarthritis. Her contribution to the paleopathology of joint and bone disease was truly outstanding. In addition, she will be remembered by all who knew her as an exceptionally warm and generous individual she will be sadly missed.

The Editors

7

Pathogenesis of osteoarthritis

7.1 Introduction: the concept of osteoarthritis as failure of the diarthrodial joint

Kenneth Brandt, Michael Doherty, and
L. Stefan Lohmander

Our view of OA and its pathogenesis continues to change. OA was previously considered a 'degenerative' disease, the inevitable accompaniment of ageing, with 'wear and tear' the principle pathogenetic mechanism. Now, OA is increasingly viewed as a metabolically active, dynamic process ... may be triggered by a variety ... view of OA needs to take

... OA. The study of ... present throughout ... he equivalent of OA ... joints in which the ... dence supports the ... species,[3,4] including

... gically, OA is often ... formation, synovial ... ocal loss of hyaline ... least initially, multi- ... nation of new cartil- ... dergoes enchondral ... n (as growing osteo- ... cartilage differ from ... turnover of many ... tin epitopes that are ... These features alone ... sease' and suggest a ... oduce new tissue in

... ms, and disability. It ... ace of OA may often ... nction.[12-14] This is ... er joints, but is not

... OA. Although the ... OA is not inevitably ... es' of symptoms, and ... is particularly likely ... lso occur at hips and ... e structural changes ... ost hyaline cartilage ... show 'improvement', ... brocartilage replace- ... e interbone distance

Such observations are all readily accommodated by the perspective of OA as a potential repair process in response to joint insult and cartilage destruction (Fig. 7.2).[9,20] In this perspective, a variety of insults may trigger the need to repair. Once the process is initiated, all the tissues in the joint are involved in what may be considered an adaptive response.[9,20,21]

The increased metabolic activity by cartilage, new bone formation, and remodelling of the joint may help keep pace with tissue loss and redistribute mechanical forces across the compromised joint; capsular thickening may help to sustain joint stability. The outcome depends on the balance between the severity and chronicity of the insult, and the effectiveness of the repair response. In many instances the repair may rectify the adverse effects of the insult ('compensated OA'), but in some cases overwhelming insult or poor tissue response lead to 'decompensated' OA, with symptoms, disability, and progression of structural damage. Such a scenario could explain the *marked heterogeneity* of OA with different sites of involvement, different numbers of joints affected, and marked variability of outcome.

If OA is, in general, a slow but successful repair process, this also explains its frequent presence in the absence of symptoms or impaired function, its

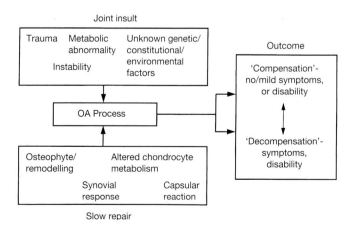

Fig. 7.1 Knee radiographs of a 68-year old patient, taken 3 years apart, showing remodelling. During this time her symptoms improved.

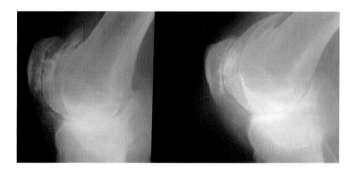

Fig. 7.2 Schematic representation of OA as a repair process triggered by a variety of insults and showing variable outcome.

generally benign natural history, and its widespread presence in man and other animals. If such a perspective is correct, the concept of OA as a single 'disease' should be replaced by the concept of OA as a *process*, with diverse triggers and outcomes. A number of consequences require emphasis:

1. Although these triggers share a common phenotypic expression as 'OA', the way in which they insult the joint may vary greatly and may involve hereditary, constitutional, metabolic, endocrine, environmental, or biomechanical mechanisms. (Fig. 7.3).

2. The site of primary insult may be any tissue in the joint (bone, cartilage, synovium, capsule, ligament, muscle), because all are essential to its health and integrity.

3. Risk factors and mechanisms involved in the development of OA need not be the same as those that determine progression or non-progression.

4. Caution must be exercised in extrapolating knowledge of the pathogenesis of OA from one joint site to another, or from one clinical form or model of OA, to OA in general.

The rationale for dividing the heterogeneous group of subjects with OA into more homogeneous subsets is to better identify these individual triggers and mechanisms. Although subsets may be defined in various ways, for example, by radiographic appearance (*atrophic* versus *hypertrophic*[22]) and by the presence of florid clinical inflammation[23] and calcium crystals (pyrophosphate arthropathy,[24] apatite-associated arthropathy[25,26]), separation at least according to the *site* and *number* of joints affected appears important.[27] Caveats to defining such subsets, however, include: the occurrence of different subsets at different sites within the same individual; evolution from one subset to another; and interaction between primary (hereditary, constitutional) and secondary (mechanical) forms of OA.[28]

An intriguing aspect of OA that remains unexplained is its *site specificity*. Only certain synovial joints show a high prevalence of OA (Fig. 7.4), with others being relatively spared. One hypothesis to explain this distribution relates to man's evolution.[29] Joints that have undergone major change in orientation and function, to permit our bipedal gait and associated liberation of the upper limb, may not yet have adapted to their new functional requirements: they may be underdesigned (that is, have poor functional reserve), and, therefore, more frequently require a reparative response in the face of insult. The distribution of OA in man and other animals is consistent with this theory, though further testing of the hypothesis is clearly problematic. Within individual joints, there is additional specificity with respect to sites of maximal cartilage loss. For large joints, this most commonly occurs at sites of maximum load bearing, supporting the importance of physical factors. Although this biomechanical explanation fits the majority of cases of large joint OA, topographical variation certainly occurs and has been used as a basis for subset classification. For example, at the hip, superior (lateral, intermediate, medial), axial, and medial patterns

of femoral head migration are recognized and have been attributed different associations.[30]

The strong association between *ageing* and OA prevalence, for all sites of involvement, also remains unexplained. Certain aspects of OA are virtually confined to the elderly, for example, marked calcium crystal deposition (calcium pyrophosphate, carbonate substituted apatite), involvement of atypical sites (glenohumeral joint, radiocarpal joint), and rapidly destructive OA of the large joints (hip, knee, glenohumeral joint). The mechanism underlying these striking age associations may relate to the age-related decline in muscle function, impairment of joint proprioception, reduction of vascular supply, and nutrition of joint tissues, or reduced regenerative potential of connective tissue. All of these factors might lower resistance to insult, tip a compensated OA joint toward decompensation, and favour more rapid progression and poor outcome. There is a dramatic decline with ageing in the biomechanical properties of cartilage matrix,[31] probably caused by subtle but cumulative changes in the structure of collagens, proteoglycans, and matrix proteins. The effect of ageing on both normal and OA tissues certainly deserves further study.

A variety of biochemical and biomechanical triggers and mechanisms have been studied in OA, particularly with respect to the cartilage. It is often difficult, however, to disentangle deleterious initiating factors from events linked to tissue response, especially when studying established, particularly end-stage, disease. Physical and biomechanical factors, though usefully separated in test systems, are likely to be inexorably linked and interdependent *in vivo*. Sharp polarization between them is likely to be artificial. Furthermore, we should not assume an 'all-or-none' or linear response, for initiating or perpetuating triggers. For example, we know that a certain

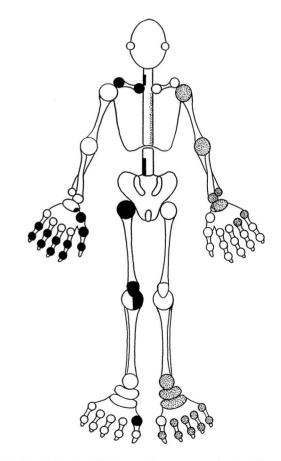

Fig. 7.4 The distribution of OA in man. Common target sites for OA are shown on the left (black). Relatively spared sites of involvement are shown on the right (stippled).

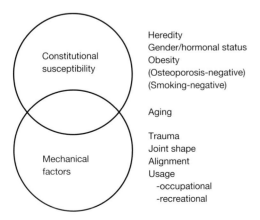

Heredity
Gender/hormonal status
Obesity
(Osteoporosis-negative)
(Smoking-negative)

Aging

Trauma
Joint shape
Alignment
Usage
  -occupational
  -recreational

Fig. 7.3 Possible risk factors for development of OA.

amount of regular loading is required for the health of both cartilage and bone, and that either too little or too much loading may result in cartilage fibrillation and thinning.[32] Such U-shaped response curves may cause problems for the unwary.

In this section, the individual component tissues of the joint are considered. The ways in which they are affected by, or contribute to, the OA process are detailed. Historically, the principal research focus has been on hyaline articular cartilage, with bone the second competing tissue of interest. However, as will be seen, all intracapsular and periarticular tissues are now coming under scrutiny, as recognition of the interdependence of joint tissues grows. Although dedicated to individual tissues, behind every chapter are the perspectives of the integrated joint and the diversity of mechanisms that may result in failure of the joint with OA.

References

1. **Ruffer, M.A. and Rietti, A.** (1911). On osseous lesions in ancient Egyptians. *J Pathol Bacteriol* **16**:439–65.

2. **Rogers, J., Watt, I., and Dieppe, P.** (1981). Arthritis in Saxon and medieval skeletons. *Br Med J* **283**:1668–70.

3. **Jurmain, R.D. and Kilgore, L.** (1995). Skeletal evidence of osteoarthritis: a palaeopathological perspective. *Ann Rheum Dis* **54**:443–50.

4. **Hutton, C.** (1987). Generalised osteoarthritis: an evolutionary problem. *Lancet* **1**:1463–5.

5. **Fox, H.** (1939). Chronic arthritis in wild mammals. *Tr Am Phil Soc* **31**:71–148.

6. **Bennett, G.A. and Bauer, W.** (1931). A systematic study of the degeneration of articular cartilage in bovine joints. *Am J Pathol* **7**:399–414.

7. **Sokoloff, L.** (1956). Natural history of degenerative joint disease in small laboratory animals. *Archives Pathol* **62**:118–28.

8. **Rothschild, B.** (1990). Radiological assessment of osteoarthritis in dinosaurs. *Ann Carnegie Mus* **59**:295–301.

9. **Bland, J.H. and Cooper, S.M.** (1984). Osteoarthritis: a review of the cell biology involved and evidence for reversibility. Management rationally related to known genesis and pathophysiology. *Sem Arthritis Rheum* **14**:106–33.

10. **Hammerman, D.** (1989). The biology of osteoarthritis. *N Engl J Med* **320**:1322–30.

11. **Caterson, B., Mahmoodian, F., Sorrell, J.M., Hardingham, T.E., Bayliss, M.T., Carney, S.L.,** *et al.* (1990). Modulation of native chondroitin sulphate structure in tissue development and in disease. *J Cell Sci* **97**:411–17.

12. **Lawrence, J.S., Bremner, J.M., and Bier, F.** (1966). Osteoarthrosis: prevalence in the population and relationship between symptoms and X-ray changes. *Ann Rheum Dis* **25**:1–23.

13. **Davis, M.A., Ettinger, W.H., Neuhaus, J.M., Barclay, J.D., and Segal, M.R.** (1992). Correlates of knee pain among US adults with and without radiographic knee osteoarthritis. *J Rheumatol* **19**:1943–9.

14. **Hadler, N.M.** (1992). Knee pain is the malady—not osteoarthritis. *Ann Intern Med* **116**:598–9.

15. **Atkinson, J.P.** (1996). A remembrance of Fred, the lowland gorilla. *Arthritis Rheum* **39**:891–3.

16. **Patrick, M., Aldridge, S., Hamilton, E., Manhire, A., and Doherty, M.** (1989). A controlled study of hand function in nodal and erosive osteoarthritis. *Ann Rheum Dis* **48**:978–82.

17. **Danielsson, L.G.** (1964). Incidence and prognosis of coxarthrosis. *Acta Orthop Scand* **64**(Suppl.):1–114.

18. **Hernborg, J.S. and Nilsson, B.E.** (1977). The natural course of untreated osteoarthritis of the knee. *Clin Orthop Rel Res* **123**:130–7.

19. **Perry, Gh., Smith, M.J.G., and Whiteside, C.G.** (1972). Spontaneous recovery of the joint space in degenerative hip disease. *Ann Rheum Dis* **31**:440–8.

20. **Radin, E.L. and Burr, D.B.** (1984). Hypothesis: joints can heal. *Sem Arthritis Rheum* **13**:293–302.

21. **Mankin, H.J.** (1974). The reaction of cartilage to injury and osteoarthritis. *N Engl J Med* **291**:1285–92.

22. **Solomon, L.** (1983). Osteoarthritis, local and generalised: a uniform disease? *J Rheumatol* **10**(Suppl. 9):13–15.

23. **Ehrlich, G.** (1972). Inflammatory osteoarthritis: I. The clinical syndrome. *J Chron Dis* **25**:317–28.

24. **Doherty, M. and Dieppe, P.A.** (1988). Clinical aspects of calcium pyrophosphate dihydrate crystal deposition. *Rheum Dis Clin NA* **14**:395–414.

25. **Dieppe, P.A., Doherty, M., MacFarlane, D.G., Hutton, C.W., Bradfield, J.W., and Watt, I.** (1984). *Br J Rheumatol* **23**:84–91.

26. **Halverson, P.B., McCarty, D.J., Cheung, H., and Ryan, L.M.** (1984). Milwaukee shoulder syndrome: eleven additional cases with involvement of the knee in seven basic calcium phosphate deposition disease. *Sem Arthritis Rheum* **14**:36–44.

27. **Kellgren, J.H. and Moore, R.** (1952) Generalised osteoarthritis and Heberden's nodes. *Br Med J* **1**:181–7.

28. **Doherty, M., Watt, I., and Dieppe, P.A.** (1983). Influence of primary generalised osteoarthritis on development of secondary osteoarthritis. *Lancet* **2**:8–11.

29. **Hutton, C.** (1987). Generalised osteoarthritis: an evolutionary problem. *Lancet* **2**:1463–5.

30. **Ledingham, J., Dawson, S., Preston, B., Milligan, G., and Doherty, M.** (1992). Radiographic patterns and associations of osteoarthritis of the hip. *Ann Rheum Dis* **51**:1111–16.

31. **Kempson, G.E.** (1991). Age-related changes in the tensile properties of human articular cartilage: a comparative study between the femoral head of the hip joint and the talus of the ankle joint. *Biochim Biophys Acta* **1075**:223–30.

32. **Buckwalter, J.A.** (1995). Osteoarthritis and articular cartilage use, disuse and abuse: experimental studies. *J Rheumatol* **22**:13–15.

7.2 Pathogenesis of structural changes in the osteoarthritic joint

7.2.1 Articular cartilage

7.2.1.1 Biochemistry and metabolism of normal and osteoarthritic cartilage

Dick Heinegård, Michael Bayliss, and Pilar Lorenzo

The clinical diagnosis of OA, as is described elsewhere in this book, depends on symptoms like pain and radiographic detection of joint space narrowing as a result of articular cartilage loss, and in many cases the presence of osteophytes. These alterations summarize some of the characteristic features of degenerative joint disease, for example, the progressive destruction of the cartilage paralleled by attempted repair responses such as osteophyte formation. Although these diagnostic features appear late in the disease, it is apparent that molecular events occur long before alterations can be observed macroscopically, or even at the microscopical level. This lack of means for the early detection of conditions leading to joint destruction in OA has hampered the development of effective therapy.

In the development of joint destruction it is clear that degradation of matrix constituents and their removal from the cartilage has to occur. It is also likely that any such process will elicit a response in the chondrocytes attempting to repair the matrix defect that develops. Therefore, the early alterations in cartilage, which might be expected as the OA process develops, should include an increased synthesis of some matrix components to compensate for the increased degradation. It is, however, unlikely that these molecular events will occur in all tissue compartments simultaneously. Since the composition of the tissue compartments, that is pericellular (closest to the cells), territorial, interterritorial (furthest away from cells), and of different zones of cartilage—surface, middle, deep—show distinct differences at the molecular level, it is plausible that the processes may start in one compartment and only later involve other compartments. Furthermore, it is possible that the cells have better means of sensing and compensating for matrix changes in their immediate environment and therefore are better fit to adequately deal with destructive events in the pericellular and territorial matrix.

This chapter deals with the alterations in matrix composition with the aging of normal cartilage and the distinctly different alterations observed during the development of OA. The characterization of such changes will not only help us to identify targets for future therapeutic intervention, but will also provide the diagnostic tools that are required for identifying and monitoring those patients that will be subject to therapy.

An understanding of such alterations depends on the knowledge of the components that form the tissue and their individual functional roles. There are several groups of such macromolecular constituents, which are described as follows.

Collagen

The major structural element of the articular cartilage is the collagen networks. One is formed from the major component in cartilage, that is, a large number of collagen II molecules assembled to form collagen fibers. These are stable and show an extremely long half-life estimated to be in the order of 100 years, compared to less than 5 years for aggrecan.[1,2] The fibers also contain small amounts of collagen XI. The very tightly regulated assembly process occurs either very close to secretion, or just outside the cells, and requires a modification of the proform of collagen produced by the chondrocyte (Fig. 7.5). Thus, specific proteolytic enzymes remove N- as well as C-terminal extensions. After removal of the extensions, the collagen molecules can associate to form fibers in a very specific manner.[3] The processed collagen molecule consists of three polypeptide chains, forming a classical triple helical structure. This is a very compact, tightly held together functional molecule that is some 3000 Å long and only 15 Å thick. The peptide backbone is resistant to proteolysis, since the side chain constituents of its amino acid residues protect it. Each end of this processed molecule, however, retains a few amino acids, forming a telopeptide structure different from the rest (Fig. 7.5). Lysine residues in this telopeptide participate in enzyme-induced cross-link formation between neighbouring collagen molecules, which further stabilizes the fibers. Cross-links constitute new stable derivatives called pyridinolines and are uniquely found in collagen. Another feature, which is rather specific to collagens, is the hydroxyproline residues constituting some ten per cent of the total. They are essential for the stability of the collagen molecule as are the hydroxylysine residues.

The collagen II that makes up the bulk of these fibers (Fig. 7.6) is quite specific for cartilage. The fibers are rather complex structures, for example in that they contain an additional collagen, collagen XI, also specific for cartilage. Current knowledge indicates that the collagen XI, which represents a few per cent of the total collagen, may have a role in determining the thickness of the collagen II fibers.[3,4] It is quite apparent that the growth of these fibers is very tightly regulated and differs between compartments in cartilage. Thus, the thinnest fibers of the tissue occur in the territorial matrix close to the cells in the superficial parts of the articular cartilage. There is a gradual increase in fiber thickness with distance from the cells, towards the interterritorial matrix. In general, fiber thickness also increases in all compartments, for example, from the superficial zones of the articular cartilage to the deep zones (Fig. 7.7). The fibers found in the superficial territorial compartment are very thin; their diameter is only a quarter of those in the deep interterritorial compartment (see Fig. 7.7). The fiber orientation is also different in various parts of the articular cartilage. Thus, those in the most superficial layer run parallel to the surface, while those in the deep parts run perpendicular. In the intermediate to upper portion of the cartilage, fibers run in variable directions,[5] illustrated in Fig. 7.7.

It is not known today what are the exact factors governing the assembly of the collagen molecules into fibers, resulting in their specific dimensions. Notably, *in vitro*, several molecules included in the family of leucine-rich repeat proteins, discussed below, have been shown to modulate fibril formation. This also includes the members of the thrombospondin family,

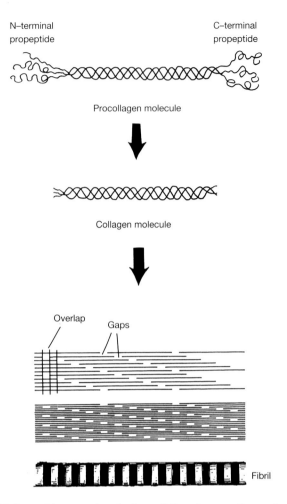

N–terminal
propeptide

C–terminal
propeptide

Procollagen molecule

Collagen molecule

Overlap

Gaps

Fibril

Fig. 7.5 Extracellular processing of collagen. Collagen is secreted in a proform that is cleaved by specific proteinases to a collagen molecule largely consisting of very compact and stable triple helical regions with non-triple helical short telopeptides in both N- and C-terminal ends. These collagen molecules are then, in a highly organized way, assembled in several steps to form the collagen fiber. Covalent crosslinks are formed over a period of years involving lysine residues in the telopeptides.

matrix closer to the cell.[3] This collagen molecule is made up of a central triple helical domain surrounded by non-triple helical regions forming a globular structure at each end. These are particularly rich in von Willebrand factor A domains, where ten are contributed by the $\alpha3(VI)$ chain.[9] These domains show capabilities of interactions among themselves and with other matrix constituents. The collagen VI molecules assemble intracellularly in an antiparallel fashion into a dimer. Two such dimers then form the tetramer that is subsequently secreted.[10] Both ends of the tetramer are thus formed from the globular N-terminal ends of pair-wise two collagen VI molecules. The tetramers align in an end-to-end fashion with their N-terminal ends facing each other. Further assembly into beaded filaments includes lateral associations.[11]

Also the collagen VI assembly appears to be promoted particularly by the leucine-rich proteoglycans decorin and biglycan, see below. These molecules remain bound to the filament in the tissue, such as to promote interactions with other structural entities. Thus, preliminary experiments (Wiberg, Heinegård, and Mörgelin, unpublished) have shown that collagen VI fibrils contain bound biglycan/decorin that in turn associates with a member of the matrilin family of proteins (see below), which then, in turn, can bind to collagen II or aggrecan (Wiberg, Heinegård, and Mörgelin, unpublished).

The collagen VI fibrillar network may have a role in protecting the cell. It is primarily found in the pericellular/territorial matrix, close to the cells, and may have functions together with other molecular assemblies. It may thus interact with the aggrecan complexes with roles in resisting compression and the collagen II fibrils with additional roles in tension. Thus, this territorial compartment may consist of several tightly knit networks, creating a very stable structure in the pericellular environment.

Aggrecan

The major non-collagenous component in articular cartilage is aggrecan. This very large molecule, Figs 7.6 and 7.8, consists of a central protein core of some 2000 amino acids with several distinct domains and different functions. Those, which are functionally most important, are the chondroitin sulfate domains, CS1 and CS2, Fig. 7.8, carrying a very large number of negatively charged glycosaminoglycan chains of chondroitin sulfate.[12,13] These chains occur as clusters in the CS2 domain, but are more randomly distributed in the CS1 domain, which has its own characteristic structure. There are some 100 such chains, each consisting of an average of 40–50 disaccharide units with two negatively charged groups in the form of sulfate on the N-acetyl galactosamine and carboxyl of the glucuronic acid, Fig. 7.8. Thus, these two domains (CS1 and CS2) contribute some 8000–10 000 negatively-charged groups to the molecules, all fixed to the protein core via xylose at one end of the chondroitin sulfate chains. An extended protein domain next to the chondroitin sulfate (CS1) region, Fig. 7.8, has a rather specific repeat structure[14] and carries a number of keratan sulfate chains. This domain is likely to confer special properties to the molecule, since the keratan sulfate chains are very closely spaced and have a structure different from other glycosaminoglycans, Fig. 7.8. Another domain with important functional properties is the N-terminal domain, G1.[15] This confers on the aggrecan molecule the ability to specifically interact with hyaluronan. This mechanism is used to link a large number of such aggrecan molecules to one molecule of hyaluronan, forming a very high molecular weight complex, as illustrated in Fig. 7.8. Although the binding of aggrecan to hyaluronan is tight, almost as strong as that between the antigen and antibody, link protein stabilizes the complex by binding both to the hyaluronan and to the G1 domain of the aggrecan.[15] This link-protein has many structural features similar to the G1 domain of aggrecan. Other globular domains have less well-defined properties. For example, the G2 domain is homologous with the major part of the G1 domain, yet its function is unknown. The C-terminal, G3 domain, contains sequences homologous to the epidermal growth factor (EGF), complement regulatory component, and a lectin,[15] illustrated in Fig. 7.8. Interestingly, more recently this lectin homology

particularly shown for COMP, as discussed below. Molecules with roles in regulating the assembly of the collagen fibers may include other constituents of the fibrillar network, for example collagen IX (Fig. 7.6). This collagen molecule contains the classical triple helical structure organized in three different collagenous domains. These are interrupted by non-triple helical domains, which is the NC-1,2,3, and 4, the latter being the N-terminal, as is illustrated in Fig. 7.6. It has been shown that the collagen IX molecule is bound to the collagen II fiber surface in the tissue. This binding is stabilized by covalent cross-links,[6] thus creating a fiber where no more collagen II molecules can be added to increase the fiber thickness and, thereby, the strength of the collagen II fiber itself, unless the collagen IX is removed by proteolysis. It is of interest to note that its NC-4 domain is rather cationic, thereby providing areas along the collagen fiber of high positive-charge density, illustrated in Figs 7.6 and 7.7.

The collagen fibrils also contain a number of other molecules bound to their surface. These include fibromodulin[7] and decorin[8] and probably others of related molecules belonging to this class of leucine-rich repeat proteins, see below. Most of these proteins contain more than one functional domain, allowing them to simultaneously interact with structures at two neighbouring collagen fibrils, as indicated in Fig. 7.6.

A distinctly different collagen network consists of thin-beaded filaments. It has collagen VI as a major constituent and is found in the territorial

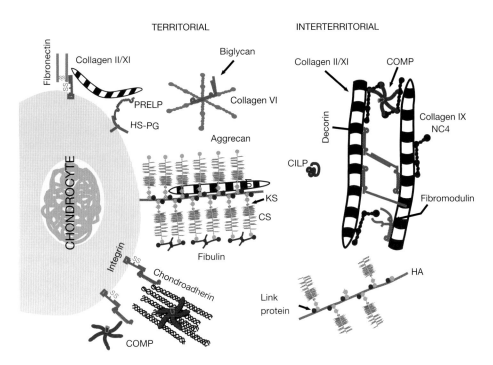

Fig. 7.6 Schematic illustration of the constituents of cartilage matrix. The spatial relationship of the various constituents to the chondrocyte is indicated by their presence in pericellular/cell associated, territorial close to the cell, and interterritorial matrix further away from the cell. The association of matrix molecules in the macromolecular organizations is indicated. HS-PG, heparan sulfate proteoglycan; KS, keratan sulfate; CS, chondroitin sulfate; HA, hyaluronan.

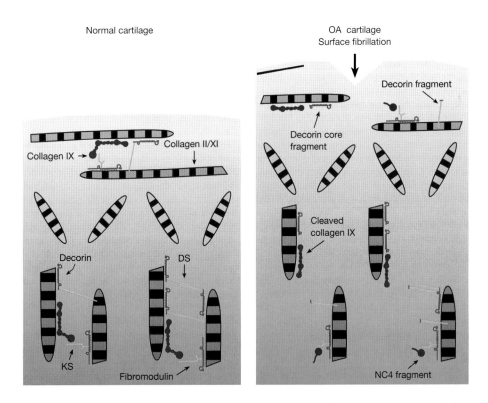

Fig. 7.7 Schematic illustration of the collagen network organization in normal and in diseased cartilage. *Normal*: the superficial part or the cartilage contains collagen fibers arranged parallel to the surface, while the deepest, major part of the tissue, contains fibers arranged perpendicular to the surface. In an intermediate layer fibers run in different directions. The collagen fibers have a number of other matrix macromolecules bound at their surface. These appear to have important roles in 'knitting' together the collagen fibers to form a network, essential for counterbalancing the swelling pressure of the aggrecan. *Disease*: the molecules at the collagen fibril surface may be cleaved in the early stages of joint disease allowing these fibrils to slip and displace in relationship to one another. Such a process would explain early swelling due to loss of the collagen counterbalance to the swelling pressure of the fixed charge groups on aggrecan, and explain the early fibrillation of the articular surface.

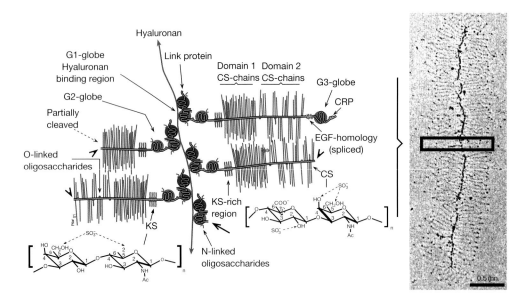

Fig. 7.8 Schematic illustration of aggrecan and its aggregate formation. A central core protein is substituted with some 100 glycosaminoglycans chains of chondroitin sulfate (CS) and keratan sulfate (KS). These chains are made of characteristic repeat disaccharides with negatively-charged groups of sulfate and uronic acid carboxyl groups. The average chondroitin sulfate chains contain some 80–100 charged groups. Specific domains of the aggrecan include an N-terminal hyaluronate binding domain G1, a homologous G2 domain, a keratan sulfate-rich region, two distinct regions of polypeptide repeats carrying the chondroitin sulfate chains, C-terminal, G3, that contains sequences constituting an EGF-like domain, a lectin homology domain, and a complement regulatory protein-like domain. Some molecules lack the C-terminal part following proteolytic cleavage. Several aggrecan molecules are bound via their N-terminal end containing a specific hyaluronate-binding domain to an extremely long hyaluronate molecule. This results in a very large complex with several hundred thousand fixed-charged groups that creates an osmotic gradient and swelling pressure. The appearance of the molecule upon electron microscopy after rotary shadowing is shown on the right. The central filament represents hyaluronate decorated with globular link protein and hyaluronate binding domains of the aggrecan molecules seen as side chain filaments. The structure of the aggrecan molecule changes with age such that most molecules have been cleaved in their C-terminal domain to become shorter, as indicated by the arrowheads in the figure. The ultimate, retained cleavage product is the HABr bold arrow bound to HA together with the link protein. Dr Matthias Mörgelin kindly provided the E-M picture.

domain has been shown to bind fibulins I and II, indicated in Fig. 7.6.[16,17] Fibulins can themselves associate to form oligomers. Thereby several aggrecan molecules can become cross-linked. This binding is mediated via EGF domains in the fibulins.[16] Similarly, the very large molecule fibrillin with a capacity to form fibrillar structures, has been shown to be able to bind to the lectin, G3 domain.[18] This lectin homology domain is cleaved off from proteoglycans resident in the matrix over a long period of time. It is thus possible that the G3 interactions are particularly important in the assembly process of the growing individual or in repair. Thus, preliminary data (Aspberg, personal communication) indicate that aggrecan molecules in the territorial matrix contain the G3 domain, which is largely lacking from those in the interterritorial matrix.

Another component interacting at this C-terminal part of the proteoglycan and with a putative role in tissue assembly is tenascin-R. This protein also has the potential to unite several proteoglycan molecules.[19]

The picture thus emerges of aggrecan being tied down both via interaction with hyaluronan in the N-terminus and via other networks involving particularly fibulins and fibrillins in the C-terminal during growth or repair. These interactions may be particularly important in tissue repair, for example, in joint disease.

The basic structural features of aggrecan described above have been determined largely from studies of molecules purified from young animal cartilage. It is clear, that a structure of this kind has the potential to generate aggregates of widely varying composition and molecular weight, to suit the mechanical and physicochemical properties of cartilage from different sources. These molecular changes are a consequence of biosynthetic and catabolic events, regulated by many cellular and extracellular processes. The extent to which these occur within articular cartilage is not uniform between species, site (which joint), zone (through the cartilage depth), tissue compartment (pericellular, territorial, and interterritorial), region of the joint (topographical distribution), as well as age. All these variables

dictate specific qualitative and quantitative changes in, for example, aggrecan structure.[20] However, it is the age of the individual that appears to have the most profound effect on the composition, stoichiometry, and stability of aggregates. Nowhere is this more evident than in normal human articular cartilage. The schematic shown in Fig. 7.8 illustrates the main structural changes that occur during the maturation and aging of the tissue. These mainly consist of an increased polydispersity and heterogeneity in the molecular size of individual aggrecan molecules, brought about by extracellular proteolytic cleavage of their core proteins. This may be confined to regions within the CS domain, but, with advancing age, an increased concentration of the G1 domain is observed, confirming that proteolytic modification of aggrecan can also be extensive, Fig. 7.8.[21,22] The average size of the hyaluronan polymer also decreases with age. Thus, structural changes in both the major components of the aggregate decrease its size in adult cartilage. Furthermore, studies have indicated that there is an age-related decrease in the concentration of the link protein relative to aggrecan, suggesting that aggregation may be less effective in adult cartilage.[23] Although these structural changes may give the impression of a molecular system that is degenerating during aging, it is important to appreciate that this is not the case and that they provide normal, mature cartilage with the properties that enable it to function in the changing biochemical and biophysical environment to which it is exposed. It should also be noted that the biosynthesis, the composition, and the structure of aggrecan in human osteoarthritic cartilage is very different from that of the adult normal cartilage: that is, OA is not an obligatory consequence of cartilage aging.

The aggregates represent an important structural unit, a key function of which is to provide a stable environment of high fixed-charge density, essential for imbibing and retaining water in the tissue by the high osmotic swelling pressure created. As is discussed elsewhere (Chapter 7.2.1.2), there are sites in the aggrecan molecules that are very sensitive to cleavage by proteinases. Consequently, during normal and pathological turnover of cartilage matrix, proteoglycan fragments are released into the synovial space.[24,25] One such cleavage point is between the G1 and G2 domains.[26] Upon this cleavage, the fragment generated, although large, is not held as tightly in the tissue and can diffuse out of the matrix. During normal turnover this process is controlled and tissue homeostasis is maintained, but in OA it leads to the disruption of the aggregate organization, loss of the fixed-charge groups from the tissue, and, thereby, reduction of its water-imbing properties.

Matrix proteins/proteoglycans

A set of molecules that is much less abundant in the cartilage is the non-collagenous matrix proteins. These include some proteins that are also proteoglycans by virtue of containing one, or a small number, of glycosaminoglycan side chains of keratan sulfate or chondroitin sulfate/dermatan sulfate (discussed below). In some instances, our understanding of the functions of these proteins is emerging, while in other cases the proteins have only just been identified. However, from their specific distribution in the cartilage, it appears that they do have different functions and could serve as indicators for different metabolic processes in the tissue.

A major family of such proteins is the leucine-rich repeat proteins (LRR-proteins), schematically illustrated in Fig. 7.9. These are made up from a central domain of characteristic repeats of some 25 amino acids.[27,28] Thus, ten to eleven repeats are surrounded by a set of disulfide loops, and in most cases there are N- as well as C-terminal extensions. The central leucine-rich repeat domain exposes a surface of so-called β-sheet structures, which are classically known to participate in protein–protein interactions. Indeed, most of the members of this family of proteins bind specifically to other constituents in the matrix and contribute to the structural network, Figs 7.6 and 7.7. Thus, the central domain represents at least one structural feature for which, in several cases, functions can be assigned. In addition, the N-terminal extension peptide in some cases has glycosaminoglycan chains attached to it and, in other cases, it contains repeated tyrosine sulfate residues,[29] and yet another variant is an extended polyaspartate sequence,[28] Fig. 7.9. Other structures of the N-terminal part range from a basic repeat sequence, adapted for interactions with, for example, heparin/heparan sulfate (PRELP—proline and arginine end leucine-rich protein),[30] to a molecule lacking this terminal extension altogether (chondroadherin).[31]

Decorin, fibromodulin, and lumican

Decorin was the first in this series of molecules to be structurally defined.[32] It contains one side chain, often dermatan sulfate. This is slightly different from the traditional chondroitin sulfate chains found in aggrecan, such that some and occasionally all the glucuronic acid residues are exchanged for iduronate within the chain sequence and there are additional sulfate groups on the uronic acid. This side chain can adopt more complex secondary structures and it appears quite likely that it can form specific interactions with other molecules in the tissue, including other dermatan sulfate chains (as indicated in Figs 7.6 and 7.7).

Thus, several members of this family, decorin, fibromodulin,[33] lumican,[34] biglycan,[35] PRELP (Bengtsson, Heinegård, and Aspberg, unpublished) and chondroadherin,[36] can interact with collagens. Although the other members have not yet been shown to interact with collagen, it is possible that all members will eventually be verified to have this capacity. In most cases these interactions include many different types of collagens, where the triple helical domain usually appears to be involved. Decorin, fibromodulin, and lumican form specific protein–protein interactions, via the leucine-rich repeat region to various collagens, including collagen II found in the cartilage. In the case of biglycan, interactions appear to be primarily directed to collagen VI.[37] Further information on the putative functions of the various molecules has been obtained in studies using gene inactivation. Thus, the mice lacking expression of the decorin show much

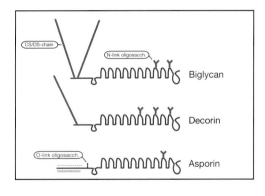

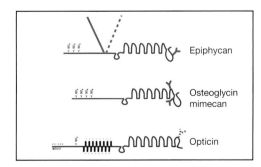

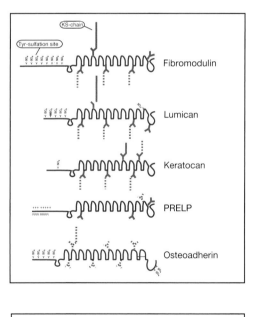

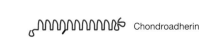

Fig. 7.9 Schematic illustration of the ECM leucine-rich repeat region LRR proteins. The molecules can be grouped in four distinct families based on gene organization and amino acid sequence homologies, as is indicated by the boxes. Functional and distinct domains are the central LRR-region and the N-terminal extension with variable character, ranging from substitution with glycosaminoglycan chains or tyrosine sulfate, to clustering of specific amino acids giving acidic alternatively basic characters.

thicker and rather irregular fibrils, particularly in the skin, when compared to the wild-type mice, causing the skin to become fragile.[38] These findings are consistent with a previously demonstrated ability of decorin to inhibit collagen fibrillogenesis.[39] Inactivation of the lumican gene also results in thicker fibrils in several tissues. Interestingly, inactivation of the fibromodulin gene results in a higher abundance of thin fibers, particularly in the tendon. At the same time, there is a higher abundance of lumican, while the mRNA level for lumican is decreased. This indicates that while the synthesis is down regulated, the elimination seems to be much less efficient.[40] Further studies have shown that lumican and fibromodulin bind to the same site on collagen, with a somewhat lower affinity for lumican.[41] It thus appears that lumican may have roles in the earlier steps in collagen fibrillogenesis and is then replaced by fibromodulin, which has a different role.

It is highly relevant that studies by electron microscopy of localization of fibromodulin,[7] and decorin[8,33] demonstrate them bound at distinct sites on the collagen in the tissue, as is indicated schematically in Figs 7.6 and 7.7. Thus, these molecules also appear to have a role in the mature fibril, particularly in the network formation, of particular importance for optimizing the tensile properties of the tissue. Thus, one of the functional domains, that is, the LRR, forms one interacting site with the collagen, while another is represented by the negatively-charged glycosaminoglycan chains that appear to be capable of either directly interacting with different collagen fibers and/or interacting with other components along the collagen. An example of such a component is the basic NC-4 domain of collagen type IX extending from the collagen fibers, which may participate in ionic interactions with the acidic glycosaminoglycan chains of decorin and fibromodulin, indicated in Figs 7.6 and 7.7.

Chondroadherin

Molecules, like chondroadherin may provide feedback information to the cells by interacting with the integrin $\alpha 2\beta 1$ receptor on the chondrocyte surface. In this way, chondroadherin may have a role in maintaining normal tissue homeostasis. There are also a number of other integrins on the chondrocyte, such as those specific for collagens ($\alpha 1\beta 1$, $\alpha 2\beta 1$, $\alpha 10\beta 1$) and those recognizing fibronectin ($\alpha 5\beta 1$).[42–44] At this stage, the exact roles of these interactions in the regulation of cellular activities is not known, although some evidence[45] indicates that chondroadherin may be involved in the regulation of cell proliferation. Chondroadherin shows a particularly high expression in the lower region of the growth plate between the zone of proliferating chondrocytes and the hypertrophic zone. It is also expressed in articular cartilage, where it is found primarily in the deeper part of the tissue.[46]

More recently, chondroadherin has been isolated from the cartilage by mild proteolysis in a complex bound at two specific locations on collagen II molecules. The binding is very tight, with a K_D in the nanomolar range.[36] The significance of this interaction that apparently occurs in the tissue is not clear. It is tempting to speculate that chondroadherin may have a role in the organization of collagen into larger aggregates in the form of fibrils close to the cell surface.

PRELP

Another molecule that has the potential to interact at the cell surface is PRELP; it contains a domain rich in arginine and proline residues specifically designed for binding to heparin/heparan sulfate.[30,47] This could influence reactions and interactions at the cell surface of the chondrocyte, where heparan sulfate appears[48] as side-chains of cell surface proteoglycans, for example, syndecan and glypican. A possible role could be to modulate the effects of fibroblast growth factor (FGF), which has potent effects on chondrocyte metabolism and which depends on heparin/heparan sulfate chains for its activity.

The leucine-rich repeat region of PRELP binds tightly to collagen like most other members of this family.[49] It is therefore possible that the protein promotes binding between collagen in the matrix and heparan sulfate containing proteoglycans at the cell surface.

Fibronectin

There are a number of other cartilage matrix proteins. Among those that are synthesized by chondrocytes is fibronectin. This molecule shows minor abundance in normal articular cartilage. There is, however, a specific splice variance found in the cartilage.[50,51] It has been shown that chondrocytes produce an increased amount of fibronectin under pathological conditions such as OA.[52]

COMP

Another abundant cartilage macromolecule, which has unique structural features, is COMP,[53] Fig. 7.6. This protein is made up of five identical subunits, linked together close to their N-terminus, via a so-called coiled-coil domain. Disulfide bonds stabilize this. Each chain is terminated at the C-terminal end with a globular structure, giving the molecule an appearance like a bouquet of tulips, Fig. 7.6. COMP is a member of the thrombospondin family and is also referred to as Thrombospondin-5. Other members of this family, particularly the trimeric Thrombospondin-1,[54] and pentameric Thrombospondin-3, have been demonstrated in the cartilage.[55] Our understanding of the functional role of these molecules in the tissue is limited. However, it is becoming increasingly clear that their C-terminal domains can bind tightly to triple helical collagens, and in some cases other matrix components. This has particularly been studied for COMP, where each of the C-terminal globular domains has the capacity to bind to one out of four specific sites, distributed rather evenly along the collagen molecules.[56] Studies, in vitro, have shown that COMP can substantially increase the rate and efficiency of collagen fibrillogenesis. This apparently occurs when each COMP molecule, simultaneously binds several collagen molecules, bringing them together and facilitating their assembly (Rosenberg, Mörgelin, and Heinegård, unpublished). It is particularly interesting to note that COMP does not bind to the collagen II fibril itself. However, it has been shown that COMP binds to any of the four non-collagenous domains of collagen IX.[57] Since this collagen is bound at the surface of collagen II fibers,[4,58] there is a possibility that COMP is another molecule that cross-links neighbouring collagen fibrils, in this case via interactions with collagen IX. It is important to note that these interactions of COMP with collagen depend on zinc. Also other divalent cations, like calcium, are of importance for the structure of the thrombospondins.[57] Further information that supports the indicated roles for COMP can be obtained from its localization. It is particularly enriched in growth cartilage, where it is synthesized and deposited by proliferating chondrocytes in the pericellular and territorial matrix. COMP expression is low in immature cartilage,[59] where the protein is found primarily close to the cells. As the articular cartilage develops, COMP protein and expression increase and, particularly in mature articular cartilage, the protein becomes primarily deposited in the interterritorial compartment in the superficial zones of the tissue.[59] Interestingly, in cartilage, showing very early superficial lesions of fibrillation at single locations, COMP expression is increased and the protein is now found primarily close to the cells rather than in the distant interterritorial matrix, where it is localized in age-matched, normal tissue (King, Lorenzo, Bayliss, and Heinegård, unpublished). This indicates that the protein has been degraded and removed from the interterritorial compartment, and is now primarily laid down in the different territorial compartment close to the cells. This can be viewed as a repair response, where COMP is produced to facilitate collagen fibril formation. However, at this time, the collagen synthesis does not seem to be significantly increased. Thus, it appears that there is an imbalance between the various components required to make a proper collagen fibril (King, Lorenzo, Bayliss, and Heinegård, unpublished observations).

Further evidence indicating that COMP has important biological properties is obtained from mutations identified in the calcium-binding domain of the molecule, which results in severe growth disturbances, that is, pseudo-achondroplasia or severe epiphyseal dysplasias.[60,61] Thus, COMP may be required for the appropriate control of cell growth and proliferation.

CILP

CILP (Cartilage Intermediary Layer Protein) is a more recently described protein[62] having little homology to previously described molecules. Interestingly, it is synthesized as a precursor protein. This is cleaved upon secretion from the cells into the 87 kDa CILP and the C-terminal of apparent weight 60 kDa protein, showing homology to an NTPPHase.[63] At this stage, little is known of the function of either protein. It is, however, to be noted that the synthesis of the protein is extensively upregulated in the early stages of OA. Thus, CILP is then found deposited close to the cells at the same time as it has been removed from its primary interterritorial location, observed in normal, age-matched cartilage. This picture is reminiscent of that of COMP (King, Lorenzo, Bayliss, and Heinegård, unpublished observations). In normal cartilage, the protein has an interesting location, primarily to the mid to lower third part of the articular cartilage.[62] This would indicate specific functional requirements for this part of the tissue, requiring the presence of this particular protein.

Perlecan

Perlecan is a proteoglycan with primary abundance in basement membranes. The protein has a large protein core that permits binding to numerous other matrix constituents ranging from laminins to cells.[64–66] The molecule is substituted, both in the N- and the C-terminals part, with a few glycosaminoglycan side-chains of heparan sulfate. In some tissues, for example cartilage, perlecan contains primarily chondroitin sulfate. Inactivation of the perlecan gene results in severe alterations of the growth plate and extensive growth disturbances.[67,68] Most of the mice, however, die during embryonic life as a result of the major defects in the heart.[68]

Matrilins

The matrilins represent a family of four oligomeric proteins. Matrilin-1 (originally named CMP for Cartilage Matrix Protein[69]) and matrilin-3 are present in the cartilage.[70] Interestingly, matrilin-1 is found in all fetal cartilages, but is then down regulated and disappears from the structures developing into articular cartilage. At the same time the protein is very prominent in, for example, tracheal cartilage.[71] Matrilin-1 is made up of three identical subunits, held together by a coiled-coil domain. A functional structure present in the members of the matrilin family is the von Willebrand factor A-domain.[72] This provides opportunities for self-interactions as well as for interactions with other matrix constituents, for example, collagens.[73] As discussed above, the matrilins appear to have a role in bridging, together with biglycan, from collagen VI-beaded filaments to other structural networks in the tissue. The variability of the matrilins is further accentuated by the identification of matrilin-1 and matrilin-3 subunits in the same molecule.[74]

Other proteins

There are a number of additional proteins in cartilage, whose functions have not been clearly defined. One of these is the matrix-Gla protein, which was originally isolated from bone.[75] Hypertrophic chondrocytes express collagen X that appears to form a network around the cells.[76] Also the hypertrophic chondrocytes express prominent bone proteins, for example, BSP (Bone Sialo Protein).[59]

Altered expression and abundance of the matrix proteins in disease

OA is a largely clinical diagnosis by patient history, X-ray, often joint instability, and pain. Since these features are only present late in the process and only then lead to patient awareness, very little is known about the early events in OA. Therefore, many studies of articular cartilage in OA have been focused on samples obtained at joint replacement surgery. Unfortunately, a misconception has made several investigators draw erroneous conclusions from studies of the cartilage with a fairly normal appearance, which is retained in severely affected joints. It is now clear that there is no normal cartilage in a diseased joint. Thus, an understanding of the early events in human OA, which may be amenable to therapeutic intervention, will only emerge from studies of other sources of diseased cartilage, that is, from non-symptomatic joints with very minor, early focal lesions.

We have recently been able to obtain such samples from the knee joints of patients undergoing amputation due to tumor in the extremities. Some of these samples from non-symptomatic patients have shown very early fibrillation and, in some cases, slight surface erosion. We could use these cartilage samples to quantitate changes in matrix constituents and also to identify altered metabolic events. It turns out that the tissue with slight surface fibrillation shows metabolic alterations similar to those in normal-looking cartilage from a severely affected joint, indicating that the biochemical abnormality affects all areas of the joint cartilage, and that these samples represent different stages of the same degenerative process (Lorenzo, Bayliss, and Heinegård, unpublished observation).

Collagen

One of the early identifiable events in developing OA appears to be an increasing volume of the tissue: that is, it swells. This can only be accomplished if the tensile properties of the collagen network become impaired, thereby preventing this structural element from resisting the swelling pressure generated by the osmotic properties of the aggrecan molecules. Thus, one of the early events in OA has to involve processes affecting the collagen network, although not necessarily the structure of the collagen fibers themselves. As is discussed below, this may emanate from processes affecting the molecules associated with the collagen fibril surface that are important for maintaining the network properties outlined in Figs 7.6 and 7.7.

Some of the initial alterations in OA, however, are found with regard to aggrecan molecules.

Aggrecan

Early in the development of osteoarthritic joint disease, the level of aggrecan in the tissue appears to change. These data are mostly inferred from histochemical studies, by staining with metachromatic and/or cationic dyes, that is, Toluidine blue, Safranin-O, or Ruthenium red. In our hands, however, although we see a pronounced reduction and altered distribution of such staining, the total amount of aggrecan in the tissue shows a rather minimal decrease (Lorenzo, Bayliss, and Heinegård, unpublished observation). At the same time, in other studies, we have shown a substantial release of proteoglycan fragments into synovial fluid in early OA.[24,77,78] Thus, it seems likely that early in OA the proteoglycans, which are lost from the tissue, are largely replaced by the chondrocytes, to maintain the overall tissue content. The altered histological staining pattern possibly indicates a redistribution of aggrecan in the various compartments, as a consequence of different rates of synthesis and degradation in each region of the tissue. It is of particular interest to note that similar alterations in staining can be obtained by simply immobilizing a joint.[79]

Another factor to take into account is that an early event in OA is tissue swelling, that is, increased tissue volume. It may be that the increased aggrecan synthesis reported does not result in higher concentrations of proteoglycans; while the total amount is higher, since it is present in a larger volume of tissue.

As is discussed elsewhere (Chapter 7.2.1.2), there is information accumulating on the character of the cleavage of aggrecan occurring in joint disease and, therefore, also the character of fragments of molecules released to the surrounding synovial fluid.

Matrix non-collagenous proteins

We have identified alterations in the metabolism of various matrix proteins occurring early in joint disease. A consistent finding is the increased synthesis of COMP, CILP, a recently described protein, (Asporin[28]), as well as of fibronectin (Lorenzo, Bayliss, and Heinegård, unpublished observations). An increased synthesis of fibronectin has previously been observed.[80] Furthermore, pronounced alterations were also observed in late disease, indicating that early changes are indeed part of the OA process. From studies of the distribution of the proteins in the cartilage, it appears that COMP is expressed by a novel population of cells in the deeper layers of the cartilage, and that these cells also express a high level of CILP (King, Lorenzo, Bayliss, and Heinegård, unpublished observations). These findings may, therefore, be an indication that some of the early responses in the OA process are initiated in the deeper layers of the cartilage rather than in the superficial zones.

It should be stressed, however, that at this stage of the disease we also find some surface fibrillation. This may result from degradation of the molecules linking the collagen fibrils, which interferes with their stability. This would result in a mechanically impaired collagen network, which in turn may yield surface fibrillations when the tissue is mechanically loaded (Fig. 7.7).

At the same time, we find alterations in the level of several matrix constituents. Thus, particularly the level of PRELP appears to decrease, whereas that of fibromodulin increases (Lorenzo, Bayliss, and Heinegård, unpublished observation). This increase would be consistent with an altered surface of the collagen fibrils and, therefore, altered tensile properties. It may be that their distribution in the tissue is altered, failing to provide the adequate properties of the various compartments.

It is apparent that studies of early events in the cartilage will provide essential information on the nature of the initial process. Thus, data are beginning to indicate that there is a fragmentation and a removal of matrix constituents from the articular cartilage at the same time as there is deposition of newly synthesized molecules to different compartments, for example, close to the cells. Also, the data suggests that there may be an unbalanced synthesis of new molecules in the attempted repair. Thus, COMP, when produced in large excesses, may actually prevent collagen fibrillogenesis impairing repair and accelerating tissue loss.

Therefore, a dual strategy in future therapeutic attempts may include prevention of fragmentation by proteinase inhibitors, concomitantly stimulating the synthesis of select matrix molecules to achieve a balance to repair attempts. This may be achieved by select growth factors, but today we are severely lacking in the knowledge necessary for us to make an educated guess about which ones are important.

One factor that should be considered in terms of modulating the progression of joint disease, is the situation with regard to the load of the joint. It is quite possible that the load produced by the normal activity of the individual may be harmful to the chondrocyte, when the tissue properties have been impaired by early events in the disease. It is apparent from published data from *in vitro* studies that the chondrocyte metabolism in the tissue can be extensively modulated by mechanical load.[81,82] Therefore, future directions should include studies of effects of mechanical load on the damaged cartilage.

Key points

1. The collagen fibrils are part of a network where individual fibers appear to contain a number of surface bound molecules that provide interactions and crossbridge to neighbouring fibrils. Turnover of collagen in cartilage is slow, while the network properties may be affected by the increased turnover of those molecules bound at the fibril surface. In pathology cartilage swelling and impaired function may be promoted by the degradation of molecules at the collagen fibril surface.

2. Aggrecan provides fixed negatively charged groups creating an osmotic active environment. Water is thereby retained and its flux is impaired conferring resistance to tissue compression.

3. Extracellular matrix proteins in cartilage have roles in modulating the assembly of structural proteins and cross linking networks formed, as well as in providing feedback to the chondrocytes on tissue structure and function.

References for further reading

D. Heinegård, A. Aspberg, A. Franzén, and P. Lorenzo. Non-collagenous glycoproteins in the extracellular matrix, with particular reference to cartilage and bone. In 'Extracellular matrix and inheritable disorders of connective tissue. 2nd edition' Eds. P. Royce and B. Steinmann. Wiley-Liss Inc, New York. In press.

An overview of matrix proteins discussing structure and functional properties. This book also contains review chapters on other aspects of matrix including collagens and cell binding proteins.

Biomechanics of diarthrodial joints. Vol I, part 2. Cartilage biomechanics. Eds. Van Mow, Anthony Ratcliffe and Savyo Woo, Springer-Verlag, New York, 1990.

This book contains a number of overview chapters on biomechanical properties of joints, including cartilage.

Kelley's textbook of rheumatology. Section I. Biology of the normal joint. Sixth edition Eds. Shaun Ruddy, Edward Harris and Clement Sledge, W.B. Saunders company, Philadelphia, 2001.

A book that contains reviews on a number of aspects of connective tissue, also extending into disease related problems.

Dynamics of bone and cartilage metabolism. Eds. Marcus Seibel, Simon Robins and John Bilezikian. Academic Press, London, 1999.

Overviews of many aspects of bone and cartilage.

References

1. Maroudas, A., Bayliss, M.T., Uchitel-Kaushansky, N., Schneiderman, R., and Gilav, E. (1998). Aggrecan turnover in human articular cartilage: use of aspartic acid racemization as a marker of molecular age. *Arch Biochem Biophys* **350**:61–71.

2. Maroudas, A., Palla, G., and Gilav, E. (1992). Racemization of aspartic acid in human articular cartilage. *Connect Tissue Res* **28**:161–9.

3. Van Der Rest, M. and Garrone, R. (1991). Collagen family of proteins. *FASEB J* **5**:2814–23.

4. Mendler, M., Eich-Bender, S.G., Vaughan, L., Winterhalter, K.H., and Bruckner, P. (1989). Cartilage contains mixed fibrils of collagen types II, IX, and XI. *J Cell Biol* **108**:191–7.

5. Aspden, R.M. and Hukins, D.W.L. (1989). Stress in collagen fibrils of articular cartilage calculated from their measured orientations. *Matrix* **9**:486–8.

6. Diab, M., Wu, J-J., and Eyre, D. (1996). Collagen type IX from human cartilage: a structural profile of intermolecular cross-linking sites. *Biochem J* **314**:327–32.

7. Hedlund, H., Mengarelli-Widholm, S., Heinegård, D., Reinholt, F., and Svensson, O. (1994). Fibromodulin distribution and association with collagen. *Matrix Biol* **14**:227–32.

8. Pringle, G. and Dodd, C. (1990). Immunoelectron microscopic localization of the core protein of decorin near the d and e bands of tendon collagen fibrils by use of monoclonal antibodies. *J Histochem Cytochem* **38**:1405–11.

9. Lamande, S.R., Sigalas, E., Pan, T.C., *et al.* (1998). The role of the α3VI chain in collagen VI assembly. Expression of an α3VI chain lacking N-terminal modules N10-N7 restores collagen VI assembly, secretion, and matrix deposition in an α3VI-deficient cell line. *J Biol Chem* **273**:7423–30.

10. Lamandé, S.R., Shields, K.A., Kornberg, A.J., Shield, L.K., and Bateman, J.F. (1999). Bethlem myopathy and engineered collagen VI triple helical deletions prevent intracellular multimer assembly and protein secretion. *J Biol Chem* **274**:21817–22.

11. Fitzgerald, J., Morgelin, M., Selan, C., *et al.* (2001). The N-terminal N5 subdomain of the α3VI chain is important for collagen VI microfibril formation. *J Biol Chem* **276**:187–93.

12. Oldberg, Å., Antonsson, P., and Heinegård, D. (1987). The partial amino acid sequence of bovine cartilage proteoglycan, deduced from a cDNA clone, contains numerous Ser-Gly sequences arranged in homologous repeats. *Biochem J* **243**:255–9.

13. Doege, K.J., Sasaki, M., Kimura, T., and Yamada, Y. (1991). Complete coding sequence and deduced primary structure of the human cartilage large aggregating proteoglycan, aggrecan. *J Biol Chem* **266**:894–902.

14. Antonsson, P., Heinegård, D., and Oldberg, Å. (1989). The keratan sulfate-enriched region of bovine cartilage proteoglycan consists of a consecutively repeated hexapeptide motif. *J Biol Chem* **264**:16170–3.

15. Heinegård, D. and Oldberg, Å. (1992). Glycosylated Matrix Proteins. In P. M. Royce and B. Steinmann (eds), *Connective Tissue and Its Heritable Disorders.* New York: Wiley-Liss, pp. 189–209.

16. Aspberg, A., Adam, S., Kostka, G., Timpl, R., and Heinegård, D. (1999). Fibulin-1 is a ligand for the C-type lectin domains of aggrecan and versican. *J Biol Chem* **274**:20444–9.

17. Olin, A.I., Mörgelin, M., Sasaki, T., Timpl, R., Heinegård, D., and Aspberg, A. (2001). The proteoglycans aggrecan and versican form networks with fibulin-2 through their lectin domain binding. *J Biol Chem* **276**: 1253–61.

18. Isogai, Z., Aspberg, A., Keene, D.R., Ono, R.N., Reinhardt, D.P., and Sakai, I.Y. (2002). Versican interacts with fibrillin-1 and links extracellular microfibrils to other connective tissue networks. *J Biol Chem* **277**:4565–72.

19. Aspberg, A., Miura, R., Bourdoulous, S., *et al.* (1997). The C-type lectin domains of lecticans, a family of aggregating chondroitin sulfate proteoglycans, bind tenascin-R by protein–protein interactions independent of carbohydrate moiety. *Proc Natl Acad Sci USA* **94**:10116–21.

20. Bayliss, M.T., Osborne, D., Woodhouse, S., and Davidson, C. (1999). Sulfation of chondroitin sulfate in human articular cartilage. *J Biol Chem* **274**:15892–900.

21. Roughley, P.J., White, R.J., and Poole, A.R. (1985). Identification of a hyaluronic acid–binding protein that interferes with the preparation of high-buoyant-density proteoglycan aggregates from adult human articular cartilage. *Biochem J* **231**:129–38.

22. Bayliss, M.T. (1990). Proteoglycan structure and metabolism during maturation and ageing of human articular cartilage. *Biochem Soc Trans* **18**:799–802.

23. Hardingham, T. and Bayliss, M. (1990). Proteoglycans of articular cartilage: changes in aging and in joint disease. *Semin Arthritis Rheum* **20**:12–33.

24. Heinegård, D., Inerot, S., Wieslander, J., and Lindblad, G. (1985). A method for the quantification of cartilage proteoglycan structures liberated to the synovial fluid during developing degenerative joint disease. *Scand J Clin Lab Invest* **45**:421–7.

25. Heinegård, D. and Saxne, T. (1991). Molecular markers of processes in cartilage in joint disease. *Br J Rheumatol* **30**(Suppl. 1):21–4.

26. Sandy, J.D., Flannery, C.R., Neame, P.J., and Lohmander, L.S. (1992). The structure of aggrecan fragments in human synovial fluid. Evidence for the involvement in osteoarthritis of a novel proteinase which cleaves the Glu 373-Ala 374 bond of the interglobular domain. *J Clin Invest* **89**:1512–6.

27. Kobe, B. and Deisenhofer, J. (1994). The leucine-rich repeat: a versatile binding motif. *TIBS* October:415–21.

28. Lorenzo, P., Aspberg, A., Önnerfjord, P., Bayliss, M., Neame, P., and Heinegård, D. (2001). Identification and characterization of asporin—a novel member of the leucine rich repeat protein family closely related to decorin and biglycan. *J Biol Chem* **276**:12201–11.

29. Antonsson, P., Heinegård, D., and Oldberg, Å. (1991). Posttranslational modifications of fibromodulin. *J Biol Chem* **266**:16859–61.

30. Bengtsson, E., Neame, P.J., Heinegård, D., and Sommarin, Y. (1995). The primary structure of a basic leucine-rich repeat protein, PRELP, found in connective tissues. *J Biol Chem* **270**:25639–44.

31. Neame, P.J., Sommarin, Y., Boynton, R.E., and Heinegård, D. (1994). The structure of a 38-kDa leucine-rich protein chondroadherin isolated from bovine cartilage. *J Biol Chem* **269**:21547–54.

32. Krusius, T. and Ruoslahti, E. (1986). Primary structure of an extracellular matrix proteoglycan core protein deduced from cloned cDNA. *Proc Natl Acad Sci* **83**:7683–7.

33. Hedbom, E. and Heinegård, D. (1993). Binding of fibromodulin and decorin to separate sites on fibrillar collagens. *J Biol Chem* **268**:27307–12.

34. Rada, J., Cornuet, P., and Hassell, J. (1993). Regulation of corneal collagen fibrillogenesis in vitro by corneal proteoglycan lumican and decorin core proteins. *Experimental Eye Research* **56**:635–48.

35. Bidanset, D.J., Guidry, C., Rosenberg, L.C., Choi, H.U., Timpl, R., and Hook, M. (1992). Binding of the proteoglycan decorin to collagen type VI. *J Biol Chem* **267**:5250–6.

36. Månsson, B., Wenglen, C., Mörgelin, M., Saxne, T., and Heinegård, D. (2001). Association of chondroadherin with collagen type II. *J Biol Chem* **276**:32883–8.

37. Wiberg, C., Hedbom, E., Khairullina, A., *et al.* (2001). Biglycan and decorin bind close to the n-terminal region of the collagen VI triple helix. *J Biol Chem* **276**:18947–52.

38. Danielson, K., Baribault, H., Holmes, D., Graham, H., Kadler, K., and Iozzo, R. (1997). Targeted disruption of decorin leads to abnormal collagen fibril morphology and skin fragility. *J Cell Biol* **136**:729–43.

39. Vogel, K.G., Paulsson, M., and Heinegård, D. (1984). Specific inhibition of type I and type II collagen fibrillogenesis by the small proteoglycan of tendon. *Biochem J* **223**:587–97.

40. Svensson, L., Aszodi, A., Reinholt, F.P., Fässler, R., Heinegård, D., and Oldberg, Å. (1999). Fibromodulin-null mice have abnormal collagen fibrils, tissue organization, and altered lumican deposition in tendon. *J Biol Chem* **274**:9636–47.

41. Svensson, L., Narlid, I., and Oldberg, A. (2000). Fibromodulin and lumican bind to the same region on collagen type I fibrils. *FEBS Lett* **470**:178–82.

42. Camper, L., Heinegård, D., and Lundgren-Åkerlund, E. (1997). Integrin $\alpha 2\beta 1$ is a receptor for the cartilage matrix protein chondroadherin. *J Cell Biol* **138**:1159–67.

43. Camper, L., Holmvall, K., Wangnerud, C., Aszodi, A., and Lundgren-Akerlund E. (2001). Distribution of the collagen-binding integrin a $\alpha 10\beta 1$ during mouse development. *Cell Tissue Res* **306**:107–16.

44. Woods Jr., V.L., Schreck, P.J., Gesink, D.S., *et al.* (1994). Integrin expression by human articular chondrocytes. *Arthritis Rheum* **37**:537–44.

45. Sommarin, Y., Larsson, T., and Heinegård, D. (1989). Chondrocyte-matrix interactions. Attachment to proteins isolated from cartilage. *Exp Cell Res* **184**:181–92.

46. Shen, Z., Gantcheva, S., Månsson, B., Heinegård, D., and Sommarin, Y. (1998). Chondroadherin expression changes in skeletal development. *Biochem J* **330**(Pt 1):549–57.

47. Bengtsson, E., Aspberg, A., Heinegård, D., Sommarin, Y., and Spillmann, D. (2000). The amino-terminal part of PRELP binds to heparin and heparan sulfate. *J Biol Chem* **275**:40695–702.

48. Sommarin, Y. and Heinegård, D. (1986). Four classes of cell-associated proteoglycans in suspension cultures of articular-cartilage chondrocytes. *Biochem J* **233**:809–18.

49. Bengtsson, E., Mörgelin, M., Sasaki, T., Timpl, R., Heinegård, D., and Aspberg, A. (2002). The Leucine-rich repeat protein PRELP binds perlecan and collagens and may function as a basement membrane anchor. *J Biol Chem* **277**:15061–8.

50. Burton-Wurster, N. and Lust, G. (1989). Molecular and immunologic differences in canine fibronectins from articular cartilage and plasma. *Arch Biochem Biophys* **269**(1):32–45.

51. Uporova, T.M., Norton, P.A., Tuan, R.S., and Bennett, V.D. (1999). Alternative splicing during chondrogenesis: cis and trans factors involved in splicing of fibronectin exon EIIIA. *J Cell Biochem* **76**:341–51.

52. Burton-Wurster, N. and Lust, G. (1985). Deposition of fibronectin in articular cartilage of canine osteoarthritic joints. *Am J Vet Res* **46**:2542–5.

53. Oldberg, Å., Antonsson, P., Lindblom, K., and Heinegård, D. (1992). COMP cartilage oligomeric matrix protein is structurally related to the thrombospondins. *J Biol Chem* **267**:22346–50.

54. DiCesare, P., Mörgelin, M., Mann, K., and Paulsson, M. (1994). Cartilage oligomeric matrix protein and thrombospondin 1. Purification from articular cartilage, electron microscopic structure, and chondrocyte binding. *Eur J Biochem* **223**:927–37.

55. Tucker, R.P., Hagios, C., Chiquet–Ehrismann, R., and Lawler, J. (1997). In situ localization of thrombospondin-1 and thrombospondin-3 transcripts in the avian embryo. *Dev Dyn* **208**:326–37.

56. Rosenberg, K., Olsson, H., Mörgelin, M., and Heinegård, D. (1998). Cartilage oligomeric matrix protein shows high affinity zinc-dependent interaction with triple helical collagen. *J Biol Chem* **273**:20397–403.

57. Thur, J., Rosenberg, K., Nitsche, D.P., *et al.* (2001). Mutations in cartilage oligomeric matrix protein causing pseudoachondroplasia and multiple epiphyseal dysplasia affect binding of calcium and collagen I, II, and IX. *J Biol Chem* **276**:6083–92.

58. Wu, J.J., Woods, P.E., and Eyre, D.R. (1992). Identification of cross-linking sites in bovine cartilage type IX collagen reveals an antiparallel type II-type IX molecular relationship and type IX to type IX bonding. *J Biol Chem* **267**:23007–14.

59. Shen, Z., Heinegård, D., and Sommarin, Y. (1995). Distribution and expression of cartilage oligomeric matrix protein and bone sialoprotein show marked changes during rat femoral head development. *Matrix Biol* **14**:773–81.

60. Briggs, M.D., Hoffman, S.M.G., King, L.M., *et al.* (1995). Pseudoachondroplasia and multiple epiphyseal dysplasia due to mutations in the cartilage oligomeric matrix protein gene. *Nat Genet* **10**:330–6.

61. Hecht, J.T., Montufar-Solis, D., Decker, G., Lawler, J., Daniels, K., and Duke, P.J. (1998). Retention of cartilage oligomeric matrix protein COMP and cell death in redifferentiated pseudoachondroplasia chondrocytes. *Matrix Biol* **17**:625–33.

62. Lorenzo, P., Bayliss, M.T., and Heinegård, D. (1998). A novel cartilage protein CILP present in the mid-zone of human articular cartilage increases with age. *J Biol Chem* **273**:23463–8.

63. Lorenzo, P., Neame, P., Sommarin, Y., and Heinegård, D. (1998). Cloning and deduced amino acid sequence of a novel cartilage protein CILP identifies a proform including a nucleotide pyrophosphohydrolase. *J Biol Chem* **273**:23469–75.

64. Hopf, M., Gohring, W., Kohfeldt, E., Yamada, Y., and Timpl, R. (1999). Recombinant domain IV of perlecan binds to nidogens, laminin-nidogen complex, fibronectin, fibulin-2 and heparin. *Eur J Biochem* **259**:917–25.

65. SundarRaj, N., Fite, D., Ledbetter, S., Chakravarti, S., and Hassell, J.R. (1995). Perlecan is a component of cartilage matrix and promotes chondrocyte attachment. *J Cell Sci* **108**(Pt 7):2663–72.

66. Iozzo, R.V., Cohen, I.R., Grassel, S., and Murdoch, A.D. (1994). The biology of perlecan: the multifaceted heparan sulphate proteoglycan of basement membranes and pericellular matrices. *Biochem J* **302**(Pt 3):625–39.

67. Arikawa-Hirasawa, E., Watanabe, H., Takami, H., Hassell, J.R., and Yamada, Y. (1999). Perlecan is essential for cartilage and cephalic development. *Nat Genet* **23**:354–8.

68. Costell, M., Gustafsson, E., Aszodi, A., *et al.* (1999). Perlecan maintains the integrity of cartilage and some basement membranes. *J Cell Biol* **147**:1109–22.

69. Paulsson, M. and Heinegård, D. (1981). Purification and structural characterization of a cartilage matrix protein. *Biochem J* **197**:367–75.

70. Klatt, A.R., Nitsche, D.P., Kobbe, B., Morgelin, M., Paulsson, M., and Wagener, R. (2000). Molecular structure and tissue distribution of matrilin-3, a filament-forming extracellular matrix protein expressed during skeletal development. *J Biol Chem* **275**:3999–4006.

71. Paulsson, M. and Heinegård, D. (1982). Radioimmunoassay of the 148-kilodalton cartilage protein. Distribution of the protein among bovine tissues. *Biochem J* **207**:207–13.

72. Deak, F., Wagener, R., Kiss, I., and Paulsson, M. (1999). The matrilins: a novel family of oligomeric extracellular matrix proteins. *Matrix Biol* **18**:55–64.

73. Tondravi, M.M., Winterbottom, N., Haudenschild, D.R., and Goetinck, P.F. (1993). Cartilage matrix protein binds to collagen and plays a role in collagen fibrillogenesis. *Prog Clin Biol Res* **383**(B):515–22.

74. Wu, J.J. and Eyre, D.R. (1998). Matrilin-3 forms disulfide-linked oligomers with matrilin-1 in bovine epiphyseal cartilage. *J Biol Chem* **273**: 17433–8.

75. Hale, J.E., Fraser, J.D., and Price, P.A. (1988). The identification of matrix Gla protein in cartilage. *J Biol Chem* **263**:5820–4.

76. LuValle, P., Daniels, K., Hay, E.D., and Olsen, B.R. (1992). Type X collagen is transcriptionally activated and specifically localized during sternal cartilage maturation. *Matrix* **12**:404–13.

77. Saxne, T., Wollheim, F., Pettersson, H., and Heinegård, D. (1987). Proteoglycan concentration in synovial fluid: predictor of future cartilage destruction in rheumatoid arthritis? *Br Med J Clin Res Ed* **295**:1447–8.

78. Dahlberg, L., Ryd, L., Heinegård, D., and Lohmander, L.S. (1992). Proteoglycan fragments in joint fluid. Influence of arthrosis and inflammation. *Acta Orthop Scand* **63**:417–23.

79. Palmoski, M., Perricone, E., and Brandt, K.D. (1979). Development and reversal of a proteoglycan aggregation defect in normal canine knee cartilage after immobilization. *Arthritis Rheum* **22**(5):508–17.

80. Lust, G., Burton-Wurster, N., and Leipold, H. (1987). Fibronectin as a marker for osteoarthritis. *J Rheumatol* **14**(Spec No):28–9.

81. Sah, R.L., Kim, Y.J., Doong, J.Y., Grodzinsky, A.J., Plaas, A.H., and Sandy, J.D. (1989). Biosynthetic response of cartilage explants to dynamic compression. *J Orthop Res* **7**:619–36.

82. Larsson, T., Aspden, R.M., and Heinegård, D. (1991). Effects of mechanical load on cartilage matrix biosynthesis in vitro. *Matrix* **11**:388–94.

7.2.1.2 Proteolytic degradation of normal and osteoarthritic cartilage matrix

John D. Sandy

Proteinases and osteoarthritis

The pathogenesis of OA can be considered[1] as a process involving changes in a synovial joint, which are due to the presence of factors (diffusional and biomechanical) that are driving degradation in focal areas of articular cartilage, and also promoting attempted repair in the cartilage, subchondral bone, and soft tissues. The main clinical problems are pain and disability, and the long-term outcome for the patient (which can vary from reasonable mobility to total loss of joint function) appears to depend on the overall balance of degradation and repair. The degradation of cartilage may first be observed macroscopically as a fibrillated surface region but in focal areas this can often progress to full depth loss of the tissue and exposure of the underlying bone.

While the end-stage of this process (involving gross loss of tissue integrity with deep surface fissuring and exposure of subchondral bone) may be aggravated by the abnormal biomechanics associated with joint deformity, it is now clear that the early- and mid-stages (before 'tissue-level' damage is evident) are characterized by a series of 'molecular-level' degradative events that are catalyzed by proteolytic enzymes with the capacity to degrade, disorganize, and release to the synovial fluid fragments of the macromolecular components of the cartilage matrix.

This chapter will review the current state of knowledge on the proteolytic enzymes involved in this early-stage molecular process. It will include a discussion of the identity of the individual proteinases present in cartilage, their known major substrates, their transcriptional control, the critical role of enzyme activation events, and the knowledge of natural inhibitors.

This review develops the theme that a very limited repertoire of proteinases is required to achieve the pathologic destruction of the cartilage matrix and irreversible loss of the tissue. Specifically, the available literature leads to the conclusion that possibly only two metallo-proteinases, ADAMTS4 (aggrecanase-1) and MMP13 (collagenase-3) are required and are indeed primarily responsible for this process.

Cartilage proteinases, cartilage matrix substrates and cleavage sites

A summary of all the proteinases which have been identified (by immunological methods and, in most cases, also by mRNA identification) in cartilage sections, cartilage extracts, cartilage-conditioned medium or primary cultures of chondrocytes, are listed in Tables 7.1–7.3. The enzymes are grouped into the MMPs (Table 7.1), the ADAMTSs (a disintegrin and metalloproteinase with thrombospondin-like motifs, Table 7.2) and all other proteinases (metallo-, cysteine, serine, and aspartic, Table 7.3). For

Table 7.1 Matrix metallo-proteinases

MMPs in cartilage (recent references)	Cleavage site(s) in human cartilage proteins followed by references to cleavage site data and recent references to substrate structures
MMP1[27,70,71] Collagenase 1	Gly975–Leu976 (primary)[72] of collagen II[73]
	Gly978–Gln979 (secondary)[7] of collagen II[73]
	Asn341–Phe342[74] of aggrecan[2,75]
	Asp441–Leu442[74] of aggrecan[2,75]
	Val447–Ala448* of aggrecan[2,75]
	Gly656–Ileu657* of aggrecan[2,75]
	His16–Ileu17[76] of link protein[77]
MMP2[27,70,71,78] Gelatinase A	Gly978–Gln979 (secondary)[7] of collagen II[73]
	Gly980–Ileu981 (tertiary)[7] of collagen II[73]
	Asn341–Phe342[74] of aggrecan[2,75]
	His16–Ileu17[76] of link protein[77]
	Leu25–Leu26[76] of link protein[77]
MMP3[27,70,71] Stromelysin 1	Gly978–Gln979 (secondary)[7] of collagen II[73]
	Ala195–Gln196 (telopeptidase)[79] of collagen II[73]
	Val198–Met199 (telopeptidase)[79] of collagen IX[73]
	Ser780–Leu781[79] of collagen IX[73]
	Ala518–Ileu519 (telopeptidase)[79] of collagen IX[73]
	Asn341–Phe342[41] of aggrecan[2,75]
	His16–Ileu17[76] of link protein[77]
MMP8[27,71] Collagenase 2	Gly975–Leu976 (primary)[72] of collagen II[73]
	Gly978–Gln979 (secondary)[7] of collagen II[73]
	Asn341–Phe342[74] of aggrecan[2,75]
	Asp441–Leu442[74] of aggrecan[2,75]
	Glu373–Ala374[80] of aggrecan[2,75]
MMP9[27,70] Gelatinase B	Gly978–Gln979 (secondary)[7] of collagen II[73]
	Gly980–Ileu981 (tertiary)[7] of collagen II[73]
	Asn341–Phe342[74] of aggrecan[2,75]
	His16–Ileu17[76] of link protein[77]
MMP10[81] Stromelysin 2	His16–Ileu17[76] of link protein[77]
MMP13[27,70,71] Collagenase 3	Gly975–Leu976 (primary)[7] of collagen II[73]
	Gly978–Gln979 (secondary)[7] of collagen II[73]
	Gly981–Ileu982 (tertiary)[7] of collagen II[73]
	Asn341–Phe342[82] of aggrecan[2,75]
	Pro384–Val385[82] of aggrecan[2,75]
MMP14 (MT1-MMP)[70,71]	Gly975–Leu976 (primary)[83] of collagen II[73]
	Gly978–Gln979 (secondary)[7] of collagen II[73]
	Asn341–Phe342[84,82] of aggrecan[2,75]
	Glu373–Ala374 (61) of aggrecan[2,75]

* Flannery, C. and Sandy, J. (unpublished)

Aggrecan residue numbers are human data and were obtained by the subtraction of 19 (leader sequence) from the numbers given in Ref. 68. Link protein numbers were obtained by the subtraction of 15 (leader sequence) from the numbers given in Ref. 69.

Table 7.2 A disintegrin and metallo-proteinase with thrombospondin-like motifs

ADAMTSs in cartilage (recent references)	Cleavage site(s) in human cartilage proteins followed by references to cleavage site data and references to substrate structures
ADAMTS1* METH-1	Glu1919–Leu1920[46] of aggrecan[2,75]
	Glu1714–Gly1715[100] of aggrecan[2,75]
	Glu1539–Gly1540[100] of aggrecan[2,75]
	Glu373–Ala374[49] of aggrecan[2,75]
	Glu441–Ala442[49] of versican V1[85]
ADAMTS2 Procollagen-N-proteinase	Ala181–Gln182[86] of collagen II[73]
ADAMTS3 Procollagen-N-proteinase	Ala181–Gln182[86] of collagen II[73]
ADAMTS4* Aggrecanase-1	Glu1919–Leu1920[47] of aggrecan[2,75]
	Glu1819–Ala1820[47] of aggrecan[2,75]
	Glu1714–Gly1715[47] of aggrecan[2,75]
	Glu1539–Gly1540[47] of aggrecan[2,75]
	Glu373–Ala374[47] of aggrecan[2,75]
	Asn341–Phe342[101] of aggrecan[2,75]
	Glu441–Ala442[49] of versican V1[85]
ADAMTS5* Aggrecanase-2	Glu373–Ala374[62] of aggrecan[2,75]

* Protein detected by Western analysis, Gao, G. and Sandy, J. (unpublished)

Aggrecan residue numbers are human data and were obtained by the subtraction of 19 (leader sequence) from the numbers given in Ref. 68. Link protein numbers were obtained by the subtraction of 15 (leader sequence) from the numbers given in Ref. 69.

Table 7.3 Other proteinases

Other proteinases in cartilage (recent references)	Cleavage site(s) in human cartilage proteins followed by references to cleavage site data and references to substrate structures
Metallo-proteinase Procollagen-C-endopeptidase BMP-1[87]	Ala1241–Asp1242[87] of collagen II[73]
Cysteine proteinases Cathepsin B[88]	Gly344–Val345[90] of aggrecan[2,75]
	Gly344–Val345 (endopeptidase)[91] of aggrecan[2,75]
	Asn341–Phe342 (exopeptidase)[91] of aggrecan[2,75]
Calpain [89]	Ala690–Ala691* of aggrecan[2,75]
	Thr447–Ala448* of aggrecan[2,75]
Serine Proteinases Plasmin[92]	Arg375–Ser376† of aggrecan[2,75]
Plasminogen activator[92]	Val378–Ileu379† of aggrecan[2,75]
Aspartic Proteinases Cathepsin D[93]	Trp680–Ileu681† of aggrecan[2,75]

* Suzuki, K., Neame, P.J., Sandy, J.D. (unpublished)

† Flannery, C. and Sandy, J. (unpublished)

Aggrecan residue numbers are human data and were obtained by the subtraction of 19 (leader sequence) from the numbers given in Ref. 68. Link protein numbers were obtained by the subtraction of 15 (leader sequence) from the numbers given in Ref. 69.

each of the 19 proteinases listed (8 MMPs, 5 ADAMTS and 6 others) the established cleavage site(s) in human cartilage proteins are also provided along with primary references to cleavage site data and recent references to substrate structures in human cartilage. The information in Tables 7.1–7.3, therefore, establishes the identity of the proteinases for which there is at least indirect evidence for a role in cartilage matrix proteolysis, and summarizes the current state of knowledge on the cleavage specificity of these enzymes for the substrates that have been studied (collagen II, collagen IX, aggrecan, link protein, and versican).

Proteolytic cleavages that have been shown by direct analysis to occur *in situ*

Demonstrating the presence of a particular proteinase and an appropriate substrate in cartilage matrix (Tables 7.1–7.3) clearly does not establish that this reaction occurs *in situ*. Determining whether a particular proteolytic event actually occurs *in vivo* has required the development of novel reagents and methods. In most cases the products have been identified by N-terminal sequencing and/or by reactivity with antibodies that have been raised to the neo-epitopes (C-terminal and/or N-terminal) generated on cleavage of the protein at the specific sites of interest.

In this regard, it appears to have been assumed widely that a particular cleavage occurs in articular cartilage matrix *in situ* if the products can be demonstrated to be present in one or more of the following situations: (1) in sections of freshly excised and fixed tissue, (2) in fresh extracts of cartilage or synovial fluid collected in the presence of proteinase inhibitors, or (3) in the products of articular cartilage explant cultures, where products were collected in the presence of proteinase inhibitors. Within these criteria, the present list of established *in situ* cleavages (four for collagen II, six for aggrecan, and one for link protein) is detailed in Table 7.4. The referenced information provided for each cleavage site (A through K) includes the methods used for detection and the source of the products analyzed.

An examination of the eleven established *in vivo* cleavages shows that in some cases (C, D, E, G, H, I, J, K) the proteolysis involved appears to be part of the biosynthetic process, in which precursor forms of the matrix protein are 'tailored' for optimal association, assembly, and function in the matrix. On the other hand, in other cases (A, B, F) the cleavages are clearly destructive since they generate products that are rendered diffusible by the cleavage and are therefore lost from the tissue. Thus, in terms of non-destructive cleavage, it is generally agreed that cleavage of procollagen II at Ala181–Gln182 (cleavage C, Table 7.4) and at Ala1241–Asp1242 (cleavage D, Table 7.4), to remove the N-terminal propeptide and C-terminal propeptides, respectively, are highly regulated processes required for the generation of the triple-helical species that can assemble into multi-molecular fibrillar structures. In a similar fashion, the heterogeneity of aggrecan core protein size in normal mature articular cartilage is clearly due to the proteolytic removal of variable amounts of the GAG-bearing domains toward the C-terminal. This heterogeneity occurs early in growth[2] and can therefore be viewed as a non-destructive 'tailoring' of aggrecan for optimal function. While this C-terminal truncation of aggrecan has been described and its origin discussed for many years[2,3] the precise C-terminii and the proteinase(s) responsible for the generation of these products still remain unsolved.[2] In this regard, a very minor percentage of the matrix aggrecan, which has been C-terminally truncated, is generated by ADAMTS activity at the Glu1714–Gly1715 site (cleavage I, Table 7.4) and the Glu1539–Gly1540 site (cleavage J, Table 7.4).[2] In the same way, normal growing and mature articular cartilages contain a significant proportion of the aggrecan in the G1-VDIPEN and G1-NITEGE forms, generated by the interglobular domain cleavage at the Asn341–Phe342 (cleavage E, Table 7.4) and Glu373–Ala374 (cleavage F, Table 7.4) sites, respectively. These species therefore appear to result from non-destructive processing during growth, although it is also clear that in adulthood they are also products of destructive proteolysis initiated by cytokines or joint injury. Link protein cleavage at the His16–Ileu17 bond (cleavage K, Table 7.4) also appears to represent a non-destructive post-translational event, which results in a product that is highly suited to its role in the stabilization of aggregates between aggrecan and hyaluronan.

In contrast to these 'tailoring' events for collagen, aggrecan, and link protein there are cleavages that are almost certainly 'destructive' and which lead to denaturation and loss of matrix components. For example, the accelerated destruction of cartilage collagen II, which accompanies ACL rupture[4] and late

Table 7.4 Proteolytic cleavage sites for cartilage matrix proteins which occur *in vivo*

A. Triple helical cleavage of collagen II by MMP1, 8, 13 and 14 at Gly975–Leu976 (Fig. 7.10)

Detected by immunoassays (COL2-3/4Cshort) for the C-terminal neo-epitope in cartilage[6], by immunoassays (9A4 and 5109) for the C-terminal neo-epitope in cartilage[94] and by N-terminal sequencing and immunodetection with N-terminal neo-epitope antisera MV-1[7] and COL2-1/4N1[6] in cartilage.

B. Triple helical cleavage of collagen II by MMP1, 2, 3, 8, 9, 13 at Gly978–Gln979 (secondary) (Fig. 7.10)

Detected by immunoassay with antibody MV-2[7] for the N-terminal neo-epitope in OA cartilage and by N-terminal sequencing in cartilage.[7,95]

C. Procollagen cleavage of collagen II at N-propeptide, Ala181– Gln182 by ADAMTS 3 (Fig. 7.10)

Detected by N-terminal sequencing of extracted cartilage collagen.[79]

D. Procollagen cleavage of collagen II by BMP-1 at C-propeptide Ala1241–Asp1242 (Fig. 7.10)

Detected by N-terminal sequencing of extracted cartilage C-propeptide.[96,97]

E. Interglobular domain cleavage of aggrecan by MMP1, 2, 3, 8, 9, 13, 14, ADAMTS4 and Cathepsin B at Asn341–Phe342 (Fig. 7.11)

Detected by immunoassays for the C-terminal neo-epitope in cartilage[98], by isolation of the C-terminal peptide in cartilage[41] and by immunoassay for the N-terminal neo-epitope in synovial fluid.[99]

F. Interglobular domain cleavage of aggrecan by MMP 8, 14 and ADAMTS1, 4, 5 at Glu373–Ala374 (Fig. 7.11)

Detected by N-terminal sequencing in cartilage explants and synovial fluid[42,45], by immunoassays for the C-terminal neo-epitope in cartilage[98] and synovial fluid[2] and by immunoassays for the N-terminal neo-epitope in cartilage explants[63] and human synovial fluid.[2]

G. Chondroitin sulfate attachment region cleavage of aggrecan by ADAMTS1, 4 at Glu1919–Leu1920 (Fig. 7.11)

Detected by N-terminal sequencing in cartilage explants[43,64], by immunoassay for the N-terminal neo-epitope in synovial fluid[2] and by immunoassay for the C-terminal neo-epitope in chondrosarcoma.[65]

H. Chondroitin sulfate attachment region cleavage of aggrecan by ADAMTS4 at Glu1819–Ala1820. (Fig. 7.11)

Detected by N-terminal sequencing in cartilage explants[43,64] and by immunoassay for the C-terminal neo-epitope in chondrosarcoma.[65]

I. Chondroitin sulfate attachment region cleavage of aggrecan by ADAMTS1, 4 at Glu1714–Gly1715 (Fig. 7.11)

Detected by N-terminal sequencing in cartilage explants[43] and by immunoassay for the C-terminal neo-epitope in chondrosarcoma[65], human cartilage[2], and synovial fluids.[2]

J. Chondroitin sulfate attachment region cleavage of aggrecan by ADAMTS1, 4 at Glu1539–Gly1540 (Fig. 7.11)

Detected by N-terminal sequencing in cartilage explants[43] by immunoassay for the C-terminal neo-epitope in chondrosarcoma[65], human cartilage[2], and synovial fluids.[2]

K. N-terminal extension region cleavage of link protein by MMP-1, 2, 3, 9, 10 at His16–Ileu17 (Fig. 7.11)

Detected by N-terminal sequencing of link protein extracted from cartilage[77] and by immunoassay of the N-terminal neo-epitope with antibody CH-3.[76]

stage human OA,[5,6] can be largely, if not entirely, attributed to cleavage at the classical collagenase-sensitive bond (Glu975–Leu976, cleavage A, Table 7.4 and Fig. 7.10). This cleavage can be catalyzed, *in vitro*, by MMPs 1, 8, 13, or 14. The secondary cleavage at Gly978–Gln979 (cleavage B, Table 7.4 and

Fig. 7.10), which has also been detected in OA cartilage,[7] has been demonstrated as generated *in vitro* with MMP13 alone and also with a combination of MMPs 1 and 3, whereas MMP-1 alone was not effective. Thus, the destructive cleavage of collagen *in vivo* could be most simply explained by the individual or combined actions of MMPs 1, 8, 13, and 14 (see Fig. 7.10).

The accelerated destruction of aggrecan, which accompanies joint injury and late stage human osteoarthritis[2] appears, at present, to be entirely due to an enhanced activity of 'aggrecanase'-mediated cleavage at Glu1919–Leu1920 (cleavage G, Table 7.4), Glu1714–Gly1715 (cleavage I, Table 7.4), Glu1539–Gly1540 (cleavage J, Table 7.4), and Glu373–Ala374 (cleavage F, Table 7.4). This 'aggrecanase' activity appears to be due to one or more members of the ADAMTS family of proteinases. Thus, all four of these cleavages are shown to be catalyzed by ADAMTS4, and both ADAMTS1 and ADAMTS5 can cleave at the highly destructive Glu373–Ala374 site (see Fig. 7.11). The products of

the fifth ADAMTS4-mediated cleavage site at Glu1819–Ala1820 (cleavage H, Table 7.4), have been detected in cartilage explants and chondrosarcoma aggrecan but so far not in human OA, probably because these products are further degraded or removed rapidly *in vivo*.

Which collagenase is actually responsible for cartilage matrix degradation?

While all of the collagenases, MMPs 1, 8, 13, and 14, can cleave collagen II at the destructive Glu975–Leu976 site there is now an accumulating body of evidence, both indirect and direct, which implicates MMP13 as the 'actual' collagenase responsible for initiating collagenolysis in articular cartilage. Before reviewing this data, it should be noted that a large number of studies

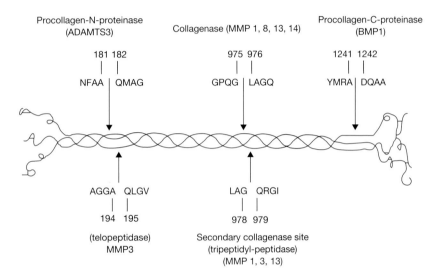

Fig. 7.10 Five proteolytic cleavage sites in collagen II are shown with the cleavage sequences, the human residue numbers, and the proteinases, which have been shown to be active at these sites. See the text, Tables 7.1–7.4 for details and references.

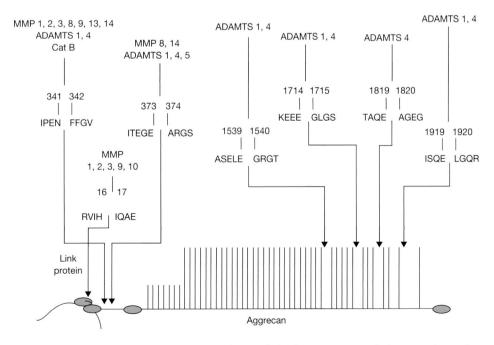

Fig. 7.11 Six proteolytic cleavage sites in aggrecan and one in link protein are shown with the cleavage sequences, the human residue numbers, and the proteinases, which have been shown to be active at these sites. See the text, Tables 7.1–7.4 for details and references.

in this area have used what are known as 'denaturation' epitopes to detect the unwinding of the triple helix of collagen II in cartilage *in situ*.[4] While it appears likely that these denaturation epitopes are exposed following cleavage at the Glu975–Leu976 bond, these papers do not provide specific details of the proteolytic events, and therefore they will not be discussed in detail here.

While each of the classical collagenases (MMP1, 8, 13, and 14) as well as MMP2, MMP3, and MMP9, may each promote cartilage collagenolysis in some situations, the weight of evidence suggesting a central and initiating role for MMP13 in the destruction of collagen II in OA is persuasive. This evidence comes from studies with proteinase inhibitors, immunolocalization of MMP proteins, and *in situ* hybridization for a range of MMP transcripts. Studies on explants of human normal and OA cartilage with an MMP inhibitor (RS102,481), which is potent for MMP8 and MMP13 but relatively ineffective against MMP-1, have suggested that MMP8 or 13, but not MMP-1, are responsible for the generation of the Gly975–Leu976 cleavage site.[5,8] While the sensitivity of MMP14 to RS102,481 was not described, this is thought to be primarily a cell-surface associated enzyme, which is therefore unlikely to be involved in cleavage of bulk collagen in the intercellular spaces of cartilage matrix. In addition, MMP14 does not appear to be involved in matrix degradation in human OA since mRNA levels were unchanged in tissues undergoing high rates of collagenolysis.[9] On the other hand, it appears that MMP13 is involved in cartilage resorption *in vivo* during bone growth[10] since it colocalizes with MMP2, which can be shown to be active by specific inhibition on gelatin histozymography. *In situ* zymography also showed collagen II degrading activity over chondrocytes in osteoarthritic cartilage, and this activity was shown to correlate in site and amount with cartilage lesion progression and in all situations to codistribute with MMP-13 mRNA expression.[11] In other work it was shown that IL13 can prevent the release of collagen from bovine nasal cartilage treated with IL-1 and that this protective effect was accompanied by a down regulation of MMP13 mRNA but an increase in MMP1 mRNA, consistent with an active role for MMP13 but not MMP1. Further, support for the central role of MMP13 has been obtained from a transgenic mouse

overexpressing MMP13 in which the end result was articular cartilage degradation and joint pathology reminiscent of human OA.[12] In summary, high levels of MMP13 mRNA and protein appear to be localized to areas of high collagenolytic activity. Moreover, hMMP13 is 5–10 times as active as hMMP1 in its ability to digest type II collagen suggesting that MMP13 has a unique role in collagen II-rich tissues such as articular cartilage.[13]

In further support of this idea, studies on the signaling events associated with MMP13 gene induction are also consistent with its involvement in cartilage pathology. Thus, in rat adjuvant-induced arthritis, a potent c-Jun N-terminal kinase (JNK) inhibitor (SP600125) suppressed both AP-1 binding and collagenase-3 mRNA accumulation and protected against radiographic joint damage.[14] This central role for the JNK pathway is supported by the finding that the hepatocyte growth factor (HGF) stimulated MMP13 production in human OA chondrocytes at the transcriptional level, and this induction was mediated by the activation of the stress-activated protein kinase (SAPK)/(JNK) pathway.[15] The conclusion that SP600125 is protective due to its blockade of MMP13 induction is also consistent with the independent observation that both JNK and NF-kappaB are required for the IL-1 induction of MMP-13.[16]

Cellular control of the activity of MMP13 *in situ*

Given the apparent central role for MMP13 in cartilage collagenolysis[5,17–20] it becomes important to review the information available on the different control mechanisms that are thought to operate *in situ* to modulate this activity (see schematic on Fig. 7.12).

It is now clear[21] that transcription of the MMP13 gene is regulated through the mitogen-activated protein kinase (MAPK) pathway, which includes the JNKs, the extracellular signal-regulated kinases (ERKs) and the p38 kinases. Indeed, the recent availability of SP 600125, a selective inhibitor of the JNKs,[14] along with PD98059 (an inhibitor of the ERK

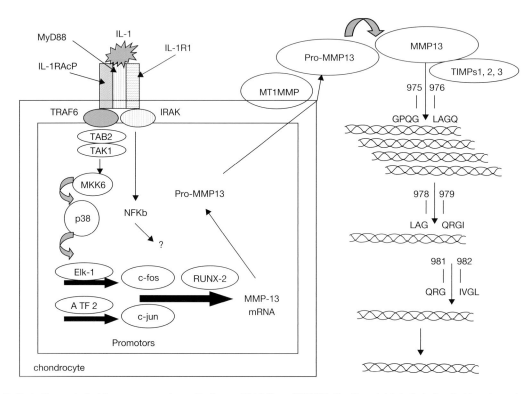

Fig. 7.12 Schematic illustrating control of the gene expression, activation, and inhibition of MMP13. The three triple helical sites that have been shown as cleaved by MMP13 are shown. See the text, Tables 7.1–7.4 for details and references.

pathway) and SB203580 (a p38 kinase inhibitor) has led to the conclusion[21] that cytokine activation of MMP13 in chondrocytic cells appears to be primarily p38 dependent (see Fig. 7.12), much as has also been shown in human fetal skin fibroblasts.[22] Upregulation of NFKb is also involved, however the precise transcriptional control events are unclear.[21] On the other hand there is increasing evidence that the p38-dependent pathway involves the DNA binding of a chondrocyte/osteoblast-specific transcription factor RUNX-2.[23,24]

Transcriptional activation of MMP13 by cytokines,[16] TGF beta or perhaps biomechanical factors[26] appears to be associated with areas of degraded cartilage matrix in osteoarthritic tissue[27] consistent with the idea that increased synthesis of MMP13 is also accompanied by an increased local activity of this proteinase in the tissue. An increased supply of pro-MMP13 will result in high activity if it is accompanied by an efficient activation process. Such activation of pro-MMP13 most likely involves a cell surface process requiring MT1MMP[28,29] so that the level of active MMP13 will likely be determined, to some extent, by the production of MT1MMP and its activation. Activation of MMP13 may indeed be part of a cascade involving not only MT1MMP but also cell surface plasmin and the interdependent activation of MMP2, MMP3, and MMP9.[29] Since MT1MMP appears to be critical to this process, work has also focused on the control of expression and the mechanism of activation of pro-MT1MMP. While OA and normal human articular chondrocytes appear to express similar message levels for MT1MMP,[9] the level of active protein on the chondrocyte surface may depend on the rate of removal of the prodomain by an unknown furin/prohormone convertase-like activity.[29] A third level of control of MMP13 activity in cartilage matrix is most likely exerted through the abundance of TIMPs 1, 2, and 3, all of which are inhibitory to MMP13.[30] There appears to be a consensus that TIMP2 is constitutively expressed by normal human chondrocytes and synoviocytes, and that its expression is not sensitive to cytokine or growth factor signaling. In contrast, both TIMP1 and TIMP3 expression appear to be upregulated in arthritic joint tissues or on treatment of cells with TGF beta.[31,32] However, in osteoarthritic cartilage the formation of active MMP13, perhaps in focal areas, appears to overwhelm the presumed protective effects of the endogenously synthesized TIMPs.

Potential for therapeutic control of MMP13 activity

Despite the biological controls which exist to limit MMP13 activity in cartilage matrix, it is clear that destructive collagenolysis does occur in the cartilage of joints of OA patients. Many studies have therefore focused on the potential to interfere with this pathway with a view to therapeutic control. Thus, recent insights into the intracellular signaling steps required to generate excess active proteinase in situ (see Fig. 7.12) have been accompanied by a recent group of papers on compounds and factors, which can negatively impact this cellular pathway (see Fig. 7.13). Three recent papers from Cawstons laboratory have shown that cytokine/growth factors such as IL-13,[33] IGF-1,[34] and TGF beta[35] all have the capacity to block collagenolysis in IL-1- or IL-1/OSM-treated cartilage cultures, and in each case this effect is associated with a down regulation of MMP13 expression. The Chinese herbal anti-rheumatic drug Tripterygium wilfordii Hook F (TWHF),[36] has now been shown, with primary human femoral head osteoarthritic chondrocytes, to inhibit cytokine-induced mRNA and protein expression of MMP13, and this inhibition operates via the AP-1 and NFKb pathways.[37] A specific inhibitor of p38 MAP kinase activity (the pyridinyl imidazole, SB203580) has been found to be an effective blocker of IL-1-induced MMP13 expression in articular chondrocytes.[16] The synthetic triterpenoid, 2-cyano-3,12-dioxoolean-1,9-dien-28-oic acid (CDDO), was shown with cytokine-treated human chondrosarcoma cells to reduce the induction of MMP-13 at the levels of messenger RNA and protein and to also reduce IL-1beta-mediated invasion of cells through a collagen matrix.[38] Recently, it has been shown that the tumor suppressor gene p53 represses promoter activity for both MMP-13 and MMP-1. Thus, individuals harboring inactive mutant forms of p53 may experience constitutive upregulation of MMP13 gene expression, which may contribute directly to cartilage loss.[39] Finally, given this intense interest in the role of MMP13 in cartilage collagen degradation the pharmaceutical industry has recently concentrated efforts on developing potent and specific inhibitors of MMP13 with a view to arthritis therapy via proteinase inhibition.[40]

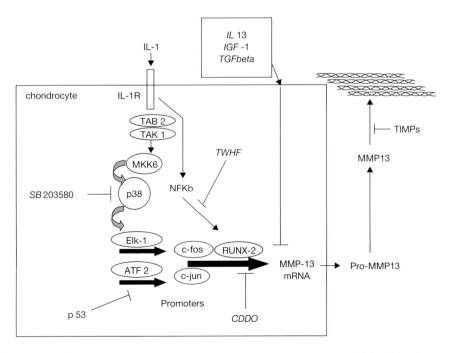

Fig. 7.13 Schematic illustrating the apparent site of action of inhibitors (bioactive peptides and small molecules), which have been shown to block the cytokine induction of MMP13 mRNA expression or synthesis/activity of the proteinase. See the text, Tables 7.1–7.4 for details and references.

Which aggrecanase is actually responsible for cartilage matrix degradation?

A central role for the aggrecanase group of proteinases (ADAMTS-1, 4, 5) in cartilage aggrecan degradation has been widely accepted in the literature only in recent years. The prevailing opinion for the majority of the past 20 years has been that one or more MMPs with aggrecan-degrading activity would be responsible for this process. The finding in human articular cartilage of large amounts of MMP3 protein along with a specific product (G1-VDIPEN341) of its action on aggrecan[41] lent strong support to the argument that MMP3 or a closely related species was responsible for aggrecanolysis in cartilage. However, in 1991, independent laboratories described the presence of an 'aggrecanase' in cartilage explants that generated products from a series of glutamyl-X endopeptidase cleavages, sites which are essentially insensitive to MMP-mediated degradation.[42,43] This was followed by the observation[44,45] that products of this same 'aggrecanase' were abundant in the synovial fluids of patients with a wide range of joint diseases. Following a long period of research into the identity of these 'aggrecanases', three proteinases (ADAMTS1, 4, and 5) were recently cloned and expressed and shown to exhibit this precise activity when incubated with aggrecan in vitro.[46,47] While the term 'aggrecanase' has in the past been used to describe any proteinase with the capacity to degrade aggrecan, it is now routinely applied only to the glutamyl-endopeptidase activity that ADAMTS1, 4, and 5 exhibit when incubated with aggrecan. Interestingly, these proteinases are members of a family (see Fig. 7.14 for schematic) that includes the procollagen-N-peptidases, ADAMTS2 and ADAMTS3, which specifically cleave the Ala181–Gln182 bond in procollagen II.

Since both normal and osteoarthritic human articular cartilage chondrocytes contain mRNA for the three aggrecanases (ADAMTS1, 4, and 5)[48] and immunoreactive protein for each enzyme is present in human cartilage extracts (Gao, G., Iruela-Arispe, L., and Sandy, J.D., unpublished), recent research has been directed toward determining which, if any, of these enzymes is actually responsible for cartilage aggrecan degradation in vivo. A summary of the current information suggests that ADAMTS4 (aggrecanase-1) is the most likely candidate; however further work is required to establish this clearly.

ADAMTS1 is considered to be an unlikely candidate due to its very low specific activity relative to ADAMTS4 and ADAMTS5. In one study on cleavage of the Glu373–Ala 374 bond[49] it was shown to exhibit about one-tenth the activity of ADAMTS4 and in another, on cleavage of the Glu1871–Leu1872 bond (bovine) it was shown to exhibit only one-hundredth of the activity of ADAMTS4 and ADAMTS5.[50] Moreover, the original purification of aggrecanase activity from IL-1 treated bovine cartilage explants[51] resulted in the isolation of ADAMTS4 and ADAMTS5, suggesting that both these enzymes are involved in the degradative process in this model. Indeed, aggrecanase assays following individual immunodepletion of ADAMTS1, 4, and 5 from the medium of IL-1 treated bovine articular cartilage explants, has suggested that ADAMTS4, and to a lesser degree ADAMTS5. is responsible.[50] On the other hand, it should be noted that analysis of transcript abundance in human arthritic fibrous tissues by real time PCR for ADAMTS1, 4, and 5 showed that ADAMTS1 was expressed at about five to ten times the level of ADAMTS4 and 5.

There is a lack of agreement on the effects of cytokines on ADAMTS4 transcript abundance in chondrocytes, although this might be due to species differences. With human cartilage explants[48] it was shown that under conditions where aggrecanase activity is induced with retinoic acid, IL-1 or TNF-alpha, there was no change in the level of mRNA for ADAMTS1, 4, or 5, all of which were constitutively expressed. A study of mRNA levels for MMP-1, 3, and 13 and ADAMTS4 and 5 in the articular cartilage and menisci of rabbits with experimentally induced OA[52] also found no change in ADAMTS expression, but a marked induction of MMPs. Constitutive expression of ADAMTS5 with no response to cytokines has also been described in human and bovine synovial membranes and joint capsule.[53] In contrast to the above, with bovine articular cartilage[50] it was found that ADAMTS5 was constitutive and unaffected by cytokines, whereas ADAMTS4 transcripts were undetectable in control tissue and markedly induced by cytokines.

It therefore appears that more work will be needed to determine the extent to which increases in aggrecanase activity in human joint disease[2,44,54] are due to the increased synthesis of ADAMTS enzyme or to a process of activation of pre-existing proteinase.

The mechanism for activation of the proteolytic activity of the ADAMTS family of proteinases has not yet been studied in detail and is not fully understood. The active forms of ADAMTS4 and ADAMTS5, purified from IL-1-treated bovine nasal cartilage, were both found in the 50–65 kDa size range, and since the full-length recombinant pro-proteins are 837 and 930 residues, respectively, (suggesting proteins in excess of 100 kDa), it is clear that generation of the active forms requires proteolytic processing events. Further, since the active 62 kDa ADAMTS4 was shown to bear an N-terminal sequence at Phe212, adjacent to the pro-hormone convertase

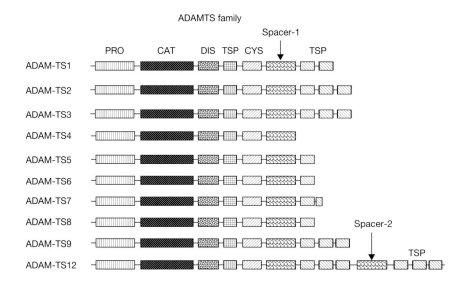

Fig. 7.14 The domain structures of the members of the ADAMTS family. The abbreviations are: PRO, prodomain; CAT, catalytic domain; DIS, disintegrin-like domain; TSP, thrombospondin-1-like domain; CYS, cysteine-rich domain. Family members which have exhibited 'aggrecanase' activity are ADAMTS1, 4, and 5.

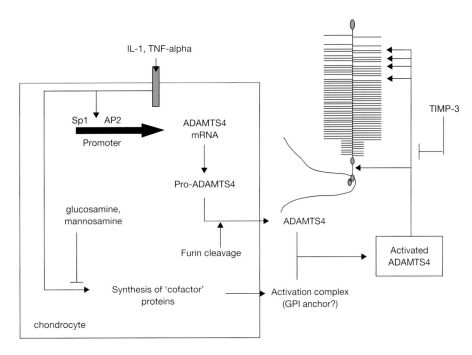

Fig. 7.15 A hypothetical scheme to explain some aspects of the control of ADAMTS4 expression, activation, and inhibition in chondrocytes. See the text for description and references.

site (RAKR), it appears that removal of the prodomain is part of the activation process. However, removal of the prodomain should result in a product of about 75 kDa, so that further processing appears to be necessary to generate the active forms observed in the cartilage explant system. Indeed, there is evidence[102] that specific C-terminal truncation events are required for the generation of active ADAMTS4. Such C-terminal processing also appears to be a feature of the control of matrix association[55] and perhaps the activity of ADAMTS1[56] and ADAMTS12.[57]

Potential for therapeutic control of ADAMTS activity in cartilage

Inhibition of the ADAMTS family of proteinases in tissues such as cartilage may be exerted through the binding of natural inhibitors. Interestingly, it has been found that while the classical MMP inhibitors, TIMP-1 and TIMP-2, are inactive against ADAMTS4, TIMP-3 is a potent inhibitor of the aggrecanase activity of both ADAMTS4 and 5.[58,59] This apparently novel TIMP specificity for inhibition of ADAMTS4 and ADAMTS5 may open possibilities for the generation of therapeutic ADAMTS-selective TIMPs.[60] In this regard it is also possible that members of the papilin family of proteins may exert potent inhibitory activity toward the aggrecanases, much as has been demonstrated with ADAMTS2.[61] The generally different inhibitor profiles for MMPs and ADAMTSs is also seen with the hydroxamate-based metalloproteinase inhibitors SE206, BB16, and XS-309. These compounds, which show inhibition of most MMPs in the low-nanomolar range, exhibited IC50 values of 137, 548, and 10 000 nM, respectively, toward ADAMTS5,[62] showing that synthesis of ADAMTS-specific inhibitors will be required before the potential for therapeutic control with low-molecular weight inhibitors can be evaluated.

In all chondrocyte and cartilage systems, which have been examined for evidence of aggrecanase activity,[43,63–65] it has been consistently observed that the endogenous activity and/or the level of active enzyme in the conditioned medium is markedly enhanced by the treatment of the chondrocytes with interleukin-1, TNF-alpha or retinoic acid. It is therefore clear

that such cytokine treatment results in the formation of increased levels of active aggrecanase (ADAMTS). This increase has been shown consistently to depend on continued cellular activity and protein synthesis[66] and it appears from Western analysis[50] that this can be at least partly explained by the increased synthesis of ADAMTS4 protein. In this regard, characterization of the 5′-flanking region of the ADAMTS4 gene has suggested that the region between −383 and +10, relative to the start site, is needed for full promoter activity and this region contains one Sp1 and three AP2 sites.[67] On the other hand, other studies have indicated that IL-1 induction of aggrecanase activity in cartilage requires the production of 'cofactor' proteins that are most likely involved in the activation of existing and/or newly synthesized ADAMTS protein. Most interesting in this regard is the finding that glucosamine and mannosamine are very effective inhibitors of the IL-1 induced process. While the mechanism of the glucosamine effect is not yet understood, it appears that the mannosamine effect can be explained by its capacity to inhibit the formation of glycosylphosphatidylinositol (GPI)-anchored proteins in a range of cell types. This appears to be important in relation to strategies for therapeutic control since it is possible that one of the 'cofactor' proteins required is MT4-MMP (or a related GPI-anchored proteinase), which might act at the cell surface to produce fully active ADAMTS proteinases. Evidence supporting this mechanism of control has been obtained with studies on a human chondrosarcoma cell line, stably transfected with ADAMTS4.[102] A schematic summarizing this hypothesis is provided in Fig. 7.15.

Key points

1. Recent research in proteolytic degradation of human cartilage matrix has suggested that the major proteinases involved in tissue destruction are collagenase-3 (MMP13) and aggrecanase-1 (ADAMTS4).

2. Control of MMP13 activity appears to be exerted by transcriptional activation by cytokines as well as cell surface activation of the proform of the proteinase. Transcriptional activation is primarily

through the p38 MAP kinase pathway but also involves NFKb. Cell surface activation involves interaction with MT1-MMP.

3. Control of ADAMTS4 activity appears to be predominantly at the level of post-transcriptional activation, which requires a furin-dependent removal of the prodomain and C-terminal truncation by an unknown proteinase.

4. Therapeutic intervention in cartilage matrix degradation may be achieved by blocking the p38-dependent transcriptional activation of MMP13 expression and controlling the extracellular activation of the secreted form of ADAMTS4.

References

(An asterisk denotes recommended reading.)

1. Dieppe, P. (1999). Osteoarthritis: time to shift the paradigm. This includes distinguishing between severe disease and common minor disability. *Br Med J* **318**:1299–300.

2. *Sandy, J.D. and Verscharen, C. (2001). Analysis of aggrecan in human knee cartilage and synovial fluid indicates that aggrecanase ADAMTS activity is responsible for the catabolic turnover and loss of whole aggrecan whereas other protease activity is required for C-terminal processing in vivo. *Biochem J* **358**:615–26.

    An extensive review of the area of aggrecan degradation in human OA is provided. The data in this paper provides a framework for understanding the proteolytic origin of aggrecan species which are present in mature articular cartilages from normal, injured and late-stage OA joints. Analysis of the synovial fluids from these same groups suggests that processing of aggrecan in normal human cartilage is dependent on MMP-like activity, whereas the destruction of aggrecan in early- and late-stage OA results from uncontrolled ADAMTS aggrecanase activity.

3. Buckwalter, J.A. and Rosenberg, L.C. (1982). Electron microscopic studies of cartilage proteoglycans. Direct evidence for the variable length of the chondroitin sulfate-rich region of proteoglycan subunit core protein. *J Biol Chem* **257**:9830–9.

4. Stoop, R., Buma, P., van der Kraan, P.M., *et al.* (2001). Type II collagen degradation in articular cartilage fibrillation after anterior cruciate ligament transection in rats. *Osteoarth Cart* **9**:308–15.

5. Dahlberg, L., Billinghurst, R.C., Manner, P., *et al.* (2000). Selective enhancement of collagenase-mediated cleavage of resident type II collagen in cultured osteoarthritic cartilage and arrest with a synthetic inhibitor that spares collagenase 1 matrix metalloproteinase 1. *Arthritis Rheum* **43**:673–82.

6. Billinghurst, R.C., Dahlberg, L., Ionescu, M., *et al.* (1997). Enhanced cleavage of type II collagen by collagenases in osteoarthritic articular cartilage. *J Clin Invest* **99**:1534–45.

7. Vankemmelbeke, M., Dekeyser, P.M., Hollander, A.P., Buttle, D.J., and Demeester, J. (1998). Characterization of helical cleavages in type II collagen generated by matrixins. *Biochem J* **330**:633–40.

8. *Billinghurst, R.C., Wu, W., Ionescu, M., Reiner, A., Dahlberg, L., Chen, J., van Wart, H., and Poole, A.R. (2000). Comparison of the degradation of type II collagen and proteoglycan in nasal and articular cartilages induced by interleukin-1 and the selective inhibition of type II collagen cleavage by collagenase. *Arthritis Rheum* **43**:664–72.

    Provides an excellent example of the use of specific MMP inhibitors to reveal the identity of the collagenase involved in cartilage collagen destruction. An inhibitor of MMP13, RS102,481, which spares MMP1, was found to effectively prevent IL-1 induced collagen degradation in cartilage cultures, providing the first definitive evidence for the central role of MMP13 in this process.

9. Buttner, F.H., Chubinskaya, S., Margerie, D., *et al.* (1997). Expression of membrane type 1 matrix metalloproteinase in human articular cartilage. *Arthritis Rheum* **40**:704–9.

10. Davoli, M.A., Lamplugh, L., Beauchemin, A., *et al.* (2001). Enzymes active in the areas undergoing cartilage resorption during the development of the secondary ossification center in the tibiae of rats aged 0–21 days. II. Two proteinases, gelatinase B and collagenase-3, are implicated in the lysis of collagen fibrils. *Dev Dyn* **222**:71–88.

11. Freemont, A.J., Byers, R.J., Taiwo, Y.O., and Hoyland, J.A. (1999). In situ zymographic localisation of type II collagen degrading activity in osteoarthritic human articular cartilage. *Ann Rheum Dis* **58**:357–65.

12. Neuhold, L.A., Killar, L., Zhao, W., *et al.* (2001). Postnatal expression in hyaline cartilage of constitutively active human collagenase-3 MMP-13 induces osteoarthritis in mice. *J Clin Invest* **107**:35–44.

13. Knauper, V., Lopez-Otin, C., Smith, B., Knight, G., and Murphy, G. (1996). Biochemical characterization of human collagenase-3. *J Biol Chem* **271**:1544–50.

14. Han, Z., Boyle, D.L., Chang, L., *et al.* (2001). c-Jun N-terminal kinase is required for metalloproteinase expression and joint destruction in inflammatory arthritis. *J Clin Invest* **108**:73–81.

15. Reboul, P., Pelletier, J.P., Tardif, G., Benderdour, M., Ranger, P., Bottaro, D.P., and Martel-Pelletier, J. (2001). Hepatocyte growth factor induction of collagenase 3 production in human osteoarthritic cartilage: involvement of the stress-activated protein kinase/c-Jun N-terminal kinase pathway and a sensitive p38 mitogen-activated protein kinase inhibitor cascade. *Arthritis Rheum* **44**:73–84.

16. Mengshol, J.A., Vincenti, M.P., Coon, C.I., Barchowsky, A., and Brinckerhoff, C.E. (2000). Interleukin-1 induction of collagenase 3 matrix metalloproteinase 13 gene expression in chondrocytes requires p38, c-Jun N-terminal kinase, and nuclear factor kappaB: differential regulation of collagenase 1 and collagenase 3. *Arthritis Rheum* **43**:801–11.

17. Wu, W., Mwale, F., Tchetina, E., Kojima, T., Yasuda, T., and Poole, A.R. (2001). Cartilage matrix resorption in skeletogenesis. *Novartis Found Symp* **232**:158–66; discussion:166–70.

18. Shingleton, W.D., Ellis, A.J., Rowan, A.D., and Cawston, T.E. (2000). Retinoic acid combines with interleukin-1 to promote the degradation of collagen from bovine nasal cartilage: matrix metalloproteinases-1 and -13 are involved in cartilage collagen breakdown. *J Cell Biochem* **79**:519–31.

19. Otterness, I.G., Bliven, M.L., Eskra, J.D., te Koppele, J.M., Stukenbrok, H.A., and Milici, A.J. (2000). Cartilage damage after intraarticular exposure to collagenase 3. *Osteoarthritis Cart* **8**:366–73.

20. Shlopov, B.V., Gumanovskaya, M.L., and Hasty, K.A. (2000). Autocrine regulation of collagenase 3 matrix metalloproteinase 13 during osteoarthritis. *Arthritis Rheum* **43**:195–205.

21. Vincenti, M.P. and Brinckerhoff, C.E. (2001). The potential of signal transduction inhibitors for the treatment of arthritis: Is it all just JNK? *J Clin Invest* **108**:181–3.

22. Ravanti, L., Toriseva, M., Penttinen, R., Crombleholme, T., Foschi, M., Han, J., and Kahari, V.M. (2001). Expression of human collagenase-3 MMP-13 by fetal skin fibroblasts is induced by transforming growth factor beta via p38 mitogen-activated protein kinase. *Faseb J* **15**:1098–100.

23. Winchester, S.K., Selvamurugan, N., D'Alonzo, R.C., and Partridge, N.C. (2000). Developmental regulation of collagenase-3 mRNA in normal, differentiating osteoblasts through the activator protein-1 and the runt domain binding sites. *J Biol Chem* **275**:23 310–8.

24. McCarthy, T.L., Ji, C., Chen, Y., Kim, K.K., Imagawa, M., Ito, Y., and Centrella, M. (2000). Runt domain factor Runx-dependent effects on CCAAT/enhancer-binding protein delta expression and activity in osteoblasts. *J Biol Chem* **275**:21 746–53.

25. Moldovan, F., Pelletier, J.P., Mineau, F., Dupuis, M., Cloutier, J.M., and Martel-Pelletier, J. (2000). Modulation of collagenase 3 in human osteoarthritic cartilage by activation of extracellular transforming growth factor beta: role of furin convertase. *Arthritis Rheum* **43**:2100–9.

26. Sun, H.B. and Yokota, H. (2001). Messenger-RNA expression of matrix metalloproteinases, tissue inhibitors of metalloproteinases, and transcription factors in rheumatic synovial cells under mechanical stimuli. *Bone* **28**:303–9.

27. Tetlow, L.C., Adlam, D.J., and Woolley, D.E. (2001). Matrix metalloproteinase and proinflammatory cytokine production by chondrocytes of human osteoarthritic cartilage: associations with degenerative changes. *Arthritis Rheum* **44**:585–94.

28. Cowell, S., Knauper, V., Stewart, M.L., *et al.* (1998). Induction of matrix metalloproteinase activation cascades based on membrane-type 1 matrix metalloproteinase: associated activation of gelatinase A, gelatinase B and collagenase 3. *Biochem J* **331**:453–8.

29. *Murphy, G., Stanton, H., Cowell, S., Butler, G., Knauper, V., Atkinson, S., and Gavrilovic, J. (1999). Mechanisms for pro matrix metalloproteinase activation. *Apmis* **107**:38–44.

   An excellent review of the area of metalloproteinase activation is provided. Potential physiological mechanisms including autoproteolysis, cell-associated plasmin, or the action of cell surface MT-MMPs are discussed as future research areas, which will need to be addressed in the search for effective disease-modifying drugs for OA.

30. Knauper, V., Cowell, S., Smith, B., *et al.* (1997). The role of the C-terminal domain of human collagenase-3 MMP-13 in the activation of procollagenase-3, substrate specificity, and tissue inhibitor of metalloproteinase interaction. *J Biol Chem* **272**:7608–16.

31. Zafarullah, M., Su, S., Martel-Pelletier, J., DiBattista, J.A., Costello, B.G., Stetler-Stevenson, W.G., and Pelletier, J.P. (1996). Tissue inhibitor of metalloproteinase-2 TIMP-2 mRNA is constitutively expressed in bovine, human normal, and osteoarthritic articular chondrocytes. *J Cell Biochem* **60**:211–7.

32. Su, S., Grover, J., Roughley, P.J., DiBattista, J.A., Martel-Pelletier, J., Pelletier, J.P., and Zafarullah, M. (1999). Expression of the tissue inhibitor of metalloproteinases TIMP gene family in normal and osteoarthritic joints. *Rheumatol Int* **18**:183–91.

33. Cleaver, C.S., Rowan, A.D., and Cawston, T.E. (2001). Interleukin 13 blocks the release of collagen from bovine nasal cartilage treated with proinflammatory cytokines. *Ann Rheum Dis* **60**:150–7.

34. Hui, W., Rowan, A.D., and Cawston, T. (2001). Insulin-like growth factor 1 blocks collagen release and down regulates matrix metalloproteinase-1, -3, -8, and -13 mRNA expression in bovine nasal cartilage stimulated with oncostatin M in combination with interleukin 1alpha. *Ann Rheum Dis* **60**:254–61.

35. Hui, W., Rowan, A.D., and Cawston, T. (2000). Transforming growth factor beta1 blocks the release of collagen fragments from boving nasal cartilage stimulated by oncostatin M in combination with IL-1alpha. *Cytokine* **12**:765–9.

36. Lai, J.H., Ho, L.J., Lu, K.C., Chang, D.M., Shaio, M.F., and Han, S.H. (2001). Western and Chinese antirheumatic drug-induced T cell apoptotic DNA damage uses different caspase cascades and is independent of Fas/Fas ligand interaction. *J Immunol* **166**:6914–24.

37. Sylvester, J., Liacini, A., Li, W.Q., Dehnade, F., and Zafarullah, M. (2001). Tripterygium wilfordii Hook F extract suppresses proinflammatory cytokine-induced expression of matrix metalloproteinase genes in articular chondrocytes by inhibiting activating protein-1 and nuclear factor-kappaB activities. *Mol Pharmacol* **59**:1196–205.

38. Mix, K.S., Mengshol, J.A., Benbow, U., Vincenti, M.P., Sporn, M.B., and Brinckerhoff, C.E. (2001). A synthetic triterpenoid selectively inhibits the induction of matrix metalloproteinases 1 and 13 by inflammatory cytokines. *Arthritis Rheum* **44**:1096–104.

39. Sun, Y., Cheung, J.M., Martel-Pelletier, J., *et al.* (2000). Wild type and mutant p53 differentially regulate the gene expression of human collagenase-3 hMMP-13. *J Biol Chem* **275**:11327–32.

40. Robinson, R.P., Laird, E.R., Donahue, K.M., *et al.* (2001). Design and synthesis of 2-oxo-imidazolidine-4-carboxylic acid hydroxyamides as potent matrix metalloproteinase-13 inhibitors. *Bioorg Med Chem Lett* **11**:1211–3.

41. Flannery, C.R., Lark, M.W., and Sandy, J.D. (1992). Identification of a stromelysin cleavage site within the interglobular domain of human aggrecan. Evidence for proteolysis at this site in vivo in human articular cartilage. *J Biol Chem* **267**:1008–14.

42. Sandy, J.D., Neame, P.J., Boynton, R.E., and Flannery, C.R. (1991). Catabolism of aggrecan in cartilage explants. Identification of a major cleavage site within the interglobular domain. *J Biol Chem* **266**: 8683–5.

43. Loulakis, P., Shrikhande, A., Davis, G., and Maniglia, C.A. (1992). N-terminal sequence of proteoglycan fragments isolated from medium of interleukin-1-treated articular-cartilage cultures. Putative site(s). of enzymic cleavage. *Biochem J* **284**:589–93.

44. Sandy, J.D., Flannery, C.R., Neame, P.J., and Lohmander, L.S. (1992). The structure of aggrecan fragments in human synovial fluid. Evidence for the involvement in osteoarthritis of a novel proteinase, which cleaves the Glu 373–Ala 374 bond of the interglobular domain. *J Clin Invest* **89**: 1512–6.

45. Lohmander, L.S., Neame, P.J., and Sandy, J.D. (1993). The structure of aggrecan fragments in human synovial fluid. Evidence that aggrecanase mediates cartilage degradation in inflammatory joint disease, joint injury, and osteoarthritis. *Arthritis Rheum* **36**:1214–22.

46. Kuno, K., Okadab, Y., Kawashimac, H., Nakamurab, H., Miyasakac, M., Ohnoa, H., and Matsushimad, K. (2000). ADAMTS-1 cleaves a cartilage proteoglycan, aggrecan [In Process Citation]. *FEBS Lett* **478**:241–5.

47. Tortorella, M.D., Pratta, M., Liu, R.Q., Austin, J., Ross, O.H., Abbaszade, I., Burn, T., and Arner, E. (2000). Sites of aggrecan cleavage by recombinant human aggrecanase-1 ADAMTS-4. *J Biol Chem* **275**:18566–73.

48. Flannery, C.R., Little, C.B., Hughes, C.E., and Caterson, B. (1999). Expression of ADAMTS homologues in articular cartilage. *Biochem Biophys Res Commun* **260**:318–22.

49. Sandy, J.D., Westling, J., Kenagy, R.D., *et al.* (2001). Versican V1 proteolysis in human aorta in vivo occurs at the Glu441–Ala442 bond, a site which is cleaved by recombinant ADAMTS-1 and ADAMTS-4. *J Biol Chem* **26**:26.

50. Tortorella, M.D., Malfait, A., Deccico, C., Arner, E., and Nagase, H. (2001). The role of ADAM-TS4 aggrecanase-1 and ADAM-TS5 aggrecanase-2 in a model of cartilage degradation. *Osteoarthritis Cart* **9**:539–52.

51. Arner, E.C., Pratta, M.A., Trzaskos, J.M., Decicco, C.P., and Tortorella, M.D. (1999). Generation and characterization of aggrecanase. A soluble, cartilage-derived aggrecan-degrading activity. *J Biol Chem* **274**:6594–601.

52. Bluteau, G., Conrozier, T., Mathieu, P., Vignon, E., Herbage, D., and Mallein-Gerin, F. (2001). Matrix metalloproteinase-1, -3, -13 and aggrecanase-1 and -2 are differentially expressed in experimental osteoarthritis. *Biochim Biophys Acta* **1526**:147–58.

53. Vankemmelbeke, M.N., Holen, I., Wilson, A.G., *et al.* (2001). Expression and activity of ADAMTS-5 in synovium. *Eur J Biochem* **268**:1259–68.

54. Sztrolovics, R., Alini, M., Roughley, P.J., and Mort, J.S. (1997). Aggrecan degradation in human intervertebral disc and articular cartilage. *Biochem J* **326**:235–41.

55. Kuno, K. and Matsushima, K. (1998). ADAMTS-1 protein anchors at the extracellular matrix through the thrombospondin type I motifs and its spacing region. *J Biol Chem* **273**:13912–7.

56. Rodriguez-Manzaneque, J.C., Milchanowski, A.B., Dufour, E.K., Leduc, R., and Iruela-Arispe, M.L. (2000). Characterization of METH-1/ADAMTS1 processing reveals two distinct active forms. *J Biol Chem* **275**:33471–9.

57. Cal, S., Arguelles, J.M., Fernandez, P.L., and Lopez-Otin, C. (2001). Identification, characterization, and intracellular processing of ADAM-TS12, a novel human disintegrin with a complex structural organization involving multiple thrombospondin-1 repeats. *J Biol Chem* **276**: 17932–40.

58. Kashiwagi, M., Tortorella, M., Nagase, H., and Brew, K. (2001). TIMP-3 is a potent inhibitor of aggrecanase 1 ADAM-TS4 and aggrecanase 2 ADAM-TS5. *J Biol Chem* **276**:12501–4.

59. Hashimoto, G., Aoki, T., Nakamura, H., Tanzawa, K., and Okada, Y. (2001). Inhibition of ADAMTS4 aggrecanase-1 by tissue inhibitors of metalloproteinases TIMP-1, 2, 3 and 4. *FEBS Lett* **494**:192–5.

60. Nagase, H., Meng, Q., Malinovskii, V., *et al.* (1999). Engineering of selective TIMPs. *Ann N Y Acad Sci* **878**:1–11.

61. Kramerova, I.A., Kawaguchi, N., Fessler, L.I., *et al.* (2000). Papilin in development; a pericellular protein with a homology to the ADAMTS metalloproteinases. *Development* **127**:5475–85.

62. Abbaszade, I., Liu, R.Q., Yang, F., *et al.* (1999). Cloning and characterization of ADAMTS11, an aggrecanase from the ADAMTS family. *J Biol Chem* **274**:23443–50.

63. Little, C.B., Flannery, C.R., Hughes, C.E., Mort, J.S., Roughley, P.J., Dent, C., and Caterson, B. (1999). Aggrecanase versus matrix metalloproteinases in the catabolism of the interglobular domain of aggrecan in vitro. *Biochem J* **344**:61–8.

64. Plaas, A.H. and Sandy, J.D. (1993). A cartilage explant system for studies on aggrecan structure, biosynthesis and catabolism in discrete zones of the mammalian growth plate. *Matrix* **13**:135–47.

65. Sandy, J.D., Thompson, V., Doege, K., and Verscharen, C. (2000). The intermediates of aggrecanase-dependent cleavage of aggrecan in rat chondrosarcoma cells treated with interleukin-1. *Biochem J* **351**:161–166.

66. Bolis, S., Handley, C.J., and Comper, W.D. (1989). Passive loss of proteoglycan from articular cartilage explants. *Biochim Biophys Acta* **993**:157–67.

67. Mizui, Y., Yamazaki, K., Kuboi, Y., Sagane, K., and Tanaka, I. (2000). Characterization of 5′-flanking region of human aggrecanase-1 ADAMTS4. gene. *Mol Biol Rep* **27**:167–73.

68. Doege, K.J., Sasaki, M., Kimura, T., and Yamada, Y. (1991). Complete coding sequence and deduced primary structure of the human cartilage large aggregating proteoglycan, aggrecan. Human-specific repeats, and additional alternatively spliced forms. *J Biol Chem* **266**:894–902.

69. Dudhia, J. and Hardingham, T.E. (1990). The primary structure of human cartilage link protein. *Nucleic Acids Res* **18**:2214.

70. Hembry, R.M., Dyce, J., Driesang, I., Hunziker, E.B., Fosang, A.J., Tyler, J.A., and Murphy, G. (2001). Immunolocalization of matrix metalloproteinases in partial-thickness defects in pig articular cartilage. A preliminary report. *J Bone Joint Surg Am* **83**(A):826–38.

71. Chubinskaya, S., Kuettner, K.E., and Cole, A.A. (1999). Expression of matrix metalloproteinases in normal and damaged articular cartilage from human knee and ankle joints. *Lab Invest* **79**:1669–77.

72. Chung, L., Shimokawa, K., Dinakarpandian, D., Grams, F., Fields, G.B., and Nagase, H. (2000). Identification of the 183.RWTNNFREY 191 region as a critical segment of matrix metalloproteinase 1 for the expression of collagenolytic activity *J Biol Chem* **275**:29610–7.

73. Eyre, D.R. and Wu, J.J. (1995). Collagen structure and cartilage matrix integrity. *J Rheumatol* **43**(Suppl.):82–5.

74. Fosang, A.J., Last, K., Knauper, V., *et al.* (1993). Fibroblast and neutrophil collagenases cleave at two sites in the cartilage aggrecan interglobular domain. *Biochem J* **295**:273–6.

75. Vilim, V. and Fosang, A.J. (1994). Proteoglycans isolated from dissociative extracts of differently aged human articular cartilage: characterization of naturally occurring hyaluronan-binding fragments of aggrecan. *Biochem J* **304**:887–94.

76. Nguyen, Q., Murphy, G., Hughes, C.E., Mort, J.S., and Roughley, P.J. (1993). Matrix metalloproteinases cleave at two distinct sites on human cartilage link protein. *Biochem J* **295**:595–8.

77. Nguyen, Q., Liu, J., Roughley, P.J., and Mort, J.S. (1991). Link protein as a monitor in situ of endogenous proteolysis in adult human articular cartilage. *Biochem J* **278**:143–7.

78. Imai, K., Ohta, S., Matsumoto, T., Fujimoto, N., Sato, H., Seiki, M., and Okada, Y. (1997). Expression of membrane-type 1 matrix metalloproteinase and activation of progelatinase A in human osteoarthritic cartilage. *Am J Pathol* **151**:245–56.

79. Wu, J.J., Lark, M.W., Chun, L.E., and Eyre, D.R. (1991). Sites of stromelysin cleavage in collagen types II, IX, X, and XI of cartilage. *J Biol Chem* **266**:5625–8.

80. Fosang, A.J., Last, K., Neame, P.J., Murphy, G., *et al.* (1994). Neutrophil collagenase MMP-8. cleaves at the aggrecanase site E373-A374 in the interglobular domain of cartilage aggrecan. *Biochem J* **304**:347–51.

81. Bord, S., Horner, A., Hembry, R.M., and Compston, J.E. (1998). Stromelysin-1 MMP-3. and stromelysin-2 MMP-10. expression in developing human bone: potential roles in skeletal development. *Bone* **23**:7–12.

82. Fosang, A.J., Last, K., Knauper, V., Murphy, G., and Neame, P.J. (1996). Degradation of cartilage aggrecan by collagenase-3 MMP-13. *FEBS Lett* **380**:17–20.

83. Ohuchi, E., Imai, K., Fujii, Y., Sato, H., Seiki, M., and Okada, Y. (1997). Membrane type 1 matrix metalloproteinase digests interstitial collagens and other extracellular matrix macromolecules. *J Biol Chem* **272**:2446–51.

84. Buttner, F.H., Hughes, C.E., Margerie, D., Lichte, A., Tschesche, H., Caterson, B., and Bartnik, E. (1998). Membrane type 1 matrix metalloproteinase MT1-MMP cleaves the recombinant aggrecan substrate rAgg1mut at the 'aggrecanase' and the MMP sites. Characterization of MT1-MMP

85. Cs-Szabo, G., Melching, L.I., Roughley, P.J., and Glant, T.T. (1997). Changes in messenger RNA and protein levels of proteoglycans and link protein in human osteoarthritic cartilage samples. *Arthritis Rheum* **40**: 1037–45.

86. Fernandes, R.J., Hirohata, S., Engle, J.M., Colige, A., Cohn, D.H., Eyre, D.R., and Apte, S.S. (2001). Procollagen II amino-propeptide processing by ADAMTS-3: Insights on dermatosparaxis. *J Biol Chem* **14**:14.

87. Hulmes, D.J., Mould, A.P., and Kessler, E. (1997). The CUB domains of procollagen C-proteinase enhancer control collagen assembly solely by their effect on procollagen C-proteinase/bone morphogenetic protein-1. *Matrix Biol* **16**:41–5.

88. Lang, A., Horler, D., and Baici, A. (2000). The relative importance of cysteine peptidases in osteoarthritis. *J Rheumatol* **27**:1970–9.

89. Szomor, Z., Shimizu, K., Yamamoto, S., Yasuda, T., Ishikawa, H., and Nakamura, T. (1999). Externalization of calpain calcium-dependent neutral cysteine proteinase in human arthritic cartilage. *Clin Exp Rheumatol* **17**:569–74.

90. Fosang, A.J., Neame, P.J., Last, K., Hardingham, T.E., Murphy, G., and Hamilton, J.A. (1992). The interglobular domain of cartilage aggrecan is cleaved by PUMP, gelatinases, and cathepsin B. *J Biol Chem* **267**:19470–4.

91. Mort, J.S., Magny, M.C., and Lee, E.R. (1998). Cathepsin B: an alternative protease for the generation of an aggrecan 'metalloproteinase' cleavage neoepitope. *Biochem J* **335**:491–4.

92. Martel-Pelletier, J., Faure, M.P., McCollum, R., Mineau, F., Cloutier, J.M., and Pelletier, J.P. (1991). Plasmin, plasminogen activators and inhibitor in human osteoarthritic cartilage. *J Rheumatol* **18**:1863–71.

93. Vittorio, N., Crissman, J.D., Hopson, C.N., and Herman, J.H. (1986). Histologic assessment of cathepsin D in osteoarthritic cartilage. *Clin Exp Rheumatol* **4**:221–30.

94. Downs, J.T., Lane, C.L., Nestor, N.B., *et al.* (2001). Analysis of collagenase-cleavage of type II collagen using a neoepitope ELISA. *J Immunol Methods* **247**:25–34.

95. Mitchell, P.G., Magna, H.A., Reeves, L.M., *et al.* (1996). Cloning, expression, and type II collagenolytic activity of matrix metalloproteinase-13 from human osteoarthritic cartilage. *J Clin Invest* **97**:761–8.

96. Van der Rest, M., Rosenberg, L.C., Olsen, B.R., and Poole, A.R. (1986). Chondrocalcin is identical with the C-propeptide of type II procollagen. *Biochem J* **237**:923–5.

97. Niyibizi, C., Wu, J.J. and Eyre, D.R. (1987). The carboxypeptide trimer of type II collagen is a prominent component of immature cartilages and intervertebral-disc tissue. *Biochim Biophys Acta* **916**:493–9.

98. Lark, M.W., Bayne, E.K., Flanagan, J., *et al.* (1997). Aggrecan degradation in human cartilage. Evidence for both matrix metalloproteinase and aggrecanase activity in normal, osteoarthritic, and rheumatoid joints. *J Clin Invest* **100**:93–106.

99. Fosang, A.J., Last, K., and Maciewicz, R.A. (1996). Aggrecan is degraded by matrix metalloproteinases in human arthritis. Evidence that matrix metalloproteinase and aggrecanase activities can be independent. *J Clin Invest* **98**:2292–9.

100. Rodriguez-Manzaneque, J.C., Westling, J., Thai, S.N., *et al.* (2002) ADAMTS1 cleaves aggrecan at multiple sites and is differentially inhibited by metalloproteinase inhibitors. *Biochem Biophys Res Commun* **293**(1): 501–8.

101. Westling, J., Fosang, A.J., Last, K., Thompson, V.P., *et al.* (2002) ADAMTS4 cleaves at the aggrecanase site (Glu373-Ala374) and secondarily at the matrix metalloproteinase site (Asn341-Phe342) in the aggrecan interglobular domain. *J Biol Chem* **277**(18):16059–66.

102. Gao, G., Westling, J., Thompson, V.P., Howell, T.D., Gottschall, P.E., and Sandy, J.D. (2002) Activation of the proteolytic activity of ADAMTS4 aggrecanase-1 by C-terminal truncation. *J Biol Chem* **277**(13):11034–41.

7.2.1.3 **Articular cartilage repair**

Ernst B. Hunziker and Jenny A. Tyler

Articular cartilage furnishes each moving, bony portion of a joint with a smooth, frictionless surface. It is unique amongst bodily tissues in being capable of reversible compression, distributing an applied load homogeneously, and minimizing contact stress to the underlying bone. The deformability and hydraulic permeability of articular cartilage tissue depend on the mutual interactions between macromolecular components of the extracellular matrix (such as the aggregating and non-aggregating proteoglycans and fibrillar collagens), water, and the composite fibrillar network within mid and deep zones.[1] Of quintessential importance is the density of the fixed negative charges associated with glycosaminoglycans whereby they become hydrated and generate a considerable swelling pressure. The tensile strength of fibrillar collagens acts as a girdle to limit tissue expansion. Since mature articular cartilage is avascular, alymphatic, and aneural, the extracellular matrix also functions as a selective permeability barrier, determining which molecules enter the tissue. The anisotropic structure (Fig. 7.19) and biochemistry of mature articular cartilage are rigorously maintained throughout life by the resident chondrocytes, which are essential for the functioning of the joint.[2] The long-term success or failure of cartilage repair depends inextricably on the ability of repair cells to re-establish a truly hyaline layer with its native mechanical properties.

Articular cartilage is subject to two main types of injury. The first, which is acute and transient, involves the temporary loss of proteoglycans and other non-collagenous molecules from the tissue, but no structural lesioning. Many environmental factors can induce such temporary matrix depletion, including abnormal mechanical loading, disruption of the synovial membrane, local infection, and anti-inflammatory drugs.[3,4] Provided that the stimulus for these changes is withdrawn within a reasonable period of time and that the collagen network is not compromised, the matrix usually recovers completely from this type of insult. The restoration process can be considered as one of active and continuous remodelling to restore matrix equilibrium.[5]

The second type of injury, which involves the mechanical severing of collagen fibrils/fibres and an accompanying loss of cells, can be caused by fracturing, frictional abrasions, penetrating lesions, or osteoarthritic processes. The outcome is extremely variable and depends on the volume/ surface area of the defect generated, and whether the subchondral bone or other peri-articular tissues are involved. As a general rule, however, such lesions do not heal.[2,6]

Osteoarthritis develops when articular cartilage chondrocytes are no longer able to maintain the balance between matrix synthesis and degradation.[5] The condition is heterogeneous with an ill-defined pathogenesis, although genetic, environmental, and mechanical influences have been implicated as initiating factors. Data derived from studies on the regulation of chondrocyte metabolism suggest that the relative concentration of mediators such as growth factors and cytokines, or an altered response of the cells to these substances during the course of degeneration, may determine

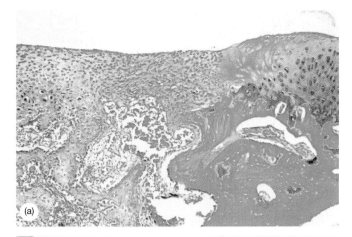

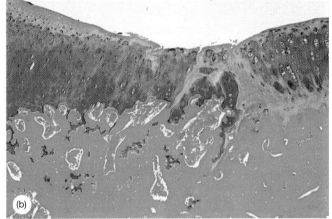

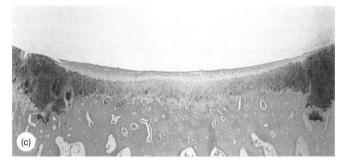

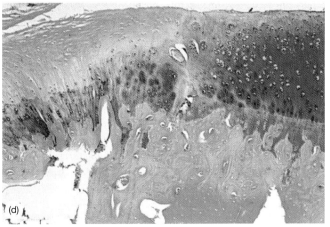

Fig. 7.16 Spontaneous repair induced by bleeding. Photomicrographs illustrating spontaneous repair of full-thickness defects in the femur of mature rabbits (18 months, 5 kg), drilled through to the subchondral bone and left without treatment: (a) 10 days; (b) 8 weeks; (c) 24 weeks; (d) 48 weeks after creation. The resin embedded sections have been processed with Safranin O, which stains proteoglycans red. (a) At 10 days, repair tissue still consists largely of undifferentiated mesenchymal cells, but there is already evidence of cartilage formation (red-stained tissue) just below the surface at the far left. (b) At 8 weeks, hyaline cartilage has formed within the defect (red-stained tissue). (c) At 24 weeks, repair tissue integrity is still maintained. (d) At 48 weeks, repair tissue shows signs of degeneration, and its affinity for Safranin O is markedly reduced.

Source: Taken from Shapiro *et al.*[11] with permission from the authors and publisher.

the rate of progress and final outcome of this disease. For reasons that are not understood, the initial transient loss of proteoglycans persists, despite increased synthesis, and progresses to the irreversible loss of collagen and cells from focal regions of the articular cartilage layer. These discrete lesions then become more extensive and ultimately penetrate the subchondral bone plate. The only predictably effective treatment for the pain and disability associated with an end-stage osteoarthritic hip or knee is the removal of both damaged and healthy cartilage from the surface of the affected joint, and its replacement with a prosthesis. The procedure restores pain-free motion within a fairly normal range and is considered to be very successful in elderly patients.[7] However, total joint arthroplasties have a limited lifespan and will not support the heavy loading or vigorous use commensurate with the needs of younger individuals.[8] Alternative treatments are therefore eagerly sought. As an interim measure, a variety of surgical interventions (described in Chapter 9) has been examined, including the grafting of fresh or cryopreserved perichondrial or periosteal tissue, osteotomy to correct angular deformity, the introduction of soft-tissue flaps to cover the damaged area, and the implantation of fibrocartilage-strengthening materials (such as carbon fibres, Dacron, or Teflon micromeshes).[9]

This chapter endeavours to outline the ways in which specific growth factors and matrices have been used to induce cartilage repair. It is not intended to be a comprehensive review of the literature in this field. Rather, it serves to furnish representative examples of novel, practical approaches currently being explored to optimize, a durable recovery of damaged cartilage in the first instance, and eventually to effect the true regeneration of this specialized tissue.

Factors contributing to the restoration of durable cartilage

Lesions that span the entire depth of the articular cartilage layer and penetrate the subchondral bone plate (full-thickness defects), induce a healing response that follows a well-defined and amply documented[10] sequence of events. These have been described in detail by Shapiro et al. for the rabbit model,[11] and may be summarized as follows:[1] a fibrin clot forms;[2] locally released growth factors induce the migration, replication, and differentiation of cells;[3] inflammatory and premesenchymal cells are recruited from the bone-marrow space;[4] these cells form a vascularized scar tissue;[5] the vascularized scar tissue undergoes enchondral ossification with the resulting formation of cartilage and bone. In some cases, this sequence of events leads to complete resurfacing of the defect with scar tissue (Fig. 7.16(a)). This material is remodelled within a couple of weeks to form a tissue that resembles cartilage in terms of cell morphology and its proteoglycan-rich matrix. By the eighth week, the defect contains cartilage-like repair tissue with subchondral bone below the tidemark (Fig. 7.16(b)). This situation can persist for up to six months (Fig. 7.16(c)), but tissue then begins to degenerate (Fig. 7.16(d)). These findings represent the best that have been obtained with small full-thickness defects in small animal models (such as the rabbit). But with larger lesions in larger species (such as the goat, Fig. 7.20), the observed sequence of events does not proceed further than the formation of a rudimentary type of fibrous connective tissue.[12]

The clinical equivalent of such lesions is generated by arthroscopic abrasive chondroplasty,[13] Pridie drilling,[14] or the application of microfracturing techniques.[15] The procedures are frequently performed on osteoarthritic knee joints as a palliative measure, in the hope that the surgically removed degenerative cartilage/bone will be replaced by spontaneously generated 'healthy' repair tissue. They have been reported to relieve patients of considerable symptomatic pain, albeit for short periods of time. However, no controlled prospective trials have been conducted to substantiate these claims. As with animal models, repair tissue formed within the surgically created defects most likely begins to disintegrate within six months to one year.[16]

There are a number of reasons why repair cartilage fails. Chondrocytes surrounding the defect do not seem to participate in the healing process, indeed, some appear to undergo necrosis and/or apoptosis.[17] Moreover, collagen fibrils do not span the interface between new and old cartilage; hence, full mechanical competence cannot be attained.[18] Integration may be further impaired by the antiadhesive properties of certain matrix proteins, particularly decorin and biglycan,[19] which prevent fibrin and incoming cells from sticking well to the defect edge.[12] A brief treatment of defect surfaces with chondroitinase or trypsin to remove these substances improves the adhesion of cells[19,20] and implanted collagen gels,[21] without being associated with adverse effects. Undoubtedly though, the main obstacle to be overcome is the inability of repair cells to remodel scar tissue into hyaline cartilage with its characteristic zonal organization of chondrocytes and macromolecular compartmentalization of the matrix. Unfortunately, we do not have a clear conception of the manner in which these zones are formed during normal development, although graded exposure to solutes from the synovial fluid, differential mechanical loading, and oxygen tension have all been implicated in creating the proper local environment. Postnatal growth activities almost certainly play a key role in this process. These cannot, of course, be duplicated in adults, whereas in foetal or early postnatal organisms with high growth activities they can.[22]

Design of matrices

The introduction of materials such as carbon fibres, Dacron, and Teflon into joints to strengthen repair tissue has been practiced for many years.[23] Recent advances in biomaterial science have now rendered possible the design of matrices to modify and guide the spontaneous repair process,[24,25] especially within large defect volumes. Matrix scaffolds can be made from a variety of polymers or co-polymers, including glycolates, lactates, alginates, collagens, and acrylates. They can be used to restore the contour of a damaged joint, to provide resilience to compression and tensile strength, to deliver cells and growth factors to a defect site, to enhance cell migration, and to furnish a template for the deposition of extracellular material. Their pore size and rate of degradation can be controlled by varying the degree of crosslinkage and the final form of the product.[26,27] A material's biocompatibility can be improved by rendering its surface slightly hydrophilic, which facilitates cell attachment and growth.[28] The mechanical properties of native cartilage can be emulated using hydrogel composites.[29]

Synthetic polymers

A hydrophilic xerogel formed from a mixture of poly(ethyl) methacrylate and tetrahydrofurturol monomers has been demonstrated to imbibe fluid from the surrounding tissues over a period of several months, when implanted within 3 mm diameter defects in mature rabbits.[30] This heterocyclic methacrylate polymer was found to gel in situ and to swell slightly, thus ensuring a tight fit with the surrounding bone. Its uptake of fluid facilitated the adsorption of matrix proteins, growth factors, and bone-derived cells. The optimal formation of cartilage, which endured for eight months, was obtained by placing the polymer just slightly below the surface of the subchondral bone: when set lower, it became surrounded by bone and no cartilage grew over its surface; when set higher, the cartilage covering was incomplete. These findings suggest that this polymer is capable of furnishing a firm but resilient substratum for the growing cartilage and at the same time is able to protect it from repeated compression.

Mono- and co-polymers of lactate and glycolate have been used extensively as scaffolds for seeded cells. The resulting products are, however, fairly hydrophobic, and need to be superficially coated with a hydrophilic layer before sufficient cells can be established to lay down a cartilaginous matrix.[31,32] Moreover, the metabolites of these polymers can sometimes generate a very acidic environment in vivo, which may elicit adverse tissue reactions. However, these matrices, which can be produced on a large scale

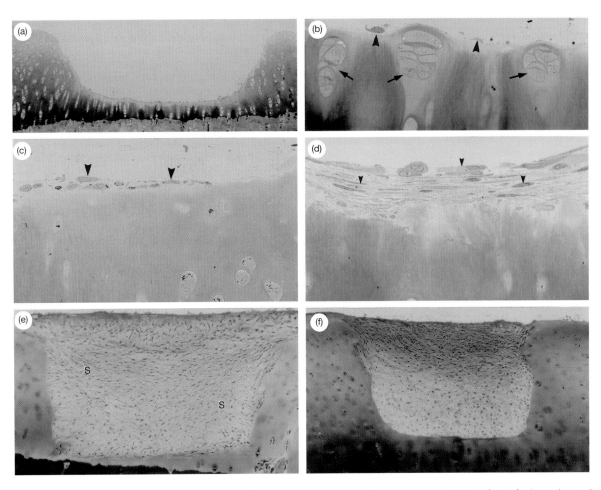

Fig. 7.17 The use of growth factors to induce chondrogenesis *in vivo*. Photomicrographs illustrating the appearance, at 4 weeks, of superficial articular cartilage defects which do not penetrate into the subchondral bone in the knee of: (a)–(d), mature rabbits (18 months; 5 kg); (e) and (f), adult miniature-pigs (3 yr, 65 kg). (a) When left untreated, such defects did not heal. (b) Proliferating chondrocyte clusters were often seen at the edge of the defect but did not migrate into the space. (c) Adhesion of cells from the synovial fluid occurred following controlled removal of surface proteoglycans with chondroitinase AC. (d) Multilayers of such cells formed following the topical application of a mitogenic growth factor (IGF-1, TGF-β; 20 ng/ml), filling about 10% of the space. (e) Complete infilling with mesenchymal cells was achieved only if the defect was filled with a biodegradable matrix (fibrin, collagen, gelatin) containing the mitogenic growth factor. These cells did not transform into chondrocytes. (f) A chondrogenic switch occurred 3–4 weeks after surgery if a growth factor from the TGF-β superfamily (200–1000 ng/ml), but not IGF-1, was incorporated into liposomes and included within the matrix in addition to the free chemotactic mitogenic growth factor. The illustration shows the beginning of this switch in the lower half of the defect. (a)–(d), semi-thin resin-embedded sections stained with toluidine blue; (e) and (f), thick, surface-polished saw cuts stained with basic fuchsine and McNeil's Tetrachrome.

in bioreactors,[33] appear to have found a potential use in the *in vitro* manufacture of cartilage plugs for grafting *in vivo* (see below).

Tissue grafts

Cartilage and osteochondral grafts,[34–36] as well as perichondrial[37] and periosteal[38] transplants, have been demonstrated experimentally to possess a promising potential to repair large cartilage defects. However, the shortage of cartilage and osteochondral grafts,[34–36] as well as the lack of an efficient means to coordinate the availability of fresh donor material with the needs of recipients, have prevented these procedures from being widely adopted. The clinical transplantation of perichondrial or periosteal tissue is associated with a number of drawbacks.[37] The great demand for alternative supplies of suitable tissue has spurred the development of tissue engineering approaches.

One such system[39] involves seeding rabbit chondrocytes onto a polyglycolic acid matrix, which is then maintained for several weeks under conditions of continuous pressurized fluid flow, to ensure the optimal diffusion of nutrients throughout the growing cartilage tissue. By this means, cartilage plugs 1 cm in diameter and up to 4 mm in thickness can be generated.

Moreover, controlled shear stresses can be applied to the developing tissue and should encourage optimal chondrocyte differentiation *in vitro*. In the foreseeable future, specifically designed functional cartilage implants derived from suitable allogeneic donor cells could be made to order within a few weeks. But such materials are, of course, subject to the same problems of transport and storage as are the freshly isolated natural cartilage and osteochondral grafts.[40,41] Storage at 4 °C in culture media helps to maintain the viability of chondrocytes for up to twenty-eight days,[42] but indefinite storage at subzero temperatures is not possible at present, since only a small proportion of cells survive the freeze/thawing process.

Collagenous polymers

Matrices composed of type I collagen are the most versatile of polymers. They are biodegradable, stimulate only a poor foreign-body reaction, and can be pulverized, gelled, spun into fibres, or woven into fabrics, braids, and meshes.[43,44] Notwithstanding these advantages, the repair results obtained after treating cartilage defects with collagen preparations alone have been very disappointing and generally less successful than those elicited by fibrin.

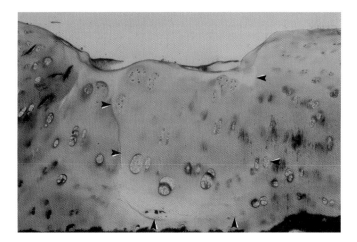

Fig. 7.18 Regeneration of cartilage tissue *in vivo* using a fibrin matrix. Partial-thickness articular cartilage defect in the femur of a miniature-pig (3 yr, 65 kg) six weeks after treatment with a fibrin matrix containing free TGF-β2 (5 n ml) and liposome-encapsulated TGF-β2 (400 n ml). Arrowheads denote the original edges of the defect. Fairly good integration has been achieved, but fibrin retracts on setting and is unsuitable for long-term repair results. (Polished saw-cut of resin-embedded tissue, surface stained with basic fuchsine and toluidine blue.)

However, as a scaffold for the seeding of transplanted cells and as a carrier for growth factors, collagen matrices may possess distinct advantages.

Identification of cells with optimal chondrogenic potential

One approach to increasing the number of cells with chondrogenic potential at the site of repair has been to isolate suitable candidates, replicate them in culture, and then implant them at high numerical density within the cartilage defect.[45] Many experimental studies and a few clinical trials have been conducted using either committed, fully-differentiated chondrocytes, or mesenchymal chondroprogenitor cells derived from periosteal tissue or bone marrow. Clear differences have been observed in the behaviour of these different cell types during the repair process.

Chondrocytes as donor cells

Adult human articular cartilage has a characteristically low ratio of cells to matrix.[2] After their isolation by enzymatic dispersal, mature differentiated chondrocytes thus have to pass through several replication cycles before sufficient cells are available for transplantation.[46,47] Traditionally, the most rapid growth is achieved when chondrocytes are cultured as adherent monolayers in the presence of serum. But they become flattened during this process and transform into non-specific fibroblast-like cells, which are capable of producing very little cartilage-specific matrix.[48] Not surprisingly, such cells fail to generate durable hyaline cartilage tissue after transplantation. However, if these modulated chondrocytes are maintained under appropriate micromass conditions or seeded within a gelatinous (three-dimensional) matrix, they gradually regain the ability to express and lay down type II collagen and aggrecan,[49] although their efficiency to do so decreases as the number of passages in culture increases. These fibroblast-like chondrocytes are very different from the fibroblastic mesenchymal cells derived from bone marrow,[50,51] synovium,[52] or periosteum.[53] Unlike these, they are not multipotential and have a very limited capacity to remodel mesenchymal scar tissue into cartilage, calcified cartilage, or bone, either *in vitro* or *in vivo*. One particular study involving such cells[54] serves to illustrate this limitation. When type I collagen gels containing isolated and expanded articular cartilage chondrocytes were implanted within osteochondral defects in rabbit

knees, they were rapidly remodelled into cartilage matrix that filled the entire lesion void, including the bony compartment. Even after six months, repair cartilage persisted within the lower part of the cavity; it had neither calcified nor transformed into bone. Ultimately therefore, this tissue probably disintegrated and failed due to mechanical overloading. In another study involving the implantation of chondrocyte-impregnated collagen gels within large equine defects,[55] a considerable influx of cells from the subchondral bone occurred, and these laid down osseous tissue within the bony compartment. However, only two-thirds of this bony matrix remained after one year, at which juncture it contained a high proportion of fibrocartilage.

A similar but more complex procedure involving chondrocytes as donor cells has been tested not only in rabbits[56,57] but also in human patients.[58] In the human trials, autologous chondrocytes were isolated from the upper medial femoral condyle of the damaged knee and expanded in monolayer cultures. A periosteal flap derived from the proximal medial tibia was sutured with its cambial layer downwards over the defect, which had been excavated to remove abnormal tissue. The modulated (i.e., fibroblast-like) chondrocytes were resuspended at high numerical density and injected beneath the flap into the defect space. Many of the patients were reported to have gained symptomatic pain-relief from this treatment for up to sixteen months. On the basis of histological analyses and immunoreactivity for type II collagen, biopsies revealed the presence of cartilage-like material at the centre of the repair tissue mass. The results were fair to moderate for femoral lesions and poor for patellar ones. Unfortunately, it is not possible to ascertain from these experiments whether the chondrocytes or the periosteal cells contributed to the neoproduction of a cartilage-like matrix. When committed chondrocytes are used as the main source of cells within lesions that impinge on or penetrate the subchondral bone plate, it is still not clear whether it is advantageous to encourage the migration of cells from the osseous layer. Future experiments, involving the use of growth factors to promote and stabilize the redifferentiation of transplanted chondrocytes, may help to clarify this point. It may well be that committed chondrocytes are useful only in the repair of lesions confined to the cartilage layer.

Osteochondral progenitor cells as donors

Osteochondral progenitor cells can be isolated from bone marrow,[51,59] periosteum,[38] or perichondrium.[37] Irrespective of their origin, such cells have been shown to form cartilage tissue when introduced into full-thickness defects. In one typical study using a rabbit model,[60] osteochondral progenitor cells derived from either bone marrow or periosteal tissue were isolated, grown in monolayer culture, resuspended within type I collagen gels, and then transplanted into large defects. Within two weeks, the autologous osteochondral progenitor cells had differentiated into chondrocytes which had laid down cartilage-like tissue within the cartilaginous portion of the defect cavity. Thereafter, the thickness of this layer progressively decreased, such that by the twenty-fourth week it was markedly attenuated and exhibited but poor hyaline-like qualities. Indentation testing of the repair cartilage revealed this to be stiffer than that formed when collagen gels were implanted in the absence of osteochondral progenitor cells, but even this was still less compliant than normal hyaline cartilage. The bony compartment of the defect space was completely filled with osseous tissue formed by the enchondral processes. Friedenstein[61] and Owen[62] have referred to these pluripotential progenitor cells as 'stromal stem cells', since they can become chondrogenic or osteogenic according to the local environment *in vitro* as well as *in vivo*, and can be distinguished from haemopoietic cells by their adherence properties in tissue culture.

Several laboratories are currently engaged in attempting to identify growth factors that promote the lineage progression, differentiation, and maturation of these connective tissue cells into tissue-specific types, which lay down cartilage, bone, muscle, tendon, ligament, or meniscus.[25,51,63]

One long-term goal of scientists interested in the design of matrices for the repair of osteochondral defects is to produce a substratum that would selectively recruit specific cell types from a non-specific source. RGD or other peptide sequences that promote cell attachments of a particular kind could be affixed to a matrix[64,65] or, alternatively, antagonists could be introduced to prevent the attachment of inappropriate cells. An improved understanding of the ligands that promote the migration and attachment of precursor cells in different lineages will undoubtedly facilitate the realization of this goal. Collagen and other matrix products bind growth factors avidly, and have already proved to be invaluable as carriers for bone-inductive materials.[66–68]

Transforming growth factors

Mature chondrocytes and their precursors produce and respond to a wide variety of growth factors. These substances are classified into groups and subgroups on the basis of homologies in the amino acid sequence, isoforms sometimes also being categorized according to the specificity of their biological activity and affinity for different cell-surface receptors. Studies relating to the response of chondrocytes to these factors have been described in detail elsewhere.[69–71] In general terms, basic fibroblast growth factors (bFGF, 1–9), epidermal growth factors (EGF, 1–6), platelet-derived growth factors (PDGF-1 and 2), insulin-like growth factors (IGF-1 and 2), transforming growth factors (TGF-β, 1–5), and bone morphogenic proteins (BMP, 1–8) have all been shown to regulate different aspects of chondrocyte migration and replication in tissue culture or during development, at each stage of their differentiation. These agents also regulate and modify each other's action whilst inducing chondrogenic differentiation and maintaining the differentiated phenotype. IGFs, BMPs, and TGFs can also promote the synthesis of cartilage matrix and decrease its degradation by mature articular chondrocytes.[72–74] However, only TGFs and BMPs are chondrogenic, in the sense that they can induce the transformation of mesenchymal precursor cells into chondrocytes, which will either produce articular cartilage or progress through the stages of enchondral ossification to hypertrophy, calcify the extracellular matrix and form bone.[75,76]

Members of the TGF-β family also include cartilage-derived morphogenic proteins (CDMP-1 and -2), activins, inhibins, and the Mullerian inhibiting substances (MIS), which share significant but varying degrees of sequence homology with the prototype TGF-β.[77,78] Growth factors from this family that have been identified in cartilage and bone are listed in Table 7.5.

Each of the BMPs thus far identified, isolated and purified[75,79] (as well as CDMPs) can induce bone formation at non-skeletal sites *in vivo*, whereas TGF-βs stimulate the production only of a fibrous, sclerotic callous.[80] However, when applied topically at skeletal sites, such as within calvariae[81] or full-thickness cartilage lesions,[82] both categories of substances induce rapid bone formation. These findings suggest that BMPs can stimulate the chondrogenic and osteogenic differentiation of stem cells at a much earlier stage in their lineage progression than TGF-βs. BMPs are pleiotropic morphogens. BMP-7, for instance, will stimulate the formation of bone when applied either to a fractured femur, to dentine, or to ligamentous tissue *in vivo*. It would thus appear that once differentiation has been initiated in a primary (probably common) stem cell, local conditions respecting oxygen tension, vascular supply (or absence of one), mechanical loading, and other factors dictate the subsequent course pursued.

TGF-βs can be mitogenic, antiproliferative, chemotactic, or inductive, the biological effects varying dramatically with dose, duration of exposure, and the stage of differentiation of the target cell.[83] Apart from variations in relative potency, the isoforms do not differ quantitatively in their range of biological effects on skeletal tissues.[82] However, temporal and regional expression patterns vary considerably. Mesenchymal cell cultures, stimulated with retinoic acid, produce TGF-β1 immediately, TGF-β2 after two to three days, and TGF-β3 after about six days.[84] Raloxifene (an anti-oestrogen) enhances the expression of TGF-β3 relative to TGF-β1 and -β2, which both decrease the recruitment of, and resorption by, osteoclasts.[85] TGF-β3 is found preferentially in the periosteum and within undifferentiated

Table 7.5 TGFβ superfamily

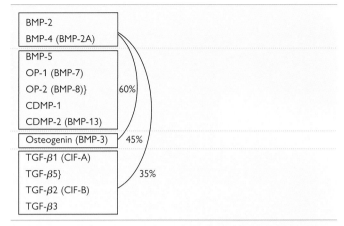

Growth factors from the TGF-β superfamily which have been identified in mammalian cartilage and bone. Isoforms shown within a box share more than 75% amino acid sequence homology and subgroups between 35–60%, as shown. Alternative names for the same growth factor are given in parenthesis.

BMP, bone morphogenic protein; OP, osteogenic protein; CDMP, cartilage-derived morphogenic protein; TGF, transforming growth factor; CIF, cartilage inducing factor.

mesenchymal tissue, adjacent to sites of intramembraneous ossification, whereas TGF-β2 is more evident within the perichondrium, precartilaginous regions, transitional chondrocytes, and the growth zones of long bones; TGF-β1 is expressed by differentiated chondrocytes and osteoblasts, and is readily detected in mature cartilage and bone.[86,87] The exact physiological significance of these complex, multiple levels of regulation is not yet fully understood, but they clearly provide a wonderful array of choices with which to attune chondrogenic differentiation. Members of the TGF-β family are perhaps the most promising candidates for the surgical induction of biological repair in articular cartilage defects.

Induction of cartilage repair in superficial defects

The failure of articular cartilage to regenerate is not due to the absence of a suitable source of cells. Mesenchymal cells derived from the margin of synovial joints can differentiate into chondrocytes that form hyaline cartilage and bone, and will always do so reproducibly and efficiently given the appropriate stimulation conditions. The reasons for failure are twofold. In the first place, the cartilage matrix surrounding a defect is antiadhesive, which means that if any floating or migrating precursor cells happen to be in the vicinity they are unable to attach themselves, and chondrocytes are too sparse to release a strong enough chemotactic signal to assist this process. Second, cartilage, being avascular, is not furnished with a supply of macrophages, which, on entering a wound, usually mount a cascade of cytokine production to attract repair cells. The full extent of the biological limitations to be overcome have gradually emerged over a number of years, and solutions to most of the problems have been found, so that the intrinsic capacity of articular cartilage to heal successfully can be harnessed without resorting to cell or tissue transplantation.[88–90]

The findings may be briefly summarized as follows. The antiadhesive nature of the defect edge can be overcome by treating it briefly with chondroitinase ABC, which induces a transient loss of proteoglycans,[20] that is, the molecules primarily responsible for inhibiting cell attachment. Cells for repair can be recruited from the synovium and stimulated to replicate by introducing a chemotactic/mitogenic growth factor (such as TGF-β1 at low concentration).[88] However, these measures do not suffice to fill the defect volume with repair cells, which require this space to be defined with a matrix scaffold (such as fibrin). These conditions being satisfied, synovium-derived

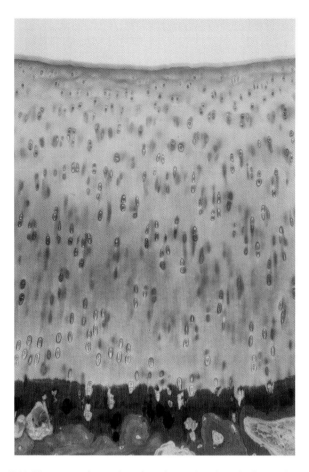

Fig. 7.19 Mature articular cartilage. Articular cartilage from the femur of a mature rabbit (18 months, 5 kg), showing typical zonal arrangement of chondrocytes. (Polished saw-cut of resin-embedded tissue, surface-stained with basic fuchsine and toluidine blue.)

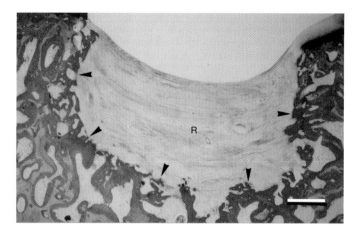

Fig. 7.20 A light micrograph of a full-thickness defect (6 mm in diameter and 4 mm in depth) created in the femoral condyle of a mature goat. At the time of surgery, this lesion underwent no treatment. Six weeks later, when this image was taken, it is incompletely filled with a vascularized, fibrous connective tissue (R). Although some neoformation of bone (arrowheads)—by intramembranous growth—has taken place along the defect edges, no cartilage tissue has been laid down and there is no evidence of enchondral ossification. Bar = 1 mm.

cells migrate, proliferate, and lay down a primitive type of mesenchymal tissue[88] (Fig. 7.17(e)). This tissue does not, however, transform into cartilage unless induced to do so by the timely application of a chondrogenic differentiation factor. The appropriate agent (such as TGF-β1 at high concentration) is encapsulated within liposomes, which are introduced together with the free chemotactic/mitogenic factor and the matrix.[90] The repair tissue thereby generated in both the rabbit and miniature pig models resembles cartilage both in terms of cell morphology and its matrix-staining characteristics (Fig. 7.17(f), 7.18). However, the cellularity of the tissue formed is still far too high,[76] and although distinct signs of a zonal stratification are apparent, the degree of sophistication achieved in native hyaline articular cartilage has yet to be achieved.

Biological adhesives

Fibrin-based glues have been used extensively in experimental orthopaedics to improve the adhesiveness of transplanted cells. In general, though, the results achieved have been unsatisfactory.[91,92] However, recent experiments conducted with transglutaminase[93] have revealed this agent to be capable of bonding pieces of cartilage more strongly than fibrin. Tissue transglutaminase occurs naturally in cartilage, where it plays a role in crosslinking the extracellular matrix during maturation.[94] Elevated amounts of this substance have also been detected within cartilage tissue near defect sites.[95]

Crosslinkage is calcium-dependent and requires the presence of a peptide-bound glutamine residue within its substrate, in order to accept an amino group within a lysine-containing peptide.[96] Type II collagen and fibronectin can both act as a glutaminyl substrate for the enzyme and form stable crosslinks with any lysine-containing protein. If transglutaminase were to be applied to the surfaces of superficial articular cartilage lesions or incorporated into a collagen matrix implanted therein, it could improve bonding between the said matrix and the defect edges without interfering with the repair process. This agent may thus prove to be extremely useful in preventing the loss of matrices from broad, shallow defects.

Induction of cartilage repair in full-thickness defects

Great care needs to be exercised when introducing growth factors of the TGF-β superfamily into a joint, with a view to inducing cartilage repair.[76] When high doses of free TGF-β, for instance, are injected intra-articularly they have been shown to promote inflammation, synovial hyperplasia, effusion, and osteophyte formation.[97–99] Fortunately, these agents can be made to bind so tightly to an implanted matrix that leakage into the synovial cavity is negligible. Nevertheless, these potent mediators of osteogenesis should not stimulate this process to such an extent that bone tissue becomes stiffer than normal or extends up into the cartilaginous compartment of the defect. In patients with penetrating lesions, it may be desirable to use a lower concentration of the agent within the matrix applied to the bony compartment than that used in the cartilaginous one. Osteogenic processes stimulated within the bony compartment can be prevented from transgressing on the cartilaginous one by inserting a structural (cell-excluding) barrier at the presumptive cartilage–bone interface (Fig. 7.21).[100] Alternatively, the functional barrier principle can be applied[101]. This involves incorporating an anti-angiogenic factor into the matrix implanted within the cartilaginous compartment of the defect void. Both of these measures inhibit the upgrowth of vessels, which are indispensable to bone formation.

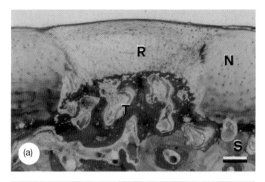

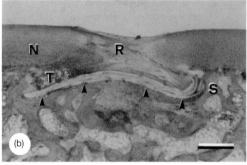

Fig. 7.21 Light micrographs of full-thickness articular cartilage defects created in Goettingen miniature pigs. (a) No structural barrier was inserted at the presumptive border between the cartilage and bone compartments. Eight weeks after surgery, repair cartilage (R) occupies the upper half of the cartilaginous defect space. This tissue has a higher numerical density of cells and is more fibrous than native cartilage (N). The lower half of the cartilaginous defect space is occupied by repair bone tissue (T), which has grown upward from and completely fills the underlying bone compartment. Repair bone (T) [dark red] is principally of the woven type, whereas native subchondral bone tissue (S) [light red] is lamellar. Bar = 100 μm. (b) Light micrograph of a full-thickness articular cartilage defect created in a Goettingen miniature pig. The bony defect space was filled with a chondrogenic matrix and a porous structural barrier membrane (Goretex®) inserted at the presumptive cartilage-bone interface. The cartilaginous defect space then was filled with the same chondrogenic matrix. Eight weeks after surgery, the primitive mesenchymal type of repair tissue initially laid down within the cartilaginous defect space has been transformed only partially into cartilage-like repair tissue (R). The bony defect space contains repair bone tissue. The Goretex® membrane (arrowheads) prevented repair bone from growing upward into the cartilaginous compartment except at the periphery on the left side (T). This encroachment is a consequence of imperfect membrane fitment against the defect wall. The Goretex® membrane has not been resorbed and it is not infiltrated with bone tissue. The membrane was inserted at a level lower than the presumptive cartilage (N)-bone (S)-interface, which led to a corresponding lowering of the border between the two repair tissue compartments. Bar = 500 μm.

Source: Reproduced from Hunziker et al.[100], with the permission of the author and the publisher.

Conclusion

Our present understanding of the basic principles involved in the successful induction of cartilage repair is such that this can now be achieved consistently in experimental model systems, which can be adapted for clinical use. Ideally, the growth factor/matrix complex would be introduced arthroscopically, in a single intervention. There is no question that, before long, such methods will enable us to intervene directly in the osteoarthritic process and thus check the progressive destruction of joint tissues by this invidious disease.

Key points

1. Superficial (partial-thickness) articular cartilage lesions do not heal.

2. The spontaneous repair of full-thickness articular cartilage lesions is limited to a small-dimensional window.

3. Repair tissue spontaneously formed within lesions induced by a number of different surgical interventions is structurally unstable and functionally less competent than normal articular cartilage.

4. Tissue engineering approaches based on the use of homogenous chondrogenic precursor cell populations or chondrocytes, combined with a scaffold and growth factors, yield experimentally promising repair results.

5. Growth-factor-based repair of partial-thickness lesions is based on the programmed release of appropriate substances from an implanted matrix.

References

(An asterisk denotes recommended reading.)

1. **Mow, V.C., Setton, L.A., Guilak, F., and Ratcliffe, A.** (1994). Mechanical factors in articular cartilage and their role in osteoarthritis. In K.E.K Kuettner and V.M. Golderg (eds), *Osteoarthritic Disorders.* Rosemont: American Academy of Orthopedic Surgeons, pp. 147–7.

2. **Hunziker, E.B.** (1992). Articular cartilage structure in humans and experimental animals. In K.E. Kuettner, R. Schleyerbach, J.G. Peyron, *et al.* (eds), *Articular Cartilage and Osteoarthritis* New York: Raven Press pp. 183–9.

3. **Helminen, H.J., Purvelin, J., Kiviranta, K.,** *et al.* (1987). Joint loading effects on articular cartilage. In H.J. Helminer (ed.), *Joint Loading, Biology and Health of Articular Structures.* Bristol: John Wright, pp. 1046–63.

4. **Hess, E.V. and Herman, J.H.** (1986). Cartilage metabolism and anti-inflammatory drugs in osteoarthritis. *Am J Med* **15**:1–32.

5. **Goldring, M.B.** (2000). The role of the chondrocyte in osteoarthritis. *Arthritis Rheum* **43**:1916–26.

6. **Ghadially, F.N., Thomas I., Oryschak A.F.,** *et al.* (1977). Long-term results of superficial defects in articular cartilage: a scanning electron microscope study. *J Pathol* **121**:213–17.

7. **Charnley, J. and Cupic, Z.** (1973). The nine- and ten-year results of low friction arthroplasty of the hip. *Clin Orthop* **95**:9–13.

8. **Chandler, H.P., Resiuck, F.T., and Wilson, R.L.** (1981). Total hip replacement in patients who are under the age of 30 at the time of arthroplasty. A five-year follow-up study. *J Bone Joint Surg* **63**(A):9–12.

9. **Messner, K.** (1994). Durability of artificial implants for repair of osteochondral defects of the medial femoral condyle in rabbits. *Biomaterials,* **15**:657–64.

10. **Convery, F.R., Akeson, W.H., and Woo, S.L-Y.** (1972). The repair of large osteochondral defects. An experimental study in horses. *Clin Orthop,* **82**:253–62.

11. *****Shapiro, F., Koide, S., and Glimcher, M.J.** (1993). Cell origin and differentiation in the repair of full-thickness defects in articular cartilage. An experimental investigation in the rabbit. *J Bone Joint Surg* **75**(A4):532–53.

    The basic biological mechanism of spontaneous repair is described in detail and the durability of the tissue formed discussed.

12. **Jackson, D.W., Lalor, P.A., Aberman, H.M., and Simon, T.M.** (2001). Spontaneous repair of full-thickness defects of articular cartilage in a goat model – A preliminary study. *J Bone Joint Surg* **83**(A):53–64.

13. **Johnson, L.L.** (1990). The sclerotic lesion: pathology and the clinical response to arthroscopic abrasion arthroplasty. In J.W. Ewing (ed.), *Articular Cartilage and Knee Joint Function, Basic Science and Arthroscopy.* New York: Raven Press, pp. 319–33.

14. **Insall, J.** (1974). The Pridie debridement operation for osteoarthritis of the knee. *Clin Orthop,* **32**(B3):302–6.

15. **Blevins, F.T., Steadman, J.R., Rodrigo, J.J., and Silliman, J.** (1998). Treatment of articular cartilage defects in athletes: an analysis of functional outcome and lesion appearance (see comments). *Orthopedics,* **21**:761–67.

16. Coletti, J.M. Jr, Akeson, W.H., and Woo, S.L-Y (1972). A comparison of the physical behaviour of normal articular cartilage and the arthroplasty surface. *J Bone Joint Surg*, 54(A):147–60.

17. Tew, S.R., Kwan, A.P.L., Hann, A., Thomson, B.M., and Archer, C.W. (2000). The reactions of articular cartilage to experimental wounding – Role of apoptosis. *Arthritis Rheum* 43:215–25.

18. Wang, C.C.B., Hung, C.T., and Mow, V.C. (2001). An analysis of the effects of depth-dependent aggregate modulus on articular cartilage stress-relaxation behavior in compression. *J Biomech* 34:75–84.

19. Rosenberg, L. and Hunziker, E.B. (1995). Cartilage repair in osteoarthritis: the role of dermatan sulphate proteoglycans. In K.E. Kuettner and V.M. Goldberg (eds), *Osteoarthritic Disorders*. Rosemont: American Academy of Orthopedic Surgeons, pp. 341–56.

20. Hunziker, E.B., and Kapfinger, E. (1998). Removal of proteoglycans from the surface of defects in articular cartilage transiently enhances coverage by repair cells. *J Bone Joint Surg* 80(B):144–50.

21. Mochizuki, Y., Goldberg, V.M., and Caplan, A.I. (1993). Enzymatical digestion for the repair of superficial articular cartilage lesions. In *Transactions of the 39th Annual Meeting, Orthopedic Research Society*, San Francisco, p. 728.

22. Namba, R.S., Meuli, M., Sullivan, K.M., Le, A.X., and Adzick, N.S. (1998). Spontaneous repair of superficial defects in articular cartilage in a fetal lamb model. *J Bone Joint Surg* 80(A):4–10.

23. Messner, K. (1994). Durability of artificial implants for repair of osteochondral defects of the medial femoral condyle in rabbits. *Biomaterials* 15(9):657–64.

24. Thomson, R.C., Wake, M.C., Yaszemski, M.J., and Mikos, A.G. (1995). Biodegradable polymer scaffolds to regenerate organs. *Adv Poly Sci* 122:245–74.

25. Martin, I., Shastri, V.P., Padera, R.F., *et al.* (2001). Selective differentiation of mammalian bone marrow stromal cells cultured on three-dimensional polymer foams. *J Biomed Mater Res* 55:229–35.

26. Thomson, R.C., Yaszemski, M.J., Powers, J.M., and Mikos, A.G. (1995). Fabrication of biodegradable polymer scaffolds to engineer trabecular bone. *J Biomater Sci, Poly Ed* 7(1):23–38.

27. Kemp, P.D., Cavallaro, J.F., and Hastings, D.N. (1995). Effects of carboiimide crosslinking and bad environment on the remodelling of collagen scaffolds. *Tissue Engineer* 1(1):71–9.

28. Downes, S., Braden, M., Archer, R.S., Patel, M., Davy, K.W., and Swai, H. (1994). Modification of polymers for controlled hydrophilicity: the effect on surface properties. In R. West and G. Batts (eds), *Surface Properties of Biomaterials*. Oxford: Butterworth-Heinemann, pp. 11–23.

29. Corkhill, P.H., Fitton, J.H., and Tighe, B.J. (1993). Towards a synthetic articular cartilage. *J Biomater Sci, Poly Ed* 4(6):615–30.

30. Downes, S., Archer, R.S., Kayser, M.V., Patel, M.P., and Braden, M. (1994). The regeneration of articular cartilage using a new polymer system. *J Mater Sci: Mater Med* 5:88–95.

31. Freed, L.E., Marquis, J.C., Nohria, A., Emmanuel, J., Mikos, A.G., and Langer, R. (1993). Neocartilage formation *in vitro* and *in vivo* using cells cultured on synthetic biodegradable polymers. *J Biomed Mater Res* 27:11–23.

32. Vacanti, C.A., Kim, W., Schloo, B., Upton, J., and Vacanti, J.P. (1994). Joint resurfacing with cartilage grown from cell-polymer structures. *Am J Sports Med* 22(4):485–8.

33. Freed, L.E., Vunjak-Novakovic, G., and Langer, R. (1993). Cultivation of cell-polymer cartilage implants in bioreactors. *J Cell Biochem* 90(3):355–74.

34. Brent, B. (1992). Auricular repair with autogenous rib cartilage grafts—two decades of experience with 600 cases. *Plastic Reconstruc Surg* 90(3):355–74.

35. Czitrom, A.A., Langer, F., McKnee, N., and Gross, A.E. (1986). Bone and cartilage allotransplantation. A review of 14 years of research and clinical studies. *Clin Orthop* 208:141–5.

36. Meyers, M.H., Akeson, W., and Convery, F.R. (1989). Resurfacing of the knee with fresh osteochondral allograft. *J Bone Joint Surg* 71(5):704–13.

37. Homminga, G.A., Bulstra, S.K., Bounmeester, P.S., and van der Linden, A.J. (1990). Perichondral grafting for cartilage lesions of the knee. *J Bone Joint Surg Br* 72(6):1003–7.

38. Moran, M.E., Kim, H.K.W., and Salter, B.B. (1992). Biological resurfacing of full-thickness defects in patellar articular cartilage of the rabbit—Investigation of autogenous periosteal grafts subjected to continuous passive motion. *J Bone Joint Surg* 74(5):659–67.

39. Dunkelman, N.S., Zimber, M.P., LeBaron, R.G., Pavelec, R., Kwan, M., and Purchio, A.F. (1995). Cartilage production by rabbit articular chondrocytes on a polyglycolic acid scaffolds in a closed bioreactor system. *Biotech Bioengineer* 46:299–305.

40. Malinin, T.I., Wagner, J.L., Pita, J.C., and Lott, K. (1985). Hypothermic storage and cryopreservtion of cartilage. An experimental study. *Clin Orthop* 197:15–26.

41. Muldrew, K., Hurtig, M., Novak, K., Schachar, N., and McGann, L.E. (1994). Localization of freezing injury in articular cartilage. *Cryobiology* 31(1):31–8.

42. Scharchar, N.S. and McGann, L.E. (1986). Investigations of low temperature storage of articular cartilage for transplantation. *Clin Orthop* 208:146–50.

43. Cavallaro, J.F., Kemp, P.D., and Kraus, K.H. (1994). Collagen fabrics as biomaterials. *Biotech Bioengineer* 49:781–91.

44. Kato, Y.P. and Silver, F.H. (1990). Continuous collagen fibres: evaluation of biocompatibility and mechanical properties. *Biomaterials* 11:169–75.

45. Nevo, Z., Robinson, D., and Halperin, N. (1992). The use of grafts composed of cultured cells for repair and regeneration of cartilage and bone. In B.K. Hall (ed.), *Bone: Fracture, Repair and Regeneration*. Boca Raton, FL: CRC Press, pp. 123–52.

46. Bentley, G. and Greer H. (1971). Homotransplantation of isolated epiphyseal and articular cartilage chondrocytes into joint surfaces of rabbits. *Nature* 230:385–8.

47. Grande, D.A., Pitman, M.I., Peterson, L., Menche, D., and Klein, M. (1989). The repair of experimentally produced defects in rabbit articular cartilage by autologous chondrocyte transplantation. *J Orthop Res* 7:208–18.

48. Benya, P.D., Padilla, S., and Nimni, M.E. (1978). Independent regulation of collagen types of chondrocytes during the loss of differentiated function in culture. *Cell* 15:1313–21.

49. Benya, P.D. and Shaffer, J.D. (1982). Dedifferentiated chondrocytes re-express the differentiated collagen phenotype when cultured in agarose gels. *Cell* 30(1):215–24.

50. Dennis, J.E., Merriam, A., Awadallah, A., Yoo, J.U., Johnstone, B., and Caplan, A.I. (1999). A quadripotential mesenchymal progenitor cell isolated from the marrow of an adult mouse. *J Bone Miner Res* 14:700–09.

51. *Pittenger, M.F., Mackay, A.M., Beck, S.C., *et al.* (1999). Multilineage potential of adult human mesenchymal stem cells. *Science* 284:143–47.

    The potential of bone-marrow-derived mesenchymal cells to differentiate into various tissue types is addressed and the tissue-specific conditions defined.

52. DeBari, C., DellAccio, F., Tylzanowski, P., and Luyten, F.P. (2001). Multipotent mesenchymal stem cells from adult human synovial membrane. *Arthritis Rheum* 44(8):1928–42.

53. DeBari, C., DellAccio, F., and Luyten, F.P. (2001). Human periosteum-derived cells maintain phenotypic stability and chondrogenic potential throughout expansion regardless of donor age. *Arthritis Rheum* 44:85–95.

54. Wakitani, S., Kimura, T., Hirocka, A., *et al.* (1989). Repair of rabbit articular surfaces with allograft chondrocytes embedded in collagen gel. *J Bone Joint Surg Br* 71(1):74–80.

55. Sams, A.E. and Nixon, A.J. (1995). Chondrocyte laden collagen scaffolds for resurfacing extensive articular cartilage defects. *Osteoarth Cart* 3:47–59.

56. Grande, D.A., Singh, I.J., and Pugh, J. (1987). Healing of experimentally produced lesions in articular cartilage following chondrocyte transplantation. *Anat Rec* 218(2):142–48.

57. Brittberg, M., Nilson, A., Peterson, L., Lindahl, A., and Isaksson, O. (1989). Healing of injured rabbit articular cartilage after transplantation with autologously isolated and cultured chondrocytes. In *Bat Sheva Seminars on Methods used in Research on Cartilagenous Tissues*, Abstracts, Vol. 1, Israel, Tel Aviv, pp. 28–9.

58. Brittberg, M., Lindahl, A., Nilsson, A., Ohlsson, C., Isaksson, O., and Peterson, L. (1994). Treatment of deep cartilage defects in the knee with autologous chondrocyte transplantation. *N Engl J Med* 331(14):879–95.

59. Benayahu, D., Kletter, Y., Zipori, D., and Wientroub, S. (1989). Bone marrow derived stromal cell line expresses osteoblastic phenotype *in vitro* and osteogenic capacity *in vivo*. *J Cell Physio* 140:1–7.

60. Wakitani, S., Goto, T., Pineda, S.J., et al. (1994). Mesenchymal cell-based repair of large full-thickness defects of articular cartilage. *J Bone Joint Surg* **76**(A):579–92.

61. Friedenstein, A. (1973). Determined and inducible osteogenic precursor cells. In K. Elliot and D. Fitzsimmons (eds), *Hard Tissue Growth, Repair, and Remineralization.* Ciba Foundation Symposium. Chichester: John Wiley, pp. 169–85.

62. Owen, M., and Friedenstein, A.J. (1988). Stromal stem cells: marrow-derived osteogenic precursors. In *Cell and Molecular Biology of Vertebrate Hard Tissues.* Ciba Foundation Symposium. Chichester: John Wiley, pp. 42–60.

63. Tsumaki, N., Tanaka, K., ArikawaHirasawa, E., et al. (1999). Role of CDMP-1 in skeletal morphogenesis: Promotion of mesenchymal cell recruitment and chondrocyte differentiation. *J Cell Biol* **144**:161–73.

64. Hubbell, J.A., Massia, S.P., and Drumheller, P.P. (1992). Surface-grafted cell-binding peptides in tissue engineering of the vascular graft. *Ann NY Acad Sci* **665**:253–8.

65. Lin, H.B., Garcia-Echeverria, C., Asakura, S., Sun, W., Mosher, D.F., and Cooper, S.L. (1992). Endothelial cell adhesion on polyurethanes containing covalently attached RGD peptides. *Biomaterials* **13**:905–14.

66. Rutherford, R.B., Sampath, T.K., Renger, D.C., and Taylor, T.D. (1992). Use of bovine osteogenic protein to promote rapid osteointegration of endosseus dental implants. *Int J Oral Maxillofacial Implant* **7**:297–301.

67. Cook, S.D., Wolfe, M.W., Salkeld, S.L., and Renger, D.C. (1995). The effect of recombinant human osteogenic protein 1 on healing of large segmental bone defects in non-human primates. *J Bone Joint Surg* **77**(A):734–50.

68. Ripamonti, U., Ma, S.S., van den Heever, B., and Reddi, A.H. (1992). Osteogenin, a bone morphogenic protein absorbed on porous hydroxy-apetite substrate induces rapid bone differentiation in calvarial defects of adult primates. *Plastic Reconstruc Surg* **90**:382–93.

69. Adolphe, M. and Benya, P. (1992). Different types of cultured chondrocytes: the *in vitro* approach to the study of biological regulation. In M. Adolphe (ed.), *Biological Regulation of the Chondrocytes.* Boca Raton, FL: CRC Press, pp. 105–39.

70. Kato, Y. (1992). Roles of fibroblast growth factor and transforming growth factor beta families in cartilage formation. In M. Adlophe (ed.), *Biological Regulation of the Chondrocyte,* Boca Raton, FL: CRC Press, pp. 141–80.

71. Trippel, S.B. (1992). Role of insulin-like growth factors in the regulation of chondrocytes. In M. Adolphe (ed.), *Biological regulation of the chondrocyte.* Boca Raton, FL: CRC Press, pp. 161–90.

72. Morales, T.I. and Hascall, V.C. (1989). Factors involved in the regulation of proteoglycan metabolism in articular cartilage. *Arthritis Rheum* **32**:1197–201.

73. Tyler, J.A. (1989). Insulin-like growth factor 1 can decrease degradation and promote synthesis of proteoglycan in cartilage exposed to cytokines. *Biochem J* **260**:543–8.

74. Luten, F.P., Chen, P., Paralkar, V., and Reddi, A.H. (1994). Recombinant bone morphogenic protein 4, transforming growth factor *b* and activin A enhance the cartilage phenotype of articular chondrocytes *in vitro*. *Exp Cell Res* **210**:224–9.

75. Reddi, A.H. (1992). Regulation of cartilage and bone differentiation by bone morphogenetic proteins. *Curr Opin Cell Biol* **4**:850–5.

76. Hunziker, E.B., Driesang, I.M.K, and Morris E.A. (2001). Chondrogenesis in cartilage repair is induced by members of the transformiong growth factor-beta superfamily. *Clin Orthop Rel Res* **391S**:S171–S181.

77. *Centrella, M., Horowitz, M.C., Wozney, J.M., and McCarthy, T.L. (1994). Transforming growth factor *b* gene family members and bone. *Endocrine Rev* **15**:27–39.
    Regulatory mechanisms involved in cartilage and bone formation are reviewed and the specific role of bone morphogenetic proteins in these processes discussed.

78. Massagué, J., Attisano, L., and Wrana, J.L. (1994). The TGF*b* family and its composite receptors. *Trends Cell Biol* **4**:172–8.

79. Wozney, J.M., Rosen, V., Celeste, A.J., Mitstock, L.M., Whitters, M.J., Kriz, R.W., et al. (1988). Novel regulators of bone formation: molecular clones and activities. *Science* **242**:1528–34.

80. Roberts, A.B., Sporn, M.B., Assoian, R.K., et al. (1986). TGF*b*: rapid induction of fibrosis and angiogenesis *in vivo* and stimulation of collagen formation *in vitro*. *Proc Nat Acad Sci* **83**: 4167–71.

81. Noda, M. and Camilliere, J.J. (1989). *In vivo* stimulation of bone formation by TGF*b*. *Endocrinology* **124**:2291–4.

82. Beck, L.S., Amman, A.J., Aufdemorte, T.B., et al. (1991). *In vivo* induction of bone by recombinant TGF*b* 1. *J Bone Miner Res* **6**:961–8.

83. Centrella, M., McCarthy, T.L., and Canalis, E. (1987). TGF*b* is a bifunctional regulator of replication and collagen synthesis in osteoblast-enriched cell cultures from fetal rat bone. *J Biol Chem* **262**:2869–74.

84. Gazit, D., Ebner, R., Kahn, A.J., and Derynck, R. (1993). Modulation of expression of cell surface binding of members of the TGF*b* superfamily during retinoic acid—induced osteoblastic differentiation of multipotential mesenchymal cells. *Mol Endocrinol* **7**:189–98.

85. Yang, N.N., Hardikar, S., Kim, J., and Sato, M. (1993). Raloxifene and 'anti-estrogen' stimulates the effects of estrogen on inhibiting bone resorption through regulating TGF*b* 3 expression on bone. *J Bone Miner Res* **8**:118.

86. Schmid, P., Cox, D., Bilbe, G., Maier, R., and McMaster, G.K. (1991). Differential expression of TGF*b*1, *b*2 and *b*3 genes during mouse embryogenesis. *Development* **111**:117–30.

87. Millan, F.A., Denhez, F., Kondaiah, P., and Akhurst, R.J. (1991). Embryonic gene expression of TFG*b*1, *b*2 and *b*3 suggest different development functions *in vivo*. *Development* **111**:131–44.

88. Hunziker, E.B. and Rosenberg, L.C. (1995). Repair of partial thickness articular cartilage defects. (Cell recruitment from the synovium.) *J Bone Joint Surg Am* **78**(A):721–33.

89. *Hunziker, E.B. (1999). Articular cartilage repair: Are the intrinsic biological constraints undermining this process insuperable? *Osteoarth Cart* **7**:15–28.
    This short review deals concisely with the problems and potential of experimental and clinical approaches to articular cartilage repair.

90. Hunziker, E.B. (2001). Growth-factor induced healing of partial-thickness defects in adult articular cartilage. *Osteoarthritis Cart* **9**(1):22–32.

91. Hendrickson, D.H., Nixon, A.J., and Grande, D.A. (1994). Chondrocyte-fibrin matrix transplants for resurfacing extensive articular cartilage defects. *J Orthop Res* **12**:485–97.

92. Kaplonyi, G., Zimmerman, I., Frenyo, A.D., Farkas, T., and Nemes, G. (1988). The use of fibrin adhesive in the repair of chondral and osteochondral injuries. *Injury* **19**:267–72.

93. Jürgensen, K., Aeschlimann, D., Cavin, V., Genge, M., and Hunziker, E.B. (1995). A new biological glue for cartilage–cartilage interfaces: tissue transglutaminase. *J Bone Joint Surg Am* **79**(A):185–94.

94. Aeschliman, D., Wetterwald, A., Fleisch, H., and Paulsson, M. (1993). Expression of tissue transglutaminase in skeletal tissues correlates with events of terminal differentiation of chondrocytes. *J Cell Biol* **120**: 1461–70.

95. Upchurch, H.F., Conway, E., Patterson, M.K. Jr, and Maxwell, M.D. (1991). Localization of cellular transglutaminase on the extracellular matrix after wounding: characteristics of the matrix bound enzyme. *J Cell Physiol* **149**:375–82.

96. Folk, J.E. and Finlayson, J.S. (1977). The e-(g-glutamyl) lysine cross-link and the catalytic role of transglutaminase. *Adv Protein Chem* **31**:1–133.

97. Allen, J.B., Manthey, C.L., and Hand, A.R. (1990). Rapid onset of synovial inflammation and hyperplasia induced by transforming growth factor *b*. *J Exp Med* **171**:231–47.

98. Elford, P.R., Graeber, M., and Ohtsu, A. (1992). Induction of swelling, synovial hyperplasia and cartilage proteoglycan loss upon intra-articular injection of TGF*b*2 in the rabbit. *Cytokine* **4**:232–8.

99. Wahl, S.M. (1992). Transforming growth factor *b* in inflammation. A cause and a cure. *J Clin Immunol* **12**:61–74.

100. Hunziker, E.B., Driesang, I.M.K., and Saager C. (2001). Structural barrier principle for growth factor-based articular cartilage repair. *Clin Orthop Rel Res* **391S**:S182–S189.

101. Hunziker, E.B., and Driesang, I.M.K. (2002). Functional barrier principle for growth-factor-based articular cartilage repair. *Clin Orthop Rel Res*, submitted for publication.

7.2.1.4 Mechanical properties of normal and osteoarthritic articular cartilage, and the mechanobiology of chondrocytes

Van C. Mow and Clark T. Hung

Articular cartilage forms a thin layer lining the articulating ends of all diarthrodial joints. The primary functions of this layer are to minimize contact stresses generated during joint loading, and to contribute to lubrication mechanisms in the joint.[1–3] When an external load is applied to the joint, the cartilage deforms to increase contact areas and local joint congruence. As a result, tensile, shear, and compressive stresses are generated in the cartilage layer in a spatially varying distribution across the joint and through the thickness of the cartilage. As a result of the specialized composition and

structural organization of the tissue, the response of the cartilage to these stresses can vary markedly.

In general, the material properties of the articular cartilage are anisotropic[4,5] (direction-dependent) and inhomogeneous[4–7] (position-dependent). Furthermore, the response of the tissue to an applied load will vary with time, giving rise to well-described viscoelastic behaviours, such as creep, stress relaxation,[4,7–9] and energy dissipation (i.e., hysteresis) (Fig. 7.22). These viscoelastic behaviours arise from the interstitial fluid flow through the porous matrix,[9] and from the time-dependent deformation of the solid macromolecules in response to loading.[4,8] Exudation and imbibition of interstitial fluid play important roles in articular cartilage, by providing a mechanism for the transport of nutrients[9,10] and for the recovery of the initial dimensions of the tissue after removal of load.[1,9] This ability of cartilage to imbibe fluid (i.e., to swell) is also important for maintaining pre-stresses in the unloaded tissue, which are important in its normal load-bearing functions.[11,12]

Although it is a relatively soft material (compared to bone), normal articular cartilage is able to withstand the large forces associated with weight-bearing and joint motion over a lifetime without damage. In OA,

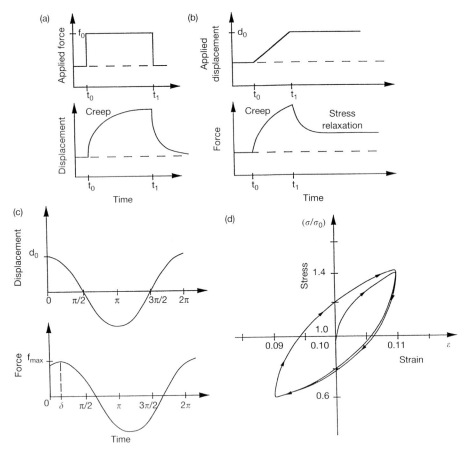

Fig. 7.22 Schematics of load-deformation behaviours of viscoelastic materials. (a) In a creep test, a step load (f_0) applied to a viscoelastic solid at t_0 results in a transient increase of deformation or creep. In articular cartilage, this transient behaviour is governed by the frictional forces generated as the interstitial fluid flows through the porous-permeable solid matrix, and by the frictional interactions between the matrix macromolecules, such as proteoglycan and collagen. Removal of f_0 at t_1 results in full recovery. In articular cartilage, recovery occurs as a result of the release of the energy stored in the elastic solid matrix that is required to overcome the frictional drag of fluid imbibition. (b) In a stress-relaxation test, a displacement is applied at a steady rate, or ramped from t_0 to t_1, until a desired level of compression is reached. This displacement results in a stress-rise followed by stress-relaxation for $t > t_1$, until an equilibrium stress value is reached. In articular cartilage, the stress rise is due to the frictional forces of fluid flow and intermolecular interactions, and stress relaxation is due to fluid redistribution within the tissue and internal rearrangement of the molecular organization. (c) In dynamic testing, a steady oscillatory displacement or force may be applied to a linear viscoelastic material. This results in an oscillatory response that lags the input by a phase-shift angle, δ. This angle is also known as the loss angle. (d) In cyclic deformation, a hysteresis loop is always generated for dissipative materials. The area enclosed within the hysteresis loop is the energy dissipated (per unit volume of material) required to execute one cycle of deformation. For articular cartilage, the energy dissipated is largely due to the friction of fluid flow through the porous-permeable solid matrix. In shear, the energy dissipated is due to intermolecular friction among the structural macromolecules, for example, collagen and proteoglycans.

however, cartilage degeneration results in the gross fibrillation of the articular surface, that is, the presence of cracks or fissures, with partial or complete loss of the tissue.[13–15] Additional signs of OA include an increase in cartilage hydration, changes in the subchondral bone, osteophytosis, altered metabolic activity of the chondrocytes, and changes in the structure and composition of the proteoglycans (PG), collagen, and other macromolecules in the affected articular cartilage, and in its mechanical and physicochemical properties.[16–18] It is known that cartilage tends to 'soften' during degeneration and in OA. This chapter provides a historical review of the study of structure-function relationships in normal articular cartilage and a contemporary understanding of how the mechanical function of the tissue may change in OA.[1,2]

Composition and structure of articular cartilage

As a material, articular cartilage is to be considered as a fibre-reinforced composite solid matrix that is saturated with water (Fig. 7.23). A detailed description of the composition and structure of articular cartilage is provided in Chapter 7.2.1.1. The water phase constitutes 65–85 per cent of the total tissue weight, and is important in controlling many of the physical properties of the tissue.[1,2,6,7,9,17,18] The dominant load-bearing structural component of the solid extracellular matrix (ECM) is type II collagen (about 75 per cent of the tissue dry weight), and the negatively charged PGs (about 20–30 per cent of the dry weight), which vary in content throughout the depth of the tissue. Accompanying the depth-dependent biochemical properties is a highly specific ultrastructure, consisting of successive 'zones' from the surface to the interface with the subchondral bone[1,6,7,19–24] (Fig. 7.23). Collagen molecules form small fibrils whose orientation and dimension varies through the depth of the cartilage.[1,4,5,19–22] The major PGs of articular cartilage consist of large numbers of aggregating macromolecules, known as 'aggrecan'. A single aggrecan molecule consists of a protein core to which numerous glycosaminoglycans (GAG) are attached.[1,12,19,23–25] These GAGs consist of repeating disaccharide units, each of which contains at least one negatively charged group (COO^- or SO_3^-). These negatively charged groups in the tissue have been quantified as a fixed charge density (FCD).[12,23] Most aggrecan molecules are bound to a long chain of hyaluronan to form large PG aggregates [molecular weight = $50–100 \times 10^6$ Da].[24,25] The large size and complex structure of the aggregates serve to immobilize and restrain the PGs within the interfibrillar space, forming the 'solid matrix' of articular cartilage. The physical response of cartilage to applied forces or deformation involves physical and chemical interactions between collagen, PGs, non-collagenous proteins, dissolved ions, and interstitial water.

The chondrocytes must ultimately maintain the composition and structure of the ECM[10,24] and provide for the biomechanical function of the cartilage layer over the lifetime of the joint. In OA, numerous changes occur in the composition and structure of the matrix molecules, and in intermolecular interactions, that adversely affect the mechanical properties of the cartilage. Under such conditions, the chondrocytes are no longer able to maintain homeostasis, either because of an alteration of the normal signal transduction pathways or cellular abnormalities, such as apoptosis or tissue necrosis. In the following sections we will review the mechanical behaviours of normal articular cartilage in tension, shear, compression, and swelling and will describe the changes that are associated with aging, cartilage degeneration, and OA.

Mechanics of articular cartilage

Tension

When cartilage is loaded or stretched in tension, the collagen fibrils and entangled PG molecules align and stretch along the axis of loading[1,4,5,19] (Fig. 7.24). For small deformations, when the tensile stress in the specimen

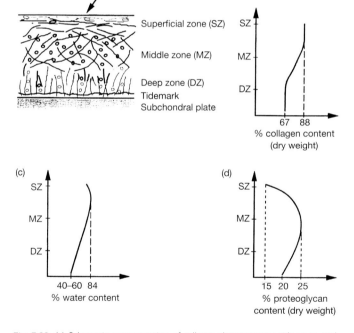

Fig. 7.23 (a) Schematic representation of collagen ultrastructure within a sagittal plane of articular cartilage. The superficial tangential zone (STZ) is a region of densely packed collagen fibrils. In the middle zone (MZ), the collagen fibrils are more loosely packed and are randomly orientated. In the deep zone (DZ), the collagen fibrils anastamose, forming larger fibre bundles that insert into the calcified zone across the tidemark. (b) The distribution of collagen, per unit of tissue dry weight, as a function of depth from the articular surface. The concentration of collagen through the depth of the tissue reflects the ultrastructural organization of the collagen. (c) The distribution of water content [(total weight minus dry weight)/total weight] as a function of depth from the articular surface. (d) Proteoglycan content per unit of tissue dry weight as a function of depth from the articular surface.

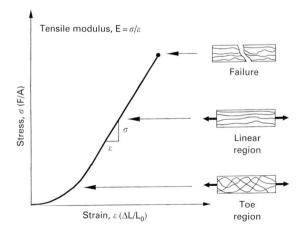

Fig. 7.24 Characteristic stress-strain relationship for articular cartilage in a steady strain-rate tensile experiment. As the cartilage is pulled in tension, the stress increases non-linearly in the toe region as randomly oriented collagen fibrils align themselves in the direction of loading. In the linear region, the tensile stress increases linearly as the collagen fibrils are stretched until failure occurs. A and L_0 are the initial cross-sectional area and length of the specimen, respectively. F and ΔL are the tensile force and change in length, and ϵ and σ are the tensile strain and stress, respectively.

is relatively small, a 'toe-region' is seen in the stress-strain curve, due primarily to the realignment of the collagen network, rather than to the stretching of the collagen fibrils. With greater deformation, the collagen fibrils are stretched and generate a larger tensile stress, due to the stiffness of the fibrils themselves.[1,4,5] The proportionality constant in the 'linear' region of the tensile stress-strain curve is known as 'Young's modulus'. This modulus is a measure of the flow-independent, or intrinsic, stiffness of the collagen-PG solid matrix, and depends on the density of the collagen fibrils, fibril diameter, type or amount of collagen cross-linking, and the strength of ionic bonds and frictional interactions between the collagen network and the more labile PG network.[1,19,26–29]

The tensile modulus of cartilage may be determined from the stress-strain relationship at equilibrium. In general, the tensile modulus of normal cartilage varies in the range 5–25 MPa, depending on the location on the joint surface (e.g., high versus low weight-bearing regions), and depth and orientation of the test specimen, relative to the surface.[1,4,5,26] In skeletally mature tissue, the surface zone of articular cartilage is much stiffer than the middle and deep zones and the tensile stiffness is greater in samples oriented parallel to the local 'split-line' direction at the surface. In human cartilage, the tensile modulus, stiffness, and failure stress correlate with the collagen content, and the ratio of collagen to PG.[26] After treatment with elastase to disrupt collagen cross-linking, reduction as great as 99 per cent in tensile stiffness and failure stress were observed, demonstrating that collagen cross-linking and fibrillar organization are significant determinants of the tensile properties of cartilage.[26] In contrast, no significant correlations have been observed between the failure or intrinsic tensile properties of the cartilage and its PG content.[27,28] In summary, these studies emphasized the role of collagen in governing the tensile stress-strain and failure behaviours of articular cartilage.

Tensile properties have been evaluated in mildly fibrillated human cartilage from cadavers, and OA cartilage obtained from patients with advanced disease undergoing joint arthroplasty. The variations in equilibrium tensile modulus among normal, mildly fibrillated, and OA human knee cartilage are shown in Table 7.6.[1,26] Decreases in the tensile modulus of femoral groove cartilage were observed in samples from patients with OA and samples with only mild fibrillation obtained from the non-arthritic cadavers. An important finding was that the grossly normal cartilage adjacent to degenerated areas exhibited decreases in tensile stiffness and failure stress similar in magnitude to those of OA cartilage. The changes in cartilage mechanics in OA appear to be secondary to micro-structural changes in the collagen network, with disorganization, or 'loosening', of the fibrillar network.[29] Age-related changes have also been reported, including a decrease in tensile stiffness and fracture stress of cartilage from surface and deep zones. In general, however, these age-related and other non-progressive degenerative changes are less severe than OA changes.[30,31]

Shear

Articular cartilage responds to shearing forces by stretching and deformation of the collagen fibrils in the solid matrix (Fig. 7.25). Under conditions of pure shear, as shown, the tissue deforms with no change in volume and, therefore, with no significant interstitial pressure gradient or fluid flow

through the matrix.[8,32,33] Viscoelastic effects, such as creep, stress-relaxation, and hysteresis, arise in shearing as a result of the frictional interactions between the collagen and PGs in the solid matrix. Shear studies of articular cartilage have been performed under equilibrium, transient, or dynamic conditions to characterize the intrinsic, or flow-independent, shear behaviours of the material. The equilibrium shear modulus for normal human, bovine, and canine articular cartilage has been found to vary in the range of 0.05–0.25 MPa.

Dynamic shear experiments are used to quantify the energy dissipation to heat resulting from the frictional interactions between macromolecules in the matrix. Values for the magnitude of the dynamic shear modulus ($|G^*|$) of normal cartilage are in the range 0.2–2.0 MPa, and vary with both the frequency and magnitude of the stress. The loss angle (δ) for cartilage in shear is a measure of the matrix dissipation, with a loss angle of 0° corresponding to a perfectly elastic material, and 90° to a perfectly dissipative material. Similarly, the values for the loss angle of normal articular cartilage depend on frequency and magnitude, but are generally in the range of 9–15°. Several studies have reported decreases in the dynamic shear modulus of bovine cartilage, as great as 50 per cent, after experimental depletion of the PG content.[32,33] In contrast, increases in the dynamic shear modulus were observed in cartilage that had been incubated with formaldehyde, which induces cross-linking of the collagen network. While the shear behaviour of cartilage clearly depends on both collagen and PG, the relatively small loss angle and large shear modulus (when compared to that of PG solutions at physiological concentrations) suggest that collagen fibrils may be the dominant determinants of the behaviour of articular cartilage in shear in Fig. 7.25.

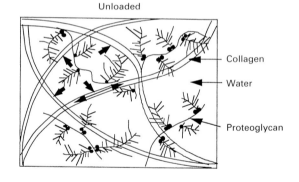

Unloaded

Collagen
Water
Proteoglycan

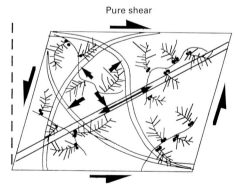

Pure shear

Fig. 7.25 When a block of material is sheared, stretching can occur throughout the sample. Maximum stretch will occur in the 45° direction, that is, the principal direction. This maximum tensile strain is equal in magnitude to the imposed shear strain. Therefore, when a block of articular cartilage is sheared, collagen fibrils can be stretched by a significant amount. Based on a comparison of the magnitude of the tensile modulus and the shear modulus, the number of collagen fibrils recruited to be stretched in this manner may be only 5–10 per cent of the fibrils available within the tissue.

Table 7.6 Equilibrium tensile modulus (mean ± SD) of normal, fibrillated, and OA human articular cartilage[26]

Site sample	Cartilage sample		
	Normal	Fibrillated	OA
Surface	7.79 (1.73)	7.15 (1.89)	1.36 (0.09)
Subsurface	4.85 (1.37)	7.47 (0.65)	0.85 (0.81)
Middle	4.00 (1.05)	4.90 (1.03)	2.11 (0.30)

All samples were harvested from the femoral condyle in an orientation parallel to the local split-line direction.

The PGs also contribute to the shear stiffness of cartilage; this is achieved indirectly by the generation of a large swelling pressure that 'inflates' the collagen network and thus provides a tensile pre-stress in the network.[11,12] The detailed variations of the dynamic complex modulus (magnitude and loss angle) as a function of frequency of excitation and amount of clamping compression used in the experiment are shown in Table 7.7.[33] These two quantities show that the shear properties of the solid matrix of articular cartilage is viscoelastic and highly non-linear.

Few shear studies have been reported for fibrillated or OA cartilage from humans. Hayes and Mockros[8] observed that degenerated cartilage was significantly more compliant in shear than normal cartilage, and attributed this to loss of the articular surface and of 'ground substance' (i.e., to a decreased PG content). The observed changes are consistent with trends demonstrated for the shear behaviour of bovine cartilage after depletion of PG or collagen.[33] Although treatment of the cartilage with formaldehyde resulted in an increase in cartilage stiffness, evidence of a role for either collagen or PG in these degeneration-induced changes has yet to be confirmed directly by studies of human OA cartilage in the shear configuration.

Compression

When cartilage is loaded in compression, changes in volume occur because of exudation and/or the redistribution of fluid within the tissue. These effects give rise to significant time-dependent viscoelastic behaviours, such as creep and stress relaxation.[1,7,9,17,18] This viscoelastic response in compression is due to the very high drag forces associated with the flow of interstitial fluid through the dense porous-permeable solid matrix, that is, the ECM, and the high fluid pressures required to cause this flow. Therefore, articular cartilage will exhibit a viscoelastic creep in response to a *constant* compressive load, that is, its compressive deformation will increase with time until an equilibrium value is reached (Fig. 7.22(a)). Conversely, if a *constant* displacement is imposed on the cartilage sample, a stress relaxation is observed, with a transient decrease in compressive stress occurring to a constant value at equilibrium (Fig. 7.22(b)).[1,9] Only at equilibrium, when no fluid flow or pressure gradients exist, is the entire applied load borne by the solid matrix. Thus, the true compressive modulus of cartilage matrix may be obtained from the relationship between compressive stress and strain at equilibrium (e.g., H_A or E), which has been shown to be linear under conditions of small strain.[9,19] Upon removal of the compressive load, articular cartilage will 'recover' its initial dimensions, largely through the elasticity of the solid matrix, and the imbibition and redistribution of fluid within the interstitium. While the dominant dissipative mechanism for the compressive viscoelastic effects in cartilage is the drag associated with interstitial fluid flow through the permeable solid matrix, flow-independent interactions between macromolecules of the solid matrix in shear will also contribute to its compression viscoelasticity.[1,8,32,33]

Movement of fluid is governed by the hydraulic permeability of the solid matrix (k), which is related to the apparent size and connectivity of its pore structure.[9,19,23] The PG concentration affects tissue permeability, because negative charges and the frictional drag of the flow of ions through the water will impede hydraulic fluid flow.[1,12,23,34] In addition, hydraulic permeability is related to the volumetric change of the porous-permeable matrix during compression, because of an increase of the FCD and a decrease of the apparent pore size associated with compaction of the tissue[1,9,19] (Fig. 7.26). As a result, both the transient and equilibrium compressive behaviours of cartilage exhibit a dependence on PG content, as demonstrated experimentally with *in situ* indentation and uniaxial, confined compression testing (Fig. 7.27).

The compressive creep behaviour of cartilage has been analysed with a constitutive model, incorporating both a fluid and a solid phase to describe the flow-dependent viscoelasticity.[1,9,19] This biphasic model has served as an important tool for determining the material properties of articular cartilage from compression tests. In addition, the biphasic theory provides a framework for interpreting and predicting the effects of flow-dependent phenomena in cartilage under more complex loading and geometric configurations.[1,19] The theoretical predictions of the compressive creep and stress-relaxation experiments have been obtained, and material properties have been determined from the experimental data. Values for the equilibrium compressive modulus ($H_A = 0.4$–1.0 MPa) for normal cartilage vary with the location on the joint surface, and between species. The hydraulic permeability in articular cartilage ($k = 0.5$–5.0×10^{-15} m^4/N-sec) is extremely small, indicating that large interstitial fluid pressures and drag-induced dissipations occur in normal articular cartilage during compressive loading. These mechanisms for fluid pressurization and flow-dependent energy dissipation provide an efficient method to shield the solid matrix of cartilage from the high stresses and strains associated with joint loading, as the pressurized fluid component provides more than 95 per cent of the load-bearing function in the cartilage layer.[2,19,35]

Values for the compressive modulus, determined using a biphasic theoretical analysis,[9] correlate with both the hydration and GAG content of articular cartilage, pointing to the importance of the physicochemical properties of the negatively charged PGs in influencing the compressive behaviours of cartilage.[1,17,19,36] During compression, the FCD increases, resulting in an increased swelling pressure and propensity of the cartilage to imbibe fluid. This increased swelling pressure is associated with an apparent stiffening of the cartilage matrix in compression.[12,36] Therefore, biologic factors that contribute to a lower FCD, such as a higher water content

Table 7.7 Variation of the mean values (± SD) of the magnitude of dynamic shear modulus, |G*| (MPa), and for the phase-shift angle δ (degrees) for skeletally mature bovine knee articular cartilage at varying frequencies (f) and compression strains (e%)[33]

	e (%)	f = 0.01 Hz	f = 0.1 Hz	f = 1.0 Hz	f = 10 Hz
|G*|, MPa	5	0.19 (0.10)	0.23 (0.15)	0.29 (0.18)	0.38 (0.20)
	10	0.57 (0.26)	0.71 (0.21)	0.87 (0.39)	1.10 (0.52)
	15	0.86 (0.35)	1.06 (0.26)	1.27 (0.47)	1.60 (0.59)
	20	1.00 (0.31)	1.20 (0.43)	1.45 (0.45)	1.79 (0.55)
δ, degrees	5	14.4 (4.13)	13.6 (3.38)	11.6 (2.06)	12.6 (4.05)
	10	14.6 (2.38)	11.5 (2.36)	10.8 (1.81)	11.6 (2.36)
	15	13.5 (2.38)	10.1 (4.73)	9.40 (1.79)	9.92 (1.86)
	20	13.1 (2.06)	9.25 (2.36)	9.07 (1.70)	9.36 (1.69)

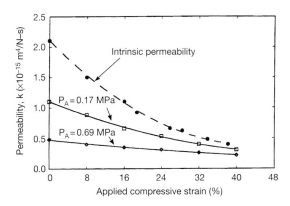

Fig. 7.26 The hydraulic permeability of normal articular cartilage decreases with increasing compression, and applied fluid pressurization (P_A). The decrease of permeability with increasing pressure is due to a phenomenon called 'drag-induced compaction', that is, as the fluid is forced to flow through the porous-permeable solid matrix, the drag exerted by the fluid on the solid matrix causes the latter to be compressed[1,9,19]. This effect has important physiologic implications, that is, it prevents the tissue from being depleted of fluid or 'wrung-out' under prolonged compression.

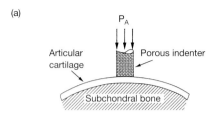

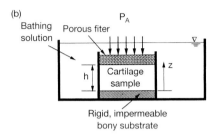

Fig. 7.27 Schema of two configurations frequently used to study the compressive behaviour of articular cartilage: (a) In the biphasic indentation configuration, a compressive load (P_A) is applied to the cartilage surface through a rigid-porous-permeable, and flat-ended, circular indenter. The porous-permeable indenter allows fluid exudation to occur freely into the indenter tip and, therefore, creep of the cartilage layer. The kinetics of creep are rate-limited by interstitial fluid flow and exudation, and, therefore, tissue permeability. This test, along with the biphasic indentation theory[1,9], permit determination of the aggregate modulus, H_A, Poisson's ratio, ν_s, and permeability, k_0. (b) In the confined compression configuration, a load (P_A) is applied to the cartilage sample via a rigid-porous-permeable loading platen. The side walls are assumed to be smooth (frictionless), impermeable, and rigid, thereby preventing lateral expansion and fluid flow. This yields a uniaxial or one-dimensional test. This test, along with the biphasic confined compression creep theory[9], permits determination of the aggregate modulus, H_A, and the intrinsic permeability coefficients, k_0 and M.

or lower GAG content, will give rise to a tissue that is more compliant in compression.

In recent years, gains have been made in our understanding of the compressive behaviour of human articular cartilage with degeneration or OA. Articular cartilage that exhibits surface fibrillation, pitting, or fraying is more compliant than normal tissue in *in situ* indentation and confined compression tests.[1,19,31,33] The compressive modulus of human patellar cartilage has been found to decrease with increasing severity of degeneration.[17–19,23] In these studies, the compressive modulus was also found to decrease with advancing age, a factor that is difficult to separate from the severity of degeneration. Hydraulic permeability, in contrast, had not been found to vary significantly with age, but can increase with degeneration. The compressive modulus and hydraulic permeability are known to depend strongly on the hydration of the tissue, which may not vary significantly with age. In summary, the changes associated with OA, such as fibrillation, increased hydration, and decreased PG content, compromise the compressive properties of articular cartilage and, therefore, disrupt the capacity of the interstitial fluid to support load.[2,9,19,35]

Recently, a constitutive law for articular cartilage was developed to incorporate the effects of negatively charged groups associated with the PGs. This triphasic theory,[1,12,34,36] provides for explicit mathematical relationships between the material coefficients of cartilage and the fundamental physicochemical parameters, such as hydration (as measured by porosity), reference FCD, and the drag coefficients between water and solid or between ions and water. This constitutive law has been used to quantify experimental observations of a direct relationship between the hydraulic permeability and water content of articular cartilage, and to finally settle a

historic controversy as to exactly how much Donnan osmotic pressure contributes to the equilibrium compressive stiffness.[1,12,23,36] Indeed, these recent studies have shown that Donnan osmotic pressure can only contribute up to approximately 50 per cent of the compressive modulus.

According to this triphasic law, the hydraulic permeability of articular cartilage will vary with the square of the porosity and inversely with the FCD, pointing to the importance of hydration in governing fluid flow, ion transport, and all other transient deformational phenomena related to hydraulic permeability.[19,34,36] The high level of agreement between the experimental data and predictions based on the triphasic theory offers promise for understanding the functional role played by the PGs in the ECM, and supports the view that fundamental mechanisms underlying the physical behaviours of normal, degenerated, and OA cartilage can now be elucidated with the use of this material model.

Swelling

Changes in the hydration of articular cartilage, or 'edema', are among the first effects detected in cartilage degeneration and OA.[1,16,17,23,37,38] With normal aging, a slight decrease in hydration occurs, so that swelling may be one of the few characteristics that distinguish age-related degeneration from OA. Swelling in cartilage arises from the presence of the high FCD associated with PG molecules.[1,11,12,19] Each PG-associated negative charge requires a 'mobile' counter-ion (e.g., Na^+) to maintain electroneutrality within the interstitium, giving rise to an imbalance of mobile ions between the interstitium and the external solution. This excess of mobile ions generates, in a colligative manner, an osmotic pressure that contributes to the swelling pressure in the tissue. When the external bathing solution is very small, by the Donnan equilibrium ion distribution law, the internal counter-ion concentration is that of the total PG charges. Using a sodium isotope method, this principle yields a simple technique to determine cartilage PG content.[12,23] With an increasing concentration of ions in the external bathing solution, the difference in ion concentration (internal minus external) will become vanishingly small, and the overall osmotic pressure will, therefore, also decrease.[12,23,24]

At equilibrium, the swelling pressure in articular cartilage will be balanced by the tensile forces generated in the collagen network[11] and the stresses developed in the solid matrix.[12] Therefore, the solid matrix is in a state of pre-stress, even when unloaded. Changes in the internal swelling pressure arising from the altered GAG content or counter-ion concentrations, result in changes in the dimensions of the tissue and in its hydration. In addition, variations in the GAG concentration and matrix stiffness throughout the cartilage will cause non-uniform swelling throughout the tissue, and will give rise to a 'warping' or 'curling' effect *ex situ*.[1,19] As a result, cartilage swells and imbibes water in hypotonic salt solutions, and loses water in hypertonic salt solutions. The amount of fluid imbibition has been shown to increase in human cartilage after the collagen network has been digested by treatment with collagenase.[27,28] Furthermore, fibrillated human cartilage has been found to imbibe more fluid than the grossly normal cartilage from OA joints.[11,12,16,23,26,37,38]

Quantification of water imbibition after equilibration in a bath, as described above, has been used extensively to study changes in cartilage swelling with aging and with OA. Immediately after excision from the bone, cartilage from grossly normal femoral heads was found to have a lower water content than fibrillated cartilage from femoral heads.[16] An important finding was that grossly normal cartilage from sites adjacent to those with 'coarse' fibrillation had a level of hydration similar to that of finely fibrillated cartilage, suggesting that the elevated water content of OA cartilage is very sensitive to collagen network damage, corroborating the experimental findings of increased hydration in cartilage after digestion with collagenase.[18,19,26,33] The swelling behaviours of articular cartilage also vary with the orientation of the tissue, due to anisotropy of the matrix.[39] When bathed in solutions with varying ion concentrations, strips of bovine cartilage were found to swell to a greater extent in the thickness dimension than in length or width. Studies of dimensional swelling effects have demonstrated that the greatest magnitude of swelling strain occurs in the deepest zone of cartilage in the length dimension, with virtually no swelling strains at the surface. The differences in swelling strain between the surface and deep zones are consistent with the differences in tissue organization and composition (Fig. 7.23).

Together, these material properties govern the ability of articular cartilage to function normally, within the highly loaded environment of a diarthrodial joint. Changes in the composition and molecular architecture of the load-carrying macromolecules of the tissue, and the amount of water present in the interstitium, will alter the normal mechanical and physicochemical properties of articular cartilage and diminish its ability to sustain these loads. Insights into this degenerative process have been gained from studies in animal models of cartilage damage that have been shown to result in OA.[15,18,29,40,41]

An experimental canine model of cartilage degeneration: transection of the anterior cruciate ligament (ACLT)

While studies of human OA have advanced our understanding of the altered mechanics of cartilage in the OA joint, they provide little information on the temporal progression of joint degeneration, particularly in the earliest stages of the disease. Studies of experimentally induced cartilage degeneration in animal models, however, provide a means of tracking the time sequence of these early events. In addition, they permit isolation of the aging factor from the degenerative process of OA, which has proved to be a major problem in the studies of human OA. Many experimental models of cartilage degeneration have been based on altered joint mechanics, including single or repetitive impact loading, and damage to ligaments or menisci[15,18,29,40,41] (see Chapter 11.3). In models that involve damage to ligaments or menisci, inhibition of these force-attenuating mechanisms will alter both the magnitude and distribution of stresses applied to the cartilage surface *in vivo*. The canine ACLT model of joint instability and OA has been the model most widely used to study degenerative changes in articular cartilage.

Alterations to cartilage composition and structure

After ACLT, morphological changes in the articular cartilage include fibrillation of the articular surface, early loss of PGs and collagen, increased cellularity and water content, degeneration of the meniscus, thickening of the joint capsule, and osteophytosis.[15–18,40–44] Biochemical and metabolic changes in the articular cartilage include increases in hydration, and in PG and collagen synthesis and breakdown, and alterations in the molecular structure of the PGs. Many of these changes occur within the first few weeks after the surgical injury, and some may be accelerated by the interruption of sensory input from the joint.[42] Finally, there is evidence that the changes in the canine knee after ACLT are progressive, and eventually closely mimic those observed in end-stage human OA.[43] The following discussion focuses on the changes in cartilage biomechanics in the tensile, compressive, shear, and swelling configurations in the canine ACLT model of OA.

Tension

In an early study of ACL in the canine knee, decreases in the equilibrium tensile modulus of the articular cartilage were observed as early as two weeks after surgery. More comprehensive studies of the tensile behaviour of articular cartilage obtained from beagle and greyhound knees, 6, 12 and 16 weeks after transection of the ACL[18,29] showed a significant decrease in the tensile modulus of the collagen network in the surface zone (average, about 64 per cent of the control values), that was independent of the site on the joint surface (Table 7.8). In addition, site-matched cartilage hydration

Table 7.8 Equilibrium tensile modulus (mean ± SD) of control dogs and of dogs that underwent ACLT 6, 12, or 16 weeks earlier

	Greyhound[1]		Beagle[2]
	Femoral groove	Femoral condyle	Femoral condyle
Control	27.4 (8.4)	23.3 (8.5)	15.5 (4.5)
6 Weeks	23.3 (8.7)	13.2 (4.4)	—
12 Weeks	12.5 (2.9)	6.7 (2.5)	—
16 Weeks	—	—	8.6 (5.0)

All cartilage was harvested from the surface and subsurface zones parallel to the split-line direction.[18,29]

was greater, and the collagen content lower, in cartilage from ACLT dogs than from controls. Also, the collagen cross-link density decreased by 11 per cent after ACLT, suggesting an accelerated turnover of the collagen network at the articular surface.

Shear

A large decrease in the dynamic shear modulus was seen 6 weeks after ACLT, with little evidence of change between 6 and 12 weeks. Evidence of an increase in the loss angle (a measure of viscous dissipation within the ECM) suggested that increased intermolecular frictional dissipation existed in the OA cartilage (i.e., loosening of the collagen–PG solid matrix).[33] Cartilage hydration generally increased after surgery (Fig. 7.28), a finding that was correlated with the decrease in the dynamic shear modulus and permeability. Consistent with the results of the tensile study of cartilage in this model (see above), the changes in shear behaviour support the concept of a disruption in the collagen–PG matrix, not unlike that observed in human OA cartilage, and emphasize the biomechanical role of collagen in reinforcing the ECM (Fig. 7.25). The magnitude of the dynamic shear modulus, and the loss angle of control cartilage and of cartilage obtained 6 and 12 weeks after ACLT is provided in Table 7.9.[44]

Compression

In studies of the canine ACLT model, decreases in the compressive modulus of knee cartilage were observed at some sites on the tibial plateau at all time points, beginning 2 weeks after surgery. We have analysed the compressive behaviour of cartilage in this model using an indentation test and the biphasic theory,[18] (Table 7.10). Decreases in the compressive modulus were observed in cartilage from sites that were covered by the meniscus *in vivo* and bare areas of the tibial plateau (average, about 24 per cent of control values), suggesting the presence of a matrix that was more compliant and deformable in compression than normal. Twelve weeks after ACLT, a significant increase in hydraulic permeability was evident that was correlated with an increase in the hydration of the cartilage (Fig. 7.28). This increase in permeability is one of the most injurious changes affecting the ability of the articular cartilage to support load after ACLT; higher permeability allows a more rapid efflux of the interstitial fluid and, hence, lower fluid pressurization. These two effects, in turn, result in greater stresses on the solid matrix and, hence, greater deformation and the increased probability of chondrocyte injury.[1,2,19,35,36] The changes in this animal model are entirely consistent with those reported in human knee OA.[17–21]

Swelling

Studies of the swelling of articular cartilage after ACLT have uniformly shown an increase in hydration, relative to controls.[18,19,41–44] After equilibration in physiological saline for up to 90 minutes, hydration increased significantly in all samples of OA cartilage from the femoral and tibial sites. Differences in swelling between control and experimental cartilage were as great as 100 per cent, consistent with the concept that disruption of the collagen network impaired the ability of the tissue to resist swelling, as

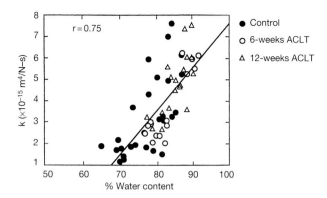

Fig. 7.28 Hydraulic permeability (k) of greyhound articular cartilage from covered and uncovered regions of the tibial plateau, plotted against water content. Tissues samples were obtained from normal knee joints, and from knees of dogs 6 and 12 weeks after transection of the anterior cruciate ligament.[18] The line shown is a linear regression line at r = 0.75.

Table 7.9 Magnitude ($\pm$ SD) of the dynamic shear modulus |G*|, and the loss angle, δ of control greyhounds and greyhounds that had undergone ACLT 6 or 12 weeks prior to sampling of the cartilage[44]

Dynamic test*	Control	Time after ACLT	
		6 weeks	**12 weeks**
|G*| (MPa)			
Posterior site	0.79 (0.25)	0.26 (0.07†)	0.24 (0.11†)
Distal site	0.44 (0.22)	0.25 (0.08†)	0.31 (0.19†)
δ (degrees)			
Posterior site	12.4 (1.72)	14.0 (1.1)	17.2 (2.9)
Distal site	13.5 (4.0)	15.1 (1.1)	17.2 (4.0)

* Dynamic testing was performed with a compressive strain of 10% and an angular displacement frequency of 10 rad/sec.

† Significantly different from the control value (p < 0.05 >).

observed in human OA cartilage.[16,17,23,37,38] The balance between swelling pressure and collagen network stress seems to be the determining factor for tissue hydration and swelling.[11,12,39]

Effects of changes in the environment of the chondrocyte

It is clear that a damaged matrix in OA, giving rise to altered physical cues during loading, has profound effects on chondrocyte metabolism. *In vitro* models have also been adopted to provide information that complements the information obtained *in vivo* with animal models. With the advantage of well-prescribed experimental boundary conditions, *in vitro* models can often provide greater precision in controlling experimental factors than *in vivo* models, in efforts to understand the mechanisms that mediate chondrocyte mechanotransduction and the progression of OA. The greatest insights may be gained by adopting a theoretical framework that describes the tissue loading behaviour and underlying load support mechanism with respect to the physically meaningful properties described above—namely, those of the solid, fluid, and ion phases,[1,2,6,7,9,12] that can be assessed more directly with biochemical assays of tissue composition and histologic studies of tissue structure.[14,16,24,25]

Explant loading studies

Although numerous *in vitro* studies have examined the effects of physiologic load levels on cartilage explants (e.g., Refs 45–48), few studies have investigated the effects of supraphysiologic loading. Load transmission beyond normal levels may result in tissue damage[15,49,50] and possibly deleterious deformation of the chondrocytes.[51] Morphologic analyses of *in vitro* cartilage injury models reveal characteristics reminiscent of the early stages of OA. Cell death and matrix changes may be initiated by a single impact load[50] or by the cumulative effects of repeated impact loading.[49] Indeed, these studies demonstrate that stress rate, loading magnitude, and duration are important determinants of cartilage damage. Impact is more destructive than a smoothly rising compression to the same peak stress.[15,49,52] Water loss from the tissue may contribute significantly to tissue damage and cell injury.[50] With increasing impact stress, a decrease in the level of PG biosynthesis and an increase in water content have been reported, with a critical threshold (15–20 MPa for moderately applied loading rates)

Table 7.10 Compressive properties (mean $\pm$ SD) of knee articular cartilage from control greyhounds and from greyhounds 6 or 12 weeks after ACLT[18]

Property	Area of plateau	Control samples	Time after ACLT	
			6 weeks	**12 weeks**
k ($\times 10^{-15}$ m⁴/Ns)	Covered	2.4 (1.3)	2.6 (0.4)	4.1 (1.0)*
	Not covered†	5.0 (1.7)	5.8 (0.4)	6.3 (1.0)*
H_A (MPa)	Covered	0.56 (0.19)	0.31 (0.10)*	0.42 (0.10)*
	Not covered	0.49 (0.19)	0.34 (0.09)*	0.36 (0.07)*
μ_s (MPa)	Covered	0.25 (0.08)	0.14 (0.03)*	0.19 (0.05)*
	Not covered	0.23 (0.07)	0.17 (0.04)*	0.18 (0.04)*
ν_s	Covered	0.07 (0.10)	0.08 (0.07)	0.09 (0.06)
	Not covered	0.05 (0.08)	0.00 (0.00)	0.04 (0.04)
Thickness (mm)	Covered	0.85 (0.17)	0.85 (0.11)	0.94 (0.24)
	Not covered†	1.7 (0.4)	1.5 (0.2)	1.4 (0.3)

Results of biphasic indentation testing of cartilage on areas of the tibial plateau covered or not covered by the meniscus.

* Significantly different from control, p < 0.05.

† Significantly different from covered sites, p < 0.05.

above which cell death throughout the matrix and apparent rupture of the collagen fibrillar network were observed.[50] Single subimpact loads (3.5–14 MPa) at higher strain rates resulted in tissue fissures and cell injury that was most pronounced near the superficial zone of the cartilage.[52,53] In contrast, loading at a low strain rate resulted in cell injury throughout the tissue without visible matrix damage.[53] Most recently, it has been found that the repetitive loading (0.5 Hz) of articular cartilage at physiological levels of stress (1 MPa) was harmful to chondrocytes only in the superficial zone, in which localized cell death occurred after 14 hours of cyclic loading

at a magnitude of 1.0 MPa and 0.5 Hz (Fig. 7.29). Cell death was likely attributed to excessive cell deformation arising from the lower mechanical properties of the superficial zone and loading-induced matrix damage.[6,7,15,50,51,53,54]

Chondrocyte Mechanotransduction

A large body of literature indicates that cartilage explants are sensitive to applied loads.[45–50] Because adult articular cartilage is avascular, alymphatic,

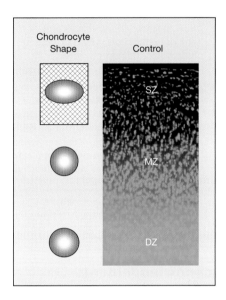
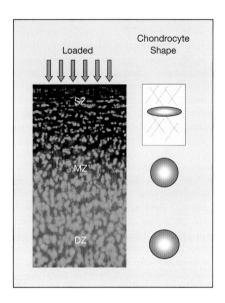

Fig. 7.29 *In vitro* mechanical cartilage explant model for the initiation of degenerative joint disease. Localized cell death has occurred in the Superficial Zone (SZ) after extensive repetitive cyclic loading (1 MPa at 0.5 Hz for 20 hours). Dead cells, not observed in the Middle Zone (MZ) or Deep Zone (DZ) are labeled red by propidium iodide staining whereas live cells are labeled green with flourescein diacetate staining. Cell death is attributed to excessive cell deformation arising from the lower mechanical properties of the SZ and load-induced matrix damage.

Source: Microscopy images courtesy of Drs. C.T. Chen and P.A. Torzilli.

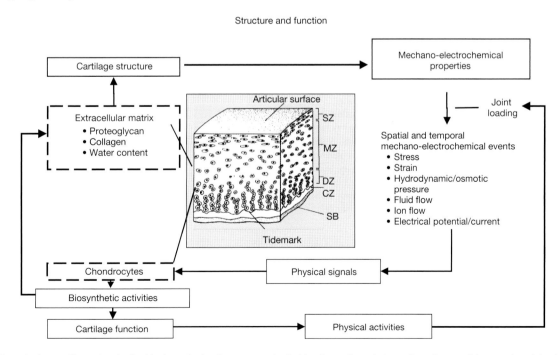

Fig. 7.30 Schematic diagram illustrating the feed-back mechanism between mechanical loading at the articular surface, the material properties of the tissue, the biosynthetic activity of the chondrocytes required to maintain the composition and organization of the ECM, and the generation of the mechanoelectrochemical stimuli necessary for the regulation of cellular activities.[7,54–56]

and devoid of nerves, these mechanical and physicochemical events occurring within the ECM during joint loading must be the signals required by chondrocytes residing deep within the matrix for control of their biosynthetic activities. Recently, a novel concept was introduced that considers the ECM as the medium for transmission of mechanical and/or physical signals necessary to stimulate and regulate chondrocyte synthetic/catabolic activities[7,24,51,54] (Fig. 7.30). It has been proposed that matrix-induced alterations in the shape and/or volume of the chondrocyte lead to changes in the nucleus and activation of signalling pathways that lead to changes in the biosynthetic activities of the cells.[54–58] Chondrocyte deformation as high as 20 per cent has been reported for physiologic levels of matrix deformation, and is associated with a decrease in chondrocyte volume.[46,58] It is clear, therefore, that the mechanical and physicochemical environment of the chondrocyte is coupled to the properties of the ECM, pericellular matrix, and cells. Greater knowledge of the changes in the ECM arising from OA (especially in view of the fact that chondrocyte stiffness seems to remain unchanged in OA) is needed to understand the cell-matrix interactions in OA.[51,58]

Recently, a new non-invasive method for determining the intrinsic tissue stiffness and FCD of a cartilage specimen was developed, utilizing a mechanical loading device, digital videomicroscopy, optimized digital image correlation technique, application of the ideal Donnan osmotic pressure law, and the theoretical framework of the triphasic theory.[12,36,59,60] In combination with microscopy-based probes, such as live-dead stains, ion sensitive indicator dyes and green fluorescent protein (GFP)-conjugated probes, this approach can provide simultaneous acquisition of real-time measurements of biological cell responses in, and the biomechanical properties of, a region within a tissue specimen. This technique will permit the concurrent study of cartilage biomechanics, distribution of PGs throughout the depth of the tissue (Fig. 7.23(d)) and chondrocyte mechanotransduction with unprecedented specificity. Knowledge gained from such innovative efforts will facilitate the development of strategies incorporating biomechanical factors in the *in vitro* development of viable biological constructs for surgical replacement of damaged cartilage.[61]

Summary

Notwithstanding the many advances over the past several decades in our understanding of cartilage degeneration, an in-depth understanding of the relationship between tissue degeneration and its effect on the mechanical behaviour and function of articular cartilage in diarthrodial joints is still lacking. Experimental animal models of joint instability have successfully recreated many of the changes in the joint that are associated with OA, and so provide a basis for studying the sequence of events during progression of early articular cartilage degeneration. In joint degeneration in humans, and in experimental animal models of joint instability, the earliest pathological changes in the articular cartilage are the deterioration of the collagen network at or near the surface, and a consequent increase in the overall water content of the tissue. The morphologic and compositional changes are associated with alterations in cartilage mechanics, including the significant loss of the tensile, compressive, and shear moduli and energy-storage capacity of the ECM; and an increase in the hydraulic permeability of the cartilage. While many studies point to disruption of the collagen-PG matrix as the initiating factor in progressive cartilage degeneration, it remains to be determined if this initial disruption is a direct result of mechanical forces, chondrocyte-derived catabolic activities, or externally-derived cytokines acting on the chondrocytes. With a better understanding of the time course of the changes in cell and tissue biology, biochemistry and biomechanics, better approaches to the prevention or treatment of cartilage degeneration and OA may be developed.

Key points

1. There is a strong structure–function relationship between the contents of collagen, proteoglycan and water in articular cartilage and the material properties and load support capabilities of the tissue.

2. Both collagen and proteoglycans have exquisitely detailed molecular structure (1–10 nm) and ultrastructural organization (1–10 μm) that endow the extracellular matrix with the strong and cohesive characteristics that allow the tissue to endure the high and repetitive loading to which it is commonly subjected, and provide a protective environment for the ensconced chondrocytes.

3. Water and proteoglycan charges play important roles in providing load support for the entire tissue. The hydrostatic pressure in the interstitial water supports 95 per cent of the loading to which articular cartilage is subjected during activities of daily living. In contrast, the proteoglycan charges provide the electromotive forces that give rise to the Donnan osmotic pressure that makes the tissue highly hydrophilic. This osmotic pressure provides less than 2.5 per cent of the total load support.

4. Articular cartilage from human OA joints or joints from animal models of OA, exhibits a high degree of swelling (i.e., it gains water content), due mainly to the destruction of the fibrillar collagen network and loss of proteoglycan content. These changes alter the mechanical properties of the extracellular matrix, increasing its hydraulic permeability, and hence preventing the tissue from performing its normal load support function.

5. Over the past several decades, numerous studies have demonstrated the validity of the canine anterior cruciate transection model for both short- and long-term *in vivo* studies of the pathoetiology of OA.

Acknowledgements

This work was sponsored in part by grants from the National Institutes of Health (AR41913; AR38733; AR46568).

References

(An asterisk denotes recommended reading.)

1. *Mow, V.C., Ratcliffe, A. (1997). Structure and function of articular cartilage and meniscus. In V.C. Mow and W.C. Hayes (eds). *Basic Orthopaedic Biomechanics* (2nd ed). Lippincott-Raven Publishers: Philadelphia, pp. 113–77.

   This general reference discusses bioengineering and biochemistry aspects of articular cartilage and other soft tissues. It addresses questions related to normal tissue structure-function relationships, and the changes that occur in diseases such as OA.

2. Mow, V.C. and Ateshian, G.A. (1997). Lubrication and wear of diarthrodial joints. In V.C. Mow and W.C. Hayes (eds). *Basic Orthopaedic Biomechanics* (2nd ed). Philadelphia: Lippincott-Raven, pp. 275–315.

3. Dowson, D. (1990). Bio-tribology of natural and replacement synovial joint. In: V.C. Mow, *et al.* (eds), *Biomechanics of diarthrodial joints*. New York: Springer, pp. 305–45.

4. Woo, S.L-Y., Akeson, W.H., Jemmott, G.F. (1976). Measurements of non-homogeneous directional mechanical properties of articular cartilage in tension. *J Biomech* 9:785–91.

5. Roth, V. and Mow, V.C. (1980). The intrinsic tensile behavior of the matrix of bovine articular cartilage and its variation with age. *J Bone Joint Surg* 62(A):1102–17.

6. Schinagl, R.M., Gurkis, D., Chen, C.C., and Sah, R.L-Y. (1997). Depth-dependent confined compression modulus of full-thickness bovine articular cartilage. *J Orthop Res* 15:499–506.

7. Wang, C.C-B., Hung, C.T., and Mow, V.C. (2000). Analysis of the effects of depth-dependent aggregate modulus on articular cartilage stress-relaxation behavior in compression. *J Biomechanics* 34:75–84.

8. Hayes, W.C. and Mockros, L.F. (1971). Viscoelastic properties of human articular cartilage. *J Appl Physiol* 31:562–8.

9. *Mow, V.C., Kuei, S.C., Lai, W.M., and Armstrong, C.G. (1980). Biphasic creep and stress relaxation of articular cartilage in compression: theory and experiments. *J Biomech Eng* **102**:73–84.

   This paper developed a theory that showed how the interstitial water in articular cartilage can influence the mechanical behavior of the tissue and enable the tissue to function in the highly loaded environment of a diarthrodial joint. This paper received the American Society of Mechanical Engineers' ASME 1981 Melville Medal—the highest honor for an original contribution to the ASME archival literature. In the two decades since its appearance, it has become the most frequently quoted paper in the J Biomech Eng. The theory and experimental methods described in it have been widely adopted and have changed the paradigm for research in soft tissue biomechanics.

10. Stockwell, R.A. (1979). In *Biology of cartilage cells.* Cambridge: Cambridge University Press.

11. Maroudas, A. (1976). Balance between swelling pressure and collagen tension in normal and degenerate cartilage. *Nature* **260**:1089–95.

12. Lai, W.M., Hou, J.S., and Mow, V.C. (1991). A triphasic theory for the swelling and deformation behaviors of articular cartilage. *J Biomech Eng* **113**:245–58.

13. Meachim, G. and Emery, I.H. (1974). Quantitative aspects of patellofemoral cartilage fibrillation in Liverpool necropsies. *Ann Rheum Dis* **33**:39–47.

14. Hough Jr., A.J. (2001). Pathology of osteoarthritis. In Moskowitz *et al.* (eds), *Osteoarthritis: Diagnosis and Medical/Surgical Management* (3rd ed). Philadelphia: WB Saunders, pp. 69–100.

15. Atkinson, T.S., Haut, R.C., and Altiero, N.J. (1998). Impact induced fissuring of articular cartilage: an investigation of failure criteria. *J Biomech Eng* **120**:191–7.

16. Maroudas, A. and Venn, M. (1977). Chemical composition and swelling of normal and osteoarthritic femoral head cartilage. II. Swelling. *Ann Rheum Dis* **36**:399–406.

17. Armstrong, C.G. and Mow, V.C. (1982). Variations in the intrinsic mechanical properties of human articular cartilage with age, degeneration, and water content. *J Bone Joint Surg* **64**(A):88–94.

18. Setton, L.A., Mow, V.C., Muller, F.J., Pita, J.C., and Howell, D.S. (1994). Mechanical properties of canine articular cartilage are significantly altered following transection of the anterior cruciate ligament. *J Orthop Res* **12**:451–63.

19. Mow, V.C., Ratcliffe, A., and Poole, A.R. (1992). Cartilage and diarthrodial joints as paradigms for hierarchical materials and structures. *Biomaterials* **13**:67–97.

20. Huang, C.Y., Ateshian, G.A., and Mow, V.C. (2001). The role of flow-independent viscoelasticity in the biphasic tensile and compressive responses of articular cartilage. *J Biomech Eng* **123**:410–17.

21. Soulhat, J., Buschmann, M.D., and Shirazi-Adl, A. (1999). A fibril-network reinforced model of cartilage in unconfined compression. *J Biomech Eng* **121**:340–7.

22. Clarke, I.C. (1971). Articular cartilage: a review and scanning electronic microscope study-1. The inter-territorial fibrillar architectural. *J Bone Joint Surg* **53**(B):732–50.

23. Maroudas, A. (1979). Physicochemical properties of articular cartilage. In M. A. R. Freeman (ed.), *Adult articular cartilage*. Kent, UK: Pitman Medical, pp. 215–90.

24. Muir, H. (1983). Proteoglycans as organizers of the extracellular matrix. *Biochem Trans* **11**:613–22.

25. Hardingham, T.E. and Fosang, A. (1992). Proteoglycans: many forms and many functions. *FASEB J* **6**:861–70.

26. Akizuki, S., Mow, V.C., Muller, F., Pita, J.C., Howell, D.S., and Manicourt, D.H. (1986). Tensile properties of knee joint cartilage. I. influence of ionic conditions, weight bearing, and fibrillation on the tensile modulus. *J Orthop Res* **4**:379–92.

27. Kempson, G.E., Muir, H., Pollard, C., and Tuke, M. (1973). The tensile properties of the cartilage of human femoral condyles related to the content of collagen and glycosaminoglycans. *Biochim Biophys Acta* **297**:456–72.

28. Schmidt, M.B., Mow, V.C., Chun, L.E., and Eyre, D.R. (1990). Effects of proteoglycan extraction on the tensile behavior of articular cartilage. *J Orthop Res* **8**:353–63.

29. Guilak, F., Ratcliffe, A., Lane, N., Rosenwasser, M.P., and Mow, V.C. (1994). Mechanical and biochemical changes in the superficial zone of articular cartilage in a canine model of osteoarthritis. *J Orthop Res* **12**:474–84.

30. Kempson, G.E. (1991). Age-related changes in the tensile properties of human articular cartilage: a comparative study between the femoral head of the hip joint and the talus of the ankle joint. *Biochim Biophys Acta* **1075**:223–30.

31. Froimson, M.I., Ratcliffe, A., Gardner, T.R., and Mow, V.C. (1997). Differences in patellofemoral joint cartilage material properties and their significance in the etiology of cartilage surface fibrillations. *Osteoarthritis Cart* **5**:377–86.

32. Hayes, W.C. and Bodine, A. (1978). Flow-independent viscoelastic properties of articular cartilage matrix. *J Biomech* **11**:407–19.

33. Zhu, W., Mow, V.C., Koob, T.J., and Eyre, D.R. (1993). Viscoelastic shear properties of articular cartilage and the effects of glycosidase treatments. *J Orthop Res* **11**:771–81.

34. Gu, W.Y., Lai, W.M., and Mow, V.C. (1998). A mixture theory for charged hydrated soft tissues containing multi-electrolytes: passive transport and swelling behaviors. *J Biomech Eng* **120**:169–80.

35. Soltz, M.A., and Ateshian, G.A. (1998). Experimental verification and theoretical prediction of cartilage interstitial fluid pressurization at an impermeable contact interface in confined compression. *J Biomech* **31**:927–34.

36. Mow, V.C., Ateshian, G.A., Lai, W.M., and Gu, W.Y. (1998). Effects of fixed charges on the stress-relaxation behavior of hydrated soft tissues in a confined compression problem. *Int J Sol Struc* **35**:4945–62.

37. *Bollet, A.J. and Nance, J.L. (1966). Biochemical findings in normal and osteoarthritic cartilage, II. Chondroitin sulfate concentration and chain length, water and ash content. *J Clin Invest* **45**:1170–7.

   This is one of the earliest papers demonstrating the important changes in articular cartilage composition, for example, glycosaminoglycan and water contents in OA joints. Other investigators subsequently correlated the composition and structure of articular cartilage with its material properties and load support capabilities.

38. Mankin, H.J., Dorfman, H., Lippiello, L., *et al.* (1971). Biochemical and metabolic abnormalities in articular cartilage from osteo-arthritic human hips: II. Correlations for morphology with biochemical and metabolic data. *J Bone Joint Surg* **53**(A):53–7.

39. Myers, E.R., Lai, W.M., and Mow, V.C. (1984). A continuum theory and an experiment for the ion-induced swelling behavior of articular cartilage. *J Biomech Eng* **106**:151–8.

40. Pond, M.J. and Nuki, G. (1973). Experimentally induced osteoarthritis in the dog. *Ann Rheum Dis* **32**:387–8.

41. McDevitt, C., Gilbertson, E., and Muir, H. (1977). An experimental model of osteoarthritis: early morphological and biochemical changes. *J Bone Joint Surg* **59**(B):24–35.

42. O'Connor, B.L., Visco, D.M., Brandt, K.D., Myers, S.L., and Kalasinski, L.A. (1992). Neurogenic acceleration of osteoarthrosis. *J Bone Joint Surg* **74**(A):367–76.

43. *Brandt, K.D., Braunstein, E.M., Visco, D.M., O'Conner, B., Heck, D., and Albrecht, M. (1991). Anterior cranial cruciate ligament transection in the dog: a bona fide model of osteoarthritis, not merely of cartilage injury and repair. *J Rheumatol* **18**:436–46.

   This important paper provides evidence that long-term study of the Pond-Nuki canine anterior cruciate ligament transaction model of OA[40,41] shows that it leads to many of the recognized pathophysiologic manifestations of OA.

44. Setton, L.A., Mow, V.C., and Howell, D.S. (1995). Changes in the shear properties of canine knee cartilage resulting from anterior cruciate transection. *J Orthop Res* **13**:473–82.

45. Sah, R.L.Y., Kim, Y.J., Doong, J-YH., Grodzinsky, A.J., Plaas, A.H.K., and Sandy, J.D. (1989). Biosynthetic response of cartilage explants to dynamic compression. *J Orthop Res* **7**:619–36.

46. Guilak, F., Meyer, B.C., Ratcliffe, A., Mow, V.C. (1994). The effects of matrix compression on proteoglycan metabolism in articular cartilage explants. *Osteoarthritis Cart* **2**:91–101.

47. Valhmu, W.B., Stazzone, E.J., Bachrach, N.M., Saed-Nejad, F., Fischer, S.G., Mow, V.C., and Ratcliffe, A. (1998). Load-controlled compression of articular

cartilage induces a transient stimulation of aggrecan gene expression. *Arch Biochem Biophys* **353**:29–36.

48. Buschmann, M.D., Kim, Y.-J., Wong, M., Frank, E., Hunziker, E.B., and Grodzinsky, A.J. (1999). Stimulation of aggrecan synthesis in cartilage explants by cyclic loading is localized to regions of high interstitial fluid flow. *Arch Biochem Biophys* **366**:1–7.

49. Radin, E.L., Ehrlich, M.G., Chernack, R., Abernethy, P., Paul, I.L., and Rose, R.M. (1978). Effect of repetitive impulsive loading on the knee joints of rabbits. *Clin Orthop* **131**:288–93.

50. Torzilli, P.A, Grigiene, R., Borrelli Jr., J., and Helfet, D.L. (1999). Effect of impact load on articular cartilage: cell metabolism and viability, and matrix water content. *J Biomech Eng* **121**:433–41.

51. Guilak, F. and Mow, V.C. (2000). The mechanical environment of the chondrocyte: A biphasic finite element model of cell-matrix interactions in articular cartilage. *J Biomech* **33**:1663–73.

52. Armstrong, C.G., Mow, V.C., and Wirth, C.R. (1985). Biomechanics of impact-induced microdamage to articular cartilage: a possible genesis for chondromalacia patella. In G.A.M. Finerman (ed.), *The knee* (Symposium on Sports Medicine). St Louis: C.V. Mosby, pp. 70–84.

53. Quinn, T.M., Allen, R.G., Schalet, B.J., Perumbuli, P., and Hunziker, E.B. (2001). Matrix and cell injury due to sub-impact loading of adult bovine articular cartilage explants: effects of strain rate and peak stress. *J Orthop Res* **19**:242–9.

54. Mow, V.C., Wang, C.B., and Hung, C.T. (1999). The extracellular matrix, interstial fluid and ions as a mechanical signal transducer in articular cartilage. *Osteoarthritis Cart* **7**:41–58.

55. Watson, P.A. (1991). Function follows form: generation of intracellular signals by cell deformations. *FASEB J* **5**:2013–19.

56. Ingber, D. (1991). Integrins as mechanochemical transducers. *Curr Opin Cell Biol* **3**:841–48.

57. Guilak, F., Tedrow, J.R., and Burgkart, R. (2000). Viscoelastic properties of cell nucleus. *Biochem Biophys Res Commun* **269**:781–6.

58. Guilak, F., Ratcliffe, A., and Mow, V.C. (1995). Chondrocyte deformation and local tissue strain in articular cartilage: a confocal microscopy study. *J Orthop Res* **13**:410–22.

59. Sun, D.N., Gu, W.Y., Guo, X.E., Lai, W.M., and Mow, V.C. (2001). The influence of inhomogeneous fixed charge density of cartilage mechano-electrochemical behaviors. *Trans Orthop Res Soc* **23**:484.

60. Wang, C.C.-B., Guo, X.E., Sun, D., Mow, V.C., Ateshian, G.A., and Hung, C.T. (2002). The functional environment of chondrocytes within cartilage subjected to compressive loading: theoretical and experimental approach. *Biorheology* **39**(1–2):39–45.

61. *Guilak, F., Butler, D.L., and Goldstein, S.A. (2001). Functional tissue engineering: The role of biomechanics in articular cartilage repair. *Clin Orthop* **39**(1S):295–305.

This important reference addresses issues that must be considered in developing tissue engineering constructs for successful functional replacement of damaged regions of diseased, for example, OA articular cartilage surfaces. The most important issue is the reliability of these artificial tissue engineered constructs in functioning satisfactorily in clinical situations.

7.2.1.5 Response of the chondrocyte to mechanical stimuli

Michael A. DiMicco, Young-Jo Kim, and Alan J. Grodzinsky

Joint loading *in vivo* causes physical perturbations of the cell

Articular cartilage is subjected to a wide range of static and dynamic mechanical loads in human synovial joints.[1,2] Peak stress amplitudes can reach 10–20 MPa (100–200 atm) during activities such as stair climbing.[3] Cartilage compressions of 15–40 per cent may occur in response to long-term or 'static' loads within the physiological range.[1] In contrast, compressions of only a few per cent occur during normal ambulation (e.g., the 'dynamic' strains that occur at walking frequencies of ~1 Hz). Clinical observations and animal studies *in vivo* have shown that joint loading can induce a wide range of metabolic responses in cartilage.[4] *Immobilization* or reduced loading can cause profound decreases in matrix synthesis and content[5] and a resultant softening of the tissue.[6] In contrast, aggrecan concentration is often higher in areas of habitually loaded cartilage,[7] and can be further increased by *dynamic* loading or remobilization of a joint,[8,9] with concomitant restoration of biomechanical properties.[6] More severe *impact*,[10] or strenuous exercise loading[11] can cause cartilage degradation with osteoarthritic changes.[11]

Many physical forces and flows that occur in cartilage during loading *in vivo* (Fig. 7.31(a)) have been identified and quantified *in vitro*. Dynamic compression of cartilage results in deformation of cells and ECM,[12,13] hydrostatic pressurization of the tissue fluid, pressure gradients and the accompanying flow of fluid within the tissue, and streaming potentials and currents induced by tissue fluid flow.[14–16] In addition, the local changes in tissue volume caused by static compression also lead to physicochemical changes within the ECM including alterations in matrix water content, fixed charge density, mobile ion concentrations, and osmotic pressure.[17–19] Any of these mechanical, chemical, or electrical phenomena in the environment of the chondrocyte may affect cellular metabolism (Table 7.11). An understanding of the spatial distribution of these forces and flows within cartilage, during compression, has been aided by the development of theoretical models for the mechanical,[20] physicochemical,[21,22] and electromechanical[15] behavior of cartilage. Such models can provide a useful framework for correlating the spatial distributions of the physical stimuli and cellular response that occur within cartilage during loading.[14,16,23,24]

The ability of cartilage to withstand physiological compressive, tensile, and shear forces depends on the composition and structural integrity of its ECM. In turn, the maintenance of a functionally intact ECM requires chondrocyte-mediated synthesis, assembly, and degradation of PGs, collagens, noncollagenous proteins and glycoproteins, and other matrix molecules. It is well known that mechanical stimuli in the microenvironment of the chondrocytes can significantly affect the synthesis and degradation of matrix macromolecules. However, the cellular transduction mechanisms that govern chondrocyte response to mechanical stimuli are not well understood. Recent data suggest that there are multiple regulatory pathways by which chondrocytes sense and respond to mechanical stimuli, including upstream signaling pathways[25–27] and mechanisms that may lead to direct changes at the level of transcription,[28–31] translation, post-translational modifications,[32,33] and cell-mediated extracellular assembly and degradation of matrix[34–36] (Fig. 7.32). Correspondingly, there may be multiple pathways by which physical stimuli can alter not only the rate of matrix production, but the quality and functionality of newly synthesized PGs, collagens, and other molecules. In this manner, specific mechanical loading regimens may either enhance or compromise the long-term biomechanical function of cartilage.

Model systems for the study of chondrocyte mechanobiology

Since the mechanisms by which chondrocytes respond to mechanical stimuli are difficult to quantify *in vivo*, models such as cartilage explant organ culture and three-dimensional (3D) chondrocyte/gel culture systems have been used. Cartilage explants preserve native tissue structure and cell-matrix interactions; therefore, they enable quantitative correlations between mechanical loading parameters and biological responses such as gene expression and biosynthesis. Geometrically defined explants can attain steady-state levels of matrix synthesis and turnover, suitable for studying

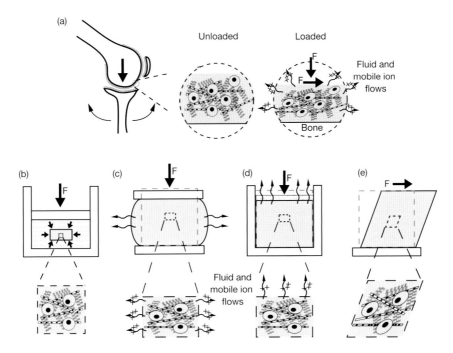

Fig. 7.31 Loading of articular cartilage causes tissue deformation and changes in the cellular microenvironment. (a) During joint motion cartilage (gray) is subjected to a complex combination of compression and shear, causing deformation of the cells and ECM, as well as fluid and ion flows. Loading can be simplified *in vitro* so that specific mechanical stimuli can be isolated and studied in cartilage explants. (b) Hydrostatic pressurization does not induce matrix strain or fluid flow. Both (c) radially unconfined and (d) confined compressions produce fluid flows and matrix deformation, while (e) simple shear induces matrix strain with little to no fluid flow.

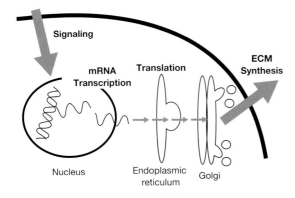

Fig. 7.32 Mechanical signals are sensed by the chondrocyte, triggering intracellular signaling cascades. These can result in altered transcription, translation of mRNA to proteins in the endoplasmic reticulum, and post-translational modifications in the Golgi. Together, these processes can lead to altered levels of matrix synthesis and secretion, as well as changes in the quality and structure of newly synthesized ECM macromolecules.

Table 7.11 Physical signals regulating cartilage metabolism

♦ Deformation of cells and matrix

♦ Intratissue fluid flow (caused by tissue deformation) (affects transport of soluble factors and nutrients; fluid shear stress)

♦ Hydrostatic pressurization of tissue fluid and pressure gradients

♦ Electrical streaming potentials and currents (caused by fluid flow)

  Physicochemical changes (caused by changes in local tissue volume) (e.g., water content, ion and fixed charge concentrations, pH, osmotic pressure)

gel culture systems have also been used to study the effects of applied mechanical compression, hydrostatic pressure, physicochemical stimuli (pH and osmolarity), and electrical currents. A variety of specialized, incubator-housed instruments for applying compression, shear, or hydrostatic pressure have been developed for *in vitro* studies using explants, isolated cells, or cell-encapsulated gel constructs (Table 7.12).[32,41]

Joint loading results in a complex combination of compression and shear forces acting on cartilage (Fig 7.31(a)). Loading can be further divided into *static* (e.g., compressive forces due to ligament tension, and weight bearing during standing) and *dynamic* (e.g., related to gait cycle) components. *In vitro*, it is possible to simplify this complex loading so that the effects of specific mechanical stimuli on chondrocytes can be studied. Hydrostatic pressurization of cartilage (Fig. 7.31(b)) results in a uniform stress throughout the tissue, and may be achieved by pressurization of the bathing medium containing the cartilage specimens[42] or by incubating the specimens in a medium containing macromolecules such as polyethylene glycol[43] that alter bath osmotic pressure. Direct mechanical compression of tissue can be performed by applying a known force ('load control') or a known displacement ('displacement control') to one surface of the

perturbations caused by applied mechanical stimuli. Muir[37] has emphasized the important but complex role of the native ECM and chondrocyte-ECM interactions in understanding the mechanisms of chondrocyte response to load. Of course, the coupling between mechanical, electrical, and chemical forces and flows within native ECM can greatly complicate the identification of specific physical stimuli, necessitating specialized experimental approaches. Investigators[37] have cautioned that the use of isolated chondrocytes that are depleted of natural matrix must be approached with care regarding the physiological interpretation of such tests and the potential for chondrocyte dedifferentiation. Therefore, 3D agarose[38] and alginate[39,40]

Table 7.12 Models for study of chondrocyte mechanobiology

- *In vivo* (animal models)
- Cartilage explants (organ culture of native animal or human tissue)
- Isolated chondrocytes in monolayer culture
- Chondrocyte-3D-gel/scaffold culture (natural or synthetic scaffolds)

specimen via a solid platen while holding the opposite platen fixed. One-dimensional ('uniaxial') unconfined compression (Fig. 7.31(c)) typically employs a nonporous compression platen, and the sample is allowed to bulge and exude fluid in the radial direction.[20] In radially-confined compression (Fig. 7.31(d)), a barrier is placed around the circumference of the sample and a porous compression platen is used; the sample is not allowed to bulge radially, and fluid flow occurs in the axial direction emulating an articular surface geometry.[15] Simple tissue shear (Fig. 7.31(e)) is achieved by displacing two plane-parallel surfaces of a specimen in opposite directions, and is characterized by the deformation of the sample with minimal intratissue fluid flow.[41] The effects of fluid shear on cells plated in monolayer culture have also been studied.[25]

Biosynthetic response of chondrocytes to mechanical stimuli

Static compression

Studies using animal and human cartilage explants have shown that static compression of up to 50 per cent can cause a dose-dependent decrease in the biosynthesis of PGs, collagens, and other ECM proteins, as assessed by the incorporation of radiolabeled precursors. This inhibition of synthesis can occur as rapidly as one hour after the onset of compression.[44] Complete recovery of biosynthesis can occur after release of compression, but is slower and depends on the duration and amplitude of loading. Interestingly, static compression and release caused differential effects on inhibition and return to normal synthetic levels for aggrecan, link protein, collagen, and small leucine-rich PGs, but did not alter the normal rate of hyaluronan production.[33] These findings provide strong evidence that the response to static compression is not a general inhibition of cellular activity, but appears to be linked to specific mechanotransduction pathways. Cell-level quantitative autoradiography has also been used to visualize the distribution of newly-synthesized matrix molecules around individual cells in response to compression.[24] Using this approach, it was discovered that static compression could stimulate directional deposition of secreted PGs around chondrocytes, superimposed on an inhibition of synthesis. Newly-synthesized PGs were deposited preferentially around cells in the equatorial plane perpendicular to the axis of compression, in regions where there was less compaction of the pericellular matrix.[24]

Dynamic compression

Dynamic compression can markedly stimulate the production of ECM molecules by chondrocytes in cartilage and in alginate and agarose gel culture systems, in a manner dependent on compression amplitude and frequency[44,45] as well as the developmental stage and the depth from the articular surface of the cartilage sample.[46–48] Compression of cylindrical calf cartilage explant disks in the 0.01–1 Hz frequency range has induced 20–100 per cent increases in PG and protein synthesis[44,49] (Fig. 7.33). Cyclic loading of adult bovine cartilage increased the synthesis of cartilage oligomeric matrix protein (COMP) and fibronectin, while static compression reduced fibronectin formation.[47] Using the unconfined geometry of Figs 7.31(c) and 7.33, dynamic compression causes fluid pressurization within the sample and a resultant fluid flow in the radial direction.

The amplitude of the hydrostatic pressure is highest in the center of the disk, while the fluid velocity is higher toward the outer tissue edges[16,23] (Fig. 7.31(c)). Compression at 0.01 Hz caused a rather uniform stimulation of biosynthesis throughout the tissue. However, at frequencies greater than 0.1 Hz, this stimulatory effect was localized to the periphery of the samples, corresponding to areas experiencing higher fluid flow velocities and cell deformation.[45] Quantitative autoradiography showed increased PG and protein deposition near cells in this outer region,[23,24] further confirming the importance of fluid flow and cell deformation in the stimulation of synthesis by dynamic compression. Recent studies[49] have shown that the application of dynamic compression and simultaneous addition of a soluble growth factor (IGF-1) to the medium enhanced protein and PG synthesis in explants almost 2-to 3-fold, respectively, greater than that achieved by either stimulus alone (Fig. 7.33(b)). In addition, compression plus IGF-1 stimulated an increase in protein synthesis at a 2-fold faster rate than that achieved by IGF-1 incubation alone (Fig. 7.33(c)). Thus, in addition to independently stimulating chondrocytes, cyclic compression appears to accelerate the transport of soluble growth factors through the dense ECM to the cells.

Dynamic tissue shear

Dynamic tissue shear of cartilage explants in the configuration of Figs 7.31(e) and 7.34(a) also stimulates chondrocyte metabolism. Application of 1–3 per cent sinusoidal shear strain over a wide frequency range (0.01–1 Hz) caused increases in matrix biosynthesis in cartilage explants[50] (Fig. 7.34(b)). This range of shear strain was estimated to be within the range experienced by cartilage during normal joint motion *in vivo*. At 0.1 Hz, this stimulation in biosynthesis increased in a dose-dependent fashion with shear strain amplitude in the 1–6 per cent range (Fig. 7.34(c)). Dynamic tissue shear causes deformation of cells and ECM but, unlike cyclic compression, shear causes little or no intratissue fluid flow (Fig. 7.31(e)). In contrast to dynamic compression, the increase in synthesis caused by tissue shear was found to be spatially uniform within the explant, as visualized by quantitative autoradiography.[50] This result was consistent with the more uniform matrix deformation and the absence of localized fluid flow produce by tissue shear. Dynamic shear in the presence of added IGF-1 stimulated cell biosynthesis in an additive fashion. However, there was no measurable increase in transport of IGF-1 produced by tissue shear, consistent with the notion that tissue shear produced little intratissue fluid flow. Contrary to dynamic compression, dynamic shear increased collagen synthesis significantly more than PG synthesis (in the presence of serum).[50] It is possible that this difference is related to the importance of collagen fibrils in providing resistance to shear loading in cartilage, suggesting that chondrocytes may recognize specific patterns of mechanical loading.

Osmotic pressure

The application of 0–800 kPa of sustained osmotic pressure to cartilage, achieved by incubating cartilage specimens in the presence of graded concentrations of polyethylene glycol, resulted in an inhibition of cellular biosynthesis similar to that seen when the specimens were subjected to static mechanical compression.[43] Although mechanical and osmotic loading methods result in different strain fields and stress distributions within the tissue,[51] both stimuli result in similar decreases in tissue hydration. These results suggest that chondrocyte response to static compression may be modulated by physicochemical factors involving tissue water content, osmolarity, and pH. The intratissue pH of cartilage (pH ~ 6.8) is always lower than the surrounding synovial fluid (pH ~ 7.4), due to the presence of negative fixed charges on the GAG chains attracting positive ions.[17] Theoretical calculations have shown that tissue pH decreases further with static compression,[18] due to increases in matrix fixed charge density and exudation of water. While chondrocyte biosynthetic responses to changes in pH are not well understood, recent studies have elucidated the role of proton pumps and other ion transporters in altering the intracellular microenvironment during cartilage compression.[19,52]

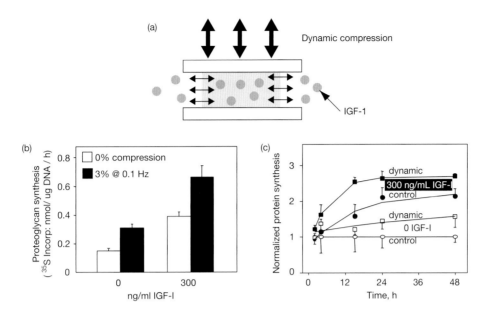

Fig. 7.33 The stimulation of PG and protein biosynthesis by dynamic compression can be enhanced by the addition of the growth factor IGF-I to the culture medium. (a) Dynamic compression enhances transport into and within cartilage by convective fluid flow. (b) Dynamic compression and IGF-I have an additive effect on PG synthesis ($n = 6$, mean ± SD). (c) The total amount of newly synthesized protein is increased with IGF-I and with dynamic compression (2 per cent at 0.1 Hz) compared with uncompressed controls, and plateaus after approximately 24 hours of treatment ($n = 6$, mean ± SD). Dynamic compression doubles the rate of transport of the growth factor into the cartilage.

Source: Adapted from Ref. 49.

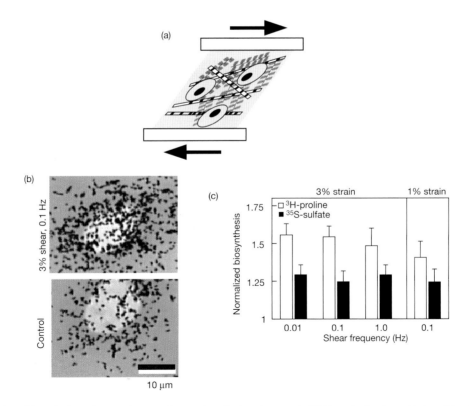

Fig. 7.34 (a) The application of dynamic tissue shear strain to cartilage explants leads to increases in PG biosynthesis, observable by cell-level quantitative autoradiography (b) of ^{35}S-labeled PGs. (c) Protein and PG synthesis were differentially upregulated by dynamic shear over controls, but this effect was not dependent on frequency (mean ± SEM, $n = 13$–21).

Source: Adapted from Ref. 50.

Effects of physical forces on chondrocyte gene expression

While initial studies focused on isolated chondrocytes due to the difficulty in extracting sufficient quantities of mRNA from tissue explants, recent advances have enabled comparative studies of gene expression using intact tissue. Such findings are useful in understanding the role of cartilage species, age, location, and the presence or absence of the surrounding ECM.

Hydrostatic pressurization

Hydrostatic pressurization (Fig. 7.31(b)) of high density monolayer cultures under moderate static[30] and intermittent loading (1–10 MPa, 0.5–1 Hz)[28] was found to increase aggrecan synthesis as well as mRNA levels of aggrecan core protein and type II collagen, by amounts that depended on the presence of serum.[28] Even subambient cyclic pressurization has been observed to stimulate aggrecan gene expression,[53] though the concomitant increase in aggrecan synthesis was abolished when chondrocyte microtubules were disrupted using nocodazole or taxol.[54] Thus, the stimulatory effect of low cyclic pressurization appears to be regulated at multiple points along the biosynthetic pathway. High levels (10–50 MPa) of static pressurization of the chondrocyte-like cell line HCS-2/8 for 4 hours had an inhibitory effect on aggrecan biosynthesis and mRNA levels for aggrecan core and TGF-β,[30,55] but increased mRNA levels of IL-6, HSP70,[30] and TNF-α. While such high levels of hydrostatic pressure may be transiently induced by mechanical compression of cartilage at high strain rates, the ensuing fluid flow within the tissue would quickly reduce the magnitude of the pressure. Thus, sustained high-pressure levels are less physiologically relevant. Such isolated chondrocyte systems are extremely important models for investigating chondrocyte mechanotransduction; however, the relevance to cellular mechanisms in native tissue must be confirmed independently due to the complex interactions that exist between the chondrocyte and the ECM *in vivo*.

Fluid shear and cell stretching

Laminar flow viscometers have been used to apply fluid shear stress to chondrocytes in monolayer culture. Fluid shear (1.6–2.2 Pa)[56] resulted in a 2-fold increase in aggrecan synthesis and nearly 10-fold increase in prostaglandin E release. Levels of mRNA for TIMP-1 increased 9-fold, 10–15-fold for IL-6 and 3-fold for MMP-9, but the mRNA for collagenase, stromelysin, 72 kD gelatinase and TGF-β did not change. The induction of MMP-9 gene appeared to be mediated via the c-Jun N-terminal kinase (JNK) signaling pathway,[57] and the aggrecan promotor via the extracellular-signal regulated protein kinases (ERK) pathway.[58] When isolated bovine and human chondrocytes were cyclically stretched on flexible membranes, aggrecan and type II collagen mRNA expression was increased.[59]

Compression

Cartilage disks from 4–6 month old bovine calves subjected to constant unconfined compressive load (0.026–0.5 MPa) showed an initial increase in aggrecan mRNA (as high as ~4-fold) within 1 hour after compression, followed by a gradual return to control levels.[29] This constant compressive load caused a transient creep strain that equilibrated to a final compressed state in 10–20 minutes. At 0.5 MPa load, there was no stimulatory effect of compression.[29] In contrast, Ragan *et al.* applied constant compression (up to 50 per cent) to specimens from 1–2 week-old calves, rather than constant load,[31] giving rise to an initial increase in compressive stress followed by stress relaxation to equilibrium in 10–20 minutes. They also found an initial increase in aggrecan and collagen type II mRNA levels by 30 min after compression;[31] however, by 24 hours after applied static compression, a significant decrease in gene expression was observed compared to uncompressed controls. Interestingly, similar static compressions caused a rapid decrease in the *synthesis* of collagen and PGs, within 1 hour.[44] Thus, although mechanical compression can rapidly alter the expression of these molecules,

the observed decrease in synthesis caused by static compression does not appear to be related solely to changes in the mRNA expression.

Effects on cell microenvironment, morphology, and intracellular signaling: clues to mechanisms

Loading of cartilage produces deformations at the tissue, cellular, and molecular length scales. For example, laser scanning confocal microscopy[12] and quantitative stereology[13] have demonstrated that compression of cartilage tissue results in similar magnitude reductions in cell height and cell volume. These decreases vary in a depth-dependent manner, consistent with the depth-varying compressive properties of the bulk tissue,[60] but do not appear to vary with radial position within a cartilage disk.[24] Deformations within the pericellular matrix also affect the physicochemical microenvironment of the chondrocyte[14,24] and may, in turn, signal the cell to modulate its biosynthetic response. Deformation-induced fluid flow in the pericellular region enhances transport of soluble factors to cell receptors, and alters the local concentration of mobile ions, leading to electrochemical changes such as shifts in pH.[17] Cell-surface connections to the ECM, including integrin receptors, enable pericellular deformations to be transmitted through the cell membrane to intracellular organelles via cytoskeletal elements such as actin microfilaments, microtubules, and intermediate filaments.[12,54,61] Deformation of the nucleus can lead to compaction of chromatin and altered molecular transport through nuclear pore complexes, processes that are important to cellular metabolism. Compression can also affect the morphology of other intracellular organelles related to matrix metabolism, such as the rough endoplasmic reticulum and the Golgi apparatus. Since the Golgi is the site of post-translational modifications of aggrecan (e.g., glycosylation and sulfation),[62] changes in Golgi morphology and function with compression may play a critical role in the known changes in GAG chain length and sulfation caused by static compression[33] (Fig. 7.35).

There is increasing evidence that connections between the chondrocyte and its pericellular matrix play a direct role in mechanotransduction signaling events. Integrins can convert extracellular mechanical stimuli into intracellular signals in a variety of cell types.[27] In chondrocytes, the alpha 5 beta 1 fibronectin-binding integrins have been implicated as part of a mechanotransduction complex that involves tyrosine protein kinases, cytoskeletal proteins, ion channels, and second-messenger signaling cascades.[63] Several recent studies have demonstrated a role for mitogen activated protein kinases (MAPKs) in the alteration of matrix gene expression and changes in matrix production by chondrocytes within cartilage under load. This family of ubiquitous signaling molecules includes ERK-1 and -2, JNK, and p38. Activated MAP kinases are thought to translocate to the nucleus, where they may induce phosphorylation of transcriptional factors and eventual upregulation of various genes. Recently, several groups have discovered the activation of MAP kinases in chondrocytes within young bovine cartilage explants subjected to radially-unconfined static, dynamic, and shear loading (Figs 7.31(c) and (e)). Isolated bovine chondrocytes exposed to fluid shear are also shown to have increased levels of activated ERK 1/2.[58] In this system, chimeric constructs containing active portions of the aggrecan gene promoter region, linked to reporter genes, showed that fluid shear could activate the aggrecan promoter, and that this activation could be eliminated by using an inhibitor of MEK, an upstream element of the MAPK pathway.

Effects of injurious mechanical loading

Acute traumatic joint injury is known to increase the risk for subsequent development of OA.[64] Furthermore, there is increasing evidence that abnormal loading seen in malaligned limbs[65] and dysplastic hip joints[66] can lead to premature arthritis. However, the mechanical and biological mechanisms

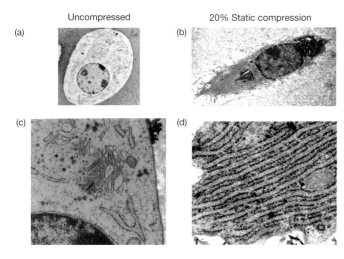

Uncompressed   20% Static compression

(a)   (b)

(c)   (d)

Fig. 7.35 The application of static compression causes deformation and altered morphology of intracellular organelles. Electron microscopy of uncompressed samples ((a) 3500×; (c) 20 000×) indicates rounded cellular morphology and normal organelle structure. Application of 20 per cent compression ((b) 3500×; (d) 20 000×) results in flattened cell shape and compaction and anisotropic organization of organelles such as the rER (d). Independent experiments showed that cells in this compressed state were alive and actively synthesizing ECM.[33]

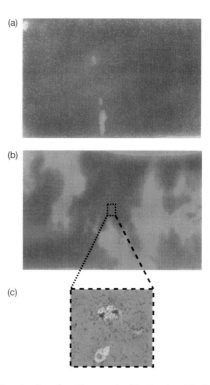

(a)

(b)

(c)

Fig. 7.36 Injurious loading of cartilage can lead to direct matrix damage and changes in cell metabolism. (a) Uncompressed control tissue. (b) Cartilage subjected to injurious compression, exhibiting macroscopic fissures. (c) Injury leads to a population of apoptotic cells showing condensed nuclei[104] as well as live cells actively synthesizing and turning over their cell-associated matrix.

Source: Adapted from Ref. 36.

responsible for these processes are not well understood. In order to quantify the events following cartilage and joint injury, investigators have turned to a variety of *in vitro* and animal models. Studies have shown that threshold levels of compressive strain, strain rate, and peak stress can cause cartilage matrix disruption, tissue swelling, cell necrosis and apoptosis, and increased loss of matrix macromolecules.[35,36,67–72] Calf cartilage explants subjected to 6 cycles of 50 per cent compression/release over 12 hours (to approximately 15 MPa peak stress) showed matrix fissuring and a population of nonviable cells with condensed nuclei on light microscopy[36] (Fig. 7.36). The remaining viable cells actively mediated an increase in PG turnover and loss, not simply due to the loosening of the collagenous matrix by the mechanical loading. Follow-on studies using multiple cycles of 1/sec strain rate compression to 30–50 per cent final strain, confirmed that a significant portion of the nonviable cells were apoptotic.[67] The induction of apoptosis, matrix swelling, and increased PG release occurred at peak stresses greater than approximately 10 MPa, though apoptotic cells could be seen even at peak stress as low as 4.5 MPa. Even a single injurious compression could increase MMP-3 mRNA levels by 10-fold.[68] Studies have also elucidated the importance of variations in strain, strain rate, and peak stress on cartilage and chondrocyte injury.[70,72] Taken together, these studies suggest that mechanical overload can cause long-term cell-mediated changes in matrix quality and turnover. Injurious compression results in a decrease in biosynthetic rates in the remaining viable cells, and these viable cells no longer respond to the stimulatory effects of moderate dynamic compression seen in normal cartilage.[72]

Collagen network disruption, however, appears primarily to be a direct result of mechanical overload. The presence of the cartilage anchorage to bone appears to be protective against matrix disruption.[69] Single ramp compressions of steer humeral head osteochondral plugs to a final strain of 68 per cent and peak stress of 14 MPa showed that matrix disruption and nonviable cells were confined to the superficial zone.[70] In contrast, injurious compression of cartilage disks without the underlying bone produced matrix disruption and apoptosis throughout the cartilage. Although the importance of viable chondrocytes in the maintenance of a healthy matrix is undisputed, the role of cell necrosis or apoptosis in catabolic degradation of ECM remains unclear.

The future: cartilage repair and tissue engineering

The role of appropriate mechanical loading in the synthesis, maintenance, and remodeling of healthy cartilage *in vivo* is well accepted, and the association of injurious mechanical loading with cartilage degradation and disease is becoming clear. Increasing attention is also being paid to the role of mechanical loading in cartilage repair and the treatment of cartilage pathologies (e.g., OA and the occurrence of focal cartilage defects in otherwise healthy joint surfaces). Short of total joint replacement, there is currently no therapy capable of resurfacing an entire joint surface. There are, however, clinical methods including osteochondral allo- and autografting and mosaicplasty that involve the transplantation of cartilage-bone specimens into a defect site. In order for such procedures to be successful in the long term, the mechanical integrity of the repair tissue must be maintained under conditions of physiological loading. Studies such as those outlined above are critical in understanding the response of repair cartilage to its mechanical environment *in vivo*. In the future, engineered tissue constructs will likely be one of the modalities used in the treatment of cartilage degeneration. Tissue engineering for cartilage repair often involves the seeding of isolated cells into a biologic or nonbiologic matrix prior to implantation, while maintaining or inducing a chondrocyte phenotype.[38,39] During the *in vitro* culture period, mechanical forces can contribute to the development of an appropriate and optimal cartilage-like ECM. Several recent studies have shown that primary chondrocytes seeded in natural and synthetic scaffolds showed modified biosynthetic rates in response to static and dynamic compression in a manner similar to that seen in native cartilage tissue.[40,73–75] In these studies, the amplitudes and frequencies required to stimulate biosynthesis were not necessarily similar to those used with native tissue, likely due to the lower intrinsic mechanical properties of the synthetic matrices. Dynamic loading regimes can also promote chondrogenic differentiation of mesenchymal stem cells.[76]

Conclusion

During the past decade, the rapidly expanding field of cartilage mechanobiology has focused attention on the ability of chondrocytes to respond to mechanical forces and other physical stimuli in their environment. Significant advances have been made in the understanding of cellular transduction mechanisms. However, many of the unique mechanobiological pathways associated with the coordinated synthesis, assembly, and degradation of the intracellular and extracellular matrices of cartilage remain to be elucidated. Progress in this field will continue to be extremely important for the further understanding of the etiology of OA in its many forms, and in improving clinical options for repair and regeneration of cartilage. This review has emphasized recent studies involving intact cartilage *in vitro* and *in vivo*, with relevance to cartilage in normal, mechanically injured, and osteoarthritic joints. Ongoing studies in many laboratories involving intact cartilage as well as isolated chondrocytes and cell-seeded scaffolds for cartilage tissue engineering should enable clinicians and researchers to take advantage of new insights at the interface between engineering and biology as applied to problems in joint disease.

Summary

Cartilage is subjected to a wide range of mechanical forces associated with joint loading *in vivo*. These mechanical forces can dramatically alter chondrocyte synthesis, assembly, and degradation of extracellular matrix (ECM) proteins and proteoglycans (PGs), in a manner dependent upon the type, magnitude, duration, and frequency of the applied load. The effects of cartilage compression and shear on the nature and kinetics of the chondrocyte response to loading are described. Recent studies suggest that there are multiple regulatory pathways by which the chondrocytes in cartilage can sense and respond to mechanical stimuli. These pathways include upstream signaling and changes at the level of gene transcription, protein translation, and post-translational modifications of newly synthesized macromolecules. Experiments have shown that chondrocyte mechanotransduction is critically important *in vivo* in the cell-mediated feedback between joint loading, the molecular structure of newly synthesized ECM collagens and PGs, and the resulting functional biomechanical properties of cartilage. In addition, threshold levels of mechanical overload injury can lead to chondrocyte death, direct matrix damage, and longer-term cell-mediated degradation of the ECM. Motivated by these findings, current approaches to creating tissue engineered cell-scaffold implants for cartilage repair are incorporating mechanical loading of the developing constructs to optimize their biological and mechanical properties.

Acknowledgements

Supported in part by NIH Grants AR33236 and AR45779.

References

(An asterisk denotes recommended reading.)

1. Herberhold, C., Faber, S., Stammberger, T., *et al.* (1999). In situ measurement of articular cartilage deformation in intact femoropatellar joints under static loading. *J Biomech* **32**:1287–95.
2. Ateshian, G.A., Kwak, S.D., Soslowsky, L.J., and Mow, V.C. (1994). A stereophotogrammetric method for determining in situ contact areas in diarthrodial joints, and a comparison with other methods. *J Biomech* **27**:111–24.
3. Hodge, W.A., Fijan, R.S., Carlson, K.L., *et al.* (1986). Contact pressures in the human hip joint measured *in vivo*. *Proc Natl Acad Sci USA* **83**:2879–83.
4. Helminen, H. (1988). *Joint Loading: Biology and Health of Articular Fractures*. Bristol: Butterworth-Heinemann Medical.
5. Behrens, F., Kraft, E.L., and Oegema Jr., T.R. (1989). Biochemical changes in articular cartilage after joint immobilization by casting or external fixation. *J Orthop Res* **7**:335–43.
6. Jurvelin, J., Kiviranta, I., Saamanen, A.M., Tammi, M., and Helminen, H.J. (1989). Partial restoration of immobilization-induced softening of canine articular cartilage after remobilization of the knee stifle joint. *J Orthop Res* **7**:352–8.
7. Slowman, S.D. and Brandt, K.D. (1986). Composition and glycosaminoglycan metabolism of articular cartilage from habitually loaded and habitually unloaded sites. *Arthritis Rheum* **29**:88–94.
8. Salter, R.B. (1993). *Continuous passive motion: a biological concept for the healing and regeneration of articular cartilage, ligaments, and tendons.* Baltimore: Williams and Wilkins.
9. Kiviranta, I., Tammi, M., Jurvelin, J., Saamanen, A.M., and Helminen, H.J. (1988). Moderate running exercise augments glycosaminoglycans and thickness of articular cartilage in the knee joint of young beagle dogs. *J Orthop Res* **6**:188–95.
10. Radin, E.L., Martin, R.B., Burr, D.B., *et al.* (1984). Effects of mechanical loading on the tissues of the rabbit knee. *J Orthop Res* **2**:221–34.
11. Saamamen, A.M., Kiviranta, I., Jurvelin, J., Helminen, H.J., and Tammi, M. (1994). Proteoglycan and collagen alterations in canine knee articular cartilage following 20 km daily running exercise for 15 weeks. *Connect Tissue Res* **30**:191–201.
12. Guilak, F. (1995). Compression-induced changes in the shape and volume of the chondrocyte nucleus. *J Biomech* **28**:1529–41.
13. Buschmann, M.D., Hunziker, E.B., Kim, Y.J., and Grodzinsky, A.J. (1996). Altered aggrecan synthesis correlates with cell and nucleus structure in statically compressed cartilage. *J Cell Sci* **109**:499–508.
14. *Guilak, F. and Mow, V.C. (2000). The mechanical environment of the chondrocyte: a biphasic finite element model of cell-matrix interactions in articular cartilage. *J Biomech* **33**:1663–73.
    This paper gives an overview of the physical environment of the chondrocyte in cartilage, and of a macroscopic continuum approach to the engineering modeling of forces and flows in the ECM and within the cell.
15. Frank, E.H. and Grodzinsky AJ. (1987). Cartilage electromechanics—II. A continuum model of cartilage electrokinetics and correlation with experiments. *J Biomech* **20**:629–39.
16. Kim, Y.J., Bonassar, L.J., and Grodzinsky, A.J. (1995). The role of cartilage streaming potential, fluid flow and pressure in the stimulation of chondrocyte biosynthesis during dynamic compression. *J Biomech* **28**:1055–66.
17. Maroudas, A. (1979). Physicochemical properties of articular cartilage. In M. A. R. Freeman (ed.), *Physicochemical Properties of Articular Cartilage.* Tunbridge Wells, England: Pitman Medical, pp. 215–90.
18. Gray, M.L., Pizzanelli, A.M., Grodzinsky, A.J., and Lee, R.C. (1988). Mechanical and physiochemical determinants of the chondrocyte biosynthetic response. *J Orthop Res* **6**:777–92.
19. Urban, J.P., Hall, A.C., and Gehl, K.A. (1993). Regulation of matrix synthesis rates by the ionic and osmotic environment of articular chondrocytes. *J Cell Physiol* **154**:262–70.
20. Mak, A.F. (1986). Unconfined compression of hydrated viscoelastic tissues: a biphasic poroviscoelastic analysis. *Biorheology* **23**:371–83.
21. Eisenberg, S.R. and Grodzinsky, A.J. (1987). The kinetics of chemically induced nonequilibrium swelling of articular cartilage and corneal stroma. *J Biomech Eng* **109**:79–89.
22. Lai, W.M., Hou, J.S., and Mow, V.C. (1991). A triphasic theory for the swelling and deformation behaviors of articular cartilage. *J Biomech Eng* **113**:245–58.
23. Buschmann, M.D., Kim, Y.J., Wong, M., *et al.* (1999). Stimulation of aggrecan synthesis in cartilage explants by cyclic loading is localized to regions of high interstitial fluid flow. *Arch Biochem Biophys* **366**:1–7.
24. Quinn, T.M., Grodzinsky, A.J., Buschmann, M.D., Kim, Y.J., Hunziker, E.B. (1998). Mechanical compression alters proteoglycan deposition and matrix deformation around individual cells in cartilage explants. *J Cell Sci* **111**:573–83.
25. Davies, P.F. (1995). Flow-mediated endothelial mechanotransduction. *Physiol Rev* **75**:519–60.
26. Das, P., Schurman, D.J., and Smith, R.L. (1997). Nitric oxide and G proteins mediate the response of bovine articular chondrocytes to fluid–induced shear. *J Orthop Res* **15**:87–93.
27. *Wang, N., Butler, J.P., and Ingber, D.E. (1993). Mechanotransduction across the cell surface and through the cytoskeleton. *Science* **260**:1124–7.
    This review focuses on the underlying mechanisms involved in cellular mechanotransduction, including extracellular, intracellular cytoskeletal, and cell membrane macromolecular constituents, relevant to chondrocytes and many other cells.

28. Smith, R., Rusk, S., Ellison, B., *et al.* (1996). *In vitro* stimulation of articular cartilage chondrocyte mRNA and extracellular matrix synthesis by hydrostatic pressure. *J Orthop Res* **14**:53–60.

29. Valhmu, W., Stazzone, E., Bachrach, N., *et al.* (1998). Load-controlled compression of articular cartilage induces a transient stimulation of aggrecan gene expression. *Arch Biochem Biophys* **353**:29–36.

30. Takahashi, K., Kubo, T., Kobayashi, K., *et al.* (1997). Hydrostatic pressure influences mRNA expression of transforming growth factor-β1 and heat shock protein 70 in chondrcyte-like cell line. *J Orthop Res* **15**:150–8.

31. Ragan, P., Badger, A., Cook, M., *et al.* (1999). Down-regulation of chondrocyte aggrecan and type-II collagen gene expression correlates with increases in static compression magnitude and duration. *J Orthop Res* **17**:836–42.

32. Parkkinen, J.J., Lammi, M.J., Pelttari, A., *et al.* (1993). Altered Golgi apparatus in hydrostatically loaded articular cartilage chondrocytes. *Ann Rheum Dis* **52**:192–8.

33. *Kim, Y.J., Grodzinsky, A.J., and Plaas, A.H. (1996). Compression of cartilage results in differential effects on biosynthetic pathways for aggrecan, link protein, and hyaluronan. *Arch Biochem Biophys* **328**:331–40.

    This paper demonstrates that the cellular response to mechanical compression can be complex, involving alterations in signaling and biosynthetic pathways for very specific ECM molecules, and not a general up- or down-regulation of synthesis.

34. Sah, R.L., Grodzinsky, A.J., Plaas, A.H., and Sandy, J.D. (1990). Effects of tissue compression on the hyaluronate-binding properties of newly synthesized proteoglycans in cartilage explants. *Biochem J* **267**:803–8.

35. Farquhar, T., Xia, Y., Mann, K., *et al.* (1996). Swelling and fibronectin accumulation in articular cartilage explants after cyclical impact. *J Orthop Res* **14**:417–23.

36. Quinn, T.M., Grodzinsky, A.J., Hunziker, E.B., and Sandy JD. (1998). Effects of injurious compression on matrix turnover around individual cells in calf articular cartilage explants. *J Orthop Res* **16**:490–9.

37. Muir, H. (1995). The chondrocyte, architect of cartilage. Biomechanics, structure, function and molecular biology of cartilage matrix macromolecules. *Bioessays* **17**:1039–48.

38. Benya, P.D. and Shaffer, J.D. (1982). Dedifferentiated chondrocytes reexpress the differentiated collagen phenotype when cultured in agarose gels. *Cell* **30**:215–24.

39. Hauselmann, H.J., Fernandes, R.J., Mok, S.S., *et al.* (1994). Phenotypic stability of bovine articular chondrocytes after long-term culture in alginate beads. *J Cell Sci* **107**:17–27.

40. Ragan, P.M., Chin, V.I., Hung, H.H., *et al.* (2000). Chondrocyte extracellular matrix synthesis and turnover are influenced by static compression in a new alginate disk culture system. *Arch Biochem Biophys* **383**:256–64.

41. Frank, E.H., Jin, M., Loening, A.M., Levenston, M.E., Grodzinsky, A.J. (2000). A versatile shear and compression apparatus for mechanical stimulation of tissue culture explants. *J Biomech* **33**:1523–7.

42. Hall, A.C., Urban, J.P., and Gehl, K.A. (1991). The effects of hydrostatic pressure on matrix synthesis in articular cartilage. *J Orthop Res* **9**:1–10.

43. Schneiderman, R., Keret, D., and Maroudas, A. (1986). Effects of mechanical and osmotic pressure on the rate of glycosaminoglycan synthesis in the human adult femoral head cartilage: an *in vitro* study. *J Orthop Res* **4**:393–408.

44. Sah, R.L., Kim, Y.J., Doong, J.Y., *et al.* (1989). Biosynthetic response of cartilage explants to dynamic compression. *J Orthop Res* **7**:619–36.

45. Kim, Y.J., Sah, R.L., Grodzinsky, A.J., Plaas, A.H., and Sandy, J.D. (1994). Mechanical regulation of cartilage biosynthetic behavior: physical stimuli. *Arch Biochem Biophys* **311**:1–12.

46. Torzilli, P.A., Grigiene, R., Huang, C., *et al.* (1997). Characterization of cartilage metabolic response to static and dynamic stress using a mechanical explant test system. *J Biomech* **30**:1–9.

47. Wong, M., Siegrist, M., and Cao, X. (1999). Cyclic compression of articular cartilage explants is associated with progressive consolidation and altered expression pattern of extracellular matrix proteins. *Matrix Biol* **18**:391–9.

48. Li, K.W., Williamson, A.K., Wang, A.S., and Sah, R.L. (2001). Growth responses of cartilage to static and dynamic compression. *Clin Orthop Rel Res* S34–48.

49. Bonassar, L.J., Grodzinsky, A.J., Frank, E.H., *et al.* (2001). The effect of dynamic compression on the response of articular cartilage to insulin-like growth factor-I. *J Orthop Res* **19**:11–7.

50. *Jin, M., Frank, E.H., Quinn, T.M., Hunziker, E.B., and Grodzinsky, A.J. (2001). Tissue shear deformation stimulates proteoglycan and protein biosynthesis in bovine cartilage explants. *Arch Biochem Biophys* **395**:41–8.

    This paper shows the effects of shear deformation of cells and matrix on chondrocyte biosynthesis, in the absence of appreciable fluid flow; that is, the effects of decoupling the complex combination of deformation and fluid flow signals occur simultaneously during the compression of the cartilage.

51. Lai, W.M., Gu, W.Y., and Mow, V.C. (1998). On the conditional equivalence of chemical loading and mechanical loading on articular cartilage. *J Biomech* **31**:1181–5.

52. *Wilkins, R.J., Browning, J.A., and Ellory, J.C. (2000). Surviving in a matrix: membrane transport in articular chondrocytes. *J Membr Biol* **177**:95–108.

    This paper summarizes mechanotransduction mechanisms related to physicochemical changes in chondrocyte environment, for example, pH, osmolarity, and the role of cell membrane channels and ion transporters in chondrocyte response and homeostasis.

53. Suh, J., Baek, G., Aroen, A., *et al.* (1999). Intermittent sub-ambient interstitial hydrostatic pressure as a potential mechanical stimulator for chondrocyte metabolism. *Osteoarthritis Cart* **7**:71–80.

54. Jortikka, M.O., Parkkinen, J.J., Inkinen, R.I., *et al.* (2000). The role of microtubules in the regulation of proteoglycan synthesis in chondrocytes under hydrostatic pressure. *Arch Biochem Biophys* **374**:172–80.

55. Lammi, M., Inkinen, R., Parkkinen, J, *et al.* (1994). Expression of reduced amounts of structurally altered aggrecan in articular cartilage chondrocytes exposed to high hydrostatic pressure. *Biochem J* **304**:723–30.

56. Smith, R., Donlon, B., Gupta, M., *et al.* (1995). Effects of fluid-induced shear on articular cartilage chondrocyte morphology and metabolism *in vitro*. *J Orthop Res* **13**:824–31.

57. Jin G., Sah R., Li Y., *et al.* (2000). Biomechanical regulation of matrix metalloproteinase-9 in cultured chondrocytes. *J Orthop Res* **18**:899–908.

58. Hung, C.T., Henshaw, D.R., Wang, C.C., *et al.* (2000). Mitogen-activated protein kinase signaling in bovine articular chondrocytes in response to fluid flow does not require calcium mobilization. *J Biomech* **33**:73–80.

59. Holmvall, K., Camper, L., Johansson, S., Kimura, J.H., and Lundgren-Akerlund, E. (1995). Chondrocyte and chondrosarcoma cell integrins with affinity for collagen type II and their response to mechanical stress. *Exp Cell Res* **221**:496–503.

60. Schinagl, R.M., Gurskis, D., Chen, A.C., and Sah, R.L. (1997). Depth-dependent confined compression modulus of full-thickness bovine articular cartilage. *J Orthop Res* **15**:499–506.

61. Lee, D.A., Knight, M.M., Bolton, J.F., *et al.* (2000). Chondrocyte deformation within compressed agarose constructs at the cellular and sub-cellular levels. *J Biomech* **33**:81–95.

62. Lohmander, L.S., Hascall, V.C., Yanagishita, M., Kuettner, K.E., and Kimura, J.H. (1986). Post-translational events in proteoglycan synthesis: kinetics of synthesis of chondroitin sulfate and oligosaccharides on the core protein. *Arch Biochem Biophys* **250**:211–27.

63. Salter, D.M., Millward-Sadler, S.J., Nuki, G., and Wright, M.O. (2001). Integrin-interleukin-4 mechanotransduction pathways in human chondrocytes. *Clin Orthop* S49–60.

64. Gelber, A., Hochberg, M., Mead, L., *et al.* (2000). Joint injury in young adults and risk for subsequent knee and hip osteoarthritis. *Ann Intern Med* **133**:321–8.

65. Sharma, L., Song, J., Felson, D., *et al.* (2001). The role of knee alignment in disease progression and functional decline in knee osteoarthritis. *JAMA* **286**:188–95.

66. Murphy, S.B., Ganz, R., and Muller, M.E. (1995). The prognosis in untreated dysplasia of the hip. *J Bone Joint Surg Am* **77**(A):985–9.

67. Loening, A., James, I., Levenston, M., *et al.* (2000). Injurious mechanical compression of bovine articular cartilage induces chondrocyte apoptosis. *Arch Biochem Biophys* **381**:205–12.

68. Patwari, P., Fay, J., Cook, M., *et al.* (2001). *In vitro* models for investigation of the effects of acute mechanical injury on cartilage. *Clin Orthop* **39**(1S):S61–S71.

69. Jeffry, J., Thomson, L., and Aspden, R. (1995). Matrix damage and chondrocyte viability following a single impact load on articular cartilage. *Arch Biochem Biophys* **322**:87–96.

70. Quinn, T., Allen, R., Schalet, B., Perumbuli, P., and Hunziker, E. (2001). Matrix and cell injury due to sub-impact loading of adult bovine articular

cartilage explants: effects of strain rate and peak stress. *J Orthop Res* **19**:242–9.

71. Chen, C.T., Burton-Wurster, N., Borden, C., *et al.* (2001). Chondrocyte necrosis and apoptosis in impact damaged articular cartilage. *J Orthop Res* **19**:703–11.

72. Kurz, B., Jin, M., Patwari, P., *et al.* (2001). Biosynthetic response and mechanical properties of articular cartilage after injurious compression. *J Orthop Res* **19**:1140–6.

73. Buschmann, M.D., Gluzband, Y.A., Grodzinsky, A.J., and Hunziker, E.B. (1995). Mechanical compression modulates matrix biosynthesis in chondrocyte/agarose culture. *J Cell Sci* **108**:1497–508.

74. Lee, D.A., Noguchi, T., Knight, M.M., *et al.* (1998). Response of chondrocyte subpopulations cultured within unloaded and loaded agarose. *J Orthop Res* **16**:726–33.

75. Mauck, R.L., Soltz, M.A., Wang, C.C., *et al.* (2000). Functional tissue engineering of articular cartilage through dynamic loading of chondrocyte-seeded agarose gels. *J Biomech Eng* **122**:252–60.

76. Elder, S.H., Goldstein, S.A., Kimura, J.H., Soslowsky, L.J., and Spengler, D.M. (2001). Chondrocyte differentiation is modulated by frequency and duration of cyclic compressive loading. *Ann Biomed Eng* **29**:476–82.

7.2.1.6 Crystals and osteoarthritis

Ann K. Rosenthal and Lawrence M. Ryan

Calcium crystals, including calcium pyrophosphate dihydrate (CPPD) crystals and the three crystals types comprising the basic calcium phosphate (BCP) crystals are common components of osteoarthritic synovial fluid.[1,2] However, 40 years after their initial description, the significance of these crystals in OA remains unclear. Progress in this area has been hampered, by an incomplete understanding of the pathogenesis of both calcium crystal disease and OA.

It is unlikely that the co-existence of calcium crystals and OA represents a chance occurrence of two common phenomena of aging. However, whether crystal deposition precedes or accompanies cartilage injury in OA, and how crystals contribute to articular damage remains unknown. Significant differences exist between CPPD and BCP crystals with regard to factors that cause their formation, their epidemiological associations, and their cellular effects. Yet, these crystals frequently co-exist in osteoarthritic joints, further muddying the waters of clinical studies. Lastly, although there is good evidence from *in vitro* studies that calcium crystals aggravate cartilage matrix degeneration, whether reducing crystal formation would ameliorate joint damage is not known.

Despite these philosophical and practical difficulties, we will present good evidence from clinical studies that calcium crystals are common components of osteoarthritic synovial fluids and may define subsets of patients with unusually severe and uniquely-distributed arthritis. We also summarize strong evidence from *in vitro* studies that calcium crystals directly injure articular tissues. We hope these findings underscore the clinical importance of identifying calcium crystals in degenerative arthritis and encourage further exploration of the role of these crystals in OA.

Clinical associations between calcium crystals and OA

CPPD crystals

CPPD crystals were originally described in 1962 by McCarty *et al.* as uricase-resistant crystals in patients with gout-like arthritis.[3] Articular

CPPD crystals form in the midzone of hyaline articular cartilage, in fibro-cartilage, and in metaplastic areas of synovium, tendons, and ligaments. They are associated with a wide spectrum of clinical disease, ranging from the acute monoarticular arthritis of pseudogout to a chronic polyarticular OA-like syndrome. Less commonly, CPPD crystals are found in patients with a polyarticular inflammatory-like arthritis resembling rheumatoid arthritis, or in neuropathic joints. CPPD crystal deposition may also be asymptomatic. Although aging is the strongest known risk factor for CPPD crystal deposition, other metabolic conditions such as hemochromatosis and hyperparathyroidism increase the frequency of articular CPPD crystals.[4]

CPPD crystals are common in OA joints. Between 30 and 60 per cent of synovial fluids from patients with OA contain some species of calcium crystal. CPPD crystals occur in one-third to one-fourth of osteoarthritic synovial fluids.[2,5,6] Gibilsco *et al.*[2] noted CPPD crystals in 42 per cent of one hundred OA synovial fluids with cell counts less than 2000/mm³. Derfus *et al.* found that 30 per cent of randomly chosen patients undergoing knee replacement had synovial fluid CPPD crystals at the time of surgery.[7] In another study, 28 per cent of knee synovial fluids from OA patients, referred to a general rheumatologist, contained CPPD crystals.[8] Histologic studies reveal a similarly high frequency of CPPD crystals in osteoarthritic joints. Sokolov *et al.* demonstrated CPPD crystals in the articular hyaline or fibro-cartilage of 33 per cent of all patients undergoing joint replacement. When only patients over the age of 75 were included, 52 per cent had cartilage CPPD crystals.[9]

CPPD crystals are significantly under diagnosed. Numerous studies suggest that even in the best of hands, CPPD crystals are commonly overlooked with polarizing light microscopy.[10] Many CPPD crystals are so small as to be below the level of detection of the light microscope.[11] These tiny crystals may be the most inflammatory.[12] The use of chondrocalcinosis, the radiologic correlate of CPPD crystal deposition, to diagnose CPPD crystal deposition also underestimates the number of patients with articular CPPD crystals[13] (Fig. 7.37). Film quality affects the rates of detection of chondrocalcinosis. Chondrocalcinosis is more difficult to discern on standing knee films and in X-rays lacking fine detail. The scarcity of intact articular cartilage in severely affected joints may also decrease the chance of detecting chondrocalcinosis. Similarly, improper handling of histologic specimens reduces the chances of CPPD crystal detection in tissues.[14]

CPPD crystals may define a subset of patients with severe OA. Ledingham *et al.* showed that CPPD crystals in osteoarthritic knees were associated with increased disability, thus suggesting a worse outcome in patients with CPPD crystal deposition.[8] Earlier studies correlated the presence of CPPD crystals in the synovial fluid of OA patients with increased joint damage as measured by radiographic scores.[5,6] Several studies, however, refute these findings.[15] In a recently described cohort of patients with hand OA, chondrocalcinosis did not worsen radiographic scores.[16] The cross-sectional design of these studies, and poor sensitivity of radiographic chondrocalcinosis as a marker for articular CPPD crystals make them less than optimal for addressing this issue. In addition, the impact of crystals on the degenerative process in smaller non-weight bearing joints may be less than in the large weight bearing joints such as the knee.

Synovial fluid studies suggest a more aggressive catabolism in osteoarthritic joints containing CPPD crystals, than in those without crystals. Biochemical markers of cartilage destruction in synovial fluid have been used as surrogates for disease severity. Patients with CPPD arthritis had higher levels of synovial fluid proteoglycan fragments and metalloproteases, than those found in synovial fluids from patients in five other disease categories.[17] The inclusion of synovial fluids from patients with acute CPPD arthritis with its attendant inflammatory cells and cytokines along with those with chronic CPPD arthritis complicates synovial fluid studies.

There is good evidence to suggest that OA patients with articular CPPD crystals have subtle differences in their disease patterns compared to those without CPPD crystals. Halverson and McCarty found that CPPD crystals in osteoarthritic synovial fluid correlated with advanced age.[1] The pattern of joint involvement may also be different. For example, CPPD crystals are often associated with degenerative arthritis in joints not typically involved

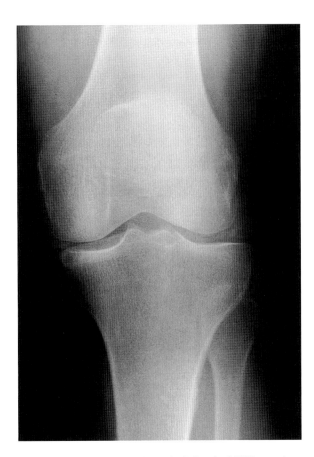

Fig. 7.37 Chondrocalcinosis, the radiographic hallmark of CPPD crystal deposition. In this knee joint, chondrocalcinosis is present in both the medial and lateral compartments.

in OA, such as the glenohumeral joint, the metacarpalphalangeal joints, and the wrist. The preference of CPPD crystals for certain joints is also confirmed by pathologic studies. Sokolof showed that CPPD crystals were significantly more common in knee than in hip OA.[9]

Several studies address radiographic differences in OA with and without CPPD crystals. Doherty and Dieppe suggest that articular CPPD crystals are associated with a 'hypertrophic' pattern of radiographic change with exuberant remodeling of bone.[18] Ledingham et al. showed that CPPD crystals in knee joint fluid correlated with bilateral disease, involvement of multiple compartments, osteophytes, attrition, and subchondral cysts.[8] In a study of radiographic OA in elderly patients with and without CPPD crystals, Sanmarti et al. found an increase in lateral knee compartment involvement and MCP joint involvement in the group with CPPD crystals.[19] Tendon calcification may also be a radiographic clue to the presence of CPPD crystals.[20]

BCP crystals

BCP crystals may be even more common in OA than CPPD, but their clinical significance is less well understood. Tricalcium phosphate, octacalcium phosphate, and carbonate-substituted apatite comprise the three crystal types included in the BCP category. BCP crystals are associated with a variety of articular and periarticular syndromes, ranging from a severe destructive arthritis known as Milwaukee Shoulder Syndrome to a periarticular inflammatory syndrome and calcific tendinitis.[21]

BCP crystals commonly occur in OA synovial fluid. Thirty to fifty per cent of synovial fluids from patients with OA will contain enough BCP crystals to allow identification by available analytical techniques.[5] Rates vary with the sensitivity and specificity of the various techniques used to identify BCP crystals. In unselected OA patients, 21/40 contained synovial

fluid BCP crystals under transmission electron microscopy.[22] Using Alizirin red and Von Kossa stains, Gibilesco et al. showed that 47 per cent of OA synovial fluids had BCP crystals.[2] Derfus et al. recently showed that BCP crystals were the most common crystal type found in knee joint fluid at the time of total knee replacement surgery.[7] Using the semiquantitative ^{14}C ethane-1-hydroxy 1,1 diphosphonate (EHDP) binding assay, they found BCP crystals in 49 per cent of patients. Histologic studies confirm the high prevalence of BCP crystals in synovial tissue at the time of joint resection. Fourteen out of 16 patients had apatite-like clumps detected by Alizirin red in the synovial samples from the hip and knee specimens taken at the time of arthroplasty for advanced OA.[23]

Our progress in understanding the clinical and pathologic significance of BCP crystals has been hampered by the lack of an accurate, reliable, and widely available assay for these crystals.[14] BCP crystals appear in the light microscope as 5–20 μm round, irregular clumps, and cannot be differentiated from debris or other particulate matter under polarizing light. Alizirin red staining is commonly used to detect BCP crystals in fresh specimens. However, this technique cannot distinguish between CPPD and BCP crystals and has a high rate of false positives. Similar problems are seen with Von Kossa used on preserved samples. A semiquantitative method based on the binding of BCP crystals to a radioactive bisphosphonate is perhaps the most accurate way to measure these crystals. Known as the EHDP binding assay, this assay is only available in a few research laboratories. Definitive identification of BCP crystals is done by X-ray diffraction or Fourier transform infrared spectroscopy. These techniques are expensive, operator-dependent, and require fairly large amounts of samples for accuracy.[14]

The presence of BCP crystals correlates with increasing severity of arthritis in OA patients. Halverson and McCarty correlated the presence of BCP crystals with radiographic severity in OA patients.[24] This was recently confirmed by others.[7] Bardin et al. showed that while 23 per cent of typical OA patients had synovial fluid BCP crystals, 83 per cent of a subset of rapidly progressive OA had articular BCP crystals. At the time of joint replacement, 80 per cent of typical OA patients and 100 per cent of patients with particularly aggressive OA had detectable quantities of BCP crystals.[25]

Whether the presence of articular BCP crystals defines a subset of OA patients with a unique pattern of disease is controversial. Involvement of the glenohumeral joint is unusual in typical OA, and yet is common in the BCP-associated syndrome: Milwaukee shoulder syndrome (MSS).[21] In MSS, there are high levels of destructive proteases and marked degradation of not only cartilage but other articular structures such as the rotator cuff.[26] However, excluding MSS, whether patients with articular BCP crystals are clinically different from those without crystals is not clear. Carroll et al. showed an association between BCP crystals and larger joint effusions in OA patients.[22] Osteophytes may be less common in OA joints with BCP crystals than in OA without BCP crystals, suggesting a difference in rates of new bone formation in the presence of BCP crystals. Higher levels of other enzymes such as 5'-nucleotidase are seen in synovial fluid with BCP crystals and may have pathologic significance.[27] Carroll et al. showed no differences in the levels of keratan sulfate, a marker of cartilage matrix degradation, in synovial fluids from OA patients with and without BCP crystals. Levels of interleukin-1β, a possible mediator of cartilage damage in arthritis, were also similar in OA synovial fluids with and without BCP crystals.[22] Preliminary work suggests a possible association between apatite clumps in the synovium and synovial fibrosis, but further studies are necessary to confirm this finding.[23]

Mixed crystal deposition

BCP and CPPD crystals frequently co-exist. Consequently, many clinical studies that identify only one crystal type probably include patients with mixed crystal deposition. This effect is exaggerated by the lack of a widely available accurate assay for BCP crystals. Halverson and McCarty showed that 30 per cent of OA synovial fluids contained both types of calcium crystals.[1] In Gibelsco's study, 48 per cent of synovial fluid samples had both CPPD and BCP crystals; while in Derfus' study of perioperative joints,

19 per cent of patients had both crystal types.[2,7] Halverson and Derfus both used the ^{14}C EHDP assay to detect BCP crystals, while Gibelsco used the Alizirin red assay. The higher rate of simultaneous CPPD and BCP crystals in Gibelsco's study may be explained by an increased rate of false positives with the Alizirin red assay. Twenty-five to 50 per cent of patients with MSS also have CPPD crystals in their knee or shoulder fluids. Patients with familial forms of calcium crystal arthritis may also have mixed crystals. Recently, a kindred was described with both MSS-like disease and synovial fluid CPPD crystals. The gene mutation had no genetic link to other characterized CPPD kindreds or gene loci, including Col 2a, 5p, or 8q.[28]

The presence of both BCP and CPPD crystals is associated with more severe arthritis than that which is seen in OA without crystals. Most studies examining OA fluids for both types of calcium crystals show a worsening radiographic grade in patients with either or both forms of calcium crystals.[2,7] However, the clinical significance of the presence of both calcium crystal types is otherwise poorly understood.

Hypotheses linking calcium crystals and OA

Three hypotheses link calcium crystals and OA (Table 7.13). Crystal deposition in cartilage may result in cartilage matrix destruction and actually cause OA. Calcium crystals may aggravate or worsen pre-existing joint damage. Lastly, calcium crystals may be inert markers of cartilage damage. Although these theories are not mutually exclusive, and crystals may have different roles in different settings, clinical studies shed some light on the interaction of calcium crystals and OA.

Hypothesis 1: Crystals cause OA

Finding asymptomatic CPPD crystals in relatively normal joints supports the idea that the crystals are not simply epiphenomena of cartilage degeneration. Histologic studies of cartilage from patients with familial CPPD suggest that CPPD deposits predate OA.[29] In menisci, the presence of CPPD crystals is not necessarily associated with fibrillation.[30] Thus, articular CPPD crystals are present before degenerative arthritis is detectable. This theory is also supported by the strong epidemiological association between CPPD crystals and joint destruction. For example, Sokoloff et al. found a six-fold increase in the frequency of CPPD crystals in OA joints compared to normal joints.[9] In addition, familial CPPD disease typically results in premature OA in most kindreds, suggesting a causative link between CPPD crystal formation and OA.[31] The rarity of finding either BCP or CPPD crystals in joints destroyed by inflammatory arthritis also supports a causative link between these crystals and OA, and refutes a simple association between calcium crystals and joint destruction.

Hypothesis 2: Crystals worsen pre-existing OA

It has been proposed by Dieppe and others that calcium crystals worsen pre-existing OA, by 'amplifying' joint damage.[32] This hypothesis is supported by the finding that 70 per cent of patients with CPPD arthritis have a pre-existing condition known to damage joints.[18,32] Furthermore, in animal models of OA, crystals seem to be an early phenomenon.[33] Fam et al. introduced large quantities of CPPD crystals into joints from animals

with early OA. They demonstrated accelerated joint degeneration in these animals compared to control animals given no additional crystals.[34]

Hypothesis 3: Crystals are simply markers for severe OA

This hypothesis states that calcium crystals are epiphenomena in OA and do not contribute to the initiation or worsening of disease. Doherty et al. suggest that CPPD crystals define a subset of OA patients with a vigorous repair response.[18] In a 5-year study, the majority of OA patients with calcium crystals showed symptomatic improvement and more remodeling compared to those without crystals.[15] Another study showed that radiographic chondrocalcinosis did not adversely affect the progression of OA.[35] This hypothesis may be particularly relevant to BCP crystals, as some believe that these crystals are essentially wear-particles or debris from bone. In its extreme, this hypothesis would suggest that calcium crystals simply co-exist with OA because of common epidemiological factors. Aging is certainly a common risk factor for both OA and calcium crystal diseases. Both have strong hereditary influences, and risks are increased after injury to the affected joint.

None of these hypotheses are mutually exclusive and most likely each is true in certain settings. Work in the laboratory, however, strongly supports a role for crystals in either initiating or worsening cartilage damage and suggests that calcium crystals are not inert particles but active participants in OA.

Laboratory studies of calcium crystals and OA

Why do calcium crystals and OA coexist?

In vitro studies not only prove the pathogenicity of these crystals, but also begin to explore their origins. Recent laboratory work suggests that OA and crystals have several common etiologic factors, which may explain their frequent coexistence. For example, chondrocyte cell death (apoptosis) and the formation of calcifying apoptotic bodies have been implicated in the pathogenesis of both OA and BCP crystal formation.[36,37] Levels of inorganic pyrophosphate (PPi), the anionic component of the CPPD crystal, are elevated in synovial fluids from patients with OA, and contribute to CPPD crystal formation.[38] Lastly, growth factors, such as TGFβ are involved in both CPPD crystal formation and in OA. High levels of TGFβ increase PPi production by chondrocytes, and induce the formation of matrix vesicles capable of making more CPPD and BCP crystals.[39] In an animal model of OA, higher TGFβ levels were associated with worsening outcome.[40]

How do calcium crystals injure articular tissues?

It was noted many years ago that, like urate crystals, calcium crystals could produce inflammation. Thus, the hypothesis that calcium crystals cause cartilage damage by invoking inflammatory mediators has been extensively explored. However, as the clinical settings and biologic behavior of these crystals are better understood, the complexity of their biologic effects becomes apparent. Mechanistic hypotheses linking calcium crystals to OA include both direct and indirect metabolic damage to cartilage, as well as detrimental mechanical effects on articular tissues (Fig. 7.38).

Hypothesis 1: Calcium crystals provoke an inflammatory response that initiates articular injury

CPPD crystals were initially noted in the setting of clinical joint inflammation,[3] and both BCP and CPPD crystals initiate an inflammatory response. Many studies, however, refute the simple hypothesis that calcium crystals only

Table 7.13 Hypotheses linking calcium crystals and osteoarthritis

- ◆ Crystals cause osteoarthritis
- ◆ Crystals worsen pre-existing osteoarthritis
- ◆ Crystals do not participate in osteoarthritis

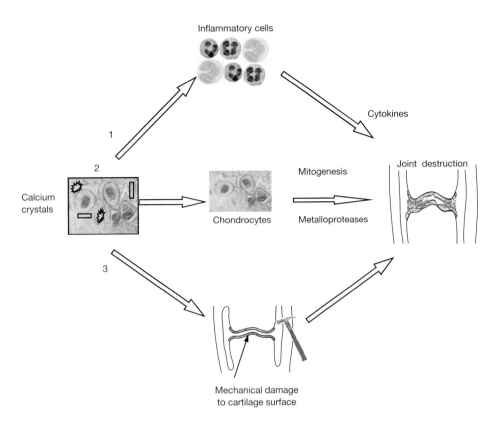

Fig. 7.38 Mechanistic hypotheses linking calcium crystals and joint degeneration.

produce damage through inflammation. For example, several studies demonstrate a strikingly poor correlation between numbers of inflammatory cells or levels of mediators in joint fluids and the presence of calcium crystals.[41] There is certainly some degree of inflammation in osteoarthritic synovium with or without crystals, but no clear correlation between evidence of inflammation in the synovial tissue and the presence of articular calcium crystals.[23]

There is good support for the hypothesis that calcium crystals initiate inflammation and that this may partially contribute to their pathogenic effects.[42] *In vitro*, both CPPD and BCP crystals induce interleukin-6 and interleukin-1 production by synovial cells. In animal models of OA, synovial changes may predate cartilage changes. These findings reinforce the often neglected but key role of the synovium in cartilage disease. Both CPPD and BCP crystals increase numbers of polymorphonuclear cells in the pouch fluid in the air pouch model of inflammation. CPPD crystals are clearly more effective inducers of inflammation than BCP crystals. Both crystal types also induce an inflammatory response in mononuclear inflammatory cells. These effects are modulated by crystal size and the types and quantities of protein bound to the crystals.

Hypothesis 2: Calcium crystals have direct effects on articular tissues independent of the inflammatory response

BCP and CPPD crystals activate fibroblasts, synoviocytes, and chondrocytes. The elegant studies demonstrating these effects and elucidating their mechanisms provide good evidence that crystals directly participate in cartilage matrix destruction.

Effect on mitogenesis. Calcium crystals induce mitogenesis in the articular cells, which ingest them. BCP-induced mitogenesis requires both endocytosis and dissolution in the acidic environment of the lysosome to induce mitogenesis.[43] Crystals exert their mitogenic effects through a complex

mechanism.[44] Calcium content is important since partial substitution of magnesium for calcium attenuates the biologic response to crystals.[45] Mitogenesis is partially dependent on phagocytosis, but also depends on the rapid response of the cell to crystal-induced membrane perturbations. The rapid response to crystals involves the phospholipase C dependent induction of protein kinase c (PKc) with elevated levels of diacylglycerol as an intermediate step. The induction of proto-oncogenes c-fos and c-myc are also involved in the BCP-induced mitogenic response, and down-regulation of PKc attenuates both the proto-oncogene response and mitogenesis. Recently, the mitogen-activated protein kinase (MAPK) signal transduction pathways, including the p42 and p44 mitogen-activated protein kinases, have been implicated in calcium crystal-induced mitogen activation.[44]

Effect on protease synthesis and secretion. Calcium crystals also induce protease synthesis from articular cells.[44] These proteases then participate directly in cartilage matrix degradation, as well as activating proenzymes and growth factors that cause further joint destruction. The first descriptions of MSS syndrome included data showing high levels of active proteinases including collagenase in synovial fluids.[26] These data have been difficult to reproduce. However, calcium crystals induce collagenase activity in the media of cultured fibroblasts. Stromelysin, which degrades proteoglycans as well as collagens, the 92 kD gelatinase, and MMP13 are also induced in fibroblasts by BCP crystals. Calcium crystals simultaneously decrease secretion of protease inhibitors such as tissue inhibitor of metalloproteinases 1 and 2, further worsening damage.[44] Transduction mechanisms for these effects are currently being delineated.

Hypothesis 3: Calcium crystals act as mechanical irritants in the joint

Although there are little data supporting the hypothesis that crystals produce mechanical damage in the joint, it remains an intriguing idea.

Hayes *et al.* exposed plugs of equine cartilage in culture to CPPD or BCP crystals and examined wear. They found an increase in sulfated compounds in the cartilage supernatant in the presence of crystals, suggesting that crystals induced proteoglycan loss from cartilage matrix, perhaps at least in part from a mechanical effect.[46]

Diagnostic and therapeutic implications of calcium crystals in OA

These clinical and laboratory studies demonstrate that a high percentage of patients with OA have articular calcium crystals, and these crystals may initiate or worsen cartilage damage through multiple mechanisms.

Before further work can proceed, there is an urgent need to improve diagnostic methods for both CPPD and BCP crystals in order to better characterize the clinical settings in which these crystals occur. The use of multiple observers or reference labs to confirm or detect crystals may improve the detection of calcium crystals. Advanced radiographic techniques such as magnetic resonance imaging may eventually be useful diagnostic tools for detecting articular calcium crystals.[14]

In vitro studies demonstrating common pathogenic factors in calcium crystal formation and OA could lead to the development of drugs, which may ameliorate cartilage degeneration in OA with and without crystals. Probenecid blocks the production or release of extracellular PPi,[47] and has been tried in a small uncontrolled clinical trials of patients with CPPD arthritis with some success.[48] Whether modifying PPi levels might also improve OA remains unknown. Phosphocitrate is another exciting discovery. This naturally occurring mitochondrial compound inhibits both crystal formation and the cellular effects of calcium crystals such as metalloprotease induction.[49] Phosphocitrate may prove to be a useful inhibitor of crystal deposition disease and might also ameliorate cartilage damage in OA.

Conclusions

CPPD and BCP crystals are commonly found in joint tissues from patients with degenerative arthritis, and may reflect more severe, more advanced, or unusually distributed disease. Although there is ample evidence from the laboratory to suggest that these crystals play an important role in either initiating or worsening cartilage damage in OA, we still have a great deal to learn about why they form and how they contribute to joint damage.

Key points for clinical practice

1. Calcium crystals are common components of osteoarthritic synovial fluids.
2. Calcium crystals likely participate in articular damage in OA.
3. Understanding why crystals form and how they contribute to joint degeneration will lead to improved treatments for osteoarthritis.

References

(An asterisk denotes recommended reading.)

1. Halverson, P. and McCarty, D. (1986). Patterns of radiographic abnormalities associated with basic calcium pyrophosphate and calcium pyrophosphate dihydrate crystal deposition. *Ann Rheum Dis* **45**:603–5.
2. Gibilisco, P., Schumacher, H.J., Hollander, J., and Soper, K. (1984). Synovial fluid crystals in osteoarthritis. *Arthritis Rheum* **28**:511–5.
3. McCarty, D., Kohn, N., and Faires, J. (1962). The significance of calcium pyrophosphate crystals in the synovial fluid of arthritic patients. 1. Clinical aspects. *Ann Intern Med* **56**:711–37.
4. Rosenthal, A. and Ryan, L. (2000). Calcium pyrophosphate crystal deposition disease, pseudogout, and articular chondrocalcinosis. In W. Koopman

(ed.), *Arthritis and Allied Conditions*. Philadelphia: Williams & Wilkens, pp. 2348–71.
5. Dieppe, P., Crocker, P., Corke, C., *et al.* (1979). Synovial fluid crystals. *Quart J Med* **48**:533–55.
6. Schumacher, H., Gordon, G., Paul, H., Reginato, A., *et al.* (1981). Osteoarthritis, crystal deposition, and inflammation. *Sem Arthritis Rheum* **11**:116–9.
7. *Derfus, B., Kurian, J., Butler, J., *et al.* (2002). The high prevalence of pathologic calcium crystals in pre-operative knees. *J Rheumatol* **29**:570–4.
   This recent addition to the literature reinforces the concept that calcium crystals are extremely common in OA.
8. Ledingham, J., Regan, M., Jones, A., and Doherty, M. (1993). Radiographic patterns and associations of osteoarthritis of the knee in patients referred to hospital. *Ann Rheum Dis* **52**:520–6.
9. Sokoloff, L. and Varma, A. (1988). Chondrocalcinosis in surgically resected joints. *Arthritis Rheum* **31**:750–6.
10. Segal, J. and Albert, D. (1999). Diagnosis of crystal-induced arthritis by synovial fluid examination for crystals: lessons from an imperfect test. *Arthritis Care Res* **12**:376–80.
11. Swan, A., Chapman, B., Heap, P., Seward, H., and Dieppe, P. (1994). Submicroscopic crystals in synovial fluids. *Ann Rheum Dis* **53**:467–70.
12. Ishikawa, H., Ueba, Y., Isobe, T., and Hirohata, K. (1987). Interaction of polymorphonuclear leukocytes with calcium pyrophosphate dihydrate crystals deposited in chondrocalcinosis cartilage. *Rheumatol Int* **7**:217–21.
13. Ryan, L. and Cheung, H. (1999). The role of crystals in osteoarthritis. *Rheum Dis Clin NA* **25**:257–67.
14. *Rosenthal, A. and Mandel, N. (2001). Identification of crystals in synovial fluids and joint tissues. *Curr Rheumatol Rep* **3**:11–6.
    This extensive review article discusses crystal identification techniques and their clinical uses.
15. Doherty, M., Watt, I., and Dieppe, P. (1984). Pyrophosphate arthropathy— a prospective study. *Br J Rheum* **23**:141–52.
16. Caspi, D., Flusser, G., Farber, I., *et al.* (2001). Clinical, radiologic, demographic, and occupational aspects of hand osteoarthritis in the elderly. *Sem Arth Rheum* **30**:321–31.
17. Lohmander, L., Hoerrner, L., and Lark, M. (1993). Metalloproteinases, tissue inhibitor, and proteoglycan fragments in knee synovial fluid in human osteoarthritis. *Arthritis Rheum* **36**:181–9.
18. *Doherty, M. and Dieppe, P. (1986). Crystal deposition disease in the elderly. *Clin Rheum Dis* **12**:97–116.
    This classic article explores the relationship between OA and calcium crystals, and delineates the issues that need be addressed to further our understanding of this relationship.
19. Sanmarti, R., Kanterewicz, E., Pladevall, M., *et al.* (1996). Analysis of the association between chondrocalcinosis and osteoarthritis:a community based study. *Ann Rheum Dis* **55**:30–3.
20. Yang, B-Y., Sartoris, D., Resnick, D., and Clopton, P. (1996). Calcium pyrophosphate dihydrate crystal deposition disease:frequency of tendon calcification about the knee. *J Rheumatol* **23**:883–6.
21. Halverson, P. (2001). Basic calcium phosphate (apatite, octacalcium phosphate, tricalcium phosphate crystal deposition diseases and calcinosis. In W. Koopman (ed.), *Arthritis and Allied Conditions*. Philadelphia: Lippincott Williams & Wilkins, pp. 2372–91.
22. Carroll, G., Stuart, R., Armstrong, J., Breidahl, P., and Laing, B. (1991). Hydroxyapatite crystals are a frequent finding in osteoarthritic synovial fluid, but are not related to increased concentrations of keratan sulfate or interleukin 1β. *J Rheumatol* **18**:861–6.
23. van Linthoudt, D., Beutler, A., Clayburne, G., Sieck, M., Fernandes, L. and Schumacher, H. Jr. (1997). Morphometric studies on synovium in advanced osteoarthritis:Is there an association between apatite-like material and collagen deposits. *Clin Exp Rheum* **15**:493–7.
24. Halverson, P. and McCarty, D. (1979). Identification of hydroxyapatite crystals in synovial fluids. *Arthritis Rheum* **22**:389–93.
25. Bardin, T., Bucki, B., Lansaman, J., Lequesne, M., Dryll, A., and Kuntz, D. (1993). Calcium crystals and rapidly destructive osteoarthritis (abstract). *Osteoarthritis Cart* **1**:15.

26. Garancis, J., Cheung, H., Halverson, P. and McCarty, D. (1981). 'Milwaukee Shoulder'-Association of microspheroids containing hydroxyapatite crystals, active collagenase, and neutral protease with rotator cuff defects.III. Morphologic and biochemical studies of an excised synovium showing chondromatosis. *Arthritis Rheum* **24**:484–91.

27. Wortmann, R., Veum, J., and Rachow, J. (1991). Synovial fluid 5'-nucleotidase activity. *Arthritis Rheum* **34**:1014–20.

28. Pons-Estel, B., Giminez, C., Sacnun, M., *et al.* (2000). Familial osteoarthritis and Milwaukee Shoulder associated with calcium pyrophosphate and apatite crystal deposition. *J Rheumatol* **27**:471–80.

29. Bjelle, A. (1981). Cartilage matrix in hereditary pyrophosphate arthropathy. *J Rheumatol* **8**:959–64.

30. McCarty, D., Hogan, J., Gatter, R., and Grossman, M. (1966). Studies on pathological calcifications in human cartilage I. Prevalence and types of crystal deposits in the menisci of two hundred fifteen cadavers. *J Bone Jt Surg* **48**(A):309–25.

31. Maldonado, I., Reginato, A., and Reginato, A. (2001). Familial calcium crystal diseases:what have we learned? *Curr Opin Rheum* **13**:225–33.

32. Dieppe, P., Alexander, G.H.J., *et al.* (1982). Pyrophosphate arthropathy:a clinical and radiologic study of 105 cases. *Ann Rheum Dis* **41**:371–6.

33. Schumacher, H., Rubinow, A., Rothfuss, S., *et al.* (1994). Apatite crystal clumps in synovial fluid are an early finding in canine osteoarthritis. *Arthritis Rheum* **37**(Suppl.):S346.

34. Fam, A., Morava-Protzner, I., Purcell, C., Young, B., Bunting, P., and Lewis, A. (1995). Acceleration of experimental lapine osteoarthritis by calcium pyrophosphate microcrystalline synovitis. *Arthritis Rheum* **38**:201–10.

35. Doherty, M., Dieppe, P. and Watt, I. (1993). Pyrophosphate arthropathy: A prospective study. *Br J Rheumatol* **32**:189–96.

36. Hashimoto, S., Ochs, R., Rosen, F., *et al.* (1998). Chondrocyte-derived apoptotic bodies and calcification of articular cartilage. *PNAS-USA* **95**:3094–9.

37. Kouri, J., Aguilera, J., Reyes, J., Iozoya, K. and Gonzalez, S. (2000). Apoptotic chondrocytes from osteoarthritic human articular cartilage and abnormal calcification of subchondral bone. *J Rheumatol* **27**:1005–19.

38. Doherty, M., Belcher, C., Regan, M., Jones, A., and Ledingham, J. (1996). Association between synovial fluid levels of inorganic pyrophosphate and short term radiographic outcome of knee osteoarthritis. *Ann Rheum Dis* **55**:432–6.

39. Rosenthal, A. (2001). Pathogenesis of calcium pyrophosphate crystal deposition disease. *Curr Rheum Rep* **3**:17–23.

40. Fahlgren, A., Andersson, B., and Messner, K. (2001). TGF-'1 as a prognostic factor in the process of early osteoarthrosis in the rabbit knee. *Osteoarthritis Cart* **9**:195–202.

41. Schumacher, H.J. (1995). Synovial inflammation, crystals and osteoarthritis. *J Rheumatol* **22**(Suppl. 43):101–3.

42. *Landis, R. and Haskard, D. (2001). Pathogenesis of crystal-induced inflammation. *Curr Rheum Rep* **3**:36–41.
   This article is an excellent discussion of the relationship between inflammation and calcium crystals in OA.

43. MCarthy, G., Cheung, H., Abel, S., *et al.* (1998). Basic calcium phosphate crystal–induced collagenase production:Role of intracellular crystal dissolution. *Osteoarthritis Cart* **6**:205–13.

44. Cheung, H. (2001). Calcium crystal effects on the cells of the joint: implications for the pathogenesis of disease. *Curr Opin Rheumatol* **12**:223–7.

45. Ryan, L., Cheung, H., and LeGeros, R., *et al.* (1999). Cellular responses to whitlockite. *Calcif Tissue Int* **65**:374–7.

46. Hayes, A., Harris, B., Dieppe, P., and Clift, S. (1993). Wear of articular cartilage:The effect of crystals. *Proc Inst Mech Eng* **207**:41–58.

47. Rosenthal, A. and Ryan, L. (1993). Probenecid inhibits transforming growth factorβ1 induced pyrophosphate elaboration by chondrocytes. *J Rheumatol* **21**:896–900.

48. Trostle, D. and Schumacher, H. (1999). Probenecid therapy of refractory CPPD deposition disease. *Arthritis Rheum* **42** (Suppl.):S160.

49. Cheung, H., Sallis, J., and Sturve, J. (1996). Specific inhibition of basic calcium phosphate and calcium pyrophosphate crystal-induction of metalloproteinase synthesis by phosphocitrate. *Biochem Biophys Acta* **131**:105–11.

7.2.2 Bone

7.2.2.1 Subchondral bone in the pathogenesis of osteoarthritis. Mechanical aspects

David B. Burr

OA is a disease not only of cartilage, but also of all the tissues of the diarthrodial joint. As the term suggests, the mineralized tissues deep below the articular cartilage are an integral part of the disease process. It is worthwhile, therefore, to review the physical properties of the mineralized tissues and their involvement in the initiation and progression of OA, as a basis for the evaluation of treatments that are directed at the bony changes as well as at the destruction of the articular cartilage.

The subchondral plate
Morphology

The subchondral plate is comprised of the subarticular mineralized tissues. It extends from the tidemark (the junction of the calcified and uncalcified cartilage) to the beginning of the marrow space (Fig. 7.39). It includes the calcified cartilage and the lamellar subchondral cortical bone, which underlie and support the articular cartilage (Fig. 7.39). The term 'subchondral bone' is also often used to refer to the primary spongiosa beneath the subchondral plate, but the changes that occur in the subchondral plate are quite different from those that occur in the cancellous trabecular bone below. The subchondral plate and trabecular bone beneath it are distinct morphologically, physiologically, and mechanically. The volume of cancellous bone is not necessarily increased in OA (indeed, it may be diminished), even though the subchondral plate may be thicker than normal.[1]

Although collagen fibres are continuous between the layers of articular hyaline cartilage and calcified cartilage, continuity has not been demonstrated at the osteochondral junction. Therefore, the osteochondral junction may represent a region of weakness, particularly to shear stresses. The subchondral plate supports the articular cartilage, directs loads to the diaphyseal cortex and may be a source of nutrients to the deeper layers of the hyaline cartilage, especially during growth.

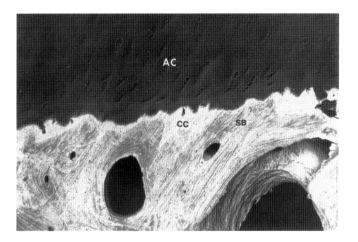

Fig. 7.39 Backscattered electron microscopic image from the infero–medial portion of a human femoral head. The calcified cartilage CC is clearly demarcated from the articular cartilage AC and adjacent subchondral bone SB. Original magnification 100×.

The thickness of the subchondral bone varies with species,[2] age,[3] gender,[4] location,[5] and function,[6] but is not related to body size.[4] The thickness of the bone undergoes changes in joint disease, but does not necessarily correlate with the density of the tissue.[7] On the convex side of a joint, the thickness of the subchondral bone is, generally, fairly constant, but on the concave side it is much greater in the central weight-bearing area than toward the margins (Fig. 7.40),[3,5] suggesting that plate thickness is influenced by weight bearing. This possibility is supported by the positive association between the thicknesses of subchondral bone, trabecular bone, and articular cartilage. Most estimates of the thickness of the subchondral bone of the tibial plateau are between 0.1–2.0 mm,[3,4,8] although thicknesses up to 3.0 mm have been reported in the weight bearing region of the tibial plateau in older individuals.[5]

Subchondral bone is highly vascular (Fig. 7.41), although many of the vessels do not reach the calcified cartilage and, except in disease, none penetrates to the articular cartilage.[5,9] The vascular pores average about 89 μm in diameter, ranging from more than 100 μm where extensions of the marrow cavity with lining cells penetrate, to 10–30 μm where vascular (Haversian) canals are surrounded by concentric lamellae. The distribution and numbers of these spaces may vary across the joint. Although the vascularity of the subchondral plate generally increases in OA, it does not change with age alone.[5] Vascular perfusion of the plate may, in fact, begin to decline by the third decade, and continues to diminish until about the age of 50–70,[10] when increases in perfusion associated with normal degenerative changes occur.

Whether these vascular spaces provide a pathway by which nutrients reach the cartilage is unclear, but the absence of vascular loops and failure to observe vessels penetrating the tidemark suggest that they do not function in a nutritional capacity. They may be more important to nutrition in younger individuals, in whom the diffusion of hydrogen ions into articular cartilage from subchondral bone can be detected, than in adults, in whom no diffusion is evident.[9] If hydrogen does not diffuse, it is unlikely that larger molecules, such as oxygen, amino acids, and glucose, would do so. The observation that avascular necrosis of subchondral bone is associated with articular cartilage deterioration in youth, but not in adults, supports the idea. More likely, the vessels supply the bone, providing a means to repair and replace the cortical bone and calcified cartilage of the subchondral plate through normal remodelling processes. This is important in the rapid densification of subchondral bone after joint overload and the bony sclerosis in joints affected by OA.

Unmyelinated nerve fibres are present in subchondral bone,[11] but nerves have not been identified in the calcified cartilage. Subchondral cysts in equine femoral heads and fetlocks fail to elicit much of a pain response, suggesting that most of the nerves in subchondral bone may be vasomotor rather than nociceptive. Recently, free nerve endings and nerve fibres which were shown immunohistochemically to contain substance P (SP, a neuropeptide that acts as both a vasodilator and a neurotransmitter in sensory nerves) were identified in the Haversian canals of the normal subchondral plate,[12] although SP-reactive fibres were not detected in either hyaline articular cartilage or calcified cartilage. Another neurotransmitter and vasodilator, calcitonin gene-related peptide (CGRP), is also frequently associated with blood vessels in the bone near the epiphysis.[13] A neurotransmitter, 5-Hydroxytryptamine, that acts as a vasoconstrictor, has also been identified in subchondral bone.[14]

Remodelling

Remodelling of the subchondral region during development results in calcification of the zone of hypertrophic cartilage in the growth plate, providing a transition between cartilage and the primary spongiosa. After maturity, remodelling of the plate probably functions to maintain joint congruity and reduce joint stresses in overloaded regions. Remodelling in the calcified bed is one of the earliest biological reactions to repetitive impulsive loading and to a single impact injury of the canine knee.

Measurements of normal remodelling in the human subchondral plate are rare, because of the difficulty of sampling non-diseased bone. Little is known, therefore, about normal turnover rates, except what can be inferred by extension from animal studies or from bone scintigraphy. In animals, bone turnover in the subchondral plate is very rapid prior to closure of the growth plate, and slows significantly with age; it is likely that bone remodelling in the human subchondral plate follows a similar pattern. Also, because bone responds to strain and high levels of strain tend to depress activation of new sites of bone turnover, it is likely that the rate of remodelling is less in the weight-bearing regions of a joint than in less loaded areas, although differences have not been detected in various regions of the tibial subchondral bone in animal studies.[2] However, a lower remodelling rate would increase the mean tissue age in the weight-bearing areas and would be reflected in a greater amount of mineralized bone underlying these areas. The situation may be reversed in end-stage OA, in which remodelling appears to be more active in weight-bearing areas of the femoral head.[15]

Rates of mineral apposition in the human femoral head range from 0.81–3.66 μm per day.[16] The lower value is comparable to the lower end of the normal range for cortical bone, but the upper value is 2–3 times greater than the highest rates found in cortical bone.[17] Higher rates occur on eburnated surfaces of OA femoral heads than in the subchondral bone underlying intact cartilage, and rates in osteopenic regions are slightly lower than those

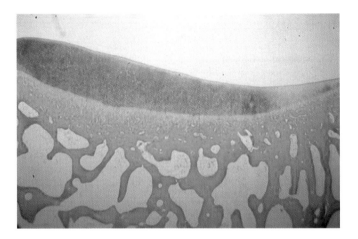

Fig. 7.40 Tibial condyle of a New Zealand White rabbit, showing thicker subchondral bone below the central weight–bearing portion of the joint, with thinning toward the joint periphery, where the overlying articular cartilage is also thinner. Stained with Safranin O. Original magnification 2.5×.

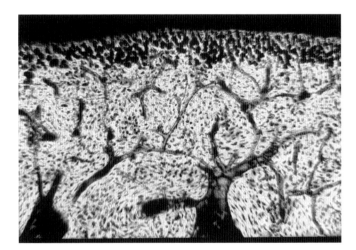

Fig. 7.41 Vascular tree in subchondral bone of the proximal tibia of a normal rabbit. Note the extensive anastomoses among the vessels. Stained with Villanueva's tetrachrome. Original magnification 125×.

in the sclerotic regions.[16] Consistent with this, fewer osteoclasts are present in the osteopenic regions than in the sclerotic regions of bone.

In a murine model of spontaneous OA, bone formation rates were as high as 3.57 μm per day in the early stages, and fell to 1.42–2.14 μm per day with advanced disease, compared to a rate of 0.71 μm per day in normal control.[18] The normal appositional rate in mice is similar to that in human iliac crest, and can probably be taken as a reasonable estimate of normal bone remodelling in humans. Interestingly, the increase in bone formation rate in OA was seen only in regions underlying cartilage degeneration; appositional rates in regions of bone underlying normal cartilage adjacent to focal OA cartilage lesions were normal.[18] Significant variations in remodelling parameters have been noted between medial and lateral tibial condyles, across each condyle, and at various distances from the joint surface.

High rates of bone turnover decrease the level of mineralization of the tissue, because the new bone is not fully mineralized. Therefore, the high turnover rate may reduce the stiffness of subchondral bone even though the bone itself increases in thickness. Grynpas et al.[15] reported both a thicker subchondral plate (compared to young and old normals) and abnormally low mineralization of subchondral bone in femoral heads from patients with OA. This reduces the material density (bone mass/bone volume) and elastic modulus of the tissue, even though its apparent density (bone mass/total volume of tissue) is increased. The material density can decrease in the presence of increased bone volume if mineralization per unit of tissue is decreased, for example, as a result of more rapid bone turnover.[19]

This demonstrates a fundamental mechanical concept that is important to understanding the role that subchondral bone plays in the process of joint degeneration: the structural properties of bone are different from its material properties. The joint responds to the overall structural stiffness of the mineralized tissues beneath the cartilage, which is determined by both the material properties and the geometry. Radiographic sclerosis of subchondral bone in OA reflects the apparent density of the structure, but is a poor indicator of the properties of the tissue. The acceleration of bone turnover in OA that results in hypomineralization of the subchondral bone reduces the elastic modulus of the tissue for a given apparent density, but when it is offset by an increase in bone volume or in plate thickness, the *overall* stiffness of the structure is increased. The subchondral plate is, in fact, thicker in subjects with OA than in controls.[15,19,20] Notably, the properties of the subchondral plate can be explained entirely on the basis of normal remodelling processes and do not support a contention that the bone itself is abnormal.

In contrast, others[20,21] have reported low rates of bone formation and resorption in human knee OA, or have been unable to detect an increase in alkaline phosphatase activity. These differences probably reflect the stage of the disease, with rapid formative processes occurring early in the disease and substantial slowing of bone turnover in late-stage OA, when sclerosis is apparent. This is consistent with the increased uptake of radioactive tracers early in the disease process[22] and the finding that uptake is greater when OA develops rapidly than when it develops more slowly. However, OA is a focal process, and the bone below degenerating cartilage may exhibit a combination of regions of high bone turnover (both formation and resorption), cystic degeneration, and osteophytosis.

Most studies of bone turnover in the human subchondral plate have been performed in samples obtained at surgery from patients with end-stage OA. This is a poor source of material for study of the pathophysiology of joint breakdown because changes detected in the subchondral bone may be secondary to the cartilage deterioration or to a reduction in weight bearing. However, normal tissue from younger arthritic subjects who have not developed full-thickness cartilage loss is difficult to obtain.

Mechanical properties

Subchondral bone is viscoelastic, that is, it deforms less, or becomes stiffer, when loading is rapid than when loading is more gradual. Deformation of the bone increases the contact area under load and minimizes stresses within the cartilage. When cartilage deformation under an impact load is limited, the contact area is minimized and high stresses can be generated in the cartilage matrix. For this reason, impact loading is detrimental to cartilage integrity.

Bone is a better shock absorber than articular cartilage, which is too thin to be effective in this capacity.[5,23,24] By attenuating force through joints, the bone underlying the articular surface can protect the cartilage from damage caused by excessive loads. Nonetheless, load transfer from the articular surface to the diaphyseal cortex creates large shear stresses in the subchondral bone,[24] particularly under the edges of the contact region. However, because of the undulations at the tidemark and osteochondral junction (Fig. 7.42), the bed of calcified cartilage transforms these shear stresses into compressive and tensile stresses,[25] which cartilage is better able to withstand. The calcified cartilage may help minimize shear stresses by providing an intermediate layer less stiff than the subchondral bone.[26]

The presence of the subchondral bone also raises the injury threshold for articular cartilage by constraining radial deformation of the cartilage under load;[25] if the cartilage is unconstrained, a 50 per cent increase in cartilage deformation will result in vertical fissures.[27] In the presence of attached subchondral bone, fissures are less likely to develop. Cartilage can withstand about 2.5–5 times the peak deformation caused by the load generated by walking, suggesting that the subchondral bone provides a large safety factor and has great capacity to protect cartilage from all but the most severe impact injuries.

Normal subchondral bone attenuates loads through the joint to a greater degree than either articular cartilage or periarticular soft tissues.[23] In normal joints, subchondral bone absorbs 30–50 per cent of the load through the joint, while cartilage attenuates only 1–3 per cent (Table 7.14).[23,28] When subchondral bone becomes sclerotic, however, it is less able to absorb and dissipate the energy of impact, increasing the force transmitted through the

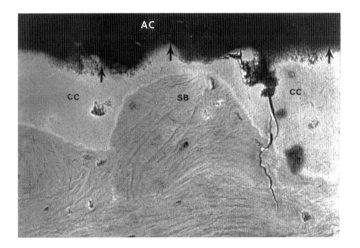

Fig. 7.42 Backscattered electron microscopic image from the infero–medial portion of a human femoral head, showing sharp undulations at the osteochondral junction and gentler undulations at the tidemark (arrows). Areas near the tidemark appear to be undergoing calcification. AC, articular cartilage; CC, calcified cartilage; SB, subchondral bone. Original magnification 400×.

Table 7.14 Force attenuation in joints

Tissue	Attenuation (%)
Subchondral bone	30
Cortical bone	30–35
Cartilage	1–3
Joint capsule/synovium	35
Synovial fluid	0

Source: Taken from Ref. 23.

joint. Because of this, the OA knee absorbs only about half as much load as the normal knee.[28]

Although subchondral bone is morphologically similar to lamellar bone, it is not as stiff as diaphyseal cortical bone.[29] Both strength and stiffness increase exponentially with apparent density and mineral content, so that a small increase in apparent density is associated with a much larger increase in stiffness. However, because the rapid turnover of bone in early OA reduces overall mineralization, subchondral bone in OA may actually be osteopenic. The younger mean tissue age,[15] and the observation that much of this new bone is woven bone,[21] may account for some observations of decreased hardness, elastic modulus, and strength of subchondral bone in OA.

The relationship of bone density to OA

Most studies show an association between increased bone density and OA. Bone mineral density is 5–15 per cent greater in patients with hip, knee, or vertebral OA than in non-arthritic controls.[30] In the Framingham Study,[31] mean bone density of the proximal femur was 5–9 per cent higher in women with grade I–II OA than in those without OA; men with OA showed similar, albeit not statistically significant, changes. Bone volume, measured histomorphometrically, may be as much as 30 per cent greater in subjects with OA.[32]

Although there are reports to the contrary, many clinical observations suggest that osteopenic women do not develop severe OA. OA and osteoporosis tend to be mutually exclusive.[33] Fewer than 1 per cent of the population have coexisting OA and osteoporosis. Severe OA is not usually seen in femoral heads removed after femoral neck fracture, and bone density in subjects with OA of the hip is greater than normal for their age group. In subjects with joint pain of OA, the risk of hip fracture is only one-third as great as in those without pain,[22] while the incidence of hip fracture in mothers of children with OA is only half as great as that in age- and sex-matched controls in the general population.[34]

The above studies included only subjects with established OA. Whether increased bone density antedated, or was secondary to, joint deterioration cannot be answered by clinical studies. Few studies have examined whether bone density is causally related to OA in a site-specific fashion. Milgram and Jasty[35] approached this question in an analysis of 21 patients with osteopetrosis. Although only three of their subjects were over 40 years old, all had OA of the hip and knee. Casden et al. also noted a high prevalence of hip OA in osteopetrotic adults.[36] These studies do not establish unequivocally that the increased density of the osteopetrotic bone caused the degeneration of the overlying cartilage, however, because the bony deformity that occurs in osteopetrosis may alter loading conditions and cause cartilage degeneration independent of bone density.

Many of the clinical studies that have concluded that an inverse relationship exists between OA and osteoporosis have failed to account for possible confounding factors, such as physical activity, obesity, and race. For example, obesity, a well-known risk factor for knee OA (see Chapter 2), is itself associated with an increase in bone density. Furthermore, the samples used in clinical studies that have demonstrated an inverse relationship between osteoporosis and OA were not random, but were subject to selection bias because only those with clinical manifestations of OA were identified as subjects. In some cases, appropriate controls for age and sex were omitted, sample sizes were extremely small, or the diagnosis of OA was based on self-report of joint pain without radiographic confirmation.

Importance of subchondral bone in the pathogenesis of OA: Initiation versus progression

Radin et al.[37] proposed that changes in subchondral bone initiate progressive joint degeneration. They suggested that impulsive loading of joints increases the density and stiffness of subchondral bone, which is then less able to attenuate and distribute forces through the joint,[38] thus increasing the stresses in the articular cartilage and promoting cartilage degeneration.

However, cartilage damage does not always lead to full-thickness cartilage loss. The initiation of cartilage damage, and its progression to full-thickness loss (that is, OA), may involve distinct pathophysiologic mechanisms. Radin and Rose[38] proposed that *initiation* of cartilage fibrillation is caused by steep stiffness gradients in the underlying subchondral bone. Focal variations in subchondral thickness have been identified in human hip joints by magnetic resonance imaging and in human patellae by micro-hardness testing. When inhomogeneity in density, or stiffness, of the subchondral bone is present, cartilage overlying the less dense bone will deform more than that over the bone with greater density. This differential deformation will 'stretch' the cartilage at the edge of the contact area in the joint, generating stresses that can tear the cartilage and initiate joint degeneration. The authors contended that *progression* to full-thickness loss occurs only in the presence of continued impulsive loading over an already stiffened subchondral plate.

The hypothesis that stiffened subchondral bone alone drives the destruction of the overlying articular cartilage has not been supported by finite element models. Mathematical modelling studies[39] show that even substantial increases in subchondral bone density will cause only modest increases in mechanical stress in the overlying cartilage. The amount of stiffening of subchondral bone required to significantly increase cartilage stresses is well beyond normal expectations. This suggests that although stiffened subchondral bone may play an important part in the OA process, it is insufficient, on a mechanical basis alone, to account for articular cartilage destruction. On the other hand, changes in the subchondral bone may have biologic effects on the overlying articular cartilage, for example, through the release of cytokines, which alter the metabolic activity of the chondrocytes (see Chapter 7.2.2.2).

Nevertheless, there is consensus that end-stage OA is characterized by remodelling of the calcified tissues of the joint and by subchondral sclerosis. Disagreements arise about whether these changes are primary, occur simultaneously with, or are secondary to, deterioration of the cartilage.

In several animal models of OA an increase in density of subchondral bone occurs early in the process that eventually leads to full-thickness cartilage loss. For example, after a 9-week period of impulsive loading in rabbits, which resulted in a 15 per cent increase in bone volume, progressive changes in the articular cartilage, leading to complete disorganization of the articular surface, followed within 6 months.[40] In a non-human primate model of OA, Carlson et al.[1] showed a high correlation between the thickness of the subchondral plate and the severity of OA. Cartilage lesions were absent in monkeys in which subchondral plate thickness was less than 400 μm but 14 per cent of female macaques and 38 per cent of male macaques with a plate thickness greater than 400 μm exhibited severe joint degeneration. However, other animal models that develop spontaneous OA do not demonstrate subchondral changes until late in the disease and, in some cases, do not show any clear relationship between OA and subchondral bone density.[41]

Such studies do not establish a cause-and-effect relationship between changes in subchondral bone and cartilage deterioration. However, in cynomolgus monkeys who develop OA spontaneously,[42] subchondral bone of the medial tibial plateau has been shown to undergo thickening well before the development of cartilage damage, and fibrillation is limited mainly to areas of cartilage that overlie the thickened subchondral bone. Similarly, when the tibia in rabbits was angulated by 30°, cartilage deterioration corresponded both spatially and temporally to the increase in density of the subchondral bone.[43] In regions in which the subchondral plate was not thickened, the cartilage remained normal. In mice with advanced OA, cartilage overlying sclerotic bone broke down, while cartilage over adjacent areas of normal bone density remained intact.[18] A progressive increase in subchondral plate thickness occurred over the 6 months following a subfracture impact to the rabbit patellofemoral joint, but changes in the cartilage were not evident for 12 months after the insult.[44] These studies suggest that subchondral sclerosis may be a necessary precondition for progression to full-thickness cartilage loss.

The contention that an increase in density of subchondral bone may be necessary for progression of OA is supported also by changes that occur in canine knee joints after transection of the anterior cruciate ligament. Bone volume in the subchondral plate is increased within 18 months after ligament transection in this model, but full-thickness loss of the articular cartilage does not develop for more than 4 years, although mild histologic changes of OA are evident in the cartilage months before the significant thickening of subchondral bone is apparent. Therefore, subchondral plate changes must not be required *for initiation* of OA in this model, although stiffening of subchondral bone may be necessary for *progression* to full-thickness loss of cartilage.

The role of the calcified cartilage and advancement of the tidemark in OA

Conventional wisdom holds that calcified cartilage provides a layer of intermediate stiffness between the articular cartilage and subchondral bone;[25] its elastic modulus is reported to be more than 10 times lower than that of subchondral bone.[26] However, backscattered electron microscopic images (Fig. 7.39) show that calcified cartilage is more mineralized and more dense than subchondral bone. This will increase its stiffness, and could have significant effects on stresses in the articular cartilage during loading of the joint. The normal undulating structure of the interfaces between the calcified and non-calcified cartilage (the tidemark), and between the calcified cartilage and underlying subchondral bone (the osteochondral junction) (Fig. 7.42), transforms shear stresses into tensile and compressive stresses, which are less destructive to cartilage.[25]

The advantage afforded by maintenance of the relative thickness of the layers of calcified cartilage and hyaline cartilage with respect to the integrity of the articular surface remains unknown. However, in normal joints the ratio of thickness of articular to calcified cartilage (approximately 10:1) is usually very highly maintained.[45]

Focal advance of the tidemark leads to thinning of the overlying hyaline articular cartilage (Fig. 7.43),[46] while concurrent changes in the subchondral bone can maintain,[47] or thicken,[48] the zone of calcified cartilage, compromising the normal proportionality between the hyaline articular cartilage and the calcified cartilage. Green et al.[47] found mild fibrillation of cartilage associated with as many as 8 reduplications of the tidemark,

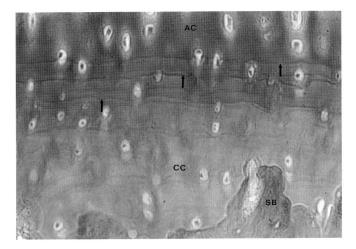

Fig. 7.43 Duplication of tidemark in proximal tibia of a New Zealand White rabbit. At least 6 tidemarks are clearly visible. AC, articular cartilage; CC, calcified cartilage; SB, subchondral bone. Stained with Safranin O. Original magnification 98×.

although reduplication also occurs in non-fibrillated and non-weight-bearing areas. A small degree of tidemark advancement can profoundly increase mechanical stress focally in the overlying articular cartilage, and could contribute to cartilage loss in OA. However, although most data show an association between tidemark advancement and cartilage fibrillation, both changes could represent independent effects of aging, rather than a cause-and-effect mechanism for progression of OA.

Repair of damage to subchondral bone

Patients in whom subchondral damage can be visualized by magnetic resonance imaging immediately after a high-impact knee injury often develop overt cartilage loss within six months, even if the cartilage is arthroscopically normal immediately after the injury. This supports the concept that damage to the subchondral tissues without overt damage to articular cartilage may lead to OA.

Microcracks in the subchondral bone and calcified cartilage can stimulate remodelling, accounting for increased vascularity and the presence of granulation tissue in degenerating joints. Microcracks, averaging 56 μm in length, have been found routinely in calcified cartilage from non-diseased femoral heads of middle-aged humans,[48] and are associated with foci of vascular remodelling in OA cartilage (Fig. 7.44). Single or repetitive high-impact loads cause microcracks in calcified cartilage,[49] which are followed by focal remodelling of the subchondral bone and deterioration of the overlying cartilage. This provides evidence that micro-damage in calcified cartilage, secondary to joint trauma, can play a role in the pathogenesis of OA. It is not known whether similar processes are implicated in the development of OA in the absence of overt trauma, nor has it been demonstrated satisfactorily that the articular cartilage itself is not damaged during the acute loading episode. It cannot be stated with certainty, therefore, that damage to calcified cartilage or subchondral bone *causes* deterioration of the overlying cartilage. Because repair of microcracks requires vascular invasion from the subchondral bone, it is probably necessary for the crack to penetrate to the osteochondral junction for repair to occur, unless some unknown form of cellular signalling exists.

Trabecular microfractures (Fig. 7.45) are distinct from microcracks in subchondral bone and calcified cartilage, but because their incidence increases with age they may be associated coincidentally with the age-related increase in the prevalence of OA. Partly for this reason, and partly because trabecular microfractures heal with fracture callous, resulting in an increase in bone volume, it has been proposed that healing microfractures increase the stiffness of the bone and contribute to the degeneration of the overlying cartilage. Finite element analyses, however, have shown that complete corticalization of the trabecular bone beneath the subchondral plate will increase stresses in the deep layers of the articular cartilage by only about 50 per cent, and that corticalization of bone at a distance greater than 1.5 mm from the tidemark probably has no effect.[39] Therefore, although densification of the subchondral plate and calcified cartilage may be associated with the initiation and/or progression of OA,[38] it is unlikely that healing trabecular microfractures in the cancellous bone below play an important role in either.

Vascular changes in subchondral bone in OA

In both clinical and experimental studies,[3] OA is associated with increased vascularity of the subchondral plate and calcified cartilage. Chondromalacia patellae is associated with a 10 per cent increase in the number of arterial capillaries.[14] This increased vascularity suggests that the subchondral plate is attempting to adapt or maintain joint geometry through normal remodelling as the OA joint becomes less congruent.[10] Foci of vascular invasion in calcified cartilage are osteon-like remodelling units, led by a tunnelling resorption front of multinucleated chondroclastic/osteoclastic cells (Fig. 7.46). Recent

(a)

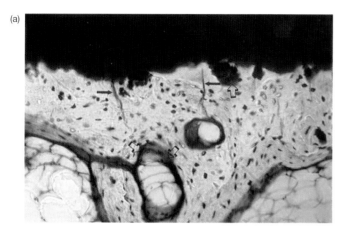

(b)

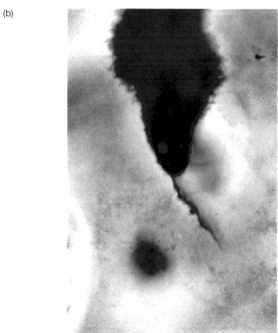

Fig. 7.44 Microcracks (solid arrows) present *in vivo* in calcified cartilage of the human femoral head. Both sections were stained *en bloc* with basic fuchsin. (a) The crack on the right is associated with a vascular bud (open arrow), presumably containing chondroclasts, while the crack on the left is associated with a resorption front (open arrow) coming from the subchondral bone. Original magnification 86×. (b) Higher magnification view showing chondroclasts leading the resorption front that is repairing a microcrack. Original magnification 312×.

Source: (a) Used with permission from Ref. 48. Copyright 1993, American Medical Association. (b) Used with permission from Burr, D.B. and Schaffler, M.B. 1995. The involvement of subchondral mineralized tissues in osteoarthrosis: quantitative microscopic evidence. *Microscopy Res Tech,* © 1997 John Wiley and Sons.

(a)

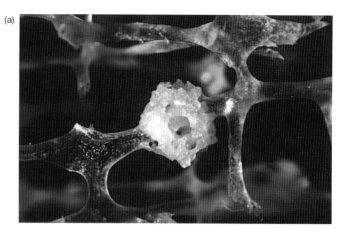

(b)

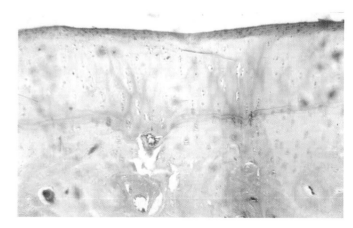

Fig. 7.45 (a) Callus formation around a trabecular microfracture. Such microfractures heal by usual fracture repair processes. Because the callus is larger than the original trabecula, it was assumed that it increased the stiffness of the trabecular architecture. However, as the callus is mineralized, it will be remodelled until the usual trabecular shape is reinstated. Original magnification 20×. (b) Polarized micrograph of a histological section, showing the presence of disorganized woven bone in the callus. Note the porosity of the callus which, in combination with the poor mechanical properties, makes it unlikely that the callus will be very stiff. Original magnification 30 ×.

Source: Courtesy of N. Fazzalari.

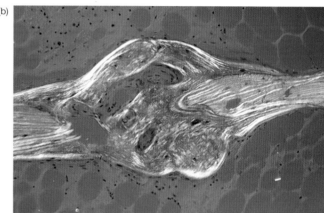

Fig. 7.46 Vascular invasion arrows of the calcified and articular cartilage in the proximal tibia of a sheep. Note that tidemark duplication is present. Stained with Safranin O. Original magnification 98×.

Source: Used with permission from Burr, D.B., Schaffler, M.B. 1995. The involvement of subchondral mineralized tissues in osteoarthrosis: quantitative microscopic evidence. *Microscopy Res Tech,* © 1997 John Wiley.

electron microscopic studies of vascular canals confirm the cutting cone-like structure of these vascular invasion foci.[5]

Vascular ingrowth in OA may be associated with angiogenesis factors, which are known to activate matrix-neutral metalloproteinases, such as prostromelysin, and to dissociate these proenzymes from complexes with metalloproteinase inhibitors. Production of angiogenesis factors by chondrocytes is associated with the resorption and calcification of cartilage in the growth plate,[50] leading to speculation that a similar relationship may occur in OA. Levels of angiogenesis factors in the synovial fluid[49] are increased in about two-thirds of all patients with OA. Failure of the chondrocytes to produce a sufficient concentration of protease inhibitors, which will also prevent vascular ingrowth, has been proposed as a pathogenetic factor in OA, but cause and effect have not yet been established.[50] The presence of high levels of angiogenesis factors in the hypertrophic zone of the growth plate has led to speculation that vascular ingrowth in OA may be a process of renewed endochondral ossification,[50] but the processes are quite different morphologically, insofar as chondrocytes do not appear to become hypertrophic or apoptotic in OA.

Although remodelling may be beneficial in OA by increasing the joint contact area and thereby reducing stress on the cartilage, it is commonly held that vascular invasion of calcified cartilage is a critical component in the progression of OA.[10] Deep fibrillation and fissuring of the cartilage matrix occur focally, with increased vascular invasion of the calcified bed. In the calcified cartilage vascular invasion, renewed mineralization around the regions of new vascular ingrowth, and focal reduplication of the tidemark are hallmarks of OA. The increased remodelling probably accounts for reports of hypomineralization of the subchondral bone in OA,[15] because it reduces the mean tissue age. These findings give rise to the hypothesis that the fate of articular cartilage is not determined solely by the stiffening of subchondral bone but, rather, by remodelling processes in both subchondral bone and calcified cartilage that cause alterations of the cartilage biologically and mechanically.

Effects of pharmacologic agents on subchondral bone in OA

Agents that reduce bone turnover could theoretically inhibit the development of progressive OA by preserving joint architecture. Treatment with bisphosphonates, which inhibit the activation of new remodelling sites in bone, results secondarily in an increase in density of the subchondral plate. If, as suggested above, dense subchondral bone is responsible for progressive OA, agents that reduce bone turnover should not prove very effective in this disease. Moreover, because bone remodelling is responsible for adapting the geometry of the joint to new conditions, anti-activation agents, such as bisphosphonates and non-steroidal anti-inflammatory drugs (NSAIDs), may, by reducing the rate of bone turnover, prevent the normal alteration in joint shape that accompanies OA and is considered to be a positive adaptation to the altered stresses associated with joint deterioration. If, however, the increased rate of remodelling is a predisposing factor for progression to OA, treatments that reduce rapid turnover may be beneficial. Administration of a bisphosphonate to dogs that were developing OA after anterior cruciate ligament transection slowed bone turnover, but did not affect the severity of articular cartilage damage.[52] However, intra-articular injection of etidronate reduced the severity of joint pathology in the canine cruciate-deficiency model of OA.[53] In the same model, carprofen was shown to decrease subchondral remodelling and to slow the progression of cartilage lesions.[54] Whether drugs that suppress subchondral bone remodelling will prove to be effective in reducing the sclerosis of bone or destruction of the overlying cartilage in humans with OA is still unclear. Such agents are more likely to be effective in inflammatory joint disease,[55] where bone loss is known to play an important role in etiopathogenesis, than in OA.

Ideally, pharmacologic agents for OA, which are designed to act on bone, should increase turnover without causing a large loss of bone through an imbalance between resorption and formation. Agents that prevent thickening of subchondral bone may be more beneficial than those that tend to preserve joint architecture. Finally, it should be kept in mind that the changes in joint architecture that occur in idiopathic OA are not primary, but secondary, and represent an attempt by the joint to adapt to changing loads. To prevent this attempt at adaptation is more likely to intensify the pathologic changes of OA than to alleviate them.

Summary

The zone of calcified cartilage and a subjacent 1–2 mm thick layer of cortical bone comprise the subchondral plate that underlies the hyaline articular cartilage. This bone is normally highly vascular; reduced vascularity of the subchondral plate with age may be associated with degeneration of the overlying cartilage. Unmyelinated nerve fibres and free nerve endings have been identified in subchondral bone. Bone remodelling rates are consistent with those in cortical bone at other sites. In OA, the rate of turnover of the subchondral bone increases, possibly in response to increased micro-damage. This results in a decrease in the average level of tissue mineralization, reducing the material density and tissue modulus, although increased thickness of the subchondral bone may offset these decreases and lead to an increase in the stiffness and apparent density of the tissue *as a whole*. The increased rate of bone turnover in OA has led to the suggestion that pharmacologic agents that depress bone turnover may be useful in the treatment of OA. However, these drugs increase bone mineral density which, typically, is already greater in patients with OA than in non-arthritic controls.

Whether the increase in bone density in OA is a cause of, or is only associated with cartilage degeneration, remains controversial, but several experimental studies have suggested that thickening of the subchondral plate may be a necessary precondition for the progression of initial cartilage damage to the loss of cartilage in OA. Thickening would exacerbate the tendencies of the subchondral bone to become stiffer and to deform less when loaded rapidly—changes which would decrease the contact area and generate higher stresses in the overlying articular cartilage. Trabecular microfractures are probably not important to this process because they have little effect on cartilage stresses when the joint is loaded.

Key points

1. Radiographic sclerosis reflects the apparent density of subchondral bone as a structure, but is a poor indicator of the properties of the tissue.

2. The apparent density and stiffness of subchondral bone increase in OA, but its tissue density and elastic modulus decrease.

3. Trabecular microfractures are unlikely to be part of the etiopathogenesis for OA, although subchondral microcracks may stimulate increased remodelling in the subchondral plate.

4. Agents that suppress bone turnover and increase subchondral density are more likely to slow the progression of structural damage in inflammatory joint disease than in OA.

References

(An asterisk denotes recommended reading.)

1. *Carlson, C.S., Loeser, R.F., Purser, C.B., Gardin, J.F., Jerome, C.P. (1996). Osteoarthritis in cynomolgus macaques. III. Effects of age, gender, and subchondral bone thickness on the severity of disease. *J Bone Min Res* **11**:1209–17.
   This paper shows that subchondral bone thickens prior to cartilage deterioration in the spontaneous development of age-related OA in non-human primates.

2. Armstrong, S.J., Read, R.A., and Price, R. (1995). Topographical variation within the articular cartilage and subchondral bone of the normal ovine knee joint: a histological approach. *Osteoarthritis Cart* **5**:25–33.

3. Milz, S. and Putz, R. (1994). Quantitative morphology of the subchondral plate of the tibial plateau. *J Anatomy* **185**:103–10.

4. Eckstein, F., Milz, S., Hermann, A., and Putz, R. (1998). Thickness of the subchondral mineralized tissue zone (SMZ) in normal male and female and pathological human patellae. *J Anatomy* **192**:81–90.

5. Clark, J.M. and Huber, J.D. (1990). The structure of the human subchondral plate. *J Bone Joint Surg* **72**(B):866–73.

6. Milz, S., Eckstein, F., and Putz, R. (1995). The thickness of the subchondral plate and its correlation with the thickness of the uncalcified articular cartilage in the human patella. *Anat Embryol* **192**:437–4.

7. Eckstein, F., Müller-Gerbl, M., and Putz, R. (1992). Distribution of subchondral bone density and cartilage thickness in the human patella. *J Anat* **180**:425–33.

8. Roux, W. (1896). Über die Dicke er statischen Elementarteile und die Maschenweite der Substantia spongiosa der Knochen. *Zeitschrift für Orthopädische Chirurgie*. IV. Band, Separatdruck.

9. Ogata, K., Whiteside, L.A., and Lesker, P.A. (1978). Subchondral route for nutrition to articular cartilage in the rabbit. *J Bone Joint Surg* **60**(A):905–10.

10. Lane, L.B., Villacin, A., Bullough, P.G. (1977). The vascularity and remodelling of subchondral bone and calcified cartilage in adult human femoral and humeral heads. *J Bone Joint Surg* **59**(B):272–8.

11. Milgram, J.W. and Robinson, R.A. (1965). An electron microscopic demonstration of unmyelinated nerves in the Haversian canals of the adult dog. *Bull Johns Hopkins Hosp* **117**:163–73.

12. Nixon, A.J. and Cummings, J.F. (1994). Substance P immunohistochemical study of the sensory innervation of normal subchondral bone in the equine metacarpophalangeal joint. *Am J Vet Res* **55**:28–33.

13. Bjurholm, A., Kreicbergs, A., Brodin, E., and Schultzberg, M. (1988). Substance P- and CGRP-immunoreactive nerves in bone. *Peptides* **9**:165–71.

14. Badalamente, M.A. and Cherney, S.B. (1989). Periosteal and vascular innervation of the human patella in degenerative joint disease. *Sem Arthritis Rheum* **18**:61–6.

15. Grynpas, M.D., Alpert, B., Katz, I., Lieberman, I., and Pritzker, K.P.H. (1991). Subchondral bone in osteoarthritis. *Calcif Tissue Int* **49**:20–6.

16. Amir, G., Pirie, C.J., Rashad, S., Revell, P.A. (1992). Remodelling of subchondral bone in osteoarthritis: a histomorphometric study. *J Clin Pathol* **45**:990–2.

17. Frost, H.M. (1969). Tetracycline-based histological analysis of bone remodeling. *Calcif Tissue Res* **3**:211–37.

18. Benske, J., Schunke, M., and Tillmann, B. (1988). Subchondral bone formation in arthrosis. Polychrome labeling studies in mice. *Acta Orthop Scand* **59**:536–41.

19. *Li, B. and Aspden, R.M. (1997). Mechanical and material properties of the subchondral bone plate from the femoral head of patients with osteoarthritis or osteoporosis. *Ann Rheum Dis* **56**:247–54.

   This is one of the clearest demonstrations of a reduction in tissue density associated with an increase in the mechanical stiffness of the subchondral cortical plate in human OA.

20. Havdrup, T., Hulth, A., and Telhag, H. (1976). The subchondral bone in OA and rheumatoid arthritis of the knee. *Acta Orthop Scand* **47**:345–50.

21. Christensen, P., Kjaer, J., Melsen, F., Nielsen, H.E., Sneppen, O., and Vang, P.-S. (1982). The subchondral bone of the proximal tibial epiphysis in osteoarthritis of the knee. *Acta Orthop Scand* **53**:889–95.

22. Cumming, R.G. and Klineberg, R.J. (1993). Epidemiological study of the relation between arthritis of the hip and hip fractures. *Ann Rheum Dis* **52**:707–10.

23. Radin, E.L., Paul, I.L., and Lowy, M. (1970). A comparison of the dynamic force transmitting properties of subchondral bone and articular cartilage. *J Bone Joint Surg* **52**(A):444–56.

24. Hayes, W.C., Swenson, L.W., Jr. and Schurman, D.J. (1978). Axisymmetric finite element analysis of the lateral tibial plateau. *J Biomech* **11**:21–33.

25. *Redler, I., Mow, V.C., Zimny, M.L., and Mansell, J. (1975). The ultrastructure and biomechanical significance of the tidemark of articular cartilage. *Clin Orthop* **112**:357–62.

   This paper shows how irregularity of the tidemark can change damaging tensile and shear stresses into less deleterious compressive stresses.

26. *Mente, P. and Lewis, J.L. (1994). The elastic modulus of calcified cartilage is an order of magnitude less than that of subchondral bone. *J Orthop Res* **12**:637–47.

   This is the only published paper presenting evidence that the stiffness of the calcified cartilage is intermediate between that of the articular cartilage and bone, and that the calcified cartilage therefore provides a mechanically stable transition between the bone and cartilage.

27. Finlay, J.B. and Repo, R.U. (1978). Cartilage impact *in vitro*: effect of bone and cement. *J Biomech* **11**:379–88.

28. Hoshino, A. and Wallace, W.A. (1987). Impact-absorbing properties of the human knee. *J Bone Joint Surg* **69**(B):807–11.

29. Brown, T.D. and Vrahas, M.S. (1984). The apparent elastic modulus of the juxtarticular subchondral bone of the femoral head. *J Orthop Res* **2**:32–8.

30. Arden, N.K., Griffiths, G.O., Hart, D.J., Doyle, D.V., and Spector, T.D. (1996). The association between osteoarthritis and osteoporotic fracture: The Chingford study. *Br J Rheumatol* **35**:1299–1304.

31. Hannan, M.T., Anderson, J.J., Zhang, Y., Levy, D., and Felson, D.T. (1993). Bone mineral density and knee osteoarthritis in elderly men and women. The Framingham Study. *Arthritis Rheum* **36**:1671–80.

32. Fazzalari, N. and Parkinson, I.H. (1997). Fractal properties of subchondral cancellous bone in severe osteoarthritis of the hip. *J Bone Miner Res* **12**:632–40.

33. Verstraeten, A., van Ermen, H., Haghebaert, G., Nijs, J., Geusens, P., and Dequeker, J. (1991). Osteoarthrosis retards the development of osteoporosis. *Clin Orthop* **264**:169–77.

34. Astrom, J. and Beertema, J. (1992). Reduced risk of hip fracture in the mothers of patients with osteoarthritis of the hip. *J Bone Joint Surg* **74**(B):270–1.

35. Milgram, J.W. and Jasty, M. (1982). Osteopetrosis. A morphological study of twenty–one cases. *J Bone Joint Surg* **64**(A):912–29.

36. Casden, A.M., Jaffe, F.F., Kastenbaum, D.M., and Bonar, S.F. (1989). Osteoarthritis associated with osteopetrosis treated by total knee arthroplasty. *Clin Orthop* **247**:202–7.

37. Radin, E.L., Paul, I.L., and Rose, R.M. (1972). Mechanical factors in osteoarthritis. *Lancet* **1**:519–22.

38. *Radin, E.L. and Rose, R.M. (1986). Role of subchondral bone in the initiation and progression of cartilage damage. *Clin Orthop* **213**:34–40.

   This paper proposes a distinction between the initiation *of cartilage damage that, the author speculates, is caused by steep gradients in stiffness and density in the subchondral bone, and the* progression *of OA, which is characterized by abnormally dense and stiff subchondral bone.*

39. Brown, T.D., Radin, E.L., Martin, R.B., and Burr, D.B. (1984). Finite element studies of some juxtarticular stress changes due to localized subchondral stiffening. *J Biomech* **17**:11–24.

40. Radin, E.L., Martin, R.B., Burr, D.B., Caterson, B., Boyd, R.D., and Goodwin, C. (1984). Effects of mechanical loading on the tissues of the rabbit knee. *J Orthop Res* **2**:221–34.

41. *Bendele, A.M. (2001). Animal models of osteoarthritis. *J Musculoskeletal Neuronal Interactions* **1**:363–76.

   This is an excellent review of current animal models of OA, including experimental models, as well as genetic and spontaneous models.

42. Carlson, C.S., Loeser, R.F., Jayo, M.J., Weaver, D.S., Adams, M.R., and Jerome, C.P. (1994). Osteoarthritis in cynomolgus macaques: a primate model of naturally occurring disease. *J Orthop Res* **12**:331–9.

43. Wu, D.D., Burr, D.B., Boyd, R.D., and Radin, E.L. (1990). Bone and cartilage changes following experimental varus or valgus tibial angulation. *J Orthop Res* **8**:572–85.

44. Newberry, W.N., Zukosky, D.K., and Haut, R.C. (1997). Subfracture insult to a knee joint causes alterations in the bone and in the functional stiffness of overlying cartilage. *J Orthop Res* **15**:450–5.

45. Muller-Gerbl, M., Schulte, E., and Putz, R. (1987). The thickness of the calcified layer in different joints of a single individual. *Acta Morphol Neerlando-Scand* **25**:41–9.

46. Karvonen, R.L., Negendank, W.G., Teitge, R.A., Reed, A.H., Miller, P.R., Fernandez-Madrid, F. (1994). Factors affecting articular cartilage thickness in osteoarthritis and aging. *J Rheum* **21**:1310–8.

47. Green, W.T., Martin, G.N., Eanes, E.D., Sokoloff, L. (1970). Microradiographic study of the calcified layer of articular cartilage. *Arch Pathol* **90**:151–8.

48. Mori, S., Harruff, R., and Burr, D.B. (1993). Microcracks in articular calcified cartilage of human femoral heads. *Arch Pathol Lab Med* **117**:196–8.

49. Vener, M.J., Thompson, R.C., Lewis, J.L., and Oegema, T.R. (1992). Subchondral damage after acute transarticular loading: An *in vitro* model of joint injury. *J Orthop Res* **10**:759–65.

50. Brown, R.A. and Weiss, J.B. (1988). Neovascularisation and its role in the osteoarthritic process. *Ann Rheum Dis* **47**:881–5.

51. Brown, R.A., Tomlinson, I.W., Hill, C.R., Weiss, J.B., Phillips, P., and Kumar, S. (1983). Relationship of angiogenesis factor in synovial fluid to various joint diseases. *Ann Rheum Dis* **42**:301–7.

52. Myers, S.L., Brandt, K.D., Burr, D.B., O'Connor, B.L., Albrecht, M. (1999). Effects of a bisphosphonate on bone histomorphometry and dynamics in the canine cruciate deficiency model of osteoarthritis. *J Rheumatol* **26**:2645–53.

53. Altman, R. and Howell, D.S. (1998). Disease-modifying osteoarthritis drugs. In K.D. Brandt, M. Doherty, and S.L. Lohmander (eds), *Textbook of Osteoarthritis*. Oxford: Oxford University Press, pp. 417–28.

54. Pelletier, J.P., Lajeunesse, D., Jovanovic, D.V., Lascau-Coman, V., Jolicoeur, F.C., Hilal, G., Fernandes, J.C., and Martel-Pelletier, J. (2000). Carprofen simultaneously reduces progression of morphological changes in cartilage and subchondral bone in experimental dog osteoarthritis. *J Rheumatol* 27:2893–902.

55. Podworny, N.V., Kandel, R.A., Renlund, R.G., Grynpas, M.D. (1999). Partial chondroprotective effects of zolendronate in a rabbit model of inflammatory arthritis. *J Rheumatol* 26:1972–982.

7.2.2.2 Subchondral bone in the pathogenesis of osteoarthritis. Biological effects

C.I. Westacott

OA is characterized by increased subchondral bone activity and focal loss of articular cartilage. Whether these changes occur independently or are linked by biochemical interactions between the two structures is not clear. Here, the evidence for alterations in bone biology and its relevance to changes in the metabolism of cartilage and other tissues is reviewed.

Subchondral bone changes in OA

Relationship with cartilage damage

Almost 40 years ago, Johnson observed changes in bone remodelling and suggested that such changes might precipitate irregularities in the integrity of articular cartilage.[1] Some time later, Sokoloff 1993[2] showed that bony changes on human hip joints could not be dissociated from cartilage fibrillation, even in early disease. However, it was Simon *et al.* 1972[3] who promoted the notion that OA begins in the bone by the demonstration that stiffening of subchondral bone, attributed to healing of the microfractures created by impulsive loading of joints, preceded cartilage damage in guinea pigs (see Chapter 7.2.2.1). Similar healing microfractures, resulting in increased subchondral bone stiffness, were reported to be the primary cause of OA in humans.[4] Bone, stiffened by callus formation during repair processes, was hypothesized to be less pliable so that the impact of loading was borne principally by the cartilage, which then degenerated. Further evidence in support of this hypothesis was lacking in humans until relatively recently. Increased subchondral bone activity, as judged by the enhanced uptake of technetium labelled diphosphonate, was shown to predict cartilage loss.[5] More importantly, the results suggested that cartilage lesions did not progress in the absence of significant subchondral bone activity. This notion gained credence from the histological and histomorphometric analyses of tibial condyles that showed cartilage degeneration to be influenced by the remodelling of underlying subchondral bone.[6]

Several animal species exhibit spontaneous OA-like changes, consistent with those seen in human disease. For example, guinea pigs of the Dunkin Hartley strain[7] and cynomolgus macaques[8] develop age-related changes in bone that precede those in cartilage. In macaques, bony changes in joints are more pronounced in the medial tibial plateau, with cartilage damage occurring mainly in areas overlying thickened subchondral bone. Similar damage to cartilage over areas of sclerotic but not normal bone is apparent in STR/1N mice,[9] suggesting that bone stiffness might be a prerequisite for cartilage damage. However, measurements of urinary markers of collagen degradation in mice of the same strain indicate that cartilage destruction precedes subchondral bone changes.[10] In animal models of OA, changes in both bone and cartilage occur as a result of mechanical or surgical alteration of joint loading. For example, impulsive loading of rabbit knees, resulting in increased bone volume, is followed by progressive changes in articular cartilage during the following 6 months,[11] as depicted in Fig. 7.47. Similar changes, over a longer time period, have been observed in canine

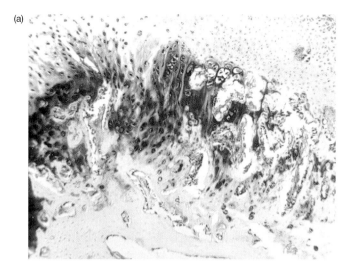

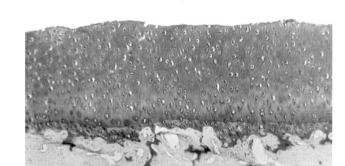

Fig. 7.47 Histological sections of rabbit knees: (a) 6 months after loading at 1.5 times body weight for one cycle per second, 40 min/day, 5 days per week for 9 weeks and (b) control animals allowed normal ambulation. (Magnification ×25, Toluidine blue stain.)

knees following anterior cruciate ligament transection. However, mild histologic changes in cartilage were evident before significant subchondral thickening was apparent,[12] suggesting that changes in bone in this model were not the initiating event. Furthermore, MRI scans of rabbit knees have revealed changes in cartilage thickness followed meniscectomy that were detectable before changes in subchondral bone remodelling.[13] Taken together these results demonstrate that subchondral bone remodelling is linked to cartilage destruction in both man and animals, although the temporospatial relationship between changes in the two structures remains elusive.

Are bone changes due to more generalized bone disease?

Rather than a direct response to mechanical injury, *per se*, Dequeker and colleagues 1997[14] have suggested that subchondral bone changes in OA, resulting in bone stiffness, are part of a more generalized alteration in bone metabolism. This notion gained credence from the observed differences in bone mass and bone metabolic parameters between patients with OA and those with osteoporosis (OP), suggesting that OA might have a protective or retarding effect on the development of OP. The increase in bone mass and change in bone quality were suggested to alter the mechanical properties of subchondral bone in OA, resulting in a reduced shock absorbing capacity leading to subchondral fracture and ultimately, cartilage degeneration. Examination of iliac crest bone composition revealed qualitative and quantitative differences in bone from patients with specific grades of OA as compared with bone from patients showing no osteoarthritic changes on hand X-rays or non-arthritic (NA) subjects. Hypermineralization was also apparent in the OA specimens, together with significantly increased osteocalcin (OC) content, suggesting altered bone cell metabolism. In addition, concentrations of insulin-like growth factor 1 (IGF-I), IGF-II, and TGFβ, growth factors with well-recognized anabolic activity on bone cells, were increased. High concentrations of such growth factors in OA bone lend support to the observation that, in general, patients with OA have a higher bone mass (see Chapter 7.2.2.3). However, whether quantitative and qualitative biochemical differences in bone only at the iliac crest, distant from joint damage, are representative of those in bone associated with OA lesions is not clear.

Evidence for altered bone metabolism in OA

Markers of bone cell activity in biological fluids

High body-mass index, together with increased bone density, suggests that new bone synthesis exceeds degradation in susceptible individuals. Such an alteration in net bone formation may occur either as a result of decreased osteoclastic activity or enhanced osteoblastic activity. Mature osteoblasts produce various non-collagenous macromolecules, a proportion of which become incorporated into bone matrix, with the remainder finding its way into the joint space and general circulation. Measurements of such bone cell products in biological fluids have been used to provide information regarding bone cell activity. Measurements of OC, a marker of bone formation, in synovial fluids from OA patients with severe scintigraphic scan abnormalities were, on average, 46 per cent higher than in patients with only mildly altered knee scans.[15] Similarly, serum concentrations of osteopontin (bone sialoprotein I (BSP)), a bone-specific matrix protein, were significantly higher in patients with bone scan abnormalities than in those without.[16] These results suggest that bone cell activity is increased in OA and, together with observations that BSP measurements increase quickly following trauma,[17] also imply that alterations in bone cell activity may occur early in disease processes.

Measurements of deoxypyridinoline, the lysine form of the collagen cross-links in bone, have been used to provide information regarding the breakdown of mature collagen, indicating bone turnover. Urinary excretion of such cross-links is higher in patients with OA,[18] and apparently increases with disease severity according to radiographic grading.[19] These studies suggest collagen degradation, and therefore bone remodelling, is enhanced and increases with disease progression in OA. Such observations support those of Mansell et al. 1997,[20] who showed increased synthesis of collagen type I, as indicated by the raised levels of immature keto-imine cross-linked collagen, together with a concomitant decrease in the mature pyridinoline cross-links of older collagen in cancellous bone from OA femoral heads. Moreover, increased local expression of alkaline phosphatase (AP), the enzyme involved in mineralization, indicated new bone synthesis whilst enhanced levels of metalloproteases, the collagen degrading enzymes, implied increased remodelling. In addition, collagen content was greatest in the subchondral bone where metabolic activity was highest.[21] Together these observations indicate that overall bone turnover is higher in OA subjects.

However, a cross-sectional evaluation of biochemical markers of tissue metabolism in patients with knee OA suggests the reverse to be true. Garnero et al. 2001,[22] showed serum OC, as well as serum and urinary C-telopeptide of type I collagen, was lower in patients than controls, implying a *decrease* in bone turnover. In addition, decreased bone formation, as assessed by bone AP measurements, has also been reported in postmenopausal women with spinal OA. Differences between observations may be explained by inherent variation within and between the patient populations studied. However, disease processes, *per se*, could also account for differences between observations. For example, remodelling processes may be

highly active in the early stages of the disease resulting in rapid bone formation and/or increased turnover, gradually slowing down or ceasing toward end stage. In normal individuals, bone loss occurs gradually with age, which may partially be explained by a reduction in the capacity of normal osteoblasts to proliferate in response to osteotropic growth factors and hormones. The results of dual-energy X-ray absorptiometry of tibial subchondral bone mineral density, however, suggest that in patients with OA, the rate at which bone loss occurs is attenuated and bone mineral density is maintained.[23] In OA bone, rather than a diminution with age, osteoblasts apparently retain their osteogenic potential.

Bone cell production of cytokines and proteases

Bone resorption and formation follow a precise sequence of events regulated by hormones and growth factors, any abnormality in expression of which may contribute to changes in bone remodelling. PCR-phenotyping of primary human osteoblasts derived from bone obtained from normal subjects and patients with OA or OP, has revealed an expression of mRNA for a wide variety of cytokines and these are summarized in Table 7.19. Despite the apparent inverse relationship between the two diseases,[14] the cytokine mRNA profiles obtained with osteoblasts from patients with OA and OP were remarkably similar, with one notable exception. mRNA for IGF-I was expressed in osteoblasts from OA, but not OP, patients. Osteoblast-like cells from OA bone produce significantly more IGF-I[24] than similar bone from NA subjects, which has been suggested to contribute to abnormal bone formation in OA. However, conflicting evidence exists regarding the involvement of IGF-I in OA. Serum measurements of IGF-I in patients with OA of the knee were lower[25] or no different to controls[26] and not linked to radiographic evidence of joint damage in knees.[25,26] Lloyd et al. 1996[27] after adjusting serum IGF-I concentrations for the effects of age, found significantly more serum IGF-I in patients with severe bilateral knee OA or distal interphalangeal disease. Moreover, a modest association was demonstrated between serum IGF-I concentrations and joint damage at these sites, but not at the spine or hip. Schouten et al. 1993[28] demonstrated a relationship between serum IGF-I measurements and osteophyte formation and growth in knee OA, which suggests that IGF-I could be associated with bony changes, but not to cartilage damage as measured by joint-space narrowing.

Further comparison of cytokine profiles in Table 7.15 reveals TNFα mRNA was detectable in OA and OP but not NA osteoblasts, implying altered remodelling in disease processes. However, Chenoufli et al. 2001[29] found neither the mRNA encoding IL-1β and TNFα, nor the protein, were detectable in osteoblasts from OA and rheumatoid arthritis (RA) patients, although osteoblasts from both patient groups produced significantly more IL-6 protein than those from NA subjects. These results were taken to imply that osteoblasts from OA bone contribute to the enhanced recruitment of osteoclast progenitors, and thereby bone remodelling, in the absence of conventional bone resorbing agents. Cytokines of the IL-6 family, which includes IL-11, oncostatin M (OSM), and leukaemia inhibitory factor (LIF), all have complex effects on bone metabolism, stimulating mesenchymal progenitor differentiation towards the osteoblastic lineage, as well as on processes that regulate osteoblast differentiation and proliferation. Lisignoli et al. 2000[30] showed OSM was only detectable at the mRNA level in osteoblasts and bone marrow stromal cells (BMSC) and was not inducible by catabolic cytokines. By contrast, both mRNA and protein for LIF, IL-11, and IL-6 were present in BMSC as well as osteoblasts from OA, RA, and post-trauma patients. Although osteoblasts from NA subjects were not examined, these results suggest the latter cytokines may play a part in the bone remodelling initiated by trauma and disease processes. In addition, IL-1β and TNFα stimulation enhanced IL-11, LIF, and IL-6 protein production in osteoblasts and BMSC from all groups,[30] implying that synergistic interaction may take place between cytokines produced within damaged joints. In addition, they suggest that over expression of LIF could lead to the accumulation of excess osteoblasts in the marrow, eventually contributing to new bone formation, whilst spontaneous production of IL-11 may also be of significance in disease processes due to the regulatory action of the cytokine on collagen metabolism.

Table 7.15 Cytokine expression profile in primary human osteoblasts

Cytokine	Activity	OA	NA	OP
IL-1β	Stimulates bone resorption	+	+	+
IL-3	Stimulates cell growth, decreases alkaline phosphatase activity	+	+	+
IL-6	Recruits osteoclasts	+#	+	+
IL-8	Chemotactic agent for neutrophils	+	+	+
IL-11	Enhances osteoclast formation	+#	?	+
TNFα	Stimulates osteoclastogenesis	+	−	+
TNFβ	Similar actions to TNFα	+	+	+
LIF	Osteoclast stimulating factor	+#	?	+
OSM	Activates osteoblasts and inhibits bone resorption	+	?	+
IGF-I	Stimulates osteoblast replication, differentiation, and matrix synthesis	+#	+#	−
TGFβ1	Differentiation of mesenchymal cells, induces osteoblast proliferation	+#	+	+
TGFβ2	Similar to TGFβ1	+	+	+
TGFβ3	Similar to TGFβ1	+	+	+
FGFβ	Potent mitogen for chondrocytes	+	?	+

OA, osteoarthritis; NA, non-arthritic; OP, osteoporotic.

+ denotes mRNA detection, # denotes protein production.

To further understand the role of cytokines and proteases in subchondral bone remodelling, Kaneko *et al.* 2001[31] compared immunohistochemical co-localization of cytokines and their respective protease products in the subchondral region of patients with RA and OA. In RA, abundant expression of cathepsins and MMPs, together with the mRNA for IL-1β and TNFα, the cytokines that induce their production, were evident in mononuclear cells and osteoclasts in subchondral bone and at the cartilage pannus junction. By contrast, no notable staining for either cathepsins or MMP-9 were apparent in OA tissue, consistent with the fact that bone erosion is not usually a feature of the disease. Little is known about osteoclast activity in OA. In mice, nitric oxide produced by osteogenic cells, such as osteoblasts and hypertrophic chondrocytes, is associated with the suppression of osteoclastic activity.[32] However, whether altered bone resorptive capacity due to changed osteoclast activity contributes to subchondral sclerosis in OA requires further attention. Normal age- and site-matched bone is not readily available, making realistic comparison of bone biology in undamaged joints with that in OA joints almost impossible. In addition, events *in vivo* are difficult to reproduce *in vitro*. Should enhanced production of cytokines, or other molecules associated with bone remodelling, contribute to altered bone cell metabolism in OA, what is the likely stimulus for their production? During osteogenic distraction, where mechanical tension–strain is applied to healing bone, human osteoblasts showed increased expression of the bone growth factors IGF-I and TGFβ.[33] Moreover, tensile stretch experiments in rats resulted in expression of mRNA for the key bone matrix proteins, OC, osteopontin, and osteonectin,[34] whilst cyclic loading stimulated production of OC, marker of osteoblast activity.[35] In addition, signalling of glutamate, normally associated with neuronal activity, is also increased in mechanically challenged bone,[36] raising the intriguing possibility that glutamate may act as an osteotropic cytokine. These results underline observations that loading accelerates the healing of bone, although how load leads to enhanced bone formation is not clear. One explanation may be that deformation of cells during loading allows architectural transcription factors to bring into alignment promoter elements that signal the production of molecules necessary for bone formation,[37] as depicted in Fig. 7.48.

Bone cell responses and altered osteoblast phenotype

Normal human osteoblasts, *in vitro*, secrete tissue inhibitor of metalloproteinases (TIMP) and gelatinase (MMP-9), but not usually interstitial collagenase (MMP-1).[38] Osteoblast-like cells from OA bone produce significantly more MMP-1 and less TIMP than similar cells from NA bone, giving rise to the notion that TIMP production in OA bone may be insufficient to negate the effects of MMP-1 (Westacott *et al.*, unpublished). In addition, raised levels of both pro and active MMP-2 have been demonstrated in OA bone, in association with abnormal collagen metabolism.[39] However, metalloproteinase production in normal human osteoblasts is under strict repression. Furthermore, the production of such enzymes diminishes with differentiation.[40] These observations therefore suggest either that osteoblasts in OA bone are not differentiated to mature osteoblasts or that bone cell phenotype in OA is altered. In order to elucidate mechanisms that could contribute to aberrant bone remodelling in OA, Hilal *et al.* 1998[24] examined the system of plasminogen activators (uPA) and their inhibitors (PIA). These molecules control the activity of plasmin, which activates latent forms of growth factors, and the proteases that initiate bone resorption. Although the uPA/PIA system functioned normally in primary osteoblasts from OA bone, the production of IGF-I was enhanced. Moreover, normal osteoblasts were relatively insensitive to IGF-I, whilst IGF-I reduced plasmin activity in OA osteoblasts. These results suggest that the enhanced production of IGF-I by OA bone cells could promote bone formation, whilst simultaneously preventing bone resorption. Later work by the same group[41] also showed a higher production of IGF-I and PGE$_2$ by OA osteoblast-like cells to be associated with resistance to parathyroid hormone-dependent catabolism. Thus, it is tempting to speculate that osteoblast-like cells from OA bone express a changed phenotype that responds differently to growth factors, allowing bone formation to proceed at the expense of resorption, resulting in an imbalance in bone turnover and ultimately bone sclerosis. Osteoblast phenotypic changes are suggested to contribute to disease processes in osteopetrosis, a condition characterized by enhanced bone formation[42] and associated with OA-like changes in the joint.[24] See Table 7.16 for a summary.

Table 7.16 Evidence for altered bone metabolism in OA

- markers of bone cell activity are increased
- production of cytokines and proteases involved in tissue remodelling are upregulated
- bone cell response to stimulus is altered

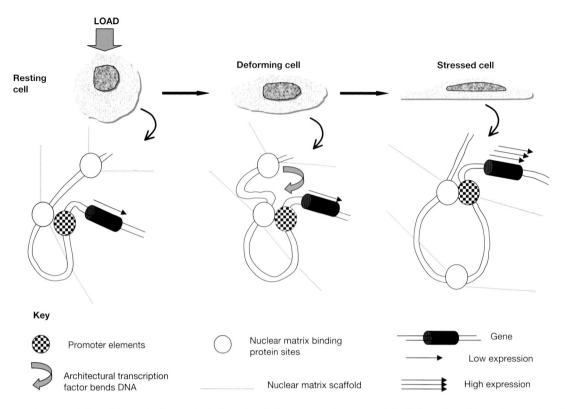

Fig. 7.48 Diagrammatic representation of the mechanism by which change in cell shape may regulate gene activity. Deformation of the nuclear matrix scaffold allows nuclear matrix proteins, which act as architectural transcription factors, to bend DNA at the promoter region. The resulting change in promoter geometry alters protein interactions and gene expression.

Are changes in bone cell biology related to altered cartilage metabolism?

Nutrition of cartilage

Subchondral bone and articular cartilage are suggested to be one functional unit, each dependent on the other.[43] This theory gives rise to the speculation that altered metabolism in bone may impinge on the activities of cartilage. If so, then direct communication between the two structures via a common blood supply would be expected. Whilst bone is well vascularized, the avascularity of articular cartilage has been acknowledged for over two hundred years. That adult articular cartilage received its nutrition from joint fluid was a commonly held belief until relatively recent times, when observations in animals[44] gave rise to suggestions that nutrients from the medullary cavity in bone may nourish cartilage. These findings were confirmed in human femoral heads by perfusion studies,[45] and later by steroscan electron microscopy, demonstrating the presence of channels running from cancellous bone through the subchondral bone plate into the basal layer of articular cartilage.[46] Since then, refinements in imaging techniques have allowed better visualization of the channels that connect bone with cartilage, as well as the blood vessels contained within them.[43]

However, the relative importance of subchondral nutrition when compared with the topical route via synovial fluid is not known. To address this question, Malinin and Ouellette 2000[47] performed a long-term study of subchondral bone-cartilage autografts in mature primates. Osteochondral plugs from femoral condyles were either replaced immediately into the original site, or into sites lined with non-toxic bone cement to prevent direct contact with the underlying bone. Abrogation of the contact between subchondral bone and autograft had little effect on cartilage during the first 5–12 months. However, by 3 years, cartilage on autografts in the cement-lined wells showed degenerative changes compatible with OA (Fig. 7.49(a)). By contrast, cartilage

on autografts placed in unlined wells was smooth and glistening and united with the surrounding articular cartilage as shown in Fig. 7.49(b). Differences were also seen in the organization of chondrocytes within autograft cartilage. Those in autografts placed in cement-lined wells were arranged in clusters in the manner of chondrocytes in OA cartilage, whereas those in autografts in unlined wells had a normal appearance (Fig. 7.50(a) and (b)). Of particular note were the presence of channels between deep layers of the cartilage and subchondral bone in autographs approximately 1 year after transplantation, as shown in Fig. 7.51. These were not found in normal cartilage, suggesting that channel formation may be an attempt to augment cartilage nutrient supply. These results therefore suggest that interruption of contact between articular cartilage and vascularized subchondral bone results in cartilage degeneration, the time course of which appears to be comparable to the slow degeneration of cartilage characteristic of OA. Thus, these results demonstrate the importance of the subchondral route for cartilage nutrition and suggest that alterations in the efficiency of the subchondral circulation may contribute to cartilage destruction in OA. In addition, attempts to improve subchondral circulation by development of hypervascularity at the free joint borders may be the stimulus for osteophyte production at the rim of cartilage in non-weightbearing areas.

Access of bone cell products to cartilage

Indirect communication between cartilage and bone is suggested by the existence of stress microfractures in bony trebeculae of the ageing skeleton. Fissures observed in histological preparations of undecalcified bone, originally considered to be artefacts, were later defined as two different types.[48] The most frequent were fine hairline microcracks in the calcified layer of cartilage that began just below the tidemark and proceeded toward the junction with bone. These occurred most often in the weightbearing

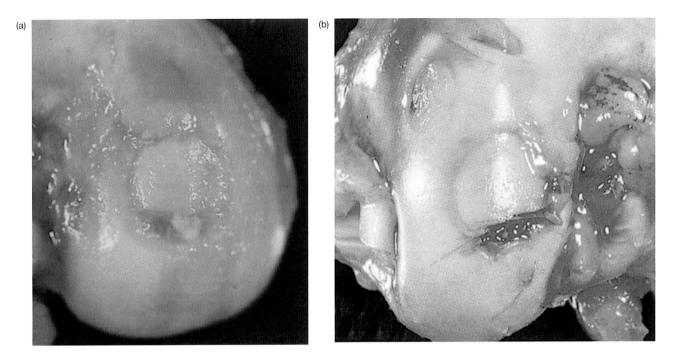

Fig. 7.49 (a) Fibrillation and pitting of the cartilage surface of an autograft, 3 years following transplantation into a cement-lined well. (b) Normal appearance of the cartilage on an autograft 3 years following implantation into an unlined well in vascularized cancellous bone.

Source: Reprinted from Osteoarthritis and Cartilage: **8**(6) Malinin and Ouellete, 2000, *Articular Cartilage Nutrition is Mediated by Subchondral Bone: A Long-Term Autograft Study in Baboons,* pp. 483–91, with the permission of the publishers WB Saunders.

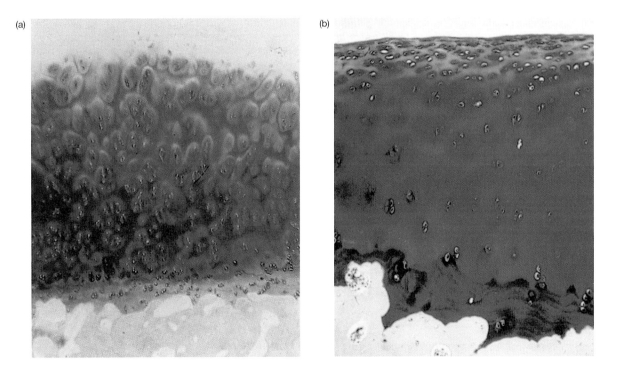

Fig. 7.50 (a) An autograft, 3 years post-transplantation into in a cement-lined well, showing chondrocytes uniformly arranged in clusters with surface fibrillation characterisitic of OA. (b) An autograft, 3 years post-transplantation into an unlined well in vascularized cancellous bone, showing normal organization of chondrocytes within the cartilage, with the deep layers of matrix showing metachromasia. (Magnification ×250, Romanowsky–Giemsa stain.)

Source: Reprinted from Osteoarthritis and Cartilage: **8**(6) Malinin and Ouellete, 2000, *Articular Cartilage Nutrition is Mediated by Subchondral Bone: A Long-Term Autograft Study in Baboons,* pp. 483–91, with the permission of the publishers WB Saunders.

regions and were attributed to mechanical fatigue. Associated with micro-cracks were 'microfractures', which were broader and protruded through gaps in the tidemark into the junction with the subchondral plate. Plugs of fibro-vascular tissue containing newly proliferated chondrocytes were often found in the microfractures that interrupted the calcified layer of cartilage. Thus, microdamage that transcends the tidemark initiates repair mechanisms, presumably via vascular invasion from the subchondral region, as suggested by the greater abundance of blood vessels in load-bearing areas

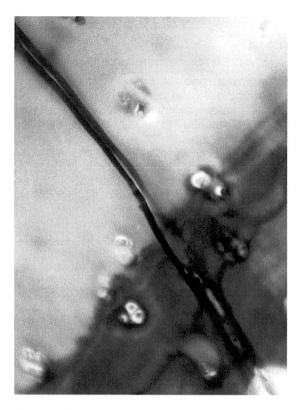

Fig. 7.51 Section of an autograft, 10 months after transplantation into a cement-lined well, showing a double-walled channel extending from the subchondral bone into the cartilage plate.

*Source: Reprinted from Osteoarthritis and Cartilage: **8**(6) Malinin and Ouellete, 2000, Articular Cartilage Nutrition is Mediated by Subchondral Bone: A Long-Term Autograft Study in Baboons, pp. 483–91, with the permission of the publishers WB Saunders).*

Table 7.17 Potential communication routes between bone and cartilage

- subchondral circulation
- hairline microcracks in subchondral bone
- microfractures across tidemark
- synovial fluid

of articular cartilage.[43] If similar damage occurs in the load bearing regions of the OA joint, molecules produced in the bone may gain access to cartilage and vice versa. See Table 7.17 for a summary.

Effects of bone cells on cartilage *in vitro*

Synovial fluid markers of bone and cartilage turnover are associated, and related to scintigraphic scan abnormalities in patients with OA.[15] These findings give rise to the supposition that in damaged joints the metabolism of bone and cartilage may be closely linked. As pathways exist between the two major structures of the joint *in vivo*, it is tempting to speculate that molecules produced by cells in one structure could alter the metabolism of cells in the adjacent structure. A co-culture system, devised to determine the effects of osteoblast-like cells on cartilage metabolism, showed for the first time that cells derived from the bone of some OA patients (38 per cent) increased GAG release from cartilage, whereas similar cells from NA bone did not.[49] Attempts to identify the soluble mediator of the effects of bone cells on cartilage revealed the presence of various cytokines in the medium

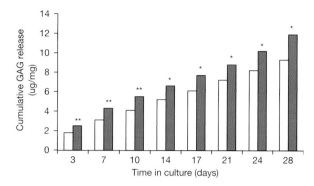

Fig. 7.52 Cumulative glycosaminoglycan (GAG) release from cartilage biopsies cultured for 28 days in medium alone or with bone cells derived from the weightbearing region of the medial femoral condyle of an OA knee. The tissue culture medium was replenished at various time points during culture and GAG released into the medium was measured by dye binding assay. White bars represent mean cumulative GAG release from 6 replicate biopsy halves cultured in medium, (control), black bars represent that from corresponding biopsy halves cultured with bone cells (test). The significance of the difference in GAG release from test biopsies as compared with that from control biopsies was assessed using Student's paired t-test (* $p < 0.05$, ** $p < 0.01$). Significant GAG release into the culture medium was observed as early as 3 days after the initiation of co-culture of cartilage with bone cells.

from cultured bone cells, although none of those measured were significantly associated with GAG loss from cartilage. These results suggest either that the effects of bone cells on cartilage were mediated by an unidentified cytokine(s), or by other molecules. Other findings suggested enzymic activity in co-culture supernatants,[50] and demonstration of aggrecanase-generated catabolites that increased with time in supernatants from cartilage incubated in the presence of bone cells,[51] lend support to this contention. These findings, therefore, imply that either bone cells produce aggrecanase(s) that directly degrades cartilage aggrecan, or that bone-cell derived cytokines act indirectly by inducing chondrocytes to produce aggrecanase. As cartilage destruction in OA proceeds from the articular surface downward,[52] it is unlikely that bone-cell derived aggrecanases contribute greatly to focal loss of cartilage. By contrast, cytokines act at specific receptors on chondrocytes and signals are transduced only in the presence of sufficient cytokine. Regional differences are apparent within and between joints in chondrocyte cytokine receptor expression,[53] whilst zonal differences in sensitivity to IL-1β suggest chondrocytes near the articulating surface are more responsive than those in deeper zones.[54] Thus, if bone cell-derived cytokines contribute to cartilage destruction *in vivo*, only cartilage in areas where chondrocytes are more sensitive to cytokines will be affected. Recent data shows that a higher proportion of bone cell cultures (79 per cent) could degrade cartilage when osteoblast-like cells were derived only from the weightbearing regions of OA joints (Westacott, unpublished), and the results of a typical experiment are shown in Fig. 7.52. Moreover, mechanical loading enhances cytokine production by osteoblasts,[55,56] whilst pressure can alter chondrocyte cytokine receptor expression.[57] Taken together these observations suggest that in overloaded joints, conditions exist whereby molecules produced by bone could exacerbate cartilage damage. Given the close association between excess loadbearing and joint damage in OA,[58] it thus becomes important to determine the mechanism by which altered bone cell metabolism may contribute to cartilage destruction.

Can cartilage products alter bone metabolism?

Potential for interaction between cells in cartilage and those in the underlying bone is provided by the subchondral circulation, which removes metabolic waste products from cartilage.[43] However, whether such products serve as signals that direct bone cell activity is not clear. Soluble products of cartilage metabolism are also deposited in the joint space, where synovial

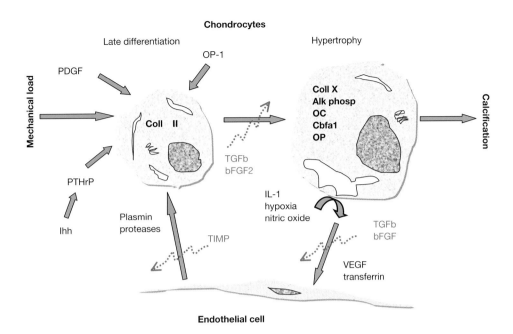

Fig. 7.53 Schematic representation of processes contributing to calcification by hypertrophic chondrocytes. Ihh, Indian hedgehog protein; PTHrP, parathyroid hormone related peptide; PDGF, platelet derived growth factor; OP-1, osteogenic protein-1; Coll II, collagen type II; TGFb, transforming growth factor-β; bFGF, basic fibroblast growth factor; Coll X, collagen type X; Alk Phosp, alkaline phosphatase; OC, osteocalcin; OP, osteopontin; IL-1, interleukin-1; VEGF, vascular endothelial growth factor; TIMP, tissue inhibitor of metalloproteinase. The negative regulators of interactions are denoted by broken lines.

fluid becomes a reservoir for a variety of anabolic and catabolic molecules produced by cells in the surrounding tissue.[59,60] Synovial fluid from OA patients can significantly stimulate proliferation of osteoblast-like cells derived from trabecular bone obtained at knee surgery.[61] These results suggest that *in vitro* at least, cartilage products may indirectly affect bone metabolism, although whether such a mechanism contributes to periarticular bone formation *in vivo* remains to be determined.

Perhaps, of more importance is evidence that suggests altered chondrocyte metabolism in OA could influence mineralization and therefore bone formation. In support of this contention, proteins normally produced by bone cells have been detected in cartilage from patients with OA. OC, alkaline phosphatase and collagen type X, thought to be involved in mineralization, were found in cartilage from patients with advanced OA,[62] whilst osteopontin expression was detected in deep zone chondrocytes and in clusters of proliferating chondrocytes in cartilage specimens with severe lesions.[63] Expression of such proteins is associated with the onset of chondrocyte hypertrophy that, in the foetal growth plate and fracture callus, is followed by mineralization. These observations imply similarities between protein expression patterns in hypertrophic chondrocytes from the epiphyseal growth plate and those from late stage OA. In the growth plate, complex signalling pathways involving several growth factors[64] and expression of Cbfa1, an osteoblast differentiation factor,[65] regulate chondrocyte differentiation to hypertrophy as depicted in Fig. 7.53. On attaining the hypertrophic state, chondrocyte secretion of VEGF and transferrin promote angiogenesis.[66] Remodelling of hypertrophic cartilage into bone results from secretion by invading endothelial cells of proteinases that upregulate expression of collagen type X, alkaline phosphatase, and factors that overrule barriers against chondrocyte differentiation. Negative regulation of the process is brought about by FGF- and TGF-mediated suppression of blood vessel invasion, whereas positive control is exerted by osteogenic protein-1 (OP-1), located in deep zone chondrocytes of OA cartilage,[67] where apoptotic chondrocytes are also thought to be involved in abnormal calcification.[68] An ordered sequence of proteolytic activity, followed by thyroid hormone signalling is thought to activate ossification. Thus, a balance between chondrocyte-derived signals repressing maturation and endothelial signals promoting differentiation of chondrocytes is essential

Table 7.18 Interactions between cells in cartilage and bone

- bone cell products alter cartilage metabolism
- chondrocyte products enhance osteoblast proliferation
- hypertrophic chondrocytes interact with endothelial cells to promote new bone formation

for normal endochondral ossification during growth and development. However, production of cytokines, growth factors, and enzymes is altered in OA.[60] In addition, osteopontin expression is upregulated by cytokines, whereas mechanical stress can stimulate expression of OC, osteopontin,[69] and other bone matrix proteins.[34] Taken together these observations suggest that an imbalance between positive and negative control mechanisms may initiate altered bone remodelling in OA.[70] Moreover, they strongly suggest that altered mechanical loading plays a major role in cartilage differentiation to hypertrophy, whilst the ensuing mineralization processes enable the calcified zone to advance at the expense of the overlying cartilage, thereby compromising the mechanical properties of the articular cartilage. See Table 7.18 for a summary.

Does bone interact with other structures?

Little information is available regarding the interaction between cells in bone and those in other components of the joint in OA. In rats, migration of bone marrow stromal cells is an early event in collagen-induced arthritis. Cells migrate from the bone marrow into the joint cavity, through the area between the articular margin and synovial insertion site.[71] Stromal cells, subsequently detected in the sublining layers of synovium in affected joints, were apparently able to promote hyperplasia. Whether migration of bone marrow cells similarly contributes to synovial hyperplasia in human joints is not known. In mouse joints, synovial cell production of TGFβ is associated with hyperplasia and marked osteophyte formation at the chondro-synovial junction.[72] Although TGFβ production is also associated with fibrosis of synovium in human joints, a similar relationship between synovial cell production of the growth factor and osteophyte formation has not been demonstrated. Cells in all major components of the joint produce TGFβ,[60] including osteophytes,[73] resulting in high concentrations of the growth factor in synovial fluids from patients with OA.[74] Thus, if TGFβ induces osteophyte formation in OA, growth factor production by cells in various structures of the joint probably contributes to their development.

Conclusion

It is now well acknowledged that the diarthrodial joint functions as a whole organ, with every tissue contributing to its mechanical stability. Changes in one component of the joint are thought to be followed by changes in an adjacent component, as the joint attempts to stabilize under the new conditions. This concept is substantiated by biochemical evidence of communication, via soluble molecules, between cells in tissues in different structures. The origins of disease activity thus become less important as all components of the joint are eventually likely to become affected to varying degrees. Better understanding of the biochemical interactions between the cells in different structures of the joint may provide valuable insight into the disease processes in OA. In addition, investigation of the mechanisms by which mechanical loading modulates cellular activity and production of key molecules, may provide important information regarding disease progression. Together, such information may lead to the identification of tissue specific molecules that indicate early disease activity and those that predict outcome.

Summary

Subchondral bone remodelling and cartilage destruction are associated in man and animals. However, whether changes in the two structures are biochemically linked is not readily apparent. Evidence suggests that bone cell metabolism is different in OA, possibly due to an altered osteoblast phenotype. Subchondral circulation, important for maintenance of cartilage integrity, provides a link between metabolic activities in cartilage and bone. Fissures that transcend the tidemark and the synovial fluid that bathes joint surfaces provide the potential for further exchange of biochemical information. *In vitro*, products of OA bone cells alter cartilage metabolism. Conversely, hypertrophic chondrocytes initiate new bone formation. In animals, bone cell migration contributes to synovial hyperplasia and osteophyte formation. Evidence suggests that interactions between the various components of the joint may be more common than previously supposed. These observations reinforce the notion that the joint should be considered as a whole organ.

Acknowledgements

Thanks are due to Professor C.J. Elson for critical review of the manuscript. The author was supported by EC contract QLK6-CT-1999-02072.

References

(An asterisk denotes recommended reading.)

1. Johnson, L.C. (1962). Joint remodelling as a basis for osteoarthritis. *J Am Vet Med Ass* **141**:1237–41.

2. Sokoloff, L. (1969). *The Biology of Degenerative Joint Disease.* Chicago: University of Chicago Press.

3. Simon, S.R., Radin, E.L., Paul, I.L., and Rose, R.M. (1972). The response of joints to impact loading II: in vivo behaviour of subchondral bone. *J Biomech* **5**:267–72.

4. Radin, E.L. (1972). The physiology and degeneration of joints. *Sem Arthritis Rheum* **2**:245–57.

5. Dieppe, P.A., Cushnaghan, J., Young, P., and Kirwan, J. (1993). Prediction of progression of joint space narrowing in osteoarthritis of the knee. *Ann Rheum Dis* **52**:557–63.

6. Matsui, H., Shimitzu, M., and Tsuji, H. (1997). Cartilage and subchondral bone interaction in osteoarthrosis of human knee joint: a histological and histomorphometric study. *Micro Res Tech* **37**:333–42.

7. Billingham, M.E.J., Meijers, M.H.M., Mahwinney, B., and Malcolm, A. (1996). Spontaneous osteoarthritis in guinea pigs: Cartilage degeneration is preceded by loss of subchondral trabecular bone (abstract). *J Rheumatol* (Suppl. 1):104.

8. Carlson, C.S., Loesser, R.F., Jago, M.J., Weaver, D.J., Adams, M.R., and Jerome, C.P. (1994). Osteoarthritis in cynomolgus macaques: a primate model of naturally occurring disease. *J Orthop Res* **12**:331–9.

9. Benske, J., Schunke, M., and Tillmann, B. (1988). Subchondral bone formation in arthrosis. Polychrome labelling studies in mice. *Acta Orthop Scand* **59**:536–41.

10. Verzijl, N., Wachsmuth, L., TeKoppele, J.M., and Raiss, R.X. (2001). Urinary collagen cross-link excretion in STR/1N mice indicates cartilage destruction as an early event in the development of spontaneous osteoarthritis. *Trans Orthop Res Soc* **26**:271.

11. Radin, E.L., Martin, R.B., Burr, D.B., Caterson, B., Boyd, R.D., and Goodwin, C. (1984). Effects of mechanical loading on the tissues of the rabbit knee. *J Orthop Res* **2**:221–34.

12. Dendrick, D.K., Goldstein, S.A., Brandt, K.D., O'Connor, B.L., Goulet, R.W., and Albrecht, M. (1993). A longitudinal study of subchondral plate and trabecular bone in cruciate-deficient dogs with osteoarthritis followed up for 54 months. *Arthritis Rheum* **36**:1460–7.

13. Calvo, E., Palacios, I., Delgado, E., *et al.* (2001). High resolution MRI detects cartilage swelling at the early stages of experimental osteoarthritis. *Osteoarthritis Cart* **9**:463–72.

14. Dequeker, J., Mokassa, L., Aerssens, J., and Boonen, S. (1997). Bone density and local growth factors in generalised osteoarthritis. *Microscopy Res Techniq* **37**:358–71.

15. Sharif, M., George, E., and Dieppe, P.A. (1995). Correlation between synovial fluid markers of cartilage and bone turnover and scintigraphic scan abnormalities in osteoarthritis of the knee. *Arthritis Rheum* **38**:78–81.

16. Petersson, I.F., Boegard, T., Dahlstrom, J., Svensson, B., Heinegard, D., and Saxne, T. (1998). Bone scan and serum markers of bone and cartilage in patients with knee pain and osteoarthritis. *Osteoarth Cart* **6**:33–9.

17. Lohmander, L.S., Saxne, T., and Heinegard, D. (1996). Increased concentrations of bone sialoprotein in joint fluid after knee injury. *Ann Rheum Dis* **55**:622–9.

18. Seibel, M.J., Duncan, A., and Robbins, S.P. (1989). Urinary hydroxy-pyridinium crosslinks provide indices of cartilage and bone involvement in arthritic diseases. *J Rheumatol* **16**:964–70.

19. Naitou, K., Kushida, K., Takahashi, M., Ohishi, T., and Inoue, T. (2000). Bone mineral density and bone turnover in patients with knee osteoarthritis compared with generalised osteoarthritis. *Calcif Tiss Int* **66**:325–9.

20. Mansell, J.P., Tarlton, J.F., and Bailey, A.J. (1997). Biochemical evidence for collagen changes in subchondral bone of the hip in osteoarthritis. *Br J Rheumatol* **36**:16–19.

21. *Bailey, A.J. and Mansell, J.P. (1997). Do subchondral bone changes exacerbate or precede articular cartilage destruction in osteoarthritis of the elderly? *Gerontology* **43**:295–304.

    Review of disease origins in OA. Based on studies in animal models, the authors suggest biochemical alterations in ligaments following trauma results in joint laxity and altered mechanical loading, and that such changes precede damage to bone and cartilage.

22. Garnero, P., Piperno, M., Gineyts, E., Christgau, S., Delmas, P.D., and Vignon, E. (2001). Cross sectional evaluation of biochemical markers of bone, cartilage, synovial tissue metabolism in patients with knee osteoarthritis: relations with disease activity and joint damage. *Ann Rheum Dis* **60**:609–26.

23. Clarke, S., Wakely, C., Duddy, J., *et al.* Dual-energy X-ray absorptiometry applied to the assessment of tibial subchondral bone mineral density in osteoarthritis of the knee. *Skeletal Radiol* (in press).

24. *Hilal, G., Martel-Pelletier, J., Pelletier, J.P., Ranger, P., Lajeunesse, D. (1998). Osteoblast like cells from human subchondral osteoarthritic bone demonstrate an altered phenotype *in vitro. *Arthritis Rheum* **41**:891–9.

    These data demonstrate changes in the activity and responsiveness of osteoblasts from OA bone, which, together with subsequent work by the same authors, suggests alterations in bone cell phenotype may contribute to disease processes in OA.

25. Hochberg, M.C., Lethbridge-Cejku, M., Scott, W.W., Reichie, R., Plato, C.C., and Tobin, J.D. (1994). Serum levels of insulin-like growth factor in subjects with osteoarthritis of the knee. Data from the Baltimore Longitudinal Study of Aging. *Arthritis Rheum* **37**:1177–80.

26. McAlinden, T.E., Teale, J.D., and Dieppe, P.A. (1993). Levels of insulin related growth factor 1 in osteoarthritis of the knee. *Ann Rheum Dis* **52**:229–31.

27. Lloyd, M.E., Hart, D.J., Nandra, D., McAlindon, T.E., Wheeler, M., Doyle, D.V., and Spector, T.D. (1996). Relation between insulin-like growth factor-I concentrations, osteoarthritis, bone density, and fracture in the general population: the Chingford study. *Ann Rheum Dis* **5**:870–4.

28. Schouten, J.S., Van den Ouweland, F.A., Valkenburg, H.A., and Lamberts, S.W. (1993). Insulin-like growth factor-1: a prognostic factor of knee osteoarthritis. *Br J Rheumatol* **32**:274–80.

29. Chenoufi, H.L., Diamant, M., Rieneck, K., Lund, B., Stein, G.S., and Lian, J.B. (2001). Increased mRNA expression and protein secretion of interleukin-6 in primary human osteoblasts differentiated in vitro from rheumatoid and osteoarthritic bone. *J Cell Biochem* **81**:66–78.

30. Lisignoli, G., Piacentini, A., Toneguzzi, S., Grassi, F., Cocchini, B., Ferruzzi, A., Gualtieri, G., and Fachini, A. (2000). Osteoblasts and stromal cells isolated from femora in rheumatoid arthritis and osteoarthritis patients express IL-11, Leukaemia inhibitory factor and oncostatin M. *Clin Exp Immunol* **119**:346–53.

31. Kaneko, M., Tomita, T., Nakase, T. *et al.* (2001). Expression of proteinases and inflammatory cytokines in subchondral bone regions in the destructive joint of rheumatoid arthritis. *Rheumatology* **40**:247–55.

32. Lowik, C.W., Nibbering, P.H., van de Ruit, M., and Papapoulos, S.E. (1994). Inducible production of nitric oxide in osteoblast-like cells and in fetal mouse bone explants is associated with suppression of osteoclastic bone resorption. *J Clin Invest* **93**:1465–72.

33. **Eingartner, C., Coerper, S., Fritz, J., Gaissmaier, C., Koveker, G., and Weise, K.** (1999). Growth factors in distraction osteogenesis. Immuno-histological pattern of TGFβ1 and IGF-I in human callus induced by distraction osteogenesis. *Int Orthop* **23**:253–9.

34. Sato, M., Yasui, N., Nakase, T., *et al.* (1998). Expression of bone matrix proteins mRNA during distraction osteogenesis. *J Bone Miner Res* **13**:1221–31.

35. Miyajima, K., Suzuki, S., Iwata, T., Tanida, K., and Iizuka, T. (1991). Mechanical stress as a stimulant to the production of osteocalcin in osteoblast-like cells. *Aichi Gakuin Dent Sci* **4**:1–5.

36. Mason, D.J., Suva, L.J., Genever, P.G., *et al.* (1997). Mechanically regulated expression of a neural glutamate transporter in bone: a role for excitatory amino acids as osteotropic agents? *Bone* **20**:199–205.

37. *Bidwell, J.P., Alvarez, M., Feister, H., Onyia, J., and Hock, J. (1998). Nuclear matrix proteins and osteoblast gene expression. *J Bone Min Res* **13**:155–6.

    Here the role of nuclear matrix proteins in the regulation of osteoblast gene expression is reviewed. The authors propose that DNA-binding proteins may act as architectural transcription factors that transduce changes in cell shape into changes in gene activity by altering promoter geometry. This hypothesis may explain how mechanical loading switches on osteoblast gene expression.

38. Rifas, L., Halstead, L.R., Peck, W.A., Avioli, L.V., and Welgus, H.G. (1989). Human osteoblasts in vitro secrete tissue inhibitor of metalloproteases and gelatinase but not interstitial collagenase as major cellular products. *J Clin Invest* **2**:686–94.

39. Mansell, J.P. and Bailey, A.J. (1998). Abnormal cancellous bone collagen metabolism in osteoarthritis. *J Clin Invest* **8**:1596–603.

40. Rifas, L., Fausto, A., Scott, M.J., Avioli, L.V., and Welcus, H.G. (1994). Expression of metalloproteinases and tissue inhibitors of metalloproteinases in human osteoblast-like cells: differentiation is associated with repression of metalloproteinase biosynthesis *Endocrinology* **134**:213–21.

41. Hilal, G., Massicote, F., Martel-Pelletier, J., Fernandes, J.C., Pelletier, J.P., and Lajeunesse, D. Endogenous prostaglandin E$_2$ and insulin-like growth factor-1 can modulate the levels of parathyroid hormone receptor in human osteoblasts. *J Bone Min Res* **16**:713–21.

42. Lajeunesse, D., Busque, L., Menard, P., Brunette, M., and Bonny, Y. (1996). Demonstration of an osteoblast defect in two cases of human malignant osteopretrosis. *J Clin Invest* **98**:1835–42.

43. *Imhof, H., Breitenseher, M., Kainberger, F., Rand, T., and Trattnig, S. (1999). Importance of subchondral bone to articular cartilage in health and disease. *Topic MagnetReson Imag* **10**:180–192.

    Using refined imaging techniques and schematic representations, the authors convincingly argue that the barrier to diffusion of nutrients between articular cartilage and subchondral bone does not exist.

44. McKibben, B. and Holdsworth, F.W. (1966). The nutrition of immature joint cartilage in the lamb. *J Bone Joint Surg* **48**(B):793–803.

45. Greenwald, A.S. and Hayes, D.W. (1969). A pathway for nutrients from the medullary cavity to the articular cartilage of the human femoral head. *J Bone Joint Surg* **51**(B):747–53.

46. Mital, M.A. and Millington, P.F. (1970). Osseous pathway of nutrition to articular cartilage of the human femoral head. *Lancet*, p. 842.

47. Malinin, T. and Ouellette, (2000). Articular cartilage nutrition is mediated by subchondral bone: a long-term autograft study in baboons. *Osteoarth Cart* **8**:483–91.

    This work shows that interruption of contact between articular cartilage and vascularized subchondral bone results in degeneration of cartilage. The onset and detection of the changes in cartilage required long time periods comparable with the time course of changes in human OA cartilage.

48. Sokoloff, L. (1993). Microcracks in the calcified layer of articular cartilage. *Arch Pathol Lab Med* **117**:191–5.

49. Westacott, C.I., Webb, G.R., Warnock, M.G., Sims, J.V., and Elson, C.J. (1997). Alteration of cartilage metabolism by cells from osteoarthritic bone. *Arthritis Rheum* **40**:1282–91.

50. Westacott, C.I., Webb, G.R., and Elson, C.J. (1998). Cells from osteoarthritic bone produce enzymes which degrade cartilage. *Trans Orthop Res Soc* **23**:919

51. Diffin, F.M., Little, C.B., Elson, C.J., and Westacott, C.I. (2001). Catabolism of aggrecan by cells derived from osteoarthritic bone. *Trans Orthop Res Soc* **26**:669.

52. Poole, A.R. (1993). Cartilage in health and disease. In: D.J. McCarty (ed.), *Textbook of Rheumatology* (chapter 15). Philadelphia: Lea and Febiger, pp. 279–333.

53. Webb, G.R., Westacott, C.I., and Elson, C.J. (1997). Chondrocyte tumor necrosis factor receptors and focal loss of cartilage in osteoarthritis. *Osteoarthritis Cart* **6**:427–37.

54. Hauselmann, H.J., Flechtenmacher, J., Michal, L., Thonar, EJ-MA., Shinmei, M., Kuettner, K.E., and Aydelotte, M.B. (1996). The superficial layer of human articular cartilage is more susceptible to interleukin-1 induced damage than the deeper layers. *Arthritis Rheum* **39**:478–88.

55. Ninomiya, J.T., Haapasalo, H.H., Staples, K., and Struve, J.A. (2001). Mechanical loading alters the expression and secretion of interleukin 6 in osteoblasts. *Trans Orthop Res Soc* **26**:233.

56. Fyhrie, D., Yeni, Y., Li, D.L., and Gibson, G. (2001). Mechanical stress driven release of TGFβ2 from mineralised cancellous bone. *Trans Orthop Res Soc* **26**:239.

57. Westacott, C.I., Urban, J.P.G., Goldring, M.B., and Elson, C.J. (2002). The effects of pressure on chondrocyte tumour necrosis factor receptor expression. *Biorheology* **39**:125–32.

58. Coggan, D., Croft, P., Kellingray, S., Barrett, D., McLaren, M., and Cooper, C. (2000). Occupational physical activities and osteoarthritis of the knee. *Arthritis Rheum* **43**:1443–49.

59. Westacott, C.I., Whicher, J.T., Barnes, I.C., Thompson, D., Swann, A.J., and Dieppe, P.A. (1990). Synovial fluid concentrations of five different cytokines in rheumatic diseases. *Ann Rheum Dis* **49**:676–81.

60. Westacott, C.I. and Sharif, M. (1996). Cytokines in osteoarthritis: mediators or markers of joint destruction? *Sem Arthritis Rheum* **25**:254–72.

61. Andersson, M.K., Anissian, L., Stark, A., Bucht, E., Fellander-Tsai, L., and Tsai, J.A. (2000). Synovial fluid from loose hip arthroplasties inhibits human osteoblasts. *Clin Orthop Rel Res* **378**:148–54.

62. Pullig, O., Weseloh, G., Ronneberger, D-L., Kakonen, S-M., and Swoboda, B. (2000). Chondrocyte differentiation in human osteoarthritis: expression of osteocalcin in normal and osteoarthritic cartilage and bone. *Calcif Tiss Int* **67**:230–40.

63. Pullig, O., Weseloh, G., Fauer, S., and Swoboda, B. (2000). Osteopontin is expressed by adult human osteoarthritic chondrocytes: protein and mRNA analysis of normal and osteoarthritic cartilage. *Matrix Biology* **19**:245–55.

64. Akiyama, H., Shigeno, C., Iyama, K., Ito, H., Hiraki, Y., Konishi, J., and Nakamura, T. (1999). Indian hedgehog in the late-phase differentiation in mouse chondrogenic EC cells, ATDC5: upregulation of type X collagen and osteprotegerin ligand mRNAs. *Biochem Biophys Res Commun* **257**:814–20.

65. Karsenty, G. (2001). Minireview: Transcriptional control of osteoblast differentiation. *Endocrinology* **142**:2731–3.

66. Carlevaro, M.F., Albini, A., Ribatti, *et al.* (1997). Transferrin promotes endothelial cell migration and invasion: implications in cartilage neovascularisation. *J Cell Biol* **136**:1375–84.

67. Chubinskaya, S., Merrihew, C., Cs-zabo, G., *et al.* (2000). Human articular chondrocytes express osteogenic protein-1. *J Histochem Cytochem* **48**:239–50.

68. Kouri, I.B., Aguilera, J.M., Reys, J., Lozoya, K.B., and Gonzalez, S. (1999). Apoptotic chondrocytes from osteoarthrotic human articular cartilage and abnormal calcification of subchondral bone. *J Rheumatol* **27**:1005–19.

69. Kubota, T., Yamauchi, M., Onozaki, J., Sato, S., Suzuki, Y., and Sodek, J. (1993). Influence of an intermittent compressive force on matrix protein expression by ROS 17/2.8 cells, with selective stimulation of osteopontin. *Arch Oral Biol* **38**:23–30.

70. Babarina, A.V., Mollers, U., Bitner, K., Vischer, P., and Bruckner, P. (2001). Role of the subchondral vascular system in endochondral ossification: endothelial cell-derived proteinases derepress late cartilage differentiation *in vitro*. *Matrix Biol* **20**:205–13.

71. Nakagawa, S., Toritsuka, Y., Wakitani, S., *et al.* (1996). Bone marrow stromal cells contribute to synovial cell proliferation in rates with collagen induced arthritis. *J Rheumatol* **23**:2098–103.

72. Bakker, A.C., van de Loo, F.A.J., van Beuningen, H.M., *et al.* (2001). Overexpression of active TGF-beta in the murine knee joint: evidence for synovial-layer dependent chondro-osteophyte formation. *Osteoarthritis Cart* **9**:128–36.

73. Uchino, M., Izumi, T., Tominaga, T., Wakita, R., Minehara, H., Sekiguchi, M., and Itoman, M. (2000). Growth factor expression in osteophytes of the human femoral head in osteoarthritis. *Clin Orthop Rel Res* **377**:119–25.

74. Schlaak, J.F., Pfers, I., Meyer Zum Buschenfelde, K.H., Marker H.E. (1996). Different cytokine profiles in the synovial fluid of patients with osteoarthritis, rheumatoid arthritis and seronegative spondylarthropathies. *Clin Exp Rheumatol* **14**:155–62.

7.2.2.3 Systemic changes in bone in osteoarthritis

David M. Reid

As highlighted in the other sections in Chapter 7, there remains controversy as to the initial pathogenesis of primary OA. Most authors believe the origins of OA to reside in initially subtle changes of articular cartilage. However, since the pioneering work of Radin and colleagues in the 1970s[1,2] there have been advocates of the 'bone' theory of pathogenesis. Recently Aspden and colleagues have reviewed the literature[3] and brought their own work to bear on this assertion (*infra vide*). They argue that a loss of density of subchondral bone is the initiating event that leads to secondary changes in articular cartilage,[4] concluding that the changes in cancellous bone may lead to an increase in bone stiffness.[5] The importance of proving or rejecting this hypothesis is the potential it brings to the treatment paradigm. If a disorder of bone were the initiating event in OA and it becomes possible to identify the disease at an early stage by serological, genetic, or imaging technology, then preventive therapy would become a distinct possibility.

A second stream of evidence links the changes in the joint with bone. The literature on the possible protective effect of OA on the prevalence of osteoporosis is extensive, with Dequeker being the main protagonist of the theory. He was among the first to suggest that patients with OA were at lesser risk of osteoporotic fractures than those with OA,[6] in part related to differences in anthropometric characteristics.[7] He hypothesized that this was due to subjects with OA being at the opposite end of the bone mass spectrum from patients with osteoporosis.[8]

These two discrete and apparently mutually exclusive hypotheses provide justification for examining the evidence for a relationship between OA and systemic effects on bone. This chapter will first describe the *in vivo* evidence that patients with established OA have changes in bone metabolism and bone mass, and will then attempt to link these data with the *in vitro* defects in subchondral bone.

In vivo bone effects

Studies have used both biochemical and biophysical assessment techniques to examine these relationships. Bone markers are indicators of systemic bone metabolism and can be assessed in both the serum and urine. They consist of enzymes or breakdown products of both formation and resorption, reflecting, respectively, the activity of osteoblasts and osteoclasts.[9] Biophysical techniques used in investigating bone in OA have primarily focused on the use of various bone mass techniques but have also included magnetic resonance imaging and isotope bone scanning.

Bone resorption markers

Excess collagen degradation products produced as part of the local biochemical changes taking place in cartilage and subchondral have been shown to appear in the urine. Initially these were detected by chromatography and were considered to be primarily hydroxyproline.[10] Subsequently the collagen cross-linking compounds pyridinoline and deoxypyridinoline were demonstrated to be elevated in subjects with OA but did not seem to be related to the grade or severity of OA.[11] Further work by MacDonald *et al.* confirmed significant elevations of both these markers in patients with OA of the knee but not in subjects with OA of the hip or nodal OA of the hands.[12] In a more recent study, pyridinoline was shown to be significantly elevated in women with hip OA awaiting joint replacement compared with normal and osteoporotic women.[13] In larger studies concentrating on patients with knee OA, urinary pyridinoline and deoxypyridinoline were found to reflect radiographic disease severity,[14] a finding especially strong in those with more widespread disease.[15] Not all investigators have confirmed increases in these cross-links in knee OA compared with normal subjects,[16] though even in the negative study by Graverand *et al.* there was a tendency for those with the most advanced disease to have higher levels.[16]

A continued concern has been whether these pyridinium cross-links are truly reflecting destruction of bone, rather than cartilage. Pyridinoline is derived from both type I collagen, the principle collagen of bone, and type II collagen in articular cartilage. In contrast deoxypyridinoline seems to be derived just from type I collagen and hence, is much more indicative of bone turnover. Initial observations suggested that while both markers were increased in OA, pyridinoline was more markedly elevated in patients with rheumatoid arthritis, reflecting more severe cartilage damage, whereas deoxypyridinoline was equally elevated in both disorders, reflecting bone turnover.[17] However, in studies examining the distribution of both markers in the tissue of patients, it has become clear that while the relative concentration of pyridinoline relative to deoxypyridinoline is greater in cartilage (50 : 1) than in bone (3 : 1), both markers are present in both tissues.[18] This raises the hypothesis that the confusion in the literature relates not to the relative contribution of the elevated markers arising from bone or cartilage, but whether bone resorption markers are increased at all in OA.

Initial pyridinium cross-link studies were undertaken using the time consuming method of high-pressure liquid chromatography. However more recent work has centred on using the newer resorption markers measured by monoclonal antibodies, including free pyridinoline cross-links.[19]

Table 7.19 Summary of bone resorption marker findings in osteoarthritis

Marker	Effect
Urinary hydoxyproline	Increase in OA[10]
Urinary pyridinoline and deoxypyrdinoline	Increase in knee OA, but not hand or hip[12]
	Increase in hip OA compared with controls[21]
	Increase in multifocal OA[14–16]
Serum and Urinary CTX–I	Decrease in knee OA compared with controls[20]

Table 7.20 Summary of bone formation marker findings in osteoarthritis

Marker	Effect
Serum and synovial fluid osteocalcin	Elevated in destructive disease[22]
Serum osteocalcin	No elevation in hip OA[13] and knee OA[15,20] compared with controls
Iliac crest osteocalcin	Elevated in women with hand OA[24]
Bone specific alkaline phosphatase	Normal[25] or decreased[26]

Relatively few studies have been reported as yet, but those that have do not support the initial promise of pyridinium cross-links as useful markers of disease extent in OA. Indeed, in a recent study by Garnero and colleagues bone resorption rates as assessed by serum and urinary C-telopeptide of type I collagen (CTX-I) were demonstrated to be *decreased* in patients with knee OA, while a panel of cartilage and types II and III collagen markers, reflecting cartilage metabolism, were increased and related to radiographic disease severity.[20] Table 7.19 presents a summary of the bone resorption marker findings in OA.

Bone formation markers

Relatively few workers have examined bone formation markers in patients with OA. Initial reports suggested that the marker, osteocalcin, which is the most abundant non-collagenous protein in bone might be elevated in those with the most destructive disease.[22] Although this suggested a secondary local cause for the elevation, synovial fluid osteocalcin levels seem to be much lower than serum levels.[23] Support was given to a systemic hypothesis by the finding that osteocalcin levels were elevated in iliac crest biopsies of elderly women with hand OA, compared to a similar aged group of women without OA, although the results were not elevated compared to those from young women.[24]

More recent and somewhat larger studies, however, have failed to show a consistent elevation in serum osteocalcin. In women with hip OA this marker was found to be present in similar amounts to patients with previous hip fracture and age-matched controls.[13] In a further group of 88 women with knee OA, osteocalcin was normal compared to matched controls whether or not they additionally had nodal hand OA,[15] and the lack of elevation was also noted in the most recent study by Garnero et al.[20]

The normal levels of serum osteocalcin in patients with knee OA is mirrored by the finding of normal levels of bone-specific alkaline phosphatase in those with spinal OA,[25] a finding disputed by Peel and colleagues who found levels to be decreased suggesting reduced bone turnover.[26] The controversy induced by these discordant results has not been helped by the observations of Sharif and colleagues who initially demonstrated a significant correlation between synovial fluid levels of osteocalcin and the cartilage marker, keratan sulphate, both of which showed a relationship with late phase isotope bone scan abnormalities.[27] A later study from the same group extended this observation by demonstrating that serum and synovial fluid osteocalcin levels were moderately correlated with those of keratan sulphate and hyaluronic acid.[23] Table 7.20 presents a summary of bone formation marker findings in OA.

Bone density

OA is strongly associated with body weight and it is therefore not too surprising that bone mineral density (BMD), which is highly correlated with body weight and frequently with height,[28] also tends to be elevated in patients with OA, especially with OA of lower limb joints. However, while early studies in subjects with OA failed to correct for body weight or body mass index (BMI),[29,30] more recent studies have corrected for this confounder with discordant results. In one small study of patients with either hip or knee OA who were awaiting surgery, correction for weight abolished the significant increase in BMD.[31] Another small study in women with nodal OA did show significant increases in BMD assessed at the spine and forearm as well as an increase in total body bone mineral, a finding that was not explained by weight.[32] Later studies with much larger groups of women with nodal OA were able to show a relationship between the radiographic score and BMD measured at multiple sites, although there was no such relationship with BMI.[33]

The viewpoint that OA and osteoporosis are at opposite ends of a spectrum has been widely proclaimed by Dequeker who contends that large epidemiological studies have demonstrated increased bone density by about 10 per cent in patients with generalized OA even after correction for body weight.[34,35] In the Framingham study, BMD of the femoral neck was found to be 5–9 per cent higher in both men and women with grades 1–3 knee OA, but surprisingly not in those subjects with grade 4 OA.[36] Further, the forearm BMD of the subjects with knee OA was not elevated compared to those without knee OA.[36]

The relationship of hip OA to BMD was examined in the Study of Osteoporotic Fractures cohort. Nearly 5000 women had a pelvic radiograph and those with grade 3 or 4 (moderate to severe) OA were found to have BMI adjusted increases in BMD of 5–9 per cent at all sites assessed (spine, proximal femur, distal radius, calcaneus) compared to the women who had grade 0–1 OA.[37]

Similarly, from the UK Chingford study, nearly 1000 women had hand and knee radiographs with BMD measurement of the spine and hip, and over 500 of the women also had spinal X-rays.[38] All OA groups (hand, knee, or spinal OA) had increased spine and femoral neck BMD after correcting for BMI,[38] although the increases were greater at the spine where osteophytes may have been a confounder (*infra vide*).

However there was no relationship between bone mass, assessed by the older technique of cortical area measurement, and the presence of hand OA in nearly 900 men examined as part of the Baltimore Longitudinal Study of Ageing.[39] In the same cohort, upper limb cortical area was not related to knee OA in men or women.[40] In a later analysis from the same study examining both men and women with knee OA, age and BMI adjusted spine BMD was elevated in relation to osteophyte formation, but hip BMD was not related to any radiographic feature of OA.[41]

Recently, using a discordant twin model, subjects with hip OA were found to have significantly increased BMD at the ipsilateral but not the contralateral hip or total body site.[42] This suggests that similar genetic factors may predispose to both OA and high BMD, and that the effect of OA itself may predispose to local BMD changes, a hypothesis supported by their finding that increased BMD in their subjects was correlated only with osteophyte formation and not joint-space narrowing. This is certainly the case in subjects with spinal OA, where osteophyte formation is clearly related to an apparent elevation in BMD values,[43] a finding which is only partly replicated at the hip[44] (see Fig. 7.54).

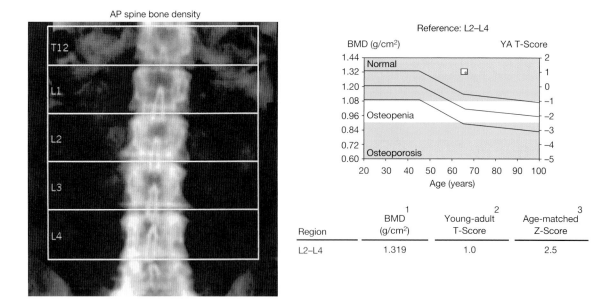

Fig. 7.54 Artificially increased spinal BMD in 65-year-old woman with lumbar vertebral osteophytes

Few longitudinal studies have examined BMD in OA subjects. However, in a group of elderly runners assessed over a 9-year period, those with knee OA had higher lumbar spine BMD measured by quantitative computed tomography throughout the study, than those without OA, but the rate of change of BMD over the period was no different.[45] Due to the aberrant effect of osteophytes on BMD, future longitudinal studies will require to consider sites where these are not part of the region of interest. Additionally the effect of buttressing causes effects on BMD at the femoral neck and Ward's triangle but not at the lateral trochanteric area, and this may be the best site for longitudinal analyses.[46]

How are we to interpret these confusing and sometimes discrepant results? Recent work has focused on more localized measurement of BMD changes at sites adjacent to affected joints. By the careful placement of regions of interest around the knee, investigators from France were able to demonstrate that the distribution of BMD was dependant on the angle of deformity suggesting, that at least some of the changes in BMD are secondary to the progression of the disease itself.[47] This finding is supported by a body of work in patients with hip OA,[48] where abnormalities of gait seem to be a particular determinant of hip BMD.[49] A further rather eclectic suggestion might be the effects of non-steroidal anti-inflammatory drugs, which have been shown to have a positive effect on bone mass even in subjects without OA.[50] The explanation for such a relationship remains obscure, but at least in the Study of Osteoporotic Fractures it does not appear to be associated with a reduction in fracture risk.[51]

Alternatively the explanation may lie in genetic factors. Polymorphisms of the vitamin D receptor gene, which do have a weak relationship to BMD,[52] may also have a role in the pathogenesis of osteophytes. However this relationship does not seem to be mediated by BMD in subjects with OA of the knee[53] or in subjects with degenerative disease of the spine.[54] On the other hand, a recent longitudinal study has demonstrated that subjects with incident knee OA, defined by the presence of osteophyte, do have higher baseline spine and hip BMD.[55] Intriguingly, the authors also demonstrated that a previous fracture protected against incident OA, independent of BMD status.[55]

While the overwhelming evidence suggests that subjects with large joint OA and probably generalized OA have increased bone mass,[56] amongst many other epidemiological factors,[57] this does not necessarily imply that sufferers are at a lower risk of fracture. Indeed, in a population study,

women with hip OA were more than twice as likely to have suffered a self-reported, but validated, fracture, despite their BMD being increased by approximately 5 per cent.[58] A similar finding was not detected in those with knee or spinal OA.[58] Similarly, self-reported OA was associated with increased age and BMI adjusted spine and hip BMD in almost 2000 men and women in the Dubbo study in Australia, but this did not reduce fracture rates perhaps due to poorer postural stability in the OA subjects counteracting the effects of increased BMD.[59] Furthermore, different types of hip OA may have a differing relationship with fracture risk, subjects with hypertrophic OA being much less likely to have vertebral fractures than those with atrophic OA or protrusio.[60]

Isotope bone scanning

Bone density measurements tell us nothing about the dynamics of bone metabolism, and bone turnover makers give an indication of the metabolism of bone only in the preceding few hours up to a few days. However, the technique of isotope bone scanning or scintigraphy, usually using a technetium labelled bisphosphonate,[61] gives a true dynamic picture of bone turnover and blood flow. Single emission photon emission tomography (SPECT) gives new options for use in a wide variety of rheumatological conditions.[62]

Scintigraphy has been used for many years to examine bone in OA.[63] The technique shows more abnormalities in the late phase of the scan (4 hours post injection of isotope) rather than the earlier phase,[64] implying bone turnover changes rather than increased blood flow. However, there is controversy concerning which pathological feature of OA is best delineated with isotope bone scans. In nodal hand OA, initial studies showed a discrepancy between the joints affected on scintigraphy and on plain radiographs,[65] but abnormal bone scans predicted the occurrence of subsequent radiographic change over 3–5 years.[66] Subsequent work suggested that growing or remodelling osteophytes seemed to best reflect increased tracer uptake.[67,68] Early-phase scan abnormalities seem to be a better reflection of pain, whereas late-phase abnormalities were a better reflection of joint tenderness.[64]

On the other hand, in knee OA abnormal bone scintigraphy was associated with radiographic deterioration primarily assessed by further joint-space narrowing. More recent comparison between scintigraphy and MRI has suggested a better correlation between high tracer uptake and joint-space narrowing than osteophytes in those with structural OA,[69] and correlation between subchondral lesions detected by MRI and chronic knee pain in subjects without radiographic OA.[70] More recent work has demonstrated a relationship between elevated levels of cartilage oligomeric matrix protein (COMP) and bone sialoprotein (BSP) and bone scan abnormalities,[71] suggesting that scintigraphy changes reflect active bone and cartilage remodelling and may therefore demonstrate early disease before radiographic changes have developed.

The unifying theory

Is it possible to bring all this somewhat contradictory evidence together to produce a unifying theory of pathogenesis and progression? The demonstration *in vitro* of reduced mineralization and increased osteoclastic activity in the subchondral bone[5] could potentially explain the increased resorption markers, especially in knee OA, noted by some authors, although it is equally feasible that the pyridinium markers in particular are reflecting cartilage metabolism more than that of the subchondral bone. Increased levels of serum osteocalcin seen by some authors may simply reflect exuberant osteophyte formation, which may in itself be related to the high levels of transforming growth factor β (TGFβ).[72]

If the hypothesis that abnormalities of lipid metabolism play a role in the pathogenesis of OA[3] is correct then the link between obesity, OA, and a tendency to high BMD would be more readily explained. Most current *in vivo* BMD techniques have either insufficient resolution to assess subchondral bone or, since they only allow a two-dimensional examination, will be assessing both cortical and subcortical bone. It remains entirely feasible therefore that subchondral bone turnover is increased in OA and predates the radiological progression. If correct the current studies underway to examine the potential effectiveness of the anti-resorptive bisphosphonate, risedronate, to inhibit radiographic deterioration[73] will prove successful.

Conclusion

Use of the term 'OA' strongly implies that bone is intimately involved in the disease process and that the changes should be associated with generalized rather than just local or subchondral effects. The evidence examined in this chapter supports this contention but does not allow a clear conclusion as to whether the changes detected in systemic 'bone markers' are related to bone or cartilage metabolism. Similarly, the increase in bone mass found in most populations of OA patients compared with controls does not necessarily prove that *bone density* is increased over and above that expected for the different body habitus and bone size of OA subjects compared with controls. Overall, however, the evidence does point to an increase in bone density in OA not entirely explained by body weight or other body habitus corrections. Whether these changes are a primary phenomenon related to the pathogenesis of the disease or secondary to the progression of disease remains unclear. Whichever is the case, increased bone mass does not appear to protect very effectively against fractures. Hopefully the results of currently progressing clinical trials of bone active anti-resorptive agents in OA will shed further light on these uncertainties.

Key clinical points

1. The elevation of some bone resorption markers in OA may reflect increased cartilage breakdown, rather than increased bone metabolism.

2. Increased bone density in OA at some sites may reflect osteophyte formation rather than underlying changes in bone mass *per se*.

3. Increases in bone density in OA are not associated with a reduction in fracture rates.

4. Isotope bone scan abnormalities in OA may reflect increased bone or cartilage remodelling.

References

(An asterisk refers to recommended reading.)

1. **Radin, E.L.** (1972–1973). The physiology and degeneration of joints. *Sem Arthritis Rheum* **2**:245–57.

2. **Radin, E.L. and Paul, I.L.** (1971). Importance of bone in sparing articular cartilage from impact. *Clin Orthop* **78**:342–4.

3. ***Aspden, R.M., Scheven, B.A., and Hutchison, J.D.** (2001). Osteoarthritis as a systemic disorder including stromal cell differentiation and lipid metabolism. *Lancet* **357**:1118–20.

   A key review of the relationship between abnormalities of the subchondral bone and the pathogenesis of OA.

4. **Li, B. and Aspden, R.M.** (1997). Mechanical and material properties of the subchondral bone plate from the femoral head of patients with osteoarthritis or osteoporosis. *Ann Rheum Dis* **56**:247–54.

5. **Li, B. and Aspden, R.M.** (1997). Composition and mechanical properties of cancellous bone from the femoral head of patients with osteoporosis or osteoarthritis. *J Bone Miner Res* **12**:641–51.

6. **Dequeker, J., Burssens, A., and Creytens, G.** (1977). Are osteoarthrosis and osteoporosis the end result of normal ageing or two different disease entities? *Acta Rhumatol Belg* **1**:46–57.

   The first of many papers from this author, summarizing the evidence that osteoporosis and OA sufferers are at opposite ends of the bone disease spectrum.

7. **Dequeker, J., Goris, P., and Uytterhoeven, R.** (1983). Osteoporosis and osteoarthrosis. osteoarthrosis. Anthropometric distinctions. *JAMA* **249**:1448–51.

8. **Dequeker, J., Franssens, R., and Borremans, A.** (1971). Relationship between peripheral and axial osteoporosis and osteoarthrosis. *Clin Radiol* **22**:74–7.

9. **Blumsohn, A. and Eastell, R.** (1997). The performance and utility of biochemical markers of bone turnover: do we know enough to use them in clinical practice? *Ann Clin Biochem* **34**(Pt 5):449–59.

10. **Macek, J. and Adam, M.** (1987). Determination of collagen degradation products in human urine in osteoarthrosis. *Z Rheumatol* **46**:237–40.

11. **Astbury, C., Bird, H.A., McLaren, A.M., and Robins, S.P.** (1994). Urinary excretion of pyridinium crosslinks of collagen correlated with joint damage in arthritis. *Br J Rheumatol* **33**:11–5.

12. **MacDonald, A.G., McHenry, P., Robins, S.P., and Reid, D.M.** (1994). Relationship of urinary pyridinium crosslinks to disease extent and activity in osteoarthritis. *Br J Rheumatol* **33**:16–9.

13. **Stewart, A., Black, A., Robins, S.P., and Reid, D.M.** (1999). Bone density and bone turnover in patients with osteoarthritis and osteoporosis. *J Rheumatol* **26**:622–6.

14. **Thompson, P.W., Spector, T.D., James, I.T., Henderson, E., and Hart, D.J.** (1992). Urinary collagen crosslinks reflect the radiographic severity of knee osteoarthritis. *Br J Rheumatol* **31**:759–61.

15. **Naitou, K., Kushida, K., Takahashi, M., Ohishi, T., and Inoue, T.** (2000). Bone mineral density and bone turnover in patients with knee osteoarthritis compared with generalized osteoarthritis. *Calcif Tiss Int* **66**:325–9.

16. **Graverand, M.P., Tron, A.M., Ichou, M.,** *et al.* (1996). Assessment of urinary hydroxypyridinium cross-links measurement in osteoarthritis. *Br J Rheumatol* **35**:1091–5.

17. **Seibel, M.J., Duncan, A., and Robins, S.P.** (1989). Urinary hydroxypyridinium crosslinks provide indices of cartilage and bone involvement in arthritic diseases. *J Rheumatol* **16**:964–70.

18. **Takahashi, M., Kushida, K., Hoshino, H.,** *et al.* (1996). Concentrations of pyridinoline and deoxypyridinoline in joint tissues from patients with osteoarthritis or rheumatoid arthritis. *Ann Rheum Dis* **55**:324–7.

19. **Gomez, Jr., B., Ardakani, S., Evans, B.J., Merrell, L.D., Jenkins, D.K., and Kung, V.T.** (1996). Monoclonal antibody assay for free urinary pyridinium cross-links. *Clin Chem* **42**:1168–75.

20. Garnero, P., Piperno, M., Gineyts, E., Christgau, S., Delmas, P.D., and Vignon, E. (2001). Cross sectional evaluation of biochemical markers of bone, cartilage, and synovial tissue metabolism in patients with knee osteoarthritis: relations with disease activity and joint damage. *Ann Rheum Dis* **60**:619–26.

    A study demonstrating that type II collagen, cartilage, markers are elevated in patients with knee OA while the type I, bone, markers are not, suggesting lack of specificity of the bone resorption markers found to be elevated in previous studies.

21. Stewart, A., Black, A., Robins, S.P., and Reid, D.M. (1999). Bone density and bone turnover in patients with osteoarthritis and osteoporosis. *J Rheumatol* **26**:622–6.

22. Campion, G.V., Delmas, P.D., and Dieppe, P.A. (1989). Serum and synovial fluid osteocalcin (bone gla protein) levels in joint disease. *Br J Rheumatol* **28**:393–8.

23. Salisbury, C. and Sharif, M. (1997). Relations between synovial fluid and serum concentrations of osteocalcin and other markers of joint tissue turnover in the knee joint compared with peripheral blood. *Ann Rheum Dis* **56**:558–61.

24. Raymaekers, G., Aerssens, J., Van den Eynde, R., *et al.* (1992). Alterations of the mineralization profile and osteocalcin concentrations in osteoarthritic cortical iliac crest bone. *Calcif Tiss Int* **51**:269–75.

25. El Miedany, Y.M., Mehanna, A.N., and El Baddini, M.A. (2000). Altered bone mineral metabolism in patients with osteoarthritis. *Joint Bone Spine* **67**:521–7.

26. Peel, N.F., Barrington, N.A., Blumsohn, A., Colwell, A., Hannon, R., and Eastell, R. (1995). Bone mineral density and bone turnover in spinal osteoarthrosis. *Ann Rheum Dis* **54**:867–71.

27. Sharif, M., George, E., and Dieppe, P.A. (1995). Correlation between synovial fluid markers of cartilage and bone turnover and scintigraphic scan abnormalities in osteoarthritis of the knee. *Arthritis Rheum* **38**:78–81.

28. Lunt, M., Felsenberg, D., Adams, J., *et al.* (1997). Population-based geographic variations in DXA bone density in Europe: the EVOS Study. European Vertebral Osteoporosis. *Osteoporos Int* **7**:175–89.

29. Jalovaara, P., Koivulsalo, F., Leppaluoto, J., Lindholm, R.V., and Vaananen, K. (1990). Mineral density of the os calcis in primary osteoarthritis of the hip and geriatric femoral neck fractures. *Ital J Orthop Traumatol* **16**:545–9.

30. Masuhara, K., Kato, Y., Ejima, Y., Fuji, T., and Hamada, H. (1994). Bone mineral assessment by dual-energy X-ray absorptiometry in patients with coxarthrosis. *Int Orthop* **18**:215–9.

31. Madsen, O.R., Brot, C., Petersen, M.M., and Sorensen, O.H. (1997). Body composition and muscle strength in women scheduled for a knee or hip replacement. A comparative study of two groups of osteoarthritic women. *Clin Rheumatol* **16**:39–44.

32. Hordon, L.D., Stewart, S.P., Troughton, P.R., Wright, V., Horsman, A., and Smith, M.A. (1993). Primary generalized osteoarthritis and bone mass. *Br J Rheumatol* **32**:1059–61.

33. Marcelli, C., Favier, F., Kotzki, P.O., Ferrazzi, V., Picot, M.C., and Simon, L. (1995). The relationship between osteoarthritis of the hands, bone mineral density, and osteoporotic fractures in elderly women. *Osteoporos Int* **5**:382–8.

34. Dequeker, J. (1997). Inverse relationship of interface between osteoporosis and osteoarthritis. *J Rheumatol* **24**:795–8.

35. Dequeker, J. (1999). The inverse relationship between osteoporosis and osteoarthritis. *Adv Exp Med Biol* **455**:419–22.

36. Hannan, M.T., Anderson, J.J., Zhang, Y., Levy, D., and Felson, D.T. (1993). Bone mineral density and knee osteoarthritis in elderly men and women. The Framingham Study. *Arthritis Rheum* **36**:1671–80.

37. Nevitt, M.C., Lane, N.E., Scott, J.C., *et al.* (1995). Radiographic osteoarthritis of the hip and bone mineral density. The Study of Osteoporotic Fractures Research Group. *Arthritis Rheum* **38**:907–16.

38. Hart, D.J., Mootoosamy, I., Doyle, D.V., and Spector, T.D. (1994). The relationship between osteoarthritis and osteoporosis in the general population: the Chingford Study. *Ann Rheum Dis* **53**:158–62.

39. Hochberg, M.C., Lethbridge-Cejku, M., Plato, C.C., Wigley, F.M., and Tobin, J.D. (1991). Factors associated with osteoarthritis of the hand in males: data from the Baltimore Longitudinal Study of Aging. *Am J Epidemiol* **134**:1121–7.

40. Hochberg, M.C., Lethbridge-Cejku, M., Scott W.W., Jr., Reichle, R., Plato, C.C., and Tobin, J.D. (1995). Upper extremity bone mass and osteoarthritis of the knees: data from the Baltimore Longitudinal Study of Aging. *J Bone Miner Res* **10**:432–8.

41. Lethbridge-Cejku, M., Tobin, J.D., Scott W.W., Jr., Reichle, R., Roy, T.A., Plato, C.C., and Hochberg, M.C. (1996). Axial and hip bone mineral density and radiographic changes of osteoarthritis of the knee: data from the Baltimore Longitudinal Study of Aging. *J Rheumatol* **23**:1943–7.

42. Antoniades, L., MacGregor, A.J., Matson, M., and Spector, T.D. (2000). A cotwin control study of the relationship between hip osteoarthritis and bone mineral density. *Arthritis Rheum* **43**:1450–5.

43. Jones, G., Nguyen, T., Sambrook, P.N., Kelly, P.J., and Eisman, J.A. (1995). A longitudinal study of the effect of spinal degenerative disease on bone density in the elderly. *J Rheumatol* **22**:932–6.

44. Liu, G., Peacock, M., Eilam, O., Dorulla, G., Braunstein, E., and Johnston, C.C. (1997). Effect of osteoarthritis in the lumbar spine and hip on bone mineral density and diagnosis of osteoporosis in elderly men and women. *Osteoporos Int* **7**:564–9.

45. Lane, N.E., Oehlert, J.W., Bloch, D.A., and Fries, J.F. (1998). The relationship of running to osteoarthritis of the knee and hip and bone mineral density of the lumbar spine: a 9 year longitudinal study. *J Rheumatol* **25**:334–41.

46. Preidler, K.W., White, L.S., Tashkin, J., *et al.* (1997). Dual-energy X-ray absorptiometric densitometry in osteoarthritis of the hip. Influence of secondary bone remodeling of the femoral neck. *Acta Radiol* **38**:539–42.

47. Hulet, C., Sabatier, J.P., Schiltz, D., Locker, B., Marcelli, C., and Vielpeau, C. (2001). Dual X-ray absorptiometry assessment of bone density of the proximal tibia in advanced-stage degenerative disease of the knee. *Rev Chir Orthop Reparatrice Appar Mot* **87**:50–60.

48. Hurwitz, D.E., Sumner, D.R., and Block, J.A. (2001). Bone density, dynamic joint loading and joint degeneration. A review. *Cells Tissues Organs* **169**:201–9.

49. Hurwitz, D.E., Foucher, K.C., Sumner, D.R., Andriacchi, T.P., Rosenberg, A.G., Galante, J.O. (1998). Hip motion and moments during gait relate directly to proximal femoral bone mineral density in patients with hip osteoarthritis. *J Biomech* **31**:919–25.

50. Morton, D.J., Barrett-Connor, E.L., and Schneider, D.L. (1998). Nonsteroidal anti-inflammatory drugs and bone mineral density in older women: the Rancho Bernardo study. *J Bone Miner Res* **13**:1924–31.

51. Bauer, D.C., Orwoll, E.S., Fox, K.M., Vogt, T.M., Lane, N.E., Hochberg, M.C., Stone, K., and Nevitt, M.C. (1996). Aspirin and NSAID use in older women: effect on bone mineral density and fracture risk. Study of Osteoporotic Fractures Research Group. *J Bone Miner Res* **11**: 29–35.

52. Gong, G., Stern, H.S., Cheng, S.C., *et al.* (1999). The association of bone mineral density with vitamin D receptor gene polymorphisms. *Osteoporos Int* **9**:55–64.

53. Uitterlinden, A.G., Burger, H., Huang, Q., *et al.* (1997). Vitamin D receptor genotype is associated with radiographic osteoarthritis at the knee. *J Clin Invest* **100**:259–63.

54. Jones, G., White, C., Sambrook, P., and Eisman, J. (1998). Allelic variation in the vitamin D receptor, lifestyle factors and lumbar spinal degenerative disease. *Ann Rheum Dis* **57**:94–9.

55. Hart, D.J., Cronin, C., Daniels, M., Worthy, T., Doyle, D.V., and Spector, T.D. (2002). The relationship of bone density and fracture to incident and progressive radiographic osteoarthritis of the knee: the Chingford Study. *Arthritis Rheum* **46**:92–9.

    A very recent paper showing that higher baseline BMD is associated with the development of incident OA of the knee.

56. Sambrook, P. and Naganathan, V. (1997). What is the relationship between osteoarthritis and osteoporosis? *Baillieres Clin Rheumatol* **11**:695–710.

57. Sowers, M. (2001). Epidemiology of risk factors for osteoarthritis: systemic factors. *Curr Opin Rheumatol* **13**:447–51.

58. Arden, N.K., Griffiths, G.O., Hart, D.J., Doyle, D.V., and Spector, T.D. (1996). The association between osteoarthritis and osteoporotic fracture: the Chingford Study. *Br J Rheumatol* **35**:1299–304.

59. Jones, G., Nguyen, T., Sambrook, P.N., Lord, S.R., Kelly, P.J., and Eisman, J.A. (1995). Osteoarthritis, bone density, postural stability, and osteoporotic fractures: a population based study. *J Rheumatol* **22**:921–5.

60. Schnitzler, C.M., Mesquita, J.M., and Wane, L. (1992). Bone histomorphometry of the iliac crest, and spinal fracture prevalence in atrophic and hypertrophic osteoarthritis of the hip. *Osteoporos Int* **2**:186–94.

61. Pauwels, E.K. and Stokkel, M.P. (2001). Radiopharmaceuticals for bone lesions. Imaging and therapy in clinical practice. *Q J Nucl Med* **45**:18–26.

62. Ryan, P.J. and Fogelman, I. (1996). Isotope imaging. *Baillieres Clin Rheumatol* **10**:589–613.

63. De Roo, M.J., Kestelijn, P., and Mulier, J.C. (1969). A critical study of the contribution of bone scintigraphy to diagnosis in orthopedic conditions. *Acta Orthop Belg* **35**:472–86.

64. Macfarlane, D.G., Buckland-Wright, J.C., Lynch, J., and Fogelman, I. (1993). A study of the early and late 99technetium scintigraphic images and their relationship to symptoms in osteoarthritis of the hands. *Br J Rheumatol* **32**:977–81.

65. Hutton, C.W., Higgs, E.R., Jackson, P.C., Watt, I., and Dieppe, P.A. (1986). 99 mTc HMDP bone scanning in generalised nodal osteoarthritis. II. The four hour bone scan image predicts radiographic change. *Ann Rheum Dis* **45**:622–6.

66. Hutton, C.W., Higgs, E.R., Jackson, P.C., Watt, I., and Dieppe, P.A. (1986). 99mTc HMDP bone scanning in generalised nodal osteoarthritis. I. Comparison of the standard radiograph and four hour bone scan image of the hand. *Ann Rheum Dis* **45**:617–21.

67. Buckland-Wright, J.C., Macfarlane, D.G., Fogelman, I., Emery, P., Lynch, J.A. (1991). Techetium 99m methylene diphosphonate bone scanning in osteoarthritic hands. *Eur J Nucl Med* **18**:12–6.

68. Buckland-Wright, J.C., Macfarlane, D.G., and Lynch, J.A. (1995). Sensitivity of radiographic features and specificity of scintigraphic imaging in hand osteoarthritis. *Rev Rhum Engl Ed* **62**:14S–26S.

69. Boegard, T. (1998). Radiography and bone scintigraphy in osteoarthritis of the knee—comparison with MR imaging. *Acta Radiol Suppl* **418**:7–37.

70. Boegard, T., Rudling, O., Dahlstrom, J., Dirksen, H., Petersson, I.F., and Jonsson, K. (1999). Bone scintigraphy in chronic knee pain: comparison with magnetic resonance imaging. *Ann Rheum Dis* **58**:20–6.

71. Petersson, I.F., Boegard, T., Dahlstrom, J., Svensson, B., Heinegard, D., and Saxne, T. (1998). Bone scan and serum markers of bone and cartilage in patients with knee pain and osteoarthritis. *Osteoarthritis Cart* **6**:33–9.

72. Uchino, M., Izumi, T., Tominaga, T., Wakita, R., Minehara, H., Sekiguchi, M., and Itoman, M. (2000). Growth factor expression in the osteophytes of the human femoral head in osteoarthritis. *Clin Orthop* 119–25.

73. Lane, N.E. and Nevitt, M.C. (2002). Osteoarthritis, bone mass, and fractures: how are they related? *Arthritis Rheum* **46**:1–4.

7.2.3 Synovium

7.2.3.1 Synovial mediators of cartilage damage and repair in osteoarthritis

Wim B. van den Berg, Peter M. van der Kraan, and Henk M. van Beuningen

Although, by definition, (OA) is not a prominent inflammatory condition, some degree of synovial hypertrophy and fibrosis is seen in the majority of symptomatic cases, whereas a moderate, but focal chronic synovitis has been noted in about 20 per cent of surgically resected specimens. Previously considered as a boring, 'degenerative' disease, a consequence of trauma or ageing, OA is now increasingly viewed as a deranged reparative process, with potential for intervention when key events or mediators can be

properly defined. The present chapter will summarize the current status of mediators and processes described in the synovial tissue of osteoarthritic conditions, with a focus on cytokines, enzymes, and growth factors. To put the relevance of the synovial reaction in perspective, the next paragraph will first briefly deal with OA characteristics and potential pathogenic pathways.

Role of synovial reaction in OA pathogenesis

OA is defined as a focal lesion of the articular cartilage, combined with a hypertrophic reaction (sclerosis) in the subchondral bone and new bone formation (osteophytes) at the joint margins. The overall picture resembles a failure in attempt at repair. It is a longstanding debate whether the initiating process originates in the bone or in the cartilage. The heterogeneous character of the ill-defined condition of OA further complicates this discussion. It is generally accepted that OA may occur as a consequence of multiple causes, ranging from blunt joint trauma, biomechanical overloading, inborn or acquired joint incongruency and genetic defects in matrix components or assembly, to an imbalance of synovial homeostasis. Probably, the joint has only a limited capacity to react to various insults and, in fact, the osteoarthritic lesion may reflect a common endpoint. On the other hand, it seems likely that the synovial reaction and mediators involved may be different in the initial stages of the various forms. As an illustration of complexity, meniscal damage or ligament rupture causes an abrupt shift in biomechanical loading of cartilage and bone, but it also generates an attempted repair reaction in the damaged tissue, be it ligamentous or cartilaginous in nature. It is now recognized, from studies in the anterior cruciate ligament transection model in dogs, that the first changes in the articular cartilage reflect a hypertrophic reaction, with enhanced synthesis of matrix and increase in content.[1] This is followed by a stage of increased matrix turnover, with net depletion of matrix components, and, finally, damage and loss of the collagen network. The hypertrophic stage clearly precedes the occurrence of the lesional stage, with its characteristic focal loss of cartilage.

There is no doubt that in late stages of OA the synovial reaction is sustained at least, in part, by wear particles and crystals released from the damaged cartilage. These triggers will stimulate synovial macrophages and fibroblasts, resulting in the generation of a broad range of inflammatory mediators, resembling those found in inflammatory joint disease such as rheumatoid arthritis (RA). This may even include an immune reaction, under conditions where the individual loses its tolerance against autoantigens from the cartilage (Fig. 7.55). The general concept in OA puts major emphasis on the direct activation of cartilage and bone, with minor involvement of the synovium. This may include a reaction of the chondrocyte to altered matrix stresses, for instance, due to shifts in loading or local

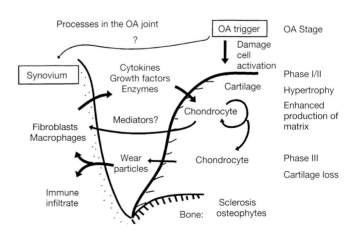

Fig. 7.55 Processes in osteoarthritic cartilage and synovial tissue.

trauma, resulting in the generation of chondrocyte mediators, which then act in the cartilage in an autocrine or paracrine fashion. In addition, diffusion to the synovium may occur, triggering synovial fibroblasts and macrophages, and contributing to perpetuation of the process. As an alternative hypothesis, direct activation and mediator generation may occur in the synovium as a consequence of disturbed homeostasis, for instance, following unsuccessful and, therefore, continued attempt at repair of ruptured ligaments, with sustained generation of growth factors. Although direct proof for the latter pathway in OA is lacking at the moment, it is now generally accepted that excessive growth factor generation is the underlying cause of tissue fibrosis in some kidney and liver diseases, and scar formation in the skin.[2] This principle is called the 'dark side of tissue repair' and may apply to OA as well.

Cytokines in OA/RA synovium

It is generally accepted that both TNFα and IL-1 are dominant cytokines in the synovial tissue of patients with RA. Evidence has accumulated that IL-1 is by far a more destructive mediator for the articular cartilage than TNFα,[3,4] but TNFα is considered as an important driving force of IL-1 production.[5] IL-1 is also produced in considerable quantities in OA synovial tissues and this may be a major source, apart from IL-1 originating from the articular cartilage, of the increased IL-1 levels in OA synovial fluid.[6,7] Of importance, IL-1 appears to be the driving force for the production of destructive enzymes (collagenase, stromelysin), and IL-6 in OA synovial tissue.[8] This is suggested by the marked inhibition of enzyme and IL-6 levels upon culture of OA synovium in the presence of IL-1 receptor antagonist (IL-1ra). The exact role of IL-6 has yet to be defined. It is considered as an upregulator of the expression of tissue inhibitor of metalloproteinase (TIMP) in synovial cells, and a pivotal stimulus of acute phase protein production by the liver. This includes several enzyme inhibitors, suggesting an important role in negative feedback control. On the other hand, IL-6 is considered a major factor in bone destruction. Its role as a potent stimulator of B cell growth seems of minor importance in OA.

Recent studies tried to identify the cellular source of the cytokines in both OA and RA, using immunohistochemistry on tissue specimens. In fact, most investigations were focused on RA synovial tissue, and OA synovial tissue was generally included as a control, in an attempt to identify disease-specific factors. Bearing in mind that the bulk of the studies refer to tissue obtained at late stages of the disease, at the time of surgery, it is demonstrated that most cytokines can be found in both OA and RA

synovium. Differences, if present, are mainly quantitative and not qualitative in nature. A study in patients with various stages of OA showed the most severe inflammatory changes and IL-1 and TNFα expression, resembling those seen in RA, in OA patients with advanced disease.[9]

A selection of destructive cytokines and regulators is summarized in Table 7.21, reflecting the general feeling of relative abundance in RA synovium. There is a tendency that TNFα is less abundant in OA synovium, whereas both IL-1α and IL-1β can be found in considerable quantities. This seems in accordance with significant levels of TNFα in synovial fluid samples of most RA patients, whereas TNFα was found only in a few OA samples.[7,10,11]

A cytokine with structural similarity to IL-1, IL-18, is found in low levels in OA synovial tissue.[12–14] The enzyme responsible for the activation of IL-1β and IL-18, ICE (Interleukin-1beta-converting enzyme), has been detected in the synovial membrane of OA patients.[15]

Remarkably, the synovial membrane expression of the proinflammatory cytokine IL-12 was found not to differ between RA and OA patients, both on the mRNA and protein level. This suggests that this cytokine might play an important role in the perpetuation of inflammation in both diseases.[16]

Leukemia inhibitory factor (LIF) is a relatively new cytokine, showing cartilage-destroying activity. It has been claimed that this is a separate action, not mediated through the generation of IL-1 and/or TNFα.[17,18] LIF can be induced by numerous cytokines and its relative role in OA remains to be identified.

The parathyroid hormone-related peptide (PTHrP) is involved in the cascade of proinflammatory cytokines. This peptide is, as most cytokines, more strongly expressed by RA synovium than by OA synovial cells.[19] However, incubation of synovial fibroblasts from OA patients with proinflammatory cytokines such as IL-1, IL-6, and TNFα, induced the production of PTHrP in those cells.[20]

A non-peptide mediator that is strongly involved in many physiological and pathological processes, nitric oxide (NO), is also spontaneously produced by synovial cells from OA patients.[21] Which cell in the synovial membrane is the main producer of NO, macrophages or fibroblasts, is still in debate.[21,22] However, since articular chondrocytes have a high capacity of NO production, these cells might contribute significantly to NO found in synovial fluid.[23]

In terms of localization of cytokines, expression seems in general more abundant in the lining layer in RA as compared with OA, but this must be viewed in relation to the more pronounced hypertrophy of the lining in RA. A final conclusion on differences in localization is, furthermore, hampered by the large variation in patterns found in different biopsies from the same patient.

Table 7.21 Synovial cytokines in OA and RA: relative abundance and major function

	OA	RA	References	Main function
IL-1	++	+++	6,7,11	Potent inducer of extracellular matrix destruction and matrix synthesis inhibition
IL-1RA	+++	++	27,28	Inhibitor of IL-1 actions
TNFα	+	+++	10,11	Induces matrix destruction and inhibits matrix synthesis. Less potent than IL-1. Induces IL-1 production
STNF-R	++	++	31,32	Inhibits TNFα
LIF	++	+++	17	Involved in synthesis inhibition of extracellular matrix components
IL-6	++	+++	7,33,34	Upregulates TIMP and IL-1RA
IL-4	−	+	26	Inhibits production of TNFα and IL-1. Upregulates IL-1RA
IL-10	+	++	24,25	Inhibits TNFα production
IL-8	++	++	35,36	Attracts inflammatory cells
IL-12	++	++	16	Stimulates TH1 lymphocytes
IL-18	+	+++	12–14	Inducer of matrix synthesis inhibition
MCP-1	++	++	35	Attracts inflammatory cells
PTHrP	+	++	19,20	Involved in inflammatory cascade

Apart from absolute levels of destructive mediators, it is of crucial importance to obtain information on the balance with natural inhibitors or regulators. TNFα and IL-1 production is under the control of cytokines like IL-4, IL-10, and IL-13. First studies in RA synovium reveal the apparent absence of IL-4, whereas IL-10 is present in variable amounts.[24–26] Information on these molecules in OA synovium is virtually lacking.

The action of the cytokines TNFα and IL-1 is under the control of cytokine-specific soluble receptors, which can be shed from connective tissue and leucocytes. In addition, IL-1 is balanced by the presence of the IL-1ra. Clear evidence is presented that IL-1ra gene expression and protein is abundant in OA synovia.[27,28] This antagonist is mainly found in the lining cells, and less so in the sublining. The inhibitor seems also more abundant in OA, as compared with RA synovium. However, it must be borne in mind that a 1000-fold excess of antagonist over IL-1 is needed to fully block the IL-1 activity,[29,30] making it doubtful whether the observed levels of IL-1ra are sufficient to really contribute to control. On the other hand, it cannot be excluded that levels in the close vicinity of cells can be extremely high.

Enzymes/inhibitors in OA synovium

As stated on the first page, IL-1 and TNFα can increase the production of proteases in synovial tissue and may be responsible for the enhanced levels of collagenase, stromelysin, and plasminogen activators found in human OA synovium. In experimental canine OA, a coordinate synthesis was noted of IL-1 and stromelysin.[37] Moreover, in human OA synovium a correlation was demonstrated between the amount of inflammatory cells and neutral protease levels.[38] In line with this, the expression of stromelysin and collagenase was less prominent in OA synovium, as compared with RA synovium.[39,40] The TIMP was easily detectable in both synovia, and levels were clearly enhanced above normal. Although the ratio protease/inhibitor was higher in RA, an unfavourable imbalance was also found in OA, suggestive for a role of these enzymes in tissue destruction.

The abundant appearance of aggrecan breakdown epitopes without the preferential cleavage sites of metalloproteinase activity has focused attention on the 'aggrecanase' enzyme. This enzyme is shown to be a member of the ADAMTS family and both ADAMTS-4 and -5 are largely responsible for aggrecan breakdown. Expression of ADAMTS-5 has been detected in human synovium, suggesting a role for this synovium-derived enzyme in joint damage in arthritic diseases.[41] From animal models it can be concluded that stromelysin plays a role in cartilage destruction. Metalloproteinase-specific degradation epitopes in aggrecan and type II collagen could not be detected in a stromelysin knockout mouse, while intense expression of these epitopes was found in wild-type mouse strains.[42]

Most of the stromelysin generated by IL-1 will be in the inactive form, needing additional proteolytic activation.[43] A potential role in activation has been attributed to the plasminogen-plasmin activator system.[44,45] Plasminogen activator inhibitors 1 and 2 (PAIs) are found in increased quantities in RA synovium, but not in OA synovium.

In addition to the metalloproteinases and aggrecanase, increasing attention has been given to other classes of enzymes. Cathepsins were found in elevated quantities in OA synovium, including the subtypes B, L, and D. The level of their specific natural inhibitors was not different in OA and normal synovium.[46,47] Moreover, cathepsins seem important in the activation of latent proteases.[48] A selection of enzymes detected in OA is summarized in Table 7.22. Further details on the role of the various enzyme systems will be addressed in the other chapters of this book.

Growth factors in OA synovium

In a broad sense, cytokines are defined as peptide regulatory factors that are produced by cells and act on cells, often in close vicinity. In that respect, the definition includes the various growth regulating mediators. However, for the moment, most authors will categorize part of the classical lymphokines and monokines under the heading 'cytokines', including a group of interleukins with clear growth-promoting activity on leucocytes, omitting yet another category of 'real' growth factors. On historical grounds, these growth factors are named after their dominant or initial mode of action, target tissue, or cellular origin. Many of these so-called growth factors can also be produced by the synovial tissue and often have a characteristic impact on synovial cells, as well as on cartilage and bone. Table 7.23 comprises a selection of growth factors, found in increased quantities in OA synovium and implicated directly or indirectly in cartilage damage and/or repair.

The colony-stimulating factors (CSFs) have their main action on bone marrow cells, stimulating hematopoietic differentiation, but are also implicated in bone resorption, through the stimulation of osteoclast generation. In synovial tissue, their main action is probably the activation of granulocyte and/or macrophage function, whereas recent data also demonstrate activation of chondrocytes (including enhanced production of IL-8). GM-CSF is a major factor in the inflamed synovium of RA patients, although increased levels are also found in most OA synovial samples. Of interest is the fact that the expression of both M-CSF and G-MCSF can be markedly enhanced in cultures of synovial fibroblasts, upon exposure to IL-1, but only M-CSF seems constitutively expressed,[52] implicating GM-CSF in acute inflammatory episodes, and M-CSF to be more important in sustained activation.

Table 7.22 Dominant synovial tissue proteinases and inhibitors in OA

Protease	References	Characteristics
Collagenase (MMP-1)	39	Produced by macrophage and fibroblast-like synoviocytes. Amount correlates with inflammation. Synthesized as an inactive pro-enzyme
Stromelysin (MMP-3)	38,49,50	Produced by macrophage and fibroblast-like synoviocytes. Amount appears to correlate with inflammatory cell infiltrate. Synthesized as an inactive pro-enzyme. Preferential cleavage site VDIPEN
Tissue Inhibitor of metalloproteinases (TIMP)	39,49,50	Produced by macrophage and fibroblast-like synoviocytes. Inhibits metalloproteinases
ADAMTS4/5 (aggrecanase)	41,43	Preferential cleavage site in aggrecan NITEGE
Plasminogen activator (PA)	44,45	Activates plasminogen
Plaminogen activator inhibitor (PAI)	44,45	Inhibits plasminogen activator
Cathepsins	46,47	Normally lysozomal enzymes
Calpain	51	Normally an intracellular enzyme but found in synovial fluid in OA
Calpastatins	51	Inhibits calpains, detected in synovial fluid

Table 7.23 Synovial tissue growth factors in OA. Detection of protein and/of message

Growth factor	References	Characteristics
Macrophage-colony stimulating factor (M-CSF)	52	Constitutively expressed by OA fibroblasts. Augments functional activities of monocytes and macrophages
Granulocyte-macrophage colony stimulating factor (GM-CSF)	52	Activates granulocytes and macrophages
Transforming growth factor β (TGF β)	57,58	Chemotactic for fibroblasts and inflammatory cells. Induces osteophyte formation and fibrosis. Modulates proteoglycan and collagen synthesis in synovium and cartilage
Insulin-like growth factor I and II (IGF)	61	Increases chondrocyte anabolism. Mitogenic for fibroblasts
Fibroblast growth factor (FGF)	53	Mitogenic for fibroblasts. Modulates proteoglycan metabolism in cartilage
Epidermal growth factor (EGF)	74	Mitogenic for fibroblasts. Modulates proteoglycan metabolism in cartilage
Platelet-derived growth factor (PDGF)	54	Mitogenic for fibroblasts. Modulates proteoglycan metabolism in cartilage
Hepatocyte growth factor (HGF)	55	Stimulates synthesis of collagenase-3 (MMP-13)

A second category of growth factors comprises PDGF, FGF, EGF, HGF, and TGFβ; all having potent mitogenic activity for synovial fibroblasts and inducing activation of cell function. The latter may include the enhanced production of destructive enzymes and generation of cytokines such as IL-1 and LIF. These factors probably contribute to the fibrotic reaction seen in OA synovial tissue. In contrast, the same set of growth factors may be involved in cartilage repair, through stimulation of chondrocyte proliferation and cartilage matrix synthesis. The relative importance of the latter action must of course be viewed in terms of the local production of similar factors by the chondrocyte itself. Both basic FGF (bFGF) as well as acidic FGF (Heparin binding GF) are found in synovial lining and sublining cells, and expression is higher in RA, as compared to OA synovium.[53] The same holds for expression of PDGF.[54] Hepatocyte growth factor (HGF) and the HGF receptor are expressed in OA synovial tissue.[55]

A factor of particular interest, but of a highly pleiotropic nature, is TGFβ. It is a potent chemotactic factor, attracting inflammatory phagocytes to the synovial tissue. In addition, it is a strong stimulus for fibroblast proliferation. However, it is rather unique amongst the growth factors in that it inhibits enzyme release and stimulates the production of enzyme inhibitors such as TIMP.[56] This effect is found with synovial cells as well as chondrocytes. In that respect, TGFβ may be viewed as an important feedback regulator of local tissue damage, following inflammatory episodes in the synovium. Finally, it stimulates matrix production by activated chondrocytes. It should be noted that TGFβ is produced in a latent form, linked to latency-associated peptide (LAP). Activation, with uncoupling from LAP, may occur under acidic conditions or by proteases. It is commonly accepted that most tissues, including synovium and cartilage, contain large amounts of latent TGFβ, which may become activated upon insults. Apart from TGFβ production by activated cells, these stores of latent TGFβ probably have a major impact on the response of a particular tissue. Significant levels of (active) TGFβ are found in the synovial fluid samples of both RA and OA patients, and enhanced production of TGFβ is demonstrated in the synovial tissue of such patients.[57] Major cell sources include macrophages and fibroblasts, and strong TGFβ immunostaining is noted in pannus tissue, at close vicinity to the articular cartilage. In fibrotic areas an exclusive expression of TGFβ is noted, in contrast to the dominant coexpression with cytokines such as IL-1 and TNFα at sites containing inflammatory infiltrates.[58] Unfortunately, such immunolocalization studies do not discriminate between latent and active TGFβ and the impact in the process of RA and OA remains largely to be identified.

A last category of important growth factors is that of the IGFs. Insulin-like growth factors, as the name implies, are growth factors that are abundant in serum and share some properties with insulin. IGF-II is an abundant factor in the embryonic stage, whereas IGF-I is the dominant factor in adult life. However, it cannot be ignored that IGF-II becomes of relevance under pathological conditions or at repair sites often showing embryonic elements.

IGF-I is a potent stimulator of chondrocyte proteoglycan synthesis and inhibits proteoglycan breakdown.[59] In that sense, it is an important homeostatic factor for cartilage and it was found that IGF-I is the main anabolic stimulus for chondrocyte proteoglycan present in serum and synovial fluid.[60] Since serum contains high levels of IGF-I, originating from the liver, it is commonly thought that the bulk of the IGF in synovial fluid is coming from the circulation. However, normal chondrocytes do make IGFs and recently, the expression of both IGF-I and -II message was demonstrated in the synovium and subsynovium of OA patients.[61] The action of IGFs is under the control of IGF-binding proteins, which can also be produced by chondrocytes. Cells isolated from OA cartilage make enhanced levels of IGF-bps,[62] but information on *in situ* production by OA synovial tissue is lacking.

The effects of synovial mediators on cartilage

As mentioned above, various cytokines, enzymes, and growth factors are found in increased quantities in OA synovium, and they can have a direct impact on cartilage and chondrocyte function. Although absolute levels of particular mediators may be indicative of their role, the net effect is mainly determined by the balance of synergizing, counteracting, and regulating mediators. The pattern of cartilage destruction is quite different in OA, as compared to RA, yet the enhanced production of numerous mediators can be found in both synovial tissues and differences, if present, seem mainly quantitative and not qualitative. This suggests that other, yet unidentified, factors are of pivotal importance, or that other aspects determine the particular cartilage response, such as local inhibitors or typical receptor expression patterns on chondrocytes in RA or OA cartilage.

In terms of their most characteristic effect on chondrocytes, cytokines can be broadly categorized into three classes: destructive cytokines, regulatory cytokines, and anabolic factors (Table 7.24). As a prime example of a destructive cytokine, IL-1 induces enhanced protease release, and inhibits chondrocyte proteoglycan and collagen synthesis. Regulatory factors like IL-4 and IL-10, inhibit IL-1 production and enhance the production of IL-ra, providing a 'double hit' to control the destructive action of IL-1. Finally, factors from the anabolic category, such as IGF-1 and TGFβ, do not really interfere with IL-1 production or action, but in fact display opposing activity; stimulation of proteoglycan and collagen synthesis, and suppression of protease action, the latter by inhibition of release and/or upregulation of inhibitors. This plain counteraction further underlines the importance of balance of the various factors.

Other members of the anabolic group worth mentioning are FGF and PDGF, which show stimulation of proteoglycan synthesis on top of the IGF-I effect,[63] and may contribute to cartilage repair by the stimulation of

Table 7.24 Cytokines in cartilage metabolism

Category	Mediator
Destructive cytokines	IL-1α, IL-1β, TNFα, TNFβ, LIF, (TGFβ)
Modulatory cytokines	IL-4, IL-6, IL-10, IL-13, TGFβ
Growth factors, chondrogenic factors…	IGF-1, PDGF, FGF, TGFβ1,2,3, BMPs…,

chondrocyte proliferation. However, a critical understanding of their role is complicated by a seemingly complex interaction with IL-1. It was demonstrated that previous exposure of chondrocytes to FGF enhances the subsequent protease release after IL-1.[64] PDGF also seems to stimulate IL-1-dependent protease release, but reduces the IL-1-mediated inhibition of proteoglycan synthesis.[65] These observations are conceivable with the notion that some growth factors can both potentiate repair, as well as enhance breakdown. More recently, a series of bone morphogenic proteins (BMPs) and specific chondrogenic factors were cloned. We are now confronted with a rapidly growing list of members showing more or less selective anabolic effects on chondrocytes. It is as yet unclear how these latter factors balance IL-1 effects, and whether the production of such factors by the synovial tissue makes a significant contribution to cartilage homeostasis and repair.

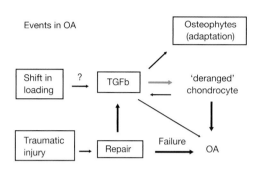

Fig. 7.56 Potential pathogenic mechanisms in osteoarthritis.

The involvement of mediators in OA cartilage pathology

To obtain insight into the key factors in OA cartilage pathology, it is imperative to identify the critical changes in the articular cartilage, and to try to fit these patterns with actions of particular mediators or combinations of mediators. Under normal conditions, cartilage maintains its homeostasis by a regulated balance of synthesis and degradative events. In theory, cartilage pathology may arise from the local overproduction of destructive mediators, or a shortage of controlling mediators, including inhibitors and anabolic growth factors. Moreover, a shift in responsiveness of the chondrocyte to these mediators may contribute to loss of homeostasis. There is no doubt that the OA chondrocyte displays an altered phenotype, which remains present after at least a number of cell passages in culture. It is as yet unclear whether this state reflects the cause or outcome of the OA process (Fig. 7.56).

An intriguing observation in human OA cartilage is the enhanced sensitivity of the chondrocytes to undergo stimulation of proteoglycan synthesis by TGFβ. Normal cartilage does not show enhanced proteoglycan synthesis upon first exposure to TGFβ. Only after a number of days in culture, in particular in the presence of TGFβ, the chondrocytes start to show this profile, probably under a TGFβ-induced shift in phenotype.[66,67] The fact that OA chondrocytes already show this pattern suggests a previous exposure to TGFβ and critical involvement of this factor in the disease process. TGFβ appears to be a crucial factor in the maintenance of cartilage integrity. Both the overexpression of a kinase-defective TGFβ type II receptor in skeletal tissues and the disruption of the TGFβ signaling mediator SMAD3 in knock-out mice, result in an accelerated terminal differentiation of chondrocytes and the development of OA.[68,69]

Further indication of a role of TGFβ in OA is provided by the marked upregulation of chondrocyte proteoglycan synthesis and the induction of osteophytes in murine knee joints, upon repeated local injection of TGFβ.[70] Osteophytes are characteristic features in OA and it was observed that repeated local injection with another growth factor, IGF-I, does not induce these hallmarks. Moreover, our group recently found that blocking of the endogenous TGFβ activity by application of a soluble form of the type II TGFβ receptor in an experimental model of OA significantly inhibited osteophyte formation.

Finally, upon prolonged exposure to TGFβ, the femoral cartilage of the murine knee joint shows typical loss of proteoglycans close to the tidemark,

and disorganization of chondrocyte spacing (Fig. 7.57). Enhanced TGFβ generation may result from the continued biomechanical overload of chondrocytes or unsuccessful and, therefore, continued repair processes in either cartilage or ligamentous tissue. The outcome of continued TGFβ exposure is a shift in the subtypes of proteoglycans made by the cartilage cells, probably resulting in impaired matrix assembly. These observations indicate that both suboptimal and supraoptimal levels of TGFβ result in cartilage pathology and eventually OA.

Although often suggested, a critical role of IL-1 in the early stages of OA seems unlikely. Observation from inflammatory models show that chondrocyte proteoglycan synthesis is markedly inhibited shortly after the induction of joint inflammation and remains suppressed in the presence of ongoing inflammation. Studies with neutralizing antibodies and IL-1ra provided convincing evidence that IL-1 is the pivotal mediator of this suppression.[3,71] In marked contrast, chondrocyte proteoglycan synthesis is enhanced in the early stages of experimental OA (Fig. 7.58). This is hardly compatible with a dominant role of IL-1, and at least suggests overkill by the generation and/or activation of anabolic factors. An OA phenomenon that may be attributable to IL-1 is the shift in phenotype of the chondrocyte. After prolonged exposure to IL-1, the production of cartilage specific collagen types such as types II and IX is reduced, whereas an increase in types I and III collagen is noted.[72] This shift may contribute to inadequate matrix repair.

Apart from the overproduction of mediators, pathology may be linked to the lack of action of anabolic growth factors. There is no evidence that IGF levels are limiting in the synovial fluid of either OA or RA patients. However, in experimental joint inflammation, IGF nonresponsiveness is noted in chondrocytes, compatible with the low level of proteoglycan synthesis in the arthritic chondrocytes. Moreover, the production of aberrant, small proteoglycans has been demonstrated in arthritic cartilage and this could be mimicked in normal cartilage, in the absence of IGF.[73] Another variant of improper IGF signalling seems to be present in OA cartilage. The chondrocytes make enhanced levels of IGF binding proteins, potentially limiting the homeostatic action of IGF. If this is the only disturbance in the IGF pathway, the lack of response may be overcome with high levels of IGF. This warrants therapeutic approaches with high doses of IGF-I. Interestingly, steroids display actions similar to IGF[73] and low doses may be applied instead of IGF, to bypass problems related to disturbed IGF receptor signalling or inhibitory binding proteins.

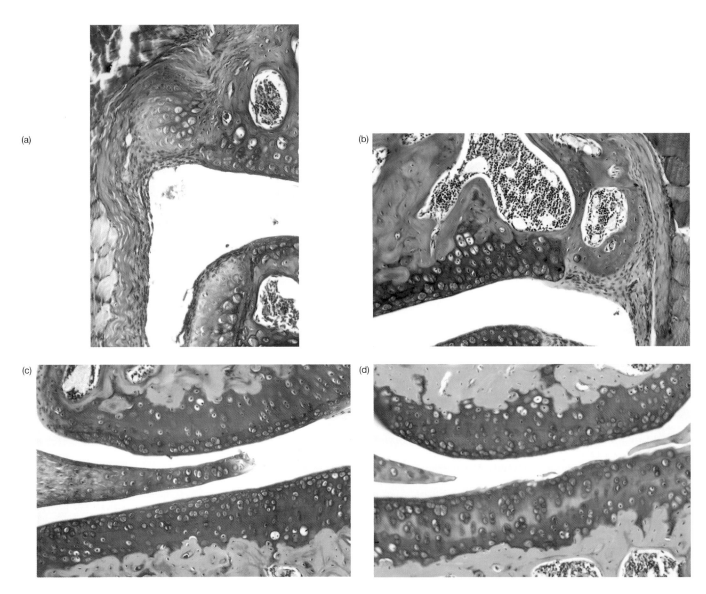

Fig. 7.57 Safranin O stained sections of the murine knee joint after local TGFβ injection: (a) outgrowth of chondroid tissue at the joint margin at day three after the last of triple TGFβ injections, given on alternate days; (b) similar treatment, but four weeks later—note the maturation into a mature osteophyte, containing bone marrow; (c) control section of tibial plateau; (d) similar region one month after six TGFβ injections, given on alternate days—note the loss of proteoglycan staining and the irregular surface and spacing of chondrocytes.

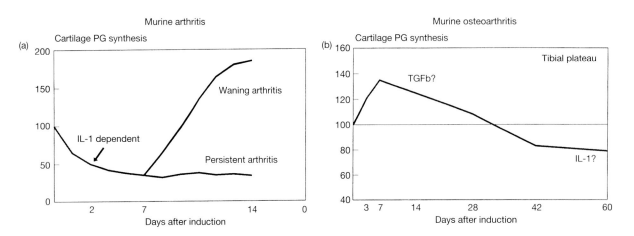

Fig. 7.58 Profile of chondrocyte proteoglycan synthesis in articular cartilage after induction of (a) joint inflammation or (b) osteoarthritis.

Final remarks

Many of the effects described in the previous sections can be ascribed to factors coming from the synovial tissue, the articular cartilage, or from both sources. To further identify key factors and the relative importance of the synovial reaction, studies are needed in various stages of proper experimental OA models, using inhibitors selectively targeting synovial tissue or cartilage. As an example, treatment with neutralizing antibodies to cytokines or growth factors will selectively touch the synovial process, since the antibody penetration of cartilage will be scant. By contrast, a smaller inhibitor such as IL-1ra will probably have sufficient access to both tissue compartments. In the near future, gene targeting, in combination with selective adhesion molecules, may provide a more elegant approach, offering interesting mechanistic tools and, hopefully, also therapeutic promises. Given the concept of failure in attempts at repair in OA, it is tempting to supply anabolic factors. However, too much growth factor may be pathologic, as suggested for TGFβ, whereas shifts in receptor expression on OA chondrocytes may skew the growth factor responses. It is anticipated that the characterization of new members of the BMPs and chondrogenic factors, in particular, may provide better tools for proper repair in due time.

Key points

1. The synovial tissue of osteoarthritic joints is a major source of mediators (cytokines, growth factors, and enzymes). These mediators are, in general, similar to the mediators found in the joints of rheumatoid arthritis patients but present in lower amounts. These mediators are major players in OA pathology, such as osteophyte formation, subchondral sclerosis, and cartilage degradation.

2. IL-1 is produced in considerable quantities in OA synovial tissues, and IL-1 appears to be an important driving force in the production of destructive enzymes. Not the absolute level of certain mediators, but the balance between the catabolic and anabolic factors will determine the final effect on joint tissues.

3. An unfavourable balance between destructive proteases and protease inhibitors is not only found in rheumatoid synovial tissue but also in OA.

References

(An asterisk denotes recommended reading.)

1. Adams, M.E. and Brandt, K.D. (1991). Hypertrophic repair of canine articular cartilage in osteoarthritis after anterior cruciate ligament transaction. *J Rheumatol* 18:428–35.

2. Border, W.A. and Ruoslahti, E. (1992). Transforming growth factor-β in disease. The dark side of tissue repair. *J Clin Invest* 90:1–7.

3. Van de Loo, A.A.J., Joosten, L.A.B., van Lent, P.L.E.M., Arntz, O.J., and van den Berg, W.B. (1995). Role of interleukin-1, tumor necrosis factor *a*, and interleukin-6 in cartilage proteoglycan metabolism and destruction. Effect of *in situ* blocking in murine antigen- and zymozan- induced arthritis. *Arthritis Rheum* 38:164–72.

4. Probert, L., Plows, D., Kontogeorgos, G., and Kollias, G. (1995). The type I IL-1 receptor acts in series with TNF to induce arthritis in TNF-transgenic mice. *Eur J Immunol* 25:1794–7.

5. Brennan, P.M., Chantry, D., Jackson, A., Maini, R., and Feldmann, M. (1989). Inhibitory effect of TNFa antibodies on synovial cell interleukin-1 production in rheumatoid arthritis. *Lancet* i:244–7.

6. Deleuran, B.W., Chu, C.Q., Field, M., *et al.* (1992). Localization of interleukin-1α, type-1 interleukin-1 receptor and interleukin-1 receptor antagonist in the synovial membrane and cartilage/pannus junction in rheumatoid arthritis. *Br J Rheumatol* 31:801–9.

7. Farahat, M.N., Yanni, G., Poston, R., and Panayi, G.S. (1993). Cytokine expression in synovial membranes of patients with rheumatoid arthritis and osteoarthritis. *Ann Rheum Dis* 52:870–5.

8. Pelletier, J.P., McCollum, R., Cloutier, J.M., and Martel-Pelletier, J. (1995). Synthesis of metalloproteinases and interleukin-6 (IL-6) in human osteoarthritic synovial membrane is an IL-1 mediated process. *J Rheumatol* 43(Suppl.):109–14.

9. Smith, M.D., Triantafillou, S., Parker, A., Youssef, P.P., and Coleman, M. (1997). Synovial membrane inflammation and cytokine production in patients with early osteoarthritis. *J Rheumatol* 24:365–71.

10. Chu, C.Q., Field, M., Feldmann, M., and Maini, R.N. (1991). Localization of tumor necrosis factor alpha in synovial tissue and at the cartilage pannus junction in patients with rheumatoid arthritis. *Arthritis Rheum* 34:1125–32.

11. Miller, V.E., Rogers, K., and Muirden, K.D. (1993). Detection of tumour necrosis factor *a* and interleukin-1β in the rheumatoid and osteoarthritic cartilage/pannus junction by immunohistochemical methods. *Rheumatol Int* 13:77–82.

12. Moller, B., Kukoc-Zivojnov, N., Kessler, U., Rehart, S., Kaltwasser, J.P., Hoelzer, D., *et al.* (2001). Expression of interleukin-18 and its monokine-directed function in rheumatoid arthritis. *Rheumatology* 40:302–9.

13. Yamamura, M., Kawashima, M., Taniai, M., *et al.* (2001). Inteferon-gamma-inducing activity of interleukin-18 in the joint with rheumatoid arthritis. *Arthritis Rheum* 44:275–85.

14. Gracie, J.A., Forsey, R.J., Chan, W.L., *et al.* (1999). A proinflammatory role for IL-18 in rheumatoid arthritis. *J Clin Invest* 104:1393–401.

15. Saha, N., Moldovan, F., Tardif, G., Pelletier, J.P., Cloutier, J.M., and Martel-Pelletier, J.M. (1999). Interleukin-1beta-converting enzyme/caspase-1 in human osteoarthritic tissues. Localization and role in the maturation of interleukin-1beta and interleukin-18. *Arthritis Rheum* 42:1577–87.

16. Sakkas, L.I., Johanson, N.A., Scanzello, C.R., and Platsoucas, C.D. (1998). Interleukin-12 is expressed by infiltrating macrophages and synovial lining cells in rheumatoid arthritis and osteoarthritis. *Cell Immunol* 188:105–10.

17. Lotz, M., Moats, T., and Villiger, P.M. (1992). Leukemia inhibitory factor is expressed in cartilage and synovium and can contribute to the pathogenesis of arthritis. *J Clin Invest* 90:888–96.

18. Bell, M.C. and Carroll, G.J. (1995). Leukemia inhibitory factor (LIF) suppresses proteoglycan synthesis in porcine and caprine cartilage explants. *Cytokine* 7:137–41.

19. Funk, J.L., Cordaro, L.A., Wei, H., Benjamin, J.B., and Yocum, D.E. (1998). Synovium as a source of increased amino-terminal parathyroid hormone-related protein expression in rheumatoid arthritis. A possible role for locally produced parathyroid hormone-related protein in the pathogenesis of rheumatoid arthritis. *J Clin Invest* 101:1362–71.

20. Yoshida, T., Horiuchi, T., Sakamoto, H., *et al.* (1998). Production of parathyroid hormone-related peptide by synovial fibroblasts in human osteoarthritis. *FEBS lett* 433:331–4.

21. *McInnes, I.B., Leung, B.P., Field, M., *et al.* (1996). Production of nitric oxide in the synovial membrane of rheumatoid and osteoarthritis patients. *J Exp Med* 184:1519–24.
    This article shows that nitric oxide is produced by the synovial membrane of osteoarthritic joints.

22. Grabowski, P.S., Wright, P.K., VanTHof, R.J., Helfrich, M.H., Ohshima, H., and Ralston, S.H. (1997). Immunolocalization of inducible nitric oxide synthase in synovium and cartilage in rheumatoid arthritis and osteoarthritis. *Br J Rheumatol* 36:651–5.

23. Melchiorri, C., Meliconi, R., Frizziero, L., Silvestri, T., Pulsatelli, L., Mazetti, and Borzi, R.M. (1998). Enhanced and coordinated in vivo expression of inflammatory cytokines and oxide synthase by chondrocytes from patients with osteoarthritis. *Arthritis Rheum* 41:2165–74.

24. Katsikis, P.D., Chu, C.Q., Brennan, F.M., Maini, R.N., and Feldmann, M. (1994). Immunoregulatory role of IL-10. *J Exp Med* 179:15–17.

25. Cush, J.J., Splawski, J.B., Thomas, R., *et al.* (1995). Elevated interleukin-10 levels in patients with rheumatoid arthritis. *Arthritis Rheum* 38:96–104.

26. Miossec, P., Naviliat, M., Dupuy D'Angeac, A., Sany, J., and Banchereau, J. (1990). Low levels of interleukin-4 and high levels of transforming growth factor β in rheumatoid synovitis. *Arthritis Rheum* 33:1180–7.

27. Firestein, G.S., Berger, A.E., Tracey, D.E., *et al.* (1992). IL-1 receptor antagonist protein production and gene expression in rheumatoid and osteoarthritis synovium. *J Immunol* **149**:1054–62.

28. Fujikawa, Y., Shingu, M., Torisu, T., and Masumi, S. (1995). Interleukin-1 receptor antagonist production in cultured synovial cells from patients with rheumatoid arthritis and osteoarthritis. *Ann Rheum Dis* **54**:318–20.

29. Arend, W.P. (1991). Interleukin I receptor antagonist. A new member of the interleukin 1 family. *J Clin Invest* **88**:1445–51.

30. Smith, R.J., Chin, J.E., Sam, L.M., and Justen, J.M. (1991). Biologic effects of an interleukin-1 receptor antagonist protein on interleukin-1-stimulated cartilage erosion and chondrocyte responsiveness. *Arthritis Rheum* **34**:78–83.

31. Roux-Lombard, P., Punzi, L., Hasler, F., *et al.* (1993). Soluble tumor necrosis factor receptors in human inflammatory synovial fluids. *Arthritis Rheum* **36**:485–9.

32. Steiner, G., Studnicka-Benke, A., Witzmann, G., Hofler, E., and Smolen, J. (1995). Soluble receptors for tumor necrosis factor and interleukin-2 in serum and synovial fluid of patients with rheumatoid arthritis, reactive arthritis and osteoarthritis. *J Rheumatol* **22**:406–12.

33. Guerne, P.A., Zuraw, B.L., Vaughan, J.H., Carson, D.A., and Lotz, M. (1989). Synovium as a source for interleukin-6 *in vitro*. Contribution to local systemic manifestations of arthritis. *J Clin Invest* **83**:585–92.

34. Field, M., Chu, C., Feldmann, M., and Maim, R.N. (1991). Interleukin-6 localisation in the synovial membrane in rheumatoid arthritis. *Rheumatol Int* **11**:45–50.

35. Seitz, M., Loetscher, P., Dewald, B., Towbin, H., Ceska, M., and Baggiolini, M. (1994). Production of interleukin-1 receptor antagonist, inflammatory chemotactic proteins, and prostaglandin E by rheumatoid and osteoarthritic synovium. Regulation by IFN-gamma and IL-4. *J Immunol* **15**:2060–5.

36. Verburgh, C.A., Hart, M.H.L., Aarden, L.A., and Swaak, A.J.G. (1993). Interleukin-8 (IL-8) in synovial fluid of rheumatoid and non-rheumatoid joint effusions. *Clin Rheumatol* **12**:494–9.

37. Pelletier, J.P., Faure, M.P., DiBattista, J.A., Wilhelm, S., Visco, D., and Martel-Pelletier, J. (1993). Coordinate expression of stromelysin, interleukin-1, and oncogene proteins in experimental osteoarthritis. *Am J Pathol* **142**:95–105.

38. Okada, Y., Shinmei, M., Tanaka, O., *et al.* (1992). Localization of matrix metalloprotease 3 (stromelysin) in osteoarthritic cartilage and synovium. *Lab Invest* **66**:680–90.

39. *Firestein, G.S., Paine, M.M., and Littman, B.H. (1991). Gene expression (collagenase, tissue inhibitor of metalloproteinases, complement, and HLA-DR) in rheumatoid arthritis and osteoarthritis synovium. *Arthritis Rheum* **34**:1094–1105.

   The authors show that osteoarthritic synovium is activated and contributes to the production of mediators in the joint.

40. Clark, I.M., Powell, L.K., Ramsey, S., Hazleman, B.L., and Cawston, T.E. (1993). The measurement of collagenase, tissue inhibitor of metalloproteinase (TIMP), and collagenase-TIMP complex in synovial fluids from 42 patients with osteoarthritis and rheumatoid arthritis. *Arthritis Rheum* **36**:372–9.

41. *Vankemmelbeke, M.N., Holen, I., Wilson, A.G., Ilic, M.Z., Handley, C.J., and Kelner, G.S. (2001). Expression and activity of ADAMTS-5 in synovium. *Eur J Biochem* **268**:1259–68.

   This article indicates that important aggrecan degrading enzymes are not only synthesized in articular cartilage but also at other joint sites.

42. Van Meurs, J.B.J., van Lent, P.L.E.M., Stoop, R., *et al.* (1999). Cleavage of aggrecan at Asn341-Phe342 site coincides with the initiation of collagen damage in murine collagen-induced arthritis. A pivotal role for stromelysin-1 in MMP activity. *Arthritis Rheum* **42**:2074–84.

43. Lohmander, L.S., Neame, P.J., and Sandy, J.D. (1993). The structure of aggrecan fragments in human synovial fluid. *Arthritis Rheum* **36**:1214–22.

44. Saxne, T., Lecander, I., and Geborek, P. (1993). Plasminogen activators and plasminogen activator inhibitors in synovial fluid. Difference between inflammatory joint disorders and osteoarthritis. *J Rheumatol* **20**:91–6.

45. Pelletier, J.P., Mineau, F., Faure, M.P., and Martel-Pelletier, J. (1990). Imbalance between the mechanisms of activation and inhibition of metalloproteinases in the early lesions of experimental osteoarthritis. *Arthritis Rheum* **33**:1466–76.

46. Martel-Pelletier, J., Cloutier, J.M., and Pelletier, J.P. (1990). Cathepsin B and cysteine protease inhibitors in human osteoarthritis. *J Orthop Res* **8**:336–44.

47. Keyszer, G.M., Heer, A.H., Kriegsmann, J., *et al.* (1995). Comparative analysis of cathepsin L, cathepsin D, and collagenase messenger RNA expression in synovial tissues of patients with rheumatoid arthritis and osteoarthritis, by *in situ* hybridisation. *Arthritis Rheum* **38**:976–84.

48. Buttle, D.J., Handley, C.J., Ilic, M.Z., Saklatvala, J., Murata, M., and Barrett, A.J. (1993). Inhibition of cartilage proteoglycan release by a specific inactivator of cathepsin B and an inhibitor of matrix metalloproteinases. *Arthritis Rheum* **36**:1709–17.

49. McCachren, S.S. (1993). Expression of metalloproteinases and metalloproteinase inhibitor in human arthritic synovium. *Arthritis Rheum* **36**:1085–93.

50. Zafarullah, M., Pelletier, J.P., Cloutier, J.M., and Martel-Pelletier, J. (1993). Elevated metalloproteinase and tissue inhibitor of metalloproteinase mRNA in human osteoarthritic synovia. *J Rheumatol* **20**:693–7.

51. Suzuki, K., Shimizu, K., Hamamoto, T., Nakagawa, Y., Hamakubo, T., and Yamamuro, T. (1990). Biochemical demonstration of calpains and calpastatin in osteoarthritic synovial fluid. *Arthritis Rheum* **33**:728–32.

52. Seitz, M., Loetscher, P., Fey, M.F., and Tobler, A. (1994). Constitutive mRNA and protein production of macrophage colony-stimulating factor but not of other cytokines by synovial fibroblasts from rheumatoid arthritis and osteoarthritis patients. *Br J Rheumatol* **33**:613–19.

53. Nakashima, M., Eguchi, K., Aoyagi, T., *et al.* (1994). Expression of basic fibroblast growth factor in synovial tissues from patients with rheumatoid arthritis. Detection by immunohistochemical staining and *in situ* hybridisation. *Ann Rheum Dis* **53**:45–50.

54. Remmers, E.F., Sano, H., Lafyatis, R., *et al.* (1991). Production of platelet derived growth factor B chain (PDGF-B/c-sis) mRNA and immunoreactive PDGF B-like polypeptide by rheumatoid synovium: coexpression with heparin binding acidic fibroblast growth factor. *J Rheumatol* **18**:7–13.

55. Nagashima, M., Hasegawa, J., Kato, K., *et al.* (2001). Hepatocyte growth factor (HGF), HGF activator, and c-met in synovial tissue in rheumatoid arthritis and osteoarthritis. *J Rheumatol* **28**:1772–8.

56. Wright, J.K., Cawston, T.E., and Hazleman, B.L. (1991). Transforming growth factor beta stimulates the production of the tissue inhibitor of metalloproteinases (TIMP) by human synovial and skin fibroblasts. *Biochim Biophys Acta* **1094**:207–10.

57. Chu, C.Q., Field, M., Abney, E., *et al.* (1991). Transforming growth factor-β in rheumatoid synovial membrane and cartilage/pannus junction. *Clin Exp Immunol* **86**:380–6.

58. Chu, C.Q., Field, M., Allard, S., Abney, E., Feldmann, M., and Maini, R.N. (1992). Detection of cytokines at the cartilage/pannus junction in patients with rheumatoid arthritis: implications for the role of cytokines in cartilage destruction and repair. *Br J Rheumatol* **31**:653–61.

59. Tyler, J.A. (1991). Insulin-like growth factor can decrease degradation and promote synthesis of proteoglycan in cartilage exposed to cytokines. *Biochem J* **260**:543–8.

60. Schalkwijk, J., Joosten, L.A.B., van den Berg, W.B., van Wijk, J.J., van de Putte, L.B.A. (1989). Insulin-like growth factor stimulation of chondrocyte proteoglycan synthesis by human synovial fluid. *Arthritis Rheum* **32**:66–71.

61. Keyszer, G.M., Heer, A.H., Kriegsmann, J., *et al.* (1995). Detection of insulin-like growth factor I and II in synovial tissue specimens of patients with rheumatoid arthritis and osteoarthritis. *J Rheumatol* **22**:275–81.

62. Dore, S., Pelletier, J.P., DiBattista, J.A., Tardif, G., Brazeau, P., and Martel-Pelletier, J.M. (1994). Human osteoarthritic chondrocytes possess an increased number of insulin-like growth factor I binding sites but are unresponsive to its stimulation. *Arthritis Rheum* **37**:253–63.

63. Verschure, P.J., Joosten, L.A.B., van der Kraan, P.M., and van den Berg, W.B. (1994). Responsiveness of articular cartilage from normal and inflamed mouse knee joints to various growth factors. *Ann Rheum Dis* **53**:455–60.

64. Chandrasekhar, S. and Harvey, A.K. (1989). Induction of interleukin-1 receptors on chondrocytes by fibroblast growth factor: A possible mechanism for modulation of interleukin-1 activity. *J Cell Physiol* **138**:236–46.

65. Smith, R.J., Justen, J.M., Sam, L.M., *et al.* (1991). Platelet-derived growth factor potentiates cellular responses of articular chondrocytes to interleukin-1. *Arthritis Rheum* **34**:697–706.

66. Lafeber, F.P.J.G., van der Kraan, P.M., Huber-Bruning, O., van den Berg, W.B., and Bijlsma, J.W.J. (1993). Osteoarthritic human cartilage is more sensitive to

transforming growth factor β than is normal cartilage. *Br J Rheumatol* **32**:281–6.

67. Inoue, H., Kato, Y., Iwamoto, M., Hiraki, Y., Sakuda, M., and Suzuki, F. (1989). Stimulation of proteoglycan synthesis by morphological transformed chondrocytes grown in the presence of fibroblast growth factor and transforming growth factor-beta. *J Cell Physiol* **138**:329–37.

68. Serra, R., Johnson, M., Filvaroff, E.H., *et al.* (1997). Expression of a truncated, kinase-defective TGF-beta type II receptor in skeletal tissue promotes terminal chondrocyte differentiation and osteoarthritis. *J Cell Biol* **139**: 541–52.

69. Yang, X., Chen, L., Xu, X., Li, C., Huang, C., and Deng, C.X. (2001). TGF-beta/SMAD3 signals repress chondrocyte hypertrophic differentiation and are required for maintaining articular cartilage. *J Cell Biol* **153**:53–46.

70. *Van Beuningen, H.M., van der Kraan, P.M., Arntz, O.J., and van den Berg, W.B. (1994). Transforming growth factor-β stimulates articular cartilage chondrocyte proteoglycan synthesis and induces osteophyte formation in the murine knee joint. *Lab Invest* **71**:279–90.
    This article demonstrates that TGFβ is a potent inducer of osteophytes in vivo.

71. Van de Loo, A.A.J., Arntz, O.J., Otterness, I.G., and van den Berg, W.B. (1992). Protection against cartilage proteoglycan synthesis inhibition by anti-interleukin-1 antibodies in experimental arthritis. *J Rheumatol* **19**:348–56.

72. Goldring, M.B., Birkhead, J., Sandell, I.J., Kimura, T., and Krane, S.M. (1988). Interleukin-1 suppresses expression of cartilage-specific types II and IX collagen and increases type I and II collagens in human chondrocytes. *J Clin Invest* **82**:2026–37.

73. Verschure, P.J., van der Kraan, P.M., Vitters, E.L., and van den Berg, W.B. (1994). Stimulation of proteoglycan synthesis by triamcinolone acetonide and insulin-like growth factor-1 in normal and arthritic murine articular cartilage. *J Rheumatol* **21**:920–6.

74. Farahat, M.N., Yanni, G., Poston, R., and Panayi, G.S. (1993). Cytokine expression in synovial membranes of patients with rheumatoid arthritis and osteoarthritis. *Ann Rheum Dis* **52**:870–5.

7.2.3.2 Synovial physiology in the context of osteoarthritis

Peter A. Simkin

Each diarthrodial joint begins early in fetal development when a cavitation event demarcates its location within the primitive, cartilaginous model of the skeletal system.[1] The cavity that is formed contains a fluid that will persist as the synovial fluid (SF) across the entire life span of the individual. Throughout those years, the SF remains in equilibrium with the perfusing plasma (P) in the synovial microvasculature. Thus, it is not a secreted product like the saliva, bile, or urine, but a fluid that resides within a basic interstitial compartment analogous in this respect to cerebrospinal, pleural, and peritoneal fluids. Each constituent of SF is in equilibrium with P, an equilibrium that may vary with local or systemic disease.

This equilibrium means, of course, that the input and outgo of each solute are in balance, that is, the flux rate of each molecule into the joint is essentially equal to its flux rate back into the P (in mg/minute or equivalent measures of mass/unit time).[2] When synovial effusions are developing or resolving there will be temporary perturbations in this balance for all solutes in the effusion.[3] Similarly, an abrupt change in the serum concentration (such as the absorption phase after ingestion of a medication or a rising glucose after a meal) or in the SF level (such as an intra-articular injection) will transiently disrupt the equilibrium for that specific solute. In general, however, the balance principle holds. In practical terms for the experimentalist, this means that a flux rate determined in one direction also yields the rate for that molecule in the opposite direction.[4–6]

The most fundamental constituent of any joint is water. Though there are significant differences between joints and between species, the normal SF volume is small. In fact, the volume is often so small that no free fluid is seen on opening the joint, but only an easily appreciated dampness of the synovial and cartilaginous surfaces. From there, the volume can range up to several hundred milliliters in pathologic effusions of capacious joints, such as the human knee.[7]

Parenthetically, this large range of volumes is a critical concern for anyone who expects to use synovial aspirates to help understand an articular disease, such as OA. Many patients with this disease experience pain and disability from joints that do not contain significant effusions. Such joints are unlikely to be aspirated and their vascular physiology is yet to be studied. Conversely, the OA patients with less troublesome symptoms may have substantial effusions, and it is only from them that we have usable information about concentrations of 'marker' molecules, volume, blood flow, and rates of solute interchange between P and SF.[8] There is essentially no physiologic information from the distal interphalangeal joints of the hands, the thumb base, or the first metatarsophalangel joint in the feet. These are the joints most often affected by OA, but they are small and yield little or no fluid on aspiration. Therefore, we know little about them.

Transport of small molecules

The P water reaches the normal knee joint through a rather rich bed of synovial microvessels at a flow rate of approximately 2 ml/min. There, it moves freely in both directions across an endothelium that is fenestrated on the lumenal side of each capillary (Fig. 7.59).[9,10] The abundant fenestrations permit bi-directional, diffusive exchange not only of water but also of other small molecules with molecular weights less than 12 000 Daltons. Lesser amounts of water also cross the endothelium through 'small' and 'large' pores that are not yet well defined but probably reflect differing degrees of separation at the junctions between adjoining endothelial cells. In addition, some bulk transport through endothelial vesicles may occur.[11]

Overall, there is a small net filtration of water across the microvessels of the normal human knee. This filtered water returns to the circulation by way of the lymphatic system. Terminal synovial lymphatics are located superficially within the normal synovial tissue. Notably, both the terminal lymphatic vessels and the postcapillary venules of the synovium, are valved to permit flow in only one direction—toward the heart.[12,13] The superficial

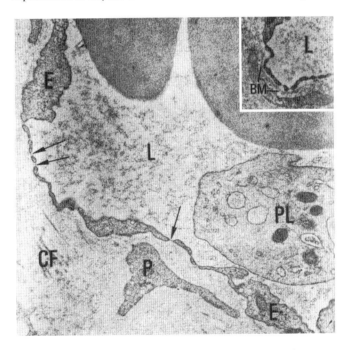

Fig. 7.59 Superficial synovial microvessel in the knee of a Cebus monkey. Fenestrations in the lining endothelial cells are marked with arrows.

Source: Taken from Ref. 10, p. 390.

location of these valves within moving joints appears to provide a propitious, pumping mechanism for moving water and solutes away from the joint and back to the central circulation. Parenthetically, the same valves presumably block the potential backflow of cytokines and proteases 'around the corner' from inflamed synovium into subchondral bone.

Given the ongoing equilibrium between the two fluids, it is only to be expected that most of the solutes in the SF are derived from the P. Studies of the exchange of the small molecules in both directions across the synovium, have found it to occur at rates consistent with simple diffusion. As those molecules that are small enough to cross the fenestrae are fully equilibrated under resting conditions, the equilibrium must be disrupted experimentally so that the re-equilibration can then be studied to quantify the kinetics of the exchange. This is easily done, by examining the clearance of radiolabelled markers from the joint, but physiologic molecules can also be measured as they re-enter a joint space in which the normal SF has been replaced by physiologic saline (Fig. 7.60).[4,8] In the normal bi-directional exchange, the rate-limiting diffusion path is thought to be the aqueous channels between adjoining cells of the synovial lining. Fat-soluble solutes (most notably, the respiratory gasses) are an apparently exception to this rule in that they can diffuse through, as well as between, the synovial cells. This thus-broadened diffusion path leads to faster trans-synovial exchange.

Glucose, too, enters a SF more rapidly than would be predicted from its molecular size.[4,14] In this case, a unidirectional transport system within the synovial lining cells is considered the most likely mechanism. Thus, the provision of abundant glucose and oxygen that is assured by the generous microvascular supply to the normal synovium, is further facilitated by the additional synovial mechanisms.

These mechanisms are relevant to the student of OA because the synovial microvasculature must meet the metabolic needs not only of synovial tissue, but also of the chondrocytes within the articular cartilage. Juvenile cartilage seems clearly able to derive nutrient needs and eliminate metabolic wastes by way of the blood supply to underlying trabecular bone.[15] In the adult, however, this route appears to become much less accessible because of a dramatic decrease in permeability of the cartilage/bone interface.[16] After this maturational change occurs, the alternative synovial source is correspondingly more important.[16] Given the size of large joints,

such as the hip and knees, the relative isolation from subchondral support means that many articular chondrocytes lie farther from their nutrient supply than do any other cells in the human body. This may be more true of chondrocytes in concave cartilage, than of the cells in their convex mates.

Motion is the business of joints and all articular structures play a role in this activity. Foremost among them is the articular cartilage that covers and cushions the opposing joint surfaces. In most joints the areas of the surfaces are disparate, in order to permit a smaller concave surface to slide across the larger opposing convexity (e.g., the tibial plateaus beneath the femoral condyles or the proximal phalanges over the metacarpal or metatarsal heads). In any one position, then, the concave member is always opposed by another cartilaginous surface, whereas a large portion of the convex surface faces synovium. Exactly which portion faces synovium will depend on the degree of flexion of the joint. These elementary principles are of practical interest for two reasons: First, the rich vasculature of the synovium may provide more effective nutritional support to the subjacent convex cartilage than to its concave mate, which could help account for the greater thickness of the convex articular cartilage that usually prevails in the central, load-bearing areas of the joint.[17] Second, the cyclic, covering and uncovering of cartilage by synovium, carries with it a threat of catching, pinching, and bleeding if the compliant synovial tissue fails to slide out of the way. Swann et al. pointed out some years ago, that the problem of synovium-on-cartilage lubrication is a low shear problem and it differs in this respect from the lubrication of the cartilage-on-cartilage interface.[18] As such, it may be particularly amenable to lubrication by SF hyaluronan (HA).

The normal motion of joints is constrained by the limits of available cartilage surface in any one axis of motion and by the corresponding ligamentous checkreins that enforce this restriction. Within the range of motion of each joint, its usage usually involves a to-and-fro reciprocity that presumably provides effective mixing of the small volume of SF it contains. It seems reasonable to presume that this convective 'stirring' greatly supplements the diffusive transport of small solutes throughout the joint space; however, this assumption has not been tested.

Convective mixing may be important not only in the transport of smaller metabolites to and from cartilage, but also in the clearance of larger molecules from the joint. Levick[19] has shown that the clearance of HA infused into stationary rabbit joints slows progressively over time and that this slowing is accompanied by a deceleration in the efflux of water. He quite reasonably attributes this phenomenon to an accumulating fiber matrix or 'filter cake' of entangled HA macromolecules that impedes access to the intrasynovial capillaries and lymphatics through the interstitial path between synovial lining cells, and likens this experience to the simple, but fruitless, task of trying to force SF through a millipore filter.[19] It seems reasonable to suspect that the normal shearing motion of surface over surface, limits the filter cake buildup in active joints, but this needs confirmation.

Transport of drugs

One group of small molecules is of special concern to students of OA. These are the pharmacologic agents that are used to alleviate the symptoms of the disease. Nonsteroidal anti-inflammatory drugs (NSAIDs) are of interest because, for the most part, they are sparingly soluble in water and highly (99 per cent or more) bound to albumin in human P. This degree of binding has been established by testing, using ultrafiltration and/or equilibrium dialysis techniques. Since, as discussed below, albumin is largely retained within the normal synovial microvessels, it would seem likely that highly bound drugs would be effectively denied access to the joint space. The issue had been examined directly for most marketed NSAIDs, however, and it is obvious that these agents do find their way into the SF of rheumatoid or OA knees with surprising rapidity (Fig. 7.61).[20,21] A compartmental re-analysis of data from 10 such studies used available measurements of blood flows and distribution volumes from presumably comparable human joints, led to an estimate that, on average, 23 per cent of each NSAID left the microcirculation and entered the SF during each passage through the

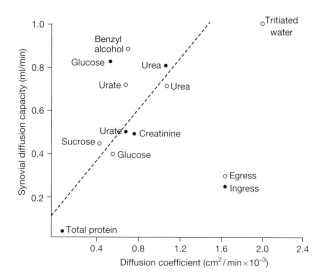

Fig. 7.60 Experimentally determined transynovial exchange. Regression is based on data for urea, creatinine, urate, and all ^{14}C-labeled molecules. Rapid rates for physiologic glucose and for benzyl alcohol are attributed to facilitated diffusion and to lipid solubility, respectively. Exchange of tritiated water falls below the regression and may be limited by synovial blood flow. Rate for total protein was plotted using the diffusion coefficient of albumin.

Source: Taken from Ref. 4, p. 585.

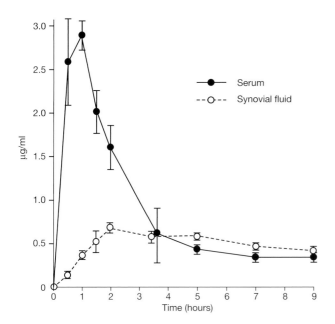

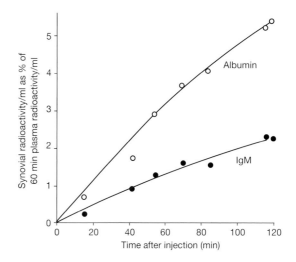

Fig. 7.61 Serial determinations of the concentration of indomethacin in serum and synovial fluid after a single 50 mg dose of the drug. Data are mean values ± SEM of 8 trials in 7 patients.

Source: Taken from Ref. 21, p. 434.

Fig. 7.62 Trace amounts of ^{131}I-labelled IgM and ^{125}I-labelled albumin were injected intravenously. Radioactivities were measured in the serum 60 minutes later and in serial synovial fluid aspirates obtained at the times indicated. The experiment shows that albumin entered the knee effusion more rapidly than IgM.

Source: Taken from Ref. 23, p. 649.

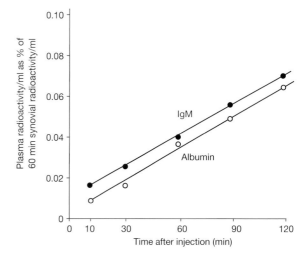

Fig. 7.63 ^{131}I-labelled IgM and ^{125}I-labelled albumin were injected into a rheumatoid knee effusion. Radioactivities were measured in a synovial aspirate 60 minutes later and in serial samples of serum obtained at the times indicated. The experiment suggests that albumin and IgM moved from the joint into the serum at the same rate.

Source: Taken from Ref. 23, p. 649.

tissue.[22] This rate is close to that which would be expected if the drug molecules did not interact with albumin.

The most probable explanation for this seeming discrepancy is that NSAIDs bind to albumin with high affinity but low avidity, that is, although most molecules of the NSAID are bound to albumin at any specific moment, any individual molecule may bind and release many times during the (approximately) one second that an aliquot of blood resides within the synovial microvasculature. Such a mechanism would give that molecule ample opportunity to escape across the endothelial barrier and begin its cycle of attachment and release with the extravascular albumin it would encounter in the interstitial space. Thus, albumin 'binding', rather than being a hindrance, may facilitate overall drug transport by greatly enhancing solubility, while interfering only minimally with access to the joint. A carrier mechanism of this type is somewhat analogous to the system by which oxygen is delivered to needy peripheral tissues by binding to intravascular (and also intracellular) hemoglobin.

Transport of proteins

The P constituents larger than approximately 12 000 Daltons cannot cross the fenestrae. Instead, they move by convection through the 'small' and 'large' apertures between endothelial cells or by transport through endothelial vessicles. The 'small' pathway is progressively more restrictive throughout the size range of most P proteins allowing albumin, for example, to enter the joint more easily than a large protein, such as α_2-macroglobulin (Fig. 7.62).[23] The situation is quite different on the outflow side of the equation, where these same proteins leave the joint at comparable rates through the lymphatic system (Fig. 7.63).[23–25] The net effect of this balance between a size-selective influx and a bulk flow efflux is that the concentration ratios of SF over P are all less than 1.0 for P proteins. In normal joints, SF/P approaches 1.0 at the small end of the molecular weight scale and nears 0 for much larger molecules, such as fibrinogen.[26] The same protein may have differing SF/P values in different normal joints, as was shown to be the case for four different P proteins in human hips and knees (Fig. 7.64).[27,28] This reflects a greater lymphatic efflux (relative to P protein influx) in the knee

than in the hip. Such between-joint differences are commonplace in studies of articular physiology. They remind us again of the dearth of data from the base of the thumb and the distal interphalangeal joints, in which OA is so common. It remains entirely plausible that normal between-joint differences play an important role in 'arthrotropism' that leads each rheumatic disease to have its own distinct pattern of spared and vulnerable joints.[29]

There has been considerable interest in the past in whether molecular charge may affect SF/P. Haptoglobin, in particular, is thought to be excluded from the joint space by its positive charge.[30] Further studies are needed in this area, but the evidence to date suggests that charge is a relatively minor factor.

Things are different when inflammatory disease affects the joint. Then, both blood flow to the synovium and lymphatic outflow from the joint

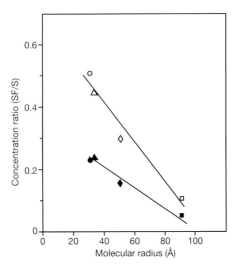

Fig. 7.64 Mean ratios of the synovial fluid to serum concentration for four plasma proteins that varied in molecular size, as indicated in the figure. Ratios for synovial fluid in normal hips are shown as open symbols and in normal knees by closed symbols. The differences between the two joint sites are highly significant and reflect underlying differences in the vascular physiology of these joints. The exact nature of those differences is not yet understood and their possible implications regarding differences in susceptibility to rheumatic diseases have not been studied.

Source: Taken from Ref. 28, p. 72.

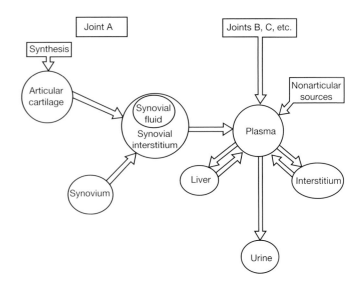

Fig. 7.65 In a hypothetical knee (joint A), cartilage matrix turnover reflects the balance between ongoing synthesis and loss. 'Lost' molecules enter the synovial fluid and equilibrate throughout the synovial interstitium. Degradation, which can potentially occur at many sites, produces putative 'marker' molecules that are cleared from the joint into the plasma by the lymphatics. In plasma, the markers mix with similar molecules from other joints as well as from nonarticular sources. From the plasma, marker molecules may redistribute into other interstitial spaces, may be further processed (primarily in the liver), or may be excreted into the urine. The literature on cartilage markers consists mainly of measurements of concentration in synovial fluid and plasma.

Source: Taken from Ref. 34, p. 349.

increase.[5,6,8] The most marked change, however, is an increase in the number of 'large' pore sites in the endothelium of synovial microvessels. The net effect is an increase in SF/P for total protein content, with much larger relative increases in the SF concentration of large rather than small proteins.[6] All inflamed joints are not alike, however, because the major determining factors of blood flow, vascular permeability, and lymphatic drainage are independent of each other. These variations occur within any one disease and between different types of arthritis. In rheumatoid arthritis (RA), for example, synovial blood flow may be significantly increased or may be so low that it fails to meet local demand, with resultant articular ischemia.[31] Concurrently, vascular permeability and lymphatic drainage may both increase markedly. In OA, the magnitude of both of these factors is usually lower than in RA, but the balance is such that SF/P in OA is not significantly different from that in RA. For this reason, the SF protein concentration holds very little diagnostic value in routine clinical practice.[32] It must be recognized, however, that this generalization is based on data from OA knees with significant effusions. Many of these joints may be altered by important, but clinically unrecognized, phlogistic factors, such as crystals of hydroxyapatite.[33] The picture might be quite different if fluid were routinely sampled from OA joints that are not swollen.

'Marker' physiology

Much current interest in OA centers around the measurement of 'markers' that may provide quantitative evidence of ongoing catabolic or anabolic processes in articular cartilage of the affected joint. The basic premise of such efforts is that tissue-specific constituents will be released as a result of local disease processes (e.g., increased synthesis or increased degradation of cartilage matrix macromolecules in quantities far in excess of those in normal tissue). In OA, the search for such markers has focused mainly on constituents of articular cartilage. Candidate markers may be measured in the SF from individual affected joints, in serum, or urine (Fig. 7.65).[34] Specific examples are discussed in Chapter 11.4.7, and will not be considered here. Rather, the following discussion will focus on the physiologic principles and experimental tools that are relevant to the interpretation of the SF data.

With rare exceptions, the marker data consist of determinations of the *concentration* of the putative marker molecule in aspirates of SF from the human knee. As such, they can be likened to snapshots of a busy intersection. They tell us what is there at the time of joint aspiration but provide no information about where it is going or how fast it is moving. Each vehicle or pedestrian in the snapshot may be stationary or may be moving at high speed, but this cannot be discerned from the still frame that one sees. So, too, the concentration of a marker in SF cannot be used alone as an indicator of the amount of that molecule entering the joint space per unit time. Consider, for example, measurements of a given marker that yield identical values in the knees of two patients. The snapshots look the same. But if one is from the knee of a typical patient with RA, the traffic will be moving essentially twice as fast as in the other knee, if the latter is the knee of a patient with OA. Furthermore, twice as much of the marker will be undergoing release from the cartilage of the RA joint, as from the OA joint. Thus, the two knee joints are very different from each other. This problem can be countered experimentally by combining the joint aspiration with the concurrent determination of articular kinetics. Radiolabeled albumin, for example, may be injected into the joint space and followed by serial external counting.[6,24,25] This simple experiment yields a trove of useful information.

After a period of time to permit distribution of the radionuclide throughout the intracapsular space (which may take as long as 8 hours in the knees of some patients with RA), the external counting data will plot as a linear monoexponential rate. The slope of this line can be expressed in min^{-1} or per cent/min as the *clearance constant* for albumin from that knee. Alternatively, the same rate may be expressed as the *half-life* for albumin. (All counts are corrected for the physical half-life of the radioactive label, so that the half-life determined experimentally is the biological half-life in that specific joint.)

When the regression line is extrapolated back to the time of injection, the intercept will yield the counts per minute per ml in the fully equilibrated joint. Because the total number of injected counts is known and the counts that have left the joint can be determined from the regression, it is a simple matter to calculate by mass balance the articular *volume* occupied by the remaining isotope. Note that the relevant volume here is not simply that of the SF but that of all the interstitial water in the intracapsular space. Since the synovium has no basement membrane to divide the joint space from the intracapsular interstitium, this is the volume that is served by the synovial microvessels and lymphatics (Fig. 7.66). This larger space, rather than the SF volume, is presumably the space throughout which marker molecules from cartilage will distribute. It is also a volume that has been found to be constant over as long as 72 hours in ambulatory patients (Fig. 7.67).[6] Therefore, the joint capsule, at least that of the human knee, defines a discrete and stable interstitial compartment.

When the articular volume (ml) is multiplied by the clearance constant (min^{-1}), the product is the *clearance* (ml/min) of that specific solute from that specific joint. Clearance is the volume of articular water that is cleared

of a marker molecule per unit time. Note the reciprocity inherent in this formulation: the clearance rate for a joint with a large effusion but a low clearance constant, that is, a long half-life, may be identical to that for a joint that is not swollen and has a high clearance constant. For albumin and other like-sized molecules having access to terminal lymphatics, the clearance values should be the same and should reflect the synovial lymph flow. Because much larger molecules (such as HA and large fragments of aggrecan) appear to have size-restricted lymphatic access, their clearance will be less than the lymph flow.[35,36] Conversely, molecules much smaller than 12 kD (e.g., many cytokines) may diffuse through fenestrae and return through the microvessels and the lymphatics. We would expect, therefore, that their clearance would be faster than the rate of lymphatic flow. The knowledge of cytokine clearance from diseased joints is of substantial interest because it would help quantify the rate of production and release of the cytokine within the joint; however, such data have not yet been obtained.

Finally, the product of the clearance (ml/min) and the concentration of a solute (mg/ml) give the *flux* (mg/min) or the mass of that solute leaving the SF to return to the circulation. Because an ongoing equilibrium is generally assumed, the flux out of the joint should equal the flux into the joint. In the case of a cartilaginous matrix molecule, this would be the 'holy grail' of marker science, that is, the mass of a specific constituent that is released into the joint per unit time. Much more would have to be known about the specific marker, of course, to know whether it comes from the breakdown of mature cartilage, from new active synthesis, or from a combination of the two. Serial quantitation of decreasing marker flux, that is, a reduction in the release rate, would confer substantial support for claims of benefit from therapeutic interventions for OA of the knee.

Articular lubrication

A quite different aspect of synovial physiology involves the remarkable system of lubrication, that enables one articular surface to slide easily across its mate at an energy cost in friction that is less than that attained by the finest comparable bearings made of polished metal on plastic or glass.[37] Even more impressive is the fact that this living bearing normally sustains and repairs itself throughout a lifespan of 100 years or more. When this system fails, however, friction increases and with that change comes wear. As the process proceeds, matrix synthesis can no longer keep pace with matrix loss, the cartilage surface is progressively destroyed, and the failed bearing develops the features that we recognize clinically as end-stage OA. This simple (and, of course, oversimplified) model implies that it is imperative for serious students of OA to understand the normal lubrication system in order to develop therapeutic strategies that will help reduce wear, promote renewal, and thus prolong the useful lifetime of the normal human joint.

The best-characterized component of the normal system of lubrication is the boundary layer lubricant, lubricin. This glycoprotein was first isolated from SF and characterized by Swann *et al.* more than 20 years ago.[18,38] Current molecular techniques have permitted full sequencing of its protein core, recognition of its parent gene, tracing its origin to synovial fibroblasts, and identification of two other products, including the SZP (superficial zone protein) of cartilage, that are derived from the same gene.[39] Still to come, one hopes, are a more complete characterization of the 'glyco' components of this glycoprotein, specific tools to assess the quantity and quality of lubricin in normal and diseased joints, a more thorough assessment of its possible interactions with HA and phospholipids, comparative studies in other species, and ultimate clinical strategies that would augment and preserve this biologic protector of normal human bearings.

Boundary layer lubricants, such as lubricin, reduce friction and wear by providing a smooth and slippery coating for the contact surfaces, just as a layer of ice may coat a winter sidewalk. Complementary to this mechanism is an important additional component: hydrodynamic lubrication. Such a system reduces friction by allowing one bearing surface to ride freely over the other on an interposed film of protecting fluid. The magnificent design of articular cartilage permits this tissue to utilize this mechanism to provide the largest measure of its own protection. Because its matrix is both

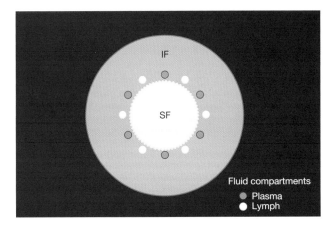

Fig. 7.66 Schematic representation of the free synovial fluid within the joint space (SF) and of the interstitial fluid within synovial tissue (IF). These adjoining spaces are best considered as a single interstitial compartment served by the same microvasculature and drained by the same lymphatic vessels.

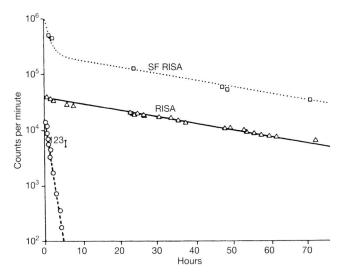

Fig. 7.67 Kinetics of isotope removal. Semilogarithmic plot of activity over time for ^{123}I and ^{131}I-labeled human serum albumin (RISA) after introduction into the stable knee effusion of an individual with OA. Externally monitored radioactivity of RISA (Δ) and ^{123}I(O) describes monoexponential plots with the intra-articular half-life of RISA approximately 36 times greater than that of ^{123}I. Synovial fluid (SF) RISA activity (□), counts/minute/ml, declined rapidly (distribution phase) and subsequently paralleled externally monitored RISA at 24 hours.

Source: Taken from Ref. 7, p. 445.

fluid-filled and compressible, loaded cartilage expresses fluid from its surface when the joint is in motion. This expressed fluid may separate each cartilage from its mate. As a femoral condyle, for instance, glides over a tibial plateau, it exudes water ahead of its own advancing contact surface, thus 'greasing the skids' for low friction service. This process was literally frozen in time by Clark and his colleagues in experiments of appealing simplicity.[40] His experimental design permits normal rabbit joints to be loaded *in vitro*, immersed in liquid nitrogen, fixed *in situ*, sectioned, and then examined by scanning electron microscopy. His studies confirm the normal compression of cartilage under load and shows that this process smooths the cartilagenous surfaces and increases the congruence of the opposing loaded areas. Most important, it reveals a continuous 100 nm thick film of fluid that separates one cartilage surface from the other and thereby prevents direct, abrasive contact.

Where does HA, a molecule synthesized in abundance by the normal synovial lining, fit in this picture? This huge molecular constituent confers the most conspicuous characteristic of normal SF—its striking viscosity. It is intuitively attractive to believe that more viscous fluids will be more slippery and, therefore, better lubricants. This is largely untrue, however, of the boundary layer mechanism. Test systems that focus on this aspect, such as the cartilage-on-glass system of Swann *et al.*[38] show that lysis of HA with hyaluronidase has no significant effect, but that friction increases substantially when the bathing SF is pretreated with proteolytic enzymes and lubricin is destroyed. When the cartilage-on-cartilage bearing of the intact joint is studied, however, HA does become important.[41] This observation seems entirely consistent with the hydrodynamic aspect of joint lubrication. Articular motion, of course, is inherently cyclic and the flow of viscous SF is much slower than the flow of water. HA would seem most valuable in minimizing outflow within the interposed film of fluid during the brief period when an area of cartilage is under a moving load.

The clinical connotations of these concepts remain confusing. We perceive friction in our patients' joints mainly through crepitus, but this measure is so coarse that most crepitant joints must already be well down the road toward bearing failure. By history, by examination, and in the laboratory, we currently have no tools that permit us to recognize those less symptomatic joints with increased friction that are likely to wear out soonest. The available evidence suggests, however, that accelerated wear will most likely occur in joints that are affected by inflammatory disease. In symptomatic joints of patients with RA, for example, metalloproteinase activity may limit the effectiveness of lubricin, while the quantity and quality of HA are obviously diminished. Perhaps the 'robust rheumatoid' patient who remains physically active but loses cartilage, exemplifies a setting in which the rheumatologist should be more concerned about articular friction and wear.

In contrast to inflammatory disease, there is less reason to expect increased friction in the OA joint, since the quantity and quality of HA are relatively preserved and lubricin seems less likely to be attacked by proteolytic enzymes. Nonetheless, it is in OA where most efforts to limit wear are now being directed. Loss of excess body weight and simple off-loading measures seem to be effective and obviously make sense in any articular disease. What, however, is the appropriate rationale for the serial HA injections that are now used so widely in treatment of patient with painful knee OA? Although this is the sole intervention intended to provide needed lubrication to diseased human joints, a serious flaw exists in the logic. The operant concept that such visco-supplementation will 'restore rheological homeostasis' seems clearly at variance with the many studies demonstrating the relatively rapid efflux and limited articular residence of the injected HA[42] (see Chapter 9.8).

In the history of any affected knee, each HA injection would seem to be little more than a very temporary patch in a long, bumpy road. Yet, this procedure has been reported to help many patients. Do the injections induce some abiding effect on the cartilage matrix, the chondrocyte, the synovium, or some other articular component that ultimately leads to less wear of cartilage and a longer bearing life? If one of these possibilities turns out to be true, this therapy will help our patients and add to our knowledge of how normal joints work and why they fail in disease.

Summary

The human synovium supports normal articular function primarily by providing vascular support to distant chondrocytes and by facilitating low-friction movement between opposing cartilaginous surfaces under load. In OA, these functions may be impaired and the synovial fluid assumes additional roles in the dispersion of therapeutic agents to cellular targets and as a pathway for clearance of catabolites from the articular cartilage. Although some progress has been made, much remains to be learned about these functions in normal and degenerating joints.

Key points

1. A simple radioisotopic technique can be used to concurrently quantify clearances of free iodide and iodinated albumin from human knees *in vivo*. As indices of synovial plasma flow and lymphatic drainage, respectively, these values provide powerful tools for assessment of microvascular pathophysiology in this tissue.

2. How can NSAIDs bind strongly to intravascular albumin and still be effective against extravascular inflammation? A compartmental analysis of kinetic data demonstrates good access of these drugs to the joint space and provides an explanation, based on the important distinction between affinity and avidity of protein–drug interactions.

3. Although the patterns of preferentially involved and spared joints vary widely among various types of arthritis, the physiologic bases for these distinctions remain unknown. Plausible working hypotheses are available for two examples: the predilection of gouty arthritis for the base of the great toe and of osteonecrosis for the head of the femur.

4. Although studies of synovial fluid and serum 'markers' of cartilage catabolism are necessary and appropriate, concentration-based analyses have important limitations in comparison with more relevant kinetics-based analyses.

5. Although intra-articular injections of hyaluronan are now used widely in the treatment of OA, their efficacy remains in question.

References

(An asterisk denotes recommended reading.)

1. **O'Rahilly, R. and Gardner, E.** (1978). The embryology of movable joints. In: L. Sokoloff (ed). *The Joints and Synovial Fluid* (Vol 1). New York: Academic Press, pp. 49–103.

2. **Simkin, P.A. and Nilson, K.L.** (1981). Trans-synovial exchange of large and small molecules. *Clin Rheum Dis* **7**:99–129.

3. **Simkin, P.A.** (1977). The pathogenesis of podagra. *Ann Intern Med* **86**:230–3.

4. **Simkin, P.A. and Pizzorno, J.R.** (1974). Transynovial exchange of small molecules in normal human subjects. *J Appl Physiol* **36**:581–7.

5. **Wallis, W.J., Simkin, P.A., and Nelp, W.B.** (1985). Low synovial clearance of iodide provides evidence of hypoperfusion in chronic rheumatoid synovitis. *Arthritis Rheum* **28**:1096–1104.

6. **Wallis, W.J., Simkin, P.A., and Nelp, W.B.** (1987). Protein traffic in human synovial effusions. *Arthritis Rheum* **30**:57–63.

7. *Wallis, W.J., Simkin, P.A., Nelp, W.B., and Foster, D.M.** (1985). Intraarticular volume and clearance in human synovial effusions. *Arthritis Rheum* **28**:441–9.

   This paper introduced a radioisotopic technique that concurrently quantifies clearances of free iodide and of iodinated albumin from human knees in vivo. As respective indices of synovial plasma flow and lymphatic drainage, these values provide powerful tools for assessment of microvascular pathophysiology in this tissue.

8. **Simkin, P.A.** (1979). Synovial permeability in rheumatoid arthritis. *Arthritis Rheum* **22**:689–96.

9. **Levick, J.R. and Smaje, L.H.** (1987). An analysis of the permeability of a fenestra. *Microvasc Res* **33**:233–56.

10. Schumacher, H.R. (1969). The microvasculature of the synovial membrane of the monkey: Ultrastructural studies. *Arthritis Rheum* **12**:387–404.

11. Levick, J.R. (1987). Synovial fluid and trans-synovial flow in stationary and moving joints. In: H. Helminen, I. Kiviranta, M. Tammia, A.M. Saamaren, K. Paukonnen, and J. Jurvelin (eds). *Joint Loading: Biology and Health of Articular Structures*. Bristol: Wright & Sons, pp. 149–86.

12. Rovensk, E. und Hüttl S. (1987). Mikrocirkul cia synovi lnej blanyultraštrúktura lymfatickej mikrovaskulatúry. *Bratsil Lek Listy* **87**:262–74.

13. Davies, D.V. and Edwards, D.A.W. (1948). The blood supply of the synovial membrane and intra-articular structures. *Ann R Coll Surg Engl* **2**: 142–56.

14. Ropes, M.W., Muller, A.P., and Bauer, W. (1960). The entrance of glucose and other sugars into joints. *Arthritis Rheum* **3**:496–513.

15. Ogata, K., Whiteside, L.A., and Lesker, P.A. (1978). Subchondral route for nutrition to articular cartilage in the rabbit. Measurement of diffusion with hydrogen gas in vivo. *J Bone Joint Surg Am* **60**:905–10.

16. McKibbin, B. and Maroudas, A. (1979). Nutrition and metabolism. In: M.A.R. Freeman, (ed.) *Adult Articular Cartilage* (2nd ed). London: Pitman Medical, pp. 461–86.

17. Kurrat, H.J. and Oberlander, W. (1978). The thickness of the cartilage in the hip joint. *J Anat* **126**:145–55.

18. Swann, D.A., Radin, E.L., Nazimiec, M., Weisser, P.A., Curran, N., and Lewinnek, G. (1974). Role of hyaluronic acid in joint lubrication. *Ann Rheum Dis* **33**:318–26.

19. Levick, J.R. and McDonald, J.N. (1995). Fluid movement across synovium in healthy joints: role of synovial fluid macromolecules. *Ann Rheum Dis* **54**:417–23.

20. Wallis, W.J. and Simkin, P.A. (1983). Antirheumatic drug concentrations in human synovial fluid and synovial tissue: observations on extravascular pharmacokinetics. *Clin Pharmocokinet* **8**:496–522.

21. Emori, H.W., Champion, G.D., Bluestone, R., and Paulus, H.E. (1973). Simultaneous pharmacokinetics of indomethacin in serum and synovial fluid. *Ann Rheum Dis* **32**:433–5.

22. *Simkin, P.A., Wu, M., and Foster, D. (1993). Articular kinetics of protein-bound antirheumatic drugs. *Clin Pharmacokin* **25**:342–50.

   How can nonsteroidal anti-inflammatory drugs bind strongly to intravascular albumin and still be effective in suppressing extravascular inflammation? This paper analyzes kinetic data demonstrating good access of these drugs to the joint space and provides an explanation based on the important distinction between affinity and avidity in protein-drug interactions.

23. Brown, D.L., Cooper, A.G., and Bluestone, R. (1969). Exchange of IgM and albumin between plasma and synovial fluid in rheumatoid arthritis. *Ann Rheum Dis* **28**:644–51.

24. Rodnan, G.P. and MacLachlan, M.J. (1960). The absorption of serum albumin and gamma globulin from the knee joint of man and rabbit. *Arthritis Rheum* **3**:152–7.

25. Sliwinski, A.F. and Zvaifler, N.J. (1969). The removal of aggregated and nonaggregated autologous gamma globulin from rheumatoid joints. *Arthritis Rheum* **12**:504–14.

26. Kushner, I. and Somerville, J.A. (1971). Permeability of human synovial membrane to plasma proteins: relationship to molecular size and inflammation. *Arthritis Rheum* **14**:560–70.

27. Reimann, I., Arnoldi, C.C., and Neilsen, S. (1980). Permeability of synovial membrane to plasma proteins in human coxarthrosis. *Clin Ortho* **147**:296–300.

28. Weinberger, A. and Simkin, P.A. (1989). Plasma proteins in synovial fluids of normal human joints. *Sem Arthritis Rheum* **19**:66–76.

29. *Simkin, P.A. (1995). Why this joint and why not that joint? *Scand J Rheumatol* **24**(Suppl. 101):13–6.

   Although the patterns of preferentially involved and spared joints vary widely among articular diseases, the physiologic bases for these distinctions remain unknown. This paper provides working hypotheses for two examples (the predilection of gouty arthritis for the base of the great toe and of osteonecrosis for the femoral head) and calls for a more careful study of differences in physiology and pathophysiology among various joint sites.

30. Sundblad, L., Jonsson, E., and Nettelbladt, E. (1961). Permeability of the synovial membrane to glycoproteins. *Nature* **192**:1192.

31. Simkin, P.A. and Wallis W.J. (1985). Microvascular physiology of the rheumatoid synovium. In: N. Zvaifler, P. Uttsinger, and G. Ehrlich (eds)

Rheumatoid Arthritis: Etiology, Diagnosis, Management. Philadelphia: Lippincott JB, pp. 181–92.

32. Shmerling, R.H., Delbanco, T.L., Tosteson, A.N. and Trentham, D.E. (1990). Synovial fluid tests. What should be ordered? *JAMA* **264**:1009–14.

33. Myers, S.L., O'Connor, B.L., and Brandt, K.D. (1996). Accelerated clearance of albumin from the osteoathritic knee: implications for interpretation of concentrations of 'cartilage markers' in synovial fluid. *J Rheumatol* **23**:1744–8.

34. *Simkin, P.A. and Bassett, J.E. (1995). Cartilage matrix molecules in serum and synovial fluid. *Curr Opin Rheumatol* **7**:346–51.

   This paper reviews several studies of biologic 'markers' in synovial fluid and plasma and discusses the limitations of concentration-based, as compared to the more relevant kinetics-based, interpretation of such data.

35. Levick, J.R. (1998). A method for estimating macromolecular reflection by human synovium, using measurements of intra-articular half lives. *Ann Rheum Dis* **57**:339–44.

36. Pitsillides, A.A., Will, R.K., Bayliss, M.T., and Edwards, J.C.W. (1994). Circulating and synovial fluid hyaluronan levels: effects of intraarticular corticosteroid on the concentration and the rate of turnover. *Arthritis Rheum* **37**:1030–8.

37. Simkin, P.A. (2000). Friction and lubrication in synovial joints. *J Rheumatol* **27**:567–8.

38. Swann, D.A., Hendren, R.B., Radin, E.L., Sotman, S.L., and Duda, E.A. (1981). The lubricating activity of synovial fluid glycoproteins. *Arthritis Rheum* **24**:22–30.

39. Jay, G.D., Britt, D.E., and Cha, C.J. (2000). Lubricin is a product of megakaryocyte stimulating factor gene expression by human synovial fibroblasts. *J Rheumatol* **27**:594–600.

40. Clark, J.M., Norman, A.G., Kaab, M.J., and Notzli, H.P. (1999). The surface contour of articular cartilage in an intact, loaded joint. *J Anat* **195**:45–56.

41. Mabuchi, K., Obara, T., Ikegami, K., Yamaguchi, T., and Kanayama, T. (1999). Molecular weight independence of the effect of additive hyaluronic acid on the lubricating characteristics in synovial joints with experimental deterioration. *Clin Biomech* **14**:352–6.

42. *Brandt, K.D., Smith, G.N. Jr, and Simon, L.S. (2000). Intraarticular injection of hyaluronan as treatment for knee osteoarthritis. What is the evidence? *Arthritis Rheum* **43**:1192–1203.

   Although hyaluronan injections are now used widely in the treatment of large joint OA, their efficacy remains in question. This critical review examines the rationale for such therapy and the evidence for and against their clinical utility.

7.2.4 Neuromuscular system

7.2.4.1 Innervation of the joint and its role in osteoarthritis

Joel A. Vilensky

The classical view pertaining to the relationship between the nervous system and joints is that neural elements simply transmit sensation, both noxious and proprioceptive, to the central nervous system (CNS). However, there is now abundant evidence that articular afferent nerves contribute to inflammatory processes within joints and, accordingly, modify the response characteristics of the nerves themselves, thereby increasing or decreasing joint pain. Similarly, evidence suggests that the sympathetic control of articular blood vessels may affect the pathologic processes associated with OA.

Joint protection is traditionally assumed to rely on afferent nerves activating surrounding muscles that act via reflexes to maintain joint movements, within the safe boundaries of excursion. Such actions presumably prevent joint instability, which may lead to the development of OA. However, data from humans with neuropathies and from deafferentation studies in animals, suggest that ipsilateral afferent nerves (and thereby joint proprioceptive output) are probably not critically important to the integrity of stable joints during normal activities. Rather, neural networks (central pattern generators, CPGs) appear capable of protecting normal joints by programming their range of excursion within 'safe' boundaries without concurrent sensory input.

Innervation of joints

Articular nerves

Articular nerves are composed of myelinated sensory axons (about 20 per cent), unmyelinated sensory axons (about 40 per cent) and vasomotor axons (about 40 per cent).[1,2] The myelinated axons (2–17 μm in diameter, with a conduction speed that is inversely correlated with the diameter) convey impulses from mechanoreceptors, specialized nerve endings within joint tissues that respond to changes in pressure and tension.[3–6] The unmyelinated axons in articular nerves consist of very small (< 2 μm) fibres that carry impulses from widely distributed free (pain) nerve endings and sympathetic efferent fibres that regulate blood flow.[5,6] Most free nerve endings are inactive during normal circumstances. They do not respond to movement, but show activity upon abnormal deformation or upon exposure to chemical agents, for example, inflammatory mediators.[7] Furthermore, vasoactive neuropeptides (e.g., substance P, calcitonin gene-related peptide) are localized within these free nerve endings, from which they are released into the intercellular space upon stimulation of the nerve. These neuropeptides are associated with the transmission of nociceptive information, and also affect the intra-articular environment by causing vasodilation and increasing venular permeability.[5]

Articular receptors

Various forms of mechanoreceptors have been described in joint tissues, and their differences in morphology and response characteristics have been related to functional specializations (e.g., type I (Ruffini) receptors are thought to function as stretch receptors, whereas type II (Pacini) receptors appear to be stimulated by compression (Figs 7.68 and 7.69 and see Ref. 5, for more details about these receptors). Although the physiologic properties of these receptors are well defined, their role in joint biomechanics is not. The difficulty in defining that role is due partly to the relative scarcity of these receptors. For example, the entire anterior cruciate ligament (ACL) of a three-year-old child was found to contain only 17 mechanoreceptors.[8] However, the scarcity of mechanoreceptors may not reflect their relative importance. Furthermore, no consensus exists on how to classify the many different types of mechanoreceptors that have been described. Some investigators have suggested that the various types simply represent a continuum, with the variability related to the specific requirements associated with each locale.[5] It is also possible that the many reports describing different types of mechanoreceptors reflect the erroneous belief that certain stains (e.g., gold chloride) are specific for neural structures, whereas they also stain other articular elements, such as vascular structures and collagen.[5,9] Therefore, although there is no doubt that joints contain receptors sensitive to various types of tissue deformation, the size, shape, and number of these structures within various tissues of the joint, and whether different articular tissues contain functionally different combinations of these structures, are unclear.

Functional aspects of nerves and receptors

How joint mechanoreceptors affect joint movements is also unclear. Most studies that have addressed this question have analysed the reflex effects on muscles surrounding the knee[5] after stimulation of sensory nerve endings in the ACL. For example, Pope et al.[10] used wire-induced traction on the ACL in an anaesthetized cat to examine reflex effects on the quadriceps and

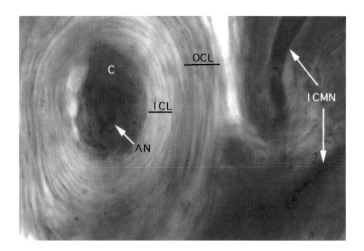

Fig. 7.68 Large type II (Pacini) nerve ending from the posterior meniscofemoral ligament of the canine knee. This ending is folded on itself. ICMN, intra-capsular myelinated axon; OCL, outer circumferential lamella; ICL, inner circumferential lamella; C, central core; AN, axis neurite (unmyelinated). Gold chloride stain. Original ×320.

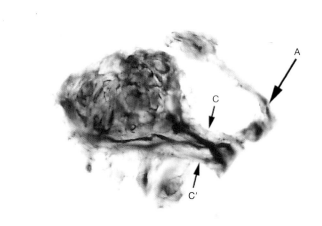

Fig. 7.69 A type I (Ruffini) nerve ending from the medial collateral ligament of knee of a cat. A, node of Ranvier of parent axon; C, C', capsule surrounding three myelinated terminal intracapsular axons. Original ×320.

hamstring muscles. Surprisingly, with forces as high as 125 newtons (4–5 times body weight) no effect on the electromyographic responses of the muscles could be demonstrated, despite evidence of normal reactivity of other reflexes (e.g., tendon taps, paw pinches). In contrast, Raunest et al.[11] found, in agreement with the results of a prior study,[12] that static and dynamic loading of the ACL in sheep resulted in significant increases in the level of activity of the quadriceps and hamstring muscles as measured by electromyography. Furthermore, recordings from articular nerves have revealed activity during movement, especially near the extremes of the range of joint excursion,[4] implying that mechanoreceptors act primarily to protect the joint from hyperflexion, hyperextension, and over-rotation. However, Johannsson et al.[4] concluded that the amount of time needed for impulses from these mechanoreceptors to activate the contraction of the muscles that could provide such protection (i.e., generate sufficient force to brake the ongoing movement) is too long to prevent the potentially damaging movements and suggested, alternatively, that mechanoreceptors assure joint stability by acting continuously to regulate the stiffness (tone) of the periarticular muscles. He noted, furthermore, that this hypothesis, which emphasizes the sensory role of ligaments of the knee joint in regulating muscle stiffness, could explain why the surgical treatment of ACL deficiency is often disappointing, that is, sensory feedback from the joint is impaired by the injury, or by the ligament repair or reconstruction.

The role of joint receptors in conscious position sense (proprioception) is also controversial, possibly because of the variability in methodologies among studies.[5] Schaible and Grubb[7] questioned whether any conscious perception of joint position originates within joints, implying that muscle and skin receptors are responsible for this sensation (see Chapter 7.2.4.3).

Theoretically, joint pain can arise from nociceptors residing in all joint tissues except articular cartilage, which is aneural. Recently, Dieppe[13] proposed that the severe joint pain associated with OA may originate primarily from the nerves located within the subchondral bone, which are stimulated by increased intraosseous pressure. Studies by Arnoldi et al.,[14] using intraosseous phlebography, provide clear evidence of the severe intraosseous statis of blood flow that may occur in OA. In other studies, the same investigators[15] documented the marked increase in intramedullary pressure in the femoral head and neck of patients with hip OA and the striking decrease in pressure that occurred promptly after intertrochanteric osteotomy.

Nevertheless, after a lower extremity injury, patients often complain of unsteadiness (giving-way) of the joint. It seems reasonable that this sensation arises in mechanoreceptors located in capsular/ligamentous structures.[5]

Inflammation greatly accentuates the transmission of pain sensation from a joint. In the presence of inflammation, articular afferent fibres exhibit increased sensitivity. Under these conditions, normally innocuous movements generate increased neural activity, which is perceived as pain. The increase in neural impulses is due to the heightened reactivity of receptors that normally respond to innocuous movements, and by the activation of nociceptors, which normally do not respond to these movements (hyperalgesia).[7] Additionally, joints appear to contain 'silent nociceptors' that become mechanosensitive in the presence of local inflammation.[7] Pain is often induced or increased when the diseased joint is loaded (weight-bearing), or with movement, although pain may occur in the immobilized or unloaded joint (rest pain[7]). Presumably, rest pain results from the responses of joint nociceptors to increased pressure or inflammatory mediators, or from an increase in the sensitivity of spinal or supraspinal neurons.[16] Because abolition or inhibition of the sensitizing process within the joint may provide a means of reducing pain, possible causes of this increased sensitivity are relevant (see below).

Increased sensitivity in joints

Intra-articular pressure

Although only a small quantity of synovial fluid can be aspirated from the normal human knee,[17] large quantities can often be aspirated from diseased joints. This increase in volume is associated with an increase in intra-articular pressure (as much as 36 mm Hg, compared to 0 mm Hg in the normal joint at rest[17]), which may enhance the sensitivity of joint afferents. Bierma-Zeinstra et al.[18] showed a significant relationship between hip pain and hip joint effusion as detected by ultrasonography.

Inflammatory mediators

A variety of inflammatory mediators (prostaglandins, thromboxanes, leukotrienes, kinins, and others) are present in synovial fluid from diseased joints. After intra-articular injection of these mediators, an enhanced response to pressure or chemical stimuli can be demonstrated in joint afferents.[7]

Nonsteroidal anti-inflammatory drugs (NSAIDs) that inhibit cyclooxygenase (COX), prevent the conversion of arachidonic acid into prostaglandins. Within the joint, prostaglandins induce and perpetuate inflammation by causing vasodilation, permitting an influx of additional inflammatory mediators. In addition, they sensitise pain receptors to other inflammatory mediators, such as histamine and bradykinin.[19] NSAIDs have been shown to reduce the levels of prostaglandins and interleukin-6 (a pro-inflammatory cytokine) in synovial fluid of OA knees.[20] This may result in a decrease in

joint pain by reducing the hypersensitivity of afferent fibres in the joint and in the spinal cord.[21,22] Because prostaglandins are also related to the central control of pain sensation, the latter action explains why NSAIDs are also believed to have a direct analgesic effect on the CNS.[19]

It is clear that NSAIDs are not effective in relieving joint pain in all patients with OA, even in those in whom efficacy can be demonstrated. Even with full therapeutic doses of NSAIDs, a substantial amount of residual pain often remains. The reasons for this are unknown. The addition of the analgesic, acetaminophen, in OA patients receiving an NSAID may further reduce the level of pain, consistent with the view that the mechanisms of action of NSAIDs and acetaminophen are different (see Chapter 9.3). Although a retrospective analysis failed to demonstrate that patients with clinical signs of inflammation (i.e., synovial tenderness, effusion) exhibited greater improvement with an anti-inflammatory dose of an NSAID than with an analgesic,[23] the current ACR Guidelines for management of OA suggest that subjects with OA who have more severe synovitis may exhibit greater relief of joint pain with an NSAID than with an analgesic.

Autonomic (sympathetic) nervous system

Joints receive sympathetic innervation, which regulates blood flow in articular arteries. Blood flow to the joint increases after elimination of sympathetic innervation and decreases when articular nerves are electrically stimulated.[7] Furthermore, recent evidence suggests that this neuronal regulation is perhaps more important in joints than in other body structures. In rabbit knees, McDougall et al.[24] demonstrated an absence of the expected reactive hyperemia after release from 5 minutes of femoral artery occulsion. Additionally, changes of systemic blood pressure produced by intravenous infusion or by phlebotomy caused a directly proportional change in blood flow to the knee joint, implying that articular arteries cannot self-regulate their resistance in response to changes in the stretching of the blood vessel wall.

The role of vasomotor control of joint blood flow has recently been investigated in relation to joint injury. McDougall et al.[25] found that after ACL transection, rabbit knees became hyperemic, in association with the early development of OA. Because prior denervation of the articular nerve supply prevented the hyperemia, the vascular changes that occur after ACL transection appeared to be neurogenically mediated.

Neuropeptides and neurogenic inflammation

Afferent fibres containing neuropeptides, such as substance P and calcitonin gene related peptide (CGRP), are commonly found in articular tissues, particularly in association with vascular structures. However, the presence of such fibres at sites in which they are not localized with blood vessels suggests that release of these neuropeptides is also directly involved in inflammatory processes, that is with, 'neurogenic inflammation'.[26] Lam and Ferrell[27] found that the severity of experimentally induced acute joint inflammation was reduced by 44 per cent (as indicated by the quantity of plasma proteins in the joint capsule; an index of vascular permeability) in animals pretreated with capsaicin, which depletes substance P from nerve endings, and by 93 per cent after pretreatment with the substance P antagonist, d-Pro[4],d-Trp[7 9 10]-SP (4–11). Neurogenic inflammation occurs partly as a result of the promotion by neuropeptides, including substance P, of inflammatory cell chemotaxis, neutrophil activation, mast cell degranulation, and fibroblast proliferation—all of which are components of the inflammatory process in joints.[27]

As described above, the presence of these neuropeptides sensitizes joint afferents, thereby increasing joint pain. It has recently been demonstrated that, in contrast to those neuropeptides that increase joint afferent sensitization, other neuropeptides decrease sensitization. In normal and acutely inflamed knee joints of rats, somatostatin (a ubiquitous hormone that inhibits many physiological functions and has anti-inflammatory effects) was shown to decrease the response of articular nerves to noxious movements.[28] In a proportion of afferents, injections of substance P or bradykinin restored the responses. Accordingly, Heppelman and Pawlak[28] hypothesized that the mechanosensitivity of articular afferents in normal joints may be regulated by a balance between pro-inflammatory neuropeptides, such as substance P, and anti-inflammatory peptides, such as somatostatin. In the inflamed joint, the pro-inflammatory peptides predominate, suggesting that the application of somatostatin or its analogues could be used clinically to reduce inflammation and the associated pain. Heppelmann *et al.*[29] demonstrated that intra-articular injection of the neuropeptide, galanin, also reduced the responses to noxious stimuli in the normal and acutely inflamed rat knee.

Joint protection

Ligaments alone cannot prevent joint dislocation during strenuous activity, when forces are generated that can exceed the mechanical strength of the ligament.[4] Coordinated muscular activity has an important role in protecting joints. However, there is some question about the role played by joint afferent nerves in this protective mechanism.

Diseases associated with impairment of joint afferentation

The occurrence of neuropathic (Charcot) arthritis suggests that joint afferent fibres do, indeed, have a protective function. Neuropathic joint disease is a destructive arthropathy usually associated with disorders affecting the peripheral nerves, such as diabetes mellitus, tabes dorsalis, leprosy, and alcoholic neuropathy (Fig. 7.70).[30] Presumably, in these conditions, as a result of a loss of proprioception, the joint is subjected to mechanical trauma, which initiates a cycle ultimately leading to joint destruction. However, an alternative hypothesis[31] for the pathogenesis of Charcot arthropathy in these disorders, suggests that joint degeneration occurs because circulatory changes (hyperemia) initiated by a neural 'reflex' associated with dorsal root disease (e.g., syphilis), spinal cord disease (e.g., syringomyelia), or nerve-trunk disease (e.g., diabetes mellitus) leads to rapid osteoclastic resorption of bone. The circulatory effects may account for the observation that a normal joint may break down within only a few weeks in a bedridden person, having been subjected to minimal activity and no overt trauma.[31] Neuropathic joints are most commonly seen today in the mid- and forefoot of patients with diabetes mellitus.[32]

Despite the intuitive logic of an association between arthropathy and loss of proprioception, upon close examination, a definitive relationship between peripheral sensory neuropathy and joint disease is not evident. Many patients with peripheral sensory disorders do not develop joint problems. For example, only 0.1 per cent of diabetics (5 per cent of those with clinically identifiable peripheral sensory neuropathy), 5 per cent of tabetics, and 25 per cent of those with syringomyelia develop neuropathic joint disease.[30,33] Often, it is not until after the occurrence of a significant episode of joint trauma that the patient with a peripheral sensory disorder develops Charcot arthropathy.[34] Furthermore, Charcot joints are more common in patients who are physically active and are usually not found in spastic patients, presumably because spasticity 'splints' the limb, protecting it from excessive joint displacement.[35]

Deafferentation studies

In accordance with the poor correlation between peripheral neuropathy and arthropathy in humans, are data from experimental deafferentation studies in animals showing that extensive limb deafferentation alone does not necessarily result in the breakdown of a stable joint.[30] Several recent long-term (up to 16 months) studies in dogs[36–39] have helped clarify the role of ipsilateral proprioception in joint protection. These studies have shown the following:

1. Extensive deafferentation of the hind limb (by L4–S1 dorsal root ganglionectomy, DRG) did not result in knee OA in active dogs that used their knees normally for as long as 16 months after the neurosurgical procedure, strongly suggesting that ipsilateral proprioceptive nerves do not play a critical role in protecting the *normal* joint from damage.

2. In contrast to the above, when DRG preceded destabilization of the knee (by ACL transection), breakdown of the unstable joint was strikingly accelerated and pathologic changes were much more severe than those in neurologically intact dogs that underwent ACL transection, providing evidence of an important role for ipsilateral proprioception in protecting the *acutely unstable joint* from rapid breakdown.

3. On the other hand, when DRG was performed 12 months *after* ACL transection, the severity of OA was no greater than that in the neurologically

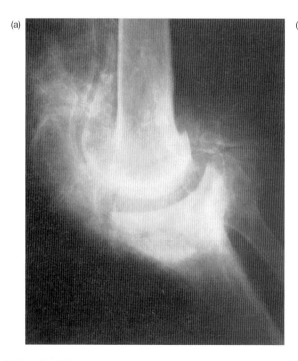
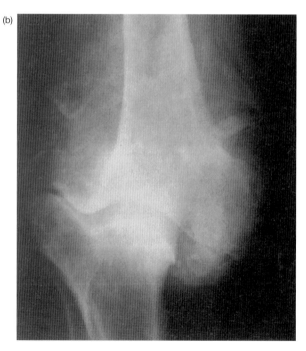

(a)   (b)

Fig. 7.70 (a) Lateral and (b) anteroposterior radiographs of the knee of a patient with Charcot arthropathy as a result of syphilis. Note the gross deformity, dislocation, extensive osteophyte formation, marked bony remodelling, and synovial osteochondromatosis.

intact cruciate-deficient dog, suggesting that ipsilateral proprioception is not necessary for protection of the *chronically unstable joint.*

How can the above observations and the weak relationship between peripheral sensory neuropathy and Charcot arthropathy be explained? O'Connor et al.[37,39] suggested that the explanation may lie in the utilization by the CNS of CPGs.

Central pattern generators

The term CPG refers to a collection of neurons or neural circuits that generate patterned motor activity, producing highly stereotyped rhythmic movements autonomously (Fig. 7.71). CPGs are located in the brain stem and spinal cord and are important for many repetitive movements, such as mastication, respiration, scratching, and locomotion. Accordingly, if external support is provided to prevent falling, an animal with a transected spinal cord can step overground or on a treadmill. CPGs are also capable of coordinating locomotor movements in the absence of movement-related afferent feedback.[40]

Presumably, in patients with sensory neuropathy, as in the deafferented dog with a stable knee (see above), CPGs are able to process sensory input from a variety of other sources (e.g., the brain, the other limbs, the back, vestibular, and visual systems) to initiate appropriate motor programmes for normal repetitive motor behaviours. Thus, the deafferented dogs continued to engage in typical repetitive canine behaviours, such as walking, galloping, and hind limb ear-scratching, suggesting that as long as sensation from other sources remained intact, their CPGs continued to function despite greatly decreased afferent input from the ipsilateral limb.

The results of the canine deafferentation studies suggest that protection of the knee in these animals occurred as a by-product of the normal usage of a normal joint.[30,36,37] CPGs in the deafferented dogs presumably interpreted 'no information' from joint afferents as an indication that 'nothing is wrong,' and controlled the excursions and loading of the joint within safe limits. However, when deafferentation preceded ACL transection, the CPGs presumably could not be 'updated' by the signalling of new joint pain and/or instability through ipsilateral proprioceptive input and coordinated movements of the unstable limb as though the limb were stable, resulting in the rapid breakdown of the joint.

To explain the lack of progression of OA in the dogs in which limb deafferentation was deferred for 12 months after ACL transection, O'Connor et al.[37,39] suggested that in the interval between ligament transection and DRG, ipsilateral sensory nerves performed two functions:

First, sensory output from the unstable joint may have directly protected it from rapid breakdown by informing the CNS that the joint was painful and/or unstable, leading to conscious modifications in use of the joint by the CNS. These modifications would have established a set of compromises between acceptable discomfort and preferred joint use for each of many behaviours (e.g., scratching, trotting, walking, sitting).[39]

Second, as each compromise was implemented and practiced, the CPGs may have been reprogrammed by the repetitive proprioceptive input defined by the new movements. Eventually, the reprogrammed CPGs protected the chronically unstable joint from excessive movements in the absence of continuous ipsilateral sensory input, in the same fashion as the normal joint is protected in the absence of such sensation.[30,39]

Summary

Although joints contain a variety of types of mechanoreceptors, their role in joint protection (via reflex muscle activity) is unclear. Similarly, the contribution of these receptors to the awareness of joint position sense is uncertain. Pain, however, is undoubtedly derived from joints, although the specific joint tissue from which joint pain originates in the patient with OA, are uncertain. The transmission of nonciceptive impulses by articular nerves is accentuated in the presence of inflammatory mediators (e.g., substance P), so that normally innocuous movements of the OA joint may be painful. In addition, substance P and other inflammatory neuropeptides are released by the nerves themselves, contributing to 'neurogenic inflammation.' However, other neuropeptides (e.g., somatostatin) are anti-inflammatory, offering the possibility of novel approaches to the treatment of joint pain and inflammation.

The relationship between OA and decreased joint proprioception is difficult to understand because the correlation between sensory neuropathy and the development of OA is poor. Furthermore, studies in dogs with a deafferented limb indicate that joint afferents are not essential for maintaining the integrity of the stable knee. Rather, neural networks (CPGs) may protect the stable joint even when ipsilateral proprioceptive output from the limb is markedly diminished. However, such afferent output appears to be important in minimizing damage to an acutely unstable joint and for reprogramming the CNS after joint injury, for example, rupture of the ACL. Thus, over time, ipsilateral sensation is no longer required to protect the joint from further damage that might result from abnormal loading during repetitive activities such as locomotion.

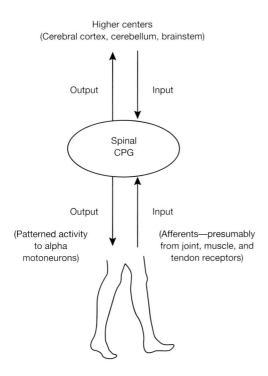

Fig. 7.71 Schematic drawing showing the input/output relationships of a theoretical spinal CPG that can organize the muscle activations associated with rhythmic activities even in the absence of movement-related feed-back. Such generators possibly 'protect' normal joints from abnormal loading by maintaining their movements within safe ranges of excursion. An alpha motor neuron is a neuron that innervates somatic muscles.

Key points

1. Joints are well-innervated structures containing a variety of anatomically and physiologically distinct nerve endings.

2. The role of such joint receptors in muscle activity and joint protection is unclear.

3. Joint pain can theoretically be derived from free nerve endings located in the ligaments, joint capsule, or subchondral bone. However, the specific source of pain in OA is not known.

4. The presence of inflammatory mediators can markedly increase and decrease the responsiveness of joint receptors that transmit sensations of pain.

5. It appears that afferent input into the CNS is not essential for the maintenance of stability of either the normal joint, or the chronically unstable joint, because neural networks (CPGs) automatically protect joints by maintaining movements within a range of excursion that does not overload the joint.

Acknowledgements

I am grateful to Dr. Brian O'Connor for providing two of the figures, reviewing earlier versions of the chapter, and insightful suggestions on how to view joint protective mechanisms. I would also like to thank Ms. Roberta Shadle for drawing Fig. 7.71 and Dr. Ethan Braunstein for providing the radiographs of the patient with Charcot arthropathy.

References

(An asterisk denotes recommended reading.)

1. O'Connor, B.L., Kunz, B., and Peterson, R.G. (1982). The composition of the medial articular nerve in the knee of the dog. *J Anat* **135**:139–45.

2. Langford, L.A. and Schmidt, R.F. (1983). Afferent and efferent axons in the medial and posterior articular nerves of the cat. *Anat Rec* **206**:71–8.

3. *Johansson, H. and Sjölander, P. (1993). The neurophysiology of joints. In: V. Wright and E.L. Radin (eds) *Mechanics of Human Joints: Physiology, Pathophysiology and Treatment*. New York: Marcel Dekker, pp. 243–90.
    This is an excellent review of joint neurophysiology, including the basis for the 'muscle stiffness' hypothesis of joint stability.

4. Johansson, H., Sjölander, P., and Sojka, P. (1991). Receptors in the knee joint ligaments and their role in the biomechanics of the joint. *Crit Rev Biomed Eng* **18**:341–68.

5. *Hogervorst, T. and Brand, R.A. (1998). Mechanoreceptors in joint function. *J Bone Joint Surg* **80**(A):1365–78.
    This is an excellent recent review of joint innervation.

6. Wyke, B. (1981). The neurology of joints: a review of general principles. *Clin Rheum Dis* **7**:223–39.

7. Schaible, H.-G. and Grubb, B.D. (1993). Afferent and spinal mechanisms of joint pain. *Pain* **55**:5–54.

8. Krauspe, R., Schmitz, F., Zoller, G., and Drenckhahn, D. (1995). Distribution of neurofilament-positive nerve fibres and sensory endings in the human anterior cruciate ligament. *Arch Orthop Trauma Surg* **114**:194–8.

9. DeAvila, G.A., O'Connor, B.L., Visco, D.M., and Sisk, T.D. (1989). The mechanoreceptor innervation of the human fibular collateral ligament. *J Anat* **162**:1–7.

10. Pope, D.F., Cole, K.J., and Brand, R.A. (1990). Physiologic loading of the anterior cruciate ligament does not activate quadriceps or hamstrings in the anesthetized cat. *Am J Sports Med* **18**:595–9.

11. Raunest, J., Sager, M., and Burgener, E. (1996). Proprioceptive mechanisms in the cruciate ligaments: an electromyographic study on reflex activity in the thigh muscles. *J Trauma* **41**:488–93.

12. Solomonow, M., Baratta, R., Zhou, B.H., *et al.* (1987). The synergistic action of the anterior cruciate ligament and thigh muscles in maintaining joint stability. *Am J Sports Med* **15**:207–13.

13. Dieppe, P. (1999). Subchondral bone should be the main target for the treatment of pain and disease progression in osteoarthritis. *Osteoarthritis Cart* **7**:325–6.

14. Arnoldi, C.C., Linderholm, H., and Müssbichler, H. (1972). Venous engorgement and intraosseous hypertension in osteoarthritis of the hip. *J Bone Joint Surg* **54**(B):409–21.

15. Arnoldi, C.C., Lemperg, R.K., and Linderholm, H. (1971). Immediate effect of osteotomy on the intramedullary pressure of the femoral head and neck in patients with degenerative osteoarthritis. *Acta Orthop Scand* **43**:357–65.

16. Neugebauer, V. and Schaible, H.-G. (1990). Evidence for a central component in the sensitization of spinal neurons with joint input during development of acute arthritis in cat's knee. *J Neurophysiol* **64**:299–311.

17. Jayson, M.I.V. and Dixon, A.S.J. (1970). Intra-articular pressure in rheumatoid arthritis of the knee. I. Pressure changes during passive joint distension. *Ann Rheum Dis* **29**:261–5.

18. Bierma-Zeinstra, S.M.A., Bohnen, A.M., Verhaar, J.A.N., Prins, A., Ginai-Karamat, A.Z., and Lameris, J. (2000). Sonography for hip joint effusion in adults with hip pain. *Ann Rheum Dis* **59**:178–82.

19. Goodwin, J.S. (1997). Anti-inflammatory drugs. In: D.P. Stites, A.I. Terr, and T.G. Parslow (eds) *Medical Immunology*. Stamford, CT: Appleton & Lange, pp. 846–60.

20. Schumacher Jr., H.R., Meng, Z., Sieck, M., *et al.* (1996). Effect of a nonsteroidal antinflammatory drug on synovial fluid in osteoarthritis. *J Rheumatol* **23**:1774–7.

21. Abramson, S.B. (1992). Treatment of gout and crystal arthropathies and uses and mechanisms of action of non-steroidal anti-inflammatory drugs. *Curr Opin Rheumatol* **4**:295–300.

22. Malmberg, A.B. and Yaksh, T.L. (1992). Hyperalgesia mediated by spinal glutamate or substance P receptor blocked by spinal cyclooxygenase inhibition. *Sci* **257**:1276–9.

23. Bradley, J.D., Brandt, K.D., Katz, B.P., Kalasinski, L.A., and Ryan, S.I. (1992). Treatment of knee osteoarthritis. Relationship of clinical features of joint inflammation to the response to a nonsteroidal anti-inflammatory drug or pure analgesic. *J Rheumatol* **19**:1950–4.

24. McDougall, J.J., Ferrell, W.R., and Bray, R.C. (1997). Spatial variation in sympathetic influences on the vasculature of the synovium and medial collateral ligament of the rabbit knee joint. *J Physiol* **503**:435–43.

25. McDougall, J.J., Ferrell, W.R., and Bray, R.C. (1999). Neurogenic origin of articular hyperemia in early degenerative joint disease. *Am J Physiol* **276**:R745–R752.

26. *Marshall, K.W. and Chan, A.D.M. (1993). Neurogenic contributions to degenerative and inflammatory arthroses. *Curr Opin Orthop* **4**:48–55.
    This is an excellent description of the role of articular nerves in 'neurogenic inflammation'.

27. Lam, F.Y. and Ferrell, W.R. (1989). Inhibition of carrageenan induced inflammation in the rat knee joint by substance P antagonist. *Ann Rheum Dis* **48**:928–32.

28. Heppelmann, B. and Pawlak, M. (1997). Inhibitory effect of somatostatin on the mechanosensitvity of articular afferents in normal and inflamed knee joints of the rat. *Pain* **73**:377–82.

29. Heppelmann, B., Just, S., and Pawlak, M. (2000). Galanin influences the mechanosensitivity of sensory endings in the rat knee joint. *Eur J Neurosci* **12**:1567–72.

30. *O'Connor, B.L. and Brandt, K.D. (1993). Neurogenic factors in the etiopathogenesis of osteoarthritis. *Rheum Dis Clin North Am* **19**:581–605.
    This paper reviews neuromuscular mechanisms that protect joints from damage, and provides a rationale for using OA as the only appropriate endpoint for the study of such mechanisms.

31. Johnson, L.C. (1964). Morphologic analysis in pathology: the kinetics of disease and general biology of knee. In: H.M. Frost (ed.) *Bone biodynamics*. Boston: Little Brown, pp. 543–654.

32. Ellman, M.A. (1993). Neuropathic joint disease (Charcot joints). In: D.J. McCarthy and W.J. Kropman (eds) *Arthritis and Allied Conditions*. Philadelphia: Lea and Febiger, pp. 1407–25.

33. Steindler, A. (1931). The tabetic arthropathies. *JAMA* **96**:250–6.

34. Johnson, J.T.H. (1967). Neuropathic fractures and joint injuries. *J Bone Joint Surg* **49**(A):1–30.

35. Bruckner, F.E. and Howell, A. (1972). Neuropathic joints. *Sem Arthritis Rheum* **2**:47–69.

36. O'Connor, B.L., Palmoski, M.J., and Brandt, K.D. (1985). Neurogenic acceleration of degenerative joint lesions. *J Bone Joint Surg* **67**(A):562–72.

37. *O'Connor, B.L., Visco, D.M., Brandt, K.D., Albrecht, M., and O'Connor, A.B. (1993). Sensory nerves only temporarily protect the unstable canine knee from osteoarthritis. Evidence that sensory nerves reprogram the central nervous system after cruciate ligament transection. *Arthritis Rheum* **36**:1154–63.
    This paper confirms the original evidence that joints are protected in the absence of ipsilateral sensory input and further suggests that the CNS is reprogrammed by ipsilateral sensory input from the unstable joint.

38. *Vilensky, J.A., O'Connor, B.L., Brandt, K.D., Dunn, E.A., and Rogers, P.I. (1994). Serial kinematic analysis of the canine knee after L4–S1 dorsal root ganglionectomy: implications for the cruciate deficiency model of osteoarthritis. *J Rheumatol* **21**:2113–17.

    This original report describes nearly normal knee kinematics in the deafferented limb.

39. *O'Connor, B.L., Visco, D.M., Rogers, P.I., Mamlin, L.A., and Brandt, K.D. (1999). Serial force plate analysis of dogs with unilateral knee instability, with and without interruption of the sensory input from the ipsilateral limb. *Osteoarthritis Cart* **7**:567–73.

    This report describes normal loading of the deafferented dog limb and suggests alternatives to the reprogramming hypothesis.

40. Leonard, C.T. (1998). *The Neuroscience of Human Movement*. St. Louis: Mosby.

7.2.4.2 Neuromuscular protective mechanisms

Michael V. Hurley

Research in OA has focused primarily on intra-articular changes to cartilage and bone. Less interest has been paid to changes of peri-articular skeletal muscles. However, muscles and joints are functionally interdependant, and well-conditioned muscles are vital for healthy joints.

Muscles effect finely controlled movement, bestow functional joint stability during physical activity, and contribute sensory information regarding limb position and movement. These motor and sensory functions of muscle are intimately interlinked and generate neuromuscular protective mechanisms that co-ordinate a smooth, efficient gait and minimize harmful loading, thus providing vital shock absorption during gait to prevent joint damage.

Rather than the usual presumption that joint damage precedes and initiates pain, disability and muscle weakness, muscle sensorimotor dysfunction that may occur due to ageing may have a significant primary role in the pathogenesis and/or progression of OA through the impairment of neuromuscular protective mechanisms. However, because muscle is an extremely plastic tissue, exercise that improves muscle sensorimotor dysfunction and restores neuromuscular protective mechanisms may have positive effects on the underlying pathology, and delay or prevent the development of further joint damage. Thus, muscle rehabilitation may have a very important role in the management of OA.

Introduction

The main focus of research in OA has been the changes to cartilage and bone, and much less attention has been devoted to changes in peri-articular skeletal muscles. In some ways it is not surprising that researchers have ignored muscle. Intuitively, changes in cartilage and bone appear more relevant to the pathological processes of OA since they comprise the 'immediate' joint milieu, whereas muscles spanning the joint seem somewhat 'detached' from the site of pathology. But this view overlooks the interdependency that muscles and joints have with each other. There is no point in having a muscle unless it crosses a joint, and a joint is functionless unless a muscle that can effect movement crosses over it.

Recently, the importance of muscle in lower limb OA has been recognized and research interest in this area has increased. This chapter presents some of the evidence that has accrued, highlighting the importance of the motor and sensory functions of muscle, the articular consequences of muscle sensorimotor dysfunction, outlines a hypothetical argument for the role of muscle

dysfunction in the pathogenesis of OA and emphasizes the potential that addressing muscle dysfunction may have in the management of OA.

Functions of skeletal muscle

Skeletal muscle has many functions, some obvious others less so. The most important are:

1. *Contraction.* To enable us to move, the excitation of α-motoneurones (α-mn) activate extra-fusal muscle fibres that contract to effect movement.

2. *Functional joint stability.* To fully benefit from the ability to move and to interact with our environment we must maintain a stable erect posture using inherently unstable lower limb and vertebral joints, so joints must possess the contradictory properties of stability and mobility. Passive joint stability is determined by the anatomy of the joint and mechanical constraints (e.g. ligaments), but these cannot prevent collapse during erect posture and movement. Stability during physical activity—functional joint stability—is determined by controlled muscle activity that enables movement, while simultaneously preventing the collapse of inherently unstable lower limb joints.[1]

3. *Proprioceptive acuity.* Golgi tendon organs and muscle spindles are proprioceptors. Muscle spindles are particularly important in signalling the rate of stretch (via Ia or primary afferents) and change in length (via II or secondary afferents) experienced by limb muscles during movement.[2–4] The sensitivity of the muscle spindles is set by excitation of γ-motorneurones (γ-mn), which activate the intra-fusal muscle fibres that comprise muscle spindles.

4. *Shock absorption.* Neuromuscular protective reflexes and mechanisms are vital for avoiding joint injury by minimizing and dissipating potentially harmful forces during weight-bearing activities, loads through finely controlled muscle activity, and accurate lower limb placement and timing.[5–7]

These motor and sensory functions of muscle are not separate but intimately interlinked. For example, during gait muscle spindles generate proprioceptive sensory information about lower limb movement, position, and loading that is used to determine an appropriate motor strategy. This is effected by controlled muscle contraction, minimizing impulsive, jarring loads being exerted on the lower limb joints (for instance at heel strike eccentric contraction of the quadriceps permits slight knee flexion), executing a smooth, efficient gait. All the while muscle spindles are continually monitoring and feeding back sensory information to the CNS to fine-tune appropriate muscle activity.

The importance of neuromuscular mechanisms in maintaining articular health and function

Optimal muscle function requires well-conditioned, non-fatigued muscles that have an intact sensory input and which are under appropriate motor control. If muscles become weak or fatigued, or their sensory acuity or motor control is impaired, the vital neuromuscular protective mechanisms are compromised. As a result the sensory input that helps determine and control appropriate motor strategies and ensures the performance of smooth, efficient movement will be impaired, resulting in excessive lower limb joint movement and instability, stress on innervated tissues eliciting pain, and jarring, impulsive joint loading that causes articular cartilage microtrauma and subchondral bone microfractures.[5,8] These subchondral microfractures heal by callus formation. Over time, this results in sclerosis of the subchondral bone, which is less resilient and dissipates impact forces poorly. Consequently, the ebonated subchondral bone becomes 'an anvil upon which the articular cartilage is pounded' causing further attrition of the articular cartilage.[5,8] Therefore optimizing neuromuscular protective reflexes and mechanisms by maintaining well-conditioned and well-controlled skeletal muscles is vital for maintaining lower limb joint health.

1. Muscles effect movement, generate proprioceptive sensory information, and stabilize joints and limbs bestowing functional stability during physical activity, and shock absorption during gait.

2. These sensorimotor functions interact to evoke neuromuscular protective mechanisms that minimize harmful, excessive joint movement and loading.

3. Muscle sensorimotor dysfunction impairs neuromuscular protective mechanisms giving rise to articular damage.

Control of motor function

Fine, accurate motor control involves the complex integration of excitatory and inhibitory input from many different sources (Fig. 7.72).[9–12] Information from descending supraspinal motor tracts in the central nervous system (CNS), segmental spinal interneurones (IN), rhythmic movement pattern generators, involuntary reflexes, and sensory input from muscle, articular, and cutaneous proprioceptors is integrated at γ-mns and efferent information is sent to the muscle spindles. Here it is integrated with information about movement in the 'parent muscle'. The resultant Ia and II afferent input is relayed back to the spinal cord where it causes *excitation* of the α-mn pool (Fig. 7.72).[9–12] This sensory information is also relayed to spinal INs where it is integrated with information from many other peripheral and central sources that may excite the IN resulting in *inhibition* of the α-mn pool (Fig. 7.72). Most factors that influence α-mn excitability will also influence γ-mn excitability and hence muscle spindle sensitivity and proprioceptive acuity.[1,13–15] The dynamic balance between inhibitory and excitatory inputs to α-mns, modulates the excitability of the α-mn pool and regulates muscle activity, movement, and joint stability.[9–12]

Effect of ageing on the neuromuscular system

Age-related changes have a profound effect on the efficient functioning of the neuromuscular system and elderly people's appreciation and control of movement. Older people have a generalized muscle weakness,[16–19] their muscles fatigue quicker, their proprioceptive acuity is impaired,[16,20,21] the time for processing sensory information takes longer, and their motor reaction times are slower. These sensorimotor changes result in postural instability[16,22–24] that contributes to the increased frequency of falls in elderly people.

Consequences of articular and muscle dysfunction

Articular receptors contribute to pre-programming muscle activity, joint range of movement and stability via their ascending projections to higher CNS centres, and peripheral pathways that converge on INs and γ-mns that control α-mn excitability. However, because joints and muscles are interdependant structures whose interplay has an important role in limb sensorimotor function and control, it is better to consider a synovial joint as a functional unit comprised of the articular structures (bone, cartilage, synovium, capsule, ligaments), the peri-articular muscles spanning the articulation, and the nerves that supply these articular structures and muscles. Alteration of the intra-articular milieu can affect muscle activity, similarly muscle dysfunction affects articular function.

The complex multiple aetiology of OA and the interdependence of the 'central' clinical features—disability, muscle sensorimotor dysfunction, and joint damage and pain—is now better appreciated though still poorly understood (Fig. 7.73). What is becoming more apparent is that

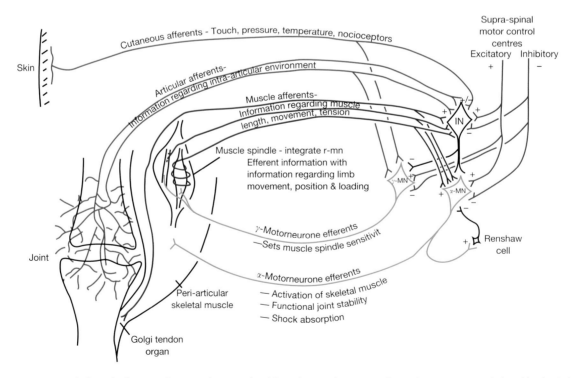

Fig. 7.72 Sensorimotor control of muscle. Sensory information from peripheral (articular, muscle, cutaneous) proprioceptors, supraspinal, and local spinal pathways convergence on INs, γ-mns, and α-mns in the spinal cord. Here the dynamic balance between excitatory (+) and inhibitory (−) input is collated. The resultant of the summation of these influences determines the excitability of the α-mns that activate extra-fusal muscle fibres that effect muscle contraction and functional joint stability. This is a diagrammatic simplification of the spinal pathways. Many other INs and input pathways will be interposed in the pathways but for clarity these have been omitted.

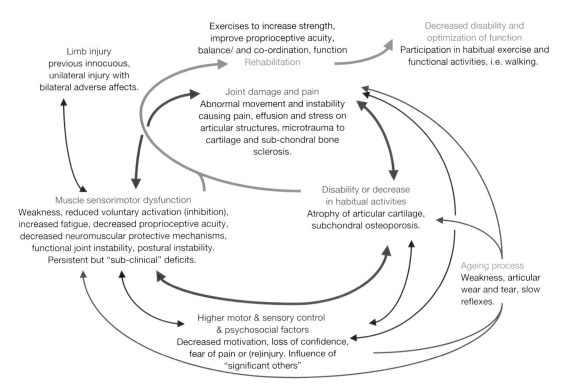

Fig. 7.73 The complex interrelationship between the 'central' clinical features of OA (muscle dysfunction, joint damage, pain and disability), physiological, and psychosocial factors in the pathogenesis and progression of OA. Arthritic changes need not necessarily be initiated by changes in joints structures that progresses (clockwise) causing disability and muscle dysfunction as usually presumed. Age-related physiological changes and/or psychosocial influences may cause muscle dysfunction and reduce participation in habitual physical activity leading to stress, forces and loading that result in structural joint damage. The pathological changes may progress in a haphazard fashion, oscillating clockwise and anti-clockwise. The direction of the arrows indicates the direction of each factor's influence.

Source: Adapted with permission from Hurley, 1999. *Rheum Dis Clin NA.*

the pathological processes that culminate in pain and joint damage may be initiated by many factors, for example ageing, physiological changes to muscle or joint, and/or psychosocial factors, that affect the balanced interdependency of the central clinical features.

The effect of articular dysfunction on muscle function. Alteration or abolition of 'normal' articular mechanoreceptor afferent discharge can be induced by joint pain, effusion, or structural damage, which alters the sensory input to α-mns, γ-mns, and Ins.[25] If this sensory input does not match expected pre-motor sensory programmes, normal postural reflex activity and motor activation patterns may be disturbed, compromising lower limb muscle strength, proprioceptive acuity, and functional joint stability and resulting in gross gait abnormalities and decreased activity.[1] This scenario reflects the usual, intuitive, presumption that arthritic damage and pain is initiated by daily mechanical wear and tear accumulated over a lifetime of 'joint abuse', which leads to reduced physical activity and muscle weakness (i.e., in Fig. 7.73 the pathology is initiated by joint damage and progresses clockwise).

The possible role of muscle dysfunction in the pathogenesis of articular damage. However the relationship between joint damage, pain, muscle dysfunction and disability, is complex and which occurs first is unknown. Rather than presuming that joint damage and pain precede muscle weakness, age-related decline in muscle function may impair neuromuscular protective mechanisms exposing joints to abnormal movement and impulsive loading, causing pain and articular cartilage attrition. This might explain the results of a cross-sectional study of a community-based population that demonstrated that in women quadriceps weakness can precede radiographic knee joint damage,[26,27] and might also explain why muscle weakness and fatigue are common, early symptoms reported by patients.[26,28–30] Thus, muscle sensorimotor dysfunction may be involved

in the pathogenesis of OA. For a more detailed review of the arguments supporting the role of muscle dysfunction in the pathogenesis of OA see Hurley 1999.[31]

The influence of psychosocial factors on muscle and articular function. Concomitant with and accentuating this age-related decline in muscle sensorimotor function are complex psychosocial factors that have profound influences on people's health beliefs and behaviour. People may begin to associate physical activity with pain and worry that physical activity will wear out their joint. They may become conscious of their muscle weakness, proprioceptive, balance, gait and functional impairments, which are not only risk factors associated with OA[16,32] but also risk factors for falling.[22,24,33] Understandably perception of neuromuscular changes, postural and joint instability will undermine people's confidence, dissuade them from participating in their normal habitual physical activities and encourage greater dependency on others, exacerbating sensorimotor dysfunction.

These cognitions, beliefs, and fears are often compounded by social factors. In general, the lay public and many healthcare professionals have a poor understanding of the causes of OA, and people with OA usually receive very poor, if any, advice about how to manage their condition.[34] Out of ignorance or convenience, OA is often explained as being the inevitable consequence of age-related joint wear and tear—giving people the choice of helping themselves by reducing their activities, or dying young! Most people take the former option and decrease their activity to prolong the life of their joint, advised and encouraged by worried, well-meaning relatives, friends, and misinformed healthcare professionals.

What is important to appreciate is that the muscle dysfunction is induced either directly through physiological changes and/or indirectly through psychosocial factors that reduce physical activities, impair neuromuscular protective mechanisms, and adversely affects joint health. It should be emphasized that much of the evidence used to construct the hypothesis that muscle sensorimotor dysfunction is involved in the pathogenesis of OA is indirect and circumstantial.[31] Moreover, muscle dysfunction may only be important as an aetiological factor for certain 'subsets' of OA, at certain joint sites, in particular the knee where most research has been performed and possibly the vertebral joints.[35–37] However, the theoretical argument and empirical support for muscle involvement in the pathogenesis of hip OA is less convincing, since the anatomy of the hip joint makes it less reliant on articular musculature for stability. In the upper limb and hand muscle dysfunction is likely to have little, if any, role.

Muscle dysfunction in the progression of OA. In their studies of community-based population Brandt *et al.* found no association between quadriceps weakness and progression of radiological OA over 2–3 years.[38] However, the authors question whether conventional standing radiographs and the Kellgren and Lawrence grading system used to assess radiological progression is sensitive enough to detect all radiological changes, and they emphasize the small number of patients observed means the power of the study is probably insufficient to rule out an association between quadriceps weakness and progression of joint damage. Thus the association between muscle weakness and joint damage is unknown.

In summary, muscle dysfunction is evident in a large majority of patients and may be involved in the pathogenesis and/or progression of joint damage through poor control of movement, impulsive lower limb joint loading, exacerbating joint damage and pain. It is also important to appreciate that the pathological processes may be initiated by many factors and may not proceed in a predictable direction, that is, clockwise as in Fig. 7.73, but oscillate backwards and forwards, at times driven by certain factors (e.g. muscle dysfunction), while at other times other factors (e.g. psychosocial factors or episodic exacerbation of pain) may have greater influences on the pathological processes. Research is needed to clarify what role, if any, muscle dysfunction has in the pathogenesis and/or progression OA.

Restoration of muscle sensorimotor function

The involvement of muscle sensorimotor dysfunction in the pathogenesis and/or progression of OA may be fortuitous. Muscle is an extremely malleable tissue, even in elderly people, and of all the tissues that comprise synovial joints, muscle is the one most easily manipulated. Therefore interventions that reverse sensorimotor deficits and restore neuromuscular protective mechanisms enable us to disrupt the viscous circle of events (Fig. 7.73), preventing the initiation of OA, or retarding or halting its progression.

There is now increasing evidence from well-conducted clinical trials for the efficacy of exercise rehabilitation in improving muscle strength, motor control, proprioceptive acuity and reaction times, restoring neuromuscular protective mechanisms, and functional joint stability,[39–41] and decreasing pain and disability without exacerbating the condition.[42] Thus exercise can restore the shock absorption properties of muscle, which should protect against further joint damage. Hence, if joint damage is caused by muscle dysfunction the onset of OA may be prevented by maintaining strong and well-conditioned muscles through 'prophylactic' exercise and maintaining a physically active lifestyle. For patients with established OA, rehabilitation that adequately addresses muscle dysfunction can improve neuromuscular protective mechanisms, decrease pain and disability, and possibly slow or halt the progression of the condition.

What is now important is to develop these efficacious research regimes into clinically effective practicable programmes that can be widely implemented, affording the large population of OA patients the opportunity to benefit. Such regimes should be integrated into education and self-management strategies that emphasize the importance of exercise and regular physical activity on a life long basis. The main challenge facing those who treat OA is to determine how best to convey the message about the importance of optimal muscle function in knee OA and how to successfully encourage participation in habitual exercise and physical activity.[34,43]

Conclusion

Muscles are integral components of synovial joints that effect movement, bestow functional joint stability, absorb harmful forces and loads generated during gait and contribute to the appreciation and control of body position and movement. Well-conditioned muscles are vital for healthy, well-functioning joints. The interrelationship between muscles, articular structures, and innervating nerves—which should all be seen as a functional unit—means that muscle motor and sensory dysfunction will cause articular dysfunction. The age-related decline in muscle function and increase in incidence of OA may not be coincidental because direct and indirect evidence could be used to argue that muscle dysfunction may be involved in the pathogenesis and/or progression of OA in some people at some (weight-bearing) joints. The validity of these hypothetical arguments can only be determined in well-designed, large, complex longitudinal studies, which are open to many confounding variables that are extremely difficult to control. Determining the role of muscle in OA is important because muscle is a physiologically 'plastic' tissue, and the benefits attained during rehabilitation—improvement of muscle sensorimotor function and restoration of neuromuscular protective mechanisms—may provide effective management strategies to prevent the onset and/or ameliorate the effects of OA.

Key points 1

1. It is intuitively presumed that mechanical 'wear and tear' causes joint pain damage leading to reduced activity and muscle weakness.

2. Indirect evidence suggests that in some people, at some lower limb weight-bearing joints muscle dysfunction may play a significant role in the development of OA.

3. Even if muscle dysfunction is not important in the pathogenesis of OA, it is an early symptom, evident in most patients, and associated with pain and disability.

4. Persistent muscle dysfunction may be a risk factor for OA progression.

Key points 2

1. Muscle is a highly adaptable tissue even in very elderly persons.

2. Exercise rehabilitation increases sensorimotor function, improves neuromuscular protective mechanisms and reduces pain and disability.

3. Rehabilitation regimes may prevent or delay the onset of joint damage, or retard or reverse the effects of OA.

4. Clinically effective rehabilitation regimes that can be widely implemented need to be developed to maintain the short-term benefits gained during efficacious research regimes.

Further Reading

Rothwell, J.C. (1994). *Control of Human Voluntary Movement* (2nd ed.). London: Chapman Hall.

Ferrell, W.R. and Proske, U. (eds). (1995). *Neutral Control of Movement.* New York: Plenum Press.

Brooks, V. (ed.) (1981). *Handbook of Physiology* (Vol II, section 1). Bethseda, Maryland: American Physiological Society.

Johansson, H. and Sjolander, P. (1993). Neurophysiology of joints. In: V. Wright, E.L. Radin (eds). *Mechanics of Human Joints.* New York: Marcel Dekker.

References

(An asterisk denotes recommended reading.)

1. *Johansson, H., Sjolander, P., and Sojka, P. (1991). A sensory role for the cruciate ligaments. *Clin Orthop* **268**:161–78.

This paper gives an in-depth description of the influence that articular receptors have on muscle function and functional joint stability and proprioceptive acuity.

2. **McClosky, D.I.** (1978). Kinaesthetic sensibility. *Physiol Rev* **58**:763–820.

3. **Matthews, P.B.C.** (1988). Proprioceptors and their contribution to somatosensory mapping: complex messages require complex processing. *Can J Physiol Pharm* **66**:430–8.

4. **Gandevia, S., D.I.M., and Burke, D.** (1992). Kinaesthetic signals and muscle contraction. *Trend Neurosci* **15**:62–5.

5. **Bland, J.H. and Cooper, S.M.** (1984). Osteoarthritis: A review of the cell biology involved and evidence for reversibility. Management rationally related to known genesis and pathophysiology. *Sem Arthritis Rheum* **14**:106–33.

6. **Jefferson, R.J., Radin, E.L., and O'Connor, J.J.** (1990). The role of the quadriceps in controlling impulsive forces around heel strike. *Proc Ins Mech Engin* **204**:21–8.

7. *****Radin, E.L., Yang, K.H., Riegger, C., Kish, V.L., and O'Connor, J.J.** (1991). Relationship between lower limb dynamics and knee joint pain. *J Orthop Res* **9**:398–405.

Healthy volunteers who suffered with intermittent knee pain have a gait that exhibited greater impact forces at heel strike. The authors coin the phrase 'microklutziness' to describe the uncoordinated gait of people who have poor neuromuscular control, and propose these people may go on to develop arthritic changes. (Heroically, they proceeded to investigate the validity of this hypothesis by analysing one of the of the authors gait before and after temporary femoral nerve paralysis, see Ref. 6.)

8. **Radin, E., Martin, B., Burr, D., Caterson, B., Boyd, R., and Goodwin, C.** (1984). Effects of mechanical loading on the tissues of the rabbit knee. *J Orthop Res*, **2**:221–34.

9. **Appelberg, B., Hulliger, M., Johansson, H., and Sojka, P.** (1983). Actions on α-motorneurones elicited by electrical stimulation of group I, II and III muscle afferent fibres in the hind limb of the cat. *J Physiol* **335**:237–92.

10. **McCrea, D.A.** (1992). Can sense be made of spinal interneuron circuits? *Behav Brain Sci* **15**:633–43.

11. **Jankowska, E. and Lundberg, A.** (1981). Interneurones in the spinal cord. *Trend Neurol Sci* **4**:230–3.

12. **Lundberg, A., Malmgren, K., and Schomburg, E.D.** (1987). Reflex pathways from group II muscle afferents. 3. Secondary spindle afferents and the FRA: A new hypothesis. *Exp Brain Res* **65**:294–306.

13. **Freeman, M.A.R., Dean, M.R.E., and Hanham, I.W.F.** (1965). The etiology and prevention of functional instability of the foot. *J Bone Joint Surg* **47**(B):678–85.

14. *****Freeman, M.A.R. and Wyke, B.** (1967b). Articular reflexes at the ankle joint: An electromyographic study of normal and abnormal influences of ankle-joint mechanoreceptors upon reflex activity in the leg muscles. *J Bone Joint Surg* **54**:990–1001.

This study established a link between what happens in the articular environment and how this affects motor control via α-motorneuones and γ-motorneurones. It demonstrated that sensory discharges from articular mechanoreceptors contribute to posture and movement by reflex co-ordination of muscle tone, and suggested muscle dysfunction might impair neuromuscular protective mechanisms and exposing joints to damage (also see Ref. 13).

15. **Ferrell, W.R., Baxendale, R.H., Carnachan, C., and Hart, I.K.** (1985). The influence of joint afferent discharge on locomotion, proprioception and activity in conscious cats. *Brain Res* **347**:41–8.

16. **Hurley, M.V., Rees, J., and Newham, D.J.** (1998). Quadriceps function, proprioceptive acuity and functional performance in healthy young, middle-aged and elderly subjects. *Age and Ageing* **27**:55–67.

17. **Bassey, E., Fiatarone, M., O'Neill, E., Kelly, M., Evans, W., and Lipsitz, L.** (1992). Leg extensor power and functional performance in very old men and women. *Clin Sci* **82**:321–7.

18. **Rutherford, O. and Jones, D.** (1992). The relationship between muscle and bone loss and activity levels with age in women. *Age and Ageing* **21**:286–93.

19. **Fiatarone, M., Marks, E. and Ryan, N.** (1990). High intensity strength training in nonagenarians: effects on skeletal muscle. *JAMA* **263**:3029–34.

20. **Ferrell, W.R., Crichton, A., and Sturrock, R.D.** (1992). Age-dependent changes in position sense in human proximal interphalangeal joints. *NeuroReport* **3**:259–61.

21. **Skinner, H.B., Barrack, R.L., and Cook, S.B.** (1984). Age-related decline in proprioception. *Clin Orthop* **184**:208–11.

22. **Tinetti, M., Speechly, M., and Ginter, S.** (1988). Risk factors for falls among elderly persons living in the community. *N Engl J Med* **319**:1701–7.

23. **Lord, S. and Castell, S.** (1994). Physical activity programme for older persons: effect on balance, strength, neuromuscular control, and balance reaction time. *Arch Phys Med Rehab* **75**:648–52.

24. **Lord, S.R., Lloyd, D.G., and Li, S.K.** (1996). Sensori-motor function, gait patterns and falls in community-dwelling women. *Age and Ageing* **25**:292–9.

25. **Hurley, M., Scott, D.L., Rees, J., and Newham, D.J.** (1997). Sensorimotor changes and functional performance in patients with knee osteoarthritis. *Ann Rheum Dis* **56**:641–8.

26. **Slemenda, C., Brandt, K.D., Heilman, D.K., Mazzuca, S., Braunstein, E.M., Katz, B.P. and Wolinsky, F.D.** (1997). Quadriceps weakness and osteoarthritis of the knee. *Ann Intern Med* **127**:97–104.

27. *****Slemenda, C., Heilman, D., Brandt, K., Katz, B., Mazzuca, S., Braunstein, E., and Byrd, D.** (1998). Reduced quadrceps strength relative to body weight a risk factor for knee osteoarthritis in women? *Arthritis Rheum* **41**:1951–9.

This cross-sectional study of a community-based population investigated the association between incident radiological knee OA and quadriceps strength. Quadriceps weakness was common in patients with and without radiological evidence of knee OA, but in women quadriceps weakness preceded and was predictive of radiological damage. Thus, quadriceps weakness might be a factor in the aetiology of knee joint damage. (Its role in progression of joint disease is less clear, see Ref. 38.)

28. **Lankhorst, G., Van de Stadt, R., and Van der Korst, J.** (1985). The relationships of functional capacity, pain, and isometric and isokinetic torque in osteoarthritis of the knee. *Scand J Rehab Med* **17**:167–72.

29. **Fisher, N.M., White, S.C., Yack, H.J., Smolinski, R.J., and Pendergast, D.R.** (1997). Muscle function and gait in patients with knee osteoarthritis before and after muscle rehabilitation. *Dis and Rehab* **19**:47–55.

30. **Hurley, M.V. and Newham, D.J.** (1993). The influence of arthrogenous muscle inhibition on quadriceps rehabilitation of patients with early, unilateral osteoarthritic knees. *Br J Rheumatol* **32**:127–31.

31. *****Hurley, M.V.** (1999). The role of muscle weakness in the pathogenesis of knee osteoarthritis. *Rheum Dis Clin North Am* **25**:283–98.

This narrative review gives a reasoned argument for the role of muscle dysfunction in the pathogenesis of OA. Greater details are provided of many studies that, directly and indirectly, support the hypothesis, than can be presented in this chapter.

32. **Hassan, B.S., Mockett, S., and Doherty, M.** (2001). Static postural sway, prioception and maximal voluntary quadriceps contraction in patients with knee osteoarthritis and normal control subjects. *Ann Rheum Dis* **60**:612–8.

33. **King, B.B. and Tinnetti, M.E.** (1995). Falls in community-dwelling older persons. *J Am Geriat Soc* **43**:1146–54.

34. **Dexter, P.A.** (1992). Joint exercises in elderly persons with symptomatic osteoarthritis of the hip or knee. Performance patterns, medical support, and the relationship between exercising and medical care. *Arthritis Care Res* **5**:36–41.

35. **Panjabi, M.M.** (1992). The stabilising system of the spine. Part 1. function, dysfunction, adaptation, and enhancement. *J Spinal Disorders* **5**:383–9.

36. **Stokes, M., Cooper, R., Morris, G., and Jaysoon, M.** (1992). Selective changes in multifidus dimensions in patients with chronic low back pain. *Euro Spine J* **1**:38–42.

37. **Hodges, S. and Richardson, C.A.** (1006). Insufficient muscular stabilisation of the lumbar spine associated with low back pain. *Spine* **21**:2640–50.

38. **Brandt, K.D., Heilman, D.K., Slemenda, C., Katz, B., Mazzuca, S.A., Braunstein, E.M. and Byrd, D.** (1999). Quadriceps strength in women with radiographically progressive osteoarthritis of the knee and those with stable radiographic changes. *J Rheumatol* **26**:2431–7.

39. **Beard, D., Dodd, C., Trundle, H., and Simpson, A.** (1994). Proprioception enhancement for anterior cruciate ligament deficiency. A prospective randomised trial of two physiotherapy regimes. *J Bone Joint Surg* **76**(B):654–9.

40. **Ihara, H. and Nakayama, A.** (1986). Dynamic control training for knee ligament injuries. *Am J Sports Med* **14**:309–15.

41. **Hurley, M.V. and Scott, D.L.** (1998). Improvements in quadriceps sensorimotor function and disability of patients with knee osteoarthritis following a clinically practicable exercise regime. *Br J Rheumatol* **37**:1181–7.

42. van Baar, M.E., Assendelft, W.J.J., Dekker, J., Oostendorp, R.A.B., and Bijlsma, J.W.J. (1999). Effectiveness of exercise therapy in patients with osteoarthritis of the hip and knee. A systematic review of randomised clinical trials. *Arthritis Rheum* **42**:1361–9.

43. Jenson, G.M. and Lorish, C.D. (1994). Promoting patient cooperation with exercise programmes: linking research, theory, and practice. *Arthritis Care Res* **7**:181–9.

7.2.4.3 Proprioception in osteoarthritis

Leena Sharma

Proprioception, that is, joint position sense, is critical to the maintenance of joint stability under dynamic conditions and, therefore, to joint protection. Proprioceptive inaccuracy may play a role in the development and/or progression of structural damage in OA, and of OA-associated disability. This chapter discusses the sources of proprioception; its role in joint protection; methods of measurement; the relationship of proprioception to age, OA and related knee conditions (hypermobility, knee effusion); evidence that proprioceptive inaccuracy can be reduced and pathogenetic pathways by which proprioceptive inaccuracy may contribute to OA.

Sources of proprioception

Proprioception, in the context used herein, is defined as the conscious and subconscious perception of the position of the joint in space, and includes awareness of both the position and movement of the joint. The coactivation of agonist and antagonist muscles needed for stabilization of a joint depends upon input to the central nervous system from the somatosensory, vestibular, and visual systems. To achieve motor control, input from these systems is processed at the level of the spinal cord, brain stem and higher centers in the brain.[1]

Proprioception derives from the integration of afferent signals from receptors in the muscles, tendons, joint capsule, ligaments, meniscal attachments, and skin. Muscle and joint receptors are major sources of joint proprioception and, because they may be activated under different conditions, are complementary.[2] Sensory receptors that contribute to proprioception include Pacinian corpuscles, Golgi joint receptors, Golgi tendon receptors, Ruffini endings, muscle spindles, and bare nerve endings. The location, stimulus specificity, and projection for each type of receptor are summarized in Table 7.25.

The distribution of mechanoreceptors within a given tissue may vary. In ligaments, mechanoreceptors are concentrated distally and proximally, near the sites of insertion of the ligament into bone.[4] Because the mid-portion of the ligament is more compliant than its attachment sites, the latter are at greater risk of injury. Triggering of the large number of receptors at the ligament insertion sites by application of load may protect these sites from injury.[4]

As shown in Fig. 7.74, the sensory input from the mechanoreceptors travels to the spinal cord and/or to structures in the brain. Input that remains at the level of the spinal cord is responsible for reflex muscle activity (Fig. 7.75). The Golgi joint receptors, Pacinian, Ruffini, and bare endings project to the thalamus and sensory cortex, to give rise to the sensation

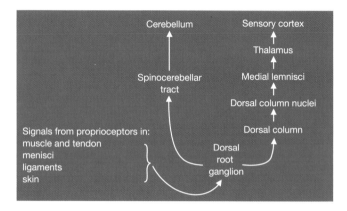

Fig. 7.74 Central pathways for proprioceptive input are shown. Projection of mechanoreceptors to the thalamus and sensory cortex gives rise to sensations of joint position, velocity, acceleration, and pressure. Projection to the cerebellum contributes to the coordination of movement and motor control.

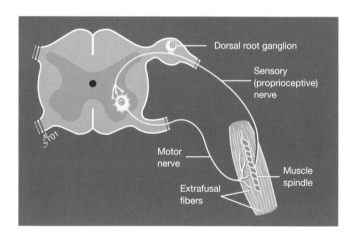

Fig. 7.75 Pathways for reflex stimulation or inhibition of muscle contraction. Mechanoreceptor input that travels to the spinal cord ascends and descends a few cord segments and is, therefore, available to periarticular muscles that are supplied by neighboring cord segments.

Table 7.25 Location, stimulus specificity, and projection of various knee mechanoreceptors

Receptor	Location	Stimulus	Projection
Bare nerve endings	Articular surfaces, ligaments	Deformation (extreme), inflammation, pain	Spinal cord, sensory cortex
Ruffini endings	Capsule, ligaments, menisci	Deformation (low level)	Spinal cord, sensory cortex
Pacinian corpuscles	Ligaments, menisci	Deformation (pressure), high forces	Spinal cord, sensory cortex
Golgi receptors	Tendons, ligaments, menisci, capsule	Extremes of force	Spinal cord, sensory cortex (for capsule and menisci), cerebellum (for tendon)
Muscle spindles	Muscles crossing joint	Muscle elongation, velocity, acceleration	Spinal cord, cerebellum

Source: Adapted from Solomonow and D'Ambrosia.[3]

of joint position, velocity, acceleration, and pressure. The spindle and Golgi tendon receptors project to the cerebellum and their input contributes to the coordination of movement and motor control.[3]

The role of proprioception in joint protection

Proprioception is critical to the maintenance of joint stability under dynamic conditions. Such sensory information constitutes the afferent limb for reflex activity: mechanoreceptor signals are transmitted to posterior horn interneurons with motor connections. Through spinal and cortical projections, the afferent system provides input necessary to drive both muscle reflexes and voluntary muscle contraction and to control movement and joint stability.[3] Muscle contraction contributes to the ability of the joint to resist dynamic disturbances and to maintain the congruity of the articular surfaces that dictates the distribution of stress. Predictable patterns of muscle activity result when ligaments are subjected to stress.

Various approaches have been applied to explore the relationship between proprioceptive input and motor output in the clinical setting. Corrigan et al.[5] found that proprioceptive accuracy in the anterior cruciate ligament (ACL)-deficient leg correlated negatively with the hamstrings/quadriceps strength ratio. Afferent input from receptors in the ACL inhibits hamstring activity. When this input is absent or aberrant because of ACL injury, this inhibitory influence is removed and hamstring activity increases, serving to stabilize the joint and to compensate for the functional absence of the ACL.

Radin et al.[6] found that, in comparison with age-matched asymptomatic controls, patients who were presumed to be pre-arthritic (based on a report of activity-related knee pain with a normal clinical examination) had a greater downward ankle velocity and higher angular shank velocity just prior to heelstrike, and a more rapid rate of loading at heelstrike, than controls. Furthermore, the symptomatic subjects exhibited a lower maximum knee flexion angle during stance and a shorter period of eccentric quadriceps contraction than the asymptomatic individuals, suggesting less efficient use of the quadriceps to control the rate of descent of the foot. Given the speed of these events during the gait cycle, it is unlikely that they are due to proprioceptive error; however, proprioceptive inaccuracy is likely to contribute to gait abnormalities and patterns of loading that predispose to OA.

Measurement of proprioception

In clinical studies, knee proprioception has been assessed using methods that may be categorized as threshold, reproduction, or visual analog (model) tests. Little is known about how these tests relate to each other. Typically, threshold testing utilizes an automated apparatus to provide slow (0.3–0.5°/second), constant, passive knee motion and to measure the difference in degrees between the onset of motion and the subject's ability to detect the motion. In contrast, reproduction tests assess a subject's accuracy in passively or actively reproducing a flexion angle at which the knee had been passively or actively placed previously. Visual analog tests require the subject to indicate the perceived flexion angle on a two- or three-dimensional model of the knee after passive or active positioning of the joint.

The relative contribution to proprioception made by the various types of muscle and joint receptors is likely to depend upon whether motion is passive or active, the angle of the joint, whether the subject is weightbearing, and the speed of movement.[7] Given the variations in test conditions and methods used, clinical studies clearly are not always assessing identical sets of receptors and pathways. It is likely that different tests reflect the status of different pathways that contribute to proprioceptive awareness under a variety of circumstances. It should be emphasized that very little is known about whether—or how—evidence of proprioceptive accuracy in these laboratory tests relates to joint position sense during the performance of activities and to protection of the joint by neuromuscular reflexes.

The relationship between age and proprioceptive accuracy

Several studies have reported reduction in the acuity of knee proprioception with age (8–14). In theory, a decline in proprioceptive accuracy, especially in the context of other age-related changes in the local environment of the joint and in the metabolism of articular cartilage chondrocytes, may contribute to the increased incidence of OA associated with aging. Correlation coefficients from studies specifically examining the relationship between age and proprioceptive acuity[9,11,14] are summarized in Table 7.26.

Kaplan et al.[10] found proprioception to be more accurate in healthy women under 30 years of age than in those more than 60 years old. Petrella et al.[12] reported that proprioception differed between young and active-old, young and sedentary-old, and active- and sedentary-old subjects. Proprioception was most accurate in the young subjects and least accurate in the sedentary-old, raising the possibility that some of the decline in proprioceptive acuity associated with aging may be due to a decline in the level of physical activity. Bullock-Saxton et al.,[15] found that proprioceptive error during partial weightbearing, but not during full weightbearing, increased with age, challenging the belief that various aspects of knee proprioception are modified in an identical fashion by age.

Because asymptomatic knee OA is prevalent in the elderly, the possibility exists that the correlation between age and decreased proprioceptive acuity is a reflection of subclinical knee OA, with impairment in proprioception occurring as a consequence of subtle OA pathology. To examine whether the decrease in proprioceptive acuity was an effect of age or of subclinical OA, we measured proprioception in 25 young controls and 29 older controls with no clinical or radiographic evidence of knee OA, and found that proprioceptive accuracy fell with increasing age in these nonarthritic subjects.[11]

Studies of proprioceptive impairment in OA

Deafferentation in the canine cruciate-deficiency model of OA

In dogs in which knee OA was induced by transection of the ACL, pathologic changes in the unstable knee were more severe and occurred more rapidly if the ipsilateral hind limb had been extensively deafferented by L4–S1 dorsal root ganglionectomy[16] or articular nerve neurectomy,[17] prior to cruciate ligament transection than changes in the unstable joint of neurologically intact cruciate-deficient dogs (see Chapter 7.2.4.1). These results illustrate that if alterations in the mechanical environment of the joint are present, interruption of the sensory input from an extremity, may accelerate joint degeneration. It should be noted, however, that proprioception was not tested specifically in the above studies and the possibility cannot be excluded that the acceleration of OA in this experimental model was due to

Table 7.26 Studies reporting a correlation between proprioceptive impairment and age

Author, year (reference)	Method of assessing proprioceptive accuracy	R for correlation with age
Skinner, 1984[14]	Threshold	0.56
	reproduction	0.57
Hurley, 1998[9]	Reproduction	0.60
Pai, 1997[11]	Threshold	0.60 (right knee)
		0.50 (left knee)

R, Pearson correlation coefficient for the strength of the relationship between age and proprioceptive inaccuracy. Each of these studies indicates the presence of a moderately strong correlation.

a reduction in pain sensation or to some other cause. Furthermore, the arthropathy produced in the canine model in some respects resembled neuropathic (Charcot) arthropathy more than it did typical OA.

Proprioceptive accuracy in patients with knee OA vs. elderly controls

As discussed above, proprioceptive accuracy decreases with age. The effect is magnified by the presence of OA. Several cross-sectional studies have shown that knee proprioception is less accurate in individuals with knee OA than in elderly control subjects[8,11,13,18–23] (see Table 7.27).

The effect of total knee arthoplasty on proprioception

Barrack et al.[18] found no difference in proprioceptive accuracy between the operated knee of patients with bilateral knee OA who had undergone unilateral total knee arthroplasty (TKA) and their contralateral OA knee. Barrett et al.[8] found that proprioception was slightly more accurate after TKA than in unoperated OA knees. Proprioceptive threshold in patients who had undergone unicondylar knee arthroplasty did not differ from that in patients who had undergone TKA.[24]

The impact of proprioceptive inaccuracy on physical function in subjects with knee OA

Although proprioception is believed to be an important component of the neuromuscular physiology of the joint, few investigations have explored the relationship between impaired proprioception and functional status in patients with knee OA.

Skinner et al.[25] found no correlation between results of either threshold or reproduction tests of proprioception and a knee score based predominantly upon pain and function. However, gait velocity and stride length decreased as proprioceptive error increased, suggesting that patients with knee OA altered their gait to compensate for their impairment.

To assess proprioception, Marks[26,27] required the subject to actively extend the knee to a random angle at about 10°/second, following which the joint was passively returned by the examiner to 90° and the subject was asked to actively reproduce the criterion angle. Among 8 women with OA, the magnitude of proprioceptive error was correlated with the score on an algofunctional index. In other relatively small studies,[28–30] in which subjects were asked to reproduce criterion angles of 20–40° (to simulate stance phase flexion during walking), an inverse relationship was noted between proprioceptive accuracy and stair climbing time,[29] and between proprioceptive accuracy and walking speed in one study.[28]

A significant, moderately strong correlation between the average value of the threshold test for both knees and the physical function score for the Western Ontario and McMaster Universities OA Index (WOMAC) was noted in patients with bilateral knee OA.[11] Hurley et al.[19] found no correlation between proprioception (active reproduction of a knee flexion angle randomly selected by the subject) and postural stability among patients with knee OA. After controlling for quadriceps strength, no relationship was detected between proprioceptive accuracy and scores on an algofunctional index, or between proprioceptive accuracy and the time required to perform a battery of knee-requiring tasks. However, in subjects without OA, proprioceptive accuracy for the knee was inversely related to the time required to perform the same tasks.[9] McChesney et al.[31] found a correlation between deceased accuracy in a proprioception threshold test at the knee and ankle and poorer postural control in elderly subjects, although proprioceptive acuity was not related to the ability of the subject to respond to threats to balance. To date, a relationship between proprioceptive inaccuracy and falls has not been described.

Table 7.27 Studies revealing a difference in proprioceptive acuity between individuals with knee OA and controls

Author, year (reference)	Method of assessing proprioceptive accuracy	Groups compared
Barrack, 1983[18]	Threshold	OA knees
		TKR
		Elderly controls
Barrett, 1991[8]	Visual analog	OA knees
		TKR
		Elderly controls
		Young controls
Sell, 1993[13]	Visual analog reproduction	OA knees
		Elderly controls
		Young controls
Hurley, 1997[19]	Reproduction	OA knees
		Elderly controls
Sharma, 1997[20]	Threshold	OA knees
		Uninvolved contralateral knee of subjects with unilateral knee OA
		Elderly controls
Pai, 1997[11]	Threshold	OA knees
		Elderly controls
		Young controls
Garsden, 1999[21]	Reproduction	OA knees
		Uninvolved contralateral knee of subjects with unilateral knee OA
		Elderly controls
Koralewicz, 2000[22]	Threshold	OA knees
		The less involved knee of subjects with bilateral knee OA
		Elderly controls
Hassan, 2000[23]	Reproduction	OA knees
		Elderly controls

TKR, total knee replacement.

Proprioception in related knee conditions

Hypermobility

Deficits in proprioception have been identified in subjects with joint hypermobility. Hall et al.[32] compared 10 women with hypermobility syndrome to age-matched controls. Proprioception was evaluated as the detection of the onset and direction of knee joint displacement at a constant angular velocity. Subjects with hypermobility syndrome had less accurate proprioception than controls. As the knee approached full extension, the controls, but not the hypermobile subjects, exhibited a more accurate proprioception, a finding that may relate to the ability to detect the extremes of motion. The authors suggested that impaired proprioception in hypermobility syndrome may result in mechanically unsound limb positions which, on a repetitive basis, could predispose to OA.

Knee effusion

To test the effect of an effusion on knee proprioception, McNair et al.[33] compared results in 10 normal men in whom 90 cc of a dextrose/saline solution had been injected intra-articularly to results in 10 controls. As one limb was moved passively, the subject was asked to actively track the movement with the other limb, on which an electrogoniometer had been placed. No difference in tracking ability was found between the two groups. As the authors noted, a knee effusion, especially if chronic, may have a greater impact on proprioceptive accuracy than experimental instillation of saline, due to mechanoreceptor damage from inflammatory mediators or stretching of tissues containing proprioceptors.

Muscle fatigue

Strenuous exercise has been shown to be associated with a temporary increase in ligamentous laxity.[34,35] This laxity may affect the function of mechanoreceptors in ligaments. As a result, individuals may be at greater risk for injury when they exercise to the point of fatigue.[36] Skinner et al.[37] found that accuracy in reproduction of the knee flexion angle in young men after induction of fatigue by repeated sprints. Lattanzio et al.[38] found that lower limb fatigue reduced the ability of healthy men and women to reproduce a knee flexion angle. In contrast, Marks et al. did not find a significant difference in proprioceptive accuracy in women before and after a fatigue protocol involving quadriceps exercise.[39]

Improvement of proprioceptive impairment

Several studies have demonstrated improvement in knee joint proprioception with the use of orthoses. Perlau et al.[40] evaluated the effect of an elastic bandage (knee sleeve) in 54 asymptomatic subjects, 22–40 years of age. In this study the knee was passively extended until a criterion angle was reached, following which the subject was required to indicate when this angle was achieved again during passive extension of the joint by the examiner. Application of the sleeve improved proprioception by 25 per cent; if baseline inaccuracy was >5°, proprioception improved by 66 per

cent with the sleeve. Improved proprioception may explain the increased sense of security afforded by such sleeves, which do not provide mechanical support. As reviewed by the authors, a sleeve predominantly affects superficial skin receptors that would react strongly to movement of the sleeve. In keeping with the belief that different sets of receptors and pathways may be involved in proprioception under various conditions, Birmingham et al.[41] found that use of a neoprene knee sleeve improved proprioceptive accuracy during voluntary active movement, but not when the subject was partially weight-bearing.

McNair et al.[42] demonstrated that use of a knee sleeve improved proprioception by 11 per cent ($p < 0.05$) in subjects with no underlying musculoskeletal or neurologic abnormalities. In a study by Barrett et al.,[8] an elastic bandage improved proprioceptive accuracy in OA, but not control, knees. Sell et al.[13] also suggested that a knee support improved proprioception in OA patients but not controls. Use of a valgus brace was associated with a significant, albeit small, improvement in accuracy of proprioception in patients with OA of the medial tibiofemoral compartment.[43]

Muscle training may lead to improvement in proprioception in patients with OA,[44] as it does in ACL deficiency or ACL reconstruction.[45] Bernauer et al.[46] studied knee proprioceptive tracking responses of 19 healthy men after a 30-day period of bedrest, during which they performed either no exercise, isotonic exercise, or isokinetic exercise for two 30-minute periods, 5 days per week. Proprioceptive accuracy after the 30 days was unchanged in the control group, and improved, albeit modestly, in both exercise groups, suggesting that exercise training can improve proprioceptive performance. In studies comparing professional ballet dancers to control subjects, proprioceptive accuracy in threshold detection was better, but accuracy in flexion angle reproduction was poorer in the dancers than in the controls.[47,48] The better threshold detection seen in the dancers may have been a consequence of muscle training; however, the reason for their poorer ability to reproduce the criterion angle than that of the controls is unclear.

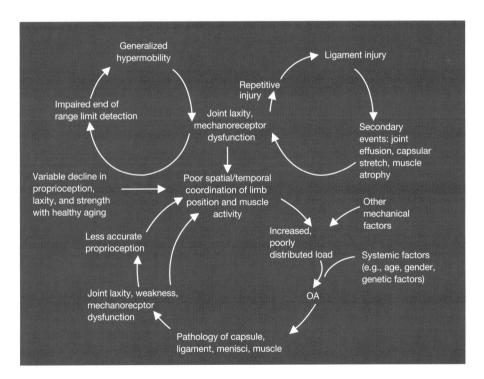

Fig. 7.76 Possible directions in the relationships between proprioception, knee OA, and related disorders are depicted. The figure includes three related cycles. In the central cycle (lowermost in the figure), proprioceptive impairment adversely affects load distribution. In conjunction with other factors, this may contribute to the development and progression of OA. In turn, damage to joint tissues in OA further reduces proprioceptive acuity. In the upper left cycle, in individuals with generalized hypermobility, joint laxity may lead to mechanoreceptor dysfunction and predispose to OA. This mechanoreceptor dysfunction may contribute to greater impairment in the ability to detect endpoints in the range of motion and to greater hypermobility. As shown in the cycle in the upper right, ligament injury may lead to secondary changes in the joint that then may lead to mechanoreceptor dysfunction.

Gait training, biofeedback, electrical stimulation, and facilitation techniques primarily used in the rehabilitation of patients with neurologic impairments have been proposed as other approaches to enhance proprioception.[27] Lephart et al.[1] have advocated rehabilitative approaches for those with proprioceptive impairment that promote motor control at all levels, that is spinal cord, brain stem, and higher brain centers.

Proprioceptive impairment in the development and progression of Knee OA: possible pathogenetic pathways

Given the cross-sectional design of the published studies of proprioception in knee OA, it is not possible to determine the direction of the relationship between impaired proprioception and knee OA. Theoretically, a proprioceptive impairment in the setting of knee OA may have contributed to, or resulted from, the disease, or both. Prior to the onset of OA, impaired proprioception may be related to normal aging, injury of mechanoreceptor-bearing structures, or hypermobility. Disturbance of the afferent component of protective muscular reflexes (see Chapter 7.2.4.2) may lead to repetitive abnormal loading across the articular surface and, thereby, to OA. Proprioceptive impairment might result also from damage to mechanoreceptors in the capsule, ligaments, menisci, muscles or tendons, by pathologic processes of OA.

To explore cause-effect directions, we examined between-knee differences in subjects who were considered to have unilateral knee OA, on the basis of clinical and radiographic criteria. The threshold for detection of slow, passive motion was higher in either the OA knee or uninvolved knee of these subjects than in knees of elderly nonarthritic subjects.[19] No difference was detected between the two knees of patients with unilateral OA, suggesting that impaired proprioception in subjects with OA may not be exclusively the result of local disease. Similarly, Garsden et al.[21] found no difference in proprioceptive acuity between the involved and uninvolved knees of subjects with unilateral OA. Although significant local pathologic changes of OA may be present without clinical manifestations, it is unlikely that changes severe enough to cause proprioceptive impairment are common in asymptomatic knees that are normal by physical exam and on radiography. In future studies, the possibility that an underlying proprioceptive defect may be a cause of OA, rather than merely the result of the disease, would be supported by the finding of reduced proprioceptive acuity also in other joint sites, for example, the elbow or wrist.

The theoretical paradigm shown in Fig. 7.76 depicts possible directions in the relationships between proprioception, knee OA, and related knee disorders. The intrinsic repair capacity of the joint and the response to structure-modifying OA drugs (DMOADs) may depend upon static and dynamic neural, mechanical, and muscular factors.[21] Treatment of proprioceptive impairment, theoretically, could have a disease-modifying effect in patients with OA.

Summary

Proprioception is critical to joint protection. Most information about proprioception in OA comes from cross-sectional studies, which reveal that proprioceptive inaccuracy increases with age, that proprioception is less accurate in subjects with knee OA than in similarly aged subjects with normal knees, and that proprioceptive acuity is correlated with some measures of physical function. Little is known about whether, or how, proprioceptive accuracy measured under laboratory conditions relates to joint position sense during the performance of activities, or to protective muscular reflexes. Proprioceptive inaccuracy may play a role in the development and/or progression of OA, and development of OA-associated disability, though this remains to be demonstrated in longitudinal studies.

Key points

1. Receptors in muscle, tendons, joint capsule, ligaments, meniscal attachments, and skin provide proprioceptive input.

2. Proprioceptive input contributes to joint-protective reflex and voluntary muscle activity.

3. Increase(s) proprioceptive inaccuracy with age.

4. Proprioception is less accurate in subjects with unilateral knee OA, even in the clinically and radiographically normal contralateral knee, than in nonarthritic subjects of similar age. This raises the possibility that a subtle subclinical neurologic defect may be an etiologic factor in some subjects with primary (idiopathic) OA.

5. Proprioceptive acuity is correlated with measures of physical function (questionnaire or performance-based) in some but not all studies.

6. Proprioception can be improved modestly through orthoses or exercise but the impact of this improvement on pain, function, or progression of OA is unclear.

References

(An asterisk denotes recommended reading.)

1. **Lephart, S.M., Pincivero, D.M., and Rozzi, S.L.** (1998). Proprioception of the ankle and knee. *Sports Med* **25**:149.

2. **Lephart, S.M., Pincivero, D.M., Giraldo, J.L.,** *et al.* (1997). The role of proprioception in the management and rehabilitation of athletic injuries. *Am J Sports Med* **25**:130–7.

3. **Solomonow, M. and D'Ambrosia, R.** (1994). Neural reflex arcs and muscle control of knee stability and motion. In W.N. Scott (ed.), *The Knee*. St. Louis: Mosby, pp. 107–20.

4. **McDougall, J.J., Bray, R.C., and Sharkey, K.A.** (1997). Morphological and immunohistochemical examination of nerves in normal and injured collateral ligaments of rat, rabbit, and human knee joints. *Anat Rec* **248**:29–39.

5. **Corrigan, J.P., Cashman, W.F., and Brady, M.P.** (1992). Proprioception in the cruciate deficient knee. *J Bone Joint Surg Br* **74B**:247–50.

6. **Radin, E.L., Yang, K.H., Riegger, C.,** *et al.* (1991). Relationship between lower limb dynamics and knee joint pain. *J Orthop Res* **9**:398–405.

7. **Guyton, A.C. and Hall, J.E.** (1996). Somatic sensation: I. General organization; the tactile and position senses. In A.C. Guyton, J.E. Hall (eds.), *Textbook of Medical Physiology*. Philadelphia: W.B. Saunders, p. 595.

8. **Barrett, D.S., Cobb, A.G., and Bentley, G.** (1991). Joint proprioception in normal, osteoarthritic and replaced knees. *J Bone Joint Surg Br* **73**(B):53–6.

9. **Hurley, M.V., Rees, J., and Newham, D.J.** (1998). Quadriceps function, proprioceptive acuity and functional performance in healthy young, middle-aged and elderly subjects. *Age Ageing* **27**:55–62.

10. **Kaplan, F.S., Nixon, J.E., Reitz, M.,** *et al.* (1985). Age-related changes in proprioception and sensation of joint position. *Acta Orthop Scand* **56**:72–4.

11. **Pai, Y.-C., Rymer, W.Z., Chang, R.W.,** *et al.* (1997). Effect of age and osteoarthritis on knee proprioception. *Arthritis Rheum* **40**:2260–5.

12. *****Petrella, R.J., Lattanzio, P.J., and Nelson, M.G.** (1997). Effect of age and activity on knee joint proprioception. *Am J Phys Med Rehabil* **76**:235–41.

    This study examines the contribution of lifestyle to the relationship between age and proprioceptive inaccuracy, and indicates that proprioception is more accurate in active elderly people than in those who are sedentary.

13. **Sell, S., Zacher, J., and Lack, S.** (1993). Proprioception decline in the osteoarthritic knee. *Z Rheumatol* **52**:150–5.

14. **Skinner, H.B., Barrack, R.L., and Cook, S.D.** (1984). Age-related decline in proprioception. *Clin Orthop* **184**:208–11.

15. *****Bullock-Saxton, J.E., Wong, W.J., and Hogan, N.** (2001). The influence of age on weight-bearing joint reposition sense of the knee. *Exp Brain Res* **136**:400–6.

    This study examines the influence of age on the accuracy of knee proprioception with full and partial weight-bearing. Age was associated with reduced accuracy only in the partial weight-bearing condition, arguing against a general decline in proprioceptive acuity with age.

16. O'Connor, B.L., Visco, D.M., Brandt, K.D., Albrecht, M., and O'Connor, A.B. (1993). Sensory nerves only temporarily protect the unstable canine knee joint from osteoarthritis. *Arthritis Rheum* **36**:1154–63.

17. O'Connor, B.L., Visco, D.M., Brandt, K.D., Myers, S.L., and Kalasinski, L. (1992). Neurogenic acceleration of osteoarthritis: The effects of prior articular nerve neurectomy on the development of osteoarthritis after anterior cruciate ligament transection in the dog. *J Bone Jt Surg* **74**(A):367–76.

18. Barrack, R.L., Skinner, H.B., Cook, S.D., et al. (1983). Effect of articular disease and total knee arthroplasty on knee joint-position sense. *J Neurophysiol* **50**:684–7.

19. *Hurley, M.V., Scott, D.L., Rees, J., et al. (1997). Sensorimotor changes and functional performance in patients with knee osteoarthritis. *Ann Rheum Dis* **56**:641–8.

   This study found no correlation between proprioception and postural stability in patients with knee OA. After controlling for quadriceps strength, no relationship was detected between proprioception and the score on an algofunctional index.

20. *Sharma, L., Pai, Y.-C., Holtkamp, K., and Rymer, W.Z. (1997). Is knee joint proprioception worse in the arthritic knee versus the unaffected knee in unilateral knee osteoarthritis? *Arthritis Rheum* **40**:1518–25.

   In this study, proprioceptive acuity in normal elderly subjects was compared with that in the uninvolved and arthritic knees of patients with unilateral knee OA. Proprioceptive accuracy was reduced to a similar degree in both the uninvolved and involved knees of the patients with OA, adding support to the concept that the impairment may be not only a result of OA but may precede OA and be a risk factor for the disease.

21. Garsden, L.R. and Bullock-Saxton, J.E. (1999). Joint reposition sense in subjects with unilateral osteoarthritis of the knee. *Clin Rehab* **13**:148–55.

22. Koralewicz, L.M. and Engh, G.A. (2000). Comparison of proprioception in arthritic and age-matched normal knees. *J Bone Joint Surg* **82**(A):1582–8.

23. Hassan, B.S., Mockett, S., and Doherty, M. (2001). Static postural sway, proprioception, and maximal voluntary quadriceps contraction in patients with knee osteoarthritis and normal control subjects. *Ann Rheum Dis* **60**:612–8.

24. Simmons, S., Lephart, S., Rubash, H., et al. (1996). Proprioception after unicondylar knee arthroplasty versus total knee arthroplasty. *Clin Orthop* **331**:179–84.

25. Skinner, H.B., Barrack, R.L., Cook, S.D., et al. (1984). Joint position sense in total knee arthroplasty. *J Orthop Res* **1**:276–83.

26. Marks, R. (1994). The reliability of knee position sense measurements in healthy women. *Physiother Can* **46**:37–41.

27. Marks, R. (1994). Correlation between knee position sense measurements and disease severity in persons with osteoarthritis. *Rev Rheum Engl* **61**:365–72.

28. Marks, R. (1993). Proprioceptive sensibility in women with normal and osteoarthritic knee joints. *Clin Rheumatol* **12**:170–5.

29. Marks, R. (1994). An investigation of the influence of age, clinical status, pain and position sense on stair walking in women with osteoarthrosis. *Int J Rehabil Res* **17**:151–8.

30. Marks, R., Quinney, A.H., and Wessel, J. (1993). Reliability and validity of the measurement of position sense in women with osteoarthritis of the knee. *J Rheum* **20**:1919–24.

31. McChesney, J.W. and Woollacott, M.H. (2000). The effect of age-related declines in proprioception and total knee replacement on postural control. *J Gerontol Biol Sci Med Sci* **55**:M658–66.

32. Hall, M.G., Ferrell, W.R., Sturrock, R.D., et al. (1995). The effect of the hypermobility syndrome on knee joint proprioception. *Br J Rheum* **34**:121–5.

33. McNair, P.J., Marshall, R.N., Maguire, K., et al. (1995) Knee joint effusion and proprioception. *Arch Phys Med Rehabil* **76**:566–8.

34. Skinner, H.B., Wyatt, M.P., Stone, M.L., et al. (1986). Exercise-related knee joint laxity. *Am J Sports Med* **14**:30–4.

35. Weisman, G., Pope, M.H., and Johnson, R.J. (1980). Cyclic loading in knee ligament injuries. *Am J Sports Med* **8**:24–30.

36. Lattanzio, P.-J. and Petrella, R.J. (1998). Knee proprioception: a review of mechanisms, measurements, and implications of muscular fatigue. *Orthopedics* **21**:463–70.

37. Skinner, H.B., Wyatt, M.P., Hodgdon, J.A., et al. (1986). Effect of fatigue on joint position sense of the knee. *J Orthop Res* **4**:112–8.

38. Lattanzio, P.-J., Petrella, R.J., Sproule, J.R., et al. (1997). Effects of fatigue on knee proprioception. *Clin J Sports Med* **7**:22–7.

39. Marks, R. and Quinney, H.A. (1993). Effect of fatiguing maximal isokinetic quadriceps contractions on ability to estimate knee-position. *Percept Mot Skills* **77**:1195–205.

40. Perlau, R., Frank, C., and Fick, G. (1995). The effect of elastic bandages on human knee proprioception in the uninjured population. *Am J Sports Med* **23**:251–5.

41. Birmingham, T.B., Inglis, J.T., Kramer, J.F., and Vandervoort, A.A. (2000). Effect of a neoprene sleeve on knee joint kinesthesis: influence of different testing procedures. *Med Sci Sports Exercise* **32**:304–8.

42. McNair, P.J., Stanley, S.N., and Strauss, G.R. (1996). Knee bracing: effects on proprioception. *Arch Phys Med Rehab* **77**:287–9.

43. *Birmingham, T.B., Kramer, J.F., Kirkley, A., Inglish, J.T., Spaulding, S.J., and Vandervoort, A.A. (2001). Knee bracing for medial compartment osteoarthritis: effects on proprioception and postural control. *Rheumatology* **40**:285–9.

   This study examines the effect of a brace designed to 'unload' the medial compartment in varus knees on measures of proprioceptive acuity and postural control. Proprioception was improved following brace application, but postural control was not improved. Some of the reported beneficial effects of 'unloading' braces may be due to the proprioceptive enhancement.

44. Hurley, M.V. and Scott, D.L. (1998). Improvements in quadriceps sensorimotor function and disability of patients with knee osteoarthritis following a clinically practicable exercise regime. *Br J Rheumatol* **37**:1181–7.

45. Pincivero, D.M., Lephart, S.M., and Henry, T.J. (1996). The effects of kinesthetic training on balance and proprioception in the anterior cruciate ligament injured knee. *J Athlet Train* **31**(Suppl. 2):S52.

46. Bernauer, E.M., Walby, W.F., Ertl, A.C., et al. (1994). Knee-joint proprioception during 30-day 6 degrees head-down bed rest with isotonic and isokinetic exercise training. *Aviat Space Environ Med* **65**:1110–5.

47. Barrack, R.L., Skinner, H.B., Brunet, M.E., et al. (1984). Joint kinesthesia in the highly trained knee. *J Sports Med Phys Fitness* **24**:18–20.

48. Barrack, R.L., Skinner, H.B., and Cook, S.D. (1984). Proprioception of the knee joint, paradoxical effect of training. *Am J Phys Med* **63**:175–81.

7.2.5 Local mechanical factors in the natural history of knee osteoarthritis. Malalignment and joint laxity

Leena Sharma

Osteoarthritis is widely believed to be the result of local factors acting within the context of a systemic susceptibility.[1–3] These local factors, specific to joint site and, in some instances, to a specific anatomic compartment within a joint, govern how load is distributed across the articular cartilage. It is the appropriate distribution of load that confers upon weight-bearing joints the ability to bear loads that are several times greater than body weight over a lifetime.[4] Because alterations in these local factors may lead to excessive stress on the joint and damage to the articular cartilage, they are receiving increasing attention in studies of the natural history of OA. This chapter examines malalignment and laxity, two local factors that may be of pathogenetic importance in OA.

Like other changes in the local mechanical environment (e.g., changes in the subchondral bone or degeneration of the meniscus), laxity and malalignment may precede and/or result from progressive OA. In a given joint, it may not be possible to differentiate cause from effect. To some extent, this has contributed to a belief that local impairments should be viewed simply as manifestations of the disease. However, whether these changes in the local environment develop before or after the onset of OA, it is likely that they alter the subsequent course of the disease. Malalignment and laxity may each be related to OA progression in a vicious cycle (Fig. 7.77). They may play a role in disease progression through direct effects on load distribution, secondary damage to other tissues, or by amplification of the effects of other risk factors (e.g., as described for obesity below). In addition, malalignment and laxity may contribute to joint pain and to a decline in physical function.

Local mechanical factors in studies of the natural history of OA

The role of malalignment and laxity in knee OA has been examined in two major types of studies: biomechanical studies, which assess the influence of the local factor on joint function or mechanics, and clinical and epidemiologic studies, which examine the relationship of the local factor to patient-relevant outcomes, such as pain, function, and the severity of structural damage (typically, as assessed radiographically). Demonstration of an effect at this second level is essential: testing the immediate or short-term mechanical impact of a local derangement is not equivalent to testing its impact on long-term structural or functional outcomes in humans. With longitudinal cohort studies, the effects of malalignment and laxity over time may be quantified.

As for any candidate risk factor for OA, there are three dimensions regarding the role of malalignment and laxity in the natural history of disease: do they contribute to: incident OA; to disease progression in those who already have OA; or to disability in those with OA? There is growing awareness that the risk factors contributing to each of these outcomes may overlap but are not identical. It is of particular importance that the effects of local mechanical factors on the risk of incident and progressive OA be examined separately, because their effect is likely to differ according to the baseline status of the joint. In theory, their effect on OA progression may be greater than that on incident OA; in the former setting, joint damage from OA may render the knee more vulnerable to alterations in load distribution or joint mechanics.

In accordance with paradigms of the pathogenesis of OA, risk factors in epidemiological studies tend to be classified as either systemic or local. However, certain systemic risk factors may act, in part, by altering the local environment of the joint. For example, in addition to its effects on chondrocyte function, the material properties of the articular cartilage, and the responses of cartilage to cytokines and growth factors, aging is associated with an increase in varus–valgus laxity[5] and declines in proprioceptive acuity[6]

(Chapter 7.2.4.3), muscle strength, and muscle mass[7–9] (Chapter 9.11.1). Similarly, gender-related effects on the development of OA may be mediated through multiple routes, including gender differences in the local environment, for example, varus–valgus laxity at the knee[5] and strength, relative to body weight.[10]

Although this chapter focuses on malalignment and laxity as prototypic local factors acting at the knee, other local factors are also likely to play a role in the evolution of OA, for example, joint position sense, strength of the periarticular musculature, torsion (rotational deformity), and subclinical or overt congenital or acquired abnormalities in joint shape or congruity.

Malalignment

Definition and effect on the local mechanical environment of the joint

Any shift from a neutral, or collinear, alignment of the hip, knee, and ankle (Fig. 7.78) will affect load distribution at the knee. In a varus knee the load-bearing axis passes medial to the knee and a moment arm is created that increases the magnitude of the forces across the medial compartment; in a valgus knee, the shift in the load-bearing axis increases the forces across the lateral compartment.[11–13] Furthermore, the severity of varus alignment correlates with the ratio of medial compartment to lateral compartment bone mineral density in patients with OA, reflecting greater bone density in the region bearing greater load.[14]

During normal gait, disproportionate transmission of load to the medial compartment results from a stance-phase adduction moment[15] that reflects the magnitude of intrinsic compressive load on the medial compartment (Fig. 7.79).[16] Varus–valgus alignment is a key determinant of this moment. Varus alignment further increases medial compartment load during gait.[17] Although valgus alignment is associated with an increase in stress in the lateral compartment,[13] until valgus deformity become(s) severe, more load is borne medially than laterally.[18,19]

Varus or valgus alignment may be either a cause or result of knee OA. Varus or valgus alignment that predates knee OA may be due to genetic, developmental, or post-traumatic factors. Studies in animal models support a link between pre-existing varus or valgus alignment and the development of knee OA.[11] Pathologic changes in knee OA that may lead to, or increase, varus malalignment include medial tibiofemoral compartment cartilage loss

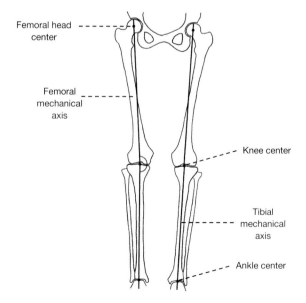

Femoral head center

Femoral mechanical axis

Knee center

Tibial mechanical axis

Ankle center

Fig. 7.78 Knee alignment is reflected by the hip-knee-ankle angle, that is the angle formed by the intersection of the femoral and the tibial mechanical axes at the center of the knee.

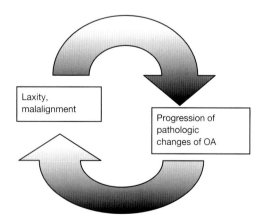

Laxity, malalignment

Progression of pathologic changes of OA

Fig. 7.77 This paradigm illustrates that the relationship of laxity and malalignment to the progression of OA is a vicious cycle.

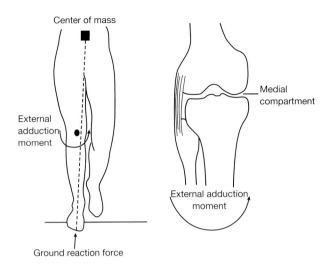

Fig. 7.79 The adduction moment at the knee occurs about an axis that moves with the tibia in the sagittal plane. The adduction moment is strongly related to the magnitude of the total intrinsic compressive load on the medial compartment. Theoretically, a greater adduction moment may contribute to the development and progression of OA in the medial tibiofemoral compartment OA. Varus–valgus alignment is a key determinant of this moment. As body weight drops onto, and moves across, the foot, forces are generated on the floor that are equal in intensity, and opposite in direction, to those experienced by the weight-bearing limb; in the figure these forces are represented as the ground reaction force.

Table 7.28 Odds ratios (OR) for progression of medial tibiofemoral compartment associated with varus alignment

Alignment	Unadjusted OR (95% CI)	OR adjusted for age, gender, BMI (95% CI)
Varus vs. non-varus	5.00 (2.77, 9.02)	4.09 (2.20, 7.62)
Varus vs. neutral/mild valgus	3.54 (1.85, 6.77)	2.98 (1.51, 5.89)

Varus, >0 degrees in the varus direction.

Mild valgus, ≤2 degrees of valgus.

Table 7.29 Odds ratios (OR) for progression of lateral tibiofemoral compartment associated with valgus alignment

Alignment	Unadjusted OR (95% CI)	OR adjusted for age, gender, and BMI (95% CI)
Valgus vs. non-valgus	3.88 (1.82, 8.24)	4.89 (2.13, 11.20)
Valgus vs. neutral/mild varus	3.23 (1.30, 8.05)	3.42 (1.31, 8.96)

Valgus, >0 degrees in the valgus direction.

Mild varus, ≤2 degrees of varus.

and bony attrition, and medial meniscus damage. Knee OA pathology that may lead to, or increase, valgus malalignment of the knee includes changes in the cartilage, meniscus, and bone of the lateral tibiofemoral compartment.

Clinical studies

Malalignment and progression of joint-space narrowing in OA knees. A very large body of literature provides evidence that alignment is an important determinant of the outcome of surgical procedures involving the knee (e.g., arthroplasty, osteotomy, meniscectomy). Considerably less attention has been paid to the role of knee alignment in the natural evolution of OA in the unoperated knee, however. Few longitudinal studies of OA have dealt with the relationship of alignment to the natural history of the disease in an unselected sample or have assessed alignment at baseline.[20–22] Because OA pathology can lead to malalignment, assessing alignment only at the *end* of the follow-up period is not a valid approach in epidemiological studies.

Schouten *et al.*[20] found that a history of bow-legs or knock-knees in childhood was associated with a 5-fold increase in the risk of progressive OA after adjustment for age, gender, and body mass index (BMI). When we examined the effect of alignment on OA progression over 18 months in 240 subjects with knee OA (based on the presence of osteophytosis and difficulty with physical function), we found that the severity of varus alignment in the dominant knee at baseline correlated with the magnitude of joint-space narrowing in the medial tibiofemoral compartment over the ensuing 18 months ($r = 0.52$, $p < 0.0001$).[22] Similarly, the severity of valgus deformity at baseline correlated with the magnitude of subsequent loss of lateral joint space width ($r = 0.35$, $p < 0.0001$). These relationships persisted after adjustment for age, gender, and BMI.

As shown in Table 7.28, the presence of varus deformity at baseline was associated with a substantial increase in the adjusted odds of progression of medial compartment OA. In recognition of the fact that medial compartment OA may be associated with either varus, valgus, or neutral alignment, the reference group for this analysis included any alignment other than varus. The odds associated with varus were elevated also when the reference group included only neutral or nearly neutral knees (Table 7.28).

Similarly, valgus malalignment at baseline was associated with an increase in the odds of progression of lateral compartment OA, regardless of whether the reference group included non-valgus knees, or only neutral/nearly neutral knees (Table 7.29). It is likely that malalignment and OA progression exist in a vicious cycle. The results of this study support the view that, regardless of whether malalignment precedes or is the result of OA, it may contribute to the progression of joint damage.

Malalignment and physical disability. In the above study, the magnitude of malalignment at baseline also predicted deterioration in physical function over the ensuing 18 months,[22] based on the change in performance of the chair-stand test. Subjects were classified into one of three groups: neither knee with >5° varus or valgus deformity; one knee with >5° varus or valgus; both knees with >5° varus or valgus. As shown in Table 7.30, no difference was apparent between the first two groups. However, subjects with bilateral knee malalignment at baseline exhibited significantly greater worsening of physical function in the subsequent 18 months, than subjects without malalignment in either knee. When functional worsening was defined as a decline of 20 per cent or greater in performance of the chair-stand test, the proportion of subjects exhibiting a decline in performance rose steadily as the number of malaligned knees increased. In comparison with subjects in whom knee alignment was normal bilaterally, malalignment >5° in one knee doubled the risk of functional decline and malalignment >5° in both knees tripled that risk.

Malalignment and patellofemoral (PF) joint OA. Valgus and varus malalignment affect forces acting on the PF joint as well as on the tibiofemoral compartment and may predispose to lateral and medial PF OA, respectively. The relatively lateral position of the tibial tubercle when the knee is in full knee extension produces the Q-angle (i.e., the angle formed by the intersection of the line of application of quadriceps force with the center line of the patellar tendon, see Fig. 7.80). The Q-angle adds a strong, laterally directed component to the contact force.[23] It is likely that this lateral vector contributes to the predominance of pathology on the lateral side of the PF joint, including dislocations, lateral pressure syndromes and, possibly, OA.[24] A decrease in the Q-angle (Fig. 7.80) results in a lateral shift of the contact area, with unloading of the medial facet; an increase in the Q-angle results in a medial shift and lateral unloading.[23]

Valgus alignment leads to a decrease in the Q-angle (Fig. 7.80), and increased stress on the lateral patellar facet; varus deformity leads to an increase in the angle and an increase in medial patellar stress. It has been theorized that alignment may influence the risk of development of OA

Table 7.30 Differences between groups (95% CI) in performance of chair-stand test between baseline and 18 months, in relation to malalignment burden at baseline

Malalignment burden at baseline	Unadjusted	Adjusted for age, gender, and BMI	Adjusted for age, gender, BMI, and pain
One knee >5° vs. neither knee >5°	0.48 (−1.40, 2.36)	0.43 (−1.44, 2.31)	0.17 (−1.66, 2.01)
Both knees >5° vs. neither knee >5°	2.88 (0.75, 5.01)	2.73 (0.52, 4.94)	2.23 (0.05, 4.41)

Units are the chair-stand rate (i.e., the number of stands per minute), estimated from the time required by the subject to complete five chair-stands. For each group, positive values indicate a decline in performant.

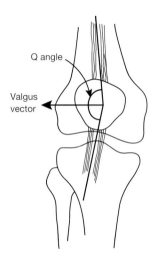

Fig. 7.80 The Q-angle is formed by the intersection of the line of application of quadriceps force with the center line of the patellar tendon. It adds a strong, laterally directed (valgus) component to the contact force (adapted from Ref. 23). Valgus deformity leads to a decrease in the Q-angle and to increased stress on the lateral patellar facet; varus deformity leads to an increase in the Q-angle and an increase in medial patellar stress.

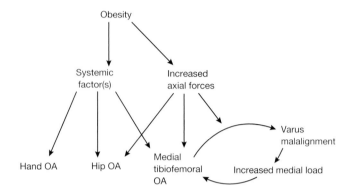

Fig. 7.81 Paradigm of the theoretical relationship between obesity and OA at different joint sites. A systemic factor that explains the effect of obesity has yet to be identified. To some extent, all lower extremity joints are subject to axial forces related to body weight. In addition, malalignment may render the knee more vulnerable than other lower extremity joints to the effect of obesity. Obesity may amplify and/or accelerate the cycle of medial tibiofemoral compartment cartilage loss and varus malalignment in OA.

of the PF joint, that is valgus and varus may increase the likelihood of lateral and medial PF OA, respectively.[25,26] In support of this possibility, Elahi et al.[27] found that knees with lateral PF OA were more likely to be valgus, that lateral PF OA was more common than medial PF OA, and that knees with isolated PF OA or mixed PF/tibiofemoral OA were more likely to exhibit valgus deformity than those with isolated tibiofemoral OA.[27]

The role of malalignment in the obesity/OA relationship. In addition to their direct effect, local factors may mediate the action of other risk factors. Knee alignment appears to act as a mediator in the relationship between obesity and OA.[28] First, a correlation between BMI and tibiofemoral compartment joint-space narrowing was detected in varus, but not valgus, knees, consistent with biomechanical evidence that body weight may be more equitably distributed between the two tibiofemoral compartments in valgus than in varus knees.[13] Second, the relationship between BMI and the radiographic severity of medial compartment OA, did not persist after controlling for varus malalignment; that is, BMI and varus deformity are linked in their effect. Varus alignment serves to focus the forces of body weight on the medial compartment, and represents a factor that helps explain why obesity is linked more strongly to OA of the knee than to OA of other lower extremity joints.

Previous epidemiological studies have failed to identify systemic metabolic factors, for example, body fat distribution, blood pressure, serum lipid, or uric acid levels, that might explain the association between obesity and knee OA, suggesting indirectly that the association may be related to local mechanical factors. Regardless of whether obesity-associated malalignment precedes or follows the onset of OA, it may amplify and accelerate a cycle of medial compartment cartilage loss and varus malalignment. This may be a mechanism underlying the progression of knee OA in obese individuals. (Fig. 7.81)[28]

Laxity

Definition and effect on the local mechanical environment of the joint

Stability is a key component of the mechanical environment of the normal joint. Knee instability, that is, laxity, may be defined as abnormal displacement or rotation of the tibia with respect to the femur.[29] In the unloaded state, knee stability is provided by the ligaments, capsule, and other soft tissues. In the loaded state it is provided by interactions between these tissues, the geometry of the femoral condyles, and contact forces generated by muscle contraction and gravity.[29] The processing of proprioceptive input by the central nervous system results in the contraction of periarticular muscles, helping to stabilize the joint.[30] During normal motion, ligament stiffness is not great. However, when the joint is subjected to large stresses, as during a sudden change in direction, soft tissue stiffness increases and limits the displacement between the femur and tibia, protecting the cartilage and other tissues from injury.[31]

As assessed clinically, joint laxity reflects an impairment for which muscle activity may not be able to compensate. Laxity results in a more abrupt motion, with larger displacements than would occur if the joint is stable. Deleterious effects of laxity include alteration of the congruence and contact regions of the opposing articular surfaces and an increase in shear and compressive stresses on the regions of the articular cartilage.[32] Bruns et al.[13] demonstrated that division of the medial or lateral collateral ligament in severely malaligned cadaver knees, resulted in further increases in peak articular pressure. Such alterations in the distribution and magnitude of contact stresses may lead to cartilage damage, diminishing the ability of the cartilage to withstand stress.[31]

In individuals who do not have arthritis, joint laxity may reflect primary capsuloligamentous laxity (related to genetic factors or age-related soft tissue changes) or prior injury. In knees with moderate to severe OA, laxity may be due to loss of articular cartilage and/or bone, chronic capsuloligamentous stretch, or combinations of ligamentous, meniscal, muscular, and capsular pathology. The ligaments and the menisci of the OA knee develop fraying similar to that seen in the articular cartilage.

Aging is associated with alterations in the material properties of ligaments. Ligament stiffness and the load at which ligament failure occurred decreased substantially with age in a study of human femur-anterior cruciate ligament (ACL)-tibia complexes.[33] The failure load was more than 300 per cent greater in specimens from younger individuals than in those from older subjects. Among subjects with no clinical or radiographic evidence of OA, a modest correlation between varus–valgus laxity and age has been described.[5] Such age-related changes may be intensified by anatomic factors and comorbid conditions.

Clinical studies

Measurement of laxity. Laxity in the frontal (varus–valgus) and sagittal (anteroposterior, AP) planes has been examined in a small number of studies of patients with knee OA. The paucity of clinical information on varus–valgus laxity in knee OA relates in part to the fact that a reliable means of measuring varus–valgus laxity is not widely available. In clinical settings, varus–valgus laxity is most commonly assessed by physical exam, which has been shown to be an unreliable method.[34,35] Sources of error during the physical exam include inadequate immobilization of the thigh and ankle, incomplete muscle relaxation, variation of the knee flexion angle, variation in the applied load, and imprecise measurement of rotation with application of load.[34–36] Previous studies assessing varus–valgus laxity utilized a computerized system (Genucom, Faro Medical Industries, Lake Mary, FL) that is no longer available[40,41] or a device designed specifically for that study.[5] However, devices that can reliably measure AP laxity are commercially available (e.g., the KT1000, KT2000 arthrometers, MEDmetric, San Diego CA).

Collateral ligament injury and OA. The literature on knee injury provides some evidence of the clinical importance of laxity, although all studies have not been equally attentive to the possible effects of concomitant injury. Lundberg *et al.*[37] found that while the majority of subjects with isolated medial collateral ligament (MCL) injury had not developed OA 10 years after the injury, combined injury to the MCL and ACL led to OA in nearly 50 per cent of subjects. Kannus[38,39] reported that 50 per cent of those with a grade III sprain of the lateral collateral ligament (LCL) developed OA within 8 years after injury, and that 63 per cent of those with a grade III sprain of the MCL developed OA within 9 years.

Varus–valgus laxity, OA severity and physical function. There is evidence that varus–valgus laxity predates the development of full-blown knee OA, that is, that laxity is not merely the result of the disease process. In support of this concept, among subjects without clinical or radiographic evidence of knee OA, we found that varus–valgus laxity correlated with age, and was greater in women than in men.[5] Additionally, varus–valgus laxity was greater in subjects with idiopathic knee OA—even in the uninvolved or only mildly involved contralateral knee—than in control subjects of comparable age who did not have clinical or radiographic evidence of knee OA.[5] Similarly, Brage *et al.*[40] found that laxity was greater in mildly arthritic knees than in knees of age-matched control subjects.

Even if laxity produces structural changes of OA, the pathologic changes of OA exacerbate varus–valgus laxity. Varus–valgus laxity was shown to increase as joint space decreased, (presumably reflecting thinning of articular cartilage and/or meniscal damage) and was greater in knees with radiographic evidence of bony attrition than in those with no bone loss.[5] Loss of bone and cartilage may increase varus–valgus laxity by approximating the points of attachment of the collateral ligaments to the femur and tibia.

As demonstrated by Pottenger *et al.*,[41] who measured varus–valgus angulation before and after removal of osteophytes in patients with advanced knee OA, it is likely that osteophytes help prevent varus–valgus laxity to some extent and contribute to knee stability. This compensation may be more successful in the earlier stages of OA. With progressive disease, however, loss of cartilage and bone appear to override the stabilizing effect of osteophytes (Fig. 7.82).

Difficulty encountered in performance of knee-requiring activities, based upon scores on the Western Ontario and McMaster Universities OA Index (WOMAC) physical function score, was significantly greater in subjects with high levels of laxity than in those with less laxity.[42]

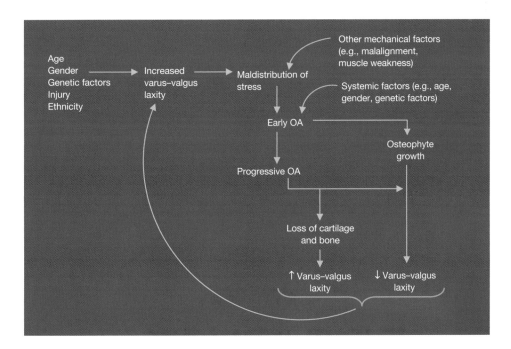

Fig. 7.82 Paradigm describing the theoretical role of varus–valgus laxity in knee OA. Several factors (shown on the left side of the figure) may increase the risk of knee OA by increasing varus–valgus laxity. The maldistribution of stress due to laxity may act in concert with other mechanical and systemic factors. Although osteophyte growth may reduce varus–valgus laxity, in the setting of OA progression, this stress is overridden by the loss of articular cartilage and bone. A vicious cycle may be initiated (adapted from Ref. 5).

Evidence exists that varus–valgus laxity may modify the relationship between muscle strength and function in patients with knee OA. In the presence of laxity, more muscle work must be directed toward stabilization of the joint. We have found that the greater the degree of laxity, the weaker the relationship between quadriceps or hamstring strength and physical function.[42] These results raise the possibility that muscle strengthening will have less impact on physical function in OA patients with knee laxity than in those with a stable knee, and that correcting varus–valgus laxity, for example, through the use of stabilizing orthotics, may improve the effects of interventions aimed at increasing the strength of the periarticular muscles in patients with knee OA.

AP Laxity and OA. In non-arthritic subjects, we found no relationship between AP laxity and age or gender.[5] Furthermore, the amount of AP translation present in knees of subjects with OA was similar to that in knees of control subjects. In our study, laxity did not appear to be associated with specific radiographic features of OA or with the global grade of OA severity.[5] In other studies however, a reduction in AP laxity was noted with increasing radiographic severity of OA.[40,43] Wada *et al.*[43] reported a decline in AP translation with increasing radiographic severity of knee OA, despite prevalent pathologic changes in the ACL among those with advanced OA.[43] It is possible that the inability to predict AP translation on the basis of the pathologic status of the ACL, is due to the fact that joint stiffness resulting from capsular changes or osteophytosis overrides the cruciate ligament insufficiency that can occur with progression of knee OA.

Summary

Thus, malalignment and laxity, common local mechanical factors that alter load distribution, are likely to influence the risk of development and progression of OA and related disability. Biomechanical evidence indicates that alignment influences the distribution of load at the knee and longitudinal data indicate that this biomechanical effect is clinically relevant to structural and functional outcomes in patients with tibiofemoral OA. Malalignment is a determinant of outcome after orthopedic surgical procedures on the knee, increases the risk of progression of tibiofemoral OA in a compartment-specific fashion, increases the risk of functional decline in people with knee OA, and in cross-sectional analyses, is associated with OA of the PF compartment. The effects of conservative interventions, such as 'unloading' braces and wedged insoles that reduce the stress imposed by knee malalignment, are under investigation. Their impact on the progression of structural damage and long-term functional outcomes is yet unknown.

Biomechanical evidence and the results of cross-sectional clinical studies indicate that varus–valgus laxity affects the course of knee OA. Laxity increases with age, has deleterious biomechanical effects that may lead to cartilage damage; is associated with a greater risk of OA in the setting of ligament injury; is worse even in the uninvolved knee of subjects with idiopathic unilateral knee OA than in knees of non-arthritic controls; is made worse by specific pathologic features of OA (e.g., loss of articular cartilage, bony attrition); alters the strength/function relationship; and is associated with deficits in physical function.

In conclusion, malalignment and laxity are local mechanical factors that alter load distribution and are likely to influence the risk of development and progression of OA disease and disability.

Key points

1. Whether malalignment and laxity develop before or after the onset of OA, it is likely that they alter the subsequent course of the disease.

2. There is some evidence that malalignment and laxity may play a role in both the progression of structural damage and the decline in physical function in OA.

3. The impact of malalignment and laxity is due to their direct effects on load distribution and their potential amplification of the action of other pathogenetic factors in OA.

References

(An asterisk denotes recommended reading.)

1. Dieppe, P. (1995). The classification and diagnosis of osteoarthritis. In: K.E. Kuettner and V.M. Goldberg (eds), *Osteoarthritic Disorders*. Rosemont: American Academy of Orthopaedic Surgeons, p. 7.

2. Kuettner, K.E. and Goldberg, V.M. (1995). Introduction. In: K.E. Kuettner and V.M. Goldberg (eds), *Osteoarthritic Disorders*. Rosemont: American Academy of Orthopaedic Surgeons, p. xxi–xxv.

3. Pelletier, J-P., Martel-Pelletier, J., and Howell, D.S. (1997). Etiopathogenesis of osteoarthritis. In: W.J. Koopman (ed.), *Arthritis and Allied Conditions: A Textbook of Rheumatology*. Baltimore: Williams and Wilkins, pp. 1969–84.

4. Woo, S.L-Y., Lewis, J.L., Suh, J-K., and Engebretsen, L. (1995). Acute injury to ligament and meniscus as inducers of osteoarthritis. In: K.E. Kuettner and V.M. Goldberg (eds), *Osteoarthritic Disorders*. Rosemont: American Academy of Orthopaedic Surgeons, pp. 185–96.

5. *Sharma, L., Lou, C., Felson, D.T., *et al.* (1999). Dunlop, D.D., Kirwan-Mellis, G., Hayes, K.W., Weinrach, D., Buchanan, T.S. Laxity in healthy and osteoarthritic knees. *Arthritis Rheum* **42**:861–70.
    This study supports the concept that varus–valgus laxity may increase the risk of knee OA and contribute to its progression in a vicious cycle.

6. Pai, Y.-C., Rymer, W.Z., Chang, R.W., and Sharma, L. (1997). Effect of age and osteoarthritis on knee proprioception. *Arthritis Rheum* **40**:2260–5.

7. Rudman, D. (1985). Growth hormone, body composition and aging. *J Am Geriatr Soc* **33**:800–7.

8. Baumgartner, R.N., Stauber, P.M., McHugh, D., Koehler, K.M., and Garry, P.J. (1995). Cross sectional age differences in body composition in persons 60+years of age. *J Gerontol* **50**(A):M307–M316.

9. Stoll, T., Huber, E., Seifert, B., Michel, B.A., and Stucki, G. (1996). Muscle strength and age: different patterns in healthy women and men (abstract). *Arthritis Rheum* **39**:S176.

10. Slemenda, C., Heilman, D.K., Brandt, K.D., *et al.* (1998). Reduced quadriceps strength relative to body weight: a risk factor for knee osteoarthritis in women. *Arthritis Rheum* **41**:1951–9.

11. Tetsworth, K. and Paley, D. (1994). Malalignment and degenerative arthropathy. *Orthop Clin NA* **25**:367–77.

12. McKellop, H.A., Llinas, A., and Sarmiento, A. (1994). Effects of tibial malalignment on the knee and ankle. *Orthop Clin NA* **25**:415–23.

13. Bruns, J., Volkmer, M., and Luessenhop, S. (1993). Pressure distribution at the knee joint: influence of varus and valgus deviation without and with ligament dissection. *Arch Orthop Trauma Surg* **133**:12–9.

14. *Wada, M., Maezawa, Y., Baba, H., Shimada, S., Sasaki, S., and Nose, Y. (2001). Relationships among bone mineral densities, static alignment, and dynamic load in patients with medial compartment knee osteoarthritis. *Rheumatology* **40**:499–505.
    This study showed that the severity of varus alignment correlates with the ratio of medial compartment to lateral compartment bone mineral density in patients with OA, reflecting greater bone density in the region bearing greater load.

15. Andriacchi, T.P. (1994). Dynamics of knee malalignment. *Orthop Clin NA* **25**:395–403.

16. Schipplein, O.D. and Andriacchi, T.P. (1991). Interaction between active and passive knee stabilizers during level walking. *J Orthop Res* **9**:113–9.

17. Hsu, R.W.W., Himeno, S., Conventry, M.B., and Chao, E.Y.S. (1990). Normal axial alignment of the lower extremity and load-bearing distribution at the knee. *Clin Orthop* **255**:215–27.

18. Johnson, F., Leitl, S., and Waugh, W. (1980). The distribution of load across the knee: a comparison of static and dynamic measurements. *J Bone Joint Surg Br* **62-B**:346–9.

19. Harrington, I.J. (1983). Static and dynamic loading patterns in knee joints with deformities. *J Bone Joint Surg Am* **65-A**:247–59.

20. Schouten, J.S.A.G., van den Ouweland, F.A., and Valkenburg, H.A. (1992). A 12 year follow up study in the general population on prognostic factors of cartilage loss in osteoarthritis of the knee. *Ann Rheum Dis* **51**:932–7.

21. Miller, R., Kettelkamp, D.B., Laubenthal, K.N., Karagiorgos, A., and Smidt, G.L. (1973). Quantitative correlations in degenerative arthritis of the knee. *J Bone Joint Surg* **55A**:956–62

22. *Sharma, L., Song, J., Felson, D.T., Cahue, S., Shamiyeh, E., and Dunlop, D.D. (2001). The role of knee alignment in disease progression and functional decline in knee osteoarthritis. *JAMA* **286**(2):188–95.
    This longitudinal study demonstrates that varus and valgus alignment increase the risk of medial and lateral knee OA progression, respectively, and that the burden of malalignment predicts decline in physical function.

23. Huberti, H.H. and Hayes, W.C. (1984). Patellofemoral contact pressures: the influence of Q-angle and tendofemoral contact. *J Bone Joint Surg Am* **66**:715–24.

24. Hungerford, D.S. and Barry, M. (1979). Biomechanics of the patellofemoral joint. *Clin Orthop* **144**:9–15.

25. Ficat, R.P. and Hungerford, D.S. (1977). Biomechanics. In R.P. Ficat and D.S. Hungerford (eds), *Disorders of the Patellofemoral Joint*. Baltimore: Williams and Wilkins, pp. 22–35.

26. Ficat, R.P. and Hungerford, D.S. (1977). Chondrosis and arthrosis, a hypothesis. In R.P. Ficat and D.S. Hungerford (eds), *Disorders of the Patellofemoral Joint*. Baltimore: Williams and Wilkins, pp. 194–232.

27. Elahi, S., Cahue, S., Felson, D.T., Engelman, L., and Sharma, L. (2000). The association between varus-valgus alignment and patellofemoral OA. *Arthritis Rheum* **43**:1874–80.

28. *Sharma, L., Lou, C., Cahue, S., and Dunlop, D.D. (2000). The Mechanism of the Effect of Obesity in Knee Osteoarthritis: the Mediating Role of Malalignment. *Arthritis Rheum* **43**:568–75.
    This study demonstrates that the relationship between obesity and OA is stronger in varus than in valgus knees, and that varus alignment mediates the relationship between obesity and medial tibiofemoral compartment OA.

29. Markolf, K.L., Bargar, W.L., Shoemaker, S.C., and Amstutz, H.C. (1981). The role of joint load in knee stability. *J Bone Joint Surg* **63**:570–85.

30. Solomonow, M. and D'Ambrosia, R. (1994). Neural reflex arcs and muscle control of knee stability and motion. In W.N. Scott (ed.) *The Knee*. St. Louis: Mosby, pp. 107–20.

31. Woo, SL-Y., Fenwick, J.A., Kanamori, A., Gil, J.E., Saw, S.S.C., and Vogrin, T.M. (2001). Biomechanical considerations of joint function. In: R.M. Moskowitz, D.S. Howell, R.D. Altman, J.A. Buckwalter, and V.M. Goldberg (eds), *Osteoarthritis, Diagnosis and Medical/Surgical Management*. Philadelphia: W.B. Saunders, pp. 145–69.

32. Buckwalter, J.A., Lane, N.E., and Gordon, S.L. (1995). Exercise as a cause of osteoarthritis. In: K.E. Kuettner and V.M. Goldberg, (eds), *Osteoarthritic Disorders*. Rosemont: American Academy of Orthopaedic Surgeons, pp. 405–17.

33. Woo, S.L., Hollis, J.M., Adams, D.J., Lyon, R.M., and Takai, S. (1991). Tensile properties of the human femur-anterior cruciate ligament-tibia complex: the effects of specimen age and orientation. *Am J Sports Med* **19**:217–25.

34. Cushnaghan, J., Cooper, C., Dieppe, P., Kirwan, J., McAlindon, T., and McCrae. F. (1990). Clinical assessment of osteoarthritis of the knee. *Ann Rheum Dis* **49**:768–70.

35. Noyes, F.R., Cummings, J.F., Grood, E.S., Walz-Hasselfeld, K.A., and Wroble, R.R. (1991). The diagnosis of knee motion limits, subluxations, and ligament injury. *Am J Sports Med* **19**:163–71.

36. Markolf, K.L., Graff-Radford, A., and Amstutz, H.C. (1978). In vivo knee stability, a quantitative assessment using an instrumented clinical testing apparatus. *J Bone Joint Surg* **60-A**:664–74.

37. Lundberg, M. and Messner, K. (1997). Ten-year prognosis of isolated and combined medial collateral ligament ruptures. *Am J Sports Med* **25**: 2–6.

38. Kannus, P. (1989). Nonoperative treatment of grade II and III sprains of the lateral ligament compartment of the knee. *Am J Sports Med* **17**:83–8.

39. Kannus, P. (1988). Long-term results of conservatively treated medial collateral ligament injuries of the knee joint. *Clin Orthop* **226**:103–12.

40. Brage, M.E., Draganich, L.F., Pottenger, L.A., and Curran, J.J. (1994). Knee laxity in symptomatic osteoarthritis. *Clin Orthop* **304**:184–9.

41. *Pottenger, L.A., Phillips, F.M., and Draganich, L.F. (1990). The effect of marginal osteophytes on reduction of varus-valgus instability in osteoarthritic knees. *Arthritis Rheum* **33**:853–8.
    In this study, varus–valgus angulation was measured before and after removal of osteophytes in patients with advanced knee OA at the time of total knee replacement. Although the amount of varus–valgus laxity in knees with osteophytes still exceeded the level of laxity in control subjects, increased prominence of osteophytosis was associated with less varus–valgus laxity (i.e., the osteophytes helped maintain normal knee alignment).

42. Sharma, L., Hayes, K.W., Felson, D.T., *et al.* (1999). Does laxity alter the relationship between strength and physical function in knee osteoarthritis? *Arthritis Rheum* **42**:25–32.

43. Wada, M., Imura, S., Baba, H., and Shimada, S. (1996). Knee laxity in patients with osteoarthritis and rheumatoid arthritis. *Br J Rheumatol* **35**:560–3.

7.3 Pathogenesis of joint pain in osteoarthritis

7.3.1 Peripheral and central pain mechanisms in osteoarthritis

Bruce Kidd

This chapter will stress the relatively poor association between osteoarthritis and pain and will illustrate the futility of searching for a unitary cause for symptoms in this disorder. A description of neurobiological events underlying osteoarthritic pain is provided and mechanisms by which changes within the joint microenvironment lead to plasticity within pain pathways are described. Finally, the relative contributions of peripheral and spinal mechanisms to OA pain are compared and the implications for pain therapy discussed.

Osteoarthritis and pain

Pain is a ubiquitous feature of life and the most common complaint of individuals with OA. It is abundantly clear from epidemiological studies, however, that in many cases radiological OA is not associated with pain. It has been quite reasonably argued that the key issue is the understanding and treatment of the pain rather than the myriad underlying cartilagenous, bony and soft tissue changes.[1]

Measurement of pain is far from straightforward, and responses to even simple enquiries can be influenced by a range of cultural, social, demographic, and environmental factors, current psychological state, previous history, as well as physical pathology.[2] It is hardly surprising that relatively subtle differences between pain questionnaires produce large differences in the reported prevalence of pain.[3] The choice of pain measure also influences the assessment of pain severity, although obesity, helplessness, and education emerge as important and potentially treatable factors for self-reported pain severity in knee OA.[4]

Symptoms in OA are generally considered to be insidious in onset and not associated with systemic disturbance. Pain may be continuous or exacerbated by activity and relieved by rest, and a diurnal pattern is often apparent.[5] Whilst symptoms are mostly experienced in or near the affected joint, referred pain and tenderness may also occur. Specific words used by individuals to describe OA symptoms include 'aching' and 'throbbing', interspersed by activity-related episodes of 'sharp' and stabbing' pain.[6,7] Attempts to discriminate between OA and other rheumatological disorders such as rheumatoid arthritis with verbal descriptions have generally proved unsuccessful however,[8] and it seems unlikely that the mechanisms underlying OA pain can be distinguished on the basis of symptoms alone.

Neurobiology of pain

Nociception and pain

An alternative approach to understanding why symptoms occur in OA is to examine the underlying nociceptive mechanisms that are associated with pain. It is important at this stage to draw a clear distinction between nociception and pain.[9] Nociception has been defined in various ways but for practical purposes may be regarded as a strictly neurophysiological process whose end result is the perception of pain. Everyday experience dictates that activity within this 'nociceptive system' most commonly arises in response to internal stress as might follow tissue injury or inflammation. Alternatively, nociceptive activity might also arise in response to, or be modified by, exogenous stress in consequence of environmental factors. (Fig. 7.83) The result of such activity includes not only pain but also the stimulation of a number of neuro-immuno endocrine mechanisms including the hypothalamic-pituitary-adrenal (HPA) axis and components of the sympathetic nervous system.[10]

In practical terms pain arises in response to injury to non-neuronal tissues (nociceptive pain) or to the nerves themselves (neuropathic pain). This division has clinical relevance insofar as nociceptive pain tends to be more responsive to anti-inflammatory drugs (NSAIDs) and opioids, whereas neuropathic pain syndromes are less so.[11] Clinical experience dictates that pain may also arise in the absence of either tissue or nerve injury and under these circumstances it is apparent that psychosocial factors are the dominant influence on nociceptive pathways (psychogenic pain).

Neural plasticity

A key advance in pain research over the last several decades has been the demonstration that the nociceptive system is capable of considerable

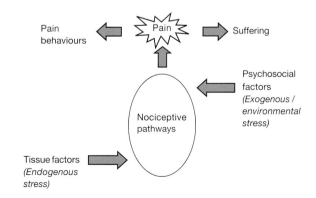

Fig. 7.83 Processes of pain.
Source: Modified from Ref. 28.

Table 7.31 Mechanisms of pain

Etiology	Neurophysiological mechanisms
Tissue injury (nociceptive pain)	Peripheral sensitization
Nerve injury (neuropathic pain)	Peripheral ectopia
Psychological stress (psychogenic pain)	Central sensitization
	Central disinhibition

Table 7.32 Pain mechanisms—key points

- In many cases radiological OA is not associated with the perception of pain.
- Symptoms in OA may arise in response to tissue factors (nociceptive pain), but a contribution from nerve fibres (neuropathic pain) and psychological stress (psychogenic pain) is also apparent.
- Pain pathways are inherently plastic and are crucially sensitive to changes within the local microenvironment as well as to previous activity. The resultant pattern of sensitization is likely to play the determining role in the final expression of OA pain.
- Sensitization of peripheral pain fibres by prostaglandins and other mediators leads to enhanced local pain, whereas accompanying changes within the central nervous system mediated by growth factors leads to more diffuse symptoms including referred pain.

functional change, or plasticity, according to different conditions. The system also retains a 'pain memory' such that previous activity determines responses to future events. A number of key neurophysiological mechanisms underlying this plasticity have been described to date and are summarized in Table 7.31.

Minor incidents experienced as part of everyday life produce short-lived excitation of specialized high threshold nociceptors with brief, spatially localized pain. More intense stimuli producing tissue damage not only activate nociceptors directly causing pain but may also modify their response properties to subsequent stimuli (peripheral sensitization).[12] This results in a decreased threshold for a response to a given stimulus leading to increased stimulus or activity—related pain. In some situations unprovoked activity might occur leading to spontaneous pain. Heightened skin sensitivity following sunburn provides a convenient example.

Injury to a peripheral nerve results in changes to the activity of its constituent neurones.[11] Abnormal expression of ion channels (most notably sodium channels) leads to abnormal input into the central nervous system from the site of injury and other proximal sites. This 'ectopic' input produces symptoms, such as parathesiae, reflecting those fibres involved. Less commonly, abnormal expression of adrenoceptors, including norepinephrine receptors, leads to sympathetically maintained pain states. Finally and at least in experimental situations, structural changes may occur with abnormal neural sprouting in both the dorsal root ganglion and dorsal horn. The functional implications of these latter changes remain unclear.

Whilst pain hypersensitivity following tissue or nerve injury is contingent to a large degree on peripheral mechanisms, other processes are also involved. Sustained or repetitive activity within peripheral fibres leads to substantial changes to the function and activity of central nociceptive pathways (central sensitization).[13] In neurophysiological terms, central sensitization results in exaggerated responses to normal stimuli together with expansion of receptive field size producing tenderness and referred pain in areas away from the site of injury. There is also reduction of the threshold for activation by novel inputs such that non-nociceptive fibres can activate central nociceptive pathways causing pain in response to trivial non-injurious stimuli.

In contrast to mechanisms that enhance neural activity others act to reduce plasticity within nociceptive pathways. Normally, these pathways are subject to powerful internal controls that operate at all levels to reduce activity. It has been speculated that suppression or dysfunction of these inhibitory systems may lead to abnormal nociceptive activity and hence pain in some chronic pain conditions (central disinhibition).[14] Table 7.32 summarizes the key points of pain mechanisms.

Tissue factors influencing OA pain

Joint innervation

The musculoskeletal system is abundantly supplied with both encapsulated receptors and free nerve endings. Three main classes of encapsulated receptor can be identified, including the cylindrical (Pacinian) corpuscles, the globular 'Ruffini' endings and the fusiform Golgi Tendon Organs.[15] These receptors are associated with rapidly conducting Ab fibres (conduction velocities greater than 30 m/s) and are found mainly in fibrous periarticular structures including ligaments, tendons, and joint capsule. They are activated by non-noxious stimuli and for the most part are mechanoreceptors.

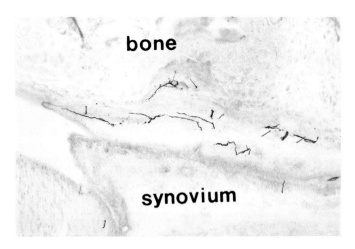

Fig. 7.84 Photomicrographs of unmyelinated fibres in osteoarthritic synovium (original magnification ×480).

In contrast to encapsulated receptors, free nerve endings are more widely distributed in fibrous capsules, adipose tissues, ligaments, menisci, and periosteum[16] (see Fig. 7.84). They are associated with small diameter fibres including Ad fibres (conduction velocities 2.5–30 m/s) and C fibres (conduction velocities less than 2.5 m/s) and respond to noxious stimuli.[17]

The 'cause' of OA pain has been variously attributed to a number of pathologies in and around the joint.[7,18,19] Potentially, pain can arise from any innervated structure including the synovium and the contiguous joint capsule, the underlying bone and periosteum, or the surrounding soft tissues including muscles tendons and ligaments. Under normal circumstances, however, structures in the immediate vicinity of the intra-articular cavity are relatively insensitive and can be mechanically stimulated in various ways without causing pain.[20] This accords with neurophysiological studies performed largely in the cat knee, showing that joint nerves contain a significant proportion of fibres that are usually unresponsive to strong pressure or to either benign or noxious movements.[21] These 'silent' or 'sleeping' nociceptors were first described in joints but have subsequently been characterized in other tissues as well.

One important conclusion to be drawn from these and similar studies is that whereas simple mechanical factors such as synovial or periosteal deformation may be associated with OA pain, they are unlikely to produce symptoms on their own. Additional factors appear to be needed to sensitize joint nociceptors to mechanical stimuli, and several lines of evidence point to the importance of mediators released from either synovium or bone.

Synovitis

Support for a synovial/capsular contribution to OA pain comes from studies in which local anaesthetic was injected into symptomatic OA knees, resulting in a significant improvement with complete abolition of pain in 60 per cent of knees at one hour.[22] The presence of inflammation, as has been convincingly demonstrated in OA and mediator-induced sensitization of articular nociceptors, provides a convincing mechanism by which symptoms might occur. Consistent with this is the presence of a generalized uptake pattern on radionuclide scintigraphic studies of knee OA that has been to shown to correlate well with self-reported pain.[23]

Bone oedema

Periosteum, subchondral, and marrow bone are richly innervated with sensory fibres and are potential sources of OA pain. Bone marrow lesions detected on magnetic resonance imaging (MRI) are shown to be much more prevalent in individuals with OA who have knee pain than those who are symptom free.[18] Large lesions were almost exclusively present in persons with knee pain although there was no association between bone lesions and pain severity. Histologically, the lesions reflect oedema of the bone marrow possibly in consequence of an inflammatory response to previous trauma.[24] It is notable that similar lesions occur in other painful musculoskeletal disorders including osteonecrosis and transient painful osteoporosis.[24]

Raised intraosseus pressure arising from impaired venous drainage has long been linked with OA pain and this is supported by the observation that fenestration of the bony cortex and osteotomy both reduce symptoms in this condition. Significantly, individuals with intraosseus hypertension have positive scitingraphic scans, which in turn correlate highly with bone marrow lesions on MRI.[25]

Peripheral nociceptive mechanisms

Nociceptors

The terminals of nociceptive fibres express multiple receptors that characteristically become active across relatively narrow ranges of stimulus intensity. To date, receptors for high intensity mechanical stimuli have not been identified but progress has been made characterizing a number of receptors for thermal and chemical stimuli. An archetypal thermal receptor that has received much recent attention is the vanilloid-1 receptor (VR-1). This is an ion channel-linked receptor that responds to temperatures above 43 °C and appears to be involved in the burning pain that accompanies thermal stimuli.[26] Interestingly, VR-1 also responds to capsaicin, which has resulted in the use of this substance as an active ingredient in hot or spicy foods for hundreds of years. More conventional G protein-coupled receptors identified on joint nociceptors include prostanoid, bradykinin, and serotonin receptors amongst others.[27]

Peripheral sensitization

The sensitivity of individual nociceptors is governed by a critical interaction with the local microenvironment as well as by factors related to previous stimuli. As an example, the response properties of the thermal receptor VR-1 are substantially modified by repeated heat stimuli or by exposure to protons, the cannabinoid receptor agonist anandamide, or the lipoxygenase product 12-(s)-hydro-peroxy-eicosatetraenoic acid (12-(S)-HPETE).[28] The cellular mechanisms by which these peripheral changes occur involve early post-translational changes to receptors/ion channels and later, longer-lasting transcription-dependant mechanisms involving changes to the chemical phenotype of the cell[27] (see Fig. 7.85).

Substances present within the extracellular space act to augment or inhibit activity in nociceptive pathways in a number of ways. Whilst some mediators such as bradykinin contribute to pain by directly activating nociceptors others are generally considered to be sensitizing agents. Prostaglandins, for example, increase cellular cAMP levels and may enhance nociceptor

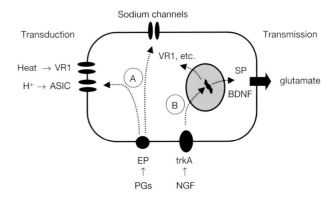

Fig. 7.85 Peripheral sensitization. A, Early phase post-translational modification of receptors/ion channels. B, Longer term transcriptional events with increased production of receptors/ion channels/central transmitters.

Source: Modified from Ref. 27.

sensitization by lowering the activation threshold for sodium channels via a protein kinase A pathway.[29] Within the joint, experimental application of prostaglandin E2 has been shown to sensitize nociceptors to mechanical and chemical stimuli with a time course that matches the development of pain-related behaviour in awake animals.[21] Other mediators on the other hand, such as the endogenous opioids and cannabinoids act at peripheral sites to reduce nociceptor activity. Opioid receptors have been demonstrated on the terminals of peripheral nerves, and local applications of opioid agonists reduce hyperalgesia in several experimental and clinical models.[30] Similarly, activation of the canabinoid CB1 receptor is negatively coupled to adenylate cyclase and blocks excitability and activation of nociceptive fibres to reduce pain.[31]

In acute situations, pro-inflammatory cytokines such as IL-1 and TNF appear to induce sensitization via receptor associated kinases and phosphorylation of ion channels, whereas in chronic inflammation, transcriptional upregulation of receptors and secondary signalling becomes more important.[32] Longer term changes to nociceptor sensitivity also involve neurotrophin growth factors, including NGF (nerve growth factor), which exert a global influence on nociceptor activity by regulating the expression of the neuropeptides, substance P, and calcitonin gene related peptide (CGRP), as well as receptors including VR1 and bradykinin B2, and ion channels such as SNS.[33]

Primary hyperalgesia

It seems highly probable that peripheral sensitization makes a significant contribution to many of the features observed in patients with OA. Under normal circumstances joint nociceptors respond only to high intensity stimuli or not at all. Peripheral sensitization, however, is associated with the increased responsiveness of nociceptors leading to local pain and tenderness (primary hyperalgesia).[12] In the joint, the responses of previously high threshold and silent nociceptors are lowered such that they become responsive to benign mechanical stimuli.[21] The episodes of sharp or stabbing pain experienced by OA patients could well be explained by such mechanisms. It is possible, but remains unproven, that activation of sensitized VR-1 receptors by body heat might result in burning discomfort in some individuals. An unresolved and highly pertinent issue is whether peripheral sensitization only occurs in the presence of inflammation or whether other, as yet unidentified, factors might also be associated with this phenomenon.

Central nociceptive mechanisms

Psychophysical studies

The clinical observation that pain may be referred away from OA joints and reports of increased tenderness over apparently normal tissues have led to speculation that changes in the central modulation of nociceptive input might contribute to symptoms in OA. Recent quantitative psychophysical studies evaluating pain mechanisms in OA lend support to this idea. Cutaneous and deep hyperalgesia to thermal and mechanical stimuli in subjects with OA has been tested over symptomatic carpometacarpal joints and control sites in the forearm.[7] Significantly, variance in movement-related pain ratings was predicted by *forearm* pain thresholds. Similar results were obtained in a study in which muscle hyperalgesia was assessed by intramuscular infusion of 6 per cent hypertonic saline.[19] OA subjects had increased pain intensity with significantly larger referred and radiating pain areas the matched controls. It is highly unlikely that local changes to nociceptive activity account for either set of results and point to the presence of enhanced central mechanisms.

Central sensitization

The central projections of peripheral nociceptive fibres terminate in the more superficial laminae of the spinal dorsal horn. The main neurotransmitter present in all primary sensory fibres is glutamate, which acts primarily on AMPA (a-amino-3-hydroxy-5-methylisoxazole) receptors to induce depolarization of 'second order' spinal neurones. Importantly, higher stimulus intensities, such as those associated with tissue damage, result in functional changes at a spinal level that facilitate nociceptive transmission. Repetitive stimulation of peripheral nociceptive fibres is associated with the functional expression of a second glutamate-responsive receptor, the NMDA (N-methy-D-aspartate) receptor, whose activation leads directly to increased excitability of spinal neurones.[13]

An increasing number of neuromodulators have been reported to augment central activity including the neuropeptide, substance P, which enhances activity of NMDA receptors and generates greater post-synaptic responses.[13] Elevated cerebrospinal fluid concentrations of substance P have been reported in patients with painful OA and a positive correlation was noted between VAS pain score and concentration of SP. Following joint replacement surgery levels were observed to fall once more.[34]

Enhanced activity within spinal pathways is offset by powerful segmental and descending inhibitory systems mediated by opioids, noradrenaline, adenosine, and other substances. Diffuse noxious inhibitory control (DNIC) is an example of one such system and clinical studies have suggested dysfunction of DNIC-like mechanisms in a number of musculoskeletal conditions including temperomandibular disorder, low back pain and OA. Quantitative sensory testing using heterotropic noxious conditioning stimulation performed in subjects with painful OA found lack of pressure pain modulation in subjects before, but not following surgery, indicating that dysfunction of DNIC had been maintained by chronic nociceptive pain in this disorder.[14]

Secondary hyperalgesia

The clinical consequences of central sensitization include enhanced pain perception at the site of injury, and development of pain and tenderness in normal tissues, both adjacent to, and removed from the primary site. Consistent with this, abolition of symptoms in one OA knee using intra-articular anaesthetic has been shown to produce a significant effect on pain perception in the contra-lateral knee not explainable by any systemic effect of the treatment.[22]

A further consequence of central sensitization is that sensory input from joint proprioceptors and other specialized nerve endings in and around the joint now gain access to nociceptive pathways, such that innocuous mechanical stimuli of such movement within the normal range now produce pain. Demonstration of the contribution from non-nociceptive Ab myelinated fibres to OA symptoms has been provided in a study of OA subjects, in which these fibres were selectively blocked resulting in increased mechanical thresholds as compared with OA subjects without the block.[35]

The phenomenon of enhanced pain away from the site of injury (secondary hyperalgesia) is characterized by enhanced responses only to mechanical stimuli.[12] A number of psychophysical studies using capsaicin have shown that whereas secondary hyperalgesia to certain mechanical

stimuli is mediated by central sensitization it remains crucially dependant on peripheral nociceptive inputs.[12] This serves to explain why OA symptoms seemingly dependent on central mechanisms in OA, such as referred pain, remit readily after joint replacement surgery.

Summary

Under normal circumstances synovial joints are relatively insensitive to noxious stimuli. Nociceptors are crucially sensitive to changes within the local microenvironment, which can lead to reduced thresholds for activation. Pain now accompanies minor traumas to which joints are exposed on a daily basis. Peripheral changes are mirrored by augmented spinal mechanisms, which further enhance nociceptive activity by allowing non-nociceptive mechanoreceptors to trigger pain. Under these circumstance pain can now arise in response to stimuli as innocuous as standing or walking. In the light of the myriad factors that are likely to impact upon the function and activity of peripheral nociceptors, it would seem to be more profitable to direct therapy towards restoration of normal neural sensitivity than by a quixotic search for a single cause for OA pain.

Key points

1. Synovial joints are relatively insensitive to pain under normal conditions and simple mechanical factors such as capsular or periosteal stretching are unlikely to trigger pain on their own.

2. Mediators released from synovium and from bone contribute to enhanced nociceptor sensitivity. Whether this occurs only in the presence of inflammation (synovitis, bone, oedema, etc.) remains unresolved. The net result of peripheral sensitization is that previously assymptomatic minor stresses and trauma now cause pain.

3. Augmented spinal mechanisms allow proprioreceptors to gain access to nociceptive pathways and trigger pain. Pain now arises in response to non-noxious stimuli such as standing or walking.

4. OA pain arises in response to a complex interaction between internal and external factors leading to enhanced nociceptor sensitivity. Under these conditions any number of previously assymtomatic stimuli produce activity within nociceptive pathways. The search for a single cause for OA pain in a given individual is ultimately futile.

References

(An asterisk denotes recommended reading.)

1. **Hadler, N.M.** (1992). Knee pain is the malady—not osteoarthritis. *Ann Intern Med* **116**:598–9.

2. **Turk, D. and Melzac, R.** (1992). The measurement of pain and the assessment of people experiencing pain. In D. Turk and R. Melzac (eds), *Handbook of Pain Assessment*. New York: The Guildford Press, pp. 3–12.

3. **O'Reilly, S.C., Muir, K.R., and Doherty, M.** (1996). Screening for pain in knee osteoarthritis: which question? *Ann Rheum Dis* **55**:931–3.

4. *****Creamer, P., Lethbridge-Cejku, M., and Hochberg, M.C.** (1999). Determinants of pain severity in knee osteoarthritis: Effect of demographic and psychosocial variables using 3 pain measures. *J Rheumatol* **26**:1785–92.
   Different pain scales (WOMAC, MPQ, VAS) measure different facets of pain in knee OA. Risk factors for activity–related pain are different from those for rest and sitting pain and point to the heterogeneous etiology of OA pain

5. **Huskisson, E.C., Dieppe, P.A., Tucker, A.K., and Cannell, L.** (1979). Another look at osteoarthritis. *Ann Rheum Dis* **38**:423–8.

6. **Wagstaff, S., Smith, O.V., and Wood, P.H.N.** (1985). Verbal pain descriptors used by patients with arthritis. *Ann Rheum Dis* **44**:262–5.

7. **Farrell, M., Gibson, S., McMeeken, J., and Helme, R.** (2000). Pain and hyperalgesia in osteoarthritis of the hands. *J Rheumatol* **27**:441–7.

8. Helliwell, P.S. (1995). The semeiology of arthritis: discriminating between patients on the basis of their symptoms. *Ann Rheum Dis* **54**:924–6.

9. Loeser, J.D. and Melzack, R. (1999). Pain: an overview. *Lancet* **353**:1607–09.

10. Besson, J.M. (1999). The neurobiology of pain. *Lancet* **353**:1610–15.

11. Bridges, D., Thompson, S.W.N., and Rice, A.S.C. (2001). Mechanisms of neuropathic pain. *Br J Anaesthesia* **87**:12–26.

12. Raja, S., Meyer, R., and Kingkamp, M. JN. C. (1999). Peripheral neural mechanisms of nociception. In P. Wall and R. Melzac (eds), *Textbook of pain*. Edinburgh: Churchill Livingstone, pp. 11–58.

13. Coderre, T., Katz, J., Vaccarino, A., and Melzack, R. (1993). Contribution of central neuroplasticity to pathological pain: review of clinical and experimental evidence. *Pain* **52**:259–85.

14. *Kosek, E. and Ordeberg, G. (2000). Lack of pressure pain modulation by heterotropic noxious conditioning stimulation in patients with painful osteoarthritis before, but not following, surgical pain relief. *Pain* **88**:69–78.

    Demonstration of the efficacy of quantitative sensory testing to probe changes within nociceptive pathways in different diseases. The study shows that changes to endogenous inhibitory systems in painful OA are reversed following joint replacement surgery.

15. Freeman, M. and Wyke, B. (1967). The innervation of the knee joint. An anatomical and histological study in the cat. *J Anat* **101**:505–32.

16. Mapp, P., Kidd, B., Gibson, S., Terry, J., Revell, P., Ibrahim, N., *et al.* (1990). Substance P-calcitonin-related peptide- and C-flanking peptide of neuropeptide Y-immunoreactive fibres are present in normal synovium but depleted in patients with rheumatoid arthritis. *Neuroscience* **37**:143–53.

17. Grigg, P., Schaible, H-G., and Schmidt, R.F. (1986). Mechanical sensitivity of group III and IV afferents from posterior articular nerve in normal and inflamed cat knee. *J Neurophysiol* **55**(4):635–43.

18. *Felson, D., Chaisson, C., Hill, C., Totterman, S., Gale, E., Skinner, K., *et al.* (2001). The association of bone marrow lesions with pain in the knee. *Ann Intern Med* **134**:541–9.

    A convincing demonstration of an association between oedema in the subchondral bone marrow and OA pain. Explores the likely relationship between findings of previous scintigraphic studies, intraosseous hypertension and the response to surgical interventions.

19. Bajaj, P., Bajaj, P., Graven-Nielsen, T., and Arendt-Nielsen, L. (2001). Osteoarthritis and its association with muscle hyperalgesia: an experimental controlled study. *Pain* **93**:107–114.

20. Kellgren, J. and Samuel, E. (1950). The sensitivity and innervation of the articular capsule. *J Bone Joint Surg* **32**(B):84–91.

21. Schaible, H-G. and Grubb, B.D. (1993). Afferent and spinal mechanisms of joint pain. *Pain* **55**:5–54.

22. Creamer, P., Hunt, M., and Dieppe, P. (1996). Pain mechanisms in osteoarthritis of the knee: Effect of intraarticular anesthetic. *J Rheumatol* **23**:1031–6.

23. McCrae, F., Shoels, J., Dieppe, P., and Watt, I. (1992). Scintigraphic assessment of osteoarthritis of the knee joint. *Ann Rheum Dis* **51**:938–42.

24. Bollet, A. (2001). Edema of the bone marrow can cause pain in osteoarthritis and other diseases of bone and joints. *Ann Intern Med* **134**(7):591–3.

25. Boegard, T., Rudling, O., Dahlstrom, J., Dirksen, H., Petersson, J., and Jonsson, K. (1999). Bone scintigraphy in chronic knee pain: comparison with magnetic resonance imaging. *Ann Rheum Dis* **58**:20–6.

26. *Caterina, M., Rosen, T., Tominaga, M., Brake, A., and Julius, D. (1999). A capsaicin receptor homologue with a high threshold for noxious heat. *Nature* **398**:436–41.

    An important milestone in the elucidation of stimulus transduction within the nociceptive system. Plus a convincing demonstration as to why chilli peppers taste hot!

27. *Wolf, C.J. and Costigan, M. (1999). Transcriptional and posttranslational plasticity and the generation of inflammatory pain. *Proc Natl Acad Sci USA* **96**:7723–30.

    A first rate review of neurological mechanisms underlying pain by one of the leaders in the field.

28. Kidd, B.L. and Urban, L.A. (2001). Mechanisms of inflammatory pain. *Br J Anaesthesia* **87**(1):1–9.

29. England, S., Bevan, S.J., and Docherty, R.J. (1996). Prostaglandin E2 modulates the tetrodotoxin-resistant sodium current in neonatal rat dorsal root ganglion neurones via the cyclic AMP-protein kinase A cascade. *J Physiol* **495**:429–40.

30. Andreev, N., Urban, L., and Dray, A. (1994). Opioids suppress spontaneous activity of polymodal nociceptors in rat paw skin induced by ultraviolet irradiation. *Neuroscience* **58**:793–8.

31. Piomelli, D., Giuffrida, A., Calignano, A., and de Fonseca, F. (2000). The endocannabinoid system as a target for therapeutic drugs. *Trends Pharmacol Sci* **21**:218–24.

32. Opree, A. and Kress, M. (2000). Involvement of the proinflammatory cytokines tumor necrosis factor-a, IL-1ß and IL-6 but not IL-8 in the development of heat hyperalgesia: effects on heat-evoked calcitonin gene-related peptide release from rat skin. *J Neurosci* **20**:6289–93.

33. Levine, J. and Reichling, D. (1999). Peripheral mechanisms of inflammatory pain. In P. Wall, R. Melzac (eds), *Textbook of pain*. Edinburgh: Churchill Livingstone, pp. 59–84.

34. Lindh, C., Liu, Z., Ordeberg, G., and Nyberg, F. (1997). Elevated cerebrospinal fluid substance P-like immunoreactivity in patients with painful osteoarthritis, but not in patients with rhizopathic pain from a herniated lumbar disc. *Scand J Rheumatol* **26**:468–72.

35. Farrell, M., Gibson, S., McKeeken, J., and Helme, R. (2000). Increased movement pain in osteoarthritis of the hands is associated with Ab-mediated cutaneous mechanical sensitivity. *J Pain* **1**:229–42.

7.3.2 Why does the patient with osteoarthritis hurt?

Nortin M. Hadler

There are flaws in the inference that coincident OA is the explanation for regional musculoskeletal disorders, such as hip, knee, or axial pain that cause people to be patients. In the community, regional disorders are far more prevalent than OA defined as pathoanatomy. This is reflected in the experience in primary care. The discordance is diminished by selection biases in rheumatologic and orthopedic practice. Furthermore, most people with the pathoanatomical features of OA are either asymptomatic or have not chosen to seek care. It has become clear that regional musculoskeletal disorders are intermittent and remittent predicaments of life that have little to do with OA as defined by contemporary imaging studies. To be well requires the wherewithal to cope with these predicaments. When coping is compromised, the sufferer may seek recourse from a health care provider. A therapeutic contract that does not include enhancement of coping skills is no longer 'state-of-the-art'.

Nearly three centuries have passed since Thomas Sydenham ushered in the era of scientific medicine. It was his genius that deduced the illness-disease syllogism;[1] symptoms and signs are the illness, which is symbolic of some underlying pathoanatomical disorder, a disease. The symbolism of symptoms and signs, a branch of philosophy known as semiotics, was not new to Sydenham. The symbolism of symptoms and signs had been appreciated since antiquity, driving a tradition of treating categories of illness according to the dictates of some abstraction or the other. Thanks to Sydenham, forevermore, the first charge to the physician is to define the disease that underlies the category of illness. Then, the physician was to design specific therapy to remedy that disease with the expectation that the illness would regress as a consequence. Without this conceptual watershed, we might still be diagnosing 'catarrh' instead of curing pneumonias, or 'dropsy' instead of designing therapy specific for each of the causes of the edematous state. The illness-disease syllogism is both the pride and the Holy Grail of western medicine. It has led to so many triumphs that we seldom question whether it has also left tragedy in its wake. In this chapter we will explore whether applying the syllogism to regional musculoskeletal illness is such a tragedy.

Every one of us has experienced musculoskeletal discomfort. Sometimes we feel compelled to seek medical care. The moment we describe our morbidity to a physician, we abdicate the station of the person who is trying to cope. We assume the role of the patient. The illness-disease syllogism is joined. What is the cause of this *regional musculoskeletal illness*?[2] For several generations, now, the usual answer has been 'OA'. More often than not, degenerative joint disease is present in the back of the patient with backache, the neck of the patient with neck pain, the knee of the patient with knee pain, and so forth. Medical science was not totally captivated by this coincidence; the age-dependent prevalence of degenerative disease of all regions had been established in necropsy surveys 60 years ago.[3] Everyone will have OA but not everyone will become a patient with regional joint pain. The mystery that remained was not whether OA was the culprit—that has been generally accepted as the given. The mystery was to define the aspect(s) of OA that afflicts the sufferer.[4] Certainly the 'ACR Criteria for Osteoarthritis' presented in the Appendix, bears witness to the fashion in which this disease-illness syllogism has commandeered thinking. In a primary care patient population, rather than highly selected patient populations, most patients with 'joint pain' do not meet ACR Criteria; they lack the radiographic features of 'OA' but are otherwise indistinguishable from those who meet the criteria.[5] Even so, few amongst us can overcome the notion that regional musculoskeletal pain and coincident OA are causal associations.

I am not suggesting that the syllogism is foolish. However, it falls short as an explanatory model for regional musculoskeletal illness today, and may never serve the vast majority of these sufferers at all. To do better, we must reconsider what we mean by 'OA' knowing that there are obvious flaws in the disease-illness syllogism with which we are imbued.

Semiotics and osteoarthritis

The title of this chapter, '*Why does the patient with OA hurt?*' is not a rhetorical device. It is a peremptory question. It constrains any response by nature of the implicit tautology; OA is painful and it is the pain of OA that is somehow responsible for causing the person to choose to be a patient with a regional musculoskeletal illness. Because of this question the clinician takes recourse in suppressing the discomfort with pharmaceuticals or trying to extirpate the putatively offending part. It is the question that seduces the pharmaceutical industry to elucidate the mechanisms of joint destruction with the expectation that therein lies the solution to the patient's dilemma.

'*People with OA hurt. Why?*' is the question that should drive molecular biology. It is less germane to the clinician, who is, traditionally, asked to minister to the small fraction of people who hurt and who also choose to be patients. But even this question is not straightforward. As has long been obvious from a close inspection of the epidemiology, OA and regional musculoskeletal discomfort have little in common—not nothing in common but surprisingly little.[6] Take the example of knee pain, where such an assertion might seem counterintuitive. The relevant data from one classical survey are presented in Table 7.34. This was a household survey undertaken by the National Center for Health Statistics in the 1970s[7] with follow-up a decade later.[8] Knee pain is most prevalent in the elderly[9] but it is highly prevalent at all ages, and at all ages more of us suffer knee pain than bear the radiographic stigmata of OA of the knee. True, those with more severe radiographic disease are somewhat more likely to experience difficulty with activities requiring mobility. However, progression of radiographic OA of the knee is slow and not predictable, whereas symptoms can exacerbate or regress regardless of radiographic progression.[10] Clearly knee pain is the malady, not OA.[11]

That insight is central to understanding the semiotics of all the regional musculoskeletal disorders. People, all people, will be forced to cope with musculoskeletal discomfort. Usually, the symptom is exacerbated by usage of the region and relieved if the region is put to rest. There are some important age-related differences in the distribution of involved regions and even

Table 7.34 The percentage of the US population that recalled having at least one month of daily knee pain in the past year compared with the prevalence of radiographic arthritis*

Age (Years)	Men		Women	
	Knee pain	Radiographic arthritis	Knee pain	Radiographic arthritis
23–34	5.7		5.2	
35–44	7.4		8.1	
45–54	12.0	2.3	11.5	3.6
55–64	11.5	4.0	15.0	7.2
65–74	14.9	8.4	19.7	17.9
25–74	9.5		10.9	

* Data are from the National Center for Health Statistics.[7]

in the quality of some regional symptoms.[12] But that does not take away the fact that each and every one of us will 'hurt' in a musculoskeletal region, and do so often and repeatedly. Coping with these predicaments is a fact of life; coping well is prerequisite to health.

This is not to belittle the fate of so many of our joints. Elegant diarthrodial joints slowly deteriorate. For some joints, such as the apophyseal joints, the process is largely genetically programmed[13,14] and therefore inexorable and unavoidable. This is the pathoanatomical process we have labeled OA. It is not linear over time, nor is it a single process across regions or in a given joint. For example, osteophytes can grow across joints with little progression in articular dissolution; this is readily demonstrable at the knee and can be so striking at the spine to warrant the designation 'ankylosing hyperostosis'. However, at no stage in the progression is the clinical consequence predictable. Osteophytes at the knee are more likely to mark a functional joint than one that has deteriorated.[15] Even people with ravaged joints need not be cognizant of that pathology, or persistently troubled, and certainly need not feel compelled to seek medical attention.

It follows that the clinically relevant question is, 'Why did this person, who may have OA and who is faced with another regional musculoskeletal predicament, choose to be a patient at this time?' This is the question that should supersede the two above. It is far more consistent with clinical reality. The task for the clinician is to assist patients in weighing the factors that have compromised their ability to cope. Certainly, the intensity of discomfort,[16] discomfort that is unfamiliar in quality, or compromise in biomechanical function[17] can contribute to their ability to cope. Occasionally, coping can be rendered effete by the magnitude of anatomical distortion consequent to OA. Importantly, coping can be confounded by myriad psychosocial stressors,[16–18] or coincident illness that further compromises health status.[19] Weighting these variables in a given patient is the art of medicine, rendered all the more challenging because seldom is causation univariate. But ignoring any places the patient at peril. Focusing on the putative inflammatory nature of OA or its anatomical stigmata is to spurn a compelling literature that offers the potential for palliation, if not remediation, of the predicament that caused the person to be a patient in the first place.

This conceptualization has been argued in the literature for decades and was the thesis of this chapter in the first edition of this book. To some the conceptualization remains counterintuitive. For those with inflexible research agendas, it causes cognitive dissonance. For others with overpowering vested interests in the pharmaceutical or surgical industries, it must seem threatening. In late 1998, the American Medical Association published a Continuing Medical Education Program for Primary Care Physicians on *Managing Osteoarthritis*.[20] A pharmaceutical firm underwrote the cost of this publication. Four rheumatologists comprised the 'Advisory Committee' for this publication all of whom avow consulting relationships with pharmaceutical companies active in the relevant marketplace, including the company that underwrote the publication costs. The 'continuing educa-tion' emphasized pathoanatomy, biochemistry, and pharmacology while retrogressively avoiding any allusion to the role of coping in the experience of the regional musculoskeletal disorders. Perhaps by the third edition of this book, such a treatment of this topic will seem counterintuitive to all seeking education and embarrassing to those who would teach. The science that drives the conceptualization regarding the role of coping in the experi-ence of regional musculoskeletal disorders is growing in scope and is ever more compelling.

Processing regional musculoskeletal symptoms

Most instances of regional musculoskeletal discomfort give us little pause. That is not to say they are trivial. During the next six weeks half of us will experience a week colored by musculoskeletal discomfort, most often in the axial skeleton.[21] But we cope—most of the time by relying on our common sense and taking recourse in over-the-counter analgesics, home advice, and home remedies. And most of the time our common sense rewards us with regression of symptoms before our confidence in our personal resources is too shaken. However, common sense is not common. It is either temporal or geographical, and is easily perturbed. In fact, industries exist in all advanced countries committed to perturbing common sense with a caco-phony of putatively well-intentioned advice. Osteopathy, the chiropractic, Christian Science, and the entire Pentecostal movement are the legacy of nineteenth-century advice.[22] Today newer alternative healers join in pro-viding recourse to a large segment of the ambulatory ill.[23] No sufferer with a regional musculoskeletal disorder is unaware of these options, all are tempted, and many take advantage. To think otherwise is naive and to ignore this aspect of a patient's experience of illness creates a barrier to com-munication, that further compromises the marginal benefits of the inter-ventions that are the purview of orthodox medicine.

At some point, some of us suffering with regional musculoskeletal illness will find our personal resources lacking and not adequately supplemented by whatever assistance we obtain from alternative providers. Fig. 7.86 is a depiction of the dynamics of coping; choosing to seek professional assist-ance is indeed a process, always anxiety-provoking and never enacted in a vacuum. For example, each year 80 per cent of Danes decide that their per-sonal resources are so inadequate that it makes sense to seek professional care for their backache promptly.[24] Americans at that time were far more persistent in coping.[21] Even though low back pain is the principle reason for seeking chiropractic or osteopathic care, and the second reason for turning to a physician,[25] Americans generally persevered for more than two weeks before they deemed it sensible to seek medical care.[26]

For the past century, the medical care provided in advanced countries has been stratified as to whether the illness arose out of the course of employment. If so, one is entitled to more comprehensive care and to wage replacement. There have been many experiments with the application of this stratification.[27] However, the most dramatic experiment, and the one most germane to our considerations, was the conceptualization of degenerative joint disease as an injury if symptoms commenced at work, or even inter-fered with work. In this fashion, and in this context, backache became 'I injured my back';[28] degenerative processes of the spine were indemnified under Workers' Compensation schemes, and processing of all regional mus-culoskeletal symptoms was changed forever (Fig. 7.86). When one's process-ing of the symptoms of a regional musculoskeletal disorder results in the decision to seek medical care, there are two alternatives: one can seek the care of a physician outside the industrial context, in which case the illness-disease syllogism is enjoined and OA comes to the fore. However, if care is sought in the industrial context, because the illness is considered to have arisen out of or in the course of, work, 'injury' subjugates OA and the patient assumes the role of a workers' compensation insurance claimant. The con-sequences of traveling these disparate pathways are dramatically different.[29] However, the thesis of this chapter is not the consequences. It is the reason for the choice between the three options in Fig. 7.86.

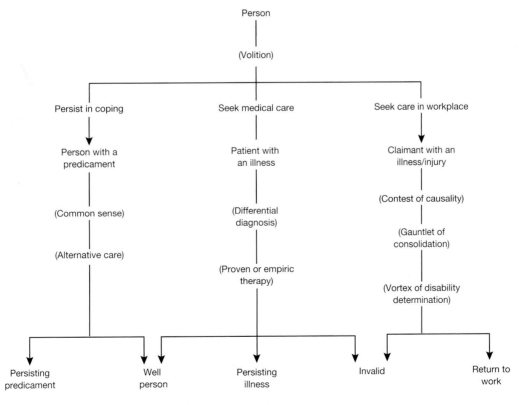

Fig. 7.86 The diagrammatic representation of a person coping with regional musculoskeletal symptoms.

Choosing to be a patient with knee pain

Nearly every western physician is convinced that the secret to evaluating the patient with knee pain is to evaluate the knee. Every medical student is taught the signs of meniscal tear, even though we have known for decades[30] that their predictive value renders them nearly useless.[31] Imaging the knee defines pathoanatomy, even elegantly, but again the predictive value of these findings is so unimpressive as to render the imaging uninterpretable in the clinical context of the illness-disease syllogism. Yet image we must. Arthroscopy adds little to the definition of pathoanatomy, and arthroscopic surgery is of no demonstrated benefit in the young and no demonstrable benefit in the old. As an upshot, in defiance of our 'standard of care', it is exceptional when we can define the disease that underlies regional knee pain and truly extraordinary when we can specifically intervene. Other chapters in this book detail the limitations of the available range of physical, pharmaceutical, and surgical options. These chapters also hold out hope for newer interventions building on the theoretical bases of those currently in use. I am no Luddite; I share the hope and encourage the effort to improve diarthrodial biology so as to diminish the likelihood that we will develop biomechanically unsound joints. But do not for a minute imagine that any such advance will eliminate, or even diminish, our need to cope with intermittent and remittent knee pain and, on occasion or even more frequently,[32] our need to turn to others for assistance in coping.

I base that prediction on the results of studies of community dwelling elderly[33] and of patients with OA, principally of the knee.[17,18,34-37] In all of these studies, quantification of radiographic OA was the measure of disease. All used standard instruments to assess pain and disability. And all assessed the psychological status of the patients by similarly standardized instruments. In all, the subject's psychological status, particularly disorders in affect, correlated better with the magnitude of pain and dysfunction than the radiographic measures. One could argue that the radiographic scores were insensitive; subtle changes in structure engender significant pain and incapacity leading to depression and other alterations in affect. There is no incontrovertible counterargument. However, we do know that enthusiastically supervised programs of 'exercise' and social support can impressively alter the patients' perception of their painful and incapacitating knee OA so that arthroplasty is no longer the only reasonable option. Other chapters in this section expand on this point.

Choosing to be a claimant with a regional back injury

The clinical consequences of the flaws in the illness-disease syllogism as it relates to knee pain, pale next to the consequences for low back pain. Low back pain was subsumed under the rubric of 'injury' 60 years ago when 'ruptured disc' was introduced into the clinical lexicon. From then on, particularly in America, any worker who experienced back pain on the job, or whose back pain interfered with function on the job, was potentially eligible for indemnification under the Workers' Compensation program.[29] The choice of the claimant role for back injury (Fig. 7.86) is seductive: there is the promise of all medical and surgical care money can buy to put the back injury right. It guarantees maintenance of wages during the healing phase and even afterward, should incapacity persist. However, the claimant risks paying a personal price in pursuit of these entitlements, a price that is inherent to the algorithm for redress promulgated under Workers' Compensation: the claimant risks aggressive surgical empiricisms and the acquisition of illness behavior in the process of disability determination. Workers' Compensation insurance underwrites an escalating numbers of workers deemed to suffer permanent partial disabilities from their regional musculoskeletal disorders, escalating medical and surgical costs, and an enormous industry that purports to be helpful. All this can be explained now that we have insight into the processing of the experience of backache that leads a worker to seek care as a 'claimant'.

It is not clear whether any worker performing any task that has been studied is more likely to experience regional backache than anyone else of similar age and sex. Certainly if the tasks in the workplace are more physically demanding, the challenge to coping is greater. Nonetheless, most cope. There is a compelling experimental literature indicating that the reason a worker with a backache chooses to be a claimant with an injury is that the job (not the task) was not accommodating when he or she was ill, and usually was not accommodating before he or she was ill.[38,39] Unfortunately, physicians, imbued with the illness-disease syllogism, are still not prepared for the possibility that a complaint of 'my back hurts' is really a complaint that 'my back hurts but I'm here because I cannot cope' in the workplace.[40] When resentment, job dissatisfaction, and the like color the illness, and medical management is constrained by an insurance paradigm that is contentious by design, the process is inherently iatrogenic. It is no surprise that long-term tragedies abound. Even if the 'injured worker' returns to work as rapidly as the 'ill' worker with a backache, he or she does so despite the perception of persisting illness.[41] No wonder workers who have previously claimed back injuries are more likely to claim again, and less likely to enjoy full health in the future.

Conclusion

The thesis of this chapter is put forth in an unwavering fashion. What happens if I am wrong, if the vaunted illness-disease syllogism really does pertain to knee and hip and axial pain? Maybe joint pain can be expunged from the human predicament if we can abrogate OA, or effectively palliate it, or postpone it for decades. Facet joints and condyles would remain pristine and articulate harmoniously throughout the days of our life.

I only wish I were wrong in this fashion. It would be far more straightforward to blithely design reductionistic experiments to hone down on the proximal molecular cause and then discover the remedy for OA. All attempts to date have fallen short. And whenever we consider the experience of joint pain, we learn that 'OA' is a minor variable. I fear I am correct. The only way we will serve the joint that hurts is to realize that it is a patient who registered the complaint.

Only then can we explore the means to enhance our patient's coping.

Key points

1. Regional musculoskeletal symptoms are intermittent and remittent predicaments of life.

2. The relationship of such symptoms to demonstrable pathoanatomy, that is OA, is tenuous at best.

3. The decision to seek care for regional musculoskeletal symptoms is more likely to be driven by psychosocial aspects of life that confound coping, than by the magnitude of joint pain or severity of anatomical changes of OA.

References

(An asterisk denotes recommended reading.)

1. **Foucault, M.** (1973). *The Birth of the Clinic: An Archeology of Medical Perception.* London: Tavistock Publications.

2. **Hadler, N.M.** (1987). *Clinical Concepts in Regional Musculoskeletal Illness.* Orlando: Grune & Stratton.

3. **Heine, J.** (1926). Über die arthritis deformans. *Virchows Arch* **260**:521–663.

4. **Sokoloff, L.** (1969). *The Biology of Degenerative Joint Disease.* Chicago: The University of Chicago Press.

5. **Bierma-Zeinstra, S., Bohnen, A., Ginae, A., Prins, A., and Verhaar, J.** (1999). Validity of American College of Rheumatology criteria for diagnosing hip osteoarthritis in primary care research. *J Rheumatol* **26**:1129–33.

6. **Hadler, N.M.** (1985). Osteoarthritis as a public health problem. *Clin Rheum Dis* **11**:175–85.

7. National Health and Nutrition Examination Survey (US). (1979). Basic data on arthritis—knee, hip, and sacroiliac joints in adults 25–74 years,

United States, 1971–1975. Hyattsville, Maryland: National Center for Health Statistics (Publication Number (PHS)79-1661. Vital and Health Statistics Series 11, No. 213).

8. **Davis, M.A., Ettinger, W.H., Neuhous, J.M., and Mallon, K.P.** (1991). Knee osteoarthritis and physical functioning: evidence from the NHANES I epidemiologic follow-up study. *J Rheumatol* **18**:591–8.

9. **Andersen, R.E., Crespo, C.J., Ling, S.M., Bathon, J.M., and Bartlett, S.J.** (1999). Prevalence of significant knee pain among older Americans: results for the Third National Health and Nutrition Examination Survey. *J Am Geritr Soc* **47**:1435–8.

10. **Massardo, L., Watt, I., Cushnaghan, J., and Dieppe, P.** (1989). Osteoarthritis of the knee joint: an eight year prospective study. *Ann Rheum Dis* **48**:893–7.

11. **Hadler, N.M.** (1992). Knee pain is the malady—not osteoarthritis. *Ann Intern Med* **116**:598–9.

12. *****Peat, G., McCarney, R., and Croft, P.** (2001). Knee pain and osteoarthritis in older adults: a review of community burden and current use of primary health care. *Ann Rheum Dis* **60**:91–7.

    Detailed discussion of the 'window' on life in the workforce provided by an analysis of the prevalence of regional musculoskeletal complaints.

13. **Videman, T. and Battié, M.C.** (1999). The influence of occupation on lumbar degeneration. *Spine* **24**:1164–8.

14. **Sambrook, P.N., MacGregor, A.J., and Spector, T.D.** (1999). Genetic influences on cervical and lumbar disc degeneration. *Arthritis Rheum* **42**:366–72.

15. **Felson, D.T., Hannan, M.T., Naimark, A.,** *et al.* (1991). Occupational physical demands, knee bending, and knee osteoarthritis: Results from the Framingham Study. *J Rheumatol* **18**:1587–92.

16. **Odding, E., Valkenburg, H.A., Algra, D., Vandenouweland, F.A., Grobbee, D.E., and Hofman, A.** (1998). Associations of radiological osteoarthritis of the hip and knee with locomotor disability in the Rotterdam Study. *Ann Rheum Dis* **57**:203–8.

17. **van Baar, M.E., Dekker, J., Lemmens, A.M., Oostendorp, R.A.B., and Bijlsma, W.J.** (1998). Pain and disability in patients with osteoarthritis of hip or knee: The relationship with articular, kinesiological, and psychological characteristics. *J Rheumatol* **25**:125–33.

18. *****Brandt, K.D., Heilman, D.K., Slemenda, C., Katz, B.P., Mazzuca, S., Braunstein, E.M., and Byrd, D.** (2000). A comparison of lower extremity muscle strength, obesity, and depression scores in elderly subjects with knee pain with and without radiographic evidence of knee osteoarthritis. *J Rheumatol* **27**:1937–46.

    This and Ref. 6 are important studies that complement the insights derived from Refs 2 and 4 above.

19. **Hopman-Rock, M., Odding, E., Hofman, A., Kraaimaat, F.W., and Bujlsma, J.W.J.** (1997). Differences in health status of older adults with pain in the hip or knee only and with additional mobility restricting conditions. *J Rheumatol* **24**:2416–23.

20. American Medical Association. (1998). *Managing Osteoarthritis.* Chicago: American Medical Association.

21. **Verbrugge, L.M. and Ascione, F.J.** (1987). Exploring the iceberg: common symptoms and how people care for them. *Med Care* **12**:264–8.

22. **Gevitz, N.** (ed.). (1988). *Other Healers: Unorthodox Medicine in America.* Baltimore: Johns Hopkins University Press, pp. 1–302.

23. **Murray, R.H. and Rubel, A.J.** (1992). Physicians and healers—unwitting partners in health care. *N Engl J Med* **326**:61–4.

24. **Biering-Sorensen, F.** (1983). A prospective study of low back pain in a general population. III. Medical service—work consequence. *Scand J Rehabil Med* **15**:89–96.

25. **Cypress, B.K.** (1983). Characteristics of physician visits for back symptoms: a national perspective. *Am J Public Health* **73**:389–95.

26. **Deyo, R.A. and Tsue-Wu, Y.-J.** (1987). Descriptive epidemiology of low-back pain and its related medical care in the United States. *Spine* **12**:264–8.

27. **Hadler, N.M.** (1995). The disabling backache. An international perspective. *Spine* **20**:640–9.

28. **Hadler, N.M.** (1987). Regional musculoskeletal diseases of the low back. Cumulative trauma versus single incident. *Clin Orthop* **221**:33–41.

29. *****Hadler, N.M.** (1999). *Occupational Musculoskeletal Disorders (2nd ed.).* Philadelphia: Lippincott Williams & Wilkins, pp. 1–433.

    This monograph offers an extensively referenced, comprehensive treatment of the fashion in which the regional musculoskeletal disorders impact on people at home, on people who choose to be patients, and on workers.

30. **Danie, D., Daniels, E., and Aronson, D.** (1982). The diagnosis of meniscal pathology. *Clin Orthop* **163**:218–24.

31. **Johnson, L.L., van Dyk, G.E., Green, J.R., Pittsley, A.W, Bays, B., Gully, S.M., and Phillips, J.M.** (1998). Clinical assessment of asymptomatic knees: comparison of men and women. *Arthroscopy* **14**:347–59.

32. **Symmons, D.P.M.** (2001). Knee pain in older adults: the latest musculoskeletal 'epidemic'. *Ann Rheum Dis* **60**:89–90.

33. **Creamer, P., Lithbridge-Cejku, M., Costa, P., Tobin, J.D., Herbst, J.H., and Hochberg, M.C.** (1999). The relationship of anxiety and depression with self-reported knee pain in the community: data from the Baltimore Longitudinal Study of Aging. *Arthritis Care Res* **12**:3–7.

34. **Summers, M.N., Haley, W.E., Reveille, J.D., and Alarcón, G.S.** (1988). Radiographic assessment and psychologic variables as predictors of pain and functional impairment in osteoarthritis of the knee or hip. *Arthritis Rheum* **31**:204–9.

35. **Salaffi, F., Cavaliere, F., Nolli, M., and Ferraccioli, G.** (1991). Analysis of disability in knee osteoarthritis. Relationship with age and psychological variables but not with radiographic score. *J Rheumatol* **18**:1581–6.

36. **Dexter, P. and Brandt, K.** (1994). Distribution and predictors of depressive symptoms in osteoarthritis. *J Rheumatol* **21**:279–86.

37. *****Steultjens, M.P.M., Dekker, J., and Bijlsma, J.W.J.** (2001). Coping, pain and disability in osteoarthritis. *J Rheumatol* **28**:1068–72.

    A multivariate analysis demonstrating the strength of the inverse association between regional musculoskeletal symptoms and coping skills.

38. **Bongers, P.M., de Winter, C.R., Kompier, M.A.J., and Hildebrandt, V.H.** (1993). Psychosocial factors at work and musculoskeletal disease. *Scand J Work Environ Health* **19**:297–312.

39. *****Hadler, N.M.** (2001). Rheumatology and the health of the workforce. *Arthritis Rheum* **44**:1971–4.

    Detailed discussion of the 'window' on life in the workforce provided by an analysis of the prevalence of regional musculoskeletal complaints.

40. **Hadler, N.M.** (1994). The injured worker and the internist. *Ann Intern Med* **120**:163–4.

41. **Hadler, N.M., Carey, T.S., and Garrett, J.** (1995). The influence of indemnification by workers' compensation insurance on recovery from acute backache. *Spine* **20**:271.

8

Clinical features of osteoarthritis and standard approaches to the diagnosis

8.1 Signs, symptoms, and laboratory tests

Sheila O'Reilly and Michael Doherty

This chapter focuses on the common clinical presentations of OA. General aspects of the symptoms and signs of OA, and the varying patterns and associations are discussed; the features of OA at individual joint sites are then detailed. Atypical features and presentations, particularly relating to serious complications, are briefly highlighted. Finally, the merits and pitfalls of routine investigations are addressed.

General clinical features

OA is a complex, heterogeneous process that may be triggered by diverse constitutional and environmental factors. It is, therefore, not surprising that the clinical presentation of OA is extremely variable in terms of timing of onset, pattern of involvement, and severity. Equally variable are the prognosis and outcome in different patients, and at different joint sites. Despite this heterogeneity, a number of generalizations about OA can be made (Key clinical points 1). For example, although rare conditions that predispose to OA may have non-locomotor manifestations, the changes of OA are confined to the musculoskeletal system. Symptoms and signs of OA are usually slow to evolve, mainly relate to joint damage rather than inflammation, and uncommonly present before middle age. Although polyarticular involvement is common, usually only one or a few joints present clinical problems at any one time.

The main clinical features of OA are *symptoms* (predominantly pain and stiffness), *functional impairment*, and *signs*. It has long been noted that there is often a marked discordance between these three, especially for smaller joints affected by OA.[1] In a clinical setting, therefore, only a good clinical history and examination, and consideration of the patient as a whole, will permit determination of the specific factors relating to pain and disability in that individual.

Symptoms of osteoarthritis

The common symptoms of OA are listed in Table 8.1.

Table 8.1 Common symptoms and signs of OA

Symptoms	Signs
Pain	Crepitus
Stiffness	Restricted movement
Alteration in shape	Tenderness
Functional impairment	—joint line
	—periarticular
± anxiety, depression	Bony swelling
	Deformity
	Muscle wasting/weakness
	± effusions, increased warmth
	± instability

Pain

This is the dominant symptom in OA and the usual reason for seeking advice. Initially, it is typically aching in nature, related to joint use, and relieved by rest. Such 'mechanical' pain is reputed to differentiate OA from inflammatory arthropathies, though formal studies only confirm the diversity of pain descriptors within each disease and the overlap between them.[2] As OA progresses, pain may become more persistent and occur also at rest and at night. Interference with restorative sleep may further compound pain severity through associated fatigue and lack of well-being.

The correlation between pain and degree of structural OA change is closest at the hip, then the knee, and is worst for hand and spinal apophyseal joints. At any site, however, joints with severe radiographic change are more likely to be painful than those with mild or no change (Fig. 8.1). Women may be more likely to report pain, though the strength of this relationship varies between studies and between joints.[3,4] Pain reporting correlates strongly with psychological variables such as anxiety and depression.[5,6]

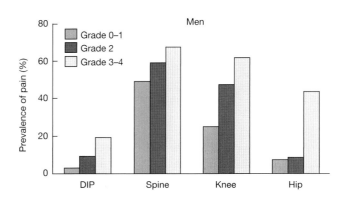

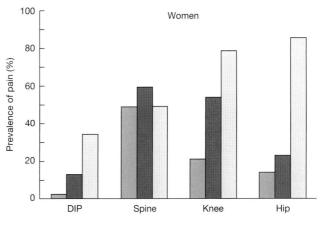

Fig. 8.1 The relationship between radiographic change and pain at various sites. The data was taken from a population survey in Northern England.

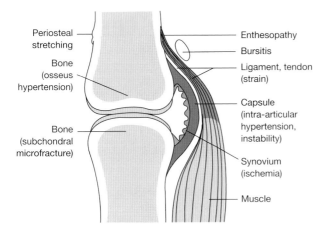

Fig. 8.2 Potential sites and mechanisms of local pain generation in OA.

The mechanisms of pain production in OA remain unclear. The OA process may affect all intracapsular and periarticular tissues of the synovial joint, resulting in many possible causes of pain (Fig. 8.2). Cartilage itself is aneural, but there is rich sensory innervation in other joint tissues. Raised intraosseous pressure, presumably secondary to venous obstruction, is well documented in large joint OA[7] and is a suggested major cause of nocturnal pain. This 'bony' pain is often associated with severe structural change and poor prognosis. Bone marrow oedema demonstrated using MRI scans has been shown to associate with pain in knee OA.[8] Periosteal stretching by bone proliferation, and subchondral microfractures may also contribute to pain. Intra-articular hypertension caused by synovial hypertrophy, excess fluid, or mechanical derangement may stimulate capsular mechanoreceptors, and ischemia from mild synovitis may excite synovial nociceptors. Periarticular involvement is common around large joint OA but is often overlooked as a cause of pain.[9] Bursitis, enthesopathy, tendinitis, and ligamentous strain probably result from altered mechanical loading across the joint due to remodelling, instability, and pain. Myalgia and cramps may accompany OA, and muscle weakness itself may indirectly contribute to pain as suggested by the demonstrable reduction in pain following training.[10]

Stiffness

For patients, 'stiffness' may vary in meaning from slowness of joint movement, to pain on initial movement such as getting up from a chair. Early morning stiffness, often interpreted as a measure of inflammation, is occasionally severe, but most patients complain more of inactivity stiffness or 'gelling' later in the day. Stiffness is generally short-lived, compared to the more prolonged, often generalized stiffness of inflammatory arthropathy. A duration of less than 30 minutes forms part of the American College of Rheumatology (ACR) diagnostic criteria for OA.[11]

Anxiety and depression

Anxiety and depression are common in patients with OA. These merit attention in their own right, in addition to the amplifying effects on pain perception and level of disability.[6] Closely allied to anxiety and depression is fibromyalgia, which, like OA, predominates in women and shows increasing prevalence with age.[12] Fibromyalgia may amplify the symptoms and disability of OA or be the principal cause of pain. It is important to recognize, since it is typically unresponsive to analgesics and requires a different management approach.

Altered joint shape, deformity

Obvious bony swelling and deformity may be a source of distress for some patients. This is particularly common with Heberden's nodes and hand OA, which may be thought unsightly.

Functional impairment

OA contributes greatly to overall disability in the community,[13] with knee OA being the greatest contributor. Disability may include poor mobility, difficulty with activities of daily living, social isolation, and loss of work opportunities with consequent financial concerns. Subsequent handicap is determined by the circumstances and aspirations of the individual. Like pain, it is a common reason for seeking medical advice. A number of validated instruments are available to assess self-reported disability and dimensions relating to general health status and quality of life. The explanation for disability and functional loss is not always clear. Pain is an important contributor and muscle weakness appears to correlate well with disability at the knee.[14] Reduced range of joint movement may be a principal feature or a contributor to overall disability. As with pain, the extent of disability is influenced by accompanying psychological factors, although it may be impossible to differentiate causation and consequence.

Signs of osteoarthritis

Common examination findings in OA are listed in Table 8.1. Many of these signs, particularly those of joint damage and remodelling, are incorporated into classification or diagnostic criteria for individual joints. Their usefulness is influenced by agreement of their presence. Several studies confirm only moderate agreement between assessors for most of these signs, crepitus appearing the least reproducible.[15] Despite this caveat, certain signs are helpful in clinical assessment.

Crepitus

Coarse crepitus, accompanying an irregular joint surface, conducts well through bone and air. It is typically palpable over a wide area of the joint, and is felt throughout the range of movement; in gross cases it may be clearly audible. Although a key feature in criteria, coarse crepitus is a non-specific sign of joint damage.

Tenderness

Tenderness to palpation along the joint-line ('capsular/joint-line tenderness') suggests a capsular/intracapsular origin of pain. Point tenderness away from the joint-line suggests a periarticular lesion; pain on resisted active movements and/or stress tests may further localize the involved periarticular structure. Periarticular lesions such as bursitis and enthesopathy commonly accompany large joint (knee, hip) OA. They may be the principal cause of pain and are often readily amenable to local treatment.

Reduced range of movement

This is extremely common in OA joints. More important than the precise reduction in movement, however, is the accompanying loss of function. This requires separate assessment of screening movements for activities of daily living to compliment self-reported disability. Reduced movement mainly results from osteophyte encroachment, remodelling, and capsular thickening, but may be accentuated by effusion and soft tissue swelling.

Deformity and instability

Deformity is a sign of advanced OA, with severe cartilage loss, osteophyte, remodelling, and bone attrition. Although deformities at individual sites may be highly characteristic of OA, none are specific. Clinically detectable instability is regarded as a late sign that may accompany severe deforming OA at certain sites such as the knee (mainly varus/valgus instability) or finger joints affected by 'erosive' OA (lateral radial-ulnar instability). Commonly, however, capsular thickening and osteophytosis maintains gross stability as OA slowly progresses. Local traumatic instability (e.g., cruciate rupture) may, of course, be a predisposing factor and predate signs of OA. Joint laxity in the hand may be a risk factor for thumb-base OA, and the role of joint laxity and malalignment in predisposing to knee OA is discussed in Chapter 7.2.5.

Muscle wasting and weakness

Wasting is often a difficult sign to assess, particularly in the elderly or obese patient. When present, it is global, affecting all muscles that act over the affected joint. Assessment of muscle weakness around a painful joint is problematic because of pain inhibition (see Chapter 7.2.3.3).

Increased warmth and effusions

Varying degrees of synovitis evidenced by warmth, synovial thickening, effusion, and stress pain (pain that worsens in the tight-pack positions) may accompany or predate signs of joint damage. Such inflammatory signs are most evident at the knee and during the early development stage of nodal finger interphalangeal OA. Effusions at the knee have been suggested as a risk factor for progression.[16] Large, warm effusions are uncommon, and the possibility of alternative pathology or associated calcium crystal deposition should be considered.

Clinical patterns ('subsets') of osteoarthritis

Several attempts have been made to subdivide the broad spectrum of OA to better define causative factors and to determine natural history and prognosis. The earliest classification was by recognised aetiology into *primary* or *secondary* OA. However, this is often unhelpful because: (1) it still leaves a large primary group in whom the predisposing factors are unclear; and (2) there is frequent overlap between the two, as shown, for example, by a higher prevalence of post-meniscectomy 'secondary' OA in subjects with a predisposition to 'primary' nodal OA.[17]

Division according to known predisposing factors (e.g., dysplasia, collagenosis, Perthe's) has been retained but principally relates to atypical and early-onset OA (see later). Further division of the larger 'primary' OA group has been attempted according to:

- the joint site involved
- the number of joints involved (one, few, many)
- associated intra-articular calcium crystal deposition

- presence of marked clinical inflammation
- the radiographic bone response (atrophic, hypertrophic).

Although 'subsets' differing in several such features have emerged, it is important to note there are no sharp distinctions. The above features change with time, so that one subset may evolve into another, and different subsets may exist at different sites within an individual. Most useful, perhaps, is simple division by site and number of involved joints. Risk factors for development and progression are increasingly attributed to specific sites or to polyarticular involvement. The common patterns (Fig. 8.3) will be described, since their recognition has some relevance for patient education and prognosis.

Nodal generalized osteoarthritis

This pattern, recognized since the nineteenth century, has been well characterized.[18] It is probably the most common, easily recognized, and best-accepted subset. Its characteristics are as follows:

- marked familial predisposition
- female preponderance
- typical onset in middle age with hand symptoms and signs
- multiple Heberden's nodes, with or without Bouchard's nodes
- polyarticular finger interphalangeal OA
- good functional outcome for hand OA
- later predisposition to OA at other common OA sites (especially knee, less frequently hip and other joints).

Presentation is usually in middle age (forties, fifties) with symptoms of pain, stiffness, and swelling in one or a few finger interphalangeal joints (IPJs). Gradually, more joints are recruited, resulting in a stuttering onset of hand IPJ polyarthritis ('monoarthritis multiplex'). Hand symptoms can persist for several years, but usually settle to leave the firm posterolateral swellings of Heberden's (distal IPJ) and Bouchard's (proximal IPJ) nodes, and typical radial or ulnar deviations (Fig. 8.4). Mild knee symptoms may accompany this slow evolution of hand OA, but it is usually in later life (sixties, seventies) that other joints become problematic. The knee is the

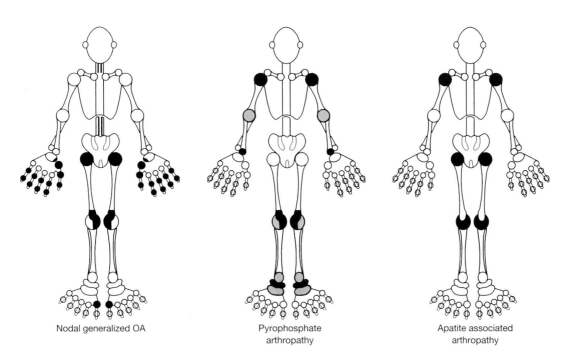

| Nodal generalized OA | Pyrophosphate arthropathy | Apatite associated arthropathy |

Fig. 8.3 Common patterns of joint pain involvement in OA.

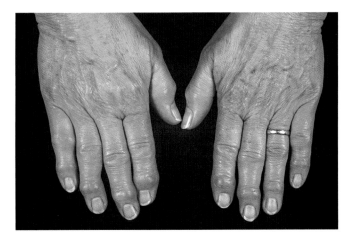

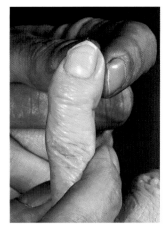

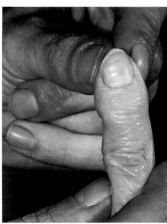

Fig. 8.4 Hand involvement in generalized nodal OA, with typical Heberden's and Bouchard's nodes.

Fig. 8.5 Instability of the DIPJ in erosive OA.

commonest large joint involved, typically with medial and patellofemoral compartment OA. The hip and other joints (glenohumeral, sterno- and acromioclavicular, first metatarsophalangeal, cervical and lumbar apophyseal joints, elbow, midtarsal joints) may also become sites of symptomatic OA in such individuals.

The existence of generalized polyarticular OA, with nodal change the marker of the subset, is supported by several studies.[18,19] Additional support for nodal generalized OA as a subset with strong constitutional, possibly autoimmune, predisposition comes from the following observations:

♦ symmetry of hand involvement,[20]

♦ strong genetic predisposition,[21] and

♦ high prevalence of IgG rheumatoid factor positivity.[22]

The problem arises, however, of when to apply the label 'nodal OA'. There are no agreed diagnostic criteria and the occurrence of just one, or a few Heberden's nodes with limited interphalangeal OA is a common, often asymptomatic finding in the elderly. One study[22] suggested a further division of 'non-nodal generalized OA', with involvement of more proximal than distal interphalangeal joint involvement, and a more equal sex distribution, than nodal OA. Clearly, distinction between nodal and non-nodal polyarticular OA is often blurred.

Erosive ('inflammatory') osteoarthritis

The presence of radiographic erosions in addition to more typical 'degenerative' changes in hands prompted differentiation of this subset from nodal OA.[24] Affected IPJs may become unstable (Fig. 8.5) and, occasionally, even ankylosed (Fig. 8.6)—both of which are further distinguishing features from more common nodal OA. Its inflammatory nature and equal involvement of proximal and distal IPJs may suggest rheumatoid arthritis. Radiographic erosions, however, are subchondral not marginal and classically evolve to a 'gulls wing' appearance combining subchondral erosion with proliferative bone remodelling (Fig. 8.6). Unlike nodal OA, it does not predispose to generalized OA, but is less favourable with regard to hand function.[25]

Existence of this uncommon subset, however, is disputed. Some authors view it merely as severe involvement within the spectrum of nodal OA.[26]

Crystal associations

Deposition of calcium crystals [calcium pyrophosphate dihydrate (CPPD) and basic calcium phosphates—mainly carbonate substituted hydroxyapatite] is a common accompaniment to the OA process, and shows a strong association with age. Crystal identification is mainly via examination of synovial fluid, though gross deposits may show on radiographs as

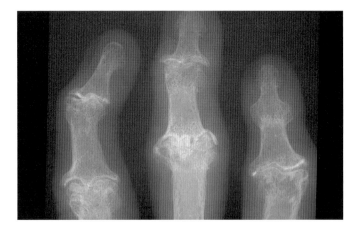

Fig. 8.6 Typical radiographic features in erosive OA with 'gull's wings' deformities and ankylosis of one DIPJ.

chondrocalcinosis (usually, but not inevitably CPPD) and, less commonly, as calcification in synovium, capsule, or periarticular structures (tendon, bursae). Whether they have a pathological role in OA remains uncertain[27] (see Chapter 7.2.1.6). Their presence, however, has been used as a means of defining certain clinical presentations and subsets of OA.

Pyrophosphate arthropathy

Acute pyrophosphate arthropathy ('pseudogout') typically presents as acute monoarthritis in an elderly patient. The knee is the usual target site (Fig. 8.7), but almost any joint may be involved. Most episodes are spontaneous, though direct trauma or stress response to intercurrent illness may be triggering factors. Pain is severe and characteristically reaches its maximum within just 6–12 hours of onset. There may be an accompanying systemic response with pyrexia and mild confusion. Examination reveals florid synovitis with marked tenderness, warmth, effusion, and restricted movement with stress pain. Overlying erythema is common and the principal differential diagnosis is gout and sepsis. Aspirated synovial fluid is inflammatory (turbid, low viscosity, high cell count with more than 90 per cent polymorphs) (Fig. 8.8) and often blood stained. Diagnosis is confirmed by the identification of CPPD crystals in synovial fluid, and exclusion of sepsis by Gram stain and culture. Attacks are self-limiting and usually resolve within one to two weeks. The mechanism of the attack is thought to be 'shedding' of preformed CPPD crystals from their origin in fibro- and hyaline cartilage. This is the one clear instance where CPPD crystals cause inflammation and arthropathy.

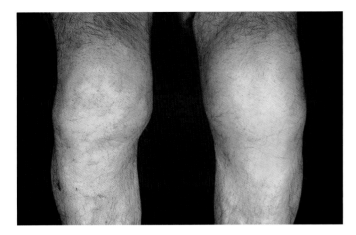

Fig. 8.7 Pyrophosphate arthropathy presenting as acute synovitis of the knee.

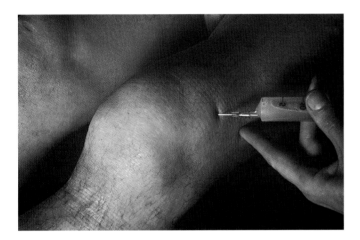

Fig. 8.8 Turbid synovial fluid obtained during an acute attack of acute pyrophosphate arthropathy.

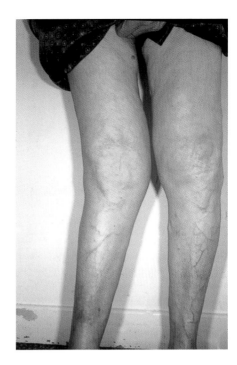

Fig. 8.9 Chronic pyrophosphate arthropathy in the knees of an elderly lady, with marked valgus deformity of the right knee.

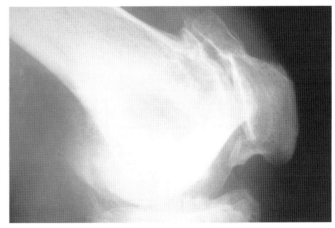

Fig. 8.10 The typical hypertrophic bone response in chronic pyrophosphate arthropathy.

Acute attacks may occur alone, but often superimpose on chronic symptomatic arthropathy. *Chronic pyrophosphate arthropathy* (CPPD deposition with structural joint changes of OA) also mainly targets knees, especially of elderly women (Fig. 8.9). Other common sites are shoulders, wrists, elbows, and metacarpophalangeal joints. Clinical and radiographic features are essentially those of OA, but possible distinctions that have been emphasized include:

♦ marked predominance in elderly women

♦ atypical distribution (glenohumeral, elbow, radiocarpal, and meta-carpophalangeal joints are not common target sites for OA)

♦ frequent marked inflammatory component (especially at knees, gleno-humeral, and radiocarpal joints)

♦ frequent 'hypertrophic' radiographic appearance with prominent osteo-phyte, cysts, and osteochondral bodies (Fig. 8.10)

♦ CPPD crystals in synovial fluid, with or without chondrocalcinosis and calcification of articular structures on radiographs

♦ association with rapidly progressive hip OA,[28] and tendency to radio-graphic progression at the knee.[29]

Many elderly OA patients with CPPD, however, have coexisting nodal OA and no clinical or radiographic features to set them apart from non-crystal associated OA. Joint damage, for example, meniscectomy, is known to pre-dispose both to localized OA and to localized CPPD deposition.[30] Furthermore, at the knee, synovial fluid positivity for CPPD increases with the severity and compartmental extent of radiographic OA.[31] It therefore seems likely that CPPD in the context of OA is more commonly a marker of the extent of the OA process (that is, joint tissue response to insult) than for a subset of OA with a specific pathogenesis.

Isolated chondrocalcinosis due to CPPD deposition may occur without the structural changes of OA, as a common age-related phenomenon, par-ticularly at the knee (Fig. 8.11). It may be asymptomatic, or result in acute pseudogout. Chondrocalcinosis *per se* is rare below the age of 55 and, par-ticularly if florid and polyarticular, should lead to the consideration of either familial CPPD deposition or predisposing metabolic disease[32] (Table 8.2). Pseudogout, arthralgia, or incidental radiographic chondrocal-cinosis may be the initial presentation of metabolic disease. Although rare, recognition is important since it may have therapeutic implications and, in the case of hemochromatosis, require screening of asymptomatic relatives.

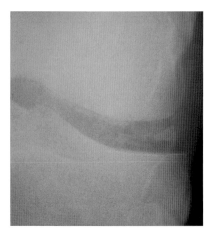

Fig. 8.11 Isolated chondrocalcinosis at the knee, with involvement of hyaline cartilage and fibrocartilage (reproduced with the kind permission of Mosby-Year Book Inc.).

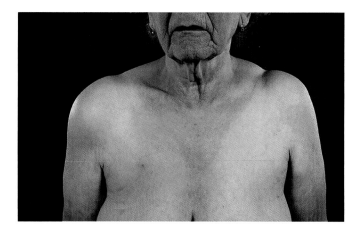

Fig. 8.12 Large, cool effusion in a 'Milwaukee shoulder' (apatite-associated arthropathy).

Table 8.2 Metabolic diseases associated with CPPD deposition

	Chondrocalcinosis	Pseudogout	Chronic arthropathy
Hyperparathyroidism	Yes	Yes	No
Hemochromatosis	Yes	Yes	Yes
Hypophosphatasia	Yes	Yes	No
Hypomagnesemia	Yes	Yes	No
Hypothyroidism	Probably	No	No
Gout	Possibly	Possibly	No
Wilson's disease	Possibly	No	No
Acromegaly	Possibly	No	No

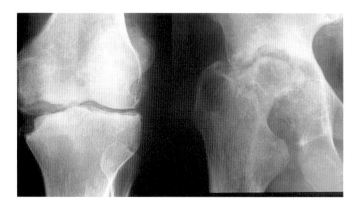

Fig. 8.13 Marked bone atrophy at the hip and knee in a patient with apatite-associated arthropathy.

Less common clinical syndromes that may arise in the context of widespread chronic pyrophosphate arthropathy include: acute tendinitis (Achilles, triceps, flexor digitorum), rarely with tendon rupture; tenosynovitis (hand flexors, extensors); and bursitis (olecranon, infrapatellar, retrocalcaneal).

Apatite-associated arthropathy ('Milwaukee shoulder syndrome')

Like CPPD, 'apatite'—basic calcium phosphates (BCP), mainly carbonate substituted hydroxyapatite, tricalcium phosphate, and octacalcium phosphate crystal aggregates—can often be identified in OA fluids and joint tissues. The origin of the apatite remains unclear, though most evidence suggests it predominantly forms within cartilage rather than being shed from subchondral bone.[33] Again, the chance of finding basic calcium crystals in knee OA fluids increases with age, and with the extent and severity of OA change.[31] However, the finding of plentiful apatite aggregates in synovial fluid and tissue has been linked to arthropathy that shows the following features:

- confinement to elderly subjects, predominantly women over 75
- localization to one or a few large joints (shoulder, hip, knee)
- subacute onset; rapid, painful progression; poor outcome
- large cool effusions (Fig. 8.12); marked instability
- 'atrophic' radiographic appearance with marked attrition of cartilage and bone (Fig. 8.13).

As with chronic pyrophosphate arthropathy, there is considerable overlap with less extreme forms of progressive OA. Furthermore, concurrence of

CPPD and apatite is common ('mixed crystal deposition'), and association with progressive, destructive knee OA is suggested.[34] However, the poor specificity of calcium crystals for distinctive arthropathy other than pseudogout, questions their use as a marker for joint *disease*. Further work is required to establish their usefulness as markers of varying aspects of the OA *process*.

OA secondary to other disease

A history of severe trauma or intra-articular mechanical derangement is, by far, the most common attributable cause of localized 'secondary' OA. Cruciate ligament damage and meniscal tears frequently lead to knee OA, the risk increasing with age and with the presence of Heberden's nodes. Generalized hypermobility is common and may be found on examination of even an elderly patient with OA, though its putative association with generalized OA[35] remains unconfirmed. There is evidence, however, that hypermobility in the hand associates with localized thumb-base (first carpometacarpal) OA but a reduced prevalence of finger interphalangeal OA.[36]

A number of defined diseases may insult synovial joints and lead to non-inflammatory arthropathy with radiographic features predominantly of OA. Despite some overlap, for clinical purposes, they are best grouped according to presentation (Table 8.3). Many are rare, and present additional clinical or radiographic features that suggest the diagnosis. Endemic and inherited conditions generally cause young-onset, polyarticular OA that is clearly unusual. Conditions that present later in life with pauciarticular OA, however, may more easily be missed. Hemochromatosis may present with arthropathy and should be recognized early before liver and other major

Table 8.3 Principal diseases predisposing to OA

Generalized, mainly polyarticular OA

(Spondylo-) epiphyseal dysplasias

Collagenoses (e.g. Stickler syndrome—progressive hereditary arthro-opthalmopathy)

Ochronosis

Hemochromatosis

Wilson's disease

Endemic OA (e.g. Kashin–Beck disease, Malmad disease)

Pauciarticular, large-joint OA

1 Knee

Epiphyseal dysplasia

Osteonecrosis (mainly medial femoral condyle)

Acromegaly

Neuropathic (Charcot) joint (classically syphilis)

2 Hip

Acetabular dysplasia

Perthes disease

Slipped femoral epiphysis

Osteonecrosis

3 Shoulder

Neuropathic (Charcot) joint (mainly syringomyelia)

Osteonecrosis (proximal humerus)

4 Elbow

Neuropathic (Charcot) joint (mainly syringomyelia)

Osteonecrosis (distal humerus)

5 Wrist

Neuropathic (Charcot) joint (mainly syringomyelia)

6 Finger interphalangeal joints

Thiemann's disease

7 Hindfoot/midfoot

Neuropathic (Charcot) joint (mainly diabetes)

organ damage is established. In general, features that should lead to consideration of a predisposing disease include:

◆ premature-onset OA (under 45 years)

◆ atypical distribution (e.g., prominent metacarpophalangeal and radio-carpal OA with florid cyst formation in hemochromatosis)

◆ short stature, abnormal body habitus, short digits

◆ premature-onset chondrocalcinosis (under 55 years)

◆ florid polyarticular chondrocalcinosis (any age).

As has already been emphasized for pain causation, only a broad-based consideration of the whole patient will permit delineation of potential predisposing disease.

Clinical features of osteoarthritis at specific sites

The predilection of OA to target certain joints is striking. This limited distribution remains unexplained, though one hypothesis suggests that joints, which have changed function in recent evolutionary history, are still 'underdesigned', with little mechanical reserve for their new functions and,

therefore, more commonly 'fail' in the face of joint insult.[37] Nevertheless, because of the high prevalence of OA even involvement of more 'protected' joint sites by OA is not uncommon. Trauma, in particular, may result in OA at almost any site.

Hand and wrist

The hand and wrist comprise many small joints acting together as a functional unit. OA selectively targets only certain of these joints, the pattern differing according to gender,[38] with women showing more common, more widespread, and more severe involvement. Although theories abound, the reasons for this remain unclear.

Proximal and distal IPJ involvement predominates in women and typically starts around middle age with symptoms of pain, stiffness, and swelling, slowly affecting one IPJ after another. Initially, there may be features of articular and periarticular inflammation, with redness and warmth. Mucous cysts, containing hyaluronan-rich jelly, form on the superolateral aspect of the IPJs and may spread quite a distance proximally or, less commonly, distally from the joint (Fig. 8.14). These herald the characteristic firm Heberden's (distal IPJ) and Bouchard's (proximal IPJ) nodes (Fig. 8.15). Fully established nodes may remain as discrete posterolateral swellings, or merge to form a posterior bar. Once fully developed, pain and stiffness usually subside, and outcome with respect to hand function, is usually excellent.[25] Concomitant to node formation is the gradual evolution of focal OA in the underlying IPJs. This may result in fixed flexion and highly characteristic fixed lateral (ulnar or radial) deviation, especially of distal IPJs—the ends of the fingers usually pointing towards the longitudinal axis of the hand (Fig. 8.16). Florid distal IPJ involvement may result in longitudinal nail ridging ('Heberden's nodes nails; Fig. 8.17). Despite the, sometimes, gross deviation, IPJ instability is not a feature; if present, 'erosive' OA changes are likely to be seen on the radiograph. Similarly, ankylosis, usually limited to just one or two IPJs, is a rare late consequence of erosive OA. Compared to nodal OA, erosive OA symptoms are often more chronic and late functional outcome less good.

First carpometacarpal joint (1st CMCJ) or thumb-base disease may occur alone or in the context of nodal generalized OA. It is generally more problematic than IPJ OA, causing pain on usage—maximal over the joint itself, but often radiating distally towards the thumb and proximally to the wrist and distal forearm (sometimes causing confusion with carpal tunnel syndrome). Common problems with daily activities include doing up buttons, lifting saucepans, opening jars, and writing. Examination may reveal

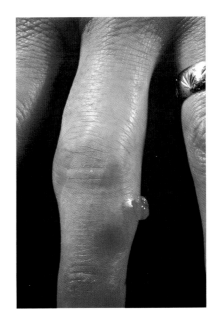

Fig. 8.14 Mucous cyst exuding hyaluronan-rich jelly extending distally.

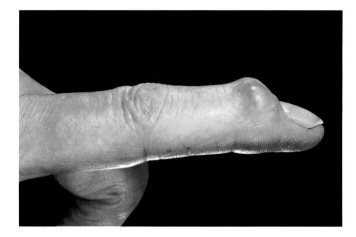

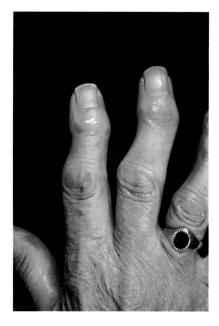

Fig. 8.16 Ulnar deviation at the DIPJs; radial deviation at the DIPJs.

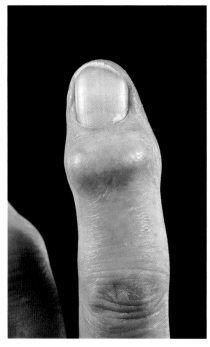

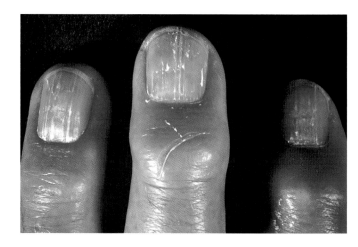

Fig. 8.15 Typical posterolateral swelling of the DIPJ.

Fig. 8.17 'Heberden's nodes nails' with longtitudinal and transverse nail ridging.

localized tenderness; restricted, painful, weak thumb movements, with or without crepitus; and difficulty with fine precision pinch. Any muscle wasting globally affects thenar muscles, unlike the selective involvement of opponens, abductor pollicis, and flexor pollicis with median nerve entrapment. In advanced OA, characteristic 'squaring' occurs due to osteophyte, remodelling, and subluxation (Fig. 8.18). The scapho-trapezial joint is an integral part of the thumb-base unit and is also commonly affected by OA, either alone or together with the 1st CMCJ. Pain is discrete, with little or no radiation; and tenderness, the principal examination finding, is well localized. Palpable osteophyte and subluxation are rare.

The radiocarpal joint may develop 'secondary' OA following wrist trauma/fracture, but it is also a common site for chronic pyrophosphate arthropathy, particularly in the elderly. Pain and tenderness are well localized to the joint-line, and signs of synovitis may be evident. Isolated median, or combined median and ulnar nerve entrapment may complicate pyrophosphate arthropathy at this site, relating more to soft tissue inflammation than articular derangement. Involvement of the mid-carpal articulation is a less common finding, again usually in association with CPPD deposition in elderly subjects.

A clinical problem that may arise in hands of elderly patients with long-standing nodal OA is superimposed tophaceous gout, secondary to chronic diuretic therapy. The joint changes that accompany OA appear to facilitate urate as well as calcium crystal deposition through a decrease in normal inhibitors or an increase in promotors of crystal formation. Presentation is with chronic or subacute pain and swelling of finger joints that may be mistaken for exacerbation or 'reactivation' of nodal OA. Typical acute attacks with lower limb predominance may be absent, and the diagnosis may be missed until the 'infected nodes' discharge pus and white material (Fig. 8.19).

Elbow

Elbow OA is uncommon in the absence of predisposing trauma or disease, but may occur as a site of CPPD deposition and in the context of nodal OA. Isolated 'primary' OA of the elbow is described in men, in association with metacarpophalangeal OA.[39] Pain is predominant at the elbow but may radiate distally into the forearm. Any, or all, of the three articulations may be

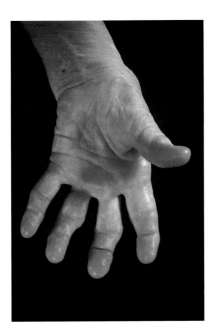

Fig. 8.18 Squaring of the first CMCJ due to osteophyte remodeling and subluxation, with consequent wasting of the thenar muscles.

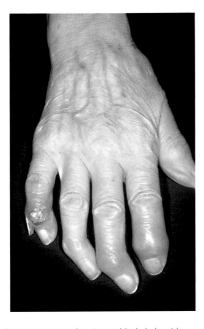

Fig. 8.19 A discharging gouty tophus in an elderly lady with pre-existing nodal OA.

involved. Reduced flexion and extension, often with fixed flexion, is usual with humeroulnar involvement, and pronation/supination may be restricted with proximal radio-ulnar OA. Crepitus and synovitis are occasionally marked. The outcome of elbow OA is usually good; function is generally retained and symptoms are often limited to a few years.

Shoulder

The acromioclavicular joint (ACJ) is commonly affected by OA. Pain is well localized (Fig. 8.20) and experienced mainly on abduction and elevation of the arm. Examination reveals localized tenderness, often with bony swelling, and crepitus on shrugging the shoulder. Typically, there is a

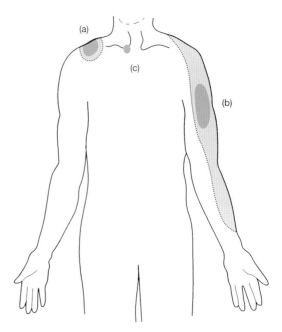

Fig. 8.20 Pattern of pain around the shoulder from OA of: (a) acromioclavicular joint; (b) glenohumeral joint; (c) sternoclavicular joint.

painful superior arc and pain on reaching for the opposite shoulder or on forced passive adduction. Associated rotator cuff pathology and/or subacromial bursitis, however, commonly coexist to present a more complex collection of regional symptoms and signs.

The glenohumeral joint (GHJ) is rarely affected by OA except in elderly women, in whom it is a common cause of shoulder pain and disability.[40] Examination reveals anterior joint-line tenderness and equally restricted active and passive movement; external rotation and abduction are the earliest and most severely affected movements. Global wasting of deltoid and rotator cuff muscles may give a bony prominence to the shoulder ('squaring') and scapula. Crepitus may be palpable anteriorly, or around the acromion if there is superior humeral migration and subacromial impingement. Again, coexisting rotator cuff disease and subacromial bursitis may amplify the disability and complicate the clinical picture.

More severe, rapidly progressive OA of the GHJ may associate with plentiful synovial fluid apatite ('Milwaukee shoulder') and/or CPPD crystals (see Chapter 7.2.1.6). Clinically, large effusions may be present, either anteriorly filling in the normal depression below the clavicle and medial to deltoid, or, more commonly, anterolaterally due to cuff rupture and free communication between the GHJ cavity, subacromial, and subdeltoid bursae. Joint rupture may result in the acute exacerbation of symptoms, followed by wide bruising around the upper arm—'epaule senile haemorrhagique'[41] (Fig. 8.21). Marked instability and occasional secondary subluxation or even dislocation may result. The outcome of such painful, debilitating arthritis is generally poor.

The sterno-clavicular joint is a common site for signs of OA (bony swelling, crepitus) in older subjects but rarely gives rise to symptoms. If present, pain is usually well localized to the joint. Pain, particularly if progressive and associated with warmth, soft tissue swelling, or erythema should lead to aspiration and consideration of sepsis and crystals (CPPD).

Hip

Attempts have been made to classify hip OA in various ways, according to recognized preceding disease (primary/secondary), bilaterality/unilaterality, the presence of generalized OA, distribution of OA within the joint, or radiographic appearance. No classification has been entirely successful and there may be a considerable overlap between patterns. The most widely used system

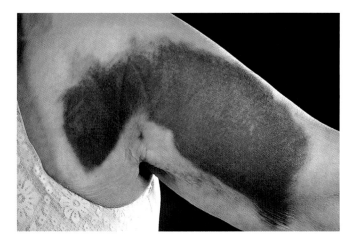

Fig. 8.21 Extensive bruising of the upper arm due to rupture of the shoulder joint—'epaule senile haemorrhagique'.

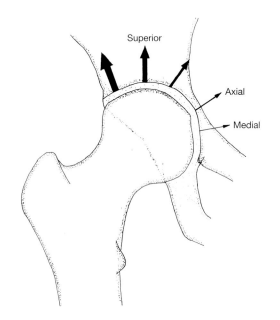

Fig. 8.22 Patterns of femoral migration around the OA hip; the arrows indicate relative frequency of each pattern.

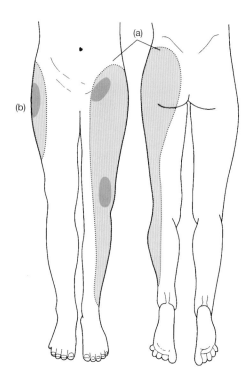

Fig. 8.23 Radiation of pain around the hip: (a) hip OA; (b) trochanteric bursitis.

is radiographic division by anatomic site (Fig. 8.22).[42] *Superior pole OA* is the commonest form and includes all types of OA secondary to structural abnormality. This is the characteristic pattern in men and is often unilateral at presentation. It may result in superolateral or superomedial femoral head migration. *Medial pole OA* is far less common and predominates in women; it is more likely to be bilateral at presentation and less likely to progress with (axial) femoral migration. A *concentric* pattern, associated with generalized OA, is also described,[43] though nodal OA, probably, more strongly associates with medial pole OA. However characterized, there is usually a striking symmetry of radiographic features in patients with bilateral hip OA. Importantly, however, in up to 30 per cent of patients, categorization according to anatomic site proves impossible ('indeterminate' pattern[16,44]).

The hip shows the best correlation between symptoms and radiographic change. Pain from the hip is typically felt maximally deep in the anterior groin (femoral nerve), but may be referred over a wide area including the lateral thigh and buttock (sciatic nerve), anterior thigh and knee (obturator nerve), and as far down the leg as the ankle (Fig. 8.23). Occasionally, pain is maximally felt at the knee, with little proximal discomfort; unlike pain

arising from the knee, this referred pain is poorly localized over a wide area, involves the distal thigh, and may be partially relieved by rubbing. Pain is usually mainly experienced during walking, but may also occur at rest and at night. Stiffness and restriction is common, and patients may have particular difficulty with bending to put on socks, tights, and shoes. Walking, manoeuvring stairs, and getting in and out of cars, becomes increasingly difficult. In women, painful hip abduction during intercourse may be an added problem.

The principal examination finding is painful restriction of hip movement (both active and passive), with internal rotation in flexion the first and most severely affected. Hip, but not knee movement, will reproduce referred pain. An antalgic gait is usual. Anterior groin tenderness, lateral to the femoral pulsation, is common; pain and tenderness over the greater trochanter, worse when lying on that side, implies secondary trochanteric bursitis. In advanced cases, wasting of gluteal and anterior thigh muscles may be apparent, with a Trendelenburg gait due to abductor weakness. A fixed flexion, external rotation deformity is the most usual end-stage result, with compensatory exaggerated lumbar lordosis and pelvic tilt. Ipsilateral leg shortening follows severe joint attrition and superior femoral migration.

Knee

The medial tibiofemoral (MTF), lateral tibiofemoral (LTF) and patellofemoral (PF) compartments share the same capsule, making the knee the largest synovial joint. This is a major target site for OA, showing associations with age, female gender, obesity, nodal OA, and CPPD deposition. As with the hip, categorization can be made by compartmental involvement. The MTF compartment is most commonly affected in terms of radiographic change (Fig. 8.24),[45] though with increasing imaging of the PF joint (Fig. 8.25) it is apparent that this is another common site, and one that may correlate more closely with symptoms.[46] Monocompartmental (MTF or PF) and bicompartmental (MTF and PF) involvement is most common. Isolated 'primary' LTF OA is rare, but the LTF compartment becomes increasingly involved as OA progresses (associating with synovial fluid CPPD and apatite).[31] Knee involvement is usually bilateral and symmetrical, particularly in women. If strictly unilateral (mainly younger men), it is usually 'secondary' to mechanical insult/trauma such as meniscectomy.

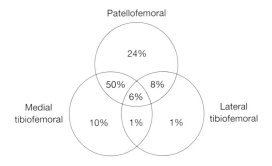

Fig. 8.24 Venn diagram showing patterns of compartmental disease in OA of the knee.

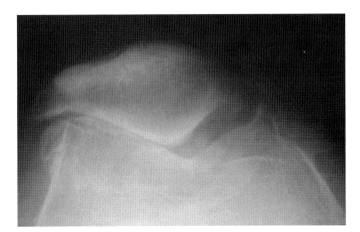

Fig. 8.25 Skyline radiograph of the knee showing severe patellofemoral OA with osteophyte, joint-space narrowing and lateral subluxation.

Pain is well localized to the originating compartment. MTF OA gives anteromedial pain, mainly on walking. PF OA causes localized anterior knee pain, worse on negotiating stairs/inclines, and a progressive aching on prolonged sitting that is relieved by standing and 'stretching' of the legs. Well-circumscribed pain, felt away from the joint line, suggests a periarticular lesion; posterior pain usually indicates a complicating popliteal cyst (Fig. 8.26). Stiffness and 'gelling' are common at this site, particularly after sitting. Loss of function, especially for walking and bending, may result in major disability. Common complaints of 'giving way', mainly relate to altered patella tracking from quadriceps weakness, severe PF OA, or altered load bearing.

Examination commonly reveals coarse crepitus with joint-line tenderness (MTF, LTF) and/or pain on PF stressing. Flexion and extension are usually restricted and painful, and weakness of the quadriceps may result in quadriceps 'lag' (more passive than active extension against gravity). Periarticular tenderness is common, particularly on the medial tibia below the MTF line (Fig. 8.27). Point tenderness at this site, with reproduction of pain on valgus stressing, suggests enthesopathy of the inferior insertion of the medial collateral ligament. More widespread tenderness, with warmth and soft-tissue swelling, suggests anserine bursitis (both lesions may coexist and distinction is often difficult). Tender medial fat pads are also common in this region, especially in obese women. Signs of synovitis (warmth, effusions, synovial swelling, stress pain) are variable, but small to modest effusions are not uncommon. Quadriceps muscle wasting is frequently present but often difficult to detect in the older patient. With time, bony swelling may be palpable and visible, especially along the anterior V-shaped contour of the bony ridges of the femoral condyles, and the lateral tibial plateaux. Severe MTF OA may result in varus angulation as the typical deformity of OA (Fig. 8.28), often accompanied by some degree of fixed flexion. Valgus deformity, however, is not rare, particularly with extensive tricompartmental disease and associated calcium crystal deposition.

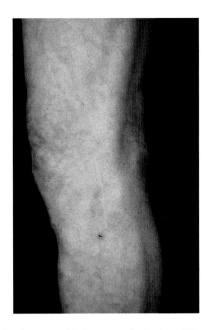

Fig. 8.26 Swelling due to a political cyst complicating knee OA.

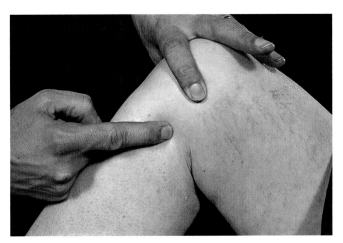

Fig. 8.27 A common periarticular tender site at the knee; the left index finger over the inferior insertion of the medial collateral ligament.

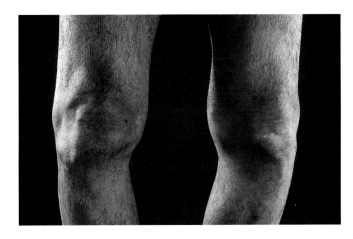

Fig. 8.28 Typical varus deformity with knee OA.

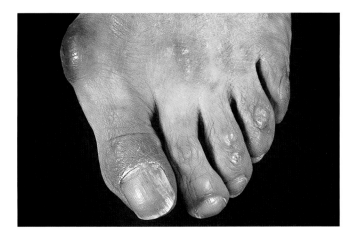

Fig. 8.29   Hallux valgus due to OA of the first MTPJ.

Table 8.4 Comparison between radiated axial pain and root entrapment

	Radiated	Root
Pain		
Maximal over or close to the spine	Yes	No
Clearly related to neck/back movement	Yes	No
Follows a dermatomal distribution	No	Yes
Eased by rubbing	Yes	No
Altered sensation		
Normal or hyperaesthetic	Yes	No
Reduced	No	±
Reduced power	No	±
Impaired reflexes	No	±

Clinically, varus and valgus are best assessed while standing, whereas fixed flexion is best assessed while lying on the couch. The presence of either varus or valgus angulation has been implicated as a factor in subsequent progression.[47] The gait is often antalgic; lateral 'thrust' during stance phase may occur with an unstable knee. Instability is not a usual consequence but may occur in advanced, destructive OA, or as a predisposing cause.

Foot and ankle

OA of the first metatarsophalangeal joint (MTPJ) is common but often asymptomatic. The usual deformity is hallux valgus, often with rotational deformity of the big toe (Fig. 8.29). Abnormal mechanical stress from inappropriate footwear may encourage this deformity (it is rare in people who do not wear shoes) as may metatarsus primus varus. Secondary problems, which cause most symptoms, include medial fibrotic bursitis ('bunion') and crossover toes. Hallux rigidus is less common and associates with large dorsal osteophytes that limit extension and thus interfere with the toe-off phase of walking.

OA changes, and nail dystrophy, similar to those in the hand, may affect the toe interphalangeal joints but are uncommon.[48] Osteophytes may develop in the talonavicular or calcaneocuboid joints, and, if large, may cause difficulties getting into shoes, and pain and stiffness when walking on uneven surfaces. Ankle and subtalar involvement is uncommon unless related to severe injury or pre-existing structural abnormality; CPPD deposition may, however, occur at this site, especially in men.

Spine

'Degenerative' change in the spine is almost invariable and particularly targets the lower cervical and lower lumbar segments. By definition, OA is limited to the apophyseal (facet) synovial joints. However, apophyseal joint OA often, though not invariably, coexists with changes of narrowing, osteophyte, and disc protrusion in nearby intervertebral joints, although the relationship between the two remains unclear. Such changes are often asymptomatic, though overall back pain is more common in those with radiographic 'degeneration'.[49]

Lumbar spine OA may associate with chronic or intermittent 'mechanical' pain, usually aggravated by movement or standing. Although predominantly close to the spine, pain is often diffuse with radiation to the buttocks or leg. Cervical involvement, similarly, causes diffuse pain, maximal in the neck, but often radiating to the shoulder, the occiput, or down the arms. Neck movements typically provoke pain. The clinical picture is often complicated by pain and stiffness from coexisting ligamentous and muscular strains. Pain radiation down limbs from lower cervical or lower lumbar spine structures requires differentiation from pain due to root entrapment (Table 8.4).

Compared to peripheral joints, examination of the spine is generally unhelpful in differentiating periarticular from articular pain. Findings may include local segmental tenderness (centrally over interspinous ligaments, paracentrally over apophyseal joints), local muscle spasm, and painful reduced movement. Tenderness over the posterior ilio-lumbar ligament region, iliac crest, or occipital ridge is common, suggesting enthesopathy. A neurological examination and examination for hyperalgesic tender sites (with negative control sites) may be required in patients with an appropriate history suggesting root entrapment, spinal stenosis, or fibromyalgia.

Warning symptoms and signs

Acute or subacute synovitis

'Flares' of OA are common in terms of temporary exacerbation of pain and stiffness, and may be accompanied by signs of mild to modest synovitis. However, florid acute or subacute synovitis, especially if accompanied by marked erythema, should not be attributed to OA, and always requires urgent investigation for an alternative cause. A common superimposed acute problem is crystal synovitis (pseudogout, less commonly urate gout), which usually causes pain and signs that are at their worst within just 12–24 hours. Sepsis, however, should always be a concern, although rheumatoid arthritis and oral steroid therapy are stronger risk factors in adults than joint damage *per se*. Sepsis is most commonly subacute in onset. Progressive pain and stiffness, additive joint involvement (e.g., a flare in a first MTPJ, followed by flares in the ipsilateral ankle and then knee), and accompanying night sweats or malaise should always suggest sepsis, especially in a compromised OA patient (e.g., with diabetes, renal impairment). In all such instances it is vital to aspirate the joint and examine fluid for sepsis (gram stain and culture) and crystals (compensated polarized microscopy). Sepsis and pseudogout may coexist and *both* investigations are mandatory.

Rapid progression

Rapidly worsening pain, or subacute onset of severe pain, is unusual in OA. Its occurrence should lead to the consideration of osteonecrosis or fracture. Osteonecrosis most commonly occurs at the distal medial femoral condyle and femoral head, causing pain on weight bearing but also often marked ('bone') pain at night. Fracture pain is mainly noticed during weight bearing. Bone malignancy (mainly secondary deposits from the lung, breast, prostate; or myeloma) adjacent to an OA joint may also cause progressive nocturnal and, eventually, persistent bone pain that is well localized and poorly correlates with joint movement. All three pathologies may be apparent on the plain radiograph; if not, however, a radionuclide scan is a useful, sensitive, and readily available second investigation as increasingly is MRI.

Locking

Sudden, painful, marked restriction on usage, usually lasting very briefly before spontaneously 'unlocking', strongly suggests an internal mechanical derangement. It is mainly limited to the knee and elbow. Osteochondral bodies, formed as part of the OA process, or a torn meniscus at the knee, are the usual causes. A history of recurrent, troublesome locking should lead to further investigation with a view to possible surgical intervention.

Usefulness and pitfalls of investigations

Radiology

The radiographic changes in OA are fully covered in Chapter 8.2. The main uses of plain radiographs in OA are:

- ◆ to support the clinical diagnosis of OA
- ◆ to assess the degree of structural change and chondrocalcinosis
- ◆ to assess the progression of structural change in large joints.

Although very helpful in these respects, the poor correlation between X-ray changes and symptoms has already been emphasized. Furthermore, radiographic OA is common in the older population and may be an incidental finding of little relevance to pain causation (e.g., from a periarticular lesion or bone malignancy). Radiographs cannot, therefore, replace a sound history and clinical examination to answer the question 'why does this patient have pain at this site at this point in time?' Over-reliance on the radiograph for clinical decision-making should be avoided.

By comparison to radiographs, other imaging techniques are rarely required for a clinical assessment of OA. MRI is particularly useful for soft tissue pathology, intracapsular derangement, and osteonecrosis; and bone scintigraphy for osteonecrosis, stress fracture, or suspected malignancy.

Laboratory tests

Blood and urine tests have no role in the diagnosis of OA. Their main use is to confirm or exclude metabolic disease that predisposes to 'OA' or chondrocalcinosis (Table 8.5). Screening for disease is only justified in the situations of young-onset OA or chondrocalcinosis, florid polyarticular chondrocalcinosis, or the presence of other suggestive clinical or radiographic features.[39] Routine screening in older subjects, other than for measurement of calcium level and thyroid function (done for other reasons in this age group), is unrewarding and not recommended. As yet, there are no biochemical 'markers' of OA for diagnosis or for the assessment of severity, progression, or prognosis (Chapter 8.3).

Although inflammatory markers and autoimmune profile are often undertaken to exclude inflammatory arthropathy, these tests are imperfect in this respect. OA itself does not trigger a readily detected acute phase response. Elevations of erythrocyte sedimentation rate (ESR), C reactive protein, and plasma viscosity may, however, occur in a patient with OA from unrelated disease in other systems, or from the mild non-specific elevation (mainly ESR) that is common in the elderly. Such tests, therefore, do not exclude a clinical diagnosis of OA. Acute pseudogout may cause a marked acute phase response, sometimes equivalent to that of septic arthritis, and only synovial fluid analysis allows correct diagnosis. Rheumatoid factors (especially IgM, low titres) are non-specific and can occur in otherwise normal subjects; their presence, therefore, does not exclude OA as the clinical problem. Similarly, elevated serum uric acid associates with obesity, diuretic use, and renal impairment (common in many OA patients) and is of little diagnostic use; gout is only confirmed by finding urate crystals in synovial fluid or tophus aspirate.

Synovial fluid analysis

Synovial fluid in OA is generally 'non-inflammatory' with retained viscosity, low turbidity, and low cell count (mainly mononuclear). However, these features show wide variation and no diagnostic specificity. The main clinical value of synovial fluid analysis is:

- ◆ to confirm the presence of CPPD crystals (to explain acute synovitis and chondrocalcinosis);
- ◆ to exclude sepsis in an acutely swollen OA joint; and,
- ◆ to confirm possible coexisting urate gout.

Conclusions

Pain is the dominant feature in OA, and may correlate poorly with structural change. The classification of OA into subsets is of limited value with the possible exceptions of nodal generalized OA and CPPD crystal associated disease. Only a comprehensive history and examination of the patient, focusing on both the locomotor symptoms and the person overall, will allow an accurate diagnosis and assessment of OA. Investigations are helpful in only a few defined situations, such as excluding metabolic diseases in florid, young-onset OA.

Key clinical points 1: General characteristics of osteoarthritis

1. There are no primary extra-locomotor manifestations.
2. Usually only one or a few joints are problematic at any time.
3. There is a slow evolution of symptoms and structural change.
4. There is a strong age association—it is uncommon before middle age.
5. Often there is poor correlation between symptoms, disability, and degree of structural change.
6. The symptoms and signs predominantly relate to joint damage rather than inflammation.

Key clinical points 2

1. Pain and restricted function are the cardinal symptoms of OA.
2. There is often a poor correlation between symptoms, disability, and degree of structural change.
3. Only a full clinical enquiry and examination will determine the cause and severity of OA-related problems.
4. Adequate patient assessment requires a holistic approach.
5. Investigations are relatively unimportant in diagnosis and decision-making; a plain radiograph is the most helpful investigation for diagnosis and for the assessment of the severity and progression of structural change.
6. Screening for underlying diseases is important in patients with florid early-onset OA.

Table 8.5 Initial biochemical investigations for metabolic disease predisposing to chondrocalcinosis or atypical, young-onset OA

Test	Disease
Serum ferritin, liver function	Hemochromatosis, Wilson's disease
Calcium, alkaline phosphatase	Hyperparathyroidism, Hypophosphatasia
Serum magnesium	Hypomagnesemia
Thyroid function	Hypothyroidism
Urine homogentisic acid	Ochronosis

References

(An asterisk denotes recommended reading.)

1. **Cobb, S., Merchant, W.R., and Rubin, T.** (1957). The relation of symptoms to osteoarthritis. *Chronic Dis* **5**:197–204.

2. **Helliwell, P.S.** (1995). The semeiology of arthritis: discriminating between patients on the basis of their symptoms. *Ann Rheum Dis* **54**:924–6.

3. **Lawrence, R.C., Everett, D., and Hochberg, M.C.** (1990). Arthritis. In R. Huntley and J. Cornoni-Huntley (eds), *Health Status and Well-being of the Elderly: National Health and Nutrition Examination—I: epidemiologic fol-low-up survey.* New York: Oxford University Press, pp. 136–5.

4. **Davis, M.A.** (1981). Sex differences in reporting osteoarthritic symptoms: a sociomedical approach. *J Health Soc Behav* **23**:298–310.

5. *Davis, M.A., Ettinger, W.H., Neuhas, J.M., Barclay, J.D., and Segal, M.R.* (1992). Correlates of knee pain among US adults with and without radi-ographic knee osteoarthritis. *J Rheumatol* **19**:1943–9.

   This was one of the first studies to differentiate between the associations with structural OA and with symptoms in OA.

6. **O'Reilly, S.C., Muir, K.R. and Doherty, M.** (1998). Knee pain and disability In the Nottingham Community: association with poor health status and psychological distress. *Br J Rheumatol* **57**:588–94.

7. **Arnoldi, C.C., Lemperg, R.K., and Linderholm H.** (1975). Intraosseous hypertension and pain in the knee. *J Bone Joint Surg* **57**B:360–3.

8. *Felson, D.T., Chaisson, C.E., Hill, C.L., Totterman, S.M.S., Gale, M.E., Skinner, K.M., Kazis, L. and Gale, D.R.* (2001). The association of bone mar-row lesions with pain in knee osteoarthritis. *Ann Intern Med* **134**:541–9.

   This study used MRI scanning to demonstrate marrow oedema and knee OA and found that its presence was associated with pain.

9. **Merrit, J.L.** (1989). Soft tissue mechanisms of pain in osteoarthritis. *Sem Arthritis Rheum* **18**(Suppl. 2):51–6.

10. **O'Reilly, S.C., Muir, K.R. and Doherty, M.** (1999). The effectiveness of home exercise on pain and disability from osteoarthritis of the knee: a randomized controlled trial. *Ann Rheum Dis* **58**:15–9.

11. **Altman, R.** (1991). Classification of disease:osteoarthritis. *Sem Arthritis Rheum* **20**(Suppl. 2):40–7.

12. **Wolfe, F., Ross, K., Anderson, J., Russell, I.J., and Hebert, L.** (1995). The prevalence and characteristics of fibromyalgia in the general population. *Arthritis Rheum* **38**:19–28.

13. **Badley, E.M.** (1995). The effect of osteoarthritis on disability on health care use in Canada. *J Rheumatol* **22**(Suppl. 43):19–22.

14. *McAlindon, T.E., Cooper, C., Kirwan, J.R., and Dieppe, P.A.* (1993). Determinants of disability in osteoarthritis of the knee. *Ann Rheum Dis* **52**:258–62.

    This community study confirmed the lack of association between disability and structural change and demonstrated a link between muscle weakness and disability in knee OA.

15. **Jones, A., Hopkinson, N., Pattrick, M., Berman, P., and Doherty, M.** (1992). Evaluation of a method for clinically assessing osteoarthritis of the knee. *Ann Rheum Dis* **51**:243–5.

16. **Ledingham, J., Dawson, S., Preston, B., Milligan, G., and Doherty, M.** (1992). Radiographic patterns and associations of osteoarthritis of the hip. *Ann Rheum Dis* **51**:1111–16.

17. **Doherty, M., Watt, I., and Dieppe, P.** (1983). Influence of primary generalised osteoarthritis on development of secondary osteoarthritis. *Lancet* **1**:8–11.

18. *Kellgren, J.H. and Moore, R.* (1952). Generalised osteoarthritis and Heberden's Nodes. *Br Med J* 181–7.

    This important paper described the relationship between Heberden's nodes and generalised OA.

19. **Hochberg, M.C., Lane, N.E., Pressman, A.R., Genant, H.K., Scott, J.C., and Nevitt, M.C.** (1995). The association of radiographic changes of osteoarthri-tis of the hand and hip in elderly women. *J Rheumatol* **22**:2291–4.

20. **Egger, P., Cooper, C., Hart, D.J., Doyle, D.V., Coggon, D., and Spector, T.D.** (1995). Patterns of joint involvement in osteoarthritis of the hand: the Chingford study. *J Rheumatol* **22**:1509–13.

21. **Stecher, R.M.** (1995). Heberden's Nodes. A clinical description of osteoarthritis of the finger joints. *Ann Rheum Dis* **14**:1–10.

22. **Hopkinson, N.D., Powell, R.J., and Doherty, M.** (1992). Autoantibodies, immunoglobulins and Gm allotypes in nodal generalized osteoarthritis. *Br J Rheumatol* **31**:605–8.

23. **Acheson, R.M. and Collart, A.B.** (1975). New Haven Survey of joint diseases. XVII. Relationships between some systemic characteristics and osteoarthro-sis in a general population. *Ann Rheum Dis* **34**:379–87.

24. **Peter, J.B., Pearson, C.M., and Marmor, L.** (1966). Erosive osteoarthritis of the hands. *Arthritis Rheum* **9**:365–88.

25. **Pattrick, M., Aldridge, S., Hamilton, E., Manhire, A., and Doherty, M.** (1989). A controlled study of hand function in nodal and erosive osteoarthritis. *Ann Rheum Dis* **48**:978–82.

26. **Cobby, M., Cushnaghan, J., Creamer, P., and Watt, I.** (1990). Erosive osteoarthritis: is it a separate disease entity? *Clin Radiol* **42**:258–63.

27. **Doherty, M. and Dieppe, P.** (1988). Clinical aspects of calcium pyrophos-phate crystal deposition. *Rheum Dis Clin North Am* **14**:395–414.

28. **Menkes, C.J., Decraemere, W., Postel, M., and Forest, M.** (1985). Chondrocalcinosis and rapid destruction of the hip. *J Rheumatol* **12**:130–3.

29. **Ledingham, J.M., Regan, M., Jones, A., and Doherty, M.** (1995). Factors affecting radiographic progression of knee osteoarthritis. *Ann Rheum Dis* **54**:53–8.

30. **Doherty, M., Watt, I., and Dieppe, P.A.** (1982). Localised chondrocalcinosis in post-meniscectomy knees. *Lancet* **1**:1207–10.

31. **Pattrick, M., Hamilton, E., Wilson, R., Austin, S., and Doherty, M.** (1993). Association of radiographic changes of osteoarthritis, symptoms, and syn-ovial fluid particles in 300 knees. *Ann Rheum Dis* **52**:97–103.

32. **Jones, A.C., Chuck, A.J., Arie, E.A., Green, D.J., and Doherty, M.** (1992). Diseases associated with calcium pyrophosphate deposition disease. *Sem Arthritis Rheum* **22**:188–202.

33. **Dieppe, P.A., Doherty, M., MacFarlane, D.G., Hutton, C.W., Bradfield, J.W., and Watt, I.** (1984). Apatite-associated destructive arthritis. *Br J Rheumatol* **23**:84–91.

34. **Dieppe, P.A., Campion, G., and Doherty, M.** (1988). Mixed crystal deposi-tion. *Rheum Dis Clin North Am* **14**:415–26.

35. **Bird, H.A., Tribe, C.R., and Bacon, P.A.** (1978). Joint hypermobility leading to osteoarthritis and chondrocalcinosis. *Ann Rheum Dis* **37**:203–11.

36. **Jónsson, H., Valtysdóttir, S.T., Kjartansson, O., and Brekkan, A.** (1996). Hypermobility associated with osteoarthritis of the thumb base: a clinical and radiological subset of hand osteoarthritis. *Ann Rheum Dis* **55**:540–3.

37. **Hutton, C.W.** (1987). Generalized osteoarthritis: an evolutionary problem? *Lancet* **1**:1463–5.

38. **Acheson, R.M., Chan, Y., and Clemett, A.R.** (1970). New Haven survey of joint diseases. XII: distribution and symptoms of osteoarthrosis in the hands with reference to handedness. *Ann Rheum Dis* **29**:275–86.

39. **Doherty, M. and Preston, B.** (1989). Primary osteoarthritis of the elbow. *Ann Rheum Dis* **48**:743–7.

40. **Chard, M. and Hazelman, B.** (1987). Shoulder disorders in the elderly. *Ann Rheum Dis* **46**:684–9.

41. **de Seze, S., Babault, A., and Ramdon, S.** (1968). L'epaule senile hemorrhag-ique. *L'Actualite Rhumatologique* **1**:107–15.

42. **Pearson, J.R. and Riddell, D.M.** (1962). Idiopathic osteoarthritis of the hip. *Ann Rheum Dis* **21**:31–7.

43. **Solomon, L.** (1976). Patterns of osteoarthritis of the hip. *J Bone Joint Surg* **41**:118–25.

44. **Croft, P., Cooper, C., Wickham, C., and Coggon, D.** (1992). Is the hip involved in generalised osteoarthritis? *Br J Rheumatol* **31**:325–8.

45. **Ledingham, J.M., Regan, M., Jones, A., and Doherty, M.** (1993). Radiographic patterns and associations of osteoarthritis of the knee in patients referred to hospital. *Ann Rheum Dis* **52**:520–6.

46. **McAlindon, T.E., Snow, S., Cooper, C., and Dieppe, P.A.** (1992). Radiograpic patterns of osteoarthritis of the knee joint in the community: the importance of the patellofemoral joint. *Ann Rheum Dis* **51**:844–9.

47. **Sharma, L., Song, J., Felson, D.T., Cahue, S., Shamiyeh, E., Dunlop, D.D.** (2001). The role of knee alignment in disease progression and functional decline in knee osteoarthritis. *JAMA* **286**:188–195.

48. **McKendry, R.J. Nodal osteoarthritis of the toes.** (1986). *Sem Arthritis Rheum* **16**:126–34.

49. **Symmons, D.P.M., van Hemert, A.M., Vandenbroucke, J.P., and Valkenburg, H.A.** (1991). A longitudinal study of back pain and radiological changes in the lumbar spines of middle aged women. II. Radiological find-ings. *Ann Rheum Dis* **50**:162–6.

8.2 Plain radiographic features of osteoarthritis

Iain Watt and Michael Doherty

The plain radiograph remains a key investigation in the clinical management of OA. It is particularly useful for:

◆ *diagnosis*—showing characteristic structural changes typical of OA and absence of features of alternative arthropathies (e.g., inflammatory erosive disease);

◆ assessment of the *severity of structural change*;

◆ identification of associated *chondrocalcinosis*.

In interpreting the plain radiograph a number of important caveats need to be remembered, most importantly:

1. The common discordance between symptoms, disability, and degree of structural OA change—the radiograph is no substitute for a thorough history and examination for determination of symptom causation.

2. The requirement of optimal views and techniques—for example, in certain joints the assessment of joint-space narrowing requires stress or loaded views.

3. Individual radiographic features are not specific.

4. The quantification of OA changes is problematic—the radiograph is relatively insensitive for detection of early OA and minor progression of cartilage and bone change (see Chapters 11.4.1, 11.4.2, and 12, as may be required for intervention studies);

5. Plain radiographs are a static, not dynamic, assessment—the radiograph provides an anatomical record of prior OA change; scintigraphy and magnetic resonance imaging (MRI) are more informative of current dynamic, physiological change (see Chapters 11.4.3 and 11.4.5).

The radiograph does, however, provide a readily available, relatively safe, and cost-effective means of assessing gross OA change. For clinical decision-making purposes it is a sufficiently reliable, informative investigation of joint structure such that other imaging modalities are required infrequently. In this chapter, the individual radiographic features of OA will be described and explained. The characteristic changes and important complications encountered at target sites will then be illustrated.

Radiographic features of osteoarthritis

The radiographic features of OA reflect the underlying pathology and involve the simultaneous occurrence of both destructive changes and attempts at repair.[1] The four main radiographic features of OA are joint-space narrowing, subchondral sclerosis, subchondral cyst formation, and osteophyte (Fig. 8.30). In addition, other features such as osteochondral body formation, synovial abnormalities, and calcium crystal deposition may be observed.

Joint-space narrowing

Loss of cartilage is a cardinal feature of OA. It is characteristically focal, and tends to predominate at sites of maximum point loading within individual joints. The focal thinning of cartilage is an important observation that

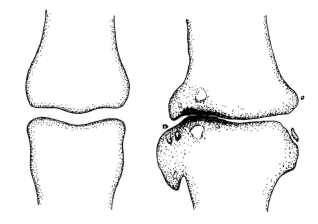

Fig. 8.30 Diagram of a normal (left) and OA (right) joint, showing focal joint-space narrowing, adjacent subchondral sclerosis, marginal osteophyte, cysts, and osteochondral bodies typical of OA.

allows differentiation of OA from other arthropathies, such as rheumatoid arthritis, which commonly cause more generalized and symmetrical cartilage loss. There are exceptions to this, such as the diffuse cartilage loss that occurs in the small interphalangeal (IP) joints of the hand, scapho-trapezial (ST) joint and, occasionally, the ankle.

Cartilage is not imaged directly on conventional radiographs. However, hyaline cartilage thickness can be estimated from the width of the interosseous distance or 'joint space'. This assumes that the opposing joint surfaces are in contact, and weight bearing or stress views may be required to ensure that this is so. The inability to demonstrate the internal structure of hyaline cartilage means that advanced pathological changes such as focal ulceration can be present without any change in radiographic joint-space width.[2] Such insensitivity is not a practical problem in diagnostic terms because other features of OA are usually present. However, it is a significant problem when joint space-width is being used as a marker of disease progression.

In addition to the lack of sensitivity to focal pathological change within cartilage, technical problems relate to precision and accuracy in the assessment of joint-space width. Errors arise from technical aspects of image production and radiographic positioning of the patient. Image resolution determines the smallest change in joint-space width that can be detected. This is reduced by geometric distortion arising from the X-ray source, variable spatial resolution of film/screen combinations, and reduced contrast from X-ray scatter within the patient. In practice these can be minimized by using X-ray tubes with a small focal spot, a Bucky grid to reduce scatter, or by using new high-resolution screen film. However, compromises need to be made and methods vary depending on the joint to be imaged. The variability in patient positioning is important as even small alterations may cause considerable error in joint-space width measurement. Custom-built adjustable positioning apparatus can be used to standardize patient position for studies of disease progression. The method can be refined further using computerized analysis of digital images. In dedicated hands, measurements with a precision of a few per cent can be obtained. However, the rate of progression of disease is so slow overall that detection of change in a short time scale of a few months is unrealistic using the current methodology. Quantitative methods using microfocal radiography, however, may be more sensitive though not generally available.[3]

Subchondral sclerosis

Changes in the thickness and biomechanical properties of hyaline cartilage during the development of OA, are associated with the increased transmission of forces to the subchondral bone. Initially, the bone responds with increased local blood flow and deposition of new bone on existing trabeculae. Sometimes this physiological response may be overwhelmed. Trabecular microfractures and then macroscopic bony collapse may ensue. This progression is identified on plain radiographs by the development of subchondral sclerosis at the sites of maximal stress. In time, frank bony collapse can be visualized. In general, subchondral sclerosis is not detectable on radiographs until cartilage thinning is present. Areas of a joint denuded of hyaline cartilage often show a striking degree of adjacent radiographic subchondral bony sclerosis. The surface of the denuded zone appears smooth and polished to the orthopaedic surgeon or pathologist (eburnation). Prolonged bone-on-bone contact can result in the grooving of the articular surface.

Physiological trabecular condensation may occur as an isolated feature at some sites and must not be confused with the pathological sclerosis of OA. It commonly occurs at the base of the proximal phalanx of the big toe (Fig. 8.31), the lateral aspect of the acetabulum at the hip, and the medial tibial plateau of the knee. Support for a normal physiological response may be gained from recognition of a normal joint-space width, and clinical evidence of increased joint stress such as an active lifestyle and increased body mass.

Subchondral cyst formation

Subchondral cysts are a typical feature of OA but also occur in other arthropathies. They are known by a multitude of other names including geodes, synovial cysts, and necrotic pseudocysts. The plethora of descriptions reflects our ignorance with respect to their causation. The term 'cyst' is used most commonly but, strictly, is erroneous because these cavities are not lined by epithelium. They occur mainly within areas of bony sclerosis at sites of increased pressure transmission. Two mechanisms of formation have been postulated and are not necessarily mutually exclusive. The synovial fluid intrusion mechanism envisages the passage of synovial fluid from the joint cavity to the subchondral bone via fissured or ulcerated cartilage, with pressure necrosis of subchondral trabeculae and subsequent cavitation. The bony contusion theory postulates direct subchondral bony injury as a consequence of diminished hyaline cartilage width, with cavities forming secondary to traumatic localized osteonecrosis.

Radiographically, cysts occur in areas of increased joint stress and are associated with bony sclerosis and joint-space narrowing (Fig. 8.32). Occasionally, communication with the articular surface can be demonstrated. They may be multiple, but are rarely more than 2 cm in diameter. Larger cysts raise the possibility of an accompanying disorder such as rheumatoid arthritis or a crystal-associated arthropathy. If typical associated radiographic features are not present, then a wider differential diagnosis for subchondral cyst formation should be considered (Table 8.6).

Osteophyte formation

Osteophytes are the hallmark of OA. These bony outgrowths occur most commonly at the margins of osteoarthritic joints, by a process of endochondral ossification at the junction of hyaline cartilage and synovium/periosteum. The stimulus causing metaplasia of synovium into cartilage and subsequent osteophyte growth is unknown, but may be related to reduced stress transmission, consequent on changes elsewhere in the joint.[4] Teleologically, osteophytes can be regarded as an attempt at repair and

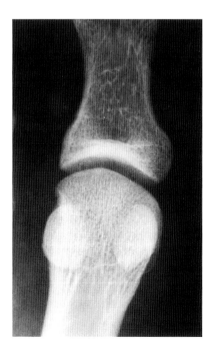

Fig. 8.31 Normal subchondral trabecular condensation at the base of the proximal phalanx in the first MTP joint.

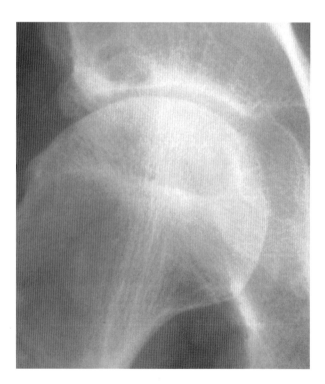

Fig. 8.32 Prominent subchondral cyst in the acetabular roof of an osteoarthritic hip. Note the accompanying sclerosis and superior joint-space narrowing.

Table 8.6 Principal causes of subchondral bone lucency

1. Arthropathies
   Osteoarthritis
   Rheumatoid arthritis
   Metabolic disorders—gout, hemochromatosis
   Hemophilia

2. Synovial proliferation
   Pigmented villonodular synovitis
   Amyloid

3. Miscellaneous (usually solitary)
   Non-neoplastic cysts—post-traumatic cysts, intraosseous ganglion
   Benign bone tumours—chondroblastoma, giant cell tumour
   Malignant bone tumours—myeloma, metastases
   Tuberculosis

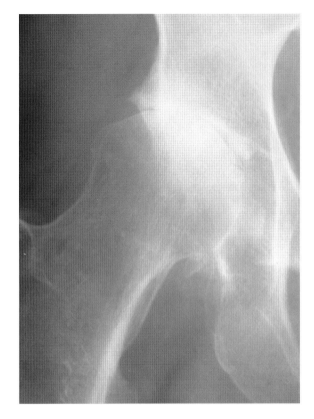

Fig. 8.34 Periosteal osteophyte of the femoral neck, visible as a line of new bone distinct from the underlying cortical margin. Note the accompanying marginal osteophyte visible on the inferior margin of the femoral head, the marked superior joint-space narrowing and supero-lateral migration of the femoral head.

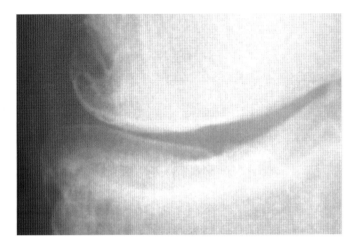

Fig. 8.33 Marginal osteophyte in the lateral compartment of an OA knee. Note that the femoral osteophyte is pointing away from the joint line, whereas the tibial osteophyte is evident as a rim of new bone pointing upwards towards the joint space.

redistribution of abnormal joint loading. One way of achieving this is by the tightening up of capsular laxity and minimizing the unloading of peripheral hyaline cartilage.

Osteophytes are recognized radiographically, most easily, as bony excrescences at joint margins tangential to the X-ray beam (Fig. 8.33). It should not be forgotten that marginal osteophytes consist of continuous lips of new bone formation around the edges of a joint. Viewed *en face* they may be seen as bands of sclerosis, or even mimic cartilage calcification. Osteophytes may develop early in the evolution of OA and can be seen prior to reduction in joint-space width. They can arise in unusual sites such as the intercondylar notch in the knee, where they are easily confused with loose bodies. Such central osteophytes arise from the endochondral ossification of residual islands of hyaline cartilage and are sometimes referred to as 'stud' or 'button' osteophytes. Certain joints demonstrate new bone formation from periosteum in contradistinction to endochondral ossification of peripheral and central osteophytes. Such periosteal osteophytes form along the femoral neck in OA of the hip. This phenomenon is known as 'buttressing' and is regarded as a response to altered mechanical stresses across the joint (see Fig. 8.34).

Identifying osteophytes on conventional radiographs is rarely a problem. Care must be taken not to confuse the normal age-related remodelling of joint anatomy, which results in the squaring of usually rounded articular

margins, with true osteophytes. Traction from joint capsules and ligamentous attachments may also result in bony spur formation, but these should not be confused with osteophyte.

Osteochondral bodies

Disintegration of the joint surface in OA results in chondral or osteochondral fragments breaking free into the joint space. These osteochondral bodies may be loose or incorporated within the synovium. They may alter in size and appearance by a process of resorption or accretion. Alternatively, chondroid metaplasia may occur *de novo* in the synovium with subsequent ossification. The composition of such bodies is variable; many show features of partial endochondral ossification, others may be more irregular and consist of dense bone only.

Radiographically, osteochondral bodies occur in the presence of established features of OA (Fig. 8.35). They vary in size and position, and can disappear completely. They often gravitate to characteristic sites within individual joints and may sometimes be difficult to visualize due to overlapping bony structures (Fig. 8.42). They may migrate into adjacent bursae such as a popliteal cyst.

Care must be taken not to confuse osteochondral bodies with normal anatomical structures such as the fabellum behind the knee (Fig. 8.35), or anatomical variants such as unfused accessory ossification sites. Other pathological conditions may give rise to osteochondral bodies, including osteochondritis dissecans or synovial osteochondromatosis. The former occurs in young people without the accompanying radiographic features of OA. Osteochondromatosis is a metaplastic condition of synovium that may result in a vast number of uniformly small cartilaginous bodies, in contrast to OA in which a small number of variably sized osseous bodies are usually seen.

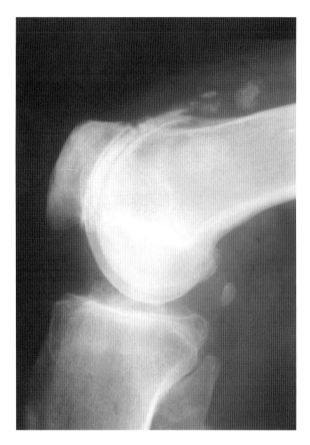

Fig. 8.35 Lateral flexion view of knee showing osteochondral bodies in the suprapatella pouch. Note the better-defined, smooth-contoured fabellum with well-defined trabeculae lying posteriorly. There is also narrowing with superior osteophyte affecting the patellofemoral compartment.

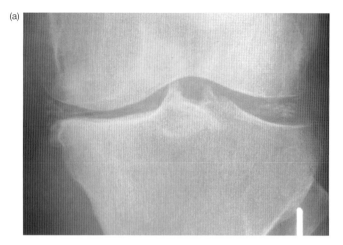

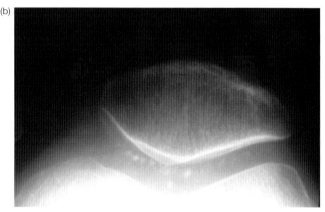

Fig. 8.36 (a) Chondrocalcinosis of medial and lateral fibrocartilage in association with medial tibiofemoral narrowing and osteophyte, and (b) a skyline view showing less common chondrocalcinosis affecting patello-femoral hyaline cartilage.

Calcification

Calcification of fibrocartilage and hyaline cartilage (chondrocalcinosis) commonly associates with OA (Fig. 8.36). Such calcification can occur as an isolated age-associated feature (Fig. 8.11), either as an asymptomatic incidental finding or in association with acute attacks of self-limiting synovitis ('pseudogout'). When chondrocalcinosis co-exists with OA, osteophyte formation may appear particularly florid and result in a hypertrophic form of OA that is sometimes termed chronic 'pyrophosphate arthropathy'. The deposited calcium crystal is usually calcium pyrophosphate, although basic calcium phosphates (mainly hydroxyapatite) may coexist. This subject is dealt with in more detail in Chapter 7.2.1.6. Chondrocalcinosis may also associate with certain metabolic diseases[5] (Table 8.2). Of these, only haemochromatosis also associates with structural changes that resemble OA, the others resulting in isolated, often polyarticular chondrocalcinosis. Conventional radiographs are insensitive in demonstrating chondrocalcinosis, although improved detection rates can be achieved with microfocal radiography. Crystal shedding and cartilage attrition may both result in reduction or loss of chondrocalcinosis.

In addition to cartilage, other structures such as synovium, capsule, entheses and, occasionally, bursae may calcify, usually in association with chondrocalcinosis rather than as an isolated phenomenon.

Additional features of advanced OA

Pathological studies demonstrate synovial thickening with some features of chronic inflammation in OA. This synovial response varies in intensity and may lead to the formation of a joint effusion. Asymmetrical loss of cartilage may result in altered joint mechanics, acceleration of joint damage, and eventual joint deformity. Rarely, extensive regional osteonecrosis of subchondral bone may occur. This is not detected initially on plain radiographs, though subsequently extensive subchondral bony collapse may be seen. Typical sites include the femoral head and the medial femoral condyle (Fig. 8.37). Idiopathic osteonecrosis in this setting is associated with OA but can also occur in its absence.

Characteristics of OA in individual joints

Interphalangeal joints

OA in the IP joints is usually symmetrical, involving multiple joints. The typical patient is a middle-aged female with predominantly distal interphalangeal (DIP) joint involvement. Proximal IP joints may be affected in addition, but only rarely in isolation, and association with DIP OA is the rule (Fig. 8.38).

Typical radiographic features include joint-space narrowing and marginal osteophytes. Small osteochondral bodies are a common additional feature. In comparison with inflammatory arthropathies, in which erosions (proliferative or non-proliferative) occur at joint margins, OA involves the full width of the articular surface to result in diffuse, though commonly eccentric, joint-space narrowing. Marginal osteophytes are prominent and are easily detected clinically due to the paucity of overlying soft tissue. They

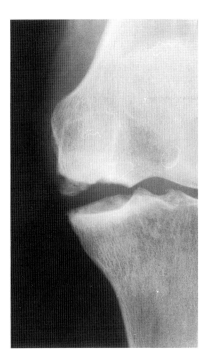

Fig. 8.37 Osteonecrosis of the medial femoral condyle. Note the destruction and fragmentation of the subchondral bone and articular surface affecting just the femoral side of the joint.

Metacarpophalangeal joints

Involvement of the metacarpophalangeal (MCP) joints with OA is unusual in the absence of involvement of the DIP and PIP joints. The typical features of OA are present and the loss of joint space may be asymmetric or more diffuse in a similar fashion to the IP joints (Fig. 8.39). The index and middle finger MCP joints are predominantly affected. Usually osteophytes and subchondral cysts are more prominent on the radial aspect of the metacarpal head, though the reason for this is unclear. MCP joint OA of the thumb can occur without accompanying changes in the IP joints.

The differential diagnosis of MCP joint OA is usually straightforward when multiple joints in the hand are involved. When MCP joints are affected in relative isolation then other diagnoses should be considered. In particular, hemochromatosis has a predilection for MCP joint involvement. It may manifest hook-like osteophytes, identical to those seen in OA (Fig. 8.39). However, hemochromatosis often produces multiple small subchondral cysts in several MCP joints and may occur at a relatively young age (less than 55 years), whilst OA creates larger and fewer geodes. Corroborating evidence of a crystal-associated arthropathy may be found elsewhere in the hand, for example, chondrocalcinosis of the triangular ligament with radiocarpal arthropathy. Other joints less frequently affected by OA, such as the ankle, may also be involved.

Wrist and carpus

The most commonly affected joints in the carpus are the carpometacarpal (CMC) joint of the thumb and the ST articulation (Fig. 8.40). The CMC joint demonstrates typical features of OA, often in association with multiple DIP joint involvement. Initially, the radiographic abnormalities are confined to the trapezium-metacarpal joint. Progression to include the remaining articulations of the trapezium may occur, especially involvement of the ST joint. Isolated OA of the ST joint is not uncommon. The main feature is joint-space narrowing. Subchondral sclerosis, appearing as a double 'tramline' may accompany the narrowing, but osteophyte is not visualized often on conventional radiographs. Radial subluxation of the metacarpal may be a feature of CMC joint OA in the thumb.

OA in the remainder of the carpus and the wrist joint is unusual in the absence of a history of trauma, preceding inflammatory arthritis or avascular necrosis. Certain patterns of joint arthritis may be recognized from the radiographs. For example, instability associated with scaphoid fractures

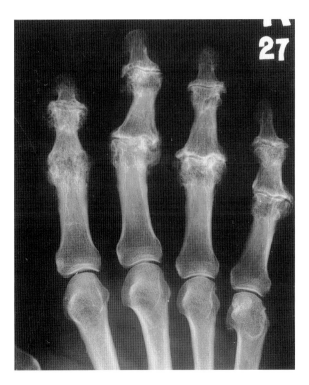

Fig. 8.38 OA of distal and proximal IP joints. Note the characteristic grooving of the distal articular surface and lateral subluxation/deviation.

are associated with Heberden's nodes in the DIP joints and Bouchard's nodes in the PIP joints. When deformity occurs it is usually in the form of radial or ulnar lateral deviation, compared to flexion/extension (swan-neck and Boutonniere) deformities in rheumatoid arthritis.

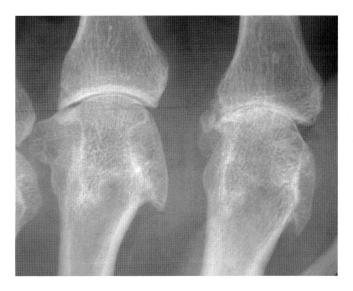

Fig. 8.39 OA of the left 2nd and 3rd MCP joints. Note the extensive radial 'hook' osteophytes and both diffuse (2nd MCP) and asymmetric (3rd MCP) loss of joint space.

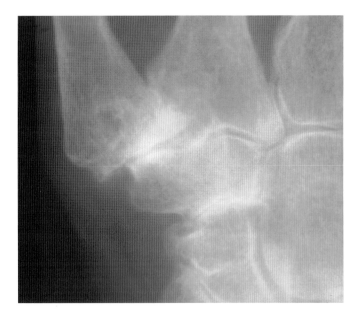

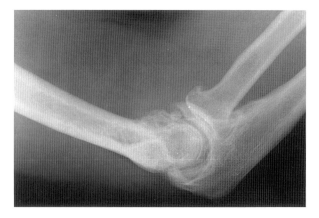

Fig. 8.42 Lateral radiograph demonstrating OA of the elbow. Features include marginal osteophytes, joint-space narrowing, and a loose osteochondral body projecting over the anterior aspect of the joint.

Fig. 8.40 OA of the CMC and ST joints of the thumb, demonstrating joint-space loss and sclerosis as the main features at both sites. At the CMC joint there is additional attrition and altered contour of the bone and a large cyst with a sclerotic margin.

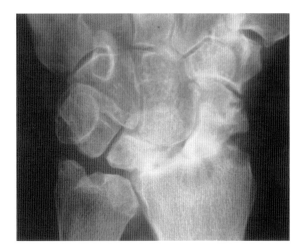

Fig. 8.41 Severe radiocarpal OA associated with non-union of a fracture of the waist of the scaphoid.

may result in radio-scaphoid arthritis (Fig. 8.41). This may progress to involve intercarpal joints and, ultimately, scapho-lunate advanced collapse (SLAC). Another example is the occurrence of radiocarpal and midcarpal joint OA that may be more common in patients with chondrocalcinosis.

Elbow

OA of the elbow is relatively unusual in the absence of trauma or other internal mechanical derangement. Typical features of repair and destruction are noted as in other joints. All three compartments may be involved but usually more severe change occurs in the radio-capitellar compartment. Elbow OA may occur in association with MCPJ OA, particularly in middle-aged men.[6] Patients with OA may complain of 'locking', caused by loose osteochondral bodies (Fig. 8.42). The reduced degree of freedom imposed by a hinge joint means that very small osteochondral fragments could cause severe functional problems. Such small loose bodies may be difficult to

identify on routine radiographs. Usually they are found in the olecranon recess of the joint cavity and may require further imaging such as air arthrography, CT, or MRI to confirm their site and presence.

Shoulder

Several pathological processes may occur in the shoulder region. OA of the acromioclavicular (AC) joint is very common with increasing age. Conversely, primary OA of the glenohumeral joint is much less frequent. However, it is not uncommon for a pre-existing condition such as rotator cuff disease to be present, which predisposes to glenohumeral joint OA or 'cuff-tear' arthropathy. Radiographic features include localized thinning of articular cartilage, initially in the postero-superior portion of the glenoid and humeral head. This corresponds to the area of contact at the point of maximal joint loading in abduction. Subchondral sclerosis and cyst formation is seen. Osteophytes may be identified around the glenoid margin; humeral head osteophytes are seen typically inferomedially in the region of the anatomical neck (Fig. 8.43). They are demonstrated to best advantage if the arm is held in external rotation. Calcification of the hyaline cartilage of the humeral head and the fibrocartilage of the glenoid labrum may be seen but is rare. In some cases, OA may progress as a more atrophic form, with rapid destruction of the femoral head as the prominent feature and little accompanying regenerative bony change.

Signs of previous trauma or associated rotator cuff disease may be detected (Fig. 8.44). Indirect evidence of rotator cuff disease includes the presence of possible sources of impingement (e.g., the presence of ACJ OA with inferior acromial osteophytes), sclerosis, and cortical irregularity of the rotator cuff insertion on the greater tuberosity and superior migration of the humeral head. Caution is advised in the use of measurements of the width of the subacromial space in the assessment of rotator cuff disease. Estimates vary depending on the angle of the X-ray beam. Optimally the subacromial space is visualized with approximately 15° of caudal angulation of the beam. In such cases, the normal subacromial space should measure at least 8 mm in width. Generalized thinning of articular cartilage, in the presence of eburnation but scanty osteophytosis, should raise the possibility of secondary reparative OA, following a previous inflammatory arthropathy such as rheumatoid arthritis.

Hip

At the hip all the cardinal signs of OA may be represented. The variation in the pattern of radiographic abnormalities suggests that patients with OA of the hip form a heterogeneous group who may have different precipitating

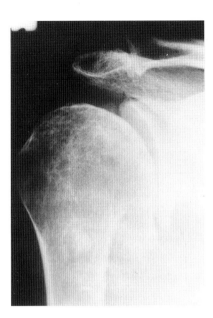

Fig. 8.43 A frontal view of the shoulder demonstrating OA of the glenohumeral joint. Note the prominent inferior head osteophyte and asymmetrical joint-space loss. There is also OA of the AC joint (narrowing plus osteophyte).

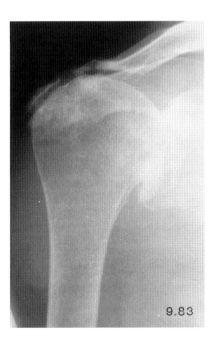

Fig. 8.44 OA of the shoulder, secondary to rotator cuff disease. Rupture of the cuff has allowed superior migration of the humeral head with subsequent pressure erosion of the acromium and lateral end of the clavicle.

factors. These radiographic patterns will be described without discussion of aetiology. Individual radiographic features of OA will be considered, with a discussion of some important points in differential diagnosis.

The hemispherical head of the femur articulates with the cup-shaped acetabulum in a ball and socket configuration. However, the articular cartilage of the acetabulum is horseshoe-shaped, rather than hemispherical, because of the presence of the acetabular notch. This deficiency, and the presence of acetabular anteversion, means that hyaline cartilage is distributed predominantly superolaterally and posteromedially (alternatively referred to as inferomedially). Thus, the pattern of joint-space narrowing in OA may vary depending on the precise location of focal hyaline cartilage loss. Such patterns are appreciated more easily early in the development of OA, classification often proving more difficult in established severe OA.

The most common site of joint-space narrowing is in the superior weight-bearing portion of the joint. Superolateral migration is the most common pattern in both sexes and is usually unilateral.[7] It incorporates superior joint-space narrowing and lateral migration of the femoral head, with accompanying widening of the posteromedial joint space. The associated features of OA such as cyst formation, osteophytosis, and sclerosis are predominantly superolateral. This pattern of migration is seen commonly in dysplastic hips (Fig. 8.45(a)). Superomedial migration is seen more commonly in women and is often bilateral (Fig. 8.45(b)). Superior joint-space narrowing occurs with resorption along the superolateral aspect of the femoral head, and osteophytosis along the femoral neck and medial/inferior aspect of the femoral head. This process results in apparent medial slipping of the femoral head.

Posteromedial migration (Fig. 8.45(c)) of the femoral head is usually bilateral and more common in women. It is difficult to explain selective joint-space narrowing in a zone of low stress—variations in acetabular design, increased varus angulation of the femoral neck, and association with generalized OA have been considered, but no definite answer exists. The radiographic appearances include narrowing of the posteromedial joint space, with associated preservation or widening of the lateral joint-space width. Lateral and medial osteophytosis may occur.

Axial migration includes features of the previously described patterns and results in concentric loss of hyaline cartilage (Fig. 8.45(d)). Associated features of OA are present and mild protrusio acetabuli may occur. It is less common than the other patterns of migration.

Florid osteophytosis is identified easily on routine images of the hip. However, even well established osteophytosis can be missed if insufficient attention is paid to analysing the radiograph. Concentric femoral head marginal osteophytes may be indicated by innocuous and easily overlooked zones of sclerosis. Acetabular osteophytes are seen along the posterior acetabular margin and can be made inconspicuous by the overlying femoral head. Central osteophytes are seen adjacent to the fovea on the femoral head and around the margin of the acetabular notch. Subchondral cyst formation in OA of the hip may be a more prominent feature than in other joints. Cysts may occur on both sides of the joint and can occur early in the disease process. Such cysts may be very large and are sometimes the earliest feature in the acetabular roof. Calcification may be seen in the acetabular labrum and may be associated with calcification of the symphysis pubis due to calcium pyrophosphate crystal deposition.

OA of the hip is routinely assessed using frontal views only; weight-bearing radiographs are not performed commonly. Lateral views may assist in detecting postero-inferior OA. If required, further details of the distribution of cartilage loss can be determined using MRI.

The differential diagnosis of OA in the older age group is usually not a problem. More careful consideration is required in premature OA, rapidly progressive disease, and when OA is secondary to previous inflammatory arthropathy or synovial disorder (see the section Considerations in the differential diagnosis of OA).

Knee

The knee is the largest joint that is affected most commonly by OA. It is a complex joint that endures considerable mechanical stresses. Many factors causing alteration in the mechanical forces acting through the knee can predispose to OA. The usual features of OA are demonstrated,[8] but the distribution of change may vary and can provide clues to the underlying cause.

The *tibio-femoral compartments* consist of medial and lateral joint spaces. OA predominantly targets the medial compartment (Fig. 8.46), though both may be involved and, occasionally, medial and lateral compartments may be affected equally. Osteophytosis is usually prominent and may be the

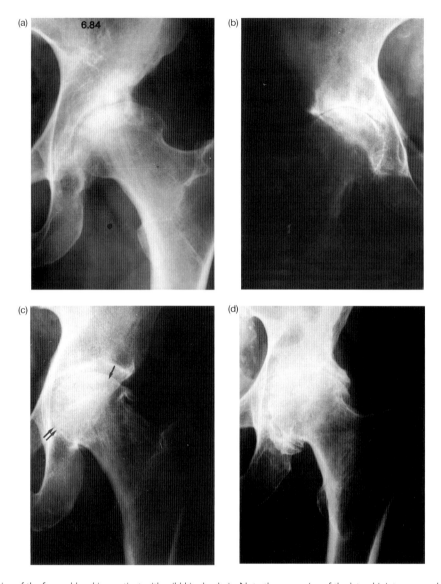

Fig. 8.45 (a) Lateral uncovering of the femoral head in a patient with mild hip dysplasia. Note the narrowing of the lateral joint space and subchondral cyst formation. (b) Typical changes of OA can be seen in the superior and medial aspects of the joint. There is almost a complete loss of hyaline cartilage with prominent acetabular cysts. (c) Posteromedial OA of the hip. Note the relative widening of the superolateral joint space (arrow), caused by the loss of posteromedial joint-space width (double arrow). (d) Concentric joint-space narrowing with florid osteophyte and a superimposed 'collar' of osteophyte around the femoral head.

earliest radiological sign of OA. Osteophytes are identified most easily at the articular margins of the tibia on the frontal view and along the margins of the femoral condyles on the lateral view. Central osteophytes arising from the mesial articular margins of the femoral condyles and the tibial spines are seen also. A prominent anterior intercondylar tibial bump may develop (Parson's third intercondylar spine; see Fig. 8.47).[9] On the frontal view osteophytes most commonly point outwards and upwards away from the joint line, except at the lateral tibial site where an upward direction is more characteristic (Figs 8.46 and 8.33).[10] Joint-space narrowing may be severe and can result in the direct apposition of femoral and tibial bone surfaces. Subchondral sclerosis and loss of hyaline cartilage occur concomitantly, with sclerosis usually more pronounced on the tibial aspect of the joint. Subchondral cysts are less common than in the hip and usually occur in the tibia rather than the femur.

The *patellofemoral compartment* is affected as commonly, if not more so, than the medial tibio-femoral compartment.[11] The patella possesses two articular facets, medial and lateral. The lateral facet is broader and is the most commonly affected by OA. This is related to the higher transmitted

forces arising from the valgus configuration of the normal knee. Joint-space narrowing, subchondral sclerosis, and osteophyte formation are the principal features (Fig. 8.48). Lateral subluxation of the patella is common. Joint-space narrowing may be difficult to judge on a lateral view, particularly when a joint effusion is present. Osteophytic lipping is identified readily at the upper and lower poles of the patella and occasionally is florid (Fig. 8.48). Eventually, bony apposition may occur between the patella and the anterior cortex of the lower femur. Anterior scalloping of the femur may ensue as a result of pressure erosion (Fig. 8.49).

Frequently, additional features of OA such as joint deformity and osteochondral body formation are seen in the knee. The fabellum possesses hyaline cartilage and articulates with the posterior surface of the lateral femoral condyle (Fig. 8.35). It may develop features of OA such as sclerosis and osteophyte formation, and may enlarge as a feature of OA.

Calcification is detected on knee radiographs with increasing frequency in older age. The most common site is in the menisci, where it may appear as rather globular, followed by the hyaline cartilage, where it usually has a linear distribution (Fig. 8.36). Such chondrocalcinosis principally results

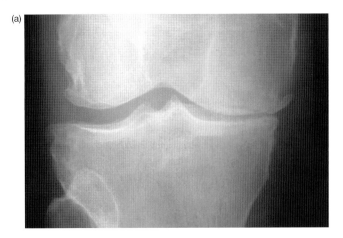

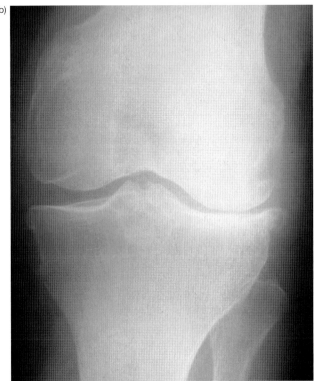

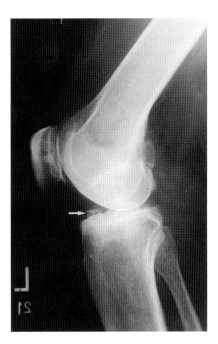

Fig. 8.47 Lateral view of knee showing Parson's bump (arrow).

Fig. 8.46 (a) Standing extended view of a right knee showing typical targeting of the medial tibiofemoral compartment with narrowing, sclerosis, and marginal osteophyte. The lateral compartment shows osteophyte only. (b) The same view of another knee showing less common predominant involvement of the lateral compartment, with marked narrowing, marginal osteophyte, and sclerosis.

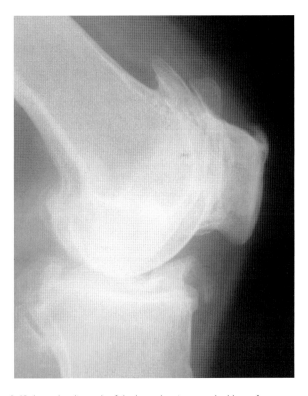

Fig. 8.48 Lateral radiograph of the knee showing a marked loss of patellofemoral joint-space width, and florid femoral and superior patellar osteophytes. An anterior enthesophyte is also evident at the quadriceps tendon insertion site. Posterior femoral osteophyte and anterior and posterior tibial osteophytes relating to the tibiofemoral joint are also clearly seen.

from calcium pyrophosphate crystal deposition. Less commonly, calcification may be noted in the synovium and ligamentous attachments.

The knee is anatomically and biomechanically complex. Consequently, the routine frontal and lateral views do not provide all the information required by clinicians for assessing disease severity and planning treatment. Specific specialized radiographic views have been developed to derive additional information.

Weight-bearing views

Routine radiographs of the knee are obtained with the patient lying on an X-ray table. Such radiographs may underestimate the extent of hyaline cartilage loss and the degree of angular deformity in the joint. Postero-anterior weight-bearing views allow the simultaneous imaging of both knees, and a more realistic assessment of lateral subluxation and varus/valgus deformity (Fig. 8.50). It has been estimated that weight-bearing views may result in an additional two to five millimetres of joint-space narrowing in affected tibiofemoral compartments.[12] Weight-bearing films in knee flexion demonstrate more narrowing than those in full extension, since the loading is then on the part of the joint that is principally targeted by cartilage loss. Rotation also influences the assessment of narrowing, and a well-positioned view for OA assessment shows the posterior and anterior borders of the tibial plateaus in close alignment and the tibial spines in the centre of the intercondylar notch. Lateral weight-bearing views are not usually performed because they are technically more difficult and add no useful additional information.

'Skyline' views

The X-ray beam passes through the patellofemoral joint from below, with the knee held in thirty degrees of flexion. This method affords an excellent assessment of patellofemoral joint space separately for both medial and lateral facets. Focal loss of hyaline cartilage, horizontal displacement of the patella, subchondral cysts, and marginal osteophytes are easily assessed (Fig. 8.51).

Tunnel views

Frontal radiographs acquired with the knee in flexion permit improved visualization of the intercondylar notch region. This view is rarely required, but may be advantageous in the evaluation of central osteophytes or in localizing possible loose osteochondral bodies.

Stress views

Joint laxity cannot be assessed on routine views. When the full extent of ligamentous laxity is required then manual stress applied during acquisition of the radiograph can provide an objective measure. In practice, these views are not requested often.

Load line views

The net vector of forces transmitted through the lower limb passes through the femoral head and the centre of the ankle mortise. The usual arrangement is for this line to intersect the knee in the intercondylar region. Abnormal skeletal design, in the form of developmental bone dysplasia or malunited fractures, may result in the excess transmission of forces to one of the tibiofemoral compartments and predispose to OA. Long-leg films, which include both legs from hip to ankle, allow the direct assessment of the load line (Fig. 8.52). This is particularly useful in the pre-operative assessment of angular deformity, prior to osteotomy or joint replacement.

Ankle

OA of the ankle is unusual in the absence of predisposing factors. The most common reason is a previous fracture, particularly if the ankle mortise is

Fig. 8.49 Lateral radiograph of the knee showing pressure erosion of the anterior surface of the lower femur in association with severe patellofemoral OA.

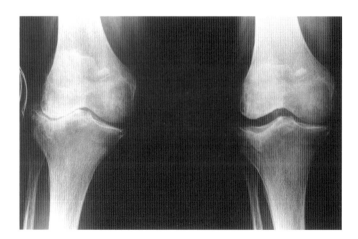

Fig. 8.50 Standing (left) and supine (right) views of the same knee with marked lateral tibiofemoral OA and valgus deformity. Note how the non weight-bearing view considerably underestimates both the degree of hyaline cartilage loss and the deformity.

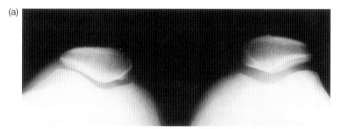
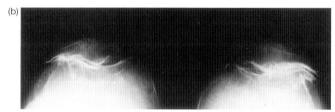

Fig. 8.51 Skyline view of the patellofemoral compartments. (a) Early lateral facet OA is demonstrated. (b) Advanced OA with complete joint-space loss, prominent grooving of the articular surfaces, and lateral patellar subluxation is evident.

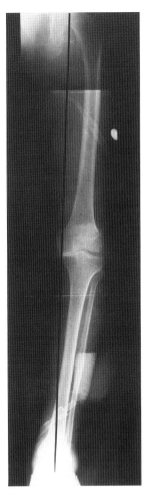

Fig. 8.52 A long-leg frontal radiograph shows the load line passing medial to the intercondylar region because of the varus deformity caused by medial compartment OA.

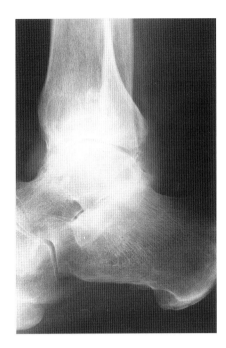

Fig. 8.53 Lateral radiograph showing severe OA of the ankle, with accompanying changes in the subtalar joint. The patient had suffered a previous ankle fracture.

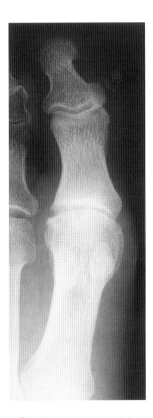

Fig. 8.54 First MTP joint OA, showing asymmetric joint-space narrowing, osteophytes, modest subchondral sclerosis, and small cysts.

involved. Abnormal biomechanics following subtalar fusion may result in secondary OA.

The typical features of OA are seen on ankle radiographs. Reduction in joint-space width may be diffuse rather than focal (Fig. 8.53). Joint-space narrowing is appreciated more easily on weight-bearing views but these are not performed routinely. Marginal osteophytes are readily recognized on frontal and lateral projections. Care must be taken not to mistake true osteophyte from capsular tug lesions and talar beaking seen in abnormal subtalar joint motion or with 'footballer's ankle'.

Great toe metatarsophalangeal joint

OA of the first metatarsophalangeal (1st MTP) joint is very common, perhaps reflecting the considerable mechanical forces transmitted through the joint during ambulation. OA at this site may occur in young people in their second or third decade. The reason for this is not clear but may be caused by unrecognized chondral or osteochondral trauma. In older patients, hallux valgus deformity, which may be associated with metatarsus primus varus, can result in OA.

Radiographic changes include joint-space narrowing, sclerosis, marginal osteophytosis, and valgus deformity (Fig. 8.54). Osteophytes are most prominent over the dorsal surface of the metatarsal head and are best demonstrated on a lateral standing view of the foot. Osteophytes are also seen around the margins of the sesamoid bones. Medial and lateral sesamoids articulate with the plantar surface of the first metatarsal head and are seen to good advantage on tangential views of the flexed forefoot. OA of sesamoids may be the principal source of pain under the toe, rather than the MTP joint itself. In addition, the sesamoids may show changes of avascular necrosis or chondromalacia.

Posterior facet joint osteoarthritis in the spine

Posterior facet joint OA becomes more frequent with increasing age and is associated commonly with intervertebral joint changes (narrowing, osteophyte, vacuum sign) though not invariably. Facet joint OA is seen often at levels different from the associated intervertebral changes. Other predisposing factors to facet joint OA include scoliosis and trauma. Facet joint configuration is variable between patients and at different levels in the spine. As a result, routine antero-posterior and lateral views visualize the joints with differing degrees of success, at different spinal levels. Facet joints are curved in space so that the X-ray beam is tangential to only a small portion of the joint in any single projection. In spite of these caveats, OA of the facet joints can be identified. Joint-space narrowing and osteophytosis may not be detected, but the accompanying sclerosis is evident usually, most commonly in the lower lumbar spine at L5/S1 (Fig. 8.55(a)). Optimal assessment of the facet joints requires computed tomography or MRI (Fig. 8.55(b)).

Patterns of osteoarthritis

OA is not a simple condition but shows considerable variation in the pattern of multiple joint involvement, the variable natural history of OA progression, and differences in the response of individual joints. Each of these factors will be considered in turn.

Patterns of joint involvement

Kellgren and Moore[13] described a particular pattern of joint involvement in primary generalized OA. Typically, in people with Heberden's nodes joints involved by OA, in addition to finger DIP joints, may include the finger proximal IP joints, the thumb CMC joint, the great toe MTP joint, the spinal apophyseal joints, and the knees. This pattern of primary nodal generalized OA is more common in middle-aged women. Subsequently, a non-nodal (that is, not associated with Heberden's nodes) type was described, favouring the involvement of wrists and hips in men.[14] It is generally accepted that subgroups of polyarticular forms of OA exist, although epidemiological studies do not all agree on the exact details of joint involvement and sex predilection.[15]

Another described variant of polyarticular OA is inflammatory or erosive OA.[16] This uncommon condition mainly afflicts middle-aged women. Usually onset is rapid, with clinical features of an inflammatory arthropathy involving the proximal and distal IP joints of the hands symmetrically, and the CMC joint of the thumb and ST articulation on the radial aspect of the hand. The radiological features include joint-space narrowing, sclerosis, and marginal osteophytes. In addition, however, subchondral erosive changes are seen, which characteristically involve the central portion of the joint at sites of hyaline cartilage thinning (Fig. 8.56). Periosteal new bone formation may accompany erosive change and, eventually, bony ankylosis can occur (Fig. 8.6). Following ankylosis, the proliferative bony response abates, and osteophytes and sclerosis may disappear. Characteristically, the end result is a joint with congruent undulating articular surfaces that create the 'seagull' sign. Such changes are seen most commonly in the distal IP joints. Other sites such as the MTP and IP joints of the feet, knees, hips, and spinal apophyseal joints may be symptomatic, but radiographic erosions at these sites are rare. The relationship of erosive to non-erosive OA is unclear. The remarkably similar pattern of joint involvement in the hand in both disorders, and variability in the degree of erosive change on radiographs, suggest that erosive OA represents one extreme of a continuum of joint response.[17]

A particular pattern of joint involvement is reported in patients with concurrent OA and chondrocalcinosis. In addition to OA of weight-bearing joints such as the knees and hips, OA may be seen more frequently in less commonly affected joints such as the radiocarpal, elbow, and glenohumeral articulations. Furthermore, there may be a tendency towards a 'hypertrophic' appearance (see below) with marked osteophyte formation, cysts, and osteochondral bodies.[18]

Natural history of disease progression

The natural history of OA varies considerably between different joints and different people. In general, most patients demonstrate slow radiographic progression with little change over many years. Disease progression tends to occur more rapidly in smaller joints, with the slowest rate of change observed in the knee. Disease activity may be episodic, with changes over

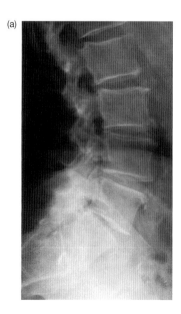
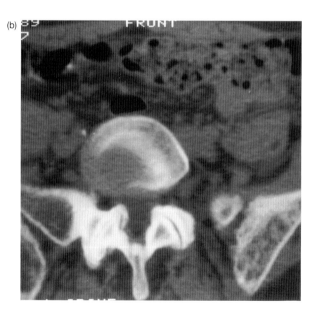

Fig. 8.55 Facet joint OA at the level of L5 S1 shown (a) on a lateral radiograph of the lumbar spine, and (b) using axial computed tomography, which demonstrates joint-space narrowing, sclerosis, and marginal osteophyte.

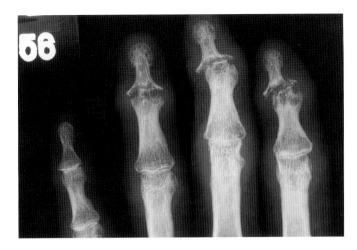

Fig. 8.56 Erosive OA in the DIP joints, showing prominent subchondral erosive changes in addition to the usual features of OA.

several months followed by a long period of stabilization during which no discernible radiographic progression may occur.

These observations hinder the use of radiographs for the quantitative assessment of disease activity. Kellgren and Lawrence[19] developed a grading system for OA that remains a standard reference for defining radiographic severity. Common to grading systems in other arthropathies, such as rheumatoid arthritis, these methods are insensitive to small changes in disease status. Furthermore, the divisions between disease stages are arbitrary. This is a particular problem in OA because disease progression may be very slow.

Variations in the response of individual joints

The degree of reparative response in OA joints varies between individuals; it may also vary within a particular individual at different times. This phenomenon has given rise to the concept of hypertrophic and atrophic forms of OA,[20] though in practice considerable overlap occurs and a spectrum of activity can be demonstrated. Hypertrophs mount a vigorous reparative response and exhibit florid osteophytosis (Figs 8.48 and 8.10), with marked sclerosis and frequent osteochondral body formation. An association with chondrocalcinosis and calcium pyrophosphate crystal deposition has been suggested.[18] Atrophs have poorly developed osteophytes and sclerosis (Figs 8.57 and 8.13). They may associate with joint effusions, often containing basic calcium phosphate crystals. Such individuals are usually elderly and female. This phenomenon reflects the variability in the response of joints to insult and contributes to the heterogeneity of the OA population. It complicates the radiographic assessment of disease activity at any one point in disease assessment.

Considerations in the differential diagnosis of osteoarthritis

Recognition of the typical features of OA on a radiograph should not signify completion of the diagnostic process. In most cases, a diagnosis of primary OA will be correct. However, consideration should be given to the available clinical and radiographic clues, so that secondary OA and coexistent medical conditions are not overlooked. This approach will be illustrated in the following scenarios.

Premature osteoarthritis

Premature OA may be defined arbitrarily as occurring before 55 years of age. This may occur without any discernible predisposing factors. Monoarticular OA in a young adult is usually explained by a preceding traumatic injury. Often this is present in the history, and evidence of previous fracture,

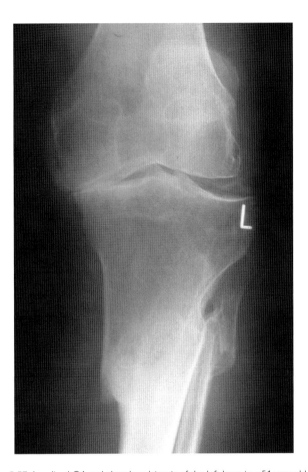

Fig. 8.57 Localized OA and chondrocalcinosis of the left knee in a 51-year-old man, secondary to a previous tibial fracture. There is marked narrowing and sclerosis of the medial tibiofemoral compartment, lateral compartment fibrocartilage calcification, lateral patellar subluxation, and the old tibial fracture that has healed with malalignment.

surgery, or osteochondritis dissecans may be visible on the radiograph (Fig. 8.57). Modelling deformities may indicate previous insults such as slipped femoral capital epiphysis or Perthe's disease in the hip.

Early OA involving several or multiple joints should lead to the consideration of developmental disorders such as multiple epiphyseal dysplasia, or an endocrine disorder such as acromegaly. It is easy to overlook mild dysplastic change (see Fig. 8.45(a)). The presence of chondrocalcinosis in the setting of premature OA particularly suggests the possibility of hemochromatosis.

Secondary reparative osteoarthritis

Osteopenia and diffuse loss of joint-space width, coexisting with other typical features of OA, should raise the possibility of secondary osteoarthritic change following a previous inflammatory arthropathy such as rheumatoid or septic arthritis (Fig. 8.58). The reparative features of OA may be so florid as to obscure evidence of a pre-existing articular disorder; this may occur in gouty arthritis and hemophilia. Both conditions produce geodes that may be confused with subarticular cysts associated with OA.

Rapidly progressive osteoarthritis

Rapidly progressive OA of the hip can occur in elderly patients after a prolonged period of stabilization and without any obvious precipitating cause (Fig. 8.59). However, this event is infrequent and warrants serious consideration of other disorders such as avascular necrosis of the femoral head, occult infection, or neuroarthropathy. Radiographic evidence of avascular necrosis may be present, such as flattening and poor definition of the cortex

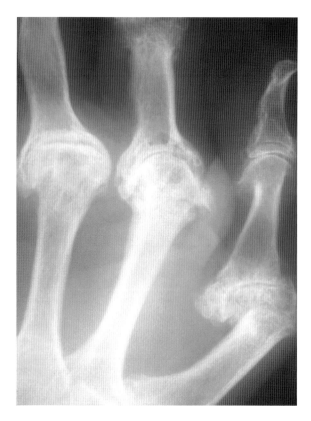

Fig. 8.58 Hand radiograph showing predominantly 'OA' changes (narrowing, osteophyte, remodelling, and cysts) in a patient with long-standing rheumatoid arthritis. The bone remodelling and osteophyte, obscure the preceding marginal erosive change, but the widespread and uniform cartilage loss is the clue to inflammatory arthropathy as the primary diagnosis.

of the sclerosed femoral head, which should shift clinical attention to include investigation of other asymptomatic joints that are at risk. Chondrocalcinosis in the hip joint, or symphysis, may suggest crystal-associated arthropathy. Joint infection in the elderly may be indolent, and the usual features of an aggressive inflammatory disorder such as intense osteopenia and erosions may be absent.

Severe pain

Severe pain in a joint with radiographic features of OA should stimulate a search for complications or alternative diagnoses. A rare complication of knee OA is osteonecrosis of the medial femoral condyle, which may represent avascular necrosis or subchondral trabecular fractures with secondary collapse in stressed or osteopenic bone. Initial radiographs may be normal or show subtle subchondral lucency with ill definition of the cortical margin. Substantial bony collapse may ensue. The presence of a large joint effusion should raise the possibility of infection or acute crystal shedding such

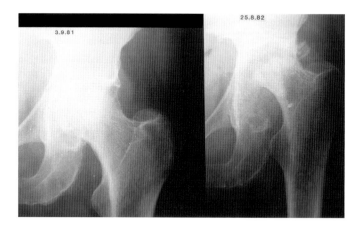

Fig. 8.59 Rapid destruction of the hip joint in an elderly lady, over just a 12-month period.

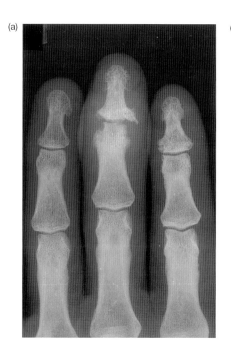

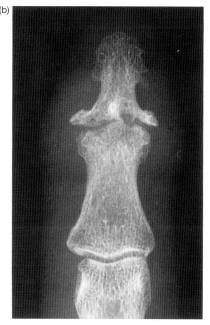

Fig. 8.60 (a) A radiograph of a patient with psoriatic arthritis, showing marginal erosions of the 'bare' areas and associated fluffy new bone ('proliferative marginal erosion'). (b) A radiograph of a patient with erosive OA demonstrating central erosion of hyaline cartilage.

as pseudogout. Severe pain in the hands of elderly patients with nodal OA of the IP joints should raise the possibility of superimposed gout secondary to chronic diuretic therapy. Radiographic clues include the presence of soft tissue tophi, erosions, and florid osteophytosis in addition to the usual features of OA.

Erosive change

The presence of erosions alongside features of OA in the hands may cause confusion with other erosive arthropathies. In fact, the characteristic symmetrical DIP distribution, coupled with the presence of central rather than marginal erosive change, means that erosive OA is readily distinguished from other erosive arthropathies such as rheumatoid arthritis and psoriasis (Fig. 8.60).[21] It should not be forgotten that radiological features of specific arthropathies may take time to develop. There may be clinical pointers to rheumatoid arthritis or gout in patients with OA, and such patients may present prior to the development of characteristic X-ray changes.

Summary

The plain radiograph remains the dominant imaging modality in the diagnosis and assessment of OA. The basic features of OA have been described, along with specific findings in individual joints. The radiographic features amount to a history of the response of the joint to previous insults. Different patterns of disease, involvement of different joint compartments, and variation in the rate of disease progression testify to the heterogeneity of this disorder.

Key clinical points

1. The key radiographic features of osteoarthritis are: focal joint-space narrowing, marginal and central osteophyte, subchondral sclerosis, cysts, osteochondral bodies.

2. These individual features lack specificity and show wide variability in terms of magnitude and rate of change.

3. The plain radiograph is helpful in confirming the clinical diagnosis of OA, assessing severity of structural change and identifying associated chondrocalcinosis, but for determining symptom causation it is no substitute for a thorough clinical assessment.

References

1. Resnick, D. (1995). *Diagnosis of bone and joint disorders* (3rd ed.), Philadelphia: W.B. Saunders, pp. 1263–371.

2. Buckland-Wright, J.C. (1994). Quantitative radiography of osteoarthritis. *Ann Rheum Dis* **53**:268–75.

3. Buckland-Wright, J.C., Macfarlane, D.G., and Lynch, J. (1992). Relationship between joint space width and subchondral sclerosis in the osteoarthritic hand: a quantitative microfocal radiographic study. *J Rheumatol* **19**:788–95.

4. Thompson, R.C. and Bassett, R.C. (1970). Histological observations on experimentally induced degeneration of articular cartilage. *J Bone Joint Surg Am* **52**:435–43.

5. Jones, A.C., Chuck, A.J., Arie, E.A., Green, D.J., and Doherty, M. (1992). Diseases associated with calcium pyrophosphate deposition disease. *Sem Arthritis Rheum* **22**:188–202.

6. Doherty, M. and Preston, B. (1989). Primary osteoarthritis of the elbow. *Ann Rheum Dis* **48**:743–7.

7. Ledingham, J., Dawson, S., Milligan, G., and Doherty, M. (1992). Radiographic patterns and associations of osteoarthritis of the hip. *Ann Rheum Dis* **51**:1111–16.

8. Boegard, T. and Jonsson, K. (1999). Radiography in osteoarthritis of the knee. *Skeletal Radiography* **28**:605–15.

9. Brossman, J., White, L.M., Stabler, A., Preidler, K.W., Andresen, R., Haghighi, P., *et al.* (1996). Enlargement of the third intercondylar tubercle of Parsons as a sign of osteoarthritis of the knee—a paleopathologic and radiographic study. *Radiology* **198**:845–9.

10. Nagaosa, Y., Lanyon, P., and Doherty, M. (2002). Size and direction of osteophyte in knee osteoarthritis: a radiographic study. *Ann Rheum Dis* **61**:319–24.

11. Ledingham, J., Regan, M., Jones, A., and Doherty, M. (1993). Radiographic patterns and associations of osteoarthritis of the knee in patients referred to hospital. *Ann Rheum Dis* **52**:520–6.

12. Leach, R.E., Gregg, T., and Siber, F.J. (1970). Weight bearing radiography in osteoarthritis of the knee. *Radiology* **97**:265–8.

13. Kellgren, J.H. and Moore, R. (1952). Generalised osteoarthritis and Heberden's nodes. *Br Med J* **1**:181–7.

14. Kellgren, J.H., Lawrence, J.S., and Bier, F. (1963). Genetic factors in generalised osteoarthritis. *Ann Rheum Dis* **22**:237–54.

15. Buchanon, W.W. and Park, W.M. (1983). Primary generalised osteoarthritis: definition and uniformity. *J Rheumatol* **10**(Suppl. 9):4.

16. Crain, D.C. (1961). Interphalangeal osteoarthritis characterised by painful inflammatory episodes resulting in deformity of the proximal and distal articulations. *JAMA* **175**:1049–53.

17. Cobby, M., Cushnaghan, J., Creamer, P., Dieppe, P.A., and Watt, I. (1990). Erosive osteoarthritis: is it a separate disease entity? *Clin Radiol* **42**:258–63.

18. Doherty, M. and Dieppe, P.A. (1988). Clinical aspects of calcium pyrophosphate dihydrate crystal deposition. *Rheum Dis Clin North Am* **14**(2):395–414.

19. Kellgren, J.H. and Lawrence, J.S. (1957). Radiological assessment of osteoarthritis. *Ann Rheum Dis* **16**:494–501.

20. Solomon, L. (1983). Osteoarthritis, local and generalised: a uniform disease? *J Rheumatol* **10**(Suppl. 9):13–15.

21. Martel, W., Stuck, K.J., Dworin, A.M., and Hylland, R.G. (1980). Erosive osteoarthritis and psoriatic arthritis: a radiologic comparison in the hand, wrist and foot. *Am J Roentgenol* **134**:125–35.

8.3 The natural history and prognosis of osteoarthritis

Elaine Dennison and Cyrus Cooper

Osteoarthritis, the most frequent joint disorder in the world today, represents a complex disease process in which a combination of systemic and local mechanisms result in characteristic pathological and radiological changes. These abnormalities are often, but not always, associated with symptoms and disability. OA has been recognized in all human populations, which have been examined to date, and can be found in skeletal remains from Neolithic times.[1] Archaeological studies also suggest that the relative frequencies of OA within and between ethnic groups at certain joint sites have changed over time.[2] However, our understanding of the aetiology, clinical features, and natural history of OA remains incomplete. This chapter reviews three aspects of the disorder: (1) approaches to definition; (2) measurement of OA and descriptive epidemiological characteristics of the disorder; and (3) the rate and determinants of progression.

Definition

Earlier this century, pathologists differentiated between two broad groups of arthritis: atrophic and hypertrophic. Atrophic disorders were characterized by synovial inflammation with erosion of cartilage and bone, and came to include rheumatoid and septic arthritis. The hypertrophic group were never subdivided, however, and gradually became synonymous with what is now termed OA. The term thus encompasses a large and heterogeneous spectrum of idiopathic joint disorders.

Techniques for the assessment of osteoarthritis

Clinical assessment

The major symptoms of OA in a joint are:

- use-related pain,
- stiffness, and
- loss of movement.

Major signs are:

- bony swelling,
- crepitus,
- joint margin tenderness,
- cool effusion,
- decreased range of movement, and
- instability.

Pain is undoubtedly the most important symptom; it tends to be use-related and associated with stiffness after inactivity. There is a documented discrepancy between radiographic grade and reporting of pain, and this relationship is influenced by gender and joint site. In the earliest epidemiological studies, women were more likely to report pain than men, and the concordance between pain and radiographic damage was strongest for the hip and weakest for the hand. With more sophisticated methods of assessing OA, it became clear that there is a gradation between the severity of radiographic disease and the prevalence of symptoms in a given joint. There are a number of potential mechanisms for pain in OA, including raised intraosseous pressure, inflammatory synovitis, periarticular problems, periosteal elevation, muscle changes, and central neurogenic changes.

Among the clinical signs of OA, bony swelling of the affected joint and crepitus are highly repeatable[3] and discriminatory between OA and other joint disorders. The usefulness of other signs, for example, soft tissue swelling, instability, and joint margin tenderness in the diagnosis and monitoring of OA currently remains uncertain. Assessment of clinical outcome in the disorder has been the subject of intensive research in the last decade. The properties of outcome measurement instruments in OA are important in determining the most appropriate methodology for studies; reliability, validity, and responsiveness to change are the three key criteria. The World Health Organisation currently recommend the use of either the Western Ontario and MacMaster Universities (WOMAC) OA index or the Lequesne algofunctional index for the monitoring of hip or knee OA. These indices are statistically more efficient than a multiplicity of unidimensional measures, and appear to detect changes in pain and physical function with greater sensitivity than either the Stamford Health Assessment Questionnaire or Arthritis Impact Measurement Scales. The Lequesne index includes assessment of pain, stiffness, walking distance, and daily-living activities for the hip and knee. Both the disease-specific instruments may be supplemented by generic health status measures, most widely used of which are the shortform 36 (SF-36), the Nottingham Health Profile, and Euroquol.

Radiographic assessment of osteoarthritis

The radiographic features currently used to assess OA were originally selected to measure various aspects of cartilage loss and subchondral bone reaction. Although several radiographic grading systems have been proposed over the last 15 years, most epidemiological studies have utilized the Empire Rheumatism Council system, first described over four decades ago.[4]

The age- and sex-specific prevalence of OA, the individual risk factors for the disorder, and the relationship between radiographic change and symptoms are all known to differ according to joint site, supporting the notion that any radiographic grading system for OA should be joint specific. However, inconsistencies in the descriptions of radiographic features of OA by Kellgren and Lawrence themselves, have led to studies being performed using criteria which are discordant.[5] Also, the prominence awarded to the osteophyte at all joint sites remains controversial. To address these issues, recent studies have broken up this overall radiographic grading system into its component features, quantified each feature more precisely, and assessed the reproducibility and clinical correlates of each.

For the knee, each of joint-space narrowing, osteophyte, and the overall Kellgren and Lawrence grade showed good within-observer reproducibility, but the scoring of osteophyte was most closely associated with knee pain.[6] At the hip, comparison of joint-space narrowing, osteophyte, sclerosis, and an overall grading system suggested that measurement of joint space was more reproducible than that of osteophyte, sclerosis, or the composite score, and was the most closely associated with reported hip pain.[7] Finally, in the hand, joint-space narrowing, osteophyte, and overall Kellgren/Lawrence grade can all be assessed reproducibly, but osteophyte appears to be more closely associated with pain.[8] Although these findings require confirmation by future studies, it is clear that a need exists for a standardized approach to the categorization of individual radiographic features at these different joint sites. Recent atlases of standard radiographs have helped in ensuring a more consistent approach to the grading of individual features and permit greater extrapolation between the results of different studies.

Radiographic measures also remain a cornerstone in the assessment of the progression of OA. A consensus meeting of the American Academy of Orthopedic Surgeons, the National Institutes of Health, and the World Health Organisation has produced recommendations for the use of radiographic measures for this purpose.[9] Careful attention must be paid to patient positioning and to inclusion of views that permit assessment of different compartments of a joint. Thus, assessment of the knee requires a weight-bearing view in the anteroposterior projection, as well as views to include the patellofemoral compartment (skyline views are superior to supine lateral in the assessment of progression of OA.[10]) For the hip joint, progression should be recorded for joint-space narrowing, both by millimetre measurements of the interbone distance and by visual grading (0–3 according to a standardized atlas). Grading appears to be influenced by the reading procedure, with higher repeatability scores obtained for paired radiographs with landmarks for joint-space width in longitudinal studies.[11] Femoral osteophytes are graded 0–3 and features such as subchondral bone cysts, sclerosis, attrition, and migration pattern can be recorded as present or absent. Radiographic features of knee disease should be recorded separately for the medial, lateral, and patellofemoral compartments. As with the hip, the narrowest point of the tibiofemoral joint space can be measured in millimetres, and both joint-space narrowing and osteophyte can be graded 0–3 in all compartments. Although advanced techniques can be used to assist assessment of the radiographs, for example, digitization of the images with computerized methods for the assessment of interbone distance or osteophyte, these techniques remain research tools and have not yet superseded radiographic assessment by eye.

Other techniques for assessing natural history

Other investigative modalities that may be of assistance in characterizing the natural history of OA, remain essentially research tools the use of which in routine clinical practice remains to be validated.

Radionuclide scintigraphy

Isotope scintigraphy using bone-seeking radionuclides such as 99 m technetium labelled methylene or hydroxymethylene diphosphonate (HDP) is a sensitive means of assessing physiological change in bone and synovium. The main role of scintigraphy in OA is to distinguish the activity of different types of process in a joint,[12] perhaps detecting change before it becomes apparent on plain radiographs.[13] This predictive capacity has been demonstrated in studies of hand OA in which the bone scan may be active before radiographic change occurs and often reverts to normal at a time when well-marked osteophytes are present, implying an altered, inactive state of the joint.[14] Such studies have also shown that hand OA is a phasic phenomenon in which each joint follows its own course.

Scintigraphic studies of knee OA have pointed to the heterogeneity of this disorder.[12] In the tibiofemoral joint, different categories of abnormality have been detected (e.g., a generalized pattern that correlates well with pain and function, and which can be suppressed by intra-articular corticosteroid injection). Other patterns include tramline activity along the joint margin, which is reported to correlate with subchondral bone sclerosis, and an extended pattern which appears to be a marker of severe disease.

Magnetic resonance imaging

Magnetic resonance imaging (MRI) provides high-contrast soft tissue images, which can be produced in any spatial plane. Despite the advantages of high resolution and this ability to produce images in any desired plane, MRI is costly and relatively unavailable. Initial studies of MRI in OA have concentrated on the anatomic features of the disorder.[15,16] These studies have highlighted a number of occult pathologies in joints that were otherwise thought to have simple OA, for example, meniscal damage and local osteochondral defects in the knee. MRI has been correlated with scintigraphic findings in the knee, and has been used in animals to visualize acute changes in cartilage. In addition, it is the investigation of choice in evaluating osteonecrosis, bony infection, periarticular pathology, and some forms of algodystrophy.

Biochemical markers

There is continual turnover of the components of healthy cartilage, with increased synthesis and degradation occurring in disorders such as OA. Some of the products of this turnover can be detected in various body fluids. Recent work in OA patients has demonstrated that candidate markers include molecules present especially during cartilage matrix synthesis and degradation, such as type II collagen degradation products and synthesis (c-propeptide) markers; cartilage oligomeric matrix protein; and two epitopes of aggrecan (a large macromolecule within cartilage): the 846 epitope (probably a synthetic marker) and keratan sulphate. In patients with accelerated disease progression, serum levels of cartilage oligomeric protein and hyaluronic acid are often elevated, perhaps reflecting the presence of synovitis in these patients. Despite increasing interest in biochemical marker assays, at present none of the available markers can be specifically recommended as providing a measure of disease progression.

Epidemiology of osteoarthritis
Prevalence of osteoarthritis

Most of the currently available information on the epidemiology of OA comes from population-based radiographic surveys. Initially, attention was focused on OA of the hand joints, or on generalized (polyarticular) OA. More recent studies from Europe and the United States of America classify rates for individual joints and permit comparison between them.

The prevalence of radiographic OA rises steeply with age at all joint sites. In a survey of 6585 inhabitants randomly selected from the population of a Dutch village,[17] 75 per cent of women aged 65–70 years had OA of their distal interphalangeal (DIP) joints. Despite the predilection for older age groups, it should be noted that even by 40 years of age 10–20 per cent of subjects had evidence of severe radiographic disease affecting their hands or feet. Knee disease appeared less frequently than hand and foot involvement. Population-based studies in the United States of America suggest comparable prevalence rates to those in Europe, rising from less than 1 per cent among people aged 25–34, to 30 per cent in those 75 years and above.[18] Both hand and knee disease appear to be more frequent in women than in men, although the female to male ratio varies among studies between 1.5 and over 4.0. Hip OA is less common than knee OA, and prevalence rates in men and women appear more similar. Some, but not all, studies have reported a male preponderance at this site. Fig. 8.61 shows the incidence of symptomatic hand, hip, and knee OA obtained from the Fallon Community Health Plan, a health maintenance organization located in the north-east of the United States of America.

Although OA is worldwide in its distribution, geographic differences in prevalence have been reported.[19] These are often difficult to interpret because of differences in sampling procedure and radiographic consistency. European and American data do not appear to differ markedly for hand and knee disease. However, hand involvement appears to be particularly frequent in Pima and Blackfoot Indian populations within the United States of America. Greater variation has been found in the distribution of hip OA, with low rates reported among the African Negroes, Asian Indians, Hong Kong Chinese, and Japanese.

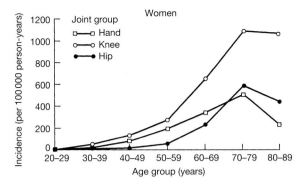

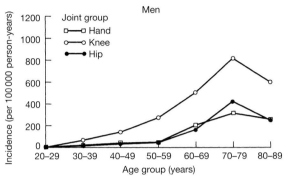

Fig. 8.61 Incidence of hand, hip, and knee OA with advancing age; data derived from Oliveria et al.[50]

Table 8.7 Epidemiological studies of incidence of OA

Study	Site	Sex	Incidence rates (per 100 000)
Wilson et al.[21]	Hip OA	M + F	47.3
	Knee OA	M + F	163.8
Kallman et al.[22]	Hand OA	M	100
Oliveria et al.[50]	Hip OA	M + F	88
	Knee OA	M + F	240
	Hand OA	M + F	100

Table 8.8 Clustering of hand joint involvement in OA among perimenopausal women

	Radiographic definition of OA	
	Grade 2 + OR	Grade 3 + OR
DIP-DIP (row)	5.0	10.0
PIP-PIP (row)	3.7	3.1
DIP-PIP (ray)	3.7	5.9
CMC-IP	1.4	1.3

The odds ratios indicate the hierarchies of association between different joint groups in OA.

DIP, distal interphalangeal; PIP, proximal interphalangeal; IP, interphalangeal; CMC, carpometacarpal (1st).

Source: Derived from Egger et al.[49]

Incidence of osteoarthritis

Table 8.7 summarizes the epidemiological studies of the incidence of OA. OA of the knee may affect the medial or lateral tibiofemoral joints, or the patellofemoral joint, or each of these areas in combination. However, isolated medial compartment, or medial plus patellofemoral disease, are the most common combinations. Different anatomically recognized subsets of hip OA also occur, and may be classified by the pattern of cartilage loss apparent on hip radiography. The most frequent pattern (superolateral) occurs in some 60 per cent of patients with hip OA, while medial and concentric cartilage loss, occur in 25 and 15 per cent of patients, respectively. The natural history of hip OA is very variable; many cases that come to surgery have a relatively short history of severe symptoms, suggesting that a progressive phase lasting between three months and three years may often precede the advanced stages of OA.

OA principally affects the DIP, proximal interphalangeal (PIP), and thumb base in the hand. Detailed studies of the distribution of hand joint involvement have been performed. Recent epidemiological data suggest that clinical and radiographic changes in hand OA are concordant in individuals, and that definition is best achieved by a combination of both measures. The evolution of hand OA is usually complete after a period of a few years; it has been studied both clinically and radiographically. Imaging studies show this evolution of change to be accompanied by sequential changes in joint anatomy and physiology. Table 8.8 illustrates the clustering of hand joint involvement that is often seen in perimenopausal women.

Progression of osteoarthritis

Disease evolution in knee OA is slow, usually taking many years. However, there is evidence that once established, the condition can remain relatively stable, both clinically and radiologically, for a further period of several years. The correlation between the clinical outcome of knee OA and its radiographic course is not strong. In a large study, Dougados et al.[23] demonstrated that although radiographic improvement was rare, overall clinical improvement at 1-year follow up was common. Longer-term studies confirmed that radiographic deterioration occurs in one- to two-thirds of patients, and that radiographic improvement is unusual (Table 8.9). A Swedish study documented that among patients with structural change, for example, tibial or femoral sclerosis, the majority experienced radiographic and symptomatic deterioration over 15 years.[24,25] Of those subjects with only osteophyte on baseline radiography, a much smaller proportion suffered deterioration. This is broadly in accord with the American College of Rheumatology Study,[26] in which joint-space narrowing was judged to be a more important determinant of progression in knee OA than was the presence of osteophyte. However, when variables were considered in combination, this study reported that a score based on joint-space narrowing, osteophyte, and sclerosis was reasonably reproducible and the best predictor of progression.

Recent British studies have also examined the progression of knee OA, both among subjects attending hospital outpatient departments and in the general population. In an 11-year follow-up study of 63 subjects who had baseline knee radiographs, the majority of knees did not show a worsening of overall grade of OA, with only 33 per cent deteriorating in Kellgren and Lawrence score over the time period.[27] When a more sensitive global scoring system was used on paired films, the proportion showing a slight deterioration increased to 50 per cent, and 10 per cent showed improvement—the latter estimate is within the limits allowed for by imprecision in radiographic grading. The visual analogue pain scores remained stable over the time period, but it was reported that those with knee pain at baseline had a greater chance of progressing, as did those with existing OA in the contralateral knee. A similar follow-up study was performed in 58 women aged 45–64, from the general population, in whom unilateral knee OA (Kellgren and Lawrence grade 2 plus) had been assigned at baseline.[28] Follow-up radiographs at 24 months revealed that 34 per cent of the women developed disease in the contralateral knee and that 22 per cent progressed radiologically in the index joint.

Table 8.10 shows the change in the radiographic score of knee OA during a 5-year follow-up period in 354 British men and women, aged 55 years

Table 8.9 Studies of the natural history of knee OA

Study		No. of subjects	Measure	Follow up (yrs)	Deterioration %
Hernborg and Nilsson[24]	1977	84 knees	C	15	55
			R	15	56
Danielsson and Hernborg[25]	1970	106 knees	R	15	33
Massardo et al.[51]	1989	31	R	8	62
Dougados et al.[23]	1992	353	C	1	28
			R	1	29
Schouten et al.[20]	1992	142	R	12	34
Spector et al.[27]	1992	63	R	11	33
Spector et al.[41]	1994	58	R	2	22
Ledingham et al.[52]	1995	350 knees	R	2	72
McAlindon[39]	1999	470	R	4	11*
Cooper et al.[46]	2000	354	R	5	22

C, clinical; R, radiographic.

* Incident OA.

Table 8.10 Change in radiographic score of knee osteoarthritis during 5-year follow up in 354 men and women aged 55 years or over*

Baseline K/L score	Follow up K/L score					
	0	1	2	3	4	All
0	148	14	16	—	—	178
1	3	32	27	2	—	64
2	—	—	59	16	1	76
3	—	—	—	28	3	31
4	—	—	—	—	5	5
All	151	46	102	46	9	354

* The analysis was based on the worst-affected knee at baseline and follow up.

Source: Reproduced with permission from Cooper et al.[46]

or over, who participated in a longitudinal study conducted by Cooper et al. Rates of incidence and progression were 2.5 and 3.6 per cent per year, respectively, in this study. Despite these studies, several questions remain about the natural history of knee OA. Some studies have excluded from follow-up, subjects whose symptoms were severe enough that they needed surgery. In other studies, many of the patients initially seen were subsequently lost for follow-up. This loss could have occurred because the patients had surgery, or because their knee symptoms had remitted.

There are fewer prospective studies of hip OA than of knee OA (Table 8.11). In a Danish follow-up study of 121 hips, over three decades ago, the majority (65 per cent) showed radiographic deterioration over a 10-year follow-up period.[29] Symptomatic improvement occurred (surprisingly) in the majority of patients in contrast to another longitudinal study that documented frequent deterioration in the clinical course of hip OA patients.[30] In a Dutch study of patients identified from the general population who had established OA in one or both hips, 29 per cent of the subjects showed a worsening of their radiographic scores over a 12-year follow-up period.[31] Nonetheless, unlike knee OA, a few patients with hip OA can experience clear-cut radiological and symptomatic recovery.[32,33] This appears to occur most often among patients who have marked osteophytosis and in those with concentric disease. Osteonecrosis is the major complication of hip OA and tends to occur late in the natural history. Rapidly progressive OA can lead to an unusual appearance with extensive bone destruction and a wide interbone distance. This appearance was initially observed among patients who ingested anti-inflammatory drugs and was termed 'analgesic hip'.[34] However, it is now recognized to also occur in groups of subjects who ingest few or no such agents.[35]

Kallman et al. reported that among men with DIP joint OA, more than 50 per cent experienced progression of radiographic disease over 10 years.[22] The progression was fastest in the DIP joints, and was slower in PIP joints and the thumb base. The presence of narrowing at baseline increased the risk that subjects would develop subsequent osteophytes, and joints with severe radiographic changes at baseline had slower progression rates than joints with milder radiographic changes. The rate of OA progression in individual subjects paralleled the rate of progression hinted at by cross-sectional studies, in which subjects are studied at different ages. The mechanisms implicated in controlling the timing of individual joint involvement remain unknown.

Similarly, Harris et al.[36] reported a study of 59 subjects with paired hand radiographs over a 10-year period. Radiographs were scored in three areas: DIP, PIP and carpometacarpal (CMC) joints using the methods of Kellgren and Lawrence and for osteophytes and narrowing. Virtually all subjects (97 per cent) deteriorated when the total scores of all joints were calculated, with new osteophytes appearing in 48 per cent of DIP joints over the follow-up period.

Determinants of progression in osteoarthritis

Just as the natural history of OA differs at different joint sites, the factors that contribute to disease progression appear to be joint specific. These determinants have been less well studied than the risk factors for prevalent disease. However, Table 8.12 summarizes the known determinants of progression at the knee and hip.

At both sites, multiple joint involvement appears to be a determinant of accelerated disease. For example, patients who sustained joint-space narrowing in the knee over a 1-year follow-up period had a larger number of joints throughout the body affected by OA than did those who experienced no joint-space narrowing.[23] Spector et al. reported that knee OA progression was more frequent in those with bilateral knee OA than in those with unilateral involvement.[27] This influence of multiple involvement extends from the knee to other joint sites. In a study of 142 subjects with baseline radiographs of the knee, Schouten et al.[20] found that a diagnosis of generalized OA (through the presence of Heberden's nodes) increased the likelihood of progressive cartilage loss in the knee by threefold. This increase in risk persisted after statistical adjustment for age, gender, and body mass index (BMI). The coexistence of Heberden's nodes with knee OA, increased the risk of knee deterioration by almost sixfold. Likewise, Doherty et al.[37] found that among patients who had undergone unilateral meniscectomy

Table 8.11 Studies of the natural history of hip OA

Study		No. of subjects	Measure	Follow up (yrs)	Deterioration %
Danielsson[29]	1964	121 hips	C	10.0	19
			R	10.0	65
Seifert et al.[30]	1969	83 hips	C	5.0	83
Van Saase[31]	1990	86	R	12.0	29
Ledingham et al.[53]	1993	136	C	2.3	66
			R	2.3	47

Table 8.12 Determinants of progression of hip and knee OA

	Strength of association	
	Knee	Hip
Generalized OA diathesis	++	+
Obesity	++	+
Joint injury	++	+
Crystal deposition	+	
Neuromuscular dysfunction	+	
Knee alignment	++	
Physical activity	++	++

previously, the presence of radiographic hand OA markedly increased the risk of developing incident knee disease. The explanation for this tendency of generalized OA to increase the rate of progression is not clear—candidates include crystal deposition, and a generalized hormonal or metabolic diathesis. Some studies have suggested that the presence of crystals in association with OA at baseline, increases the risk of progressive disease.[37] Thus, in one study,[38] 10 subjects with rapidly progressive OA were, over 1 year, compared with 84 subjects with more slowly progressive OA. The prevalence of synovial fluid crystals (hydroxyapatite or calcium pyrophosphate) was substantially higher in those with progressive disease. However, other epidemiological studies[23,20] have failed to document chondrocalcinosis as a risk factor for progression of disease, although the relatively small number of subjects with coexistent knee OA and chondrocalcinosis at baseline has limited the power of these investigations.

Another factor consistently associated with progression of OA is obesity. Several longitudinal studies[23,28,37,40–43] have reported that obese patients are more likely to experience progressive disease than non-obese patients. The evidence that weight loss slows progression of disease is less clear-cut. In the Dutch population study,[20] weight loss did not appear to slow progression. These findings contrast with the data from a clinical study of obese patients who underwent rapid weight loss, and an US epidemiological study, both of which pointed to an improvement in joint symptoms. Obesity has also been documented as a risk factor for progression in hip OA.[43]

Varus or valgus knee alignment acts to increase medial or lateral load through the knee joint, respectively, and increases the risk of disease progression four- to fivefold.[44] Similarly, joint injury, muscle weakness, and joint instability have also been demonstrated to be determinants of disease progression. Disruption of the neurological input from structures around the joint (at its most extreme a 'Charcot joint') also appears important in predisposing to accelerated damage.

Physical activity has been associated with OA in many studies. Coggon et al. reported a case-control study utilizing patients waiting for hip replacement, to study associations with lifting and other occupational activities.[42] After adjustment for potential confounders, the risk in men increased progressively with the duration and heaviness of occupational lifting. In another

case-control study reported from Hong Kong,[40] lifting heavy weights or climbing 15 flights of stairs each day were associated with increased risk of hip OA in both sexes, while women who performed gymnastics regularly were at a sixfold increased risk of hip OA, and those who performed kung fu had an odds ratio of 22 for OA of the knee. In a study of incident knee OA in Framingham, the United States of America, heavy physical activity was associated with an increased risk of knee OA in both sexes; adjustment for BMI, weight loss, knee injury, health status, calorie intake, and smoking strengthened the association.[39] A cross-sectional study of participants in the Study of Osteoporotic Fractures[43] found that the risk of moderate to severe radiographic hip OA in elderly women was modestly increased in women who had performed more physical activity as a teenager.

It would appear that the most currently recognized risk factors for knee OA (obesity, injury, physical activity, Heberdens nodes) influence incidence rather than progression,[45] but that patients with peripheral joint OA of sufficient severity to require hospital referral have high levels of physical disability over an 8-year follow-up.[46] For example, 44 per cent of Bristol rheumatology patients with lone hand disease acquired significant knee or hip OA 8 years later.[47]

By contrast, several studies have suggested that hormone replacement therapy (HRT) is associated with a reduction in the risk of hip and knee OA, particularly in long-term users.[48] Although these studies report on prevalent disease, further work is now indicated to determine an effect on OA progression.

Conclusions

OA is firmly established as a public health problem. There have been advances in defining the disorder, measuring its component features clinically, radiographically, and by other investigative techniques. The descriptive epidemiological characteristics of OA, have been elucidated, and the risk factors for prevalent disease are clearly understood for the knee, hip, and hand. Epidemiological information on the rate and determinants of progression of the disorder remains less detailed. However, it is clear that progression is a joint-specific phenomenon and there may be disease subsets at each site in which progression depends on different groups of factors, which may include increasing age, obesity, crystal deposition, the presence of polyarticular OA, joint instability, muscle weakness, knee malalignment, and neurogenic dysfunction. The challenge of identifying subjects at risk of rapid progression, through a variety of diagnostic modalities, is currently the subject of intensive research. With the completion of studies examining the efficiency of biochemical markers, scintigraphy, and newer imaging techniques such as magnetic resonance, it is likely that the processes underlying progressive disease will be better understood and developed.

Summary

Osteoarthritis (OA) is the most common joint disorder in the world today. Characteristic pathological and radiographic changes are variably associated with symptoms and disability. Pain is typically use related and associated with stiffness after inactivity, and is poorly correlated with radiographic grade. Several radiographic grading systems have been proposed and recommendations exist for the use of radiographic measures to assess progression of OA. Other investigative modalities (which largely remain research tools at present) include isotope bone scans, magnetic resonance imaging, and use of biochemical markers.

The prevalence of OA rises steeply with age at all joint sites. Hand and knee OA is more common in women than men, but there is little sex difference in the incidence of hip OA. Radiographic improvement with time is uncommon, and several longitudinal studies of the incidence and progression of OA have now been performed. Determinants of progression include obesity, joint injury, and physical activity.

Key points

1. OA is the most common joint disorder in the world today.
2. Characteristic pathological and radiographic changes occur.
3. Pain correlates poorly with radiographic grade.
4. Several radiographic grading systems have been proposed.
5. Other investigative modalities include isotope bone scans, MRI, and use of biochemical markers.
6. Prevalence of OA rises with age at all joint sites.
7. Hand and knee OA is more common in women than men.
8. Radiographic improvement with time is uncommon.

Acknowledgements

The authors thank the Medical Research Council for research support.

Further reading

Felson, D.T. and Zhang, Y. (1998). An update on the epidemiology of knee and hip osteoarthritis with a view to prevention. *Arthritis Rheum* **41**:1343–55.

Dieppe, P.A., Hirsch, R., Helmick, C.G., Jordan, J.M., Kington, R.S., Lane, N.E., *et al.* (2000). In D.T. Felson (ed.) *Osteoarthritis: new insights Part 1: The disease and its risk factors. Ann Intern Med* **133**:635–46.

References

(An asterisk denotes recommended reading.)

1. Rogers, J., Dieppe, P., and Watt, I. (1981). Arthritis in Saxon and medieval skeletons. *Br Med J* **283**:668–71.

2. Inoue, K., Hukuda, S., Fardellon, P., Yang, Z.Q., Nakai, M., *et al.* (2001). Prevalence of large-joint osteoarthritis in Asian and Caucasians skeletal populations. *Rheumatology* **40**:70–3.

3. Cushnaghan, J., Cooper, C., Dieppe, P., Kirwan, J., McAlindon, T., and McCrae, F. (1990). Clinical assessment of osteoarthritis of the knee. *Ann Rheum Dis* **49**:68–70.

4. *Kellgren, J.K. and Lawrence, J.S. (1957). Radiological assessment of osteoarthritis. *Ann Rheum Dis* **15**:494–501.
   A historical paper describing the conventional OA grading system.

5. Spector, T.D. and Cooper, C. (1993). Radiographic assessment of osteoarthritis in population studies: whither Kellgren and Lawrence? *Osteoarthritis Cart* **1**:203–6.

6. Spector, T.D., Hart, D.J., Byrne, J., Harris, T.A., Dacre, J.E., and Doyle, D.D. (1993). Definition of osteoarthritis of the knee for epidemiological studies. *Ann Rheum Dis* **52**:790–4.

7. Croft, P., Cooper, C., Wickham, C., and Coggon, D. (1990). Defining osteoarthritis of the hip for epidemiologic studies. *Am J Epidemiol* **132**:514–22.

8. Kallman, D.A., Wigley, F.M., Scott, W.W., Hochberg, M., and Tobin, J.D. (1989). New radiographic grading scales of osteoarthritis of the hand. *Arthritis Rheum* **32**:1584–91.

9. Dieppe, D.A. (1995). Recommended methodology for assessing the progression of osteoarthritis of the hip and knee joints. *Osteoarth Cart* **3**:73–7.

10. Lanyon, P., Jones, A., and Doherty, M. (1996) Assessing progression of patellofemoral osteoarthritis: a comparison between two radiographic methods. *Ann Rheum Dis* **55**:875–9.

11. Auleley, G.R., Giraudeau, B., Dougados, M., and Ravaud, P. (2000) Radiographic assessment of hip osteoarthritis progression: impact of reading procedures for longitudinal studies. *Ann Rheum Dis* **59**:422–7.

12. McCrae, F., Shoels, J., Dieppe, P., and Watt, I. (1992). Scintigraphic assessment of osteoarthritis of the knee joint. *Ann Rheum Dis* **51**:938–42.

13. Dieppe, P.A., Cushnaghan, J., Young, P., and Kirwan, J. (1993). Prediction of the progression of joint space narrowing and osteoarthritis of the knee by bone scintigraphy. *Ann Rheum Dis* **52**:557–63.

14. Hutton, C.W., Higgs, E.R., Jackson, P.C., Watt, I., and Dieppe, D.A. (1986). 99TC-HMDP bone scanning in generalised nodal osteoarthritis. 2. The 4-hour bone scan image predicts radiographic change. *Ann Rheum Dis* **45**:622–6.

15. McAlindon, T.E., Watt, I., McCrae, F.M., Goddard, P., and Dieppe, P.A. (1991). Magnetic resonance imaging in osteoarthritis of the knee: correlation with radiographic and scintigraphic findings. *Ann Rheum Dis* **50**:14–19.

16. Hutton, C.W. and Vennart, W. (1994). Osteoarthritis and magnetic resonance imaging: potential and problems. *Ann Rheum Dis* **54**:237–43.

17. *Van Saase, J.L.C.M., Van Romunde, L.K.S., Cats, A., *et al.* (1989). Epidemiology of osteoarthritis: Zoetermeer Survey. Comparison of radiological osteoarthritis in a Dutch population with that in ten other populations. *Ann Rheum Dis* **48**:271–80.
    One of the first epidemiological studies to document the prevalence of OA in difference populations.

18. *Felson, D.T., Naimark, A., Anderson, J., *et al.* (1987). The prevalence of knee osteoarthritis in the elderly. The Framingham osteoarthritis study. *Arthritis Rheum* **30**:914–18.
    An important paper documenting the prevalence of knee OA in an US population.

19. Lawrence, J.S. and Sebo, M. (1979). The geography of osteoarthrosis. In G. Nuki (ed.) *The aetiopathogenesis of osteoarthritis.* London: Pitman Medical, pp. 155–83.

20. Schouten, J.S.A.G., Van den Ouweland, F.A., and Valkenburg, H.A. (1992). A twelve-year follow-up study in the general population on prognostic factors of cartilage loss in osteoarthritis of the knee. *Ann Rheum Dis* **51**:932–7.

21. Wilson, M.G., Michet, C.J., Ilstrup, D.M., and Melton, L.J. (1990). Idiopathic symptomatic osteoarthritis of the hip and knee: a population based incidence study. *Mayo Clin Proc* **65**:1214–21.

22. Kallman, D.A., Wigley, F.M., Scott, W.W., Hochberg, M.C., and Tobin, J.D. (1990). The longitudinal course of hand osteoarthritis in a male population. *Arthritis Rheum* **33**:1323–32.

23. Dougados, M., Gueguen, A., Nguyen, M., *et al.* (1992). Longitudinal radiologic evaluation of osteoarthritis of the knee. *J Rheumatol* **19**:378–83.

24. Hernborg, J.S. and Nilsson, B.E. (1977). The natural course of untreated osteoarthritis of the knee. *Clin Orthop* **123**:130–7.

25. Danielsson, L. and Hernborg, J. (1970). Clinical and roentgenologic study of knee joints with osteophytes. *Clin Orthop* **69**:224–6.

26. Altman, R.D., Fries, J.F., Bloch, D.A., *et al.* (1987). Radiographic assessment of progression in osteoarthritis. *Arthritis Rheum* **30**:1214–25.

27. Spector, T.D., Dacre, J.E., Harris, P.A., and Huskisson, E.C. (1992). The radiological progression of osteoarthritis: an eleven-year follow-up study of the knee. *Ann Rheum Dis* **51**:1107–10.

28. Hart, D.J., Doyle, D.V., and Spector, T.D. (1999). Incidence and risk factors for radiographic knee osteoarthritis in middle-aged women: the Chingford study. *Arthritis Rheum* **42**:17–24.

29. Danielsson, L.G. (1964). Incidence and prognosis of coxarthrosis *Acta Orthop Scand* **66**(Suppl.):1–87.

30. Seifert, M.H., Whiteside, C.G., and Savage, O. (1969). A five-year follow-up of 50 cases of idiopathic osteoarthritis of the hip (abstract). *Ann Rheum Dis* **28**:325–6.

31. Van Saase, J.L.C.M. (1990). *Osteoarthrosis in the general population: a follow-up study of osteoarthrosis of the hip*, Ph.D. Thesis, Leiden State University, Netherlands.

32. Bland, J.H. and Cooper, S.M. (1984). Osteoarthritis: a review of the cell biology involved and evidence for reversibility. *Sem Arthritis Rheum* **14**:106–33.

33. Perry, G.H., Smith, M.J.G., and Whiteside, C.J. (1979). Spontaneous recovery of the joint space in degenerative hip disease. *Ann Rheum Dis* **31**:440–8.

34. Newman, N.M. and Ling, R.S.M. (1985). Acetabular bone destruction related to non-steroidal anti-inflammatory drugs. *Lancet* **2**:11–14.

35. Rashad, S., Revell, P., Hemingway, A., *et al.* (1989). The effect of non-steroidal anti-inflammatory drugs on the course of osteoarthritis. *Lancet* **2**:519–22.

36. Harris, P.A., Hart, D.J., Dacre, J.E., Huskisson, E.C., and Spector, T.D. (1994). The progression of radiological hand osteoarthritis over 10 years: a clinical follow-up study. *Osteoarthritis Cart* **2**:247–52.

37. *Doherty, M., Watt, I., and Dieppe, P. (1983). Influence of primary generalised osteoarthritis on development of secondary osteoarthritis. *Lancet* **2**:8–11.

   An important paper describing the role of generalized OA as an aetiological factor in the development of secondary OA.

38. Bardin, T., Bucki, B., Lequesne, M., *et al.* (1985). Crystals in the synovial fluid of osteoarthritic joints are associated with rapid disease progression. *Br J Rheumatol* **27**(Suppl. 2):94.

39. McAlindon, T.E., Wilson, P.W.F., Aliabadi, P., Weissman, B., and Felson, D.T. (1999). Level of physical activity and the risk of radiographic and symptomatic knee osteoarthritis in the elderly: The Framingham study. *Am J Med* **106**:151–7.

40. Lau, E.C., Cooper, C., Dam, D., Chan, V.N.H., Tsang, K.K., and Sham, A. (2000). Factors associated with osteoarthritis of the hip and knee in Hong Kong chinese: obesity, joint injury, and occupational activities. *Am J Epidemiol* **152**:855–62.

41. Spector, T.D., Hart, D.J., and Doyle, D.V. (1994). Incidence and progression of osteoarthritis in women with unilateral knee disease in the general population: the effect of obesity. *Ann Rheum Dis* **53**:565–8.

42. Coggon, D., Kellingray, S., Inskip, H., Croft, P., Campbell, L., and Cooper, C. (1998). Osteoarthritis of the hip and occupational lifting. *Am J Epidemiol* **147**:523–8.

43. Lane, N.E., Hochberg, M.C., Pressman, A., Scott, J.C., and Nevitt, M.C. (1999). Recreational physical activity and the risk of osteoarthritis of the hip in elderly women. *J Rheumatol* **26**:849–54.

44. *Sharma, L., Song, J., Felson, D.T., Cahue, S., and Shamiyeh, E. (2001). The role of knee alignment in disease progression and functional decline in knee osteoarthritis. *JAMA* **286**:188–195.

   The first longitudinal paper to discuss biomechanical factors and their clinical relevance to the development of lower limb OA.

45. Olsen, D.T., Zhang, Y., Anthony, J.M., Naimark, A., and Anderson, J.J. (1992). Weight loss reduces the risk for symptomatic knee osteoarthritis in women: the Framingham study. *Ann Intern Med* **116**:535–9.

46. Cooper, C., Snow, S., McAlindon, T.E., Kellingray, S., Stuart, B., Coggon, D., and Dieppe, P.A. (2000). Risk factors for the incidence and progression of radiographic knee osteoarthritis. *Arthritis Rheum* **43**:995–1000.

47. Dieppe, P., Cushnaghan, J., Tucker, M., Browning, S., Shepstone, L. (2000). The Bristol 'OA500 study': Progression and impact of the disease after 8 years. *Osteoarthritis Cart* **8**:63–8.

48. Nevitt, M.C., Cummings, S.R., Lane, N.E., Hochberg, M.C., Scott, J.C., Pressman, A.R., Genant, H.K., *et al.* (1996). Association of estrogen replacement therapy with the risk of osteoarthritis of the hip in elderly white women. *Arch Intern Med* **156**:2073–80.

49. Egger, P., Cooper, C., Hart, D.J., Doyle, D.V., Coggon D., and Spector, T.D. (1995). Patterns of joint involvement in osteoarthritis of the hand: the Chingford study. *J Rheumatol* **22**:1509–13.

50. Oliveria, S.A., Felson, D.T., Reed, J.I., Cirillo, P.A., and Walker, A.M. (1995). Incidence of symptomatic hand, hip and knee osteoarthritis among patients in a health maintenance organisation. *Arthritis Rheum* **38**:1134–41.

51. Massardo, L., Watt, I., Cushnagan, J., *et al.* (1989). Osteoarthritis of the knee joint: an eight year prospective study. *Ann Rheum Dis* **48**:893–7.

52. Ledingham, J., Regan, M., Jones, A., and Doherty, M. (1995). Factors affecting radiographic progression of knee osteoarthritis. *Ann Rheum Dis* **54**:53–8.

53. Ledingham, J.M., Dawson, S., Preston, B., and Doherty, M. (1993). Radiographic progression of hospital referred hip osteoarthritis. *Ann Rheum Dis* **52**:263–7.

9

Management of osteoarthritis

9.1 Introduction: the comprehensive approach

*Kenneth Brandt, Michael Doherty, and
L. Stefan Lohmander*

The importance of holistic assessment of the patient

The assessment and management of patients with OA is a challenge to the clinical skills and judgement of any health professional. The main problems for which the patient with OA seeks advice are pain and functional impairment. However, the correlation between pain severity, disability, and the extent of structural OA changes is not always strong, and the consequences of pain and impairment vary greatly from person to person, depending on factors such as personality, affect, occupational and recreational aspirations, coexistent disease and disability, and the expectations of available health care delivery.[1–3] Assessment of the patient with symptomatic OA is, therefore, potentially complex and must occur on at least two levels:

1. assessment of *the joint*—for example, which joint is involved, articular versus periarticular pain, degree of structural damage, instability, inflammation, restriction, and disability;

2. assessment of *the person*—for example, impact and severity of pain, affect, level of distress, handicap, other medical problems, social support, quality of life, and beliefs and knowledge of arthritis and its treatment.

This requires a global, holistic approach if a successful management plan, with realistic goals, is to be developed with the patient. Full account must be taken of the individual seeking advice, as well as of the severity of the OA afflicting their joints.

Management objectives

There is general agreement[4–6] that the central objectives of management are to:

- educate the patient,
- control pain,
- optimize function,
- reduce handicap, and
- beneficially modify the OA process.

These clearly interrelate and overlap. To achieve these aims, there are a wide variety of interventions from which to choose.[4–8]

Issues in treatment selection

When deciding on the appropriate management strategy for an individual patient, the following general considerations are pertinent:

1. Any management plan must be *individualized and patient-centred*. The selection of treatments and the order in which they are tried is determined by the individual requirements and characteristics of the patient (the person and the joint, as above). The patient's perceptions and knowledge of OA and their preferences for certain forms of therapy require consideration and discussion. If the plan does not accord with the patient's beliefs, modified or not by the information they have received, adherence is likely to be jeopardized.[9,10]

2. The *site of OA involvement* determines in part the selection of interventions, because some treatments, such as intra-articular injections or topical creams, are limited in suitability or efficacy to one, or only a few, sites.

3. In general, *simple and safe interventions are tried first*, before more complex, potentially injurious, treatments. In addition to the balance of safety and efficacy, the costs, local availability, and logistics of delivery of individual treatments will also influence decision-making.

4. The status and requirements of the patient will change with time, usually slowly but sometimes rapidly. This necessitates *regular review* and *readjustment of treatment options*, rather than the rigid continuation of a single plan.

5. The wide variety of treatment approaches may require the expertise of a number of different health professionals. A *coordinated multidisciplinary team approach* is often required to deliver health care efficiently and to present coherent, rather than contradictory, management advice.

The core and options approach

Although management is individualized to each patient, certain evidence-based interventions should be considered for every patient with OA, especially those with knee or hip involvement. This is not only because these interventions can be effective,[4–8] but also because they are safe. These core interventions, which largely involve *life-style changes*, include the following.

Education

This is central to any management plan. It is a primary responsibility of every doctor and allied health professional to inform patients and care givers about the nature of their condition and its investigation, treatment, and prognosis. Knowing about OA helps patients manage and cope with their condition and make informed choices between treatment options. However, in addition to being a professional responsibility, education itself improves the outcome. Although the mechanisms are unclear, provision of access to information and contact with a therapist may reduce pain and disability in patients with large joint OA, improve self-efficacy, and reduce health care costs.[11–18] Such benefits are modest but long-lasting and safe.[16,18] The content and format of such 'education' requires discussion and tailoring to the individual, but can take many forms, including group classes,[15,16,18] educational literature, interactive computer programmes,[14] and regular management reviews conducted over the telephone[12,13] or by mail.[17]

OA is often considered a uniformly progressive 'wear and tear' disease, the inevitable consequence of ageing, for which there is little effective therapy other than the eventual surgical replacement of the arthritic joint. This negative attitude, based on the 'doomsday scenario' of worn-out joints,[19] is widespread not only in the community,[9] but among doctors and other health care professionals. In reality, however, OA is not inevitably progressive. Many intervention strategies can reduce symptoms and improve function.[4–8] An optimistic, rather than a fatalistic, approach is, therefore, justified.

Exercise

Many patients with OA are concerned that continued physical activity may further damage their joints. The musculoskeletal system, however, is designed to move, and reduced activity is detrimental to all its component tissues. Furthermore, poor aerobic fitness, a consequence of reduced activity, is associated with a low sense of 'well-being' and more reporting of pain and handicap from OA. Therefore, patients with OA should be encouraged to exercise, using 'small amounts often' to increase general fitness, improve muscle strength, and maintain or increase the range of joint movement. There is good evidence that such exercise can reduce pain and disability from knee and hip OA.[19–25] Even simple, unsupervised exercise undertaken at home can prove effective and safe.[25] In addition to its effects on pain and disability from OA, increased aerobic fitness encourages restorative sleep, improves psychological health, promotes functional independence, and benefits common co-morbidities such as obesity, diabetes, chronic heart failure, and hypertension.[26] There are very few contra-indications, even in elderly subjects, to a 'prescription of exercise' that combines stretching ('warm-up'), strengthening, and aerobic routines.[26] There is good evidence that such exercise not only reduces pain and disability but also improves the reduced muscle strength, proprioception, standing balance, and abnormal gait patterns associated with large joint OA,[25–29] thus fundamentally influencing the physiological parameters of joint function.

Reduction of adverse mechanical factors

Encouraging patients to 'pace' their activities through the day, rather than attempting too much at one go, may allow them to accomplish more in a given period. The use of a walking stick[30] is a simple way of reducing symptoms from hip or knee OA. Other mechanical approaches include wedged insoles for patients with knee OA and varus deformity,[31] shock-absorbing insoles for hip or knee OA, and taping of the patella for patellofemoral OA.[32] Modification of the patient's home or work environment can further minimize 'external' adverse mechanical factors. The patient may already be utilizing strategies to cope with the consequences of their OA, but such strategies may be improved, or new ones adopted, with the assistance of a therapist.[15,16]

Obese patients with large joint OA should be encouraged to lose weight. Obesity is a risk factor for knee OA and its associated pain and disability, and increases the risk of radiographic progression.[33] It may also be a weaker risk factor for the development and progression of hip OA.[33] In patients who are overweight, weight loss can improve symptoms of established knee OA[34] and reduce the risk of developing knee OA.[35] Weight loss, however, is notoriously difficult to achieve. Dietary restriction may be more effective when combined with exercise.[34] Importantly, as with other lifestyle changes, the person must have the 'willingness to change' if the programme is to be successful.[36,37]

Simple analgesia

Paracetamol (acetaminophen) is the traditional oral drug of first choice and, if effective, is the preferred long-term analgesic.[4,6] This is because of its efficacy, lack of contra-indications or drug interactions, long-term safety, availability, and low cost. The previous American College of Rheumatology (ACR) guidelines for knee and hip OA[38,39] also favoured paracetamol. In the ACR 2000 update,[5] however, it was argued that an oral non-steroidal anti-inflammatory drug (NSAID) is an alternative initial oral drug in those with moderate-to-severe pain or with clinical signs of inflammation. This issue has fuelled considerable debate[40,41] and is fully discussed in Chapters 9.2, 9.3, and 9.4. However, in Europe at least, paracetamol remains the oral analgesic to try first, certainly in preference to oral NSAIDs.[4,6,42]

A wide variety of other non-pharmacological, drug and surgical interventions that may be considered as *additional options*, are selected and added, as required, to the above core interventions (Table 9.1). It is very difficult to rank treatments in order of OA 'severity' because of the numerous ways in which severity can be defined (e.g., X-ray change, pain, disability) and the fact that different assessment measures do not necessarily progress in parallel. Pragmatically, therefore, the above effective and safe treatments are given initial, equal priority for all patients, irrespective of severity. Other drug treatments, and more invasive measures, are considered second in order. Surgery, of course, is the 'final option' that is reserved for patients with persistent pain and disability, significant to that individual, and clearly resistant to conservative interventions. The lives of patients who are severely incapacitated by hip or knee OA can be transformed by successful joint replacement.[43,44] Surgery, however, is not without its risks. Furthermore, there are no clear guidelines for deciding the timing of surgery or selecting those who might benefit most.[44] As always, a global assessment is paramount, with patients actively involved in determining their own outcome.

The evidence for efficacy and the advantages and drawbacks of all currently available interventions for OA are fully discussed in Chapters 9.2–9.21.

Table 9.1 Available management options for OA

Core	Options
• Education, coping	• Other non-pharmacological
Self-management	interventions
Telephone contact	Walking stick, aids, appliances
• Exercise:	Patella taping
Aerobic conditioning	Local physical treatments
Strengthening	Heat, cold
Range of movement	Pulsed electrical stimulation
• Avoidance of adverse	• Local and systemic drug therapies
mechanical factors	Topical creams/gels
Pacing of activities	Topical NSAIDs
Appropriate footwear	Topical capsaicin
Weight loss if obese	Local injection therapies
• Simple analgesics (acetaminophen)	Intra-articular corticosteroid
	Periarticular corticosteroid
	Intra-articular hyaluronan
	Oral drugs
	Opioid derivatives
	Oral NSAIDs
	Coxibs
	Low-does amitriptyline
	Diacerhein
	Nutripharmaceuticals
	Glucosamine,
	Chondroitin sulphate
	• Operative interventions
	Invasive physical interventions
	Arthroscopic lavage (knee)
	Closed tidal irrigation (knee)
	Capsular distension (hip)
	Surgery
	Osteotomy
	Joint replacement
	Arthrodesis

The exciting possibility of pharmacological modification of the OA process is considered in Chapter 11.

Published guidelines for effective management of OA

It is apparent that generic decision trees for management of OA are difficult to formulate, given the variability of OA and the individual characteristics of each patient. Nevertheless, recent guidelines have been proposed for the management of OA at the knee[4–6] and hip,[5,6] the two joint sites that contribute the largest community burden of OA pain, disability, and health care requirements.

Clinical guidelines were defined in 1995 by the Institute of Medicine in Washington as 'systematically developed statements to assist practitioner and patient decisions about appropriate health care for specific clinical decisions'. The ACR recommendations of 2000[5] are an update of previous guidelines for hip and knee OA published in 1995.[38,39] Unlike the 1995 guidelines, which reflected the consensus opinion of eight experts in OA and included an algorithm for OA management, the 2000 update amalgamated guidelines for hip and knee into one article, attempted a more systematic review of published clinical trials, replaced 'guidelines' with 'recommendations' and presented no algorithm.

The European League Against Rheumatism (EULAR) recommendations for knee OA[4] differed from previous OA guidelines in adopting an evidence-based guideline format, combined with expert consensus, focused on key management questions. Some of the strengths and weaknesses of the ACR and EULAR approaches are summarized in Table 9.2. Notwithstanding such differences in approach, there is substantial agreement between these two documents. In particular, the importance of full patient assessment, education, and support are highlighted in both. Similar recommendations are echoed in guidelines that are aimed at general practitioners, who manage the majority of patients with OA.[6]

Guidelines, of course, will modify patient care only if they are read and discussed by relevant health care deliverers and if action is taken as a consequence. Their main purpose is to highlight treatment options, to suggest minimum standards of care and to stimulate debate.[45] Any guidelines require regular review and alteration to take into account the perspective of all interested parties (including patients), new research evidence, and changes in health care delivery.

Table 9.2 Comparison of the ACR[5] and EULAR[4] 2000 Recommendations for OA management

ACR	EULAR
Recommendations on management of knee and hip OA	Recommendations on management of knee OA only
Four American expert contributors	23 experts from 12 European countries
Expert consensus format	Evidence-based guideline format examining key clinical questions, plus expert consensus
Included studies up to 2000	Included trial data up to December 1998 (e.g. no data on coxibs)
Included data relevant to US practitioners (e.g., no data on topical NSAIDs)	Included all published data on 23 intervention modalities
No clear distinction between trial-based evidence and expert opinion	Clear distinction between trial-based evidence and expert opinion

From the systematic literature review undertaken for the EULAR recommendations,[4] examining clinical trials in knee OA published from 1966–98, it was noteworthy that:

1. The majority of trials assessed pharmacological interventions.
2. Over half (54 per cent) of all trials were of NSAIDs.
3. Quality scores were in the low-mid range for most studies.
4. Efficacy of only 16 of the 23 treatment modalities examined was supported by evidence from at least one randomized controlled trial (RCT) permitting grading of 1A or 1B category of evidence.
5. Among the surgical interventions, only arthroscopic debridement and patella replacement were supported by evidence from at least one RCT—osteotomy and joint replacement were supported only by grade 3 evidence, that is, descriptive studies.
6. Because insufficient summary statistics were presented, the standardized effect size, true effect size and Number Needed to Treat (for 20 per cent reduction in baseline pain above placebo) could be calculated in only 9, 2, and <1 per cent of publications, respectively.

The EULAR Task Force concluded that the evidence base for knee OA treatment was far from complete, especially for non-pharmacological and surgical interventions. Such a review, though disappointing in terms of a firm evidence base to guide clinical decisions, is clearly helpful in informing the future research agenda.

The generalizability of clinical trial data

It is often difficult to extrapolate RCT or other research data to routine clinical practice. For example:

1. OA has different risk factors and outcomes at different joint sites. Though rarely studied, it is possible that the treatment response also varies between sites. Extrapolation of trial data from one joint site to another is often made, but may not be justified.
2. A large number of exclusions usually apply in clinical trials (e.g., degree of radiographic change, comorbidity, concurrent medications, concurrent calcium pyrophosphate crystal deposition, presence of knee effusion). This conveniently produces a study population that is relatively homogeneous for factors that may influence outcome, restricting the number of patients required. The disadvantage, however, is that the subjects who are enrolled in such trials may be unrepresentative of many patients in clinical practice. Whether such treatments are likely to be effective in more typical, but complex, patients is often unanswered by such trials.
3. The homogeneity of study populations means that the possible predictors of response cannot be readily examined. In clinical practice, however, we all want to know if certain patient characteristics can help guide in the selection of the most appropriate treatment options. When formally studied, the evidence is not always what we might have predicted. For example, contrary to popular opinion,[4,5] the presence of clinical inflammation at the knee may not predict a better response to an NSAID[40,46] or an intra-articular injection of corticosteroid.[47]
4. An inclusion criterion for many NSAID or coxib studies is for the patient to show a 'flare' of symptoms following withdrawal of their current oral drugs. Such a selection bias towards drug-responsive patients increases the likelihood of a trial treatment response (beneficial for the pharmaceutical sponsor) but limits the generalizability of the findings.
5. Most clinical trials are relatively short-term (6 weeks to 6 months) and only a very few extend to 18–24 months. Many patients with OA, however, have chronic symptoms and disability and more long-term efficacy data are needed. When available, long-term data (e.g. for oral NSAID[48,49]) are often far less positive than data from short-term studies.
6. Most trial evidence for interventions relates to their use as monotherapy and few investigate combination therapy or the possible additive effects

Table 9.3 Ways in which clinical trials in OA may be improved

- More consistency in clinical outcome measures—use of a smaller number of well-validated instruments that assess core outcome measures[50]
- Longer duration of study
- Examination of clinical predictors of response—for example degree of structural change, presence of knee effusion, pain at night or at rest versus pain only on usage, age, obesity
- Adherence to the CONSORT agreement for a more uniform reporting of clinical trials[51]
- In addition to the summary results for treatment groups, incorporation of the effect size, Numbers Needed to Treat or overall treatment 'responders', to afford a better idea of the clinical usefulness of a treatment.
- More use of factorial designs to efficiently investigate the individual and combined effects of two or more treatments.

of treatments. In practice, however, several treatments are given concurrently as a package of care.

There are, of course, different forms of evidence. The incidence of side effects, costs, logistics of delivery, and personal experience all influence opinion concerning the overall clinical usefulness and effectiveness of specific treatments. The EULAR recommendations[4] noted the frequent discordance between the research evidence and the opinion of the experts, who were drawn from 12 European countries. It appears that our clinical practice is governed as much by our own experience, local situation, and personal bias as by the balance of published research evidence.

There are a number of ways in which both the design and the reporting of clinical trials could improve the quality and clinical relevance of the data obtained (Table 9.3). Hopefully, in the future we will obtain more clinically relevant evidence for existing, as well as for novel treatments, to facilitate their more efficient and targeted use in individual patients.

References

1. Davis, M.A., Ettinger, W.H., Neuhaus, J.M., Barclay, J.D., and Segal, M.R. (1992). Correlates of knee pain among US adults with and without radiographic knee osteoarthritis. *J Rheumatol* 19:1943–9.
2. Hadler, N.M. (1992). Knee pain is the malady—not osteoarthritis. *Ann Intern Med* 116:598–9.
3. Creamer, P., Lethbridge-Cejku, M., and Hochberg, M.C. (2000). Factors associated with functional impairment in symptomatic knee osteoarthritis. *Rheumatology* 39:490–6.
4. Pendleton, A., Arden, N., Dougados, M., Doherty, M., Bannworth, B., Bijlsma, J.W.J., *et al.* (2000). EULAR recommendations for the management of knee osteoarthritis: report of a task force of the Standing Committee for International Studies Including Therapeutic Trials (ESCISIT). *Ann Rheum Dis* 59:936–44.
5. American College of Rheumatology Subcommittee on osteoarthritis Guidelines (2000). Recommendations for the medical management of osteoarthritis of the hip and knee. 2000 update. *Arthritis Rheum* 43:1905–15.
6. Walker-Bone, K., Javaid, K., Arden, N., and Cooper, C. (2000). Medical management of osteoarthritis. *Br Med J* 321:936–40.
7. Dieppe, P., Chard, J., Faulkner, A., and Lohmander, S. (2000). Osteoarthritis. In F. Godlee (ed.) *Clinical Evidence. A Compendium of the Best Evidence for Effective Health Care.* London: BMJ, Issue 4 (www.evidence.org).
8. Felson, D.T. (2000). Osteoarthritis: New insights. Part 2: Treatment approaches. *Ann Intern Med* 133:726–37.
9. Goodwin, J.S., Black, S.A., and Satish, S. (1999). Aging versus disease: the opinion of older black, Hispanic and non-Hispanic white Americans about the causes and treatment of common medical conditions. *J Am Geriat Soc* 47:973–9.
10. Horne, R. (1999). Patients' beliefs about treatment: the hidden determinant of treatment outcome? *J Psychosom Res* 47:491–5.
11. Weinberger, M., Tierny, W.M., Booher, P., and Katz, B.P. (1989). Can the provision of information to patients with osteoarthritis improve functional status? *Arthritis Rheum* 32:1577–83.
12. Rene, J., Weinberger, M., Mazzuca, S.A., Brandt, K.D., and Katz, B.P. (1992). Reduction of joint pain in patients with knee osteoarthritis who have received monthly telephone calls from lay personnel and whose medical regimens have remained stable. *Arthritis Rheum* 35:511–5.
13. Weinberger, M., Tierney, W.M., Booher, P., and Katz, B.P. (1993). Cost-effectiveness of increased telephone contact for patients with osteoarthritis: a randomised controlled trial. *Arthritis Rheum* 36:243–6.
14. Rippey, R.M., Bill, D., Abeles, M., Day, J., Downing, D.S., Pfeiffer, C.A., *et al.* (1987). Computer-based patient education for older persons with osteoarthritis. *Arthritis Rheum* 30:932–5.
15. Lorig, K.R., Lubeck, D., Kraines, R.G., Seleznick, M., and Holman, H.R. (1985). Outcomes of self-help education for patients with arthritis. *Arthritis Rheum* 28:680–5.
16. Lorig, K.R., Mazonson, P.D., and Holman, H.R. (1993). Evidence suggesting that health education for self-management in patients with chronic arthritis has sustained health benefits while reducing health care costs. *Arthritis Rheum* 36:439–46.
17. Fries, J.F., Carey, C., and McShane, D.J. (1997). Patient education in arthritis: randomised controlled trial of a mail delivery program. *J Rheumatol* 27:1378–83.
18. Superio-Cabuslay, E., Ward, M.M., and Lorig, K.R. (1996). Patient education interventions in osteoArthritis rheumatoid arthritis: a meta-analytic comparison with non-steroidal anti-inflammatory drug treatment. *Arthritis Care Res* 9:292–301.
19. Hurley, M.V. (1995). Conservative management of osteoarthritic knees. *Br J Therapeutic Rehab* 2:179–83.
20. Kovar, P.A., Allegrante, J.P., MacKenzie, C.R., Petersen, M.G.E., Gutin, B., and Charlson, M.E. (1992). Supervised fitness walking in patients with osteoarthritis of the knee. *Ann Intern Med* 116:529–34.
21. Westby, M.D. (2001). A health professional's guide to exercise prescription for people with arthritis: a review of aerobic fitness activities. *Arthritis Care Res* 45:501–11.
22. van Baar, M.E., Dekker, J., Oostendorp R.A.B., Bijl, D., Voorn, T.B., Lemmens, J.A.M., *et al.* (1998). The effectiveness of exercise therapy in patients with osteoarthritis of the hip or knee: a randomised clinical trial. *J Rheumatol* 25:2432–9.
23. van Baar, M.E., Assendelft, W.J.J., Dekker, J., Oostendorp, R.A.B., and Bijlsma, W.J. (1999). Effectiveness of exercise therapy in patients with osteoarthritis of the hip or knee: a systematic review of randomised controlled trials. *Arthritis Rheum* 42:1361–9.
24. Ettinger, W.H., Burns, R., Messier, S.P., Applegate, W., Rejeski, J., Morgan, T., *et al.* (1997). A randomised trial comparing aerobic exercise and resistance exercise with a health education program in older adults with knee osteoarthritis: The Fitness, Arthritis, and Seniors Trial (FAST). *JAMA* 277:25–31.
25. O'Reilly, S.C., Muir, K.R., and Doherty, M. (1999). The effectiveness of home exercise on pain and disability from osteoarthritis of the knee: a randomised controlled trial. *Ann Rheum Dis* 58:15–19.
26. American Geriatrics Society Panel on Exercise and Osteoarthritis. (2001). Exercise Prescription for older adults with osteoarthritis pain: consensus practice recommendations. *J Am Geriat Soc* 49:808–23.
27. Hurley, M.V. and Scott, D.L. (1998). Improvements in sensorimotor function and disability of patients with knee osteoarthritis following a clinically practicable exercise regime. *Br J Rheumatol* 37:1181–7.
28. Messier, S.P., Royer, T.D., Craven, T.E., O'Toole, M.L., Burns, R., and Ettinger, W.H. (2000). Long-term exercise and its effect on balance in older, osteoarthritic adults: results from the Fitness, Arthritis, and Seniors Trial (FAST). *J Am Geriat Soc* 48:131–8.
29. Messier, S.P, Thompson, C.D., and Ettinger, W.H. (1997). Effects of long-term aerobic or weight training regimens on gait in an older osteoarthritic population. *J Appl Biomech* 13:205–25.

30. **Blount, W.P.** (1956). Don't throw away the cane. *J Bone Joint Surg* **38**(A):695–8.

31. **Sasaki, T. and Yasuda, K.** (1987). Clinical evaluation of the treatment of osteoarthritic knees using a newly designed wedged insole. *Clin Orthop* **221**:181–7.

32. **Cushnaghan, J., McCarthy, C., and Dieppe, P.A.** (1994). Taping the patella medially: a new treatment for osteoarthritis of the knee joint? *Br Med J* **308**:753–5.

33. **Felson, D.T.** (chair) (2000). Osteoarthritis: New insights. Part 1: The disease and its risk factors. *Ann Intern Med* **133**:635–46.

34. **Huang, M-H., Chen, C-H., Chen, T-W., Weng, M-C., Wang, W-T., and Wang, Y-L.** (2000). The effects of weight reduction on the rehabilitation of patients with knee osteoarthritis obesity. *Arthritis Care Res* **13**:398–405.

35. **Felson, D.T., Zhang, Y., Anthony, J.M., Naimark, A., and Anderson, J.J.** (1992). Weight loss reduces the risk for symptomatic knee osteoarthritis in women: the Framingham Study. *Ann Intern Med* **116**:535–9.

36. **Prochaska, J.O., DiClemente, C.C., and Norcross, J.C.** (1992). In search of how people change. *Am Psychol* **47**:1102–14.

37. **Keefe, F.J., Lefebvre, J.C., Kerns, R.D., Rosenberg, R., Beaupre, P., Prochaska, J.,** *et al.* (2000). Understanding the adoption of arthritis self-management: stages of change profiles among arthritis patients. *Pain* **87**: 303–13.

38. **Hochberg, M.C., Altman, R.D., Brandt, K.D., Clark, B.M., Dieppe, P.A., Griffin, M.,** *et al.* (1995). Guidelines for the medical management of osteoarthritis. Part I. Osteoarthritis of the hip. *Arthritis Rheum* **38**:1535–40.

39. **Hochberg, M.C., Altman, R.D., Brandt, K.D., Clark, B.M., Dieppe, P.A., Griffin, M.,** *et al.* (1995). Guidelines for the medical management of osteoarthritis. Part II. Osteoarthritis of the knee. *Arthritis Rheum* **38**:1541–6.

40. **Brandt, K.D. and Bradley, J.D.** (2001). Should the initial drug used to treat osteoarthritis pain be a nonsteroidal antiinflammatory drug? *J Rheumatol* **28**:467–73.

41. **Felson, D.T.** (2001). The verdict favours nonsteroidal antiinflammatory drugs for treatment of osteoarthritis a plea for more evidence on other treatments. *Arthritis Rheum* **44**:1477–80.

42. **Eccles, M., Freemantle, N., and Mason, J.** (1998). Evidence based guideline development project: summary guideline for non-steroidal anti-inflammatory drugs versus basic analgesia in treating the pain of degenerative arthritis. *Br Med J* **317**:526–30.

43. **Wiklund, I. and Romanus, B.** (1991). A comparison of quality of life before and after arthroplasty in patients who had arthrosis of the hip joint. *J Bone Joint Surg* **73**(A):765–9.

44. **Dieppe, P., Basler, H.D., Chard, J., Croft, P., Dixon, J., Hurley, M.,** *et al.* (1999). Knee replacement surgery for osteoarthritis: effectiveness, practice variations, indications and possible determinants of utilization. *Rheumatology* **38**:73–83.

45. **Woolf, S.H., Grol, R., Hutchinson, A., Eccles, M., and Grimshaw, J.** (1999). Potential benefits, limitations and harms of clinical guidelines. *Br Med J* **318**:527–30.

46. **Bradley, J.D., Brandt, K.D., Katz, B.P., Kalasinski, L.A., and Ryan, S.I.** (1991). Comparison of an anti-inflammatory dose of ibuprofen, an analgesic dose of ibuprofen, and acetaminophen in the treatment of patients with osteoarthritis of the knee. *N Engl J Med* **325**:87–91.

47. **Jones, A. and Doherty, M.** (1996). Intra-articular corticosteroids are effective in osteoarthritis but there are no clinical predictors of response. *Ann Rheum Dis* **55**:829–32.

48. **Williams, H.J., Ward, J.R., Egger, M.J., Neuner, R., Brooks, R.H., Clegg D.O.,** *et al.* (1993). Comparison of naproxen and acetaminophen in a two-year study of treatment of osteoarthritis of the knee. *Arthritis Rheum* **36**: 1196–206.

49. **Dieppe, P.A., Cushnaghan, J., Jasani, M.K., McCrae, F., and Watt, I.** (1993). A two-year, placebo-controlled trial of non-steroidal anti-inflammatory therapy in osteoarthritis of the knee joint. *Br J Rheumatol* **32**:595–600.

50. A task force of the Osteoarthritis Research Society. (1996). Design and conduct of clinical trials in patients with osteoarthritis. *Osteoarthritis Cart* **4**:217–43.

51. **Altman, D.G., Schulz, K.F., Moher, D., Egger, M., Davidoff, F., Elbourne, D.,** *et al.* (2001). The revised CONSORT statement for reporting clinical trials: explanation and elaboration of reporting of randomised controlled trials. *Ann Intern Med* **134**:663–94.

9.2 Systemic analgesics

John D. Bradley

In most cases, pain leads the individual with OA to consult a physician, and it is relief of pain that the OA patient desires most. Furthermore, pain is a major determinant of disability and quality of life in OA. While treatment of the underlying cause of the joint pain is desirable, treatment of the pain itself is incumbent on the physician. For many patients with OA, this treatment frequently begins and ends with non-steroidal anti-inflammatory drugs (NSAIDs), which have been the mainstay of therapy for this disease for over 50 years. Aspirin has been supplanted by newer, 'safer' NSAIDs, but these newer drugs are prescribed frequently for patients with OA at the upper end of their dose range, with the intent of suppressing inflammation as well as providing pain relief.[1]

Although inflammation is often detectable in OA,[2] the clinical importance of suppressing joint inflammation has been called into question by studies demonstrating that for many patients with OA, the efficacy of simple analgesics (drugs devoid of clinically significant anti-inflammatory effects) is comparable to that of NSAIDs. For example, in a 4-week randomized clinical trial by Bradley et al.,[3] acetaminophen, 4000 mg per day, was as effective as either an analgesic dose (1200 mg per day) or anti-inflammatory dose (2400 mg per day) of ibuprofen in subjects with knee OA. Signs of inflammation, that is joint swelling and tenderness, did not correlate with the response to these therapies.[4] Similarly, relief of knee pain after treatment with the analgesic nefopam, was comparable to that seen after treatment with the NSAID flurbiprofen.[5] Previous evidence indicated that ibuprofen, 1200 mg/d, which has a minimal anti-inflammatory effect,[6] was as effective as the very potent anti-inflammatory drug, phenylbutazone, 400 mg/d, in relieving joint pain in patients with OA.[7] A long-term comparison of acetaminophen, 2600 mg/d, and naproxen, 750 mg/d, showed no difference between the two treatment groups with respect to pain relief.[8] Schumacher et al.[9] found that ibuprofen, 2400 mg/d, was superior to acetaminophen, 2600 mg/d, in relief of knee OA pain, and noted a positive correlation between the synovial fluid leukocyte count and the clinical response. However, in a subsequent study the same group found no correlation between the clinical response to treatment with the NSAID, etodolac, and of synovial fluid levels cytokines, the synovial fluid leukocyte count, or the presence of crystals in the joint fluid.[10] Thus, a significant proportion of OA pain may not be attributable to inflammation or inflammation may be an important cause of OA pain but may not respond adequately to NSAIDs (or both).

Origins of joint pain in osteoarthritis

Pain may be broadly classified according to its origin. Pain that is caused by the stimulation of peripheral afferent nociceptors, for example, by stretch, pressure, thermal, electrical or chemical stimuli, local inflammation, or damage, is referred to as 'nociceptive' pain. This is differentiated from pain attributed to the malfunction of the peripheral nerves and dorsal root ganglia, that is, 'neuropathic' pain; and for pain that is attributable to central nervous system (CNS) pain processing disorders, that is, 'central' pain; and that due to psychiatric problems, that is, 'psychogenic' pain. While pain

Table 9.4 Pain types and examples

Pain type	Examples
Nociceptive	Arthritis, gastric ulcer, cardiac ischemia
Neuropathic	Diabetic peripheral neuropathy, post-herpetic neuralgia, lumbar radiculopathy
Central	Multiple sclerosis, post-stroke pain
Psychogenic	Depression, somatization disorder

Table 9.5 Origins of pain in OA

- Synovium
- Periosteum
- Subchondral bone
- Joint capsule
- Intra- and para-articular ligaments
- Menisci
- Para-articular tendons and associated muscles

syndromes associated with OA may involve multiple mechanisms, OA pain is generally considered to be nociceptive (Table 9.4).

Because articular cartilage, the tissue that generally exhibits the most striking pathologic changes in OA, is aneural, OA pain must originate in other articular and periarticular tissues. Candidates include the synovium and joint capsule, which are richly innervated by neurons with nociceptor and mechanoreceptor functions.[11] Synovial inflammation in OA may be induced by degraded proteoglycans or cartilage fragments released from the damaged articular surface, or by calcium-containing crystals, which can cause the release of proinflammatory mediators, such as bradykinin and prostaglandins, which sensitize peripheral nociceptors. Potential sites of origin of OA pain include the synovium, periosteum, subchondral bone, joint capsule, intra- and para-articular ligaments, menisci, para-articular tendons, and associated muscles[12] (Table 9.5).

Does joint pain protect against joint damage in osteoarthritis?

Concerns have been expressed about the possible acceleration of joint damage by analgesic therapy in patients with OA. Analgesics may impair protective muscle reflexes that are triggered by joint pain, with a resultant increase in loading of the damaged joint. Schnitzer et al.[13] demonstrated an increase in joint loading in subjects with medial compartment knee OA treated with the NSAID, piroxicam. Most subjects experienced considerable reduction in joint pain during treatment, but this was associated with significant increases in knee adductor and maximum quadriceps moments. The increase in loading most likely resulted from the analgesic effect of the NSAID; treatment with acetaminophen resulted in similar loading changes at the knee.[14] Additional studies are required to determine whether the increase in loading that occurs as a result of the relief of joint pain accelerates the progression of OA.

Acetaminophen

Mechanism of analgesia

Acetaminophen readily penetrates the CNS at therapeutic doses; its central action may be mediated through activation of the diffuse noxious inhibitory control pathway.[15] Acetaminophen has minimal effect on the activity of cyclooxygenase (COX), regardless of whether the constitutive or inducible isoform of the enzyme is tested. Although COX is present in the CNS, particularly in the glial cells, there is no evidence that COX in the CNS is more sensitive to inhibition by acetaminophen than COX at peripheral sites.[16] Furthermore, even if prostaglandins are administered centrally during treatment with acetaminophen, an analgesic effect is evident.[17] Spinal administration of acetaminophen produces analgesia that is not reversed by the opioid antagonist, naloxone; concomitant supraspinal administration produces synergistic analgesia, which is partially blocked by naloxone.[18] Therefore, a component of the central analgesic effect of acetaminophen appears to involve endogenous opioid pathways.

Clinical considerations

Because it is readily available, inexpensive, well tolerated, and effective, acetaminophen deserves a place at the top of the list of initial drug therapies for OA (see Chapter 9.3). Acetaminophen remains the sole agent in the class of simple non-narcotic analgesics available in the United States of America; others, such as nefopam and dipyrone, are available in other countries. Like aspirin, acetaminophen shows a nearly linear dose-response curve for analgesia that reaches a plateau at about 1000 mg.[19] The maximum recommended dose is 4000 mg/d, in divided doses. Although product-labeling information indicates that acetaminophen is appropriate for the treatment of mild-to-moderate pain, it is effective also in OA patients with moderate-to-severe joint pain.[20] Unfortunately, many older patients take acetaminophen no more than once a day despite persistent and severe pain.[21] Possible barriers to the patient's optimal use of acetaminophen include memory and attention deficits, depression, and a sense of resignation and even futility.

Analgesic nephropathy was first associated with the habitual use of phenacatin-containing analgesics. Chronic renal insufficiency has been reported to occur also in patients who consumed acetaminophen 'regularly.' In 1989, Sandler et al.[22] reported an association between chronic use of acetaminophen and endstage renal disease. As pointed out in the accompanying editorial,[23] however, numerous flaws existed with respect to the experimental design (e.g., patient selection; disproportionate use of proxies to obtain histories of analgesic abuse from patients, relative to controls) and interpretation of the results, limiting the conclusions that could be drawn from that study. Fored et al.,[24] in a study in which patients were enrolled relatively early in the course of their renal disease and photographs of acetaminophen products and their packaging were used to improve the subjects' recall, recently suggested a dose-dependent association between chronic intake of acetaminophen and chronic renal failure. Although the results were consistent with the presence of a dose-dependent exacerbation of chronic renal failure by acetaminophen (and also by aspirin), the authors acknowledged the impossibility of excluding bias caused by consumption of the analgesic for symptoms due to the underlying conditions that predisposed to renal failure.

A recent analysis of the Physicians' Health Study cohort, in which the possibility of recall bias was reduced by ascertaining information about exposure to analgesics before the diagnosis of renal failure was made, failed to reveal a positive association between acetaminophen use and the risk of moderate renal insufficiency.[25] However, the level of exposure was ascertained retrospectively, after a follow-up period of 14 years. Although the Physicians' Health Study may have been underpowered to detect an association between the heavy use of analgesics and the risk of clinically significant renal failure,[26] it supports the finding that persons without pre-existing renal disease who use acetaminophen have only a small risk of endstage renal disease. The mechanisms and specific metabolites responsible for renal injury due to acetaminophen are not well characterized. Acute overdoses of acetaminophen, usually greater than 6 g, can cause, occasionally, acute renal tubular necrosis.

It is well known that overdoses of acetaminophen may result in acute hepatic necrosis, liver failure, and death. Furthermore, it has been claimed that even when taken in the recommended doses (i.e., not exceeding 4 g/d), acetaminophen may cause hepatic necrosis. These claims, however, are based essentially only on case reports and retrospective analyses. In many instances, extrapolation of the blood acetaminophen concentration obtained upon arrival of the patient in an emergency room indicates that the quantity of acetaminophen ingested exceeded the therapeutic dose (often by a large amount), and/or evidence exists that additional potential hepatotoxins were consumed along with acetaminophen.

It has also been suggested that the use of acetaminophen by those who drink alcohol is relatively contraindicated. Ethanol induces the hepatic cytochrome P-450 enzymes responsible for the metabolism of acetaminophen, enhancing the production of a toxic metabolite, N-acetyl-benzoquinoneimine. This metabolite, which is normally inactivated by conjugation with glutathione, may become problematic when glutathione stores are depleted as a result of a pre-existing condition, such as alcoholism, or an acetaminophen overload, such as an overdose. In such cases, hepatotoxicity can be prevented by the timely administration of N-acetyl-cysteine, which repletes intracellular glutathione.

Caution is recommended when acetaminophen is used in therapeutic doses by individuals consuming alcohol. The current edition of the Physicians' Desk Reference[27] carries the following warning for acetaminophen: 'If you consume 3 or more alcoholic drinks every day, ask your doctor whether you should take acetaminophen or other pain relievers/fever reducers.' However, the evidence supporting that recommendation is not clear-cut. Kuffer et al.[28] found that the administration of acetaminophen, 4000 mg/d for 2 days, to alcoholic subjects who had been drinking heavily resulted in increases in serum transaminase levels no greater than those seen after the administration of a placebo.

The view that use of acetaminophen is relatively contraindicated in patients with chronic liver disease also does not appear to have a solid basis. In a study of 20 patients with various forms of chronic liver disease, Benson et al.[29] found no elevation of hepatic enzymes after a relatively brief period of administration of acetaminophen, 4 g/d. It should be noted, however, that no prospective long-term studies of the effects of chronic ingestion of acetaminophen in therapeutic doses by subjects with chronic liver disease or by alcoholics have been published.

NSAIDs

Mechanisms of analgesia

Although NSAIDs have been classified as peripheral-acting analgesics, they have substantial effects in the spinal cord and brain. The ability of NSAIDs to penetrate the CNS is variable, and dependent largely on their pKa and lipophilicity. NSAIDs that penetrate the CNS (e.g., indomethacin, ketoprofen, diclofenac) may inhibit COX centrally. Because prostaglandins can inhibit the pain-suppressing influences of spinal noradrenergic synapses, NSAIDs may reduce pain by eliminating the prostaglandin-mediated disinhibition of pain messages.[30]

However, the effectiveness of NSAIDs as analgesics correlates poorly with their potency as COX inhibitors.[31] In patients with hip or knee OA, only a weak correlation was noted between the magnitude of pain relief and the serum concentrations of either total ibuprofen or its biologically active S-enantiomer.[32] The effectiveness of some NSAIDs as analgesics may be attributable to mechanisms unrelated to inhibition of COX, such as, inhibition of central hyperalgesia induced by glutamate and substance P.[33] The analgesic effect of some NSAIDs is inhibited by naloxone, implying a mechanism involving opioid receptors.[34]

The role of lipoxygenase inhibition in NSAID-induced analgesia is unclear. While 8,15-diHETE, a leukotriene produced by stimulated neutrophils, induces hyperalgesia by sensitization of primary afferent nociceptors, most NSAIDs have little effect on the production of 8,15-diHETE.

Clinical considerations

Relief of OA pain by NSAIDs is often apparent within a few days of initiation of therapy, and tends to increase over 4 or more weeks if therapy is continued—an observation unexplained by the pharmacokinetics. Some NSAIDs, especially propionic acid derivatives, produce maximal analgesia at doses much lower than those needed for their optimal anti-inflammatory effect. Non-acetylated salicylates, for example, salsalate, choline magnesium trisalicylate, are weak COX inhibitors, yet are as effective as aspirin (an irreversible COX inhibitor) in relieving OA pain.

Aspirin is inexpensive, but the direct cost of treatment with this agent, as is the case for most NSAIDs (see Chapter 9.5), is compounded by the cost of treatment of its complications. Gastrointestinal symptoms, ulcers, and bleeding make aspirin a poor choice for most OA patients. Hearing loss, tinnitus, bruising, and hyperuricemia may also occur, even with subtherapeutic doses of salicylate. Ibuprofen, which is available as an over-the-counter (OTC) preparation, is relatively safe and effective in low doses (less than 1600 mg/d). Considering the overall costs of treatment, it is preferable to aspirin if an NSAID is required for analgesia in patients with OA pain (see Chapter 9.3). Naproxen, which is also available OTC in the United States of America, offers the advantage of less frequent dosing (twice daily, compared to 3–4 times daily for ibuprofen). Naproxen is effective in treating OA pain in the range of 500–750 mg per day. Chapter 9.3 reviews in detail the adverse effects associated with NSAID use.

Other generic and proprietary NSAIDs are comparably effective for the treatment of OA symptoms. Some have more favorable side effect profiles and some are more convenient, permitting once-daily dosing. These factors, and patient preference, may provide justification for the selection of one of these agents. In a recent study employing a cross-over design[35] that compared diclofenac/misoprostol with acetaminophen in the treatment of symptomatic knee OA, even though the NSAID provided clear superior relief of joint pain and improvement in the quality of life, only slightly more than half of the subjects indicated they preferred that treatment, perhaps due to the significantly higher incidence of gastrointestinal distress associated with diclofenac/misoprostol. Studies comparing the newer, better tolerated COX-2 selective NSAIDs with acetaminophen are in progress.

Patients frequently experience an initial response to an NSAID which then 'wears off', resulting in the serial prescription of multiple other NSAIDs. It is not clear whether this loss of effectiveness is due to a change in pharmacodynamics or attenuation of a placebo effect. In any event, because of either this limited duration of efficacy, or side effects, only 5–20 per cent of patients with OA who are started on an NSAID are still using the same NSAID one year later.[36]

Opioids

Mechanisms of analgesia

Opioids are often referred to as 'centrally acting' analgesics, but they are shown to be effective when administered intra-articularly (that is, peripherally) in low doses.[37] Indeed, the primary afferent nociceptor cell body synthesizes opioid receptors and transports them centrally and peripherally.[38] Opioids inhibit the sensitization of nociceptors by inflammatory mediators, such as, prostaglandins and leukotrienes, and elevate the threshold for nociceptor activation.[39] Activation of δ and κ opioid receptors not only produces analgesia, but also alters sympathetic nerves to prevent the release of nociceptor-sensitizing agents, such as prostanoids.[40] Activation of μ and δ opioid receptors can inhibit the release of substance P from peripheral afferent nociceptors.[41]

In general, commercially available opioid analgesics interact predominantly with μ-receptors, as does the predominant pain-modulating endogenous opioid, β-endorphin. Other endogenous opioids, such as enkephalins and dynorphins, interact chiefly with δ and κ opioid receptors, respectively. High concentrations of these opioid receptors are found along the central neural pathways involved in nociception, such as the dorsal horn of the spinal cord, periaqueductal gray matter, and thalamus. Because of the relatively high density of opioid receptors in the central nervous system and the permeability of that region to exogenous opioids, central mechanisms probably predominate over peripheral effects when exogenous opioids are administered systemically.

Clinical considerations

Unlike acetaminophen and NSAIDs,[42] opioids do not demonstrate a 'ceiling effect'; opioid analgesia continues to increase with higher doses, without a clear plateau. However, opioids are associated with *tolerance, dependence,* and *addiction* (Table 9.6), whereas acetaminophen and NSAIDs are not. Fear and misunderstanding of tolerance, dependence, and addiction on the part of patients, physicians, and society are largely responsible for the limited use of opioid analgesics in the treatment of chronic non-cancer pain, including OA pain.

Tolerance refers to the requirement for increasing doses of the drug over time to produce a clinically observable effect. This can be beneficial, because adverse effects of opioids limit their use and most adverse effects improve over about 1–2 weeks with continued treatment.[43] Constipation must be dealt with pro-actively, as it is common with essentially all opioids, and tolerance does not develop to this side effect. In clinical trials involving opioid analgesics for OA pain, a stable clinical response and opioid dose have been achieved within a few weeks after initiation of treatment.[44,45] Requirements for dose increases are usually due to worsening of the underlying disease, sometimes referred to as *pseudo-tolerance.*

Dependence refers to the requirement for continuation of opioid therapy to maintain function, and the exacerbation of symptoms that occurs upon withdrawal. This is greatly feared by patients, who must be advised that physiological dependence on opioids is not equivalent to addiction. Withdrawal reactions are uncomfortable, but are generally mild and brief in duration,[43] and can be avoided by the gradual reduction of the opioid dose over a few weeks.

Addiction refers to drug-seeking behavior that is independent of the medical indication for the drug, is 'compulsive', and is associated with physical, psychological, occupational, or interpersonal difficulties. As few as 0.03 per cent of patients, for whom opioids are prescribed, become addicted.[39]

Table 9.6 Glossary of terms related to opioid dependency

- ◆ **Tolerance:** requirement for increasing dose to maintain an effect.
- ◆ **Pseudo-tolerance:** increasing dose requirement due to worsening of underlying condition.
- ◆ **Dependency:** requirement for continued drug use to maintain function.
- ◆ **Addiction:** compulsive drug-seeking that is independent of the medical indication for use, with associated physical, psychological, occupational, or interpersonal difficulties.
- ◆ **Pseudo-addiction drug-seeking behavior:** compulsive drug-seeking that appears excessive, but is attributable to inadequate relief of pain

Pseudo-addiction refers to drug-seeking behavior that may seem excessive to the physician, but is driven by the patient's pursuit of adequate relief of pain. Such drug-seeking behavior disappears when adequate analgesia is provided. The physician's prescribing behaviors, for example, providing too few tablets and/or indicating an excessively long dosing interval, particularly for short-acting opioids,[46] may cause pseudo-addiction behaviors.

Before prescribing an opioid analgesic for chronic OA pain the physician should seek other means of controlling the symptoms, including use of non-pharmacologic modalities[47] and non-opioid analgesics, which might include acetaminophen, NSAIDs, topical therapy, and intra-articular therapy. Opioids may be used in combination with non-opioid drugs. Some additive benefit has been demonstrated with acetaminophen[48] and with NSAIDs.[44,45,49] Goals for therapy should be defined and agreed upon by the patient and physician. The patient and physician must agree on the pattern of opioid use. While activity-related pains may be treated with a short-acting analgesic *post hoc*, prevention of the pain exacerbation with prophylactic use of analgesics may be a superior strategy, resulting in less pain, impairment, limitation of activity, and affectual abnormalities.

Patients with chronic and severe OA pain may benefit from a long acting or sustained-release opioid, dosed at regular intervals, but may require 'rescue' analgesia with a short-acting opioid for exacerbations of pain. Regular patterns of 'rescue' analgesic use indicate that modification of the long-acting/sustained-release opioid dosing regimen is needed.[50]

Long-acting/sustained-release opioids cause less nausea and cognitive dysfunction than comparable doses of short-acting opioid analgesics.[45] Alertness and coordination are not significantly impaired by chronic stable opioid therapy.[51] Nonetheless, an increased risk of falls has been noted in opioid-treated elderly patients.[52] The overall incidence and spectrum of adverse effects from opioids is not significantly altered in elderly patients,[50] but the adverse effects may be more problematic. Elderly patients appear to be more sensitive to the analgesic effects of opioids than younger persons.[53]

The tolerability and effectiveness of opioids in managing chronic OA pain have been evaluated in several recent studies, as described below.

Tramadol is a short-acting analgesic with both μ-opioid receptor agonist activity and serotonin and norepinephrine reuptake inhibitory activity, both of which contribute to its analgesic effects. Administered in a dose of 50–100 mg up to four times a day, as needed, it provides pain relief comparable to that of one or two tablets of acetaminophen, 325 mg/codeine, 30 mg, taken up to four times a day (up to 240 mg codeine).[54] Fleischmann et al.[55] found tramadol to be superior to a placebo in controlling knee OA pain for at least 12 weeks. Schnitzer et al.[44] demonstrated that patients with OA who were naproxen responders tolerated naproxen dose reduction better when tramadol was co-administered. In contrast, among naproxen non-responders, tramadol was not significantly superior to a placebo.

The adverse event profile of tramadol is similar to that of proxyphene or codeine. When titrated to approximately equi-analgesic doses, tramadol caused more nausea, and resulted in more discontinuation of treatment because of adverse events, than a codeine/acetaminophen formulation.[54] Nausea and vomiting can be minimized by gradually phasing in the full dose of tramadol, with incremental increases of 25 mg/d every 3 days.[56]

Seizures have been reported in patients taking tramadol within the recommended dose range. The seizure risk is increased in subjects who exceed the recommended dose; those with a history of seizures, or at risk for seizure (such as patients with head trauma, metabolic disorders, ethanol or drug withdrawal); and those taking tramadol concomitantly with a selective serotonin reuptake inhibitor, tricyclic antidepressant, opioid, monoamine oxidase inhibitor, or other drug that reduces the seizure threshold.

Tolerance to the analgesic effects of tramadol has not been demonstrated, and its abuse and addiction potential are very low. Given that its efficacy and side-effect profile are similar to those of codeine/acetaminophen, and that the difference in cost between these two therapeutic agents is considerable, the only advantage of tramadol, relative to codeine/acetaminophen, would seem to be that it is not regulated as a controlled substance.

A combination tablet containing tramadol 375 mg/acetaminophen 325 mg has recently become available. In a study comparing this product with capsules of a codeine/acetaminophen combination (30 mg/300 mg) for management of chronic low back pain, OA pain, or both, the mean double-blind daily dose over a 22-day treatment period was 3.5 tablets of the tramadol formulation and 3.5 capsules of the codeine formulation. Maximum daily doses were 5.5 tablets and 5.7 capsules, respectively. Efficacy of the two treatments was similar and the overall incidence of adverse events was comparable. A significantly greater proportion of patients in the codeine/acetaminophen group reported somnolence and/or constipation, while a greater proportion of the tramadol group reported headaches.[57]

Propoxyphene is a relatively weak opioid analgesic that generally causes minimal effects on mood and mentation and, therefore, has low abuse potential. The effectiveness of propoxyphene as an analgesic is enhanced by combination with acetaminophen. Such combinations usually contain propoxyphene napsylate (100 mg) or propoxyphene hydrochloride (65 mg) and acetaminophen (650 mg) formulated in a tablet that may be taken as often as every 4–6 hours, as needed. In a four-week randomized comparison of slow-release diclofenac (100 mg/d) versus dextropropoxyphene (180 mg/d)/acetaminophen (1.95 g/d), improvement in joint pain and mobility were significantly greater in the diclofenac group.[58] A higher proportion of those in the propoxyphene/acetaminophen group developed work performance problems and lost time from work, in comparison with the diclofenac treatment group.

Codeine is also a more effective analgesic when combined with acetaminophen. The analgesic effectiveness of codeine, 30 mg/acetaminophen, 325 mg, dosed 1–2 tablets every 4–6 hours, as needed, is comparable to that of propoxyphene/acetaminophen. However, intolerable side effects, such as nausea, constipation, dizziness, dysphoria, and sedation are more common with the codeine combination.[59] Although a long-term study showed sustained efficacy of codeine/acetaminophen, adverse effects severely limited its usefulness.[60] In a recent four-week, placebo-controlled study of monotherapy with controlled-release codeine for treatment of hip or knee OA, reduction in pain scale scores was nearly linear over the dose range tested. The final mean codeine dose, 159 mg per day, resulted in 36 mm reduction on a 100 mm visual analog pain scale. Fifteen of the 51 subjects randomized to codeine, but only 4 of the 52 in the placebo group, discontinued treatment because of adverse effects. Subjects completing the study expressed a strong preference for the codeine regimen.[61]

Oxycodone is a potent short-acting opioid analgesic that is often combined with acetaminophen, or compounded into a sustained-release formulation as a single agent. Caldwell et al.[45] titrated treatment in subjects with painful OA using open-label acetaminophen/oxycodone over the first 30 days, and then randomized subjects to receive a double-blinded placebo, acetaminophen/oxycodone, or sustained-release oxycodone for an additional 30 days. The proportion of subjects who dropped out of the study because of inadequate pain control was higher in the placebo group than in either of the active treatment groups, and no difference was apparent among the three groups with respect to discontinuation because of adverse events. Nausea was more frequent among oxycodone-treated subjects than in the placebo group; nausea and dry mouth were more frequently reported with immediate-release oxycodone, and constipation with the sustained-release formulation. Adverse events reported among subjects ≥65 years old were similar to those in younger subjects, except for lesser headaches and pruritis and more vomiting among the latter. The mean oxycodone dose was 40 mg/d, which provided approximately 40–50 per cent reduction in global pain intensity and substantially improved the quality of sleep.

Roth *et al.* evaluated sustained-release oxycodone at two doses, 10 and 20 mg twice daily, in comparison with a placebo, for the treatment of OA pain.[49] While the 40 mg/d dose provided superior analgesia, 14 of 44 subjects randomized to this treatment discontinued due to adverse effects; only 5 withdrew due to inadequate pain control. In contrast, 22 of 45 subjects in the placebo group discontinued due to inefficacy, and only 2 dropped out due to adverse events. Subjects ≥65 years old experienced more somnolence with oxycodone than with the placebo. During an 18-month open-label extension, all subjects were titrated to maximize benefit and tolerability of oxycodone. Pain control remained stable despite no significant rise in the oxycodone dose. During planned discontinuations of oxycodone only two subjects reported withdrawal reactions (daily doses of 60 and 70 mg per day). Except for constipation, the prominence of common opioid side effects declined with continued therapy.

Morphine is the standard for management of cancer-related pain, and was evaluated in non-malignant musculoskeletal pain by Moulin *et al.*[62] who treated patients who were refractory to NSAIDs and tricyclic antidepressants, and naïve to high-potency opioids. After titration of morphine to a mean daily dose of 83.5 mg, pain relief was superior to the placebo; however, the morphine dose escalation was limited by side effects in 28 per cent of subjects. Morphine did not cause significant changes in psychological or physical functioning, memory, attention, concentration, or planning. Another study evaluating morphine, dihydrocodeine, and buprenorphine for chronic non-cancer pain demonstrated a correlation between pain relief and improvement in function.[63] Functional improvement was optimized with achievement of pain reduction of 50 per cent compared to baseline. Subjects who experienced greater pain relief reported fewer adverse effects.

Fentanyl a very highly potent opioid that can be delivered transdermally, has recently been compared to sustained-release morphine in the treatment of chronic non-cancer pain.[64] Most subjects suffered from back and lower limb pain of musculoskeletal and/or neurological origin and were receiving high potency oral opioids at the time of their enrolment. After unblinded, cross-over 28-day treatment periods, subjects reported a preference for fentanyl over sustained-release morphine. However, dose titration was substantially greater with fentanyl than with morphine, and subjects used more immediate-release morphine as a rescue analgesic during fentanyl treatment periods than during treatment with sustained-release morphine. Furthermore, fentanyl treatment was associated with more nausea and twice as many treatment discontinuations for adverse effects.

The effectiveness of narcotic analgesics may be improved, and the dose thereby minimized, by combination with dextromethophan, an N-methyl D-aspartate receptor antagonist.[65] Co-therapy with an antidepressant may also enhance the efficacy of opioids in some patients.[66]

Antidepressants

Although no antidepressant has been approved by the United States Food and Drug Administration for the treatment of pain, antidepressants are often prescribed for management of chronic pain syndromes. Pain threshold and tolerance are increased by these agents. Their efficacy is best documented in the treatment of neuropathic pain, such as diabetic peripheral neuropathy, post-herpetic neuralgia, and post-stroke pain. Few antidepressants have been formally tested in patients with arthritis pain, in general, or OA pain, in particular.

Some antidepressants exhibit multiple mechanisms of action. Chronic pain and depression frequently coexist (see Chapter 9.13), and may share neurochemical mechanisms.[67] Improvement in depressive symptoms correlates with reduction in pain, and both may correlate with the serum concentration of the antidepressant and its active metabolites. However, several observations suggest that the analgesic and antidepressant effects of these agents are separable:

- the analgesic dose is often substantially lower than that needed to treat the depression;
- the onset of analgesia is rapid, whereas antidepressant effects require weeks;
- some effective antidepressants are relatively poor analgesics.

The most extensively tested and widely utilized antidepressants for the management of chronic arthritis pain are amitriptyline and imipramine, both of which are tricyclic heterocyclic antidepressants. Low doses, that is, 10–25 mg, may be administered up to three times daily, with a similar or larger dose at bedtime, especially if sleep is disturbed by pain. The analgesic effect should be apparent within 2–4 weeks, following which the dose may be adjusted accordingly. Imipramine is less sedating than amitriptyline, but both may cause anticholinergic side effects, for example, dry mouth, constipation, urinary retention.

In the United States of America, S-adenosyl methionine (SAM) is available as an OTC supplement, and in some countries in Europe and South America as a prescription drug. SAM has been shown to be an effective anti-depressant, and reduces OA pain.[68] The optimum dose is probably 600–1200 mg/d. SAM has no significant anticholinergic or anti-dopaminergic adverse effects, which are common with the older heterocyclic antidepressants. SAM may trigger hypomania or mania in bipolar affective disorder patients.

Conclusion

The future will undoubtedly witness the availability of new classes of analgesics. Pain control is the primary objective of the currently available systemic-acting pharmacologic agents used to treat patients with OA. Function and quality of life can be improved by adequate control of joint pain, but are impaired by the adverse effects of many of the currently available analgesics. This is especially true in the elderly—the population at greatest risk for OA. Because of marked inter-individual variations in efficacy and side effects, the choice of an analgesic agent (or combinations of multiple agents) must be individualized. Pain management must not begin and end with the prescription of an analgesic, but must include a careful evaluation of the patient's physical, psychological, and social problems and needs and appropriate utilization of non-pharmacological management strategies.

Key points

For pain related to OA:

1. Acetaminophen is effective, even for moderately severe pain, and is safe when dosed appropriately.
2. NSAIDs are effective at low doses; higher doses confer greater risk of toxicity.
3. Opioids are an appropriate component of a management strategy for patients with severe and refractory pain.
4. Fear of dependency and addiction impedes the appropriate use of opioids.
5. Combination drug regimens may provide additive pain relief.

References

(An asterisk denotes recommended reading.)

1. Mazzuca, S.A., Brandt, K.D., Katz, B.P., Stewart, K.D., and Li, W. (1993). Therapeutic strategies distinguish community-based primary care physicians from rheumatologists in the management of osteoarthritis. *J Rheumatol* **20**:80–6.
2. Baddour, V.T. and Bradley, J.D. (1999). Clinical assessment and significance of Inflammation In knee osteoarthritis. *Curr Rheumatol Reports* **1**:59–63.
3. Bradley, J.D., Brandt, K.D., Katz, B.P., Kalasinski, L.A., and Ryan, S.I. (1991). Comparison of an anti-inflammatory dose of ibuprofen, an analgesic dose of ibuprofen and acetaminophen in the treatment of patients with osteoarthritis of the knee. *N Engl J Med* **325**:87–91.
4. Bradley, J.D., Brandt, K.D., Katz, B.P., Kalasinski, L.A., and Ryan, S.I. (1992). Treatment of knee osteoarthritis: relationship of clinical features of joint inflammation to the response to a nonsteroidal anti-inflammatory drug or pure analgesic. *J Rheumatol* **19**:1950–4.
5. Stamp, J., Rhind, V., and Haslock, I. (1989). A comparison of nefopam and flurbiprofen in the treatment of osteoarthritis. *Br J Clin Prac* **43**:24–6.

6. Huskisson, E.C., Hart, F.D., Shenfield, G.M., *et al.* (1971). Ibuprofen: a review. *Practitioner* **207**:639–43.

7. Moxley, T.E., Royer, G.L., Hearron, M.S., *et al.* (1975). Ibuprofen versus buffered phenylbutazone in the treatment of osteoarthritis: Double-blind trial. *J Am Geriatr Soc* **23**:343–9.

8. Williams, H.J., Ward, J.R., Egger, M.J., Neuner, R., Brooks, R.H., Clegg, D.O., *et al.* (1993). Comparison of naproxen and acetaminophen in a two-year study of treatment of osteoarthritis of the knee. *Arthritis Rheum* **36**:1196–206.

9. Schumacher, H.R. Jr, Stineman, M., Rahman, M., Magee, S., and Huppert, A. (1990). The relationship between clinical and synovial fluid findings and treatment response in osteoarthritis (OA) of the knee (abstract). *Arthritis Rheum* **33**:S92.

10. Schumacher, H.R. Jr, Meng, Z., Sieck, M., *et al.* (1996). Effect of non-steroidal antiinflammatory drug on synovial fluid in osteoarthritis. *J Rheumatol* **23**:1774–7.

11. Kidd, B.L., Mapp, P.I., Blake, D.R., Gibson, S.J., and Polak, J.M. (1990). Neurogenic influences in arthritis. *Ann Rheum Dis* **49**:649–52.

12. Altman, R. and Dean, D. (1989). Introduction and overview: pain in osteoarthritis. *Sem Arthritis Rheum* **18**(Suppl. 2):1–3.

13. Schnitzer, T.J., Popovich, J.M., Andersson, G.B.J., and Andriacchi, T.P. (1993). Effect of piroxicam on gait in patients with osteoarthritis of the knee. *Arthritis Rheum* **36**:1207–13.

14. Schnitzer, T.J., Andriacchi, T.P., Feddor, D., and Lindeman, M. (1990). Effect of NSAIDs on knee loading in patients with osteoarthritis (OA). *Arthritis Rheum* **33**:592.

15. Tjolson, A., Lund, A., and Hole, K. (1991). Antinociceptive effect of para-cetamol in rats is partly dependent on spinal serotonergic systems. *Eur J Pharmacol* **193**:193–201.

16. Bruchhausen, F.V. and Baumann, J. (1982). Inhibitory actions of desacetyla-tion products of phenacetin and paracetamol on prostaglandin synthetases in neuronal and glial cell lines and rat renal medulla. *Life Sci* **30**:1783–91.

17. Piletta, P., Porchet, H.C., and Dayer, P. (1991). Central analgesic effect of acetaminophen but not of aspirin. *Clin Pharmacol Ther* **49**:350–4.

18. Raffa, R.B., Stone, D.J. Jr, and Tallarida, R.J. (2000). Discovery of 'self-synergistic' spinal/supraspinal antinociception produced by acetaminophen (paracetamol). *J Pharmacol Exp Ther* **295**:291–4.

19. Cooper, S.A. (1981). Comparative analgesic efficacies of aspirin and aceta-minophen. *Arch Intern Med* **141**:282–5.

20. Bradley, J.D., Katz, B.P., and Brandt, K.D. (2001). Severity of knee pain does not predict a better response to an antiinflammatory dose of Ibuprofen than to analgesic therapy in patients with osteoarthritis. *J Rheumatol* **28**:1073–6.

21. Pahor, M., Guralnik, J.M., Wan, J.Y., Ferruci, L., Penninx, B.W.J.H., Lyles, A., Ling, S., and Fried, L.P. (1999). Lower body osteoarticular pain and dose of analgesic medications in older disabled women: The Women's Health and Aging Study. *Am J Public Health* **89**:930–4.

22. Sandler, D.P., Smith, J.C., Weinberg, C.R., Buckalew, V.M. Jr., Dennis, V.W., Blythe, W.B., *et al.* (1989). Analgesic use and chronic renal disease. *N Engl J Med* **320**:1238–43.

23. Gates, T.N. and Temple, A.R. (1989). Analgesic use and chronic renal disease (letter). *N Engl J Med* **321**:1125.

24. Fored, C.M., Ejerblad, E., Lindblad, P., Fryzek, J.P., Dickman, P.W., Signorello, L.B., *et al.* (2001). Acetaminophen, aspirin, and chronic renal failure. *N Engl J Med* **345**:1801–8.

25. Rexrode, K.M., Buring, J.E., Glynn, R.J., Stampfer, M.J., Youngman, L.D., and Gaziano, J.M. (2001). Analgesic use and renal function in men. *JAMA* **286**:315–21.

26. USRDS ADR/reference tables. (2001). A. Incidence. Minneapolis: USRDS Coordinating Center, 2001. (Accessed October 24 2001, at http://www.usrds.org/reference.htm)

27. Physicians' Desk Reference (56th ed.). (2002). Montvale, NJ: Medical Economics, p. 2002.

28. Kuffner, E.K., Dart, R.C., Bogdan, G.M., Hill, R.E., Casper, E., and Darton, L. (2001). Effect of maximal daily doses of acetaminophen on the liver of alcoholic patients: A randomised, double-blind, placebo-controlled trial. *Arch Intern Med* **161**:2247–52.

29. Benson, G.D. (1983). Acetaminophen in chronic liver disease. *Clin Pharmacol Ther* **33**:95–101.

30. Taiwo, Y.O. and Levine, J.D. (1988). Prostaglandins inhibit endogenous pain control mechanisms by blocking transmission of spinal nonadrenergic synapses. *J Neurosci* **8**:1346–9.

31. *McCormack, K. and Brune, K. (1991). Dissociation between the antinoci-ceptive and antiinflammatory effects of the nonsteroidal anti-inflammatory drugs. A survey of their analgesic efficacy. *Drugs* **41**:533–47.

    Although somewhat dated, this is a comprehensive overview of the pharmaco-therapeutic characteristics of NSAIDs as analgesics and anti-inflammatory agents.

32. Bradley, J.D., Rudy, A.C., Katz, B.P., Ryan, S.I., Kalasinski, L.A., Brater, D.C., *et al.* (1992). Correlation of serum concentrations of ibuprofen stereoiso-mers with clinical response in the treatment of hip and knee osteoarthritis. *J Rheumatol* **19**:130–4.

33. Urquhart, E. (1993). Central analgesic activity of nonsteroidal anti-inflammatory drugs in animal and human pain models. *Sem Arthritis Rheum* **23**:198–205.

34. Björkman, R., Hedner, J., Hedner, T., and Henning, M. (1990). Central, naloxone-reversible antinociception by diclofenac in the rat. *Nauyn-Schmiedeberg's Arch Pharmacol* **342**:171–6.

35. Pincus, T., Koch, G.G., Sokka, T., *et al.* (2001). A randomized, double-blind, crossover clinical trial of diclofenac plus misoprostol versus acetaminophen in patients with osteoarthritis of the hip or knee. *Arthritis Rheum* **44**:1587–98.

36. Scholes, D., Stergachis, A., Penna, P.M., Normand, E.H., and Hansten, P.D. (1995). Nonsteroidal antiinflammatory drug discontinuation in patients with osteoarthritis. *J Rheumatol* **22**:708–12.

37. Stein, C., Comisel, K., Haimerl, E., Yassouridis, A., Lehrberger, K., Herz, A., *et al.* (1991). Analgesic effect of intra-articular morphine after arthroscopic knee surgery. *N Engl J Med* **325**:1123–6.

38. Basbaum, A.I. and Levine, J.D. (1991). Opiate analgesia: how central is a peripheral target? *N Engl J Med* **325**:1168–9.

39. Levine, J.D. and Taiwo, Yo. (1989). Involvement of the mu-opiate receptor in peripheral analgesia. *Neuroscience* **32**:571–5.

40. Taiwo, Y.O. and Levine, J.D. (1991). κ- and δ-opioids block sympathetically dependent hyperalgesia. *J Neurosci* **11**:928–32.

41. Levine, J.D., Fields, A.L., and Basbaum, A.I. (1993). Peptides and the pri-mary afferent nociceptor. *J Neurosci* **13**:2273–86.

42. Beaver, W.T. (1981). Aspirin and acetaminophen as constituents of analgesic combination. *Arch Intern Med* **141**:293–300.

43. *Pappagallo, M. and Heinberg, L.J. (1997). Ethical Issues In the manage-ment of chronic nonmalignant pain. *Sem Neurol* **17**:203–11.

    This is an excellent appraisal of the issues surrounding the use of opioids in the treatment of chronic non-malignant pain.

44. Schnitzer, T.J., Kamin, M., and Olson, W.H. (1999). Tramadol allows reduc-tion of naproxen dose among patients with naproxen-responsive osteo-arthritis pain: A randomized, double-blind, placebo-controlled study. *Arthritis Rheum* **42**:1370–7.

45. Caldwell, J.R., Hale, M.E., Boyd, R.E., Hague, J.M., Iwan, T., Shi, M., and Lacouture, P.G. (1999). Treatment of osteoarthritis pain with controlled release oxycodone or fixed combination oxycodone plus acetaminophen added to nonsteroidal antiinflammatory drugs: A double blind, random-ized, multicenter, placebo controlled trial. *J Rheumatol* **26**:862–9.

46. Weissman, D.E. and Haddox, J.D. (1989). Opioid pseudoaddiction-an iatro-genic syndrome. *Pain* **36**:363–6.

47. Perkins, P.J. and Doherty, M. (1999). Nonpharmacologic therapy of osteoarthritis. *Cur Rheumatol Reports* **1**:48–53.

48. Jaffe, J.H. and Martin, W.R. (1990). Opioid analgesics and antagonists. In A.G. Gilman, T.W. Rall, A.S. Nies, and P. Taylor (eds) *The Pharmacological Basis of Therapeutics* (8th ed.). New York: MacMillan, pp. 485–521.

49. Roth, S.H., Fleischmann, R.M., Burch, F.X., Dietz, F., Bockow, B., Rapoport, R.J., Rutstein, J., and Lacouture, P.G. (2000). Around-the-clock, controlled-release oxycodone therapy for osteoarthritis-related pain. *Arch Intern Med* **160**:853–60.

50. AGS Panel on Chronic Pain In Older Persons. (1998). The management of chronic pain in older persons. *J Am Geriatr Soc* **46**:635–51.

51. Sjogren, P., Olsen, A.K., Thomsen, A.B., and Dalberg, J. (2000). Neuropsychological performance in cancer patients: the role of oral opioids, pain and performance status. *Pain* **86**:237–45.

52. *Ebly, E.M., Hogan, D.B., and Fung, T.S. (1997). Potential adverse outcomes of psychotropic and narcotic drug use in Canadian seniors. *J Clin Epidemiol* **50**:857–63.

    This paper provides an assessment of the risks associated with opioid analgesics in elderly patients.

53. Bellville, J.W., Forrest, W.H. Jr., Miller, E., and Brown, B.W. (1971). Influence of age on pain relief from analgesics. A study of postoperative patients. *JAMA* **217**:1835–41.

54. Rauck, R.L., Rouff, G.E., and McMillen, J.I. (1994). Comparison of tramadol and acetaminophen with codeine for long-term pain management in elderly patients. *Curr Ther Res* **55**:1417–31.

55. Fleischmann, R.M., Kamin, M., and Olson, W.H. (1999). Safety and efficacy of tramadol for the signs and symptoms of osteoarthritis. *Arthritis Rheum* **42**(Suppl.):S144.

56. Petrone, D., Kamin, M., and Olson, W. (1999). Slowing the titration rate of tramadol HCl reduces the incidence of discontinuation due to nausea and/or vomiting: A double-blind randomized trial. *J Clin Pharm Ther* **24**:115–23.

57. Mullican, W.S. and Lacy, J.R. (for the TRAMAP-ANAG-006 Study Group). (2001). Tramadol/acetaminophen combination tablets and codeine/acetaminophen combination capsules for the management of chronic pain: a comparative trial. *Clin Therapeutics* **23**:1429–45.

58. Parr, G., Darekar, B., Fletcher, A., and Bulpitt, C.J. (1989). Joint pain and quality of life; results of a randomized trial. *Br J Clin Pharmac* **27**:235–42.

59. Boissier, C., Perpoint, B., Laporte-Simitsidis, P., Hocquart, J., Gayel, J.L., Rambaud, C., *et al.* (1992). Acceptability and efficacy of two associations of paracetamol with a central analgesic (dextropropoxyphene or codeine): comparison in osteoarthritis. *J Clin Pharmacol* **32**:990–5.

60. Kjaersgaard-Andersen, P., Nafei, A., Skov, O., Madsen, F., Andersen, H.M., Krøner, K., *et al.* (1990). Codeine plus paracetamol versus paracetamol in longer-term treatment of chronic pain due to osteoarthritis of the hip. A randomized, double-blind multicentre study. *Pain* **43**:309–18.

61. Peloso, P.M., Bellamy, N., Bensen, W., Glen, T.D., Harsanyi, Z., Babul, N., and Darke, A.C. (2000). Double blind randomized placebo control trial of controlled release codeine in the treatment of osteoarthritis of the hip or knee. *J Rheumatol* **27**:764–71.

62. Moulin, D.E., Iezzi, A., Amireh, R., Sharpe, W.K.J., Boyd, D., and Merskey, H. (1996). Randomised trial of oral morphine for chronic non-cancer pain. *Lancet* **347**:143–7.

63. Zenz, M., Strumpf, M., and Tryba, M. (1992). Long-term oral opioid therapy in patients with chronic non-malignant pain. *J Pain Symptom Manage* **7**:69–77.

64. Allan, L., Hays, H., Jensen, N.-H., de Wroux, B.L.P., Bolt, M., Donald, R., and Kalso, E. (2001). Randomised crossover trial of transdermal fentanyl and sustained release oral morphine for treating chronic non-cancer pain. *Br Med J* **322**:1–7.

65. Katz, N.P. (2000). MorphiDex (MS:DM) double-blind studies in chronic pain patients. *J Pain Symptom Manage* **19**(Suppl. 1):S37–S41.

66. *Levy, M.H. (1996). Pharmacologic treatment of cancer pain. *N Engl J Med* **335**:1124–32.

    This is an excellent approach to comprehensive pain management, including non-pharmacologic modalities and combination pharmacotherapy.

67. Feinmann, C. (1985). Pain relief by antidepressants: possible modes of action. *Pain* **23**:1–8.

68. Bradley, J., Flusser, D., Katz, B., Schumacher, H.R. Jr, Brandt, K., Chambers, M., *et al.* (1994). A randomized double-blind, placebo-controlled trial of intravenous loading with S-adenosylmethionine (SAM) followed by oral SAM therapy in patients with knee osteoarthritis. *J Rheumatol* **21**:905–11.

9.3 The role of NSAIDs in the treatment of osteoarthritis

Steven B. Abramson

Non-steroidal anti-inflammatory drugs (NSAIDs) are among the most widely prescribed medications throughout the world. Their use is indicated for a variety of painful musculoskeletal conditions, including OA and rheumatoid arthritis (RA), as well as for other pain syndromes, including dysmenorrhea and headache. Despite a generally favorable benefit-to-risk ratio, long-term NSAID use can be limited by the development of peptic ulcer disease or renal insufficiency, particularly in elderly populations. Both the therapeutic benefit and potential toxicity of these drugs are, in a large measure, due to their capacity to inhibit the synthesis of prostaglandins (PGs) by the cyclooxygenase (COX) enzymes[1] (Fig. 9.1). There are at least two distinct isoforms of PGH synthase, or COX: COX-1 and COX-2. COX-1 is constitutively expressed in many tissues, where it regulates physiological functions. COX-2, an inducible form, is not normally expressed by most tissues, but is upregulated at sites of inflammation and within certain neoplasms.[2,3] This concept, although useful to conceptualize

the COX paradigm, should be understood to be an oversimplification. For example, COX-2 is expressed constitutively in normal tissue, such as kidney and brain, and such expression may increase in response to physiological stress. Conversely, although COX-1 functions as a 'housekeeping' enzyme in many tissues, its expression can also be upregulated in disease.[2,3]

Soon after the discovery of COX-2, it was hypothesized that drugs that selectively inhibited COX-2 would have the beneficial properties of conventional NSAIDs without the disadvantage of their associated gastrointestinal (GI) side effects.[4] This led to the development and introduction of COX-2 selective agents, the coxibs, which have been studied extensively in multicenter randomized clinical trials over the past decade.[5,6] However, despite the burgeoning amount of scientific and clinical information about the coxibs, fundamental questions remain, and new ones have emerged, that have a direct impact on clinical practice. This chapter addresses recent

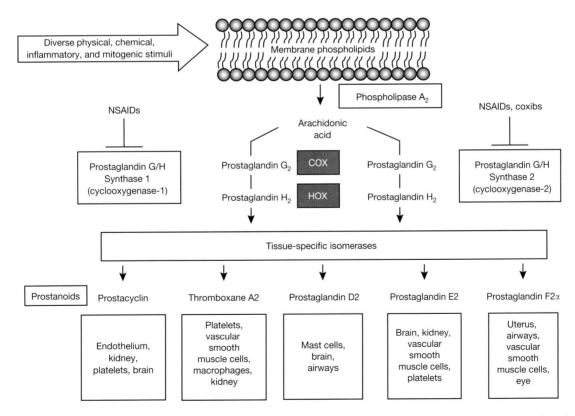

Fig. 9.1 Production of prostaglandins and thromboxane. Upon exposure to a variety of stimuli, arachidonic acid is released from cell membranes through the action of phospholipases. Cyclooxygenases, also known as prostaglandin G/H synthases, metabolize arachidonate to intermediate eicosanoids. The end products vary and are determined by tissue specific terminal enzymes, called isomerases. NSAIDs and coxibs inhibit COX-1 and/or COX-2, as shown. Although COX-2 is induced by cytokines at inflammatory sites, this isoenzyme is also 'constitutively' expressed in a variety of tissues (see Table 9.7).

advances in our understanding of the biology of the COXs and the role of NSAIDs in the treatment of OA.

Biology and regulation of COX-1 and -2

Until the mid-1980s, it was believed that PG formation was limited solely by the activation of phospholipases, which released arachidonate from cell membranes as substrate for a constitutively expressed COX enzyme. In 1988, an interleukin-1 (IL-l)-dependent transcriptional up-regulation of COX was identified in cultured dermal fibroblasts.[1–3] This suggested the existence of second, novel COX isoenzyme, which was synthesized *de novo* in the presence of inflammatory stimuli. A major breakthrough occurred by 1992 with the molecular cloning and characterization of a previously unrecognized COX isoform, designated COX-2 (or PGH synthase-2) that, like COX-1, had an apparent molecular weight of 70 kd.[2,3] COX-1 and -2 share approximately 60 per cent amino acid sequence homology.[2] The promoter region of the COX-2 gene contains response elements that are sensitive to inflammatory mediators, which accounts for its rapid inducibility, while the gene for COX-1 has features consistent with a 'housekeeping' gene product involved in physiologic homeostatic processes. Despite these differences between the COX genes, the domains important for the enzymatic function for arachidonate metabolism are remarkably similar.[2] The COX-2 substrate access channel is larger than the COX-1 channel, however, primarily due to the presence of a side pocket in the COX-2 molecule (Fig. 9.2).[7] This difference can be utilized to develop COX-1 or -2 specific agents.

The most important difference between the two isoforms is their pattern of tissue expression and regulation.[2–4] COX-1 is constitutively expressed in most tissues, notably platelets, endothelial cells, GI tract, renal microvasculature, glomerulus, and collecting ducts.[2,3] Its expression can increase 2- to 4-fold under stimulatory conditions and is little affected by glucocorticoids. COX-2, on the other hand, is typically undetectable in most tissues under basal conditions, but its expression in many cell types, including macrophages, fibroblasts, chondrocytes, epithelial, and endothelial cells, is augmented 10- to 80-fold upon stimulation by inflammatory cytokines, growth factors, or endotoxin. Moreover, COX-2 expression is inhibited by glucocorticoids.[2]

Since the original discovery of COX-2 in cytokine-stimulated cells, it has become apparent that COX-2 is also expressed in a variety of non-inflammatory tissues, including kidney, brain, neoplasms, bone, and cartilage,[2,3] particularly under 'physiologic stress' conditions (Table 9.7). In the kidney, PGs modulate vascular tone and salt and water homeostasis.[2,8] 'Constitutive' expression of COX-2 has been detected in the vasculature, cortical macula densa, and medullary interstitial cells of the kidney, and its expression increases with age.[1,8] COX-2 mRNA and protein are increased by salt and water restriction, suggesting that physiologically important renal PGs derive from both COX-1 and -2 activity. Therefore, it is not surprising that clinical studies indicate that selective COX-2 agents, like conventional NSAIDs, impair compensated renal function in the setting of congestive heart failure or volume depletion.[1,8,9]

COX-2 is also expressed constitutively in the central nervous system (CNS). Selective COX-2 inhibitors are antipyretic, indicating a role for this isoform in the febrile response. COX-2 mRNA and protein are constitutively expressed in excitatory neurons in the brain of rats, predominantly in forebrain neurons in the cortex and hippocampus, and in dendritic spines, which are intimately involved in synaptic signaling. There is evidence that CNS COX-2 plays a role in learning and memory.[2,3] Moreover, there is evidence for separate central analgesic actions of NSAIDS, mediated by the inhibition of CNS COX-2 activity.[10] Finally, with regard to CNS COX expression, there is epidemiological and observational evidence that NSAIDs reduce the incidence and may provide therapeutic benefit in patients with Alzheimer's disease.[11,12] However, it should also be noted that NSAID therapy has been associated with decreased cognition, particularly in the elderly, including longitudinal memory loss.[13]

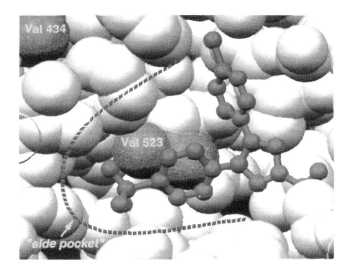

Fig. 9.2 A view of the 'side pocket' in the vicinity of Val 523 present at the active site of COX-2, but not of COX-1. COX-2 selective agents, such as the coxibs, fit into this side pocket, as illustrated, but are too large to be accommodated by the active site of the COX-1 enzyme (from Ref. 7).

Table 9.7 Constitutive expression of COX-2*

Tissue	COX-2 expression	Possible function(s)
Kidney	Macula densa (juxtaglomerular apparatus)	Regulation of intravascular volume
	Medullary interstitial cells	
Brain	Endothelial cells	Febrile response
	Cortical excitatory neurons	Pain
		Neuronal connectivity
		CNS development
		Learning and memory
Bone	Osteoblasts	Osteoclast differentiation
		Regulation of bone remodelling
Colon cancer	Mucosal epithelium	Adhesion of epithelium to extracellular matrix
		Resistance to apoptosis
Female reproductive system	Ovary	Ovulation (follicular rupture)
	Uterus	Embryo implantation
Gastrointestinal tract	Intestinal epithelium	Mucosal fluid secretion
		Bacterial clearance
	Gastric ulcers	Ulcer healing
Blood vessels	Endothelium	Anti-thrombotic (?)

* See reviews in Refs 2 and 4.

COX-2 expression in arthritis

PGs produced by cells within the inflamed joint contribute to the classical inflammatory signs of heat, redness, swelling, and pain. One of the earliest reports of the production of PGs in human arthritis was by Dayer *et al.*,[14] who reported the production of collagenase and PGs by isolated adherent rheumatoid synovial cells. Since the introduction of COX-2 selective agents for the treatment of arthritis, interest has focused upon the distribution of the COX-2 isoform in joint tissues. Crofford and co-workers, in an immunohistologic analysis of COX expression in synovium from patients with RA, observed extensive and intense intracellular COX-2 staining in mononuclear cells and vascular endothelium, with weaker staining in the synovial lining layer.[15] Siegle et al.,[16] analysed sections of synovial tissue from patients with inflammatory arthritides (RA, psoriatic arthritis (PsA), ankylosing spondylitis (AS)) and from patients with OA, using COX-1 and -2-specific antisera for immunostaining. They found that strong COX-2 immunostaining was present in the synovial endothelium, lining cells, fibroblast-like cells, and chondrocytes, in samples from patients with inflammatory arthritis, whereas staining of OA synovial tissue was scant. COX-1 staining was confined to synovial lining cells and no significant differences in staining were apparent among the different arthritides. The detection of COX-1 expression by synovial lining cells was unexpected, and the role of COX-1 derived prostanoids produced by the synovial lining is unknown.

The data from studies by Siegle et al., indicate that the intensity of COX-2 staining is much greater in RA than in OA synovial tissue. In contrast to synovium, however, OA cartilage produces a prodigious amount of PGs, comparable to that observed in RA.[17] OA cartilage explants cultured ex vivo spontaneously release PGE_2 at levels 50-fold times higher than normal cartilage and 18-fold higher than those produced by normal cartilage stimulated with cytokines and endotoxin.[17] This superinduction of PGE_2 coincides with the upregulation of chondrocyte COX-2 mRNA and protein. The addition of IL-1 antagonists to OA explant cultures, inhibits the spontaneous production of PGE_2 by these cultures, indicating that IL-1 derived from chondrocytes induces COX-2 expression and stimulates the production of PGs.[18] Dexamethasone, non-selective NSAIDs and coxibs inhibit the production of PGE_2 by OA cartilage.

The existing literature is contradictory with respect to the potential effects of eicosanoid overproduction on cartilage metabolism. For example, it has been reported that PGE_2 reverses proteoglycan degradation induced by IL-1 in bovine and human cartilage explants, inhibits IL-l-induced matrix metalloprotease (collagenase, stromelysin) expression in human synovial fibroblast and enhances collagen type II and PG synthesis.[18] Conversely, Robinson and colleagues reported in 1978 that PGs produced by rheumatoid explant tissues inhibited cartilage proteoglycan synthesis.[19] In addition, PGE_2 activates metalloproteinases, as has been reported in epithelial cells, human synoviocytes, and human OA cartilage explants.[2] Thus, eicosanoids released by chondrocytes and synovial cells, may exert both anabolic and catabolic effects on matrix metabolism, with the net result on cartilage integrity being uncertain at present.

The use of NSAIDs in osteoarthritis

Evidence for inflammation in osteoarthritis

OA is not classified as inflammatory arthritis. Neutrophils, the cellular hallmark of an acute inflammatory response, do not generally accumulate in OA synovial fluid. Classical signs and symptoms of inflammation—heat, redness, swelling, and pain—are also not typically present. Moreover, as noted above, the expression of COX-2, a marker of inflammatory events in tissue, is not a characteristic feature of OA synovium. COX-2 derived eicosanoids produced by OA chondrocytes embedded within the avascular cartilage, are more likely to play an autocrine/paracrine role in modifying cartilage metabolism than in provoking signs and symptoms of inflammation. Based upon these observations, the inhibition of COX-2 by NSAIDs, selective or non-selective, is not expected to be an important component of therapeutic strategies for OA. Indeed, for many patients, NSAIDs are no more effective than simple analgesics, as will be discussed below.

However, in selected patients inflammatory processes do play a role in provoking signs and symptoms—and, although the data are preliminary, may contribute to the progression of disease[20–23] (Fig. 9.3). For example, individuals may have episodes of recurrent synovitis characterized by increased effusion, warmth, and tenderness of the joint. Such episodes can

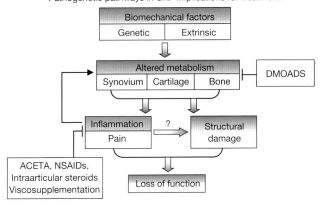

Pathogenetic pathways in OA: Implications for treatment

Fig. 9.3 Schema of the pathogenesis of OA. Current treatments, including acetaminophen (ACETA), NSAIDs, viscosupplementation (see Chapter 9.8) and intra-articular steroid injections, relieve pain and/or inflammation. Putative disease-modifying OA drugs (DMOADs) (discussed in Chapter 11.2.2) target the metabolic abnormalities that contribute to the structural deterioration of cartilage or changes in the subchondral bone. The question mark indicates that whether inflammation promotes the progression of structural damage in patients with OA is unproved.

result from local synovial reactions to cartilage debris or calcium crystal deposition, although precipitating factors in the majority of patients are unknown.[24] Elevations of serum CRP, a marker of inflammation, have been reported in patients with OA and may identify a subset at risk for more rapid disease progression.[20] Areas of increased radionuclide uptake ('hot spots' on bone scintigraphy) have also been reported to identify joints that are more likely to show radiographic progression of OA or to require surgical intervention[21] (see Chapter 11.4.5).

Arthroscopy has provided new insights to the presence of inflammation in OA and the possible implications for disease progression. Studies of patients with knee pain indicate that as many as 20 per cent exhibit evidence of hyperplastic synovitis.[22] The histological findings in these patients include hyperemia, proliferation of the lining cells, and a moderate infiltration of mononuclear cells in the subintimal layers.[22,23] Unlike the inflamed synovium of RA, osteoarthritic synovitis is localized, often to the region of the cartilage lesion. Work by Dougados and co-workers suggests that arthroscopic evidence of synovitis in OA is a risk factor for progressive cartilage degeneration.[22,23] These intriguing arthroscopy findings need corroboration and their correlation with routine radiographs, serum biomarkers such as CRP, MRI, and bone scintigraphy remains to be determined.

Simple analgesics versus anti-inflammatory drugs in osteoarthritis

Efficacy of acetaminophen versus NSAIDs. In choosing specific pharmacotherapy, it is important to keep in mind that the reduction of joint pain for most patients with OA is modest, in the order of 20–30 per cent.[25] Therefore, treatment programs should ensure that non-pharmacological therapy is optimized, including proper exercise, weight loss, and the use of assisting devices, as needed.[26–28] Strategies for drug treatment need to take into account the heterogeneity of the disease among patients, which can affect large and small joints, as well as articulations of the axial skeleton. The course of disease will also vary among individuals. Typically, symptomatic OA is characterized by chronic pain, worsened by activity, which can range from mild to severe. Symptoms often deteriorate over time as the structural damage to articular cartilage progresses. As noted above, chronic symptoms may be punctuated by acute exacerbations, sudden increases in pain or swelling, that may require therapeutic intervention with anti-inflammatory drugs, such as intra-articular corticosteroids or brief courses of NSAIDs.

Notwithstanding the heterogeneity of the patients described above, attempts have been made by professional organizations to establish treatment guidelines for OA. It is generally accepted that the initial drug treatment for most patients with symptomatic OA is simple analgesia, using agents such as acetaminophen. This is the formal recommendation in the guidelines published by the European League Against Rheumatism (EULAR) in 2000[29] and the American College of Rheumatology (ACR) in 1995.[28] The revised ACR guidelines, published in 2000, state that 'the prescription of an NSAID merits consideration as an alternative initial therapeutic approach' in patients with severe pain.[27] These revised recommendations have been the subject of debate that has focused on several issues: (1) the evidence that NSAIDs are more effective than acetaminophen as initial therapy in selected OA populations (e.g., those with inflammation); (2) the evidence that the clinician's criteria for 'severe' or inflammatory disease can predict NSAID responders; (3) the uncertainty that the COX-2 selective NSAIDs have a safety profile comparable to simple analgesics; and (4) the socioeconomic cost-benefit of simple analgesic versus the more expensive COX-2 selective agents or coxibs. Despite the merits of the debate, it is noteworthy that since the introduction of the selective COX-2 agents, the use of NSAIDs for the treatment of OA has markedly increased, so that more than 50 per cent of all NSAID prescriptions for patients over 65 years old who are 'new' to NSAID therapy are now written for a coxib, rather than for a non-selective NSAID.[25]

What is the evidence that informs this debate? Clinical trials evaluating NSAIDs clearly demonstrate a short-term symptomatic effect that is superior to placebo, and most indicate a safer GI profile for coxibs than for non-selective NSAIDs. However, the cost of the coxibs is substantially higher than simple analgesics or most non-selective NSAIDs and concerns for cardiovascular safety have emerged, as discussed below, which make it important to evaluate the benefit-to-risk of NSAIDs versus simple analgesia with acetaminophen. In the classical studies by Bradley and Brandt in patients with mild to moderate knee OA, anti-inflammatory doses of ibuprofen (2400 mg/day) were not more effective than either analgesic doses of ibuprofen (1200 mg/day) or acetaminophen (4 g/day).[30,31] Subset analysis, however, did suggest that the anti-inflammatory dose of ibuprofen was superior to acetaminophen in patients with rest pain. Based on this and other studies the EULAR recommendations state that acetaminophen (or paracetamol) 'is the oral analgesic to try first and, if successful, is the preferred long-term oral analgesic'.[29,30]

While these and other studies indicate that acetaminophen *can be* as effective as NSAIDs in many patients with OA, there are also data to indicate that NSAIDs provide superior efficacy in subsets of patients.[32,33] A meta-analysis conducted by the North of England Non-steroidal Anti-inflammatory Drug Guideline Development Group[34] showed that patients taking NSAIDs had significantly greater improvement in both pain at rest and pain on motion than those taking acetaminophen. Wolfe et al.,[32] examining the opinions of patients with hip or knee OA about the effectiveness of their own treatment with NSAIDs and acetaminophen, found that a greater percentage of those surveyed reported that NSAIDs were more effective than acetaminophen than vice versa. Nonetheless, nearly half of those who responded to the survey reported that acetaminophen was at least effective, and as satisfactory, as the NSAIDs they had received.

For patients with mild to moderate joint pain, some studies have indicated that the difference in efficacy between NSAIDs and acetaminophen is negligible but that differences between these two treatments emerge among patients with more severe symptoms or, possibly, in those with disease of the hip.[33,35] The sum of the evidence suggests that although NSAIDs are more efficacious than acetaminophen in some OA patients, it is reasonable to use acetaminophen as an initial treatment, particularly in patients who have no prior experience with either NSAIDs or acetaminophen, or who have risk factors associated with NSAID-induced GI adverse events (Table 9.8). However, patients who report a previous lack of benefit from a full dose of acetaminophen (i.e., 4 g/day) or, as suggested by the recent American College of Rheumatology Guidelines,[36] who present with a flare of disease accompanied by the recent onset of signs of inflammation, might rationally

Table 9.8 Risk factors for serious GI or renal adverse events in patients taking NSAIDs

Gastro-intestinal	Renal
Age over 65	Age over 65
History of previous peptic ulcer disease	History of hypertension
History of upper GI bleeding	Congestive heart failure
Anticoagulants, including aspirin	Diuretic use
Oral corticosteroids	Angiotensin converting enzyme inhibitors (ACE)
Comorbid medical conditions	

be treated with an NSAID. In retrospective analyses, however, neither the presence of a knee effusion nor the severity of knee pain predicted a better response to an anti-inflammatory dose of ibuprofen than to acetaminophen.[31,37] Prospective clinical trials of NSAIDs versus acetaminophen, in which patients are randomized on the basis of signs of inflammation or severity of joint pain, have not been performed.

In any case, clinical guidelines should not be rigid. The judgment of the physician, the effectiveness of non-pharmacologic measures, and observations made during timely follow-up assessments should all factor into therapeutic decisions about the care of the individual patient.

Safety of acetaminophen versus NSAIDs. Given the data that suggest that NSAIDs may have superior efficacy in selected OA populations, it should be noted that expert recommendations that favor acetaminophen as initial therapy are influenced by its lesser cost and perceived greater safety. While there is little doubt that the economics favor acetaminophen use, two questions have emerged regarding adverse events: (1) is full-dose acetaminophen (4 g/day) associated with more toxicity than previously appreciated and (2) does the improved GI safety profile of the coxibs change the benefit-to-risk ratio that had previously favored acetaminophen over non-selective NSAIDs?

Acetaminophen is generally considered to be safe and well tolerated. Acute hepatotoxicity, with liver failure, may occur with overdose, however, and has been observed with doses in excess of 150 mg/kg/day (>10 g/d).[38] The risk of hepatotoxicity, even with therapeutic doses of acetaminophen, is reported to increase in patients with excessive alcohol consumption.[38,39] However, a systematic review of the effect of therapeutic doses of acetaminophen in patients with chronic alcoholism showed that serious confounding conditions that could have caused hepatotoxicity were present in nearly all reported cases.[40] Furthermore, administration of acetaminophen to chronic alcoholics shortly after their admission to a detoxification center resulted in no greater increase in serum transaminase levels than placebo.[41]

Whether patients with non-alcoholic chronic liver disease are at risk for acetaminophen hepatotoxicity is unknown at present. Benson[42] reported that administration of acetaminophen, 4 g/d, to subjects with a variety of chronic liver diseases increased the mean half-life of the drug, but did not result in an increase in liver damage. However, these observations reflect an experience in only 20 subjects studied for less than two weeks and must be interpreted with caution. No prospective studies examining the risk of hepatotoxicity from chronic administration of therapeutic doses of acetaminophen in patients with underlying liver disease have been performed.

An additional area that merits consideration is the potential association of analgesic drugs and chronic renal insufficiency. In a recent nation-wide, case-controlled study, Swedish investigators demonstrated that regular use of either aspirin or acetaminophen was associated, in a dose-dependent manner, with an increased risk of chronic renal failure.[43] The authors acknowledged the possibility of bias caused by consumption of the analgesics because of symptoms related to the underlying condition that predisposed to renal failure.

Based on the above and prior studies and earlier reports, it is recommended that clinicians carefully consider the use of aspirin, acetaminophen, and NSAIDs in patients with chronic renal disease.[44] Caution is required in recommending the restriction of moderate doses of acetaminophen that might induce patients to change to other medications, such as NSAIDs, whose safety is more questionable than that of acetaminophen. A National Kidney Foundation position paper states that 'acetaminophen … remains the non-narcotic analgesic of choice for episodic use in patients with underlying renal disease …, but habitual consumption of acetaminophen should be discouraged (and if) indicated medically, long-term use of this drug should be supervised by a physician' (see Chapter 9.2).[45]

The most serious adverse events seen with the use of non-selective NSAIDs are related to NSAID-associated peptic ulcer disease and its complications (e.g., hemorrhage, perforation, gastric outlet obstruction). Notably, many patients who incurred a serious GI complication from use of an NSAID have not had prior GI symptoms.[46] Furthermore, GI hemorrhage appears to be associated not only with prescription use of aspirin and other NSAIDs, but also with OTC use of these agents. In a recent study of more than 400 patients undergoing evaluation for upper GI hemorrhage, use of OTC aspirin or non-aspirin NSAID during the week prior to admission was reported by 35 and 9 per cent, respectively, while prescription use of aspirin or a non-aspirin NSAID was reported in 6 and 14 per cent, respectively.[47] Given the very common use of OTC agents, short-term NSAID use may be a major cause of ulcer-related GI hemorrhage.

Clinical trials that have compared acetaminophen with NSAIDs in the treatment of OA have generally been short-term (less than 12 weeks), using 4 g/d of acetaminophen. In these studies the risk of adverse GI events associated with the use of non-selective NSAIDs has been greater than that with acetaminophen, resulting in a benefit-to-risk ratio that favored acetaminophen. However, a recent nested case-control study by García Rodríguez et al.,[48] using the United Kingdom General Practitioners Research database, indicated that after adjustment for age, sex, ulcer history, smoking and the use of steroids, anticoagulants, gastroprotective drugs, aspirin and prescription (but not OTC) NSAIDs, doses of acetaminophen greater than 2 g/d conferred a risk for upper GI complications as great as that with traditional NSAIDs. If that observation is correct, the mechanism underlying upper GI toxicity of high-dose acetaminophen could theoretically be related to its ability to function as a weak inhibitor of COX-1.[49,50] It should be noted that these recent findings by García Rodríguez[44] require further investigation. Direct comparisons between COX-2 specific inhibitors and acetaminophen in large outcome trials exceeding 6 months duration are not available, but are needed to determine the most appropriate initial pharmacological therapy of patients with OA.

Safety of COX-2 selective NSAIDs versus non-selective NSAIDs. Non-selective NSAIDs are not only associated with an increased risk for serious upper GI complications, but also with nephrotoxicity, including renal insufficiency, hypertension, peripheral edema and congestive heart failure.[8,46,51,52] Epidemiological studies indicate that the risk of serious upper GI complications is greater in certain patient groups, particularly in the elderly.[46,51,52] (Table 9.8)

Soon after the discovery of COX-2, it was hypothesized that an NSAID that selectively inhibited COX-2 would have the beneficial properties of NSAIDs without the associated GI side effects. Endoscopic studies have shown that the coxibs are associated with a lower incidence of gastroduodenal ulcers than comparator non-selective NSAIDs.[53–55] Moreover, there is evidence that the coxibs are better tolerated than non-selective NSAIDs with respect to the incidence of non-specific abdominal pain and dyspepsia.[56] On the other hand, Langman et al.,[57] in an analysis of eight double-blind randomized clinical trials of rofecoxib in patients with OA, found that the cumulative incidence of non-specific GI adverse events, such as dyspepsia, epigastric pain, nausea, and diarrhea, was less prevalent with this coxib than with comparator NSAIDs over 6 months. However, the magnitude of the difference, although statistically significant ($p = 0.02$), was small (23.5 vs. 25.5 per cent, respectively) and not *clinically* significant and the incidence rates converged after 6 months.

Two Phase IV large outcome studies of at least 6 months duration, published in the fall of 2000, indicate that the use of coxibs is accompanied by a lower incidence of serious GI toxicity than that seen with comparator NSAIDs.[5,6] The Celecoxib Long-term Arthritis Safety Study (CLASS) compared celecoxib at a dose of 400 mg twice daily to diclofenac 75 mg twice daily, and to ibuprofen, 800 mg three times daily, in a study which randomized more than 8000 patients, approximately 75 per cent of whom had OA and 25 per cent RA. Analysis of data from more than 4400 patients who received treatment for 6 months showed that celecoxib did not significantly reduce the frequency of ulcer complications (0.76 vs. 1.45 per cent, $p = 0.09$) in comparison with the non-selective NSAIDs,[5] although the difference with respect to the combination of symptomatic ulcers and ulcer complications was statistically significant (2.08 vs. 3.54 per cent, $p = 0.02$). Furthermore, no superiority of celecoxib, relative to the comparator NSAIDs, was apparent in those subjects who received low-dose aspirin for cardiovascular prophylaxis during the study (approximately 20 per cent of all subjects enrolled) and there was no significant difference between treatment groups with respect to either ulcer complications or the combination of ulcer complications and symptomatic ulcers among those who remained on treatment for 13 months.[58]

The Vioxx® Gastrointestinal Outcomes Research (VIGOR) Trial compared rofecoxib, 50 mg once daily, to naproxen, 500 mg twice daily, in nearly 9000 patients with RA; none of them were taking low-dose aspirin. In this study, in which the median duration of follow-up was 9 months, the incidence of confirmed upper GI events was significantly reduced in patients receiving rofecoxib.[6]

The CLASS and VIGOR trials were not designed to demonstrate that the risk of hemorrhage or perforation in patients using coxibs is equivalent to that of subjects receiving placebo. However, the results of these studies, and of other randomized clinical trials that preceded them, make it reasonable to recommend the use of a coxib when an NSAID is indicated for patients who are at increased risk for serious upper GI complications[4] (Table 9.8), at least in subjects who are not taking low-dose aspirin. Co-administration of a gastroprotective agent, such as a proton pump inhibitor or misoprostol, has been shown to reduce the incidence of GI adverse events in patients taking a non-selective NSAID.[59–61] The merit of combining a gastroprotective agent with a coxib in at-risk patients is unknown.

An unanticipated finding in the VIGOR trial was an apparent increase in the incidence of myocardial infarction in the rofecoxib group, relative to the naproxen group. Specifically, 20 of the 4047 subjects in the rofecoxib group (0.5 per cent), but only 4 of 4029 (0.1 per cent) in the naproxen group, had a myocardial infarction during the study. In contrast to the CLASS trial, low-dose aspirin use was an exclusion criterion in the VIGOR study. However, even if subjects who were candidates for secondary cardiovascular prophylaxis (e.g., those with a history of myocardial infarction, cerebral vascular accident, transient ischemic attacks, angina, a coronary artery bypass graft or angioplasty) were excluded, the incidence of myocardial infarction in the rofecoxib group remained higher than that in the naproxen group (12 of 3877 (0.3 per cent) versus 4 of 3878 (0.1 per cent), respectively).[58]

Because the absolute number of cardiovascular events in the VIGOR trial was low and the study was not powered to examine the incidence of cardiovascular events, additional studies are needed to determine whether this observation was due to an increased risk for thrombosis imparted by rofecoxib, to a protective effect of the comparator drug, naproxen, or to chance alone. Interpretation of the VIGOR data is also complicated by the fact that the patients enrolled in this study had RA, a disease that may, itself, increase the risk of coronary thrombosis.[62]

Unopposed COX-1 activity has become the focus of current debate regarding the possible thrombogenic potential of the coxibs. Physiologically, thromboxane derived from platelets promotes vasoconstriction and platelet aggregation, while prostacyclin (PGI$_2$) derived from vascular endothelium has opposite effects, promoting vasodilation and inhibiting platelet aggregation. The consequences of a reduction in prostacyclin production by vascular endothelial cells, resulting from selective inhibition of COX-2 in the presence of unopposed thromboxane production, mediated by unopposed COX-1 activity in the platelets have led to questions about the cardiovascular safety of coxibs.[1,6] In a canine model of coronary artery thrombosis, celecoxib abolished the prolongation of the time to artery occlusion, which resulted from the administration of aspirin and the vasodilatation that normally occurs in response to the production of prostacyclin by vascular endothelium.[63] Conversely, other data raise the possibility that inhibition of COX-2 could be *beneficial* in atherosclerotic disease. COX-2 is expressed in macrophage-rich areas of atherosclerotic plaques. Pharmacologic inhibition of COX-2 is accompanied by a decrease in the levels of matrix matalloproteinases (MMPs) in the atherosclerotic plaques.[64] It has been suggested that local synthesis of COX-2 by activated macrophages may be associated with acute ischemic syndromes, perhaps as a result of the rupture of plaques induced by the action of MMPs.[64]

Until more information is available, it is prudent to prescribe low-dose aspirin (≤325 mg daily) or another anti-platelet agent in patients treated with coxibs who are at risk for cardiovascular events. Certainly, because they do not inhibit platelet aggregation, it should be recognized that coxibs alone confer no cardiovascular protection.[65] To further add to the complexity of the current clinical decision, a new question has emerged regarding the concomitant use of NSAIDs and aspirin: namely, do non-selective NSAIDs, which may compete for aspirin at the COX-1 catalytic site, interfere with its cardioprotective activity? A report by Catella-Lawson and colleagues has indicated that the concomitant administration of ibuprofen (400 mg), but not rofecoxib (25 mg) or diclofenac (75 mg), antagonized the irreversible platelet inhibition (platelet aggregation and thromboxane B2 production) induced by low-dose aspirin (81 mg).[50] In these studies, acetaminophen (1000 mg), was shown to be a weak non-specific COX inhibitor, but did not antagonize the aspirin effect. Future studies will need to address these unanswered questions regarding the interaction among aspirin, non-selective NSAIDs, and coxibs, with respect to both gastrointestinal and cardiovascular safety.

Can the cardiovascular findings in the VIGOR study be generalized to all patients taking COX-2 selective inhibitors? The answer is not known. Although the absolute incidence of myocardial infarction in the VIGOR trial was comparable to that in CLASS, the VIGOR study excluded patients with angina pectoris or symptomatic congestive heart failure, while CLASS did not. Hence, patients in the CLASS study may have been at greater risk for myocardial infarction than those in the VIGOR trial. On the other hand, as noted above, the VIGOR study excluded subjects taking low-dose aspirin or other antiplatelet agents, such as ticlopidine (surrogates for coronary artery disease). Therefore, several key questions remain unanswered:

1. Does rofecoxib increase the risk of thromboses, and if so, is this a property of the class of highly selective COX-2 inhibitors?

2. Should risk factors for cardiovascular disease or thrombosis (e.g., hypertension, diabetes, obesity, antiphospholipid antibodies, total knee replacement surgery) be considered relative contraindications to therapy with a selective COX-2 inhibitor?

3. Does the use of low-dose aspirin nullify the gastroprotective advantage of COX-2 selective NSAID over conventional NSAIDs, as suggested, but not proven, by the CLASS trial?

These key clinical questions cannot be answered unequivocally on the basis of the current evidence, and require further intensive study.[66]

GI complications are not the only risks of NSAID therapy. Other adverse events include alterations in renal function, effects on blood pressure, and fluid retention, including increased risk for congestive heart failure. Because renal sodium excretion is at least partially mediated by COX-2, fluid retention and hypertension occur with both non-specific and COX-2 specific inhibitors.[1] In the CLASS trial, the percentage of patients having the adverse event of peripheral edema was similar for those receiving celecoxib and those receiving non-selective NSAIDs.[5] In the VIGOR trial, the incidence of adverse effects related to renal function in the rofecoxib group was similar to that in naproxen-treated patients.[6] There is no convincing evidence that COX-2 in vascular endothelium, kidney, or elsewhere, is inhibited more effectively by coxibs than by conventional NSAIDs. However, it is unclear whether unopposed COX-1 activity resulting from selective COX-2 inhibition will result in yet undetermined toxicity. At present, the data indicate

that COX selectivity confers neither an advantage nor disadvantage with respect to the development of renal side effects.

An additional concern regarding NSAID therapy pertains to potential effects on fracture healing. Emerging evidence suggests that NSAID administration in patients undergoing spinal fusion surgery may increase non-union rates.[67,68] Similarly, in a recent study of fractures of the diaphysis of the femur in 92 patients, there was a marked association between non-union and the use of NSAIDs after fracture, and delayed healing was noted in patients who took NSAIDs and whose fractures had united.[69] Whether differences exist between selective and non-selective COX-2 inhibitors with respect to their effects on bone healing and repair is unknown.

Other anti-inflammatory agents in OA

The above discussion has focused on the role of NSAIDs in relieving the signs and symptoms of OA. Additional drugs are under investigation, which may prove useful in the future therapy of symptomatic OA. These include diacerein, glucosamine, and nitric oxide-releasing NSAIDs.

Nitric-oxide releasing NSAIDs (NO-NSAIDs) are chemical entities obtained by adding a nitroxybutyl moiety to a conventional NSAID. NO-NSAIDs inhibit inflammation via COX-dependent and -independent effects. These compounds retain the anti-inflammatory, analgesic, and antipyretic activity of the parent compound but appear to have less GI toxicity.[70,71] Epidemiological studies have also shown that nitric oxide donor drugs reduce the risk of upper GI bleeding, which might be important in patients receiving low-dose aspirin. In a study by Lanas *et al.*[70] in patients taking any type of NSAID, the use of nitrovasodilator therapy was independently associated with a decreased risk of bleeding. Experimental evidence indicates that NO-releasing NSAIDs may act, in part, by enhancing the production of PGs by gastric mucosa.[71] There is also experimental evidence to indicate an inhibition of neutrophilic infiltration that characterizes acute ulcer formation.

Finally, it should be noted that, in contrast to simple analgesics and NSAIDs, agents such as hyaluronan, glucosamine, and diacerhein have been reported not only to relieve joint pain and improve function, but also to have structure-modifying effects in OA (although, in each case, reservations exist with respect to the latter conclusion) (see Chapters 9.8, 9.9, and 11.2.2). Studies are required to determine whether these compounds should be combined with acetaminophen or NSAIDs to provide optimal efficacy in patients with OA.

Summary

NSAIDs are among the most widely prescribed drugs used for the treatment of OA. While simple analgesics, such as acetaminophen, are indicated in the initial pharmacological therapy of OA, some patients will obtain insufficient benefits from acetaminophen and will require treatment with NSAIDs for symptomatic improvement. In some instances, symptomatic improvement with an NSAID is greater than with acetaminophen, perhaps due to the presence of synovitis, caused by deposition of calcium crystals, fragments of cartilage or bone, or by unknown stimuli. The use of NSAIDs has been associated with serious adverse events in 1–4 per cent of patients, including GI hemorrhage and perforation, congestive heart failure, and renal insufficiency. The introduction of selective COX-2 inhibitors has improved the benefit-to-risk ratio, in comparison with non-selective COX inhibitors, because of the decreased incidence of serious GI adverse events. However, the coxibs offer no apparent advantage over conventional NSAIDs with respect to other toxicities, such as hypertension, fluid retention, and congestive heart failure, presumably because COX-2 is expressed not only at the sites of inflammation, but also in normal tissue, often in response to conditions of physiological stress. Because they do not confer the anti-platelet effects associated with COX-1 inhibitors, there is some concern that selective COX-2 inhibitors may increase the risk for cardiovascular thrombotic events. Large clinical outcome trials will be needed to determine the validity of this concern. In contrast to simple analgesics and NSAIDs, agents such as hyaluronan, glucosamine, and diacerein may not only relieve joint pain and improve function, but may also prove to have structure-modifying effects in OA.

Key points

1. At least two distinct isoforms of cyclooxygenase exist. COX-1 is constitutively expressed in many tissues, where it regulates physiological functions. COX-2, an inducible form is upregulated at sites of inflammation. COX-2 is also expressed in normal tissue, often in response to conditions of physiological stress.

2. Inflammatory synovitis occurs in a subset of patients with OA and may contribute to the disease process in these patients, such as may occur in response to calcific deposits, cartilage fragments, or unknown stimuli.

3. For most patients with symptomatic OA, initial drug treatment should be a simple analgesic, such as acetaminophen. Prescription of an NSAID merits consideration as an alternative initial therapeutic approach in selected patients with severe pain and clinical evidence of acute inflammation.

4. The introduction of selective COX-2 inhibitors (coxibs) has improved the GI benefit-to-risk ratio, in comparison with that seen with non-selective COX inhibitors.

5. The coxibs offer no apparent advantage over conventional NSAIDs with respect to other toxicities, such as hypertension, fluid retention, or congestive heart failure.

6. Because it is unclear whether coxibs increase the risk of thrombosis, it is prudent to prescribe low-dose aspirin ($=325$ mg daily) or another anti-platelet agent in patients treated with coxibs who are at risk for cardiovascular thrombotic events.

References

(An asterisk denotes recommended reading.)

1. *Fitzgerald, G.A. and Patrono, C. (2001). The coxibs: selective inhibitors of cyclooxygenase-2. N Engl J Med 345:433–42.

    This comprehensive review of the literature regarding the benefit-to-risk ratio of treatment with coxibs versus non-selective NSAIDs, addresses the theoretical basis for concerns about potential consequences of unbalanced COX-2 inhibition.

2. *DuBois, R.N., Abramson. S.B., Crofford, L.J., et al. (1998). Cyclooxygenase in biology and disease. FASEB J 12:1063–73.

    This article by an international group of investigators, the COX-2 Study Group, reviews the expression and regulation of the cyclooxygenases. The expression of COX-2 in normal tissue and under conditions of physiological stress provides insight into the non-gastrointestinal toxicities of selective COX-2 inhibitors.

3. Smith, W.L. and Langenbach, R. (2001). Why there are two cyclooxygenase isozymes. J Clin Invest 107:1491–5.

4. Lipsky, P.E., Abramson, S.B., Breedveld, F.C., et al. (2000). Analysis of the effect of COX-2 specific inhibitors and recommendations for their use in clinical practice. J Rheumatol 27:1338–40.

5. Silverstein, F.E., Faich, G., Goldstein, J.L., et al. (2000). Gastrointestinal toxicity with celecoxib vs. nonsteroidal anti-inflammatory drugs for osteoarthritis and rheumatoid arthritis. The CLASS Study: a randomized controlled trial. JAMA 284:1247–55.

6. Bombardier, C., Laine, L., Reicin, A., et al. (2000). A double-blind comparison of rofecoxib and naproxen on the incidence of clinically important upper gastrointestinal events: the VIGOR trial. N Eng J Med 343:1520–8.

7. Fitzgerald, G.A. and Loll, P., COX in a crystal ball (2001). Currrent status and future promise of prostaglandin research. J Clin Invest 107:1335–7.

8. Brater, D.C., Harris, C., Redfern, J.S., and Gertz, B.J. (2001). Renal effects of COX-2 selective inhibitors. Am J Nephrol 21:1–15.

9. Swan, S.K., Rudy, D.W., Lasseter, K.C., et al. (2000). Effect of COX2 inhibition on renal function in elderly persons receiving a low salt diet. Ann Int Med 133:1–9.

10. Cashman, J.N. (1996). The mechanisms of action of NSAIDs in analgesia. Drugs 52:13–23.

11. Stewart, W.F., Kawas, C., Corrada, M., et al. (1997). Risk of Alzheimer's disease and duration of NSAID use. Neurology 48:626–32.

12. Bas, A., Ruitenberg, A., Hoffman, A., et al. (2001). Nonsteroidal antiinflammatory drugs and the risk of Alzheimer's disease. N Eng J Med 345:1515–21.

13. Saag, K.G., Rubeinstein, L.M., Chrischilles, E.A., et al. (1995). Nonsteroidal antiinflammatory drugs and cognitive decline in the elderly. J Rheumatol 22:2142–7.

14. Dayer, J.M., Krane, S.M., Russell, R.G., and Robinson, D.R. (1976). Production of collagenase and prostaglandins by isolated adherent rheumatoid synovial cells. Proc Natl Acad Sci USA 73:945–9.

15. Crofford, J. (1999). COX-2 in synovial tissues. Osteoarthritis Cart 7:406–8.

16. Siegle, I., Klein, T., Backman, J.T., Saal, J.G., Nusing, R.M., and Fritz, P. (1998). Expression of cyclooxygenase 1 and cyclooxygenase 2 in human synovial tissue. Arthritis Rheum 41:122–9.

17. Amin, A.R., Attur, M., Patel, R.J., et al. (1997). Superinduction of cyclooxygenase-2 activity in human osteoarthritis-affected cartilage. J Clin Invest 99:1231–7.

18. Pelletier, J.-P., Martel-Pelletier, J., and Abramson, S.B. (2001). Osteoarthritis, an inflammatory disease. Potential implication of new therapeutic targets. Arthritis Rheum 44:1237–47.

19. Lippiello, L., Yamamoto, K., Robinson, D., and Mankin, H.J. (1978). Involvement of prostaglandins from rheumatoid synovium in inhibition of articular cartilage metabolism. Arthritis Rheum 21:909–17.

20. Spector, T.D., Hart, D.J., Nandra, D., et al. (1997). Low-level increases in serum c-reactive protein are present in early osteoarthritis of the knee and predict progressive disease. Arthritis Rheum 40:723–7.

21. Dieppe, P.A., Cushnaghan, J., Young, P., and Kirwan, J. (1993). Prediction of the progression of joint space narrowing of the knee by bone scintigraphy. Ann Rheum Dis 52:557–63.

22. Ayral, X., Dougados, M., Listrat, V., Bonvarlet, J.P., Simonnet, J., and Amor, B. (1996). Arthroscopic evaluation of chondropathy in osteoarthritis of the knee. J Rheumatol 23:698–706.

23. Ayral., X., Pickering, E.H., Woodworth, T.J., McKillop, N., Loose, L., and Dougados, M. (2001). Synovitis predicts the arthroscopic progression of medial tibiofemoral knee osteoarthritis (OA) (abstract). Ann Rheum Dis 60:57.

24. Concoff, A.L. and Kalunian, K.C. (1999). What is the relation between crystals and osteoarthritis? Curr Opin Rheumatol 11:436–40.

25. *Brandt, K.D. and Bradley, J.D. (2001). Should the initial drug used to treat osteoarthritis pain be a nonsteroidal antiinflammatory drug? J Rheumatol 28:467–73.

    This thoughtful and provocative response to the recent OA treatment guidelines published by the American College of Rheumatology raises important clinical, commercial, and pharmacoeconomic issue that affect therapeutic decision-making.

26. Mazzuca, S.A., Brandt, K.D., Katz, B.P., Chabers, M., Byrd, D., and Hanna, M. (1997). Effects of self-care education on the health status of inner-city patients with osteoarthritis of the knee. Arthritis Rheum 40:1466–74.

27. *American College of Rheumatology Subcommittee on Osteoarthritis Guidelines. (2000). Recommendations for the medical management of osteoarthritis of the hip and knee: 2000 Update. Arthritis Rheum 43:1905–15.

    This article and the EULAR recommendations[29] indicate the position of two leading professional organizations attempting to formulate evidence-based guidelines for treatment of OA.

28. Hochberg, M.C., Altman, R.D., Brandt, K.D., et al. (1995). Guidelines for the medical management of osteoarthritis. Part I: Osteoarthritis of the Hip; and Part II: Osteoarthritis of the Knee. Arthritis Rheum 38:1535–46.

29. Pendleton, A., Arden, M., Dougados, M., and Lequesne, M. (2000). EULAR recommendations for the management of knee osteoarthritis: Report of a task force of the Standing Committee for International Clinical Studies Including Therapeutic Trials (ESCISIT). Ann Rheum Dis 59:936–44.

30. Bradley, J.D., Brandt, K.D., Katz, B.P., Kalasinski, L.A. and Ryan, S.I. (1991). Comparison of an anti-inflammatory dose of ibuprofen, an analgesic dose of ibuprofen, and acetaminophen in the treatment of patients with osteoarthritis of the knee. *N Engl J Med* **325**:87–91.

31. Bradley, J.D., Brandt, K.D., Katz, B.P., Kalansinski, L.A. and Ryan, S.I. (1992). Treatment of knee osteoarthritis: relationship of clinical features of joint inflammation to the response to a nonsteroidal anti-inflammatory drug or pure analgesic. *J Rheumatol* **19**:1950–4.

32. Wolfe, F., Zhao, S., and Lane, N. (2000). Preference for nonsteroidal antiinflammatory drugs over acetaminophen by rheumatic disease patients. *Arthritis Rheum* **43**:378–85.

33. Pincus, T., Koch, G.G., Sokka, T., et al. (2001). A randomized, double-blind, crossover clinical trial of diclofenac plus misoprostol versus acetaminophen in patients with osteoarthritis of the hip or knee. *Arthritis Rheum* **44**:1587–98.

34. Eccles, M., Freemantle, N., and Mason, J. (2001). North of England Evidence Based Guideline Development Project: summary guideline for non-steroidal anti-inflammatory drugs versus basic analgesia in treating the pain of degenerative arthritis. *Br Med J* **1998**:317–526.

35. *Felson, D.T. (2001). The verdict favors nonsteroidal antiinflammatory drugs for the treatment of osteoarthritis and a plea for more evidence on other treatments. *Arthritis Rheum* **44**:1477–80.

   This editorial presents the views of a leading clinical epidemiologist with respect to the evidence regarding the use of NSAIDs and simple analgesics in OA.

36. Altman, R.D., Hochberg, M.C., Moskowitz, R.W., and Schnitzer, T.J. (2000). Recommendations for the medical management of osteoarthritis of the hip and knee. *Arthritis Rheum* **43**:1905–15.

37. Bradley, J.D., Katz, B.P., and Brandt, K.D. (2001). Severity of knee pain does not predict a better response to an antiinflammatory dose of ibuprofen than to analgesic therapy in patients with osteoarthritis. *J Rheumatol* **28**:1073–6.

38. Tanaka, E., Yamazaki, K., and Misawa, S. (2000). Update: the clinical importance of acetaminophen hepatotoxicity in non-alcoholic and alcoholic subjects. *J Clin Pham Ther* **25**:325–32.

39. McClain, C.J., Price, S., Barve, S., Devalarja, R., and Shedlofsky, S. (1999). Acetaminophen hepatotoxicity. An update. *Curr Gastroenterol Rep* **1**:42–9.

40. Dart, R.C., Kuffner, E.K., and Rumack, B.R. (2000). Treatment of pain or fever with paracetamol (acetaminophen) in the alcoholic patient: a systematic review. *Am J Med* **7**:123–34.

41. Kuffner, E.K., Dart, R.C., Bogdan, G.M., Hill, R.E., Casper, E., and Darton, L. (2001). Effect of maximal daily doses of acetaminophen on the liver of alcoholic patients. *Arch Intern Med* **161**:2247–52.

42. Benson, G.D. (1983). Acetaminophen in chronic liver disease. *Clin Pharmacol Ther* **33**:95–101.

43. Fored, C.M., Ejerblad, E., Lindblad, P., et al. (2001). Acetaminophen, aspirin and chronic renal failure. *N Eng J Med* **345**:1801–9.

44. Crofford, L. (2001). Rational use of analgesic and anti-inflammatory drugs. *N Eng J Med* **345**:1844–6.

45. Henrich, W.L., Agodoa, L.E., Barrett, B., et al. (1996). Analgesics and the kidney: summary and recommendations to the Scientific Advisory Board of the National Kidney Foundation from an ad hoc committee of the National Kidney Foundation. *Am J Kidney Dis* **27**:162–1.

46. Singh, G., Ramsey, Dr. R., Morfeld, D., Shi, H., Hatoum, H.T., and Fries, J.F. (1996). Gastrointestinal tract complications of nonsteroidal anti-inflammatory drug treatment in rheumatoid arthritis. *Arch Intern Med* **156**:1530–6.

47. Wilcox, C.M., Shalek, K.A., and Cotsonis, G. (1999). Striking prevalence of over-the-counter nonsteroidal antiinflammatory drug use in patients with upper gastrointestinal hemorrhage. *Arch Intern Med* **154**:42–6.

48. Garcia-Rodriguez, L.A. and Hernandez-Diaz, S. (2001). The relative risk of upper gastrointestinal complications among users of acetaminophen and non-steroidal anti-inflammatory drugs. *Epidemiology* **12**:570–6.

49. Ouellet, M. and Percival, M.D. (2001). Mechanism of acetaminophen inhibition of cyclooxygenase isoforms. *Arch Biochem Biophys* **387**:273–80.

50. Catella-Lawson, F., Reilly, M.P., Kapoor, S.C., et al. (2001). Cyclooxygenase inhibitors and the antiplatelet effects of aspirin. *N Eng J Med* **345**:1809–17.

51. Hernandez-Diaz, S. and Garcia Rodriguez, L.A. (2001). Epidemiological assessment of the safety of conventional nonsteroidal anti-inflammatory drugs. *Am J Med* **110**(3A):20S–7S.

52. Singh, G. and Triadafilopoulos, G. (1999). Epidemiology of NSAID induced gastrointestinal complications. *J Rheumatol* **26**:18–24.

53. Laine, L., Harper, S., Simon, T., et al. (1999). A randomized trial comparing the effect of rofecoxib, a cyclooxygenase-2 specific inhibitor, with that of ibuprofen on the gastroduodenal mucosa of patients with osteoarthritis. *Gastroenterology* **117**:776–83.

54. Hawkey, C., Laine, L., Simon, T., et al. (2000). Comparison of the effect of rofecoxib (a cyclooxygenase 2 inhibitor), ibuprofen, and placebo on the gastroduodenal mucosa of patients with osteoarthritis: a randomized, a double-blind, placebo-controlled trial. *Arthritis Rheum* **43**:370–7.

55. Goldstein, J.L., Correa, P., Zhao, W.W., et al. (2001). Reduced incidence of gastroduodenal ulcers with celecoxib, a novel cyclooxygenase-2 inhibitor, compared to naproxen in patients with arthritis. *Am J Gastroenterol* **96**:1019–27.

56. Feldman, M. and McMahon, A.T. (2000). Do cyclooxygenase-2 inhibitors provide benefits similar to those of traditional nonsteroidal anti-inflammatory drugs, with less gastrointestinal toxicity? *Ann Int Med* **132**:134–43.

57. Langman, M.J., Jensen, D.M., Watson, D.J., et al. (1999). Adverse upper gastrointestinal effects of rofecoxib compared with NSAIDs. *JAMA* **282**:1929–33.

58. FDA Arthritis Advisory Committee Meeting. (2001). Gaithersburg, Maryland, February 7, 2001. *FDA Arthritis Advisory*, February 7.

59. Garcia Rodriguez, L.A. and Ruigomez, A. (1999). Secondary prevention of upper gastrointestinal bleeding associated with maintenance acid-suppressing treatment in patients with peptic ulcer bleed. *Epidemiology* **10**:228–32.

60. Yeomans, N.D., Tulassay, Z., Juhasz, L., et al. (1998). A comparison of omeprazole with ranitidine for ulcers associated with nonsteroidal anti-inflammatory drugs: Acid Suppression Trial: Ranitidine versus Omeprazole for NSAID-associated Ulcer Treatment (ASTRONAUT) Study Group. *N Eng J Med* **338**:719–26.

61. Silverstein, F.E., Graham, D.Y., Senior, J.R., et al. (1995). Misoprostol reduces serious gastrointestinal complications in patients with rheumatoid arthritis receiving nonsteroidal anti-inflammatory drugs. A randomized, double-blind, placebo-controlled trial. *Ann Int Med* **123**:241–9.

62. Del Rincon, I., Williams, K., Stern, M.P., Freeman, G.L., and Escalante, E. (2001). High incidence of cardiovascular events in a rheumatoid arthritis cohort not explained by traditional cardiac risk factors. *Arthritis Rheum* **44**:2737–45.

63. Hennan, J.K., Huang, J., Barrett, T.D., et al. (2001). Effects of selective cyclooxygenase-2 inhibition on vascular responses and thrombosis in canine coronary arteries. *Circulation* **104**:820–5.

64. Cippollone, F., Prontera, C., Pini, B., et al. (2001). Overexpression of functionally coupled cyclooxygenase-2 and prostaglandin E synthase in symptomatic atherosclerotic plaques as a basis of prostaglandin E_2-dependent plaque instability. *Circulation* **104**:921–7.

65. Lanas, A. (2001). Nonsteroidal anti-inflammatory drugs, low-dose aspirin, and potential ways of reducing the risk of complications. *Eur J Gastroenterol Hepatol* **13**:623–6.

66. Catella-Lawson, F. and Crofford, L.J. (2001). Cyclooxygenase inhibition and thrombogenicity. *Am J Med* **110**(Suppl.):12S–32.

67. Dumont, A.S., Verma, S., Dumont, R.J., and Hurlbert, R.J. (2000). Nonsteroidal anti-inflammatory drugs and bone metabolism in spinal fusion surgery: a pharmacological quandary. *J Pharmacol Toxicol Methods* **43**:31–9.

68. Glassman, S.D., Rose, S.M., Dimar, J.R., Pruno, R.M., Campbell, M.J., and Johnson, J.R. (1998). The effect of postoperative nonsteroidal anti-inflammatory drug administration on spinal fusion. *Spine* **23**:834–8.

69. Giannoudis, P.V., MacDonald, D.A., Matthews, S.J., Smith, R.M., Furlong, A.J., and De Boer, P. (2000). Nonunion of the femoral diaphysis. The influence of reaming and non-steroidal anti-inflammatory drugs. *J Bone Joint Surg* **82**:655–8.

70. Lanas, A., Bajador, E., Serrano, P., et al. (2000). Nitrovasodilators, low-dose aspirin, other nonsteroidal antiinflammatory drugs, and the risk of upper gastrointestinal bleeding. *N Eng J Med* **21**:834–9.

71. Uchida, M., Matsueda, K., Shoda, R., Muraoka, A., and Yamato, S. (2001). Nitric oxide donating compounds inhibit HCl-induced gastric mucosal lesions mainly via prostaglandin. *Jpn J Pharmacol* **85**:133–8.

9.4 Economic considerations in pharmacologic management of osteoarthritis

Aslam H. Anis, Carlo A. Marra, and Jolanda Cibere

Approximately US$245 billion was spent (11 per cent annual growth) on pharmaceuticals in North America, Europe, South America, and Japan in 2000/2001.[1] Musculoskeletal drugs accounted for US$13.1 billion, the biggest growth (19 per cent) in any one therapeutic category. Much of this growth was due to COX-2 selective inhibitors, which are now being used by more than 50 per cent of OA consumers.[2] Because of the availability of acetaminophen and several generic NSAIDs, the treatment of OA has traditionally been relatively inexpensive. While pharmacotherapy for OA will continue to provide good value for money relative to the considerable burden of disease, the cost-effectiveness of new therapies must be unequivocally established using rigorous scientific methods.[3,4]

As a result of the increasing pressures faced by health care systems with static budgets, decision-makers and practitioners are faced today with new challenges. For example, new drugs must pass the cost-effectiveness hurdle before they are made available by drug plans or hospital formularies.[5] Evaluation processes and submission guidelines for new prescription pharmaceuticals seeking formulary inclusion have been published,[6,7] and publicly funded health care systems, private insurers, and preferred provider organizations, such as HMOs, have adopted these strategies.[8] This requirement for these data, often referred to as 'pharmacoeconomics' or 'economic evaluations,' is new. The objective of using economic evaluations in formulary decision-making is based on optimal resource allocation, which relies on 'cost-benefit' or 'cost-effectiveness' analyses (see below) as its criterion to maximize the health benefits accruing to beneficiaries, given the operating budget.[9]

It is important to note the distinction between adopting such an optimizing framework and implementing strategies that aim merely to contain costs. To support such a mandate of 'benefit maximization', cost-effectiveness data must be evaluated and an implicit rank ordering of the relevant drugs must be made, based on their cost-efficiency.[10] Only then should a plan spend its budget by going down the list until all funds are exhausted. No other criteria for allocation of drug plan resources will maximize total health benefits.[11]

Economic evaluation models

Economic evaluation methodologies are broadly classified as: (1) cost minimization analysis, (2) cost-effectiveness analysis, (3) cost utility analysis, and finally (4) cost benefit analysis.[12] These methodologies have been summarized in Table 9.9. Because most economic evaluations of the pharmacotherapy of OA have been cost-effectiveness and cost-utility analyses, the remainder of this section will focus on these two types of studies.

Cost-effectiveness analysis is appropriate when the assumption of equivalent health effects is not valid, that is, two interventions, when compared, may produce differing degrees of health benefits and costs. Thus, cost-effectiveness analysis evaluates the incremental difference in costs over the incremental differences in effects produced. A range of outcome measures, such as laboratory tests, symptoms, function, mortality, quality of life, and quantity of life are available. In OA, effectiveness can be measured clinically by evaluating joint pain or the patient's global assessment of health. Validated disease-specific instruments, such as the Health Assessment Questionnaire (HAQ), the Western Ontario and McMaster Universities Osteoarthritis Index (WOMAC), and the Lequesne Index are also available.[13]

Under *cost utility* analysis, the effectiveness of the health interventions in question is measured, using a metric known as 'utility,' which ranges in value from 0 (dead) to 1 (perfect health). Health utilities can be measured directly among the population in question using techniques such as the standard gamble or the time trade-off method, or indirectly, using pre-scaled instruments, such as the European Quality of Life (EQ5D), Health

Table 9.9 Types of methodologies for economic evaluation

Type of study	Measurement/valuation of costs in the treatment strategies compared	Identification of consequences	Measurement/valuation of consequences
Cost-minimization analysis	Dollars	Identical in all relevant respects	None
Cost-effectiveness analysis	Dollars	Single effect of interest, common to both alternatives	Natural units (e.g., joint pain or the patient's global assessment of health)
Cost-utility analysis	Dollars	Single or multiple effects, not necessarily common to both alternatives	Quality-adjusted life years
Cost-benefit analysis	Dollars	Single or multiple effects, not necessarily common to both alternatives	Dollars

Source: Adapted from Ref. 12.

Utilities Index (HUI), Quality of Well-being Index, and the SF6D.[14] Cost utility analysis is a specific type of cost-effectiveness analysis, in which the outcomes are presented as the incremental costs divided by the incremental difference in utilities. Often, cost utility analyses are reported as cost per quality-adjusted life years (QALY) gained, which is calculated by weighting the life expectancy by the utility weight derived from the outcome of that health intervention. Cost per QALY gained is a unique and preferred measure of the economic value of different interventions, because it permits comparison across disease groups, thereby facilitating funding allocation decisions.

Measuring costs

Once the appropriate measurement of costs has been specified, the 'perspective' of the analysis is the key to undertaking a proper economic evaluation of health care interventions.[15,16] The perspective may be societal, in which all costs, regardless of who bears them, are included; alternatively, only the costs incurred by the relevant payer, for example, the health care system, health maintenance organization, ministry of health, etc., may be identified and included.

An essential step is the identification of the unit costs of the individual resources used in the delivery of health care, such as physician time, nursing time, medications, laboratory procedures, physical therapy, etc. The quantities of these resources must then be measured. The total dollar value of the costs may then be determined from the product of the quantity of resources and their respective prices.

In calculating these costs, one must distinguish between *accounting costs* and *economic costs*. Accounting costs are the nominal value of all expenditures incurred, as recorded in the balance sheets (e.g., all salary and wages payments, cost of laboratory supplies, and medications). In contrast, economic costs are the costs of producing health outcomes (e.g., cost per patient treated). An associated concept is that of *opportunity costs*. In determining economic costs, economic principles dictate that the next best alternative use of resources, (i.e., the opportunity cost) be used. Opportunity costs are defined as the 'value of the benefits foregone because the resource is not available for its best alternative use'.[12]

Given standard accounting practices, accounting costs are often accumulated by departments, rather than at the patient level, and their analysis often results in large inaccuracies. Accounting costs may be assigned to departments other than the one in which consumption of the resources has occurred, and often give rise to charges that cover expenses related to items such as expansion, bad debts, and disallowed reimbursement costs. While economic costs tend to be marginal costs (the extra amount of resource consumption for provision of service, compared to not providing that service), accounting costs tend to be average costs. The nuances associated with these differences are explained in greater detail by Finkler.[17]

A distinction is often made also between direct and indirect costs. Direct costs are those associated with provision of the health intervention; indirect costs are those associated with productivity gains or losses due to changes in the patient's ability to work because of illness. When a health intervention involves cost outlays that continue over several years, the present value of the intervention must be calculated by discounting the future costs required.[18]

Sensitivity analysis

The last important step is the conduct of extensive sensitivity analyses. Sensitivity analysis accounts for uncertainties related to the measurement of health outcomes and the health care resources utilized. Sensitivity analysis can be performed using the confidence intervals of the estimated costs and benefits. In addition, because the final number presented is a ratio of costs and effects, one must also consider that these may be correlated. Methods have been developed that take into account the interdependence of costs and effects and permit probabilistic sensitivity analysis.[19]

Internal/external validity of pharmacoeconomic evaluations

The economic evaluation of drug therapy can be classified under two broad study designs.[20] The first is the 'piggybacking' of an economic evaluation onto a randomized controlled trial (RCT). Although this design has the highest internal validity for both clinical and economic effects, it suffers from the lack of generalizability. In designing an economic evaluation that is to be appended to a clinical trial, methodologic issues, such as the choice of comparators, sample size, and collection of data on resource utilization and outcomes must be considered.[19] Also, since the time horizon of interest is often longer than that captured by the clinical trial, other techniques, such as modeling, must be adopted to estimate the long-term costs and outcomes.

The other approach that is often employed is decision analysis, that is, the use of modeling techniques to map probabilities for clinical events, costs, and outcomes that have been reported in the literature or are derived from expert opinion. This design permits the investigator to estimate long-term costs and outcomes and effectiveness (rather than efficacy) data from several sources. Efficacy refers to whether, under ideal conditions, a drug has the ability to bring about the effect intended; effectiveness refers to whether, in the usual clinical setting, a drug, in fact, achieves the effect intended. However, this approach is frequently limited by the high degree of uncertainty of the parameter estimates and requires many assumptions. For the economic evaluation of treatments for OA, the decision-analytic or modeling approach has been utilized more often than the piggybacking of economic evaluations onto RCTs.

Interpreting the results

Economic evaluations are useful to decision-makers who must allocate resources to maximize health benefits under budgetary restraints.[10] However, clinicians are mainly concerned with the effectiveness of drug therapy for individuals. Therefore, cost-effectiveness analysis has a limited role in bedside decision-making.[10] Nonetheless, an understanding of the principles of economic evaluations will permit clinicians to understand these decisions so that they can advise patients and policy makers when they feel that funding decisions do not apply to a particular case. A brief checklist for the evaluation of economic evaluations is provided in Table 9.10.

Table 9.10 Brief checklist for pharmacoeconomic evaluations

Was a well-defined study question posed in an answerable format?
Was a comprehensive description of the competing alternatives given?
Was the effectiveness of the alternatives established?
Were all the important and relevant costs and consequences for each alternative identified?
Were costs and consequences measured accurately in appropriate physical units (e.g., number of physician visits, lost work-days, gained life-years)?
Were costs and consequences valued credibly?
Were costs and consequences adjusted for differential timing (i.e., discounting)?
Was an incremental analysis of costs and consequences of alternatives performed?
Was allowance made for uncertainty in the estimates of costs and consequences (statistical and/or sensitivity analyses)?
Did the presentation and discussion of study results include all issues of concern to users (e.g., incremental cost-effectiveness ratios, comparison with other studies, generalizability to other groups)

Source: Adapted from Ref. 12.

Summary of the OA pharmacoeconomic literature

Therapeutic guidelines for OA

Recommendations for the management of knee and hip OA have recently been published by the American College of Rheumatology (ACR),[20] the European League Against Rheumatism (EULAR),[21] and North of England Guideline Development Group.[22] The first line pharmacotherapeutic recommendations for management of OA include acetaminophen, non-selective NSAIDs and selective COX-2 inhibitors.[20–22] These recommendations have been based primarily on efficacy data derived from RCTs. Only the North of England Guidelines Development Group considered economic merit.[22] Despite the recent recognition of the importance of economic considerations, in general, no evaluations comparing the cost-effectiveness of older NSAIDs and acetaminophen are available. Only the newer non-selective NSAIDs, nabumetone and meloxicam, and the newer COX-2 specific inhibitors, celecoxib and rofecoxib, have been evaluated from an economic perspective.

Acetaminophen

The first line therapy recommended for treatment of OA is acetaminophen.[20–22] The analgesic efficacy of acetaminophen, 4 g/d, was shown to be comparable to that of ibuprofen, 1200 or 2400 mg per day.[23] In addition, acetaminophen is generally considered to be safer than branded non-selective NSAIDs, and is less expensive, although the cost difference between acetaminophen and generic NSAIDs may be minimal.

However, on the basis of a *post hoc* analysis, it has recently been suggested that the efficacy of acetaminophen is not as great as that of NSAIDs in patients with severe OA pain.[24] In contrast, however, in a retrospective analysis of their RCT, Bradley *et al.*[25] concluded that greater pain severity at baseline did not predict a better response to an anti-flammatory dose of ibuprofen than to an analgesic dose of that NSAID or to acetaminophen in patients with knee OA. A prospective RCT in which patients are stratified on the basis of baseline pain severity to treatment with an NSAID or acetaminophen is needed.

Furthermore, the safety of acetaminophen has been brought into question by a recent study that reported a 1.3-fold increased risk of gastrointestinal complications in current acetaminophen users, in comparison with non-users, and a 1.9-fold increased risk in those who take ≥2000 mg/d.[26] Although the data were analysed in detail, the information obtained from the general practitioners' computerized database that was used by the authors did not include over-the-counter NSAID use. As a result, the authors were unable to adjust for this major confounding variable, which could have explained, at least in part, the elevated risk of GI complications among acetaminophen users. Because of the uncertainty of the efficacy and safety of acetaminophen, from an economic perspective, a need exists for prospective studies that provide a direct comparison between acetaminophen and non-selective NSAIDs and the newer COX-2 inhibitors, so that the relative cost-effectiveness of the agents can be measured. To date, no economic evaluations of acetaminophen have been published.

Non-selective NSAIDs

For those who fail to respond to acetaminophen, anti-inflammatory drugs are recommended. The specific agent to be used depends on the risk for GI complications. In low-risk patients, non-selective NSAIDs are recommended.[20,22] Within this group of drugs many individual NSAIDs are available that appear to have equivalent efficacy.[27] Ibuprofen is associated with a lower rate of toxicity, including GI bleeding,[27–29] even when dosage is taken into account.[28] It has similar efficacy and a low cost in comparison with other non-selective NSAIDs. However, ibuprofen has not been directly evaluated for its cost-effectiveness in comparison with other non-selective NSAIDs, with the exception of nabumetone,[30] a newer NSAID claimed to have fewer GI adverse effects than other non-selective NSAIDs. When the direct medical costs associated with nabumetone, ibuprofen, and ibuprofen plus misoprostol were compared, an economic benefit was found in favor of nabumetone.[30] However, because the results were based on a small number of patients and endoscopic outcomes, it is possible that clinically significant events were overestimated.

Another recent cost-effectiveness study reported a cost per life-year gained for nabumetone compared to ibuprofen of £2517 (US$4335, 1998 value) and £1880 (US$3100, 1998 value), depending on the model used. However, the 95 per cent confidence intervals were large, ranging from £-104 to 28 346 and £-463 to 24 566, respectively, suggesting a very imprecise point estimate that is dependent on underlying model assumptions.[31] In addition, this study did not include indirect costs, but was otherwise well conducted, based on a large trial, and included appropriate sensitivity analyses. The cost-effectiveness of nabumetone was considered comparable to that of other therapies currently available in most western health care systems.[31]

The cost-effectiveness of meloxicam, an NSAID that has been reported to have fewer non-specific GI adverse effects (e.g., epigastric pain, nausea, dyspepsia, diarrhea) than other non-selective COX-2 inhibitors, was recently compared to that of diclofenac.[32] The decision analysis model was based on adverse effect data from a RCT in OA, while resource utilization and cost data were obtained from other sources. Meloxicam was found to be cost-saving, compared to diclofenac, because of its improved GI safety. A study applying this model to data from France and Italy reached the same conclusion, although the sensitivity analyses showed that the models were susceptible to variation in the probability of GI adverse events.[33] Both meloxicam studies[32,33] assumed equivalent efficacy and did not include an evaluation of indirect costs, quality of life, or patient preferences. In addition, these analyses were based on a low dose of meloxicam, 7.5 mg per day, potentially biasing the results.

Topical NSAIDs

A recent systematic review[34] concluded that topical NSAIDs are efficacious and they were recommended in the recent ACR treatment guidelines for OA.[20] The potential cost-effectiveness due to the reduced risk of GI effects associated with this treatment option has been evaluated only in one study, which compared topical piroxicam with oral ibuprofen.[35] This cost minimization analysis led to the conclusion that a substantial reduction in cost (£34.55, that is approximately US$54 in 1994) per patient could be achieved with piroxicam in comparison with oral ibuprofen, over a 3-month treatment period. Although the cost reductions varied in the sensitivity analyses, topical piroxicam remained cost saving.

Although these recent analyses have suggested cost-effectiveness, or even cost-savings, with the newer non-selective NSAIDs, nabumetone and meloxicam, caution must be used in interpreting these findings. As pointed out previously, a comparison based on non-equivalent drug dosages will lead to biased conclusions, particularly since the tolerability and safety of NSAIDs is dose-dependent. Rochon *et al.*[36] found that manufacturer-supported trials of NSAIDs were frequently of poor quality and that claims of superiority, particularly with respect to side effect profiles, were often not supported by evidence. Most of the above studies were either directly supported by the drug manufacturer or included secondary authors who were affiliated with the manufacturer. In addition, most of the economic analyses of NSAIDs were based on hypothetical models, rather than an outcomes data, a third-party payer perspective was employed in most cases, and indirect costs were usually not included.

Selective COX-2 inhibitors

The recent introduction of the selective COX-2 inhibitors has changed the treatment of OA. In Canada, during 1995–8, on average, about 1.7 million prescriptions were written annually for NSAIDs, resulting in annual expenditures of about Canadian $44 million. After the introduction of selective COX-2 agents, these figures increased to almost 1.9 million prescriptions and $78 million in expenditures.[2] Approximately 50 per cent of all COX-2 specific inhibitor use in Canada is for OA.[2] Authors of recent editorials have attempted to place the new selective COX-2 inhibitors in clinical perspective.[37–39] The International COX-2 Study Group outlined specific instances in which selective COX-2 inhibitors should be used in preference to non-selective NSAIDs, based on expert opinion derived from epidemiological studies that evaluated the risks of serious GI complications.[37] In addition, a recent editorial by Brandt and Bradley[40] provides some insight into the relative roles of different types of pharmacotherapy for OA. Based on a comprehensive review of the evidence, these authors concluded that despite the fact that selective COX-2 inhibitors represent an 'important extension of the pharmacologic options available for the treatment of OA symptoms,' acetaminophen remains the drug of choice for initial management of OA pain.

The efficacy of COX-2 selective inhibitors is equivalent to that of non-selective NSAIDs for the treatment of OA.[41,42] However, there has been much speculation and debate about the relative risk of their GI and other toxicities, compared to those of non-selective NSAIDs. Recently, as described in detail in Chapter 9.3, the results of two large prospective RCTs, the CLASS[43] and the VIGOR trials,[44] both of which were designed as GI safety studies, were reported. For the purposes of this discussion it is notable that no significant differences were observed between subjects receiving celecoxib and those who received comparator non-selective NSAIDs (ibuprofen or diclofenac) with respect to symptomatic ulcers, complicated ulcers, or serious adverse events, and the only significant difference between treatment groups was a reduction favoring celecoxib in the incidence of withdrawal from the study due to adverse effects.

Notably, in the CLASS trial,[43] no significant differences between treatment groups were observed with respect to the risk of myocardial infarction. However, the prevalence of various cardiovascular risk factors was not described, making evaluation of this endpoint difficult. This point is relevant because, in contrast to the CLASS study,[43] in the VIGOR trial,[44] although a significant gastroprotective effect of rofecoxib was demonstrated, the rofecoxib treatment group exhibited a 4-fold increase in the risk of myocardial infarction. This unexpected increase in the incidence of cardiac events in patients treated with a COX-2 selective inhibitor has prompted further investigation: the authors of a recent analysis[45] of four randomized trials (including the CLASS and VIGOR trials) comparing either celecoxib or rofecoxib to non-selective NSAIDs, concluded that myocardial infarction rates in both the CLASS and VIGOR trial were much higher than those previously reported in a meta-analysis that examined aspirin use for the primary prevention of myocardial infarction in more than 23 000 individuals. Notably, however, a significant proportion of the individuals from the meta-analysis were physicians, who may have been more health conscious (e.g., less likely to be smokers) than the patients in the selective COX-2 inhibitor groups. Without baseline data regarding cardiovascular risk factors in the CLASS and VIGOR trials, it is difficult to determine if this is an appropriate comparison. However, because much of the proposed economic benefit of selective COX-2 inhibitors is derived from the avoidance of adverse events, it remains to be demonstrated whether the apparent GI benefits will be experienced in clinical practice and if these will be overshadowed by an increase in cardiac events.

The publication of the results of the VACT trial has supplied additional data on the relative efficacy of the selective COX-2 inhibitors and acetaminophen in the treatment of OA.[46] This study was a randomized, parallel-group, double-blind trial in which 382 patients with OA of the knee who had previously been treated with NSAIDs or acetaminophen were enrolled. Patients were randomly assigned to receive rofecoxib, 12.5 mg/day; rofecoxib, 25 mg/day; celecoxib, 200 mg/day; or acetaminophen, 4000 mg/day for 6 weeks. The results indicated that for all outcome measures, all strategies employing the selective COX-2 inhibitors were superior to acetaminophen treatment. Specifically, rofecoxib, 25 mg/day, provided statistically significant efficacy advantages over acetaminophen, 4000 mg/day, celecoxib, 200 mg/day, and rofecoxib, 12.5 mg/day. However, because this short-term clinical trial did not assess economic endpoints, it is difficult to comment on the relative cost-effectiveness of these regimens.

Economic analyses have compared selective COX 2 specific inhibitors with non-selective NSAIDs alone, or with an NSAID/misoprostol formulation or H$_2$ receptor antagonist, mostly by utilizing decision analysis to model outcomes and costs.[47–49] These analyses, all of which were similar, were supported by pharmaceutical companies and included their employees as authors. Each study concluded that celecoxib use would result in a significant reduction in the morbidity associated with GI toxicity. In addition, from the Swiss healthcare perspective, the model predicted that use of celecoxib would be the least costly and most effective strategy.[50] Similar results have been generated by investigators using a similar model (the Arthritis Cost Consequence Evaluation System, ACCES).[50] Application of this model to data from Norway[51] and Sweden[52] also led to the conclusion that celecoxib was preferable to non-selective NSAIDs in the economic analyses.

Another pharmaceutical industry-initiated analysis examined the cost-effectiveness of rofecoxib, in comparison with non-selective NSAIDs.[53] Decision-modeling was done to determine the economic impact, from the perspective of the National Health Service, of switching to rofecoxib, all patients with OA in the United Kingdom currently being treated with a non-selective NSAIDs. The investigators constructed three models: the first model considered only observed perforations, symptomatic ulcers and bleeds, while the second and third models considered silent endoscopic ulcerations occurring with a rate of 85 and 40 per cent, respectively. Results with the first model, the most conservative of the three, indicated a cost of approximately £15 600 (approximately US$22 940, 2000) per life year gained with rofecoxib treatment. In contrast, the other two models concluded that rofecoxib was cost-saving.

Importantly, none of the above analyses factored in the additional costs of the increased incidence of cardiac events that may be associated with the use of selective COX-2 inhibitors, as suggested by the VIGOR Study,[47] and, therefore, may have over-estimated the cost-effectiveness of rofecoxib. Furthermore, the models considered only direct medical costs from the perspective of a third party payer and did not consider the impact on health-related quality of life. In addition, the use of acetaminophen or topical NSAIDs as treatment comparators was ignored, so that the results cannot be extended to include these therapies. Considering the limitations of these analyses, their results should be considered as preliminary until they can be verified by studies utilizing better research designs and sources of data.

Maetzel et al.[54] recently published a decision-analysis based, cost-effectiveness study that was performed from the perspective of a provincial Canadian Ministry of Health, that is, a third party payer perspective. The COX-2 selective inhibitors, celecoxib and rofecoxib, were compared to non-selective NSAIDs over a 5-year period. The authors attempted to address the limitations of earlier analyses by incorporating the risk and costs of developing cardiovascular complications (specifically, myocardial infarction) and the impact of the drugs on health-related quality of life (as assessed by utility values). Findings were based on the efficacy of the coxibs observed in the CLASS[43] and VIGOR[44] trials. In assessing the cost-effectiveness of the coxibs, subjects were classified as being of 'average risk' (i.e., those who had not experienced an upper GI event—defined as major bleeding, perforation, obstruction, or endoscopically confirmed symptomatic ulcer) or being of 'high risk' (i.e., those who had experienced an upper GI event). Celecoxib was compared to diclofenac and ibuprofen; rofecoxib to naproxen.

Among patients who were not taking low-dose aspirin for the prevention of cardiovascular disease, coxib was neither cost-effective in average risk patients or in a population with a typical mix of average and high risk patients. However, among elderly subjects who did not have additional risk factors, rofecoxib appeared to be cost-effective among those older than 76 years, and celecoxib among those older than 81 years. Among high risk patients, rofecoxib and celecoxib were both found to be cost-effective, relative to the comparator non-selective NSAIDs. However, they were not cost-effective when the not-selective NSAID was given in combination with a proton pump inhibitor. It is a limitation of this analysis that acetaminophen was not included as a comparator in the OA patient groups and that only direct medical costs were considered.

Therapies for GI protection

Because NSAIDs are associated with a variety of GI side effects that include both non-life threatening symptoms (including epigastric pain, dyspepsia, nausea, and diarrhea) and life-threatening events (hemorrhage, perforation, and death), gastroprotective agents are often co-prescribed. Whereas the non-life threatening symptoms are often ignored, they can lead to substantial resource utilization including gastroprotective pharmacotherapy, and expensive investigations to rule out the presence of an ulcer or gastric cancer (such as endoscopy or X-rays). The economic importance of the prevention of catastrophic GI events is underscored by the high cost of their management. In Canada, a recent evaluation of the average hospital stay and the case costs for bleeding peptic ulcer were 5.73 days and $2953 (1998 Canadian, equivalent to approximately US$2002, 1998), respectively.[55] Another study evaluated the excess costs from gastrointestinal disease associated with NSAIDS from a Medicaid perspective.[56] The investigators found that there was an excess of $111 (US, 1989) per patient in mean annual costs for gastrointestinal disorders between regular users of NSAIDs and non-users. Although costs of treatment are likely to vary greatly between demographic locations, these figures illustrate the relative economic impact of NSAID-induced gastropathy in OA.

The relative effectiveness of different gastroprotective modalities was recently evaluated in a meta-analysis.[57] Whereas misoprostol, 400–800 μg/day, proton pump inhibitors, and H2 receptor antagonists were all effective in reducing the risk of endoscopically apparent gastric and duodenal ulcers, only misoprostol, 800 μg/day, reduced the risk of clinically significant ulcerations (although this regimen was associated with a higher risk of diarrhea than the other gastroprotective agents studied).

Another recent meta-analysis of 21 placebo-controlled, randomized trials examining the relative efficacy of gastroprotective agents in preventing severe, acute NSAID-induced gastroduodenal damage found both misoprostol and proton pump inhibitors to be superior to histamine-2 receptor antagonists.[58] Therefore, research has focused on the economic evaluation of misoprostol either as a single product[59–62] or in combination with diclofenac[63,64] for the prevention of NSAID-induced ulcer complications. Most of these analyses conclude that use of misoprostol results in a reduction of GI ulceration, but at a higher incremental cost. Similarly, authors of a recent systematic review[65] of the cost-effectiveness of prophylaxis of NSAID-induced gastropathy in OA or RA concluded that high-quality evidence existed to recommend the economic superiority of misoprostol as a single product over other strategies, but low-quality evidence to support the cost-effectiveness of the NSAID/misoprostol combination product. Thus, misoprostol may be cost-effective when compared to other strategies (including placebo) and its economic attractiveness increases in older or high-risk patients. While proton-pump inhibitors appear to be efficacious for the prevention of NSAID-induced adverse events, there is little economic information evaluating their use in this role.

Other therapies for OA

Second line pharmacologic treatments for OA recommended by the ACR guidelines[20] include intra-articular injection of hyaluronan and glucocorticoids, tramadol, codeine, and topical agents, such as capsaicin and methylsalicylate. To date, no economic evaluations of any of these therapies has been published.

Summary

In terms of expenditure, pharmaceutical products continue to be one of the fastest growing sectors of health care. This is true especially for musculoskeletal agents. Because of the introduction of recent innovations, this class of drugs has been among the fastest growing worldwide. Policy makers need to consider the relative cost-effectiveness of both new and old agents within this class to maximize health benefits from a finite budget. Well-conducted pharmacoeconomic analyses are of paramount importance in making funding decisions for the pharmacotherapy of OA. Recommendations of various professional bodies for first-line drugs for the management of OA include acetaminophen, non-selective anti-inflammatory drugs (NSAIDs) and selective cyclooxygenase-2 (COX-2) inhibitors. However, among these, the available cost-effectiveness literature does not provide much useful information from which to draw decisions. Because of its relatively low incidence of toxicity, effectiveness, and low cost, acetaminophen should be the first-line agent used. For those in whom acetaminophen is not effective, a non-selective NSAID, with or without misoprostol (depending on the risk for GI complications), should be utilized.

Given the emergence of several new, expensive agents with limited benefits relative to conventional therapy for the treatment of OA, it is notable that economic evaluations of these agents have been performed only sporadically and without the systematic evaluation of available comparative therapies. Specifically, a paucity of information exists regarding the cost-effectiveness of acetaminophen, older or topical NSAIDS, and second-line treatments. Economic evaluations of recently introduced non-selective NSAIDs and selective COX-2 inhibitors have, to a certain extent, been industry-driven as the manufacturers seek reimbursement eligibility by third party payers. Methodological issues must be resolved before a recommendation can be made for preferred use of these agents based upon their economic merit.

Key points

1. There is no adequate pharmacoeconomic evidence comparing acetaminophen and older or topical NSAIDs with newer NSAIDs or with selective COX-2 inhibitors in treatment of OA. Therefore, the relative cost-effectiveness of the latter is unknown.

2. Pharmacoeconomic comparisons of non-selective NSAIDs and selective COX-2 inhibitors are generally of poor quality or not sufficiently comprehensive. It is difficult, therefore, to determine which is more cost-effective. Economic analyses have not incorporated the increased incidence of cardiac events that appears to be associated with selective COX-2 inhibitors.

3. Analyses of misoprostol are of reasonable quality and show that the drug is cost-effective as a single entity, in comparison with placebo or other gastroprotective modalities. However, a paucity of economic data is available on the combination product of misoprostol/diclofenac.

4. Future economic analyses on the pharmacotherapy of OA should concentrate on the gaps in the literature identified above.

5. Because acetaminophen is effective, inexpensive, and relatively free of toxicity, from an economic perspective it is reasonable to initiate OA therapy with this agent. In patients who do not respond, an NSAID, with or without misoprostol, depending on age and risk factors is a cost-effective alternative. In those patients who require a gastroprotective agent, but cannot tolerate misoprostol, proton pump inhibitors are likely to be efficacious but the data evaluating their cost-effectiveness in this role are limited.

Acknowledgements

Carlo Marra is supported by an Arthritis Society/Canadian Institutes of Health Research Fellowship. Jolanda Cibere is supported by a Canadian Institutes of Health Research Clinician Scientist Award.

References

(An asterisk denotes recommended reading.)
1. Drug Monitor, IMS HEALTH Global Services. (2001). Global Pharma sales up 11% in June 2001. Retrieved August 25, 2001. http://www.imshealth.com

2. Marra, C.A., Esdaile, J.M., Sun, H.Y., and Anis, A.H. (2000). Cost of COX inhibitors: How selective should we be? *J Rheumatol* **27**:2731–3.

3. MacLean, C.H., Knight, K., Paulus, H., Brook, R.H., and Shekelle, P.G. (1998). Costs attributable to osteoarthritis. *J Rheumatol* **25**:2213–8.

4. Canadian Coordinating Office for Health Technology Assessment (1997). *Guidelines for economic evaluations of pharmaceuticals: Canada* (2nd ed.). Ottawa: CCOHTA.

5. Anis, A.H., Rahman, T., and Schecter, M. (1998). Using pharmacoeconomic analysis to make drug insurance coverage decisions. *Pharmacoeconomics* **13**:119–26.

6. Siegel, J.E., Torrance, G.W., Russell, L.B., Luce, B.R., Weinstein, M.C., and Gold, M.R. (1997). Guidelines for pharmacoeconomic studies. Recommendations from the panel on cost effectiveness in health and medicine. *Pharmacoeconomics* **11**:159–68.

7. Commonwealth Department of Human Services (1995). *Guidelines for the pharmaceutical industry on preparation of submissions to the pharmaceutical benefits advisory committee including major submissions involving economic analyses.* Canberra: Australian Government Publishing Service.

8. Hatoun, H.T. and Freeman, R.A. (1994). The use of pharmacoeconomic data in formulary selection. *Top Hosp Pharm Management* **13**:47–53.

9. Granata, A.V. and Hillman, A.L. (1998). Competing practice guidelines: Using cost-effectiveness analysis to make optimal decisions. *Ann Intern Med* **128**:56–63.

10. *Detsky, A.S. and Naglie, I.G. (1990). A clinician's guide to cost-effectiveness. *Ann Intern Med* **113**:147–54.

    This review is an excellent introduction to cost-effectiveness analysis and allocation of budgets on the basis of economic principles. In addition, it contains a section outlining the role of cost-effectiveness analysis in bedside decision-making.

11. *Weinstein, M.C., Siegel, J.E., Gold, M.R., Kamlet, M.S., and Russell, L.B. (1996). Recommendations of the panel on cost-effectiveness in health and medicine. *JAMA* **276**:1253–8.

    This review outlines recommendations for the conduct of economic evaluations in medicine, at a level appropriate for both the researcher and the clinical practitioner conducting or critically appraising such studies.

12. *Drummond, M.F., O'Brien, B., Stoddart, G.L., and Torrance, G.W. (eds) (1997). *Methods for the economic evaluation of health care programmes* (2nd ed.). Oxford: Oxford Medical Publications.

    This text is an excellent introduction to economic evaluation in health care. The authors have intended it to be 'a well-equipped toolkit' that would provide readers the skills necessary to critically appraise economic evaluations that appear in the literature. It is highly recommended for those who seek more information about the methodology used for the economic evaluation of health care.

13. Brazier, J.E., Harper, R., Munro, J., Walters, S.J., and Snaith, M.L. (1999). Generic and condition-specific measures for people with osteoarthritis of the knee. *Rheumatology* **38**:870–7.

14. Coons, S.J., Rao, S., Keininger, D.L., and Hays, R.D. (2000). A comparative review of generic quality of life instruments. *Pharmacoeconomics* **17**:13–35.

15. Task Force on Principles for Economic Evaluation. (1995). Economic analysis of health care technology. A report on principles. *Ann Intern Med* **122**:61–70.

16. O'Brien, B.J., Heyland, D., Richardson, W.S., Levine, M., and Drummond, M.F. (for the Evidence-Based Medicine Working Group) (1997). How to use an article on economic analysis of clinical practice. *JAMA* **277**:1552–7.

17. Finkler, S.A. (1982). The distinction between costs and charges. *Ann Intern Med* **96**:102–9.

18. Krahn, M. and Gafni, A. (1993). Discounting in the economic evaluation of health care interventions. *Medical Care* **31**:403–18.

19. Drummond, M.F. and Davies, L. (1991). Economic analysis alongside clinical trials. Revisiting the methodological issues. *Int J Tech Assess Health Care* **7**:561–73.

20. American College of Rheumatology subcommittee on osteoarthritis guidelines. (2000). Recommendations for the medical management of osteoarthritis of the hip and knee. *Arthritis Rheum* **43**:1905–15.

21. Pendleton, A., Arden, N., Dougados, M., Doherty, M., Bannwarth, B., Bijlsma, J.W.J., *et al.* (2000). EULAR recommendations for the management of knee osteoarthritis: report of a task force of the standing committee for international clinical studies including therapeutic trials (ESCISIT). *Ann Rheum Dis* **59**:936–44.

22. Eccles, M., Freemantle, N., and Mason, J. (North of England Non-steroidal Anti-Inflammatory Drug Guideline Development Group) (1998). North of England evidence based guideline development project: summary guideline for non-steroidal anti-inflammatory drugs versus basic analgesia in treating the pain of degenerative arthritis. *Br Med J* **317**:526–30.

23. Bradley, J.D., Brandt, K.D., Katz, B.P., Kalasinski, L.A., and Ryan, S. (1991). Comparison of an antiinflammatory dose of ibuprofen, an analgesic dose of ibuprofen, and acetaminophen in the treatment of patients with osteoarthritis of the knee. *N Engl J Med* **325**:87–91.

24. Pincus, T., Koch, G.G., Sokka, T., Lefkowith, J., Wolfe, F., *et al.* (2001). A randomized, double-blind, crossover clinical trial of diclofenac plus misoprostol versus acetaminophen in patients with osteoarthritis of the hip or knee. *Arthritis Rheum* **44**:1587–98.

25. Bradley, J.D., Katz, B.P., and Brandt, K.D. (2001). Severity of knee pain does not predict a better response to an antiinflammatory dose of ibuprofen than to analgesic therapy in patients with osteoarthritis. *J Rheumatol* **28**:1073–6.

26. Garcìa Rodrìguez, L.A. and Hernandez-Diaz, S. (2001). Relative risk of upper gastrointestinal complications among users of acetaminophen and nonsteroidal anti-inflammatory drugs. *Epidemiology* **12**:570–6.

27. Wynne, H.A. and Campbell, M. (1993). Pharmacoeconomics of non-steroidal anti-inflammatory drugs (NSAIDs). *Pharmacoeconomics* **3**:107–23.

28. Fries, J.F., Williams, C.A., and Bloch, D.A. (1991). The relative toxicity of nonsteroidal antiinflammatory drugs. *Arthritis Rheum* **34**:1353–60.

29. Langman, M.J.S., Weil, J., Wainwright, P., Lawson, D.H., Rawlins, M.D., Logan, R.F.A., Murphy, M., Vessey, M.P., and Colin-Jones, D.G. (1994). Risks of bleeding peptic ulcer associated with individual non-steroidal anti-inflammatory drugs. *Lancet* **343**:1075–8.

30. Bentkover, J.D., Baker, A.M., and Kaplan, H. (1994). Nabumetone in elderly patients with osteoarthritis. Economic benefits versus ibuprofen alone or ibuprofen plus misoprostol. *Pharmacoeconomics* **5**:335–42.

31. McCabe, C.J., Akehurst, R.L., Kirsch, J., Whitfield, M., Backhouse, M., Woolf, A.D., Scott, D.L., Emery, P., and Haslock, I. (1998). Choice of NSAID and management strategy in rheumatoid arthritis and osteoarthritis. The impact on costs and outcomes in the UK. *Pharmacoeconomics* **14**:191–9.

32. Jansen, R.B., Burrell, A., Nuijten, M.J.C., and Hardens, M. (1996). An economic evaluation of meloxicam 7.5 mg versus diclofenac 100 mg retard in the treatment of osteoarthritis in the UK: a decision analysis model based on gastrointestinal complications. *Br J Med Econ* **10**:247–62.

33. Jansen, R.B., Capri, S., Nuijten, M.J.C., Burrell, A., Marini, M.G., and Hardens, M. (1997). Economic evaluation of meloxicam (7.5 mg) versus sustained release diclofenac (100 mg) treatment of osteoarthritis: a cross-national assessment for France, Italy and the UK. *Br J Med Econ* **11**:9–22.

34. Moore, R.A., Tramer, M.R., Carroll, D., Wiffen, P.J., and McQuay, H.J. (1998). Quantitative systematic review of topically applied non-steroidal anti-inflammatory drugs. *Br Med J* **316**:333–8.

35. McKell, D. and Stewart, A. (1994). A cost-minimisation analysis comparing topical versus systemic NSAIDs in the treatment of mild osteoarthritis of the superficial joints. *Br J Med Econ* **7**:137–46.

36. Rochon, P.A., Gurwitz, J.H., Simms, R.W., Fortin, P.R., Felson, D.T., Minaker, K.L., and Chalmers, T.C. (1994). A study of manufacturer-supported trials of nonsteroidal anti-inflammatory drugs in the treatment of arthritis. *Arch Intern Med* **154**:157–63.

37. Lipsky, P.E., Abramson, S.B., and Breedveld, F.C. (for the International COX-2 Study Group) (2000). Analysis of the effect of COX-2 specific inhibitors and recommendations for their use in clinical practice. *J Rheumatol* **27**:1338–40.

38. Freemantle, N. (2000). Cost-effectiveness of non-steroidal anti-inflammatory drugs (NSAIDs)—what makes a NSAID good value for money. *Br J Rheumatol* **39**:232–4.

39. Peterson, W.L. and Cryer, B. (1999). COX-1 sparing NSAIDS—Is the enthusiasm justified? *JAMA* **282**:1961–3.

40. Brandt, K.D. and Bradley, J.D. (2001). Should the initial drug used to treat osteoarthritis pain be a nonsteroidal antiinflammatory drug? *J Rheumatol* **28**:467–73.

41. Bensen, W.G., Fiechtner, J.J., McMillen, J.I., Zhao, W.W., Yu, S.S., *et al.* (1999). Treatment of osteoarthritis with celecoxib, a cyclooxygenase 2 inhibitor: A randomized, controlled trial. *May Clin Proc* **74**:1095–105.

42. Day, R., Morrison, B., Luza, A., Castaneda, O., Strusberg, A., *et al.* (2000). A randomized trial of the efficacy and tolerability of the COX-2 inhibitor rofecoxib vs. ibuprofen in patients with osteoarthritis. *Arch Intern Med* **160**:1781–7.

43. Silverstein, F.E., Faich, G., Goldstein, J.L., *et al.* (2000). Gastrointestinal toxicity with celecoxib versus nonsteroidal anti-inflammatory drugs for osteoarthritis and rheumatoid arthritis. The CLASS study: A randomized controlled trial. *JAMA* **284**:1247–55.

44. Bombardier, C., Laine L., Reicin A., *et al.* (for the VIGOR Study Group) (2000). Comparison of upper gastrointestinal toxicity for rofecoxib and naproxen in patients with rheumatoid arthritis. *N Engl J Med* **343**:1520–8.

45. Mukherjee, D., Nissen, S.E., and Topol, E.J. (2001). Risk of cardiovascular events associated with selective COX-2 inhibitors. *JAMA* **286**:954–9.

46. Geba, G.P., Weaver, A.L., Polis, A.B., Dixon, M.E., Schnitzer, T.J., *et al.* (for the VACT investigators) (2002). Efficacy of rofecoxib, celecoxib, and acetaminophen in osteoarthritis of the knee. A randomized trial. *JAMA* **287**:64–71.

47. Burke, T.A., Zabinski, R.A., Pettit, D., Maniadakis, N., Maurath, C.J., and Goldstein, J.L. (2001). A framework for evaluating the clinical consequences of initial therapy with NSAIDs, NSAIDs plus gastroprotective agents, or celecoxib in the treatment of arthritis. *Pharmacoeconomics* (Suppl. 1):33–47.

48. Zabinski, R.A., Burke, T.A., Johnson, J., Lavoie F., Fitzsimon, C., Tretiak, R., and Chancellor, J.V.M. (2001). An economic model for determining the costs and consequences of using various treatment alternatives for the management of arthritis in Canada. *Pharmacoeconomics* (Suppl. 1):49–58.

49. Chancellor, J.V.M., Hunsche, E., de Cruz, E., and Sarasin, F.P. (2001). Economic evaluation of celecoxib, a new cyclo-oxygenase 2 specific inhibitor, in Switzerland. *Pharmacoeconomics* (Suppl. 1):59–75.

50. Pettit, D., Goldstein, J.L., McGuire, A., Schwartz, S., Burke, T., *et al.* (2000). Overview of the Arthritis Cost Consequence Evaluation System (ACCES): a pharmacoeconomic model for celecoxib. *Rheumatology* **39**(Suppl. 2):33–42.

51. Svarvar, P. and Aly, A. (2000). Use of the ACCES model to predict the health and economic impact of celecoxib in patients with osteoarthritis or rheumatoid arthritis in Norway. *Rheumatology* **39** (Suppl. 2):43–50.

52. Haglund, U. and Svarvar, P. (2000). The Swedish ACCES model: Predicting the health economic impact of celecoxib in patients with osteoarthritis or rheumatoid arthritis. *Rheumatology* **39** (Suppl. 2):51–6.

53. Moore, R.A., Phillips, C.J., Pellissier J.M., and Kong, S.K. (2001). Health economic comparisons of rofecoxib versus conventional nonsteroidal antiinflammatory drugs for osteoarthritis in the United Kingdom. *J Med Econ* **4**:1–17.

54. Maetzel, A., Krahn, M.D., and Naglie, G. (2002). Economic assessment: celecoxib and rofecoxib for patients with osteoarthritis or rheumatoid arthritis. Ottawa: Canadian Coordinating Office for Health Technology Assessment, Technology Overview no 6.

55. Marshall, J.K., Collins, S.M., and Gafni, A. (1999). Demographic predictors of resource utilization for bleeding peptic ulcer disease: the Ontario GI Bleed Study. *J Clin Gastroenterol* **29**:165–70.

56. Smalley, W.E., Griffen, M.R., Fought, L.R., and Ray, W.A. (1996). Excess costs for gastrointestinal disease among nonsteroidal anti-inflammatory drug users. *J Gen Intern Med* **11**:461–9.

57. Rostom, A., Wells, G., Tugwell, P., Welch, V., Dube, C., *et al.* (2000). The prevention of chronic NSAID induced upper gastrointestinal toxicity: A Cochrane collaboration meta-analysis of randomized controlled trials. *J Rheumatol* **27**:2203–14.

58. Leandro, G., Pilotto, A., Franceschi, M., Bertin, T., Lichino, E., and Di Mario, F. (2001). Prevention of acute NSAID-related gastroduodenal damage: a meta-analysis of controlled clinical trails. *Digest Dis Sci* **46**:1924–36.

59. Maetzel, A., Bosi Ferraz, M., and Bombardier, C. (1998). The cost-effectiveness of misoprostol in preventing serious gastrointestinal events associated with the use of nonsteroidal antiinflammatory drugs. *Arthritis Rheum* **41**:16–25.

60. Hillman, A.L. and Bloom, B.S. (1989). Economic effects of prophylactic use of misoprostol to prevent gastric ulcer in patients taking nonsteroidal anti-inflammatory drugs. *Arch Intern Med* **149**:2061–5.

61. Jönsson, B. and Haglund, U. (1992). Cost-effectiveness of misoprostol in Sweden. *Int J Technol Assess Health Care* **8**:234–44.

62. Gabriel, S.E., Jaakkimainen, R.L., and Bombardier, C. (1993). The cost-effectiveness of misoprostol for nonsteroidal antiinflammatory drug associated adverse gastrointestinal events. *Arthritis Rheum* **36**:447–59.

63. Al, M.J., Michel, B.C., and Rutten, F.F.H. (1996). The cost-effectiveness of diclofenac plus misoprostol compared with diclofenac monotherapy in patients with rheumatoid arthritis. *Pharmacoeconomics* **10**:141–51.

64. Knill-Jones, R. (1992). An economic evaluation of Arthrotec in the treatment of arthritis. *Br J Med Econ* **5**:51–8.

65. van Dieten, H.E.M., Korthals-de Bos, B.C.K., van Tulder, M.W., Lems, W.F., Dijkmans, B.A.C., and Boers, M. (2000). Systematic review of the cost-effectiveness of prophylactic treatments in the prevention of gastropathy in patients with rheumatoid arthritis or osteoarthritis taking non-steroidal anti-inflammatory drugs. *Ann Rheum Dis* **59**:753–9.

9.5 Topical NSAIDs

Michael Doherty and Adrian Jones

Topical delivery of salicylate and, subsequently, the newer non-steroidal anti-inflammatory drugs (NSAIDs) has been investigated for over 70 years.[1] It is claimed that this method of delivery is effective in relieving locomotor pain and avoids the serious side effects associated with oral NSAIDs. Although topical products are popular with patients, many physicians remain sceptical of such efficacy and safety claims, largely due to the paucity of published controlled trials, the marked placebo response associated with topical application, and perceived high cost.[2,3]

Nevertheless, despite the reservations of many physicians and government licensing agencies, an increasing number of topical NSAIDs have been marketed. They now form a significant proportion of total NSAID sales, in some countries their market share represents over 50 per cent of all anti-rheumatic agents. In many countries they are largely obtained 'over the counter' without a prescription. Available topical NSAIDs include salicylate, benzydamine, diclofenac, felbinac, flurbiprofen, ibuprofen, indomethacin, ketoprofen, and piroxicam. All have oral equivalents except benzydamine. Felbinac (biphenylacetic acid) is the active form of the prodrug fenbufen. As with oral NSAIDs, the major market for topical NSAIDs is for regional soft tissue pain. Few studies relate to OA, and only a minority of topical NSAIDs are specifically licensed for use in OA. Once topical NSAIDs are available, however, their usage is often extended to OA and to other forms of arthritis.

In this chapter we review the potential advantages and disadvantages of topical NSAIDs and examine data relating to their use in OA.

Theoretical suitability of topical NSAID delivery

At first sight, there seem several potential advantages to topical compared to oral NSAIDs (Table 9.11). For patients with only one, or a few, painful joints—the usual situation with OA—it seems appropriate to target the site where analgesia is required, thereby avoiding unnecessary systemic exposure. Topical products are generally well tolerated; from a patient perspective it makes intuitive sense to apply a treatment where it is needed so compliance is usually high. Such popularity may partly relate to self-efficacy—the patient participating in, and controlling, their own treatment. The massage required to apply topical creams or gels may itself alleviate pain. Importantly, compared to oral delivery, topical NSAIDs result in lower blood levels. Since the risk of major adverse events, especially gastrointestinal (GI), is dose- and blood-level related, topical NSAIDs should be safer.

Local application, however, may also have its problems. It may be less suitable than oral delivery for multiple regional pain, for relatively inaccessible sites such as the spine, or for pain arising from deep structures such as the hip or glenohumeral joint. Patients with compromised hand function may have difficulty applying topical agents, and some products are messy and discolour clothing. Side effects may still occur—local reactions to the NSAID or carrier (reddening, itching, photosensitivity); more widespread hypersensitivity reactions (bronchoconstriction, extensive skin/mucous membrane reactions); or even severe renal adverse reactions such as interstitial nephritis and renal failure following excessive[4] or normal[5] application. Whether topical agents penetrate locally and achieve adequate periarticular and joint tissue levels has also been questioned. Furthermore, many topical NSAIDs cost more per day than the equivalent oral drug. Whether they are better or safer than cheaper 'over the counter' rubefacients or embrocations (themselves not formally tested in OA) remains unknown.

Given these various considerations, what is the evidence for their efficacy and safety in man?

Pharmacokinetics and mode of action

The skin presents a barrier through which only a limited amount of active substance from a given preparation will penetrate, for example, approximately 25 per cent for ibuprofen. Several factors, such as dose, fat solubility, and ionized state of the drug determine penetration into the stratum

Table 9.11 Theoretical advantages and disadvantages of topical application of NSAIDs

Advantages

- Makes sense for single regional pain syndromes
- Very popular with patients
- Well tolerated
- Good adherence
- Self-efficacy—shift of locus of control to patient
- Possible concomitant benefit from massage
- Lower serum levels—therefore safer (especially with respect to gastrointestinal and renal/cardiovascular side effects)

Disadvantages

- Inappropriate for multiple regional pain syndromes
- May be difficult or messy to apply
- Possible local skin reactions
- Systemic (especially hypersensitivity) reactions may still occur despite low serum levels
- May not achieve adequate tissue (especially deep tissue) levels for therapeutic effect
- Cost
- May be no better than cheaper rubefacients

corneum, with lipid soluble, unionized drugs penetrating best. Diffusion through skin is accelerated by occlusive dressings and local hyperaemia. Some additives induce hyperaemia and, thus, influence absorption as well as exerting possible effects from hyperaemia *per se*. Topical NSAIDs come in a variety of delivery systems including creams, gels, foams, patches, and sprays. Pre-medicated patches offer better standardization of the dose of NSAID delivered, but all other modalities give variable self-administered dosing. This itself presents special problems for efficacy and costing studies.

For many drugs that penetrate the skin, rapid clearance via the skin capillaries prevents local drug accumulation. Such rapid clearance explains the systemic efficacy of transdermal nitrates and oestrogen. However, rapid clearance may not be inevitable and there are limited data from animal and human studies to support high local tissue levels of salicylate and certain NSAIDs, with only minor uptake into the systemic circulation, after topical delivery. For example, in dogs, topical salicylate achieves higher concentrations than oral aspirin in cartilage, fascia, ligament, muscle, and tendon, despite much lower blood levels.[6] In one study of felbinac applied to human knees six hours prior to orthopaedic surgery[7] the relative drug concentrations in different tissues were: skin 750; subcutaneous fat 230; muscle 220; synovium 100; synovial fluid 3; and serum 1. Similarly, topical ibuprofen and piroxicam may reach several hundred-fold higher concentrations in periarticular tissues compared to plasma.[8–10] However, not all data support such high tissue concentrations from topical delivery. Another study that involved pre-dosing of orthopaedic patients with felbinac or oral fenbufen prior to knee surgery[11] found that oral fenbufen gave higher concentrations in periarticular tissues and synovial fluid than topical felbinac; all tissue concentrations were lower than those reported in the previous study.[7] It is clear that meticulous technique is required to avoid contamination during sampling of contiguous periarticular/articular tissues, and methodological differences may account for the disparity between these studies.[11]

Because of the relative ease of collection, there are more data on synovial fluid and plasma levels than periarticular tissues. All studies concur in showing low plasma levels after topical salicylate or NSAID. Such levels are in the order of 20–100 times lower than those following oral administration of the identical or equivalent drug at recommended doses.[6–12] With few exceptions,[12] drug concentrations in synovial fluid after topical application are significantly lower than those following oral administration.[6,7,10,11] When it has been examined, for example for diclofenac,[13] fenbufen,[14] and piroxicam,[10] similar synovial fluid concentrations are found in both the topically treated knee and the contralateral untreated knee of the same patient, suggesting that synovial fluid NSAID concentrations, rather than resulting from direct penetration down from skin, primarily result from secondary reperfusion into synovium after absorption into the blood stream. However, in one study of topical salicylate, synovial fluid levels were achieved that were 60 per cent of those following oral aspirin even though plasma levels were several hundred-fold lower,[6] supporting local penetration as well as blood-borne delivery.

The balance of evidence, therefore, confirms low plasma concentrations following topical delivery, but questions whether adequate levels are achieved in target tissues. Such inconclusive pharmacokinetic evidence of efficacy, fuels the scepticism on topical NSAIDs.[2,3] However, the issue of tissue drug levels is clouded since:

- 'adequate' therapeutic levels of NSAIDs in periarticular and joint tissue sites are not established;

- much pharmacokinetic data on topical NSAIDs is unpublished as 'data on file' in pharmaceutical houses;

- synovial fluid data are only available for the knee and extrapolation to smaller, more superficial joints such as finger interphalangeal joints is problematic.

Of course, 'adequate' synovial fluid levels may not be required for symptom benefit in OA. Mechanisms of pain production in OA are complex. Much of the pain that associates with OA may originate in periarticular rather than intracapsular structures.[15] Furthermore, it is possible that drug-induced effects on afferent nociceptor fibers in the skin might influence spinal cord

handling of afferent impulses from adjacent joints.[16] Neurovascular interactions between skin and underlying deep structures might also modulate pain.[17] The relevance of synovial fluid drug concentrations to the clinical efficacy of topical NSAIDs has not been formally examined, though it is apparent that serum levels of NSAID following topical delivery do not correlate with clinical efficacy.[18] The relevance of serum and synovial fluid concentrations to the clinical efficacy of topical NSAIDs is therefore open to question and should not be a major reason for denying their use. Wider investigation of the possible local extracapsular effects of topical NSAIDs is certainly warranted.

Data on clinical efficacy in osteoarthritis

Most clinical data on topical NSAIDs relate to studies of soft-tissue lesions. A number of problems exist for most such studies:

- poor definition of acute regional pain syndrome, often with pooling of different conditions;

- short observation periods, mainly 7–14 days;

- the self-limiting nature of many lesions;

- questionable assessments of pain, function, or clinical signs;

- a marked placebo response in all studies (up to 40–70 per cent).

Few such studies appear in peer-reviewed journals. Nevertheless, despite these caveats there are randomized placebo-controlled studies that attest to the efficacy of topical NSAIDs, including piroxicam,[19] diclofenac,[20] indomethacin,[21] flurbiprofen,[22] and felbinac,[23] in acute and chronic soft tissue injury.

Relatively fewer, particularly placebo-controlled, studies relate to OA. Again, there are problems common to many of these studies including:

- variable definitions of OA;

- short observation periods, usually 14 days and a maximum of 4 weeks;

- a very high placebo response, averaging about 60–70 per cent;

- often inappropriate primary and secondary outcome measures;

- inadequate power to determine a good estimate of efficacy.

Such paucity of data has limited the licensing of topical agents for use in OA, particularly in the United States of America.

Placebo-controlled studies in osteoarthritis

In one double-blind cross-over study of 50 patients with hand OA,[24] topical trolamine salicylate gave better relief of pain and stiffness than placebo cream, a benefit that largely went within two hours of application. The placebo in this study had no counterirritant action, and benefit from massage alone probably lasted for approximately 30 minutes.

A randomized double-blind study of piroxicam versus placebo gel, applied three or four times daily to the most symptomatic knee of 246 OA patients, demonstrated greater efficacy with piroxicam at two weeks.[25] Global patient opinion showed improvement in 80 versus 68 per cent of patients, with marked-moderate improvement in 51 versus 33 per cent. Interestingly, improvement in the contralateral OA knee occurred to a lesser but equal extent in piroxicam (31 per cent) and placebo (36 per cent) patients, suggesting no clinical benefit at distant sites following single joint treatment.

A randomized, double-blind, parallel-group study of topical 2 per cent diclofenac gel conducted in 70 patients with symptomatic knee OA and only modest radiographic change, showed clinical superiority over the placebo gel at the end of the two-week study period, significant differences being observed for the aggregated and individual subscale (pain, stiffness, function) scores of the WOMAC.[26] A 15-day randomized placebo-controlled study of diclofenac plasters (180 mg active drug) applied twice daily in 155 patients with knee OA also showed superiority of the treatment plaster over placebo at all three assessments (days 4, 7, and 15), significant differences being observed for the primary outcomes of pain visual analogue scale (VAS) and the Lequesne Index.[27] Retrospective estimation of the effect size of this treatment[28] showed it to be impressive at 0.91.

Two randomized placebo-controlled multi-centre studies have also reported on eltenac, an NSAID showing structural similarity to diclofenac but with one benzene ring being substituted by a thiophen ring, a modification that improves absorption following topical application. The first study compared topical eltenac gel (1 per cent) to oral diclofenac (50 mg bd) and placebo over a four-week period in 290 patients with knee OA using a three arm double-dummy design.[29] No significant differences were observed between groups in terms of the Lequesne Index and pain VAS, though GI side effects were more common in the oral diclofenac group and skin reactions more common in the eltenac group. However, post-hoc subgroup analysis showed significant, similar clinical benefit for both active agents compared to placebo (Lesquesne Index), in those with moderate to severe baseline pain—a similar finding was reported for intra-articular hyaluronan.[30] The second study compared three strengths of eltenac gel (0.1, 0.3, 1 per cent) to placebo gel over a four-week period in 237 patients with knee OA.[18] Again, although there were non-significant differences in the Lequesne Index in favour of the three eltenac limbs, only subanalysis of those with highest baseline pain showed significantly better efficacy for the 1 per cent gel compared to placebo. Several problems inherent in topical NSAID studies are well illustrated by this study. For example, almost half the patients (102/234) were protocol violators through use of too little or too much of the un-metered gel as judged by the weight of returned tubes (an intention-treat analysis was appropriately used); the standardized effect size of 0.5 used in the power calculation was not achieved; up to 2 g of paracetamol was permitted daily in all groups, perhaps masking the independent effect size of the gel; the ability to fully explore predictors of response was not incorporated into the design; and the pre-study notion that better efficacy might be seen in those with milder pain was not realized. Such aspects merit consideration in future studies.

Comparative studies in osteoarthritis

Several studies report similar efficacy when the topical is compared to the parent or alternative oral NSAID. For example, in a double-blind double-dummy study of 275 patients with mild-moderate knee OA, felbinac was as effective over a two-week period as oral fenbufen, with a similar low incidence of side effects.[31] Parity was also demonstrated in a similarly designed study of 235 patients with mild knee OA, comparing piroxicam gel and oral ibuprofen (1200 mg per day) thrice daily over a four-week period.[32] Both active agents appeared comparable in the 290 patient study comparing oral diclofenac (100 mg daily) and 1 per cent eltenac gel to placebo.[29] In three smaller (40–50 patient) double-blind double-dummy studies of patients with various diagnoses, including OA, equal efficacy after one week was found with salicylate cream or oral aspirin (2600 mg daily) at various peripheral and axial sites.[33,34] Topical salicylate, however, had advantages of faster pain relief and fewer side effects.

The ability to substitute topical for oral NSAID has been demonstrated in one open UK study.[35] One hundred and ninety-one elderly subjects on oral NSAID for OA (mainly knee) were randomized to continue their NSAID for four weeks, or to use piroxicam gel plus half their oral NSAID dose for two weeks, and then gel alone for a further two weeks. Both groups improved from baseline, but the gel group showed greater improvements in joint tenderness and movement, and in AIMS (Arthritis Impact Measurement Scale) scores.

When topical NSAIDs have been directly compared in OA, there are little or no differences in efficacy between products. The design of such studies, however, is often questionable,[36,37] with a strong likelihood of type II error One interesting recent study[38] compared topical piroxicam gel (0.5 per cent) to a homeopathic gel (containing comfrey, poison ivy and marsh-tea extracts) that is widely used in Europe (Spiroflor SRL®) and the United States of America (Triflora®). This four-week, randomized, double-blind study in 184 knee OA patients showed improvements from baseline with both gels (applied 3 times daily) but no significant difference between them using a pain-on-walking VAS and a single joint Ritchie Index. As with other studies,[36,37] however, this trial did not have an appropriately powered equivalence study design and is weakened by the absence of a placebo control. Possible differences between various topical agents that are in current use, therefore, have yet to be adequately examined.

Systematic reviews

A quantitative systematic review of topical NSAIDs, was undertaken by Moore et al. in 1998.[39] They separated data relating to acute and chronic conditions. They defined a clinically relevant successful outcome for chronic conditions, mainly single joint OA, as at least 50 per cent pain relief, in terms of patient global opinion (excellent/good), pain on movement or at rest (no pain, slight pain), or observer global opinion (excellent/good)—patients not in these categories were considered treatment failures. Only information available in dichotomous form was used and the denominator was the number of patients randomized (i.e., intention to treat analysis). The efficacy at two weeks was estimated. From the 12 placebo-controlled trials with dichotomous data (giving information on 1097 patients) the relative benefit over placebo was calculated as 2.0 (95 per cent, confidence interval 1.5–2.7) and the number needed to treat (NNT) was 3.1 (2.7–3.8). In other words, three patients need to be treated for one of them to achieve a successful outcome where they would not have done so with placebo. Sensitivity analysis by quality score or treatment group size did not alter these results. Significant superiority over placebo was demonstrated in 7 of the 12 studies. However, in all 12 studies the proportion of patients with a successful outcome favoured the topical NSAID over placebo (Fig. 9.4). In both acute and chronic conditions, involving 25 controlled trials and 10 160 patients, the incidence of local and systemic adverse events and study withdrawals related to treatment was low and the relative risk was no different from placebo. The conclusion from the review was that topical NSAIDs are effective in relieving pain and apparently safe.

Safety and economic considerations

Short-term studies in OA all report a very low incidence of side effects from topical NSAIDs, similar to,[24,25,31,32,35] or lower[29,33,34] than, oral NSAIDs.

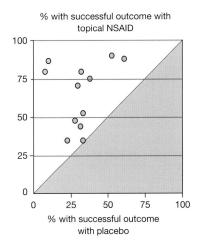

% with successful outcome with topical NSAID

Fig. 9.4 L'Abbé plot showing proportions of patients that achieved successful outcomes (at least 50% pain relief) on either topical or placebo treatment in each of 12 placebo-controlled clinical trials analysed by Moore et al.[39]

Source: Adapted with permission from www.eBandolier.com

Large surveillance studies in general practice appear to confirm their safety. For example, in 23 590 patients given felbinac for two weeks for locomotor pain (22 per cent for OA or arthritis), only 1.5 per cent developed adverse events, mainly local reactions.[40] However, six adverse events relating to the upper GI tract were attributed to felbinac. Other case reports of upper GI events in patients using topical NSAIDs suggest that the risk from these products, although low, may not be negligible.

A large case-control study has evaluated the risk of a major upper GI event associated with topical NSAID use.[41] Using a record-linkage database, 1103 patients, hospitalized for upper GI bleeding or perforation, were each compared to matched community and hospital controls (eight controls per case) for prior drug exposures. After adjusting for the confounding effect of concomitant exposure to oral NSAIDs and ulcer-healing drugs, no association between topical NSAIDs and upper GI events was discerned.

A number of studies have estimated the economic benefits of topical versus oral NSAIDs, using various models of comparative efficacy, GI ulcer rates, and clinical decision-making. Although generally considered an expensive alternative to oral NSAIDs,[2,3] two studies, at least, suggest that topical piroxicam should be more cost-effective than oral ibuprofen for the treatment of mild OA,[42] as would felbinac compared to a combination product containing diclofenac and misoprostol.[43]

The place of topical NSAIDs in management guidelines

Three recent publications have provided guidelines on the management of OA.[28,44,45]

Although the American College of Rheumatology recommendations[44] support the consideration of topical analgesics for mild-moderate pain, only topical methylsalicylate is specified and it is placed, with capsaicin, after paracetamol and oral NSAIDs in order of preference for pharmacological therapy. Such brief consideration primarily reflects the fact that topical NSAIDs are not approved for the reimbursement of OA treatment in the United States of America. A recent UK review of medical management of OA[45] found 'reasonably strong evidence to conclude that topical NSAIDs are effective and safe for patients with OA'. However, as with the ACR recommendations, the use of topical NSAIDs was positioned with capsaicin below paracetamol, stronger (opioid) analgesia, oral NSAIDs, and COXIBs. The EULAR recommendations[28] listed 1B category evidence in favour of topical NSAIDs and reported the two effect sizes that could be calculated from the published data as 0.91 for diclofenac[27] and −0.05 for eltenac,[29] noting the suggested significant benefit from eltenac in those with more severe pain. One of the ten clinical propositions addressed by the EULAR Task Force was 'NSAIDs (oral or topical) should be considered in patients (with effusion) unresponsive to paracetamol'. From the data available at that time, the Task Force concluded that both oral and topical NSAIDs are efficacious in the management of knee OA but the statement, as echoed in the ACR recommendations, that they should be used in those patients in whom paracetamol has failed, though attractive, was not supported by research evidence. Also, they did not find good evidence that the presence of clinical inflammation was a predictor of better response from NSAID.

The three most recent published guidelines, ranging from expert opinion to evidence-based formats, therefore concur in considering topical NSAIDs as effective, safe analgesics that should be included within the treatment options of OA, especially knee OA.

Conclusions

Several observations already support the positioning of topical NSAIDs within the commonly used drug options for OA, and above oral NSAIDs in the preference order of symptomatic agents for knee OA:

1. Topical NSAIDs achieve only low blood levels and appear very safe in comparison to oral NSAIDs.

2. Several placebo-controlled studies attest to the clinical efficacy of topical NSAIDs for knee, and possibly hand OA.

3. The few comparative studies suggest similar efficacy of topical NSAIDs to oral NSAIDs.

4. Topical NSAIDs may prove more cost-effective than oral NSAIDs.

There are still, however, relatively few published studies in this area and a number of outstanding issues remain to be resolved:

1. Further well-designed studies are required to confirm clinical efficacy and effect size.

2. Further studies are required to establish the cost-effectiveness of topical NSAIDs at common OA sites.

3. Further studies are required to clarify the mechanisms of action via this route of delivery.

4. All clinical trials need to be adequately powered, include clinical predictors of response within the study design, and assess long-term (many months rather than just a few weeks) treatment.

Key points

1. Topical NSAIDs are popular with patients and account for a significant proportion of world-wide analgesic sales ('over-the-counter' and prescribed).

2. Most randomised placebo-controlled trials report efficacy of topical NSAIDs in OA.

3. A quantitative systematic review in 1998 suggested a relative benefit over placebo of 2.0 (95% CI 1.5–2.7) and an NNT of 3.1 (95% CI 2.7–3.1) for chronic locomotor pain.

4. Efficacy of topical NSAIDs can be equivalent to oral NSAIDs.

5. Topical NSAIDs are safe, with no increased risk of gastrointestinal bleeding or perforation.

6. Topical NSAIDs may be cost-effective.

References

(An asterisk denotes recommended reading.)

1. **Nothmann, M. and Wolff, M.** (1933). The absorption of salicylic acid by human skin. *Klin Wochscht* **12**:345–6.

2. **Anonymous.** (1989). Topical NSAIDs: a gimmick or a godsend? *Lancet* **2**:779–80.

3. **Anonymous.** (1997). Topical NSAIDs for joint disease. *Drug Therapeut Bull* **37**:87–8.

4. **O'Callaghan, C.A., Andrews, P.A., and Ogg, C.S.** (1994). Renal disease and use of topical non-steroidal anti-inflammatory drugs. *Br Med J* **308**:110–11.

5. **Fernando, A.H.N., Thomas, S., Temple, R.M., and Lee, H.A.** (1994). Renal failure after topical use of NSAIDs. *Br Med J* **308**:533.

6. **Rabinowitz, J.L., Feldman, E.S., Weinberger, A., and Schumacher, H.R.** (1982). Comparative tissue absorption of oral 14 C-aspirin and topical triethanolamine 14 C-salicylate in human and canine knee joints. *J Clin Pharmacol* **22**:42–8.

7. **Sugawara, Y.** (1985). Percutaneous absorption and tissue absorption of L-141 topical agent. *Jpn Med Pharmacol* **13**:183–94.

8. **Peters, H., Chlud, K., Berner, G.,** *et al.* (1987). Percutaneous kinetics of ibuprofen. *Akt Rheumatol* **12**:208–11.

9. **Kanazawa, M., Ito, H., Shimooka, K., and Mase, K.** (1987). The pharmacokinetics of 0.5 per cent piroxicam gel in humans. *Eur J Rheumatol Inflamm* **8**:117.

10. **Sugawara, S., Ohno, H., Ueda, R.,** *et al.* (1984). Studies of percutaneous absorption and tissue distribution of piroxicam gel. *Jpn Med Pharmacol Sci* **12**:1233–8.

11. *Bolten, W., Salzman, G., Goldmann, R., and Miehlke, K. (1989). Plasma and tissue concentrations of biphenylacetic acid following one week oral fenbufen medication and topical administration of felbinac gel on the knee joint. *J Rheumatol* **48**:317–22.

A well-conducted study that discusses the technical problems involved in sampling locomotor tissues for drug level estimations.

12. Riess, W., Schmid, K., Botta, L., et al. (1986). Percutaneous absorption of diclofenac. *Arzneimittel Forschung Drug Res* **36**:1092–6.

13. Radermacher, J., Jentsch, D., Scholl, M.A., Lustinetz, T., and Frolich, J.C. (1991). Diclofenac concentrations in synovial fluid and plasma after cutaneous application in inflammatory and degenerative joint disease. *Br J Clin Pharmacol* **31**:537–41.

14. Dawson, M., McGee, C.M., Vine, J.H., et al. (1988). The disposition of biphenylacetic acid following topical application. *Eur J Clin Pharmacol* **33**:639–42.

15. Creamer, P., Lethbridge-Cejku, M., and Hochberg, M.C. (1998). Where does it hurt? Pain localisation in osteoarthritis of the knee. *Osteoarthritis Cart* **6**:318–23.

16. Woolf, C.J. and Wall, P.D. (1986). Relative effectiveness of C primary fibres of different origins in evoking a prolonged facilitation of the flexor reflex in the rat. *J Neuroscience* **6**:1433–42.

17. Kidd, B.L., Mapp, P.I., Blake, D.R., Gibson, S.J., and Polak, J.M. (1990). Neurogenic influences in arthritis. *Ann Rheum Dis* **49**:649–52.

18. *Ottillinger, B., Gomor, B., Michel, B.A., Pavelka, K., Beck, W., and Elsasser, U. (2001). Efficacy and safety of eltenac gel in the treatment of knee osteoarthritis. *Osteoarth Cart* **9**:273–80.

A randomized placebo-controlled study that suggests better efficacy in those with more severe pain. Some of the problems inherent in the study of topical treatments are highlighted.

19. Russell, A.L. (1991). Piroxicam 0.5 per cent topical gel compared to placebo in the treatment of soft tissue injuries: a double blind study comparing efficacy and safety. *Clin Invest Med* **14**:35–43.

20. Schapira, D., Linn, S., and Scharf, Y. (1991). A placebo-controlled evaluation of diclofenac diethylamine salt in the treatment of lateral epicondylitis of the elbow. *Curr Ther Res* **49**:162–8.

21. Ginsburgh, F. and Famaey, J-P. (1991). Double-blind, randomised crossover study of the percutaneous efficacy and tolerability of a topical indomethacin spray versus placebo in the treatment of tendinitis. *J Int Med Res* **19**:131–6.

22. Poul, J., West, J., Buchanan, N., and Grahame, R. (1993). Local action transcutaneous flurbiprofen in the treatment of soft tissue rheumatism. *Br J Rheumatol* **32**:1000–3.

23. Hosie, G. and Bird, H. (1994). The topical NSAID felbinac versus oral NSAIDs: a critical review. *Eur J Rheumatol Inflamm* **14**:21–8.

24. Rothacker, D., Difigilo, C., and Lee, I. (1994). A clinical trial of topical 10% trolamine salicylate in osteoarthritis. *Curr Ther Res* **55**:584–97.

25. Kageyama, T. (1987). A double blind placebo controlled multicenter study of piroxicam 0.5% gel in osteoarthritis of the knee. *Eur J Rheumatol Inflamm* **8**:114–15.

26. Grace, D., Rogers, J., Skeith, K., and Anderson, K. (1999). Topical diclofenac versus placebo: a double blind, randomised clinical trial in patients with osteoarthritis of the knee. *J Rheumatol* **26**:2659–63.

27. Dreiser, R.L. and Tisne-Camus, M. (1993). DHEP plasters as a topical treatment of knee osteoarthritis—a double-blind placebo-controlled study. *Drugs Exp Clin Res* **19**:117–23.

28. Pendleton, A., Arden, N., Dougados, M., Doherty, M., Bannworth, B., Bijlsma, J.W.J., et al. (2000). EULAR recommendations for the management of knee osteoarthritis: report of a task force of the Standing Committee for International Clinical Studies Including Therapeutic Trials (ESCISIT). *Ann Rheum Dis* **59**:936–44.

29. *Sandelin, J., Harilainen, A., Crone, H., Hamberg, P., Forsskahl, B., and Tamelander, G. (1997). Local NSAID gel (Eltenec) in the treatment of osteoarthritis of the knee. A double blind study comparing eltenac with oral diclofenac and placebo gel. *Scand J Rheumatol* **26**:287–92.

A randomized placebo-controlled study that shows better efficacy in those with more severe pain and no major difference in efficacy between topical and oral NSAID. Problems in study design for topical agents are highlighted and discussed.

30. Lohmander, L.S., Dalen, N., Englund, G., Hamalainen, M., Jensen, E.M., Karlsson, K., et al. (1996). Intra-articular hyaluronan injections in the treatment of osteoarthritis of the knee: a randomised, double-blind, placebo-controlled multicentre trial. *Ann Rheum Dis* **55**:424–31.

31. Tsuyama, N., Kurokawa, T., Nihei, T., Nagano, A., Tachibana, N., and Hanaoka, K. (1985). Clinical evaluation of L-141 topical agent on osteoarthrosis deformans of the knees. *Clin Med* **1**:697–729.

32. Dickson, D.J. (1991). A double-blind evaluation of topical piroxicam gel with oral ibuprofen in osteoarthritis of the knee. *Curr Ther Res* **49**:199–207.

33. Shamszad, M., Perkal, M., Golden, E.L., and Marlin, R. (1986). Two double-blind comparisons of a topically applied salicylate cream and orally ingested aspirin in the relief of chronic musculoskeletal pain. *Curr Ther Res* **39**:470–9.

34. Golden, E.L. (1978). A double-blind comparison of orally ingested aspirin and a topically applied salicylate cream in the relief of rheumatic pain. *Curr Ther Res* **24**:524–9.

35. Browning, R.C. and Johnson, K. (1994). Reducing the dose of oral NSAIDs by use of feldene gel: an open study in elderly patients with osteoarthritis. *Adv Ther* **11**:198–207.

36. Giacovazzo, M. (1992). Clinical evaluation of a new NSAID applied topically (BPAA gel) versus diclofenac emulgel in elderly osteoarthritic patients. *Drugs Exptl Clin Res* **18**:201–3.

37. Rau, R. and Hockel, S. (1989). Piroxicam gel versus diclofenac gel in activated gonarthrosis. *Fortschr Med* **22**:485–8.

38. Van Haselen, R.A. and Fisher, P.A.G. (2000). A randomised controlled trial comparing topical piroxicam gel with a homeopathic gel in osteoarthritis of the knee. *Rheumatology* **39**:714–9.

39. *Moore, R.A., Tramer, M.R., Carroll, D., Wiffen, P.J., and McQuay, H.J. (1998). Quantitive systematic review of topically applied non-steroidal anti-inflammatory drugs. *Br Med J* **316**:333–8.

The only systematic review of topical NSAID clinical efficacy. The review gives quantitative estimates with respect to the relative benefit and the NNT (number needed to treat) for clinical efficacy relative to placebo.

40. Newbery, R., Shuttleworth, P., and Rapier, C. (1992). A multicentre post marketing surveillance study to evaluate the safety and efficacy of felbinac 3% gel in the treatment of musculoskeletal disorders in general practice. *Eur J Clin Res* **3**:139–50.

41. *Evans, J.M.M., McMahon, A.D., McGilchrist, M.M., et al. (1995). Topical non-steroidal anti-inflammatory drugs and admission to hospital for upper gastrointestinal bleeding and perforation: a record linkage case-control study. *Br Med J* **311**:22–6.

Best available evidence to confirm the safety of topical NSAIDs. This large case control study showed no increased risk of major gastrointestinal bleeding or perforation requiring hospitalization, after adjustment for potential confounders.

42. McKell, D. and Stewart, A. (1994). A cost-minimisation analysis comparing topical versus systemic NSAIDs in the treatment of mild osteoarthritis of the superficial joints. *Br J Med Econ* **7**:137–46.

43. Peacock, M. and Rapier, C. (1993). The topical NSAID felbinac is a cost effective alternative to oral NSAIDs for the treatment of rheumatic conditions. *Br J Med Econ* **6**:135–42.

44. American College of Rheumatology Subcommittee on osteoarthritis guidelines. (2000). Recommendations for the medical management of osteoarthritis of the hip and knee. *Arthritis Rheum* **43**:1905–15.

45. Walker-Bone, K., Javaid, K., Arden, N., and Cooper, C. (2000). Medical management of osteoarthritis. *Br Med J* **321**:936–40.

9.6 Topical capsaicin cream

Kenneth D. Brandt and John D. Bradley

Capsaicin (*trans*-8-methyl-*n*-vanillyl-6-nonenamide) (Fig. 9.5) is an alkaloid derived from the seeds and membranes of the Nightshade family of plants, which includes the common pepper plant. It is the active ingredient in Tabasco sauce (Fig. 9.6).

Capsaicin has received attention as a topical analgesic agent.[1] Initially, it was believed that capsaicin worked by a 'counterirritant' mechanism,[2] that is, by the stimulation of faster conducting nociceptors that activated the descending diffuse noxious inhibitory control system which, in turn, inhibited the more slowly conducting pain signals transmitted along small diameter unmyelinated fibers in the spinal cord. (This 'gate control' concept may also be relevant to the mechanism of action of transcutaneous electrical nerve stimulation (TENS) and acupuncture.)[3] Subsequently, however, it was shown that capsaicin, when applied topically, stimulates the release of the neuropeptide, substance P, from the peripheral nerves and prevents its re-accumulation from cell bodies and nerve terminals in both the central and peripheral nervous system. Substance P is an important chemical mediator responsible for the transmission of pain from the periphery to the central nervous system.

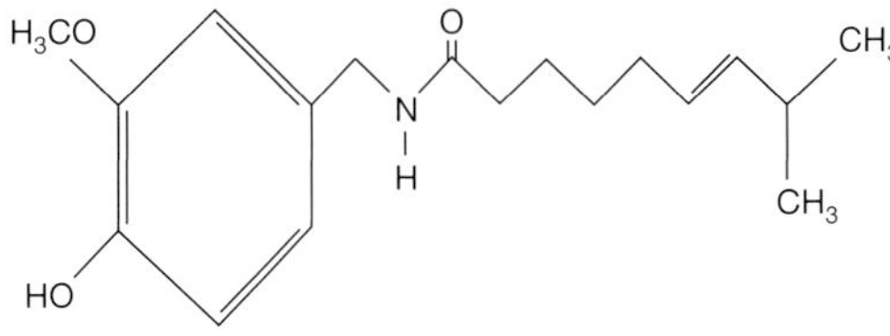

Capsaicin has been used in the treatment of a variety of painful disorders, including postherpetic neuralgia, cluster headaches, diabetic neuropathy, phantom limb pain, and postmastectomy pain.[4–7] Local application of capsaicin results in the depletion of substance P from the entire neuron, so that branches from the peripheral nerves to deeper structures, such as the joint, are effectively depleted.[1,8] Initially, external transport of substance P is blocked; with continued treatment, synthesis of substance P is reduced.

Although normal articular cartilage has no nerve supply and, therefore, cannot be a source of pain, histologic studies of joint innervation have shown that the joint capsule, tendons, ligaments, subchondral bone, and periosteum are extensively innervated.[9–11] Furthermore, as the pathologic changes of OA progress, capillaries originating in the medullary spaces of the subchondral bone and carrying nerve endings within their walls invade the normally avascular articular cartilage. Small diameter nerve fibers in the synovium[12] and subchondral plate[13] have been shown to stain immunohistochemically for substance P, as has sclerotic bone[14] and areas of bony eburnation[15] and of fibrillated cartilage[15] in OA joints. Synovial concentrations of substance P are increased in patients with OA.[16,17]

There is some evidence that, in addition to modulating pain, substance P may mediate inflammation within the joint. Intra-articular infusion of substance P in rats with adjuvant arthritis increased the severity of joint inflammation, and this effect could be blocked by infusion of a substance P antagonist.[18] Intra-articular injection of substance P increases blood flow to the joint, transudation of plasma proteins, and release of lysosomal enzymes.[19] In addition, substance P is a chemoattractant for neutrophils and monocytes,[19] and stimulates synovial cells to produce prostaglandins and collagenase, mediators associated with joint damage.[18,20] Although the importance of substance P in the pathogenesis of joint inflammation in OA is not clear, and mediators other than substance P are undoubtedly involved, substance P may play an important role in mediating joint pain in OA and pharmacological inhibition of substance P may be useful in the symptomatic management of OA.

In 1991, Deal *et al.*[21] reported the results of a randomized, double-blind, placebo-controlled multi-center trial involving patients with moderate to very severe pain due to knee OA. Patients in the active treatment group applied either 0.025 per cent capsaicin cream, or the vehicle, four times daily to anterior, posterior, and lateral aspects of the most severely affected knee. The results are shown in Table 9.12.

Improvement in joint pain was significantly greater ($p = 0.02$) in subjects who received capsaicin than in the placebo group. After four weeks of treatment, the evaluation of the physician and the pain score of the patient both showed a mean reduction of 22 per cent ($p = 0.05$) for those using the active cream, but of only 14 per cent ($p = 0.05$) and 10 per cent ($p = 0.06$), respectively, for those using the placebo cream.

A local burning sensation was noted by 44 per cent of patients using the capsaicin preparation and by one patient in the placebo group. However, burning diminished with continuation of treatment, and 94 per cent of patients in the active treatment group and 88 of those in the placebo group

H_3CO HO — (*trans*-8-methyl-*n*-vanillyl-6-nonenamide)

Fig. 9.5 Chemical structure of capsaicin.

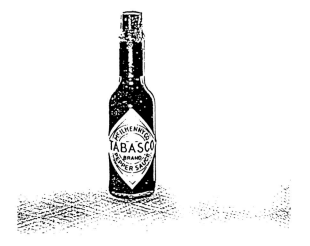

Fig. 9.6 Capsaicin is derived from the pepper plant and is the active ingredient in Tabasco sauce. (Photo by Kathie Lane.)

Table 9.12 Results of placebo-controlled trials of capsaicin cream in patients with OA

Study	OA joint site	Capsaicin strength (%)	Duration of study (weeks)	Number of subjects treated	Decrease in joint pain at end of study (%)	
					Capsaicin 0.25%	Capsaicin 0.025%
Deal et al.[21]	Knee	0.025	4	36 Capsaicin 34 Placebo	22	14
McCarthy et al.[22]	DIP, PIP, MCP	0.075	4	7 Capsaicin 7 Placebo	60	20
Altman et al.[23]	Various (70% knee)	0.025	12	57 Capsaicin 56 Placebo	53	27
Schnitzer et al.[24]	Various (approx. 80% knee)	0.25 vs 0.025	4	31 Capsaicin 29 Placebo	74	66

DIP, distal interphalangeal joints; PIP, proximal interphalangeal joints; MCP, metacarpophalangeal joints.

completed the study. Although the burning, which occurred at the site of application, obviously affected blinding of the study, and may have favored a positive response to the capsaicin, the authors attempted to take this into account by comparing the results in patients treated with capsaicin who experienced burning, with those in capsaicin-treated patients who did not have this side effect. No difference in drug response was apparent between the two groups.

In 1992, McCarthy and McCarty reported a more potent formulation of capsaicin (0.075 per cent) in a placebo-controlled, four-week, double-blind randomized trial involving 14 subjects with painful OA of the distal or proximal interphalangeal joints or first carpometacarpal joint[22] (Table 9.12). By week four, the topical application of capsaicin had reduced joint pain by nearly 60 per cent and joint tenderness by approximately 40 per cent, in comparison with the baseline values, while improvement in these parameters in patients treated with topical application of the vehicle alone was only about 20 and 10 per cent, respectively. No changes were noted, however, with respect to grip strength, joint swelling, duration of morning stiffness, or joint function. As in the study by Deal et al.,[21] all patients who received capsaicin reported a burning sensation in the skin. However, none discontinued treatment because of this side effect, and the local discomfort diminished over the first week and became increasingly tolerable with continued treatment.

In both of the above studies, patients were permitted to continue their usual treatment with NSAIDs or analgesics; capsaicin was used as an adjunct to the usual therapy. In contrast, Altman et al. has reported a clinical trial of 0.025 per cent capsaicin cream as *monotherapy* for OA[23] (Table 9.12). In this double-blind study, NSAIDs and the other medications that the patients were receiving for the treatment of OA were discontinued, before entry into the study. Use of acetaminophen was permitted during the study but was restricted to three days per month, and patients were given only 12 tablets of acetaminophen per month, to be used for non-arthritic pain or fever. Patients were evaluated for 12 weeks, that is, considerably longer than in either of the two trials cited above. Although subjects had OA at a variety of joint sites, 70 per cent of those treated with capsaicin and 79 per cent of those treated with the vehicle had knee OA. Among the 113 patients included in the study, 57 received capsaicin and 56 were treated with the vehicle.

Baseline pain scores in the two groups, measured on a visual analog scale, were comparable (57 mm for capsaicin, 56 mm for vehicle). Based on global evaluation of the patients, those who received capsaicin reported significantly greater reduction of pain at weeks 4, 8, and 12, than the controls. At week 12, mean improvement in pain in the capsaicin group was about 53 per cent, while that in the placebo group was about 27.4 per cent ($p = 0.02$) (Fig. 9.7) (Table 9.12).

This study is important insofar as it shows that improvement in joint pain can occur with capsaicin as the *sole* analgesic therapy and can be sustained. Indeed, pain relief was as great after 12 weeks of treatment as after

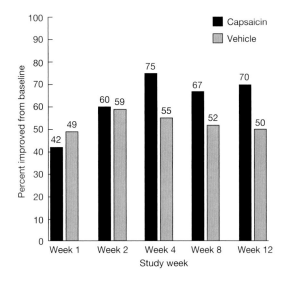

Fig. 9.7 Mean per cent change in pain intensity over 12 weeks of therapy with capsaicin, 0.025 per cent, or vehicle in 89 evaluable patients with OA.

VAS, visual analog scale; $^{*}p < 0.05$ vs vehicle.

Source: Taken from Altman, R.D., Aven, A., Holmburg, C.E., *et al.* 1994. *Sem Arthritis Rheum* **23**(Suppl. 3):25–33.

only four weeks. Furthermore, the magnitude of improvement in joint pain was as great as that seen with NSAIDs.

In a recent single-blind study of patients with OA at a variety of joint sites,[24] a high-strength (0.25 per cent) capsaicin cream (not currently available in the United States of America), applied only twice a day, provided greater pain relief, with a considerably more rapid onset of action, than 0.025 per cent capsaicin cream applied four times daily. It is unclear, however, whether the fact that the dosing regimens were not comparable may have affected outcomes in the two treatment groups. As in the study by Altman et al.,[23] medications that might have interfered with the efficacy evaluation (e.g., NSAIDs, systemic analgesics) were withdrawn prior to randomization, that is, capsaicin was employed as the *only* analgesic agent during the study. Furthermore, only one patient in the high-strength capsaicin treatment group discontinued therapy because of a sensation of burning at the site of application. Although the incidence of burning was initially greater with the high-strength formulation, by day seven, and subsequently for the remainder of this 28-day study, the number of patients who reported burning was no greater in the high-strength capsaicin group than in the 0.025 per cent capsaicin group.

Table 9.13 Mean daily analgesic use at week 6, number of tablets taken per day[*]

Treatment group	Mean daily analgesic use	Standard error
Placebo	4.00	0.20
GTN	3.52[†]	0.16
Capsaicin	3.72[#]	0.16
Capsaicin/GTN	3.25[†]	0.18

GTN, glyceryl trinitrate.

Source: Taken from McCleane G. 2000. *Eur J Pain* **4**: 355–60.

[*] Pretreatment mean analgesic consumption was 4 tablets per day.

[†] $p = < 0.01$.

[#] $p = < 0.05$.

Topical capsaicin therapy appears to be safe and effective, and warrants initial consideration in the management of OA pain. Patients should apply the medication in a thin film to all sides of the involved joint and should be instructed to wash their hands immediately after application of the cream, to avoid contact with eyes and mucus membranes, and broken or inflamed skin. In all of the studies cited above, the topical burning sensation caused by capsaicin generally subsided with continued treatment and seldom resulted in discontinuation of treatment. Intolerance may also be managed by temporarily switching to a lower-strength preparation (if the 0.025 per cent formulation is not the initial choice). A higher potency cream may then be used, if necessary, after tolerance to the skin irritating effect of the lower-strength preparation has developed.

A recent 6-week study of patients with radiographically confirmed OA of the hip, knee, shoulder, or hand indicated that the addition of glyceryl trinitrate to capsaicin (0.025 per cent) resulted in less local discomfort than capsaicin alone and a greater decrease in the use of concurrent analgesic than either agent alone[25] (Table 9.13).

Key points

Use of topical capsaicin for treatment of OA pain

1. Is safe
2. May be employed as an adjunct to systemic analgesic/NSAID treatment
3. May be effective as monotherapy
4. The magnitude of response may be as great as with NSAIDs or acetaminophen
5. Somewhat inconvenient: irritating to eyes and mouth, requires 3–4 applications per day, and improvement may not occur until 3–4 weeks after use.

References

(An asterisk denotes recommended reading.)

1. **Virus, R.M. and Gebhart, G.F.** (1979). Pharmacologic actions of capsaicin: apparent involvement of substance P and serotonin. *Life Science* **25**:1273–84.
2. **Kantor T.** (1989). Concepts in pain control. *Sem Arthritis Rheum* **18**:94–9.
3. **Gunn, C.C.** (1978). Transcutaneous neural stimulation, acupuncture, and the current of injury. *Am J Acupuncture* **6**:191–6.
4. **Bernstein, J.E., Korman, N.J., Bickers, D.R., Dahl, M.V., and Millikan, L.E.** (1989). Topical capsaicin treatment of chronic postherpetic neuralgia. *J Am Acad Dermatol* **21**:265–70.
5. **Sicuteri, F., Fusco, B., Marabini, S., and Fanciullacci, M.** (1988). Capsaicin as a potential medication for cluster headache. *Med Sci Res* **16**:1079–80.
6. **Ross, D.R. and Varipapa, R.J.** (1989). Treatment of painful diabetic neuropathy with topical capsaicin. *N Engl J Med* **321**:474–5.
7. **Raynor, H.C., Atkins, R.L., and Westerman, R.A.** (1989). Relief of local stump pain by capsaicin cream. *Lancet* **2**:276–7.
8. **Fitzgerald, M.** (1983). Capsaicin and sensory neurones—a review. *Pain* **15**:109–30.
9. **Samuel, E.P.** (1952). The autonomic and somatic innervation of the articular capsule. *Anat Rec* **113**:84–93.
10. **Ralson, H.J., Miller, M.R., and Kasahara, M.** (1960). Nerve endings in human fasciae, tendons, ligaments, periosteum and joint synovial membrane. *Anat Rec* **136**:137–47.
11. **Milgram, J.W. and Robison, R.A.** (1965). An electron microscopic demonstration of unmyelinated nerves in the Haversian canels of the adult dog. *Bull Johns Hopkins Hosp* **117**:163–73.
12. **Kidd, B.L., Mapp, P.I., Blake, D.R., Gibson, S.J., and Polak, J.M.** (1990). Neurogenic influences in arthritis. *Ann Rheum Dis* **49**:649–52.
13. **Nixon, A.J. and Cummings, J.F.** (1994). Substance P immunohistochemical study of the sensory innervation of normal subchondral bone in the equine metacarpophalangeal joints. *Am J Vet Res* **55**:28–33.
14. **Badalamente, M.A. and Cherney, S.B.** (1989). Periosteal and vascular innervation of the human patella in degenerative joint disease. *Sem Arthritis Rheum* **18**:61–6.
15. **Wojtys, E.M., Beaman, D.N., Glover, R.A., and Janda, D.** (1990). Innervation of the human knee joint by substance-P fibers. *Arthroscopy: J Arth Rel Surg* **6**:254–63.
16. **Menkes, C.J., Mauborgne, A., Loussadi, S., et al.** (1991). Substance P (SP) levels in synovial tissue and synovial fluid from rheumatoid arthritis (RA) and osteoarthritis (OA) patients. In *Scientific Abstracts of the 54th Annual Meeting of the American College of Rheumatology, Seattle, WA, October 27–November 1*.
17. **Marshall, K.W., Chiu, B., and Inman, R.D.** (1990). Substance P and arthritis: analysis of plasma and synovial fluid levels. *Arthritis Rheum* **33**:87–90.
18. **Levine, J.D., Clark, R., Devor, M., Helms, C., Moskowitz, M.A., and Basbaum, A.I.** (1984). Intraneuronal substance P contributes to the severity of experimental arthritis. *Science* **226**:547–9.
19. **Kimball, E.S.** (1990). Substance P, cytokines and arthritis. *Ann NY Acad Sci* **594**:293–308.
20. **Lotz, M., Carson, D.A., and Vaughan, J.H.** (1987). Substance P activation of rheumatoid synoviocytes: Neural pathway in pathogenesis of arthritis. *Science* **235**:893–5.
21. **Deal, C.L., Schnitzer, T.J., Lipstein, E., et al.** (1991). Treatment of arthritis with topical capsaicin: a double-blind trial. *Clin Ther* **13**:383.
22. **McCarthy, G.M., McCarty, D.J.** (1992). Effect of topical capsaicin in the therapy of painful osteoarthritis of the hands. *J Rheumatol* **19**:604.
23. *****Altman, R.D., Aven, A., Holmburg, C.E., et al.** (1994). Capsaicin cream 0.025% as monotherapy for osteoarthritis: a double-blind study. *Sem Arthritis Rheum* **23**:25–33.

    This is the first report of efficacy of capsaicin cream as monotherapy for OA pain, that is, in patients who were not concomitantly to taking NSAIDS/analgesics.
24. *****Schnitzer, T., Posner, M., and Lawrence, I.** (1995). High-strength capsaicin cream for osteoarthritis pain: rapid onset of action and improved efficacy with twice daily dosing. *J Clin Rheumatol* **1**:268–73.

    This paper presents results of a comparative clinical trail of two doses of capsaicin cream, 0.25 and 0.025%, both of which were employed as monotherapy in patients with OA of various joint sites, but mostly of the knee. The higher strength formulation was applied only twice daily and the lower strength, four times daily. Results showed much more rapid pain relief with the higher strength formulation and, at the end of this 4-week study, favored the higher strength formulation but the difference was not significant. The high-dose group reported burning sensations at the application site, relative to low dose, but the frequency of reports of local discomfort subsided rapidly and on day seven of treatment the two groups were virtually identical.
25. **McCleane, G.** (2000). The analgesic efficacy of topical capsaicin is enhanced by glyceryl trinitrate in painful osteoarthritis: a randomized, double blind, placebo controlled study. *Eur J Pain* **4**:355–60.

9.7 Intra-articular glucocorticoids and other injection therapies

Adrian Jones and Michael Doherty

As a rheumatic disease the effects of OA are localized to the joint with none of the systemic symptoms and pathology as seen, for example, with rheumatoid disease. It would seem logical, therefore, when considering interventions to concentrate on the ones that deliver the therapeutic agent directly to the target joint and thus bypass the potential problems of systemic administration. Many of the joints principally affected by OA, especially the knee, are readily accessible and thus amenable to intra-articular injection. This chapter principally concentrates on glucocorticoids, which are widely available and used, but other agents are briefly considered. Some intra-articular therapies such as hyaluronans (Chapter 9.8), possible disease-modifying OA drugs (DMOADs; Chapter 11.2.1) and joint lavage (Chapter 9.17) are considered elsewhere.

Historical considerations

The history of intra-articular therapy is surprisingly long. Following the observations in the 1930s that synovial fluid in osteoarthritic joints is characterized by an alkaline pH, and the resultant hypothesis that acidity might stimulate joint repair, some workers attempted to treat OA by intra-articular injection of various acids, including lactic acid[1] and phosphoric acid.[2] Although encouraging results were reported from a large series of patients,[3] the studies were uncontrolled and the practice slowly faded. It was not really until the discovery of the power of factor F (adrenal extract) to ameliorate the effect of rheumatoid arthritis that interest in intra-articular agents was rekindled. Thorn is generally credited with the first use of intra-articular factor F but it was Hollander who reported the first large series in OA.[4] This demonstrated promising efficacy in terms of symptomatic relief and, as will be discussed later such agents have been subjected to a number of placebo controlled, double-blind randomized trials that demonstrate efficacy albeit of short duration. The short duration of action and concerns about safety means that the use of corticosteroids in OA remains an often hotly debated issue.

Following clinical observations of improvement in osteoarthritic joints subjected to arthroscopy, the use of arthroscopic and later percutaneous irrigation was subjected to randomized trial. Benefit was again demonstrated although perhaps of a longer duration.

The known changes in OA in the synovial fluid—reduced viscosity, altered macromolecules—has also led to attempts to alter the rheological and biochemical properties of the fluid initially with silicone oils, which was unsuccessful[5] and more recently with hyaluronans. These are discussed elsewhere (Chapter 9.8).

In recent years the emergence of 'evidence-based medicine' has led to a re-evaluation of many established therapies such as corticosteroids. Whilst these studies have generated new confirmatory experiments that establish the role of intra-articular steroids, they have also caused investigators to reconsider the role and efficacy of other elements of intra-articular injection. These include the effect of placebo and peri-articular injection, local anaesthetics, and opiates. It has also encouraged attempts to define predictors of response to the injection in order to enable clinicians to more precisely define the role of an injection in an individual.

Finally, as discussed elsewhere, our better understanding of OA has also led to a search for other intra-articular agents that might alter symptomatic outcome (e.g. the super-oxide dismutase inhibitor, orgotein). In addition, the development of strategies that might alter structural outcome in OA (e.g. the DMOADs, tissue engineering, cytokine administration) often involve intra-articular administration.

Intra-articular administration—practical considerations

Although intra-articular injection is widely practised, some recent studies have called into question the ability of operators to accurately localize such injections with almost a third of knee injections being inaccurate.[6] As will be discussed below, this may have an effect on efficacy and must be taken into account when considering the results of clinical trials. Attempts to improve accuracy using radiographic[7] or ultrasonographic techniques have been studied[8–10] but as yet not widely adopted for most peripheral joints, for example, the knee, hand, and shoulder. For deeper joints such as the hip and the spinal apophyseal (facet) joints, imaging is crucial and many techniques are described.[11,12]

Glucocorticoids

These are the most widely employed agents in the intra-articular management of OA. Most controlled data relates to their use in the knee, and although benefit is described at other sites including the hip, thumb-base, spine, and interphalangeal joints, controlled data are lacking.

Efficacy

A number of older and now more recent studies have attempted to evaluate the efficacy of intra-articular corticosteroids. A Cochrane review group has been established to look at this question but has not yet published its findings. In the studies that have been conducted using a wide number of steroids, the general findings are that intra-articular corticosteroids reduce pain (Table 9.14). This effect is, however generally short-lived (<6 weeks) and there are issues, therefore, regarding the frequency of repeat injections, which relate to logistical and safety arguments. The timing and frequency of injection remains, in our opinion, a matter for discussion between the patient and the operator, taking into account issues of safety, cost, co-morbid conditions that may limit the use of other therapies, and the magnitude and duration of response in the individual patient.

One small double-blind study comparing 10 ml 0.5 per cent bupivicaine + triamcinolone versus 10 ml 0.5 per cent bupivicaine or 10 ml saline in patients awaiting hip joint replacement, demonstrated a worse deterioration in symptoms in the patients receiving triamcinolone compared to the other two groups.[21]

Table 9.14 Studies comparing intra-articular corticosteroids to placebo injection in patients with knee osteoarthritis

Steroid	Dose (mg)	Total patients	Design	Duration of benefit (weeks)	Ref.
Hydrocortisone acetate	50	59	Parallel group	Nil	13
Hydrocortisone acetate		25 (38 knees)	Cross-over	Nil	14
Hydrocortisone tertiary butylacetate		25 (38 knees)	Cross-over		14
Triamcinolone hexacetonide	20	34	Parallel group	<4 weeks	15
Triamcinolone hexacetonide	20	12	Between knees	1	16
Triamcinolone hexacetonide	20	16	Cross-over	?4	16
Triamcinolone hexacetonide	20	84	Parallel group	<6	17
Triamcinolone hexacetonide	20	60	Parallel group	6	18
Dexamethasone	4	26	Parallel group	7	19
Cortivazol	3.75	53	Parallel group	4	20

The choice of agent to use is unclear as few direct comparisons of agents have been made. In general, it is considered that longer acting, more hydrophobic steroids are more effective. For example, in a study comparing hydrocortisone tertiary butylacetate versus hydrocortisone acetate (short-acting) or placebo, only the patients receiving hydrocortisone tertiary butylacetate showed statistically significant benefit.[14] Similarly 20 mg triamcinolone hexacetonide was significantly more effective that 6 mg betamethasone.[22]

Animal models have suggested that corticosteroids may have a favourable effect on the osteoarthritic process. This is discussed elsewhere but the evidence for such an effect in humans is lacking.

Predictors of response

The targeting of corticosteroid injections towards patients in whom the benefit is likely to be greatest is desirable and some studies have attempted to clarify if this can be done. Although many guidelines suggest that corticosteroid injection should be targeted at patients experiencing a 'flare' of symptoms, there is little objective evidence to suggest that the efficacy is any greater in this setting. In a placebo controlled double-blind study comparing triamcinolone to placebo injection, no predictors of response could be identified.[18] The possible predictors that were studied included: effusion, age, gender, and degree of radiographic change. Another study did suggest that the presence of a joint effusion might predict a more favourable response[17] but it is possible that the presence of an effusion predicts accuracy of the injection, which is itself a predictor of response.[6] An earlier study failed to demonstrate a benefit from the presence of an effusion.[15]

At the hip, one study of 45 patients, 27 of whom had OA has suggested that night pain and a predominant hypertrophic pattern of bone response might predict a more favourable response to an injection with 4 ml 1% lidocaine + 80 mg methylprednisolone.[23] In the spinal apophyseal joints, a radionuclide SPECT scan demonstrating increased isotope uptake in a facet joint may predict patients with back pain who will respond more favourably to corticosteroid injection and allow more precise targeting of the injection.[24]

Adverse effects

Sepsis

The most feared complication, septic arthritis, appears to be rare although most studies examining this are often problematic because of difficulties with: precise identification of the denominator (number of injections and the type of arthritis involved); the background risk of sepsis (increased in OA); the elimination of protopathic bias (the flare of OA for which the injection is given actually resulting from prior sepsis); and standard approaches to establishing the diagnosis of sepsis. A recent estimate derived from a retrospective survey in France suggests an overall risk of sepsis of 13 per million injections with the incidence being much lower if prepackaged steroid-filled syringes are used (6 v 48).[25] In a retrospective 10-year survey of septic arthritis in Nottingham (population 600 000), only 3 cases of septic arthritis possibly related to corticosteroid injection were identified.[26] Overall the risk of infection appears low.

Local reactions

A flare of synovitis in a joint, following injection, may also be due to a post-injection synovitis. The mechanism underlying this is unclear. A crystal synovitis is often invoked but the fact that it may also occur after placebo injection with normal saline makes the mechanism seem more uncertain than a simple steroid crystal synovitis. The incidence of this reaction is unclear but rates of 12–24 per cent following steroid injection[15,17,18,27,28] have been observed, compared to a rate of 10 per cent following placebo injection.[17] In the event of a flare the crystalline nature of many steroids can cause problems of attribution if such crystals are wrongly identified by compensated polarizing light microscopy as calcium pyrophosphate dihydrate crystals.

Skin atrophy may also occur, particularly with fluorinated steroids and if the injected steroid leaks from the joint usually in the situation where a small superficial joint is injected. Precise figures for the incidence of this are not available. Tendon rupture after injection of an arthritic joint has also been described, particularly at the thumb base.[29] Peri-articular injections are more likely to result in this complication (Fig. 9.8).

Systemic effects of corticosteroid injections

Absorption of injected steroid from the joint has been long recognized. Peak plasma levels after an intra-articular injection of 80 mg methylprednisolone are of the order of 169 ng ml^{-1} and this is achieved 8 hours post-injection.[30] A measurable effect on the pituitary-adrenal axis has been observed with injections of 40 mg methylprednisolone[31] or after >40 mg triamcinolone diacetate.[32] Whether such adrenal suppression has any long-term sequelae is unclear. Although immunosuppression has been implicated in incidental case reports as a problem (e.g. reactivation of tuberculosis[33]) the link is tenuous and at the frequency of injections generally proposed (i.e. no more than three-monthly), it would seem unlikely to be a significant problem.

The propensity of absorbed glucocorticoids to upset diabetic control is often cited[27] but we are unaware of any substantial data quantifying this as a real clinical problem, and although like others we warn patients of the risk in practice we have not seen problems. On the other hand menstrual irregularity after injection is sometimes observed.

Facial flushing, presumably due to altered vascular tone, is seen in some patients following intra-articular corticosteroid injection (Fig. 9.9). One prospective study has estimated the risk at 40 per cent of injections with severe effects occurring in 12 per cent.[34] It seems prudent to warn patients of the possibility and if it occurs to consider changing to a different steroid preparation as this may reduce the risk.[34] Anaphylaxis after intra-articular steroid injection has been reported but is rare[35,36] as is steroid psychosis.[37]

One case report has suggested a possible fat embolism syndrome following injection of a rheumatoid hip with methylprednisolone and hyaluronate.[38]

Cartilage and bone

Since glucocorticoids were first used there have been concerns over possible resulting joint damage. A Charcot-like arthropathy was initially described with hydrocortisone,[39] and animal models particularly in rabbits seemed to

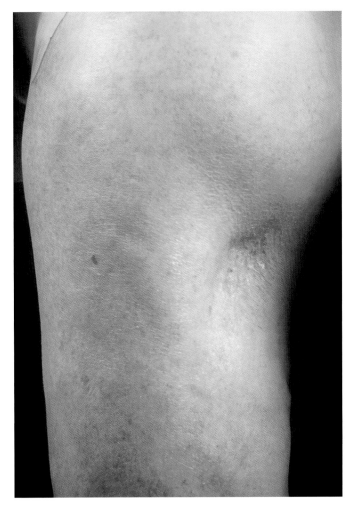

Fig. 9.8 Local skin atrophy following fluorinated corticosteroid injection of an anserine bursa.

provide experimental support for such changes, but animal experiments using larger joints has often suggested a possible beneficial role of glucocorticoids. A rapidly destructive arthropathy may be seen in OA in any case and the specificity and attribution of such changes is unclear. Large case series of long-term follow-up of children with juvenile idiopathic arthritis who have received multiple injections have failed to demonstrate any adverse effect of the joint with the exception of one patient with avascular necrosis of the hip.[40] A small case-control study of patients awaiting hip replacement has, however, suggested more rapid symptomatic deterioration in the group receiving the steroid injection.[21] In addition a recent study of temporomandibular joint OA has suggested worse cartilage and bone changes in joints treated with intra-articular corticosteroids.[41] The relevance of both these findings remains unclear and to date we are not persuaded that glucocorticoids when used at the current levels are detrimental in man.

Para-articular injection

Although pain in OA may arise from the joint, it is also possible that peri-articular structures may also be important. It is therefore probable that injecting peri-articular structures may also be effective. Peripatellar injection of corticosteroids in one study produced benefits equivalent to that seen with articular injection.[42] Anserine bursitis may also be common in knee OA and may respond well to local injection.[43] The danger of

(a)

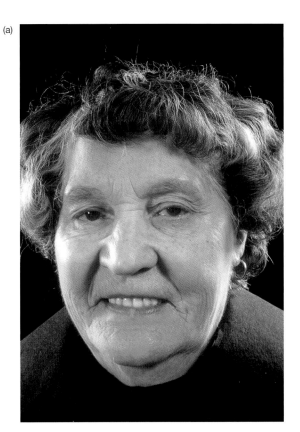

(b)

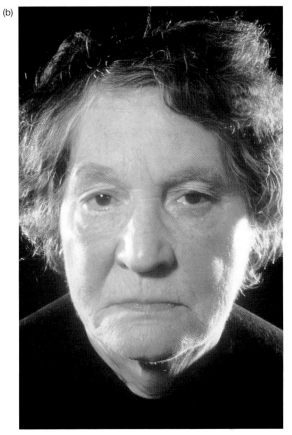

Fig. 9.9 (a) Facial appearance before and (b) after intra-articular injection of steroid for knee osteoarthritis.

peri-articular injection with regard to tendon rupture has also been empha-sized, although the magnitude of this risk is hard to determine.

Regional nerve blocks

The blockade of nerves supplying a joint might well be expected to give good pain relief, and techniques have been described for accomplishing this for most joints. Animal models of OA have suggested that denervation may carry a risk of accelerating the osteoarthritic process.[44] Such concerns have also been suggested in man although this must be weighed against the fact that such techniques are usually advocated for those unfit for surgery. The risk of structural deterioration in this context must be borne against the efficacy of pain relief, which in some cases may be considerable.

Radiosynovectomy

Intra-articular injection of radiocolloids, such as [90]Yt or chemical toxins such as Osmium, has for many years been used in patients with painful knee effusions due to a variety of arthritis. Although enthusiasts have claimed great success, randomized trials demonstrating benefit in OA are few.[45] Although a number of case series contain patients with OA, the benefit seems marginal with one retrospective case series reporting only a 10 per cent improvement rate at one year in patients with OA[46] and a prospective series reporting that only two out of four patients with knee OA showed improvement at 1 year.[47]

Orgotein

Orgotein, a bovine Cu-Zn super-oxide dismutase, has been subject to a number of clinical trials. The rationale of its use is unclear but it is thought that the drug will inhibit phagocytic response to hydroxyapatite crystals as well as ameliorate the effect of any hypoxic-reperfusion injury.

In a 24-week, double-blind, placebo-controlled trial in 45 patients with knee OA, 12 fortnightly injections of 2 mg orgotein was superior to placebo in decreasing pain and improving function. Effects were somewhat slow in onset, occurring at 8–14 weeks.[48] Six of the 29 patients receiving orgotein (21 per cent) experienced a post-injection 'flare'.

In a randomized double-blind comparison of 40 mg of methylpred-nisolone and either 8 or 16 mg orgotein, no statistically significant difference was seen between the groups except at 24 weeks, when 16 mg of orgotein appeared to be more efficacious.[28] A dose-ranging study in 139 patients with knee OA of orgotein (8×3, 16×2, or $32 \, mg \times 1$) versus three placebo injec-tions demonstrated more withdrawals due to inefficacy in the placebo group and higher efficacy ratings in the orgotein group, but with no differences between the doses used.[49]

In a study of 419 patients with knee OA, randomized to receive either 4 mg orgotein, 8 mg orgotein, or betamethasone, a faster onset of action was observed in the betamethasone group.[50] However, blinding was not adequate since only the dose of orgotein was masked; patients and physi-cians knew who was receiving corticosteroids.

Although published work suggests that orgotein may be of symptomatic benefit in knee OA, to date the agent is not widely available or licensed.

Other therapies

Although some clinicians add local anaesthetic to corticosteroid injections, evidence for this practice is lacking. Local anaesthetics may, however, be useful on their own. In a study of 20 patients with bilateral painful knee OA, subjects were randomized to receive either 5 ml of 0.23 per cent bupivicaine or an equivalent volume of saline. Although principally designed as a study to investigate pain mechanisms in OA (i.e. was the pain principally arising from structures in intimate contact with the joint cavity) it did demonstrate

marked improvements in pain at 1 hour in the bupivicaine group. Although a statistically significant reduction in the visual analogue pain score was not observed beyond this time, prolonged changes in the McGill pain question-naire were observed up to seven days. Also of interest was the fact that sim-ilar improvements were observed in the contralateral non-injected knee but only in the local anaesthetic group.[51] The mechanism behind this is unclear but has also been observed with other agents including corticosteroids and hyaluronans.[52]

Risks of local anaesthetic injection are few although convulsions have been described. Since the duration of action of glucocorticoids is short, it may be that local anaesthetics if giving a similar duration of action may be deemed safer, particularly with regard to cartilage damage and sepsis. However, the animal studies demonstrating the possible effect of denerva-tion on deterioration of OA need to be borne in mind.

Guanethidine is an agent often used for regional sympathetic blockade in conditions such as complex regional pain syndrome. It is been assessed for use in the painful shoulder. In a small randomized study of 18 patients with chronic shoulder pain, five of whom were considered to have glenohumeral OA, statistically significant symptomatic benefit was demonstrated com-pared to saline injection.[53] However, the number of OA patients was small and the significance of these data is unclear.

Since pain in OA might be mediated in part by prostaglandins and since non-steroidal anti-inflammatory drugs are effective in OA, it would seem logical to consider intra-articular injection of such agents. Some benefit was claimed in one open study of a small group of fifteen patients with knee OA receiving intra-articular phenylbutazone (190 mg) and 5 ml 1 per cent procaine although most patients required three injections.[54] Tenoxicam was successfully studied as an intra-articular agent but its withdrawal from the market means that it has not been adopted as a clinical agent.[55] Hip joint distension with or without intra-articular indoprofen failed to demonstrate any additional benefit from the addition of the non-steroidal anti-inflammatory drug.[56]

In a small randomized double-blind cross-over study of 23 patients with knee OA 1 mg of intra-articular morphine provided a significantly more prolonged relief of pain compared to intravenous morphine + intra-articular saline placebo.[57] In a parallel group study comparing 4 mg intra-articular dexamethasone, 3 mg intra-articular morphine, and saline placebo, both the morphine and dexamethasone groups demonstrated a similar reduction in pain over a 7-day period.[19] Given the prejudices against opiate use it remains to be seen whether this will become a more widespread therapy. Similarly the 5-HT blocking agent, tropisteron, has also demonstrated benefit in OA in one small pilot study. It remains to be seen whether this will become a readily available clinical agent.[58]

Joint distension alone has been postulated to be effective in OA although a double-blind, placebo-controlled study in 38 patients with hip OA failed to demonstrate any benefit.[59] Attempts to ameliorate the osteoarthritic process by the intra-articular administration of dextrose have also been attempted.[60] The rationale of this approach is that dextrose will promote healing of the tissues damaged by the OA process. One randomized double-blind controlled study compared injections of 9 ml 10 per cent dextrose (in bacteriostatic water and 0.75 per cent lidocaine), to a control injection (9 ml bacteriostatic water and 0.75 per cent lidocaine) in 111 knees in 68 patients.[60] Injections were administered twice monthly. Pain was improved in both the control and active treatment groups with no clear preference in favour of the active treatment. Other outcome measures were also not convincingly different between the two groups.

Summary

Intra-articular glucocorticoids are effective in OA but their duration of action is short, with more hydrophobic agents such as triamcinolone ace-tonide and hexacetonide being more effective. Currently it is not possible to predict which patients will respond, and individual patient responses and preferences will need to be taken into account to determine use. The safety of intra-articular corticosteroids is good but patients should be warned about flushing, post-injection flare, and a small risk of sepsis. Pre-packaged syringes may be preferable.

Although other agents have been evaluated, few of them are currently used in clinical practice.

Key clinical points

1. Intra-articular glucocorticoids produce symptomatic benefit in OA at many sites.

2. The duration of benefit is short-lived (<6 weeks).

3. Hydrophobic corticosteroids (triamcinolone acetonide and triamcinolone hexacetonide) are more effective than hydrocortisone acetate.

4. Toxicity of glucocorticoids is low but patients should be warned regarding flushing (12 per cent), post-injection flare (15 per cent), and sepsis (1 : 78 000 risk).

5. There may be an increasing role for intra-articular analgesics and other locally delivered disease-modifying agents (DMOADs, gene vectors, cytokine therapy).

References

(An asterisk denotes recommended reading.)

1. Waugh, W.G. (1938). Treatment of certain joint lesions by injection of lactic acid. *Lancet* (i):487–9.

2. Crowe, H.W. (1944). Treatment of arthritis with acid potassium phosphate. *Lancet* (i):563–4.

3. Waugh, W.G. (1945). Mono-articular osteo-arthritis of the hip. *Br Med J* (i):873–4.

4. Hollander, J.L., Brown, E.M., and Jessar, R.A. (1951). Hydrocortisone and cortisone injected into arthritic joints. *JAMA* 147:1629–35.

5. Wright, V., Haslock, D.I., Dowson, D., Seller, P.C., and Reeves, B. (1971). Evaluation of silicone as an artificial lubricant in osteoarthrotic joints. *Br Med J* 2:370–3.

6. *Jones, A., Regan, M., Ledingham, J., Pattrick, M., Manhire, A., and Doherty, M. (1993). Importance of placement of intra-articular steroid injections. *Br Med J* 307:1329–30.

   An interesting small study challenging the accuracy of routine non-radiographically guided peripheral joint injections.

7. Bliddal, H. (1999). Placement of intra-articular injections verified by mini air-arthrography. *Ann Rheum Dis* 58:641–3.

8. Bliddal, H. and Torp-Pedersen, S. (2000). Use of small amounts of ultrasound guided air for injections. *Ann Rheum Dis* 59:926–8.

9. Fredberg, U., van Overeem Hansen, G., and Bolvig, L. (2001). Placement of intra-articular injections verified by ultrasonography and injected air as contrast medium. *Ann Rheum Dis* 60:542.

10. Qvistgaard, E., Kristoffersen, H., Tersler, L., Danneskiold-Samsøe, B., Torp-Pedersen, S., and Bliddal, H. (2001). Guidance by ultrasound of intra-articular injections in the knee and hip joints. *Osteoarth Cart* 9:512–7.

11. Dory, M. (1981). Arthrography of the lumbar facet joints. *Radiology* 140:23–7.

12. Glémarec, J., Guillot, P., Laborie, Y., Berthelot, J-M, Prost, A., and Maugas, Y. (2000). Intraarticular glucocorticosteroid injection into the lateral atlantoaxial joint under fluoroscopic control. *Joint Bone Spine* 67:54–61.

13. Miller, J.H., White, J., and Norton, T.H. (1958). The value of intra-articular injections in osteoarthritis of the knee. *J Bone Jt Surg Br* 40-B:636–43.

14. Wright, V., Chandler, G.N., Monson, R.A.H., and Hartfall, S.J. (1960). Intra-articular therapy in osteoarthritis. *Ann Rheum Dis* 19:257–61.

15. Friedman, D.M. and Moore, M.E. (1980). The efficacy of intraarticular steroids in osteoarthritis: a double-blind study. *J Rheumatol* 7:850–6.

16. Dieppe, P.A., Sathapatayavongs, B., Jones, H.E., Bacon, P.A., and Ring, E.F.J. (1980). Intra-articular steroids in osteoarthritis. *Rheumatol Rehab* 19:212–17.

17. *Gaffney, K., Ledingham, J., and Perry, J.D. (1995). Intra-articular triamcinolone hexacetonide in knee osteoarthritis: factors influencing the clinical response. *Ann Rheum Dis* 54:379–81.

    The largest most recent study of the efficacy of intra-articular steroid injections, which also attempts to define predictors of response.

18. Jones, A. and Doherty, M. (1996). Intra-articular corticosteroids are effective in osteoarthritis but there are no clinical predictors of response. *Ann Rheum Dis* 55:829–32.

19. Stein, A., Yassouridis, A., Szopko, C., Helmke, K., and Stein, C. (1999). Intra-articular morphine versus dexamethasone in chronic arthritis. *Pain* 83:525–32.

20. *Ravaud, P., Moulinier, L., Giraudeau, B., Ayral, X., Guerin, C., Noel, E., Thomas, P., Fautrel, B., Mazieres, B., and Dougados M. (1999). Effects of joint lavage and steroid injection in patients with osteoarthritis of the knee. *Arthritis Rheum* 42:475–82.

    A well-conducted large study not only of the efficacy of intra-articular steroids but more importantly of the superior efficacy of joint lavage.

21. Flanagan, J., Thomas, T.L., Casale, F.F., and Desai, K.B. (1988). Intra-articular injection for pain relief in patients awaiting hip replacement. *Ann Royal Coll Surg Eng* 70:156–7.

22. Valtonen, E.J. (1981). Clinical comparison of triamcinolone hexacetonide and betamethasone in the treatment of osteoarthrosis of the knee joint. *Scan J Rheumatol* (Suppl.):S41:1–7.

23. Plant, M.J., Borg, A.A., Dziedzic, K., Saklatvala, J., and Dawes, P.T. (1997). Radiographic patterns and response to corticosteroid hip injection. *Ann Rheum Dis* 56:476–80.

24. Dolan, A.L., Ryan, P.J., Arden, N.K., Stratton, R., Wedley, J.R., Hamann, W., Fogelman, I., and Gibson, T. (1996). The value of SPECT scans in identifying back pain likely to benefit from facet joint injection. *Br J Rheumatol* 35:1269–73.

25. *Seror, P., Pluvinage, P., Lecoq d'Andrade, F., Benamou, P., and Attuil, G. (1999). Frequency of sepsis after local corticosteroid injections (an inquiry on 1 160 000 injections in rheumatological private practice in France) *Rheumatology* 38:1272–4.

    Although flawed by its retrospective nature the best current evidence of the true risk of sepsis following intra-articular injection.

26. Weston, V.C., Jones, A.C., Bradbury, N., Fawthrop, F., and Doherty, M. (1999). Clinical features and outcome of septic arthritis in a single UK Health District 1982–1991. *Ann Rheum Dis* 58:214–9.

27. Clemmesen, S. (1971). Triamcinolone hexacetonide for intraarticular and intramuscular therapy. *Acta Rheum Scand* 17:273–8.

28. Gammer, W., and Broback, L.-G. (1984). Clinical comparisons of orgotein and methylprednisolone acetate in the treatment of osteoarthrosis of the knee joint. *Scand J Rheumatol* 13:108–12.

29. Tonkin, M.A. and Stern, H.S. (1991). Spontaneous rupture of the flexor carpi radialis tendon. *J Hand Surg Br* 16(B):72–4.

30. Bertouch, J.V., Meffin, P.J., Sallustio, B.C., and Brooks, P.M. (1983). A comparison of plasma methylprednisolone concentrations following intra-articular injection in patients with rheumatoid arthritis and osteoarthritis. *Aust N Z J Med* 13:583–6.

31. Lazerevic, M., Skosey, J.L., Djordjevic-Denic, G., Swedler, W.I., Zgradic, I., and Myones, B.L. (1995). Reduction of cortisol levels after single intra-articular and intramuscular steroid injection. *Am J Med* 99:370–3.

32. Shuster, S. and Williams, I.A. (1961). Adrenal suppression due to intra-articular corticosteroid therapy. *Lancet* (i):171–2.

33. Courtman, N.H. and Weighill, F.J. (1992). Systemic tuberculosis in association with intra-articular steroid therapy. *J R Coll Surg Ed* 37:425.

34. Pattrick, M. and Doherty, M. (1987). Facial flushing after intra-articular injection of steroid. *Br Med J* 295:1380.

35. Larsson, L. (1989). Anaphylactic shock after administration of triamcinolone acetonide in a 35 year old female. *Scand J Rheumatol* 18:441–4.

36. Hopper, J.M. and Carter, S.R. (1993). Anaphylaxis after intra-articular injection of bupivicaine and methyl-prednisolone. *J Bone Joint Surg (Br)* 75(B):505–6.

37. Robinson, D.E., Harrison-Hanley, E., and Spencer, R.F. (2000). Steroid psychosis after an intra-articular injection. *Ann Rheum Dis* 59:927.

38. Famularo, G., Liberati, C., Sebastiani, G.D., and Polchi, S. (2001). Pulmonary embolism after intra-articular injection of methylprednisolone and hyaluronate. *Clin Exp Rheumatol* 19:355.

39. Chandler, G.N., Jones, D.T., Wright, V., and Hartfall, S.J. (1959). Charcot's arthropathy following intra-articular hydrocortisone. *Br Med J* (**i**):952–3.

40. *Sparling, M., Malleson, P., Wood, B., and Petty, R. (1990). Radiographic followup of joints injected with triamcinolone hexacetonide for the management of childhood arthritis. *Arthritis Rheum* **33**:821–6.
    The best current data on the safety of repeated corticosteroid injections as regards joint integrity and progression.

41. Haddad, I.K. (2000). Temporomandibular joint osteoarthrosis. *Saudi Med J* **21**:675–9.

42. Sambrook, P.N., Champion, G.D., Browne, C.D., Cairns, D., Cohen, M.L., Day, R.O., *et al.* (1989). Corticosteroid injection for osteoarthritis of the knee: peripatellar compared to intra-articular route. *Clin Exp Rheumatol* **7**:609–13.

43. Kang, I. and Han, S.W. (2000). Anserine bursitis in patients with osteoarthritis of the knee. *Southern Med J* **93**:207–9.

44. O'Connor, B.L. and Brandt, K.D. (1992). Neurogenic acceleration of osteoarthrosis. *J Bone Joint Surg Am* **74**(**A**):367–76.

45. Doherty, M. and Dieppe, P.A. (1981). Effect of intra-articular yttrium-90 on chronic pyrophosphate arthropathy of the knee. *Lancet* (**ii**):1243–6.

46. Taylor, W.J., Corkill, M.M., and Rajapaske, C.N.A. (1997). A retrospective review of Yttrium-90 synovectomy in the treatment of knee arthritis. *Br J Rheumatol* **36**:1100–5.

47. Jahangier, Z.N., Moolenburgh, J.D., Jacobs, J.W.G., Serdijn, H., and Bijlsma, J.W.J. (2001). The effect of radiation synovectomy in patients with persistent arthritis: A prospective study. *Clin Exp Rheumatol* **19**:417–24.

48. Lund-Oleson, K. and Menander-Huber, K.B. (1983). Intra-articular orgotein therapy in osteoarthritis of the knee. *Arzneim Forsch* **33**:1199–203.

49. Mcllwain, H., Silverfield, J.C., Cheatum, D.E., Poiley, J., Taborn, J., Ignaczak, T., *et al.* (1989). Intra-articular orgotein in osteoarthritis of the knee: a placebo-controlled efficacy, safety, and dosage comparison. *Am J Med* **87**:295–300.

50. Mazieres, B., Masquelier, A.-M., and Capron, M.-H. (1991). A French controlled multicenter study of intraarticular orgotein versus intraarticular corticosteroids in the treatment of knee osteoarthritis: a one-year followup. *J Rheumatol* **18**(Suppl. 27):134–7.

51. Creamer, P., Hunt, M., and Dieppe, P. (1996). Pain mechanisms in osteoarthritis of the knee: effect of intra-articular anesthetic. *J Rheumatol* **23**:1031–6.

52. Jones, A.C., Pattrick, M., Doherty, S., and Doherty, M. (1995). Intra-articular hyaluronic acid compared to intra-articular triamcinolone hexacetonide in inflammatory knee osteoarthritis. *Osteoarthritis Cart* **3**:269–73.

53. Gado, K. and Emery, P. (1996). Intra-articular guanethidine injection for resistant shoulder pain: a preliminary double blind study of a novel approach. *Ann Rheum Dis* **23**:1031–6.

54. Moens, B. and Moens, C. (1986). Intra-articular injection of phenylbutazone in gonarthrosis. *Ann Rheum Dis* **44**:788–91.

55. Papathanassiou, P. (1994). Intra-articular use of tenoxicam in degenerative osteoarthritis of the knee joint. *J Int Med Res* **22**:332–7.

56. Egsmose, C., Lund, B., and Andersen, R.B. (1984). Hip joint distension in osteoarthrosis. A triple-blind controlled study comparing the effect of intra-articular indoprofen with placebo. *Scand J Rheumatol* **13**:238–42.

57. Likar, R., Schäter, M., Paulak, F., Sittl, R., Pipam, W., Schalk, H., Geissler, D., and Bernatsky, G. (1997). Intraarticular morphine analgesia in chronic pain patients with osteoarthritis. *Anesth Analg* **84**:1313–7.

58. Stratz, T. and Muller, W. (2000). The use of 5-HT3 receptor antagonists in various rheumatic diseases. *Scand J Rheumatol* **29**(Suppl. 113):66–71.

59. Høilund-Carlsen, P.F., Meinicke, J., Christiansen, B., Karle, A.K., Stage, P., and Uhrenholdt, A. (1985). Joint distension arthrography for disabling hip pain. *Scand J Rheumatol* **14**:179–83.

60. Reeves, K.D. and Hassanein, K. (2000). Randomized prospective double-blind placebo-controlled study of dextrose prolotherapy for knee osteoarthritis with or without ACL laxity. *Alternative Therapies* **6**:68–80.

9.8 Intra-articular hyaluronan injection

Kenneth D. Brandt

Hyaluronan (HA) is a large, polydisperse linear glycosaminoglycan composed of repeating disaccharides of glucuronic acid and N-acetyl glucosamine (Fig. 9.10). Synoviocytes, fibroblasts, and chondrocytes all synthesize HA.[1] Synovial fluid is an ultrafiltrate of plasma, modified by addition of a high concentration of HA, which is synthesized and secreted by Type B cells of the synovial lining.[2–4] The molecular weight (mw) of HA in normal human synovial fluid is $6–7 \times 10^6$ Da and the concentration 2–4 mg/ml.[2]

High mw HA is viscoelastic, that is, it behaves as a viscous liquid at low shear rates and elastic solid at high shear rates. Because of its HA content, joint fluid acts as a viscous lubricant during slow movement of the joint, as in walking, and as an elastic shock absorber during rapid movement, as in running. Synovial fluid HA lubricates the soft tissues (e.g., adjacent fronds of synovial villi) and provides a surface layer on the articular cartilage.

HA has a variety of effects on cells *in vitro* that may relate to its reported effects on joint disease: it inhibits PGE-2 synthesis induced by interleukin-1 (IL-1);[5] protects against proteoglycan (PG) depletion, and cytotoxicity induced by oxygen-derived free radicals, IL-1, and mononuclear cell-conditioned medium;[6,7] suppresses cartilage matrix degradation by fibronectin fragments,[8,9] and reduces leukocyte adherence, proliferation, migration, and phagocytosis.[3] HA increases mRNA expression for IL-1β, tumour necrosis factor -α (TNF-α), and insulin-like growth factor-1 (IGF-1).[10] Such *in vitro* studies, however, have compared the effects of the HA only with those of the culture medium or vehicle, but not with that of solutions that would more closely simulate synovial fluid from patients with OA, in which the endogenous HA concentration may average 1.5 mg/ml.

Inflammation increases the rate of clearance of HA and protein from the joint.[11] It has been suggested that HA acts as a chemical sponge, binding or entangling macromolecules and particulate debris, and that the rapid clearance of injected HA facilitates the removal of these deleterious substances from the joint space.[12] However, injection of exogenous HA had no effect on the rate of clearance of radiolabelled albumin from the canine knee joint[13] and little evidence exists that injection of exogenous HA promotes clearance of metabolites and debris or significantly augments fluid flow through the joint.

In OA, the concentration and mw of synovial fluid HA are reduced.[14,15] The original rationale for use of intra-articular (IA) HA in treatment of OA[2] was to increase the viscosity of the synovial fluid.[2] Investigators have contended that altered properties of synovial fluid contributed importantly to the progression of joint destruction in OA and that transient supplementation of joint fluid led to long-lasting increases in the mw and concentration of endogenous HA,[16,17] with improved joint function and reduction in joint pain. As indicated below, however, the evidence in support of HA therapy is not wholly convincing.

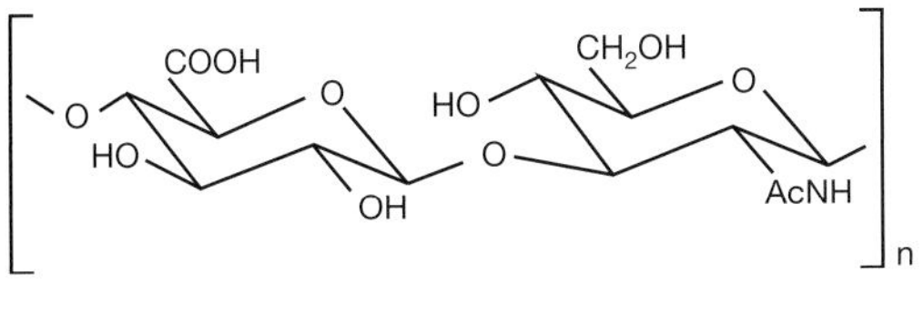

HA preparations marketed for IA injection range from $0.25–2 \times 10^6$ Da and have been purified from rooster comb or human umbilical cord or synthesized by bacteria. To increase the average mw and synovial half-life, HA has been chemically cross-linked to form hylans, whose average mw may be as high as 23×10^6 Da. In the United States of America, one non-crosslinked preparation of HA, from rooster combs, Hyalgan® (mw = $5–7.5 \times 10^5$ Da), and one hylan, Synvisc® (hylan G-F20), have been approved for use in humans with knee OA whose joint pain has not responded to non-medicinal measures and analgesic drugs. Synvisc® is a highly purified formulation of rooster comb HA, the major portion of which is cross-linked with formaldehyde and the remainder with vinyl-sulfone to form a highly viscous gel (mw = $6–7 \times 10^6$ Da).[18] The American College of Rheumatology Guidelines for the Medical Management of Osteoarthritis recommend the use of IA HA injections for treatment of joint pain in patients with knee OA who have failed to respond adequately to conservative non-pharmacologic therapy and simple analgesics.[19]

Does injection of exogenous HA lead to a sustained increase in the viscoelasticity of the synovial fluid?

Injected HA has a short residence time in the joint. For Hyalgan®, the half-life is 17 hours;[20] the smaller component of Synvisc® (90 per cent of the preparation) has a half-life of 1.5 days: the half-life of larger component is 8.8 days.[21] In a study of 7 patients with knee OA, each of whom received a single IA injection of human umbilical cord HA (Healon®, mw = 2×10^6 Da), although the mean concentration of HA in samples obtained 2–22 days after the injection rose by about 10 per cent, pre- and post-treatment values were both well within the range of normal for the human joint.[14] The mw of HA from the OA joint was lower than normal before treatment and, although it increased somewhat after treatment, remained considerably lower than normal (Table 9.15).[22] Because injected HA would have been cleared from the joint by the time the post-treatment sample was obtained and post-treatment values were higher than those for the HA injected, the authors concluded that injection of exogenous HA favourably alters the molecular parameters of the HA synthesized by the OA synovium. However, no statistical analysis of the results was provided and the measurements of mw were performed on samples obtained no longer than about a week after the injection.

In animal studies, no consistent effect of IA HA injection has been observed.[23] For example, in horses with bilateral carpal osteochondral defects in which one carpus was injected with the above HA preparation and the other with saline, no differences were noted between the concentration of HA or protein, or the specific viscosity, of synovial fluid from the

Fig. 9.10 Chemical structure of HA. The molecule is a long-chain polymer consisting of repeating units of D-glucuronic acid and N-acetylglucosamine.

Table 9.15 Effects of intra-articular injection of Healon® on the hyaluronan (HA) concentration and limiting viscosity of HA in synovial fluid from humans

Sample	HA Concentration (mg/ml)		Limiting viscosity (cc/g)	
	Mean ± SD	Range	Mean ± SD	Range
Healon®	10	10	NA	2000–2500
Normal synovial fluid[†]	2.26 ± 0.13	1.45–2.94	5230 ± 140	4500–6000
OA Synovial Fluid[‡]				
Pre-treatment	1.56 ± 0.36	1.14–1.99	3325 ± 650	3000–4300
Post-treatment	1.73 ± 0.29	1.38–2.14	3825 ± 512	3300–4500
Improvement with treatment	0.17 ± 0.27	− 0.39–0.42	500 ± 316	200–900

NA, not available; OA, osteoarthritis.

[†] Values obtained on 71 joints from 42 donors, collected as 10 pooled samples and 3 individual samples.[14]

[‡] HA concentration values are from all 7 patients enrolled in this study.[22] Limiting viscosity values are from 4 of the 7 patients, in whom intrinsic viscosity was measured 1 week after injection of Healon®.

two carpi obtained serially for as long as 35 days after injection.[24] In a canine cruciate-deficiency model of OA in which HA was injected weekly for 5 weeks into the unstable knee, beginning the day after anterior cruciate ligament transection (ACLT), the HA concentration of synovial fluid aspirated before each injection was lower than that in samples obtained from either the contralateral knee 12 weeks after ACLT or the ipsilateral knee prior to ACLT.[25] The mean concentration of HA in synovial fluid from the HA-injected knees was no greater than joint fluid from that in saline-injected controls.

Although synoviocyte cell lines derived from patients with OA synthesized more HA, and HA of higher mw, when exogenous HA was added to the medium,[26] the highest concentration added, 0.4 mg/ml, was lower than that in synovial fluid from most OA joints, and much lower than that in normal human synovial fluid. In primary cultures of synoviocytes from horses with osteochondral fractures, neither the rate of HA synthesis nor the mw of the HA which was synthesized were altered by addition to the medium of HA preparations for therapeutic use in horses at concentrations as high as 1.5 mg/ml.[27]

Evidence that *intravenous* (IV) administration of HA was effective in horses with an intercarpal joint osteochondral fragment raises further doubt that this therapy works by local viscosupplementation.[28] Seventy-two days after surgery, lameness scores were lower, synovial histopathologic changes less severe, and synovial fluid concentrations of protein and prostaglandin E_2 lower in horses that had received an IV injection of 40 mg of HA on days 13, 20, and 27 after surgery, than in horses that had received IV saline injections as a control. However, no effect of HA on pathologic changes of OA or on the PG concentration or net rate of PG synthesis in articular cartilage from the damaged joint was noted.

The half-life of HA after IV administration in rats, rabbits, and sheep, is only minutes, with uptake occurring primarily in the reticuloendothelial cells of the liver.[29,30] Although no information is available concerning the effects of IV HA administration on synovial membrane biology, there is no a priori reason to believe that the small quantity of HA injected IV in the horse would stimulate HA production by the synovium. Confirmation of the above findings and examination of the effects of IV HA on synovium are needed; if the results are validated, it would be difficult to understand the rationale for use of multiple IA injections of HA in doses much higher, relative to body weight, than those required for a beneficial effect.

Effects of IA HA injection on OA pain

Several investigators have concluded that HA injection relieves joint pain and improves function in humans with knee OA (e.g., see Refs 31–33). In 1997, Kirwan and Rankin[31] reviewed published studies of the effects of IA HA therapy and compared outcomes with those obtained after IA injection of placebo or corticosteroid. More recently, Hochberg published an updated summary of clinical trials of IA HA in patients with knee OA and concluded that this therapy resulted in improvement in knee pain and function greater than that produced by placebo and comparable to that achieved with nonsteroidal antiinflammatory drugs (NSAIDs); further, that it offered significant advantage over aspiration alone or placebo injections for up to 6 months, and that it may have an advantage over IA glucocorticoid injection.[34] On the other hand, a review of the limitations in the experimental design and/or interpretation of published clinical trials of IA therapy in humans have also been published recently.[23] HA injections appear to result in improvement, which is similar in magnitude to that of arthrocentesis or placebo, but of a somewhat greater duration. The magnitude of improvement after a series of IA HA injections appears comparable to that after corticosteroid injection.[35] The latter produces improvement more rapidly, but the benefit appears to be more short-lived than after IA HA. Whether improvement after HA injection is real or is due to a placebo effect or regression to the mean (i.e., patients who are selected for IA injection have symptoms that are more severe than average and their pain would improve even without treatment) is unresolved.[23]

The pivotal double-blind trial of Hyalgan® serves to emphasize the vigour of the placebo response to IA injections.[32] In this study, patients were treated with five weekly IA injections of HA or saline or naproxen, 500 mg/bid. Subjects who received IA injections were given dummy tablets, as a control for the naproxen, while those in the naproxen arm received five weekly subcutaneous injections of lidocaine, as a blind for the IA injections. Among those who completed the study (approximately 67 per cent), a decrease in knee pain after a 50-foot walk ≥20 mm on a visual analogue scale (VAS), was seen in 56 per cent of those who received HA and 41 per cent of the placebo group (Fig. 9.11). Twenty-six weeks after initiation of treatment, about 47 per cent of patients in the HA group, but only 33 per cent of those in the saline group, were 'pain-free' or reported only 'mild pain' ($p = 0.039$).

Results in the HA group were similar to those in the naproxen group, leading the authors to conclude that treatment with HA was as effective as naproxen for patients with knee OA and had fewer side effects. However, an intention-to-treat analysis of all subjects randomized to treatment (rather than of only the completers) showed that the series of IA saline injections was as effective as the positive control, naproxen (Table 9.16). Although this study was not powered specifically to detect the difference between Hyalgan® and IA saline, more than 100 patients were randomized in each treatment arm of this study, affording sufficient power to have permitted detection of a difference as small as 10 per cent between the HA and saline groups, had one existed. Furthermore, although consumption of rescue acetaminophen in the HA treatment group was about the same as in the saline group, in both it was some 40 per cent greater than in the naproxen group.

Although it has been claimed that the efficacy of IA HA is comparable to that of NSAIDs in patients with knee OA,[32,33] and that HA therapy could reduce the need for NSAIDs (and thus the risks associated with the systemic inhibition of cyclooxygenase) there is no evidence that, in clinical practice, HA therapy is followed by a reduction in NSAID dose or discontinuation of NSAID treatment.

Direct comparisons of hylans and non-crosslinked HA formulations are limited. A recent report of a study[36] in which hylan G-F 20 was compared with a non-crosslinked hyaluronan, concluded that patients treated with the hylan experienced greater improvement in joint pain. However, although the authors described the results of a 2-arm clinical trial, the data were extracted from a 4-arm study; that is, results for two of the treatment

groups were omitted from the published manuscript. The full study, in fact, compared denatured hylan G-F 20 (to eliminate viscoelasticity), hylan G-F 20, and two non-crosslinked hyaluronans.[37,38] Notably, results with *none* of the active HA formulations were significantly different from those with the denatured Synvisc® control. Similarly, in a clinical trial whose results, however, have been presented to date only in abstract form, no differences between placebo, hylan G-F 20, and a non-crosslinked HA preparation was apparent 26 weeks after the onset of treatment.[39]

Likewise, in a double-blinded placebo-controlled trial of the HA preparation, Artzal®,[40] no difference between the two treatment groups was apparent in intention-to-treat, per protocol or area-under-the-curve analyses. *Post hoc* analyses favoured the HA in subjects older than age 60 and those who had worse scores on an algofunctional index. However, subgroup analysis of the Hyalgan® study described above[32] did not reveal such differences.

No information is available to establish the optimal number of IA injections or the dose necessary for a successful therapeutic outcome. However, injections of hylan G-F 20, given one week apart, were more effective in relieving knee pain than two injections administered two weeks apart.[41] Nor does much information exist to permit a direct comparison of the efficacy and adverse effects of the two HA preparations currently approved by the FDA for use in humans.

Although the robust and sustained placebo response in clinical trials raises questions about the true efficacy of this procedure in humans, several studies in animals provide indirect evidence that exogenous HA may relieve joint pain in OA, arguing that a placebo effect cannot fully explain the benefit of this treatment in humans. Most of these pre-clinical studies have assessed joint pain through use of a surrogate, such as gait analysis; in racehorses, relief of pain has been judged by the ability of the horse to race. (It should be recognized, however, that lameness in racehorses may result from tendonitis, epiphysitis, osteochondritis dissecans, and not only from OA, and that the underlying cause of lameness in the reported studies has generally not been established.) Furthermore, studies that have controlled for concomitant interventions, such as use of phenylbutazone or corticosteroid, have not been reported. Nevertheless, lameness in racehorses has been treated with IA injection of HA for almost 30 years and forceplate data from horses with lameness due to osteochondral fractures suggest the HA injection promotes weight-bearing on the injected limb, lending credence to an analgesic effect of this treatment.[42] In support of that possibility, when the OA knee of sheep was injected weekly for five weeks with either 2×10^6 Da HA, 0.8×10^6 Da HA, or saline, the rate of loading and peak vertical ground reaction force (GRF) generated by the arthritic extremity were significantly greater in the group that had received the higher mw HA preparation than in that which had received the lower mw product. GRF values for both HA treatment groups were higher than those for the saline control.[43]

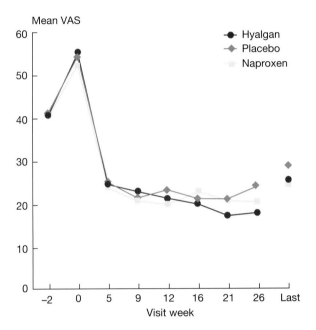

Fig. 9.11 Mean pain experienced during 50-foot walk by subjects in each of the three treatment groups during the study. The ordinate reflects pain scores, in mm, on a 100 mm visual analogue scale (VAS). Data presented are for those subjects who completed the study (approximately 67% of those who were randomized to treatment).

Visit week-2 (screening visit), visit week 0 (baseline visit after washout of analgesic/antiinflammatory drugs).

Source: Taken from Ref. 32.

Table 9.16 Level of pain after 50-foot walk, measured in millimetres on a 100-mm visual analogue scale[*]

Study group *n* Mean (SD)	Study week					% Improvement in pain, compared to baseline		
	Baseline	12	16	26	Last observation	Week 12	Week 26	Last observation
HA	163	115	109	105	160	57	67	50
	54 (29)	23 (25)	21 (24)	18 (21)	27 (27)			
Placebo	167	129	123	113	163	56	56	49
	55 (29)	24 (26)	22 (25)	24 (27)	28 (30)			
Naproxen	162	125	119	111	160	61	61	54
	54 (28)	21 (25)	24 (28)	21 (25)	25 (28)			

HA, hyaluronan.

[*] Data are from all patients randomly assigned to study groups.

Source: Adapted, with permission, from Ref. 32.

When the effect of HA on nociception was assessed in the anesthetized cat by direct measurement of impulses in an exposed articular nerve after production of synovitis, it was found that the rate of firing of afferent impulses, which increased significantly after injection of the irritant, was reduced by IA injection of an elastoviscous hylan, whereas injection of chemically degraded hylan had no effect.[44] The authors speculated that the high mw hylan solution buffered the transmission of mechanical signals to the nerve terminals or provided a diffusion barrier for ions and algogenic molecules in the joint. However, the brief duration of this experiment ($5\frac{1}{2}$ hours) does not permit conclusions regarding the mechanism underlying the long lasting relief of joint pain reported after IA HA injection in some humans.

Receptors for HA have been identified and characterized on many connective tissue cells. The analgesic effect of 860 kDa HA in a rat model of joint pain was blocked by prior injection of 6.8 kDa HA or of an octa-saccharide of HA, both of which bind to HA receptors.[45,46] In contrast, injection of an HA tetrasaccharide, which does not bind to HA receptors, did not interfere with the analgesic response to the HA. The pain response to injection of a mixture of bradykinin, the bradykinin antagonist Des-Arg^9-(Leu^8)-bradykinin, and HA was no different from that after injection of only bradykinin and the antagonist,[46] suggesting that the analgesic effect of HA requires interaction between HA and its receptors on neurons or other cells, but does not involve direct interaction of HA with bradykinin or its receptors.

Structure-modifying effects of IA HA injection

In animal models, studies attempting to ascertain whether IA injection of HA significantly modifies structural damage in the OA joint have produced conflicting results. For example, studies in beagles and in rabbits have suggested that IA HA injection reduced cartilage damage.[47–52] However, when dogs that had undergone ACLT were treated prophylactically with a series of IA injections of HA, no effect on morphologic changes of OA was apparent. Indeed, a striking reduction in the PG concentration in the articular cartilage was seen in every dog seven weeks after the last HA injection,[53] raising a concern that HA treatment could *accelerate* joint damage in OA. In support of this possibility, HA injection in sheep, which had undergone menis-cectomy, resulted in *increases* in osteophytosis and cartilage fibrillation and reduction in the rate of PG synthesis by the OA cartilage.[44,54]

As indicated above, forceplate data have shown that the increase in severity of joint pathology after injection of the knee with HA is associated with an increase in loading of the arthritic knee, consistent with 'analgesic arthropathy'. Hurwitz *et al.*[55] reported that the adductor moment at the knee in patients with medial compartment knee OA was greater when they were taking an NSAID than after withdrawal from the drug, when their knee pain was more severe, that is, pharmacologic amelioration of joint pain resulted in an increase in mechanical loading of the damaged joint.

In humans, data relative to a structure-modifying effect of HA are sparse. On the basis of arthroscopic observations at baseline and again one year later, Listrat *et al.*[56] concluded that HA treatment slowed the progression of chondropathy. However, that conclusion must be tempered by the relatively small number of patients studied, the fact that the HA group exhibited less severe chondropathy at baseline than those treated conventionally, and the fact that the proportion of patients who required an NSAID during the study was twice as great among the controls as in the HA group. Furthermore, although arthroscopy is useful for observation of damage to menisci, ligaments, and the articular surface, it is not a good tool with which to detect anatomic or biochemical changes in the OA joint. Cartilage thickness and the mechanical quality of the cartilage cannot be assessed well by arthroscopy unless a striking loss of cartilage has occurred. Arthroscopy is not an accurate, sensitive, reproducible, and validated outcome measure for evaluation of chondropathy in OA.

Safety of HA treatment

In general, HA therapy seems safe. It carries none of the concerns associated with systemic inhibition of prostaglandin synthesis by NSAIDs. Local reactions at the injection site (pain, tenderness, erythema) may occur but are generally transient and require little more than reassurance of the patient and an ice pack. A retrospective study of 336 patients treated over $2\frac{1}{2}$ years (1537 injections involving 458 knees) suggested that the incidence of local adverse events after injection of hylan G-F 20 was relatively low and was influenced by the injection technique:[57] with a medial approach and a par-tially flexed knee, the incidence was 5.2 per cent; with a straight medial approach, 2.4 per cent; and with a straight or lateral approach, 1.5 per cent.

Some reports, however, have suggested a considerably higher incidence of local reactions following treatment with hylan G-F 20. In a study of 22 patients who received a total of 88 injections into 28 knees, post-injection 'flares' occurred in 27 per cent of patients and after 11 per cent of injec-tions.[58] In some patients, joint swelling lasted as long as three weeks and the synovial fluid leucocyte count exceeded 50 000 cells per mm^3, raising a concern about the presence of acute bacterial infection, although cultures of the synovial fluid and crystal analysis have been negative in these cases. In some cases, the synovial fluid leukocyte count may exceed 100 000 cells/mm^3.[59] The intensity of the synovitis has led physicians to treat the flare in some patients with an IA steroid injection. In a recent placebo-controlled 52 week clinical trial comparing hylan G-F 20 with the non-crosslinked hyaluronan Artzal® (see above), no serious adverse reactions due to either HA treatment were noted (Lohmander, S.L., personal communication).

In a few cases, IA injection of HA has been followed promptly by an acute attack of pseudogout, confirmed by evidence of crystals of calcium pyrophosphate in the synovial fluid.[60,61] However, Daumen-Legre *et al.*[62] recently observed no local flares after injection of courses of HA in 30 knees (26 patients) with chondrocalcinosis. No direct comparisons are available of the incidence of local reactions after injection of hylan G-F 20, other HA preparations, arthocentesis alone, or corticosteroid.

As noted above, forceplate studies in animals have suggested that over-loading of the damaged joint may occur after IA injection of HA, which may lead to depletion of PGs in articular cartilage and an increase in structural damage. Given the increasing use of HA on humans, this is an important area for further study.

Key points

1. Data with respect to the superiority of intra-articular HA injections, relative to placebo, are contradictory.

2. There is no evidence that higher molecular weight formulations (e.g., hylans) are more effective than non-crosslinked HA formula-tions in symptomatic treatment of OA in humans.

3. The evidence that intra-articular HA therapy slows progression of joint damage in humans with OA is not convincing.

4. The concept that the clinical response to intra-articular HA injection is due to 'viscosupplementation' is tenuous.

5. Except for infrequent episodes of acute synovitis after intra-articular HA injection, the treatment seems safe.

Summary and conclusions

Although the concept that viscosupplementation by IA injection of HA is useful in the treatment of OA is promoted heavily by manufacturers of the HA preparations that are marketed, few data exist to support this mechanism of action. Data from humans, in particular, are scarce. No evidence exists that this treatment restores the concentration or mw of synovial fluid HA to normal levels for a sustained period. Furthermore, effects attributed to viscosupplementation have not been seen by all investigators and there is no evidence that joint damage in OA is caused by a change in *any* of the properties of synovial fluid.

Several clinical trials indicate that IA injection of HA can result in relief of joint pain in patients with knee OA and that this effect may last for months. Similar results may be seen with placebo, however, and it is not clear that the difference between HA and placebo is *clinically* significant. Neither the clinical nor pre-clinical data to date convincingly support a distinction between lower molecular weight HAs and chemically cross-linked hylans in treatment of OA in humans. Nonetheless, pre-clinical studies suggest an analgesic effect that cannot be readily attributed to a placebo response, although they provide no insight into possible underlying mechanisms. Relief of joint pain for months after the injected material has been cleared from the joint is difficult to explain by *any* mechanism, whether it is biochemical, physicochemical, or mechanical.

The pre-clinical data are contradictory with respect to whether IA injection of HA modifies progression of joint damage in OA and, if so, whether treatment is beneficial or detrimental. Numerous methodological differences exist among the published animal studies: in addition to the species used, the duration of treatment, source, and mw of the HA, timing of the intervention (prophylactic or therapeutic) and the outcome measures employed, may all influence the results. Insufficient information is available to permit a conclusion concerning the effect of this treatment, if any, on the progression of OA in humans.

Acknowledgments

Supported by NIH grants AR20582 and AR39250. We thank Deborah Jenkins and Kathie Lane for their assistance in the preparation of this manuscript.

References

(An asterisk denotes recommended reading.)

1. **Balazs, E.A.** (1982). The physical properties of synovial fluid and the special role of hyaluronic acid. In A. Helfet (ed.), *Disorders of the Knee* (2nd ed.). Philadelphia: JB Lippincott, pp. 61–74.

2. **Balazs, E.A. and Denlinger, J.L.** (1993). Viscosupplementation: a new concept in the treatment of osteoarthritis. *J Rheumatol* **39**:S3.

3. **Ghosh, P.** (1996). The role of hyaluronic acid (hyaluronan) in health and disease: interactions with cells, cartilage and components of the synovial fluid. *Clin Exp Rheumatol* **12**:75–82.

4. **Laurent, T.C., Laurent, U.B.G., and Fraser, J.R.E.** (1996). The structure of hyaluronan: An overview. *Immunol Cell Biol* **74**:A1–7.

5. **Yasui, T., Adatsuka, M., Tobetto, K., Hayaishi, M., and Anto, T.** (1992). The effect of hyaluronan on interleukin-1-a-induced prostaglandin-E_2 production in human osteoarthritis synovial cells. *Agents Actions* **37**:155–6.

6. **Larsen, N.E., Lombard, K.M., Parent, E.G., and Balazs, E.A.** (1992). Effect of hylan on cartilage and chondrocyte cultures. *J Orthop Res* **10**:23–32.

7. **Presti, D. and Scott, J.E.** (1994). Hyaluronan mediated protective effect against cell damage caused by enzymatically generated hydroxyl radicals is dependent on hyaluronan molecular mass. *Cell Biochem Function* **12**:281–8.

8. **Homandberg, G.A., Hui, F., Wen, C., Kuettner, K.E., and Williams, J.M.** (1997). Hyaluronic acid suppresses fibronectin fragment mediated cartilage chondrolysis: I. In vitro. *Osteoarthritis Cart* **5**:309–19.

9. **Williams, J.M., Plaza, V., Hui, F., Wen, C., Kuettner, K.E., and Homandberg, G.A.** (1997). Hyaluronic acid suppresses fibronectin fragment mediated cartilage chondrolysis: II. In vitro. *Osteoarthritis Cart* **5**:235–40.

10. **Noble, P.W., Lake, F.R., Henson, P.M., and Riches, D.W.** (1993). Hyaluronate activation of CD44 induces insulin-like growth factor-1 expression by a tumor necrosis factor-alpha-dependent mechanism in murine macrophages. *J Clin Invest* **91**:2368–77.

11. **Myers, S.L., Brandt, K.D., and Eilam, O.** (1995). Even low-grade synovitis significantly accelerates clearance of protein from the canine knee. Implications for measurement of synovial fluid 'markers' of osteoarthritis. *Arthritis Rheum* **38**:1085–91.

12. **Engstrom-Laurent, A.** (1997). Hyaluronan in joint disease. *J Internal Med* **242**:57–60.

13. **Myers, S.L. and Brandt, K.D.** (1995). Effects of synovial fluid hyaluronan concentration and molecular size on clearance of protein from the canine knee. *J Rheumatol* **22**:1732–9.

14. **Balazs, E.A., Watson, D., Duff, I.F., and Roseman, S.** (1967). Hyaluronic acid in synovial fluid. I. Molecular parameters of hyaluronic acid in normal and arthritis human fluids. *Arthritis Rheum* **10**:357–76.

15. **Dahl, L.B., Dahl, I.M.S., Engstrom-Laurent, A., and Granath, K.** (1985). Concentration and molecular weight of sodium hyaluronate in synovial fluid from patients with rheumatoid arthritis and other arthropathies. *Ann Rheum Dis* **44**:817–22.

16. **Iwata, H.** (1993). Pharmacologic and clinical aspects of intra-articular injection of hyaluronate. *Clin Orthop* **289**:285–91.

17. **Mensiteri, M., Ambrosio, L., Innace, S., Perbellini, A., and Nicolais, L.** (1995). Viscoelastic evaluation of different knee osteoarthritis therapies. *J Mat Sci: Mat Med* **6**:130–7.

18. **Wobig, M., Dickhut, A., Maier, R., and Vetter, G.** (1998). Viscosupplementation with hylan G-F20: A 26-week controlled trial for efficacy and safety in the osteoarthritis knee. *Clin Ther* **20**:410–423.

19. **Altman, R.D., Hochberg, M.C., Moskowitz, R.W., and Schnitzer, T.J.** (2000). Recommendations for the medical management of osteoarthritis of the hip and knee. *Arthritis Rheum* **43**:1905–15.

20. **Fiorentini, R.** (1996). Proceedings of the United States Food and Drug Administration Advisory Panel on Orthopaedic and Rehabilitation Devices Panel, 11/21/96. CASET, Fairfax, VA, p. 8.

21. **Berkowitz, D.** (1996). Proceedings of the United States Food and Drug Administration Advisory Panel on Orthopaedic and Rehabilitation Devices Panel, 11/20/96. CASET, Fairfax, VA, p. 87.

22. **Peyron, J.G. and Balasz, E.A.** (1974). Preliminary clinical assessment of Na-hyaluronate injection into the human knee. *Pathol Biol* **22**:731–6.

23. *****Brandt, K.D., Smith, G.N., and Simon, L.S.** (2000). Intraarticular injection of hyaluronan as treatment for knee osteoarthritis. What is the evidence? *Arthritis Rheum* **43**:1192–1203.

    This paper reviews limitations in the evidence that 'viscosupplementation' accounts for the long-standing symptomatic relief seen in some patients after IA HA injection; that the clinical response to IA HA is greater than a placebo effect; and that IA HA injections may modify the progression of joint damage in OA.

24. **Hilbert, B.J., Rowley, G., Antonas, K.N., McGill, C.A., Reynoldson, J.A., and Hawkins, C.D.** (1985). Changes in the synovia after intra-articular injection of sodium hyaluronate into normal horse joints after arthrotomy and experimental cartilage damage. *Austr Vet J* **62**:182–4.

25. **Smith, G.N. Jr., Mickler, E.A., Myers, S.L., and Brandt, K.D.** (2001). Effect of intraarticular hyaluronan injection on synovial fluid hyaluronan in the early stage of canine post-traumatic osteoarthritis. *J Rheumatol* **28**:1341–6.

26. **Smith, M.M. and Ghosh, P.** (1987). The synthesis of hyaluronic acid by human synovial fibroblasts is influenced by the nature of the hyaluronate in the extracellular environment. *Rheumatol Int* **7**:113–22.

27. **Lynch, T.M., Caron, J.P., Arnoczky, S.P., Lloyd, J.W., Stick, J.A., and Render, J.A.** (1998). Influence of exogenous hyaluronan on synthesis of hyaluronan and collagenase by equine synoviocytes. *Am J Vet Res* **59**:888–92.

28. **Kawcak, C.E., Frisbie, D.D., Trotter, G.W.,** *et al.* (1997). Effect of intravenous administration of sodium hyaluronate on carpal joints in exercising horses after arthroscopic surgery and osteochondral fragmentation. *Am J Vet Res* **58**:1132–40.

29. **Fraser, J. and Laurent, T.** (1989). Turnover and metabolism of hyaluronan. In: The biology of hyaluronan-Ciba Foundation symposium. Chichester, Sussex, United Kingdom: John Wiley, pp. 41–59.

30. **Ericksson, J., Fraser, R., Laurent, T.,** *et al.* (1983). Endothelial cells are a site of uptake and degradation of hyaluronic acid in the liver. *J Exp Cell Res* **144**:223–8.

31. *****Kirwan, J.R. and Rankin, E.** (1997). Intra-articular therapy in osteoarthritis. *Baillière's Clin Rheumatol* **11**:769–94.

    A good review of IA HA therapy in patients with knee OA. This and Ref. 34, provide a good general background and a good anthology.

32. *****Altman, R.D., Moskowitz, R., and the Hyalgan Study Group.** (1998). Intraarticular sodium hyaluronate (Hyalgan®) in the treatment of patients with osteoarthritis of the knee: A randomized clinical trial. *J Rheumatol* **25**:2203–12.

This paper describes the results of a pivotal clinical trial of a hyaluronan, in which results among subjects completing the study showed statistically significant superiority of HA over placebo, but an intent-to-treat analysis showed that IA injections of saline (the placebo) were as effective as naproxen, 500 mg bid.

33. Adams, M.E., Atkinson, M.H., Lussier, A.J., *et al.* (1995). The role of viscosupplementation with hylan G-F 20 (Synvisc) in the treatment of osteoarthritis of the knee: a Canadian multicenter trial comparing hylan G-F 20 with non-steroidal anti-inflammatory drugs (NSAIDs) and NSAIDs alone. *Osteoarthritis Cart* 3:213–26.

34. *Hochberg, M.C. (2000). Role of intra-articular hyaluronic acid preparations in medical management of osteoarthritis of the knee. *Sem Arthritis Rheum* 30:2–10.

   This is a recent review of clinical trials of IA HA injection in patients with knee OA.

35. Jones, A.C., Pattrick, M., Doherty, S., and Doherty, M. (1995). Intra-articular hyaluronic acid compared to intra-articular triamcinolone hexacetonide in inflammatory knee osteoarthritis. *Osteoarthritis Cart* 3:269–73.

36. Wobig, M., Dickhut, A., Maier, R., and Vetter, G. (1998). Viscosupplementation with hylan G-F 20: A 26-week controlled trial of efficacy and safety in the osteoarthritic knee. *Clin Ther* 20:410–23.

37. Allard, S. and O'Regan, M. (2000). Letters to the Editor. *Clin Ther* 22:792–93.

38. Wobig, M. and Balazs, E.A. (2000). The authors reply. *Clin Ther* 22:793–95.

39. Karlsson, J. and Selin-Sjogren, L. (1999). A comparison of two-hyaluronan drugs and placebo in patients with mild to moderate osteoarthritis of the knee—a controlled, randomized, parallel-design multicenter study. *Acta Orthop Scand* 70(Suppl. 287):62.

40. Lohmander, L.S., Dalen, N., Englund, G., *et al.* (1996). Intra-articular hyaluronan injections in the treatment of osteoarthritis of the knee: a randomised, double blind, placebo controlled multicentre trial. Hyaluronan Multicentre Trial Group. *Ann Rheum Dis* 55:424–31.

41. Scale, D., Wobig, M., and Wolpert, W. (1994). Viscosupplementation of osteoarthritic knee with hylan: a treatment schedule study. *Curr Ther Res* 55:220–32.

42. Auer, J.A., Fackelman, G.E., Gingerich, D.A., and Fetter, A.W. (1980). Effect of Hyaluronic Acid in naturally occurring and experimentally induced osteoarthritis. *Am J Vet Res* 41:568–74.

43. *Ghosh, P., Read, R., Armstrong, S., Wilson, D., Marshall, R., and McNair, P. (1993). The effects of intraarticular administration of hyaluronan in a model of early osteoarthritis in sheep. I. Gait analysis and radiological and morphological studies. *Sem Arthritis Rheum* 22(6 Suppl. 1):18–30.

   In this study, injection of HA in an ovine model of OA resulted in increases in loading of the arthritic extremity and severity of pathologic changes of OA.

44. Pozo, M.A., Balazs, E.A., and Belmonte, C. (1997). Reduction of sensory responses to passive movements of inflamed knee joints by hylan, a hyaluronan derivative. *Exp Brain Res* 116:3–9.

45. Cher, E.C. and Underhill, C. (1992). The hyaluronate receptor is a member of the CD44 (HCAM) family of cell surface glycoproteins. *J Cell Biol* 116:2765–74.

46. Gotoh, S., Miyazaki, K., and Onaya, J. (1988). Experimental knee pain model in rats and analgesic effect of sodium hyaluronate. *Folia Pharmacol Jpn* 92:17–27.

47. Kikuchi, T., Yamada, H., and Shimmei, M. (1996). Effect of high molecular weight hyaluronan on cartilage degeneration in a rabbit model of osteoarthritis. *Osteoarthritis Cart* 4:99–110.

48. Yoshioka, M., Shimizu, C., Harwood, F.L., Coutts, R.D., and Amiel, D. (1998). Long-term effects of hyaluronan on experimental osteoarthritis in the rabbit knee. *Osteoarthritis Cart* 6:1–10.

49. Shimizu, C., Yoshioka, M., Coutts, R.D., *et al.* (1997). The effects of hyaluronan during the development of osteoarthritis. *Osteoarthritis Cart* 5:251–60.

50. Takahashi, K., Goomer, R.S., Harwood, F., Kubo, T., Hirasawa, Y., and Amiel, D. (1999). The effects of hyaluronan on matrix metalloproteinase-3 (MMP-3), (interleukin-1∃), and tissue inhibitor of metalloproteinase-1 (TIMP-1) gene expression during the development of osteoarthritis. *Osteoarthritis Cart* 7:182–90.

51. Abatangelo, G., Botti, P., Del Bue, M., *et al.* (1989). IA sodium hyaluronate injections in the Pond-Nuki experimental model of osteoarthritis in dogs. I. Biochemical results. *Clin Orthop Rel Res* 241:278–85.

52. Schiavinato, A., Lini, E., Guidolin, D., *et al.* (1989). IA sodium hyaluronate injections in the Pond-Nuki experimental model of osteoarthritis in dogs. II. Morphological findings. *Clin Orthop Rel Res* 241:286–99.

53. Smith, G.N. Jr, Myers, S.L., Brandt, K.D., and Mickler, E.A. (1998). Effect of IA hyaluronan injection in experimental canine osteoarthritis. *Arthritis Rheum* 41:976–85.

54. Ghosh, P., Read, R., Numata, Y., Smith, S., Armstrong, S., and Wilson, D. (1993). The effects of intraarticular administration of hyaluronan in a model of early osteoarthritis in sheep. II. Cartilage composition and proteoglycan metabolism. *Sem Arthritis Rheum* 22(6 Suppl. 1):31–42.

55. Hurwitz, D.E., Sharma, L., and Andriacchi, T.P. (1999). Effect of knee pain on joint loading in patients with osteoarthritis. *Curr Opin Rheumatol* 11:422–6.

56. Listrat, V., Ayral, X., Patarnello, F., *et al.* (1997). Arthroscopic evaluation of potential structure modifying activity of hyaluronan (Hylgan) in osteoarthritis of the knee. *Osteoarthritis Cart* 5:153–60.

57. Lussier, A., Cividino, A.A., McFarlane, C.A., Olszynski, W.P., Potashner, W.J., and De Médicis R. (1996). Viscosupplementation with hylan for the treatment of osteoarthritis: findings from clinical practice in Canada. *J Rheumatol* 23:1579–85.

58. Puttick, M.P.E., Wade, J.P., Chalmers, A., Connell, D.G., and Rangno, K.K. (1995). Acute local reactions after intra-articular hylan for osteoarthritis of the knee. *J Rheumatol* 22:1311–14.

59. Pullman-Mooar, S., Mooar, P., Sieck, M., Clayburne, G., Schumacher, Jr., H.R. (1999). Are there distinctive inflammatory flares of synovitis after hyalgan GF intraarticular injections? (Abstract). *Arthritis Rheum* 42:S9.

60. Luzar, M.J. and Altawil, B. (1998). Pseudogout following intraarticular injection of sodium hyaluronate. *Arthritis Rheum* 41:939–40.

61. Maillefert, J.F., Hirschhorn, P., Pascaud, F., Piroth, C., and Tavernier, C. (1997). Acute attack of chondrocalcinosis after intraarticular injection of hyaluronan. *Rev Rheum Engl Ed* 64:593–4.

62. Daumen-Legre, V., Pham, T., Acquaviva, P.C., and Lafforgue, P. (1999). Evaluation of safety and efficacy of viscosupplementation in knee osteoarthritis with chondrocalcinosis (Abstract). *Arthritis Rheum* 42:S9.

9.9 Nutritional therapies

Timothy E. McAlindon

Nutritional products are widely promulgated, and used, as remedies for OA, but are rarely tested in controlled clinical trials. Although few of these have been adequately tested, glucosamine and chondroitin sulfate have been evaluated in manufacturer-sponsored clinical trials in Europe. A meta-analysis of these trials suggested efficacy for OA symptoms, but found methodological problems and possible publication bias, suggesting that the effect sizes may be exaggerated. A recent 3-year clinical trial of glucosamine confirmed efficacy for symptoms and also suggested the possibility that glucosamine might influence radiographic progression. All trials have demonstrated the remarkable safety of these products. Because of this, glucosamine and chondroitin offer potential as adjunctive therapies in the treatment of OA. Although results from independent trials are awaited, it seems reasonable to recommend a trial of such therapies to individuals with OA.

Glucosamine and chondroitin sulfate

The idea that glucosamine and chondroitin might have therapeutic effects in treating OA by providing substrate for reparative processes in cartilage has been around since at least the 1960s. In fact, glucosamine has been used for decades in veterinary medicine for the symptomatic relief of arthritis. Two enticing properties of these 'nutraceuticals' are (1) their excellent safety profile and (2) the assertion that they may reduce progression of cartilage damage.[1]

Laboratory studies

Laboratory studies have suggested that both glucosamine and chondroitin can be absorbed through the gastrointestinal tract.[2] Radio-isotope studies of glucosamine show rapid distribution throughout the body with selective uptake by articular cartilage.[3,4] In-vitro studies have indicated that glucosamine can stimulate GAG and proteoglycan synthesis.[5–7] The biologic fate of orally administered chondroitin sulfate is less clear, but some evidence exists to suggest that the compound may be absorbed, possibly as a result of pinocytosis.[8] Chondroitin sulfate is able to cause an increase in RNA synthesis by chondrocytes,[9] which appears to correlate with an increase in the production of proteoglycans and collagens.[10–13] Such effects may partly result from the competitive inhibition of degradative enzymes.[14] In addition, there is evidence that chondroitin sulfate partially inhibits leukocyte elastase.[15] While these data are encouraging, it is clear that these compounds have not been subjected to the systematic level of research and development enjoyed by pharmaceutical products, and that many important questions remain unaddressed. It is uncertain whether these compounds are absorbed *intact*, whether they are metabolized to any degree, and what role they actually play *in vivo*. Currently, there remains no theoretical or empirical evidence to support the original supposition that these compounds provide substrate for articular cartilage repair.

Clinical studies

Placebo-controlled trials

In contrast, the clinical efficacy of both glucosamine and chondroitin has been tested in numerous clinical trials. One meta-analysis and quality evaluation has been the undertaking of trials of glucosamine and chondroitin products for symptoms due to knee and/or hip OA.[16] This involved a search for published or unpublished double-blind randomized placebo-controlled trials, of four or more weeks duration, that reported extractable data on the effect of treatment on symptoms. Six eligible glucosamine and 9 chondroitin trials were found (Table 9.17). Quality scores ranged from 12.3–55.4 per cent of maximum possible with mean 35.5 per cent. Only two studies described adequate allocation concealment, while three reported an intent-to-treat analysis. A manufacturer supported them all, to some extent. Statistical evaluation suggested publication bias resulting due to under-representation of small null, or negative trials ($p < 0.02$). The aggregated effect sizes were moderate for glucosamine and large for chondroitin, but were diminished when only high quality trials or large trials were considered. It was concluded that trials of these preparations for OA symptoms demonstrate moderate to large effects, but that quality issues, and likely publication bias, suggest that these effects are, at best, exaggerated.

A number of further trials have emerged since the publication of the meta-analysis, some of which have had less compelling results. Houpt's 2-month double-blind randomized placebo-controlled trial (RCT) of glucosamine hydrochloride among 118 participants with knee OA found trends in favor of active treatment, but did meet the primary endpoint (statistically significant change in the WOMAC pain scale).[17] A six-month placebo-controlled RCT of glucosamine among 80 participants with knee OA in the United Kingdom found no difference at all between the groups.[18] Rindone *et al.* also concluded from their 2-month RCT among 98 VA patients with knee OA that glucosamine was no better than placebo in reducing knee pain.[19] In contrast, a 2-month RCT of a glucosamine/chondroitin combination among a group of 34 military recruits with knee or spinal OA found significantly greater improvements in selected outcome measures.[20] Most recently, Reginster *et al.* published the results of a three-year industry-sponsored placebo-controlled clinical trial of glucosamine, whose primary focus was the influence of treatment on radiographic progression of knee OA. This high quality trial of 200 participants used the WOMAC questionnaire to assess the effect of glucosamine on pain and function. While the magnitude of effect on symptoms was modest, it is notable that this benefit was present even after three years of treatment.[1]

Comparator trials: glucosamine

Glucosamine has been compared to an NSAID in the treatment of OA in a number of trials.[21–23] Muller-Fassbender *et al.* enrolled 199 hospitalized patients with knee OA into a 4-week randomized trial of glucosamine sulfate 500 mgs three times/day, versus ibuprofen 400 mgs, three times/day.[22] Participants receiving ibuprofen responded more quickly to treatment, but, by the 4-week time-point, both groups had experienced an identical reduction in their baseline Lequesne Index score. Most notable is the difference in

Table 9.17 Clinical trials of glucosamine and chondroitin included in a meta-analysis[16*]

Author	Study no.	Type	Mode of administration	Joint studied	Primary outcome[†]	Effect size[‡]
Glucosamine trials						
29	155	Manuscript	Oral	Knee	Lequesne	0.37
30	329	Abstract	Oral	Knee	Lequesne	0.69
31	54	Manuscript	I/A	Knee	Pain	0.54
32	20	Manuscript	Oral	Knee	Pain	1.28
33	101	Abstract	Oral	Knee	WOMAC	0.34
34	252	Manuscript	Oral	Knee	Lequesne	0.23
Chondroitin trials						
35	127	Supplement	Oral	Knee	Lequesne	0.64
36	80	Supplement	Oral	Knee	Pain	0.87
37	46	Supplement	Oral	Knee	Pain	1.04
38	140	Supplement	Oral	Knee	Pain	1.16
39	125	Manuscript	Oral	Knee	Pain	0.98
40	17	Manuscript	I/M	Knee	Mobility	1.47
41	120	Manuscript	Oral	Knee/hip	NSAID use	0.53
42	40	Manuscript	I/M	Knee	Pain	4.56
43	104	Manuscript	Oral	Knee	Lequesne	0.61

* This study was a significant outlier and was dropped from the final analysis.

† Lequesne, Lequesne Algofunctional Index; Pain, global pain score (Likert or Visual Analog); WOMAC, WOMAC Osteoarthritis Index; Mobility, mobility score.

‡ Effect size from the intergroup difference in mean outcome value at trial end, divided by the standard deviation of the outcome value in the placebo group (0.2, small effect, 0.5, moderate; 0.8, large).

adverse experience rates between the two groups—35 in the ibuprofen group reported adverse effects (with 7 drop-outs) compared with only 6 in the glucosamine group (1 dropout). Most of these were gastro-intestinal in nature. The authors concluded that glucosamine and ibuprofen have comparable short-term efficacy, albeit with a slower onset for glucosamine. No power calculations were performed to determine the magnitude of difference that this size of study might be able to detect, nor is information presented about how the 4-week study duration was determined.

Qiu *et al.* compared glucosamine with ibuprofen in a 4-week double blind RCT of 178 patients with knee OA.[23] Both groups responded equally to the treatments, with an approximately 50 per cent reduction in scores. Adverse event and dropout rates were strikingly greater ($p = 0.002$) in the ibuprofen arm. Lopes-Vaz compared the efficacy of oral glucosamine 1.5 g/day with ibuprofen 1.2 g/day in an 8-week double-blind RCT among 38 patients with knee OA.[21] Both groups improved, but the scores intersected at the 4-week time-point, such that significantly greater improvement was seen in the glucosamine arm by the end of the trial ($p < 0.05$). There were no power calculations presented in the report. Based on number projections in other NSAID trials,[24] it is, perhaps, surprising that any difference was found in this small clinical trial.

Comparator trials: chondroitin

Morreale *et al.* performed a 6-month RCT comparing chondroitin sulfate with diclofenac in 146 patients with knee OA.[25] The design was rather complex in that participants assigned to the chondroitin took this for three months, while those assigned to the NSAID group received diclofenac for one month only. All participants took placebo during months 3–6. A double-dummy approach was used to preserve blinding, with all participants observed for the full 6-month period. Participants were allowed acetaminophen for breakthrough pain. During the first month, both groups showed a fall in the Lequesne Index score, but this was significantly greater in the diclofenac group. The Lequesne Index scores then rebounded following cessation of diclofenac in the NSAID group, but continued to decline in those receiving chondroitin such that there were significant differences at days 60 and 90 favoring chondroitin. This benefit appeared to persist for

2–3 months after the chondroitin had been stopped. There were three adverse events in each group thought possibly or probably related to treatment, all of mild or moderate severity. These results contribute to the description of chondroitin as a 'symptomatic slow acting drug' for treating OA.

Human disease-modification studies

Glucosamine

Probably the most enticing aspect of these compounds is the claim that they may have disease-modifying properties in OA. Reginster *et al.* recently published the results of the first human RCT designed to investigate this possibility.[1] They enrolled 200 knee OA patients into a 3-year placebo controlled trial whose primary outcome measure was joint-space width (JSW) in the medial compartment of the knee, evaluated from standardized straight-leg weight-bearing radiographs. At trial end they measured a mean decrease in JSW of 0.31 (95 per cent confidence limits 0.48–0.13) among those receiving placebo, compared to 0.06 (0.22–0.09) among the treated group (p for difference = 0.04). While these results are intriguing, there remain a number of puzzling aspects to this study. In the first place, the relationship between joint-space width at the knee and the clinical impact of the disease has consistently been shown to be poor. Thus, the clinical implications of modest retardation of joint-space loss remain to be fully understood. Another problem is that adequacy of radiographic positioning could be influenced by knee symptoms resulting in an underestimation of JSW in those with more severe pain. The absence of further relevant radiographic data (e.g. osteophytosis, global severity) in this paper is, therefore, unfortunate. There is also considerable variability around each of the mean JSW estimates, which will reduce expected statistical power in future trials hoping to replicate their findings.

Chondroitin

Uebelhart *et al.* performed a 1-year randomized placebo-controlled study of chondroitin sulfate 800 mgs daily among 42 participants with knee OA.[26] Computer-generated joint-space measurements were used to evaluate radiographic progression. They found progression of joint-space loss among the placebo group but no change in those taking chondroitin sulfate. This study has been criticized for the short duration of follow-up. Verbruggen *et al.* evaluated progression of radiographic hand OA during a 3-year period among 34 patients taking chondroitin sulfate 400 mgs three times/day, compared to 85 patients taking placebo.[27] They found reduced development of erosive OA in the treated group. Limitations of this study include small numbers of participants, unbalanced treatment assignment and questions about the methodology used to obtain radiographs.

Safety issues

The more rigorous controlled clinical trials of oral glucosamine and chondroitin preparations published as manuscripts in peer-reviewed journals include 600 participants taking oral glucosamine or chondroitin sulfate,[16] for up to three years duration.[1] These have shown minor or moderate adverse rates to be similar to those taking placebo. Reported adverse events have generally been gastro-intestinal in nature. Comparator studies suggest that Glucosamine is substantially safer than NSAIDs, particularly in respect of GI toxicity. Perhaps more problematic is the suggestion that glucosamine may interfere with glucose tolerance. This observation is based on studies administering intravenous glucosamine to laboratory animals.[28] Exacerbation, or development, of diabetes has not been reported in clinical trials of oral glucosamine. In particular, no evidence was found of any influence of glucosamine on fasting blood glucose levels in the recent 3-year trial.[1] Thus, it remains doubtful that the laboratory findings are relevant to oral therapy in humans. Further research is needed into the influence of long-term oral glucosamine ingestion on glucose tolerance.

Other nutritional products

Piascledine (avocado/soybean unsaponifiables)

A large number of nutritional products are touted for their purported benefits in arthritis and it is encouraging that some of these are now being scientifically evaluated. Piascledine is an emulsion derived from the unsaponifiables fractions of Avocado and Soybean oils that has *in-vitro* effects on articular chondrocytes that could ameliorate osteoarthritic processes. It has been tested in two large randomized placebo-controlled clinical trials.[44,45] The first of these included 164 individuals with OA of the hip or knee and used post-treatment withdrawal NSAID requirements as the primary efficacy measure. By day 90 (45 days after treatment withdrawal) 70 per cent of the placebo group were using NSAIDs compared with only 43 per cent of the treated group ($p = 0.001$).[45] The second was a multicenter randomized placebo-controlled 6-month trial that compared Piascledine with placebo among 164 enrollees with OA of the hip or knee.[44] A divergence in efficacy outcomes between the two groups was evident as early as one-month, at which point the difference in LFI (the primary outcome measure) was statistically significant ($p = 0.04$). By the 6-month timepoint, significant differences were also found in the intent-to-treat analyses for global pain visual analog scales, functional disability visual analog scales, and participant overall assessment.

Conclusions

The question arises as to what might be reasonable advice about nutritional products for an individual with OA, given the incomplete state of current knowledge. Current evidence supports modest efficacy for glucosamine and chondroitin in the treatment of OA *symptoms*. One recent trial also raised the possibility that glucosamine might reduce the rate of radiographic progression. The products are safe and could play a valuable role in the management of this disorder. Nevertheless, further independent studies are needed to confirm these findings and to determine the clinical applicability of these compounds. Physicians need to become involved in these treatment decisions, but are obfuscated by wide variability in the formulation and purity of the numerous preparations available to consumers.

Key points

1. Glucosamine and chondroitin sulfate products are widely promulgated, and used as remedies for OA.

2. The efficacy of glucosamine and chondroitin sulfate for OA symptoms has been tested in numerous controlled clinical trials. These have shown efficacy but have also manifested methodological problems that would be expected to lead to exaggerated estimates of benefit.

3. A recent 3-year trial of glucosamine also demonstrated efficacy for symptoms and suggested the possibility of reduction of radiographic progression.

4. A multicenter NIH-funded study of glucosamine and chondroitin is currently in progress.

Further reading

Towheed, T.E., Anastassiades, T.P., Shea, B., Houpt, J., Welch, V., and Hochberg, M.C. (2001). Glucosamine therapy for treating osteoarthritis (Cochrane Review). *Cochrane Database Syst Rev* 1.

References

1. Reginster, J.Y., Deroisy, R., Rovati, L.C., *et al.* (2001). Long-term effects of glucosamine sulphate on osteoarthritis progression: a randomised, placebo-controlled clinical trial. *Lancet* **357**(9252):251–6.

2. Tesoriere, G., Dones, F., Magistro, D., and Castagnetta, L. (1972). Intestinal absorption of glucosamine and N-acetylglucosamine. *Experientia* **28**(7):770–1.

3. Setnikar, I., Giachetti, C., and Zanolo, G. (1984). Absorption, distribution and excretion of radio-activity after a single I.V. or oral administration of [14C]glucosamine to the rat. *Pharmatherapeutica* **3**:358.

4. Setnikar, I., Giachetti, C., and Zanolo, G. (1986). Distribution of glucosamine in animal tissues. *Arzneimittel forschung/Drug Res* **36**:729.

5. Vidal, Y., Plana, R.R., Bizzarri, D., and Rovati, A.L. (1978). Articular cartilage pharmacology: in vitro studies on glucosamine and NSAIDs. *Pharmacol Res Commun* **10**:557.

6. Vidal, Y., Plana, R.R., and Karzel, K. (1980). [Glucosamine: its importance for the metabolism of articular cartilage. 2. Studies on articular cartilage]. *Fortschr Med* **98**(21):801–6.

7. Karzal, K. and Domenjoz, R. (1971). Effects of hexosamine derivatives on glycosaminoglycan metabolism of fibroblast cultures. *Pharmacology* **5**:337.

8. Theodore, G. (1977). Untrsuchung von 35 arhrosefallen, behandelt mit chondroitin schwefelsaure. *Schweiz Rundschaue Med Praxis* **66**.

9. Vach, J., Pesakova, V., Krajickova, J., and Adam, M. (1984). Effect of glycosaminoglycan polysulfate on the metabolism of cartilage RNA. *Arzneim Forsch/Drur Res* **34**:607–9.

10. Ali, S.Y. (1964). The degradation of cartilage matrix by an intracellular protease. *Biochem J* **93**:611.

11. Baici, A., Salgam, P., Fehr, K., and Boni, A. (1979). Inhibition of human elastase from polymorphonuclear leucocytes by a GAG-polysulfate. *Biochem Pharm* **29**:1723–7.

12. Hamerman, D., Smith, C., Keiser, H.D., and Craig. R. (1982). Glycosaminoglycans produced by human synovial cell cultures collagen. *Rel Res* **2**:313.

13. Knanfelt, A. (1984). Synthesis of articular cartilage proteoglycans by isolated bovine chondrocytes. *Agents Actions* **14**:58–62.

14. Bartolucci, C., Cellai, L., Corradini, C., Corradini, D., Lamba, D., and Velona, I. (1991). Chondroprotective action of chondroitin sulfate. Competitive action of chondroitin sulfate on the digestion of hyaluronan by bovine testicular hyaluronidase. *Int J Tissue React* **13**(6):311–7.

15. Bartolucci, C., Cellai, L., Iannelli, M.A., *et al.* (1995). Inhibition of human leukocyte elastase by chemically and naturally oversulfated galactosaminoglycans. *Carbohydr Res* **276**(2):401–8.

16. McAlindon, T.E., LaValley, M.P., Gulin, J.P., and Felson, D.T. (2000). Glucosamine and chondroitin for treatment of osteoarthritis: a systematic quality assessment and meta-analysis. *JAMA* **283**(11):1469–75.

17. Houpt, J.B., McMillan, R., Wein, C., and Paget-Dellio, S.D. (1999). Effect of glucosamine hydrochloride in the treatment of pain of osteoarthritis of the knee. *J Rheumatol* **26**(11):2423–30.

18. Hughes, R.A. and Carr, A.J. (2000). A randomized double-blind placebo-controlled trial of glucosamine to control pain in osteoarthritis of the knee. *Arthritis Rheum* **43**(Suppl. 9):S384.

19. Rindone, J.P., Hiller, D., Collacott, E., Nordhaugen, N., and Arriola, G. (2000). Randomized, controlled trial of glucosamine for treating osteo-arthritis of the knee. *West J Med* **172**(2):91–4.

20. Leffler, C.T., Philippi, A.F., Leffler, S.G., Mosure, J.C., and Kim, P.D. (1999). Glucosamine, chondroitin, and manganese ascorbate for degenerative joint disease of the knee or low back: a randomized, double-blind, placebo-controlled pilot study. *Mil Med* **164**(2):85–91.

21. Lopes Vaz, A. (1982). Double-blind clinical evaluation of the relative efficacy of ibuprofen and glucosamine sulphate in the management of osteoarthrosis of the knee in out-patients. *Curr Med Res Opin* **8**(3):145–9.

22. Muller-Fassbender, H., Bach, G.L., Haase, W., Rovato, L.C., and Setnikar, I. (1994). Glucosamine sulfate compared to ibuprofen in osteoarthritis of the knee. *Osteoarth Cart* **2**:61–9.

23. Qiu, G.X., Gao, S.N., Giacovelli, G., Rovati, L., and Setnikar, I. (1998). Efficacy and safety of glucosamine sulfate versus ibuprofen in patients with knee osteoarthritis. *Arzneimittelforschung* **48**(5):469–74.

24. Bellamy, N., Buchanan, W.W., Chalmers, A., *et al.* (1993). A multicenter study of tenoxicam and diclofenac in patients with osteoarthritis of the knee. *J Rheumatol* **20**(6):999–1004.

25. Morreale, P., Manopulo, R., Galati, M., Boccanera, L., Saponati, G., and Bocchi, L. (1996). Comparison of the antiinflammatory efficacy of chondroitin sulfate and diclofenac sodium in patients with knee osteoarthritis. *J Rheumatol* **23**(8):1385–91.

26. Uebelhart, D., Thonar, E.J., Delmas, P.D., Chantraine, A., and Vignon, E. (1998). Effects of oral chondroitin sulfate on the progression of knee osteoarthritis: a pilot study. *Osteoarthritis Cart* **6**(Suppl. A):39–46.

27. Verbruggen, G., Goemaere, S., and Veys, E.M. (1998). Chondroitin sulfate: S/DMOAD (structure/disease modifying anti- osteoarthritis drug) in the treatment of finger joint OA. *Osteoarthritis Cart* **6**(Suppl. A):37–8.

28. Giaccari, A., Morviducci, L., Zorretta, D., *et al.* (1995). In vivo effects of glucosamine on insulin secretion and insulin sensitivity in the rat: possible relevance to the maladaptive responses to chronic hyperglycaemia. *Diabetologia* **38**(5):518–24.

29. Reichelt, A., Forster, K.K., Fischer, M., Rovati, L.C., and Setnikar, I. (1994). Efficacy and safety of intramuscular glucosamine sulfate in osteoarthritis of the knee: A randomized, placebo-controlled, double-blind study. *Drug Res* **44**:75–80.

30. Rovati, L.C. (1997). The clinical profile of glucosamine sulfate as a selective symptom modifying drug in osteoarthritis: current data and perspectives. *Osteoarthritis Cart* **5**(Suppl. A):72.

31. Vajaradul, Y. (1981). Double-blind clinical evaluation of intra-articular glucosamine in outpatients with gonarthrosis. *Clin Ther* **3**(5):336–343.

32. Pujalte, J.M., Llavore, E.P., and Ylescupidez, F.R. (1980). Double-blind clinical evaluation of oral glucosamine sulphate in the basic treatment of osteoarthrosis. *Curr Med Res Opin* **7**(2):110–114.

33. Houpt, J.B., McMillan, R., Paget-Dellio, D., Russell, A., and Gahunia, H.K. (1998). Effect of glucosamine hydrochloride (GHcl) in the treatment of pain of osteoarthritis of the knee. *J Rheumatol* **25**(Suppl. 52):8.

34. Noack, W., Fischer, M., Forster, K.K., Rovati, L.C., and Setnikar, I. (1994). Glucosamine sulfate in osteoarthritis of the knee. *Osteoarthritis Cart* **2**:51–9.

35. Bourgeois, P., Chales, G., Dehais, J., Delcambre, B., Kuntz, J.L., and Rozenberg, S. (1998). Efficacy and tolerability of chondroitin sulfate 1200 mg/day vs chondroitin sulfate 3 × 400 mg/day vs placebo. *Osteoarthritis Cart* 1998;**6**(Suppl. A):25–30.

36. Bucsi, L. and Poor, G. (1998). Efficacy and tolerability of oral chondroitin sulfate as a symptomatic slow-acting drug for osteoarthritis (SYSADOA) in the treatment of knee osteoarthritis. *Osteoarthritis Cart* **6** (Suppl. A):31–6.

37. Uebelhart, D., Thonar, E.J., Zhang, J., and Williams, J.M. (1998). Protective effect of exogenous chondroitin 4,6-sulfate in the acute degradation of artic-ular cartilage in the rabbit. *Osteoarthritis Cart* **6** (Suppl. A):6–13.

38. Pavelka, K., Bucsi, L., and Manopulo, R. (1998). Double-blind, dose effect study of oral CS 4&6 1200 mg, 800 mg, 200 mg against placebo in the treat-ment of femorotibial osteoarthritis. *Rheumatol Eur* **27**(Suppl. 2):63.

39. L'Hirondel, J.L. (1992). Klinische doppelblind-studie mit oral verabre-ichtem chondroitinsulfat gegen placebo bei der tibiofemoralen gonarthrose (125 patienten). *Litera Rhumatol* **14**:77–84.

40. Kerzberg, E.M., Roldan, E.J., Castelli, G., and Huberman, E.D. (1987). Combination of glycosaminoglycans and acetylsalicylic acid in knee osteo-arthrosis. *Scand J Rheumatol* **16**(5):377–80.

41. Mazieres, B., Loyau, G., Menkes, C.J., *et al.* (1992). [Chondroitin sulfate in the treatment of gonarthrosis and coxarthrosis. 5-months result of a multi-center double-blind controlled prospective study using placebo]. *Rev Rhum Mal Osteoartic* **59**(7–8):466–72.

42. Rovetta, G. (1991). Galactosaminoglycuronoglycan sulfate (matrix) in ther-apy of tibiofibular osteoarthritis of the knee. *Drugs Exptl Clin Res* **17**:53–7.

43. Conrozier, T. (1998). Anti-arthrosis treatments: efficacy and tolerance of chondroitin sulfates (CS 4&6). *Presse Med* **27**(36):1862–5.

44. Maheu, E., Mazieres, B., Valat, J.P., *et al.* (1998). Symptomatic efficacy of avocado/soybean unsaponifiables in the treatment of osteoarthritis of the knee and hip: a prospective, randomized, double-blind, placebo-controlled, multicenter clinical trial with a six-month treatment period and a two-month followup demonstrating a persistent effect. *Arthritis Rheum* **41**(1):81–91.

45. Blotman, F., Maheu, E., Wulwik, A., Caspard, H., and Lopez, A. (1997). Efficacy and safety of avocado/soybean unsaponifiables in the treatment of symptomatic osteoarthritis of the knee and hip. A prospective, multicenter, three-month, randomized, double-blind, placebo-controlled trial. *Rev Rhum Engl Ed* **64**(12):825–34.

9.10 Mechanisms by which micronutrients may influence osteoarthritis

Timothy E. McAlindon

Enormous public interest exists in the relationship between diet and arthritis. Speculative lay publications on this subject abound, and shelves of health food stores are filled with nutritional supplements touted for their putative ability to help arthritis sufferers. However, until recently, traditional scientific studies seldom examined the relationship between nutritional factors (other than obesity) and OA. This is, perhaps, surprising insofar as many mechanisms exist by which certain micronutrients can be hypothesized to influence pathogenetic processes in OA. These mechanisms include antioxidant effects of micronutrients, their participation in metabolic processes, and their anti-inflammatory actions.

Antioxidants

There is considerable evidence that continuous exposure to oxidants contributes to the development or exacerbation of many of the common human diseases associated with aging.[1] Such oxidative damage accumulates with age and has been implicated in the pathophysiology of cataract,[2] coronary artery disease[3] and certain forms of cancer.[5] As the prototypical age-related 'degenerative' disease, OA may also be, in part, a product of oxidative damage to articular tissues.

Reactive oxygen species are chemicals with unpaired electrons. They are formed continuously in the tissues by endogenous, and some exogenous, mechanisms.[1] For example, it has been estimated that 1–2 per cent of all electrons that travel down the mitochondrial respiratory chain leak, forming a superoxide anion ($O_2^{\bullet -}$).[5] Other endogenous sources of reactive oxygen species include the oxidative burst of phagocytes, mixed function oxidase enzymes, and hypoxia-reperfusion events.[6] These reactive oxygen species are capable of damaging large molecules, such as lipoproteins, proteins, and DNA.[7] Because reactive oxygen species are identical to those generated by irradiation of H_2O, 'living' has been likened to being continuously irradiated.[1]

There is evidence that cells within joints produce reactive oxygen species, and that oxidative damage is physiologically important.[8] In laboratory studies, animal and human chondrocytes have been found to be potent sources of reactive oxygen species.[8] Hydrogen peroxide production has been demonstrated in aged human chondrocytes after exposure to the pro-inflammatory cytokines, interleukin-1, and tumor necrosis factor-α, and has been observed in live cartilage tissue.[9] Superoxide anions have been shown to adversely affect collagen structure and integrity *in vitro*, and appear to be responsible, *in vivo*, for depolymerization of synovial fluid hyaluronan.[8,9]

The human body has extensive and multi-layered antioxidant defense systems.[1] Intracellular defense is provided primarily by antioxidant enzymes, including superoxide dismutase, catalase and peroxidases. In addition to these enzymes, there are a number of small molecule antioxidants, which play an important role, particularly in the extracellular space, where antioxidant enzymes are sparse.[10] These include the micronutrients, alpha-tocopherol (vitamin E), beta-carotene (a vitamin A precursor), other carotenoids, and ascorbate (vitamin C). The concentrations of these antioxidants in the blood are primarily determined by dietary intake. The concept that micronutrient antioxidants might provide further defense against tissue injury when intracellular enzymes are overwhelmed has led to the hypothesis that high dietary intake of these micronutrients might protect against age-related disorders. Because some studies have shown that higher intake of dietary antioxidants appears to protect against other age-related disorders, such as cataracts and coronary artery disease, it is plausible that antioxidants might also protect against the development of OA.[2–4]

Effects of micronutrients on articular cartilage metabolism

In addition to being an antioxidant, vitamin C has several functions in the biosynthesis of cartilage molecules. First, through the vitamin C-dependent enzyme, lysylhydroxylase, vitamin C is required for the post-translational hydroxylation of specific prolyl and lysyl residues in procollagen, a modification essential for stabilization of the mature collagen fibril.[2–4,11–13] Vitamin C also appears to stimulate collagen biosynthesis by pathways independent of hydroxylation, perhaps through lipid peroxidation.[14] In addition, by acting as a carrier of sulfate groups, vitamin C participates in glycosaminoglycan biosynthesis.[15] Therefore, deficiency of vitamin C may impair not only the production of cartilage, but also its mechanical properties.

The results of *in-vitro* and *in-vivo* studies are consistent with this possibility. Addition of ascorbic acid to cultures of adult bovine chondrocytes resulted in a reduction in levels of degradative enzymes and in increased synthesis of type II collagen and proteoglycans.[16] Peterkovsky *et al.*[17] observed decreased synthesis of articular cartilage collagen and proteoglycan in guinea pigs deprived of vitamin C. In addition, in the presence of vitamin C deficiency,[17] these authors found high blood levels of insulin-like growth factor-1 (IGF-1) binding proteins, which normally inhibit the anabolic effects of the potent growth factor, IGF-1. This suggests that vitamin C may also influence growth factors through pathways that remain to be elucidated.

Vitamin D may have direct effects on chondrocytes in osteoarthritic cartilage. During bone growth, vitamin D regulates the transition of growth plate cartilage to bone. Normally, chondrocytes in developing bone lose their vitamin D receptors with the attainment of skeletal maturity. It has recently become apparent, however, that the hypertrophic chondrocytes in osteoarthritic cartilage can redevelop vitamin D receptors.[18] These chondrocytes are metabolically active and may play an important role in the pathophysiology of OA. Although this evidence is indirect, it raises the possibility that vitamin D may influence pathologic processes in OA through effects on these cells.

Effects of micronutrients on bone

Reactive changes in the bone underlying, and adjacent to, damaged cartilage are an integral part of OA.[19–25] Sclerosis of the underlying bone, trabecular microfractures, attrition of bone and subchondral cyst formation are all likely to accelerate the degenerative process as a result of adverse biomechanical changes[26] (see Chapter 7.2.2.1). Other phenomena, such as osteophytes (bony spurs) may represent attempts to repair or stabilize the process.[27] It has also been suggested that bone mineral density may influence the skeletal expression of the disease, with a more erosive form occurring in individuals with 'softer' bone.[28] Although some cross-sectional studies have suggested a modest inverse relationship between OA and osteoporosis, recent prospective studies have suggested that individuals with lower bone mineral density are at increased risk for both incident OA and progression of the disease.[29] The hypothesis that the nature of bony response in OA may determine outcome has been further advanced by the recent demonstration that patients with bone scan abnormalities adjacent to an osteoarthritic knee have a higher rate of progression than those without such changes.[30]

Normal bone metabolism is contingent on the presence of vitamin D, a compound that is derived largely from the diet or from cutaneous exposure to ultraviolet light. Suboptimal vitamin D levels may have adverse effects on calcium metabolism, osteoblast activity, matrix ossification, and bone density.[31] Low tissue levels of vitamin D may, therefore, impair the ability of bone to respond optimally to pathophysiological processes in OA, and may thereby predispose to disease progression.

Anti-inflammatory effects of micronutrients

Vitamin E has diverse influences on the metabolism of arachadonic acid, an anti-inflammatory fatty acid found in all cell membranes. Vitamin E blocks the formation of arachidonic acid from phospholipids and inhibits lipoxygenase activity, although it has little effect on cyclooxygenase.[32] It is, therefore, possible that vitamin E reduces the modest level of synovial inflammation that may accompany OA.

Studies of nutritional factors in OA

Obesity and OA

Overweight people are at considerably increased risk for the development of OA in their knees, and may also be more susceptible to hip and hand joint involvement[33] (see Chapter 2). Furthermore, weight loss appears to reduce the risk for development of knee OA and to improve symptoms in those with prevalent disease.[33] Because overweight individuals do not necessarily have increased load across their hand joints, investigators have wondered whether systemic factors, such as dietary factors or other metabolic consequences of obesity, may mediate some of this association. Indeed, early laboratory studies using strains of mice and rats appeared to suggest an interaction between body weight, genetic factors, and diet, although attempts to demonstrate a direct effect of dietary fat intake proved inconclusive.[34]

Evidence that vitamin C and other antioxidant micronutrients might be beneficial in OA

Animal studies

OA can be induced in animals by various surgical procedures. When Schwartz and Leveille[35] treated guinea pigs with either a high (150 mg/day) or low (2.4 mg/day) dose of vitamin C prior to such surgery, those treated with the higher dose of vitamin C (which would correspond to a dose in humans of at least 500 mg/day) showed 'consistently less severe joint damage than animals on the low level of the vitamin.' Furthermore, features of OA were significantly less frequent in the animals treated with the high dose of vitamin C. Similar findings were reported by Meacock et al.[36] in a study in surgically-induced guinea pig model of OA, in which the feed of half of the animals was supplemented with vitamin C after the surgical procedure. The authors reported, 'Extra ascorbic acid appeared to have some protective effect ($p = 0.008$) on the development of spontaneous [OA] lesions. ...'

Epidemiological studies

We investigated the association of self-reported dietary intake of antioxidant micronutrients among participants followed longitudinally in the Framingham Knee OA Cohort Study,[37] a population-based group derived from the Framingham Heart Study Cohort. Participants had knee radiographs taken at a baseline examination performed in 1983–5, and again approximately eight years later, in 1992–3. Knee OA was classified using the Kellgren and Lawrence grading system.[22] Knees without radiographic evidence of OA at baseline (Kellgren and Lawrence grade ≤1) were classified as developing *incident* OA if they exhibited grade 2 or greater changes by follow-up. Knees with radiographic evidence of OA at baseline were classified as exhibiting *progressive* OA if the Kellgren and Lawrence grade increased by 1 or more.

Nutrient intake, including dietary supplements, was calculated from dietary habits reported at the mid-point of the study, using a food frequency questionnaire. In our analyses, we ranked micronutrient intake into sex-specific tertiles and asked specifically whether higher intakes of vitamin C, vitamin E, and beta(β)-carotene, compared with a panel of non-antioxidant 'control' micronutrients, were associated with reduced incidence or reduced progression of knee OA. The lowest tertile for each dietary exposure was used as the reference category. Odds ratios were adjusted for age, sex, body mass index, weight change, knee injury, physical activity, total calorie intake, and health status.

Complete assessments were available for 640 participants (mean age = 70.3 years). Incident and progressive knee OA occurred in 81 knees and 68 knees, respectively. We found no significant association of *incident* radiographic knee OA with any micronutrient (adjusted odds ratio, OR, for highest vs lowest tertile of vitamin C intake = 1.1; 95 per cent confidence limits 0.6–2.2). On the other hand, for *progression* of radiographic knee OA, we found a three-fold reduction in risk for those in the middle and highest tertiles for vitamin C intake (adjusted OR for highest vs lowest tertile = 0.3; 95 per cent confidence limits 0.1–0.6). Notably, those in the highest tertile for vitamin C intake also exhibited a reduced risk of developing knee pain during the course of the study (OR = 0.3; 0.1–0.8). Although knee pain can bias the assessment of joint-space measurements by impairing the subject's ability to fully extend the knee during radiographic examination (see Chapter 11.4.2), the apparent 'protective' associations we found in our analyses were present even among those subjects who did not report joint pain during the observation period. It is also of note that the difference between the lowest and middle tertile for vitamin C intake was relatively modest, approximately 60 mgs. Although it is difficult to make such estimates with precision from a food frequency questionnaire, it nevertheless suggests that an individual might decrease their risk for progression through a relatively modest consistent increase in dietary intake of vitamin C.

Reduction in risk of OA *progression* was seen also for β-carotene (OR = 0.4; 0.2–0.9) and vitamin E, but was less consistent, insofar as that the β-carotene association diminished substantially after adjustment for vitamin C, and the vitamin E effect was seen only in men (OR = 0.07; 0.01–0.6). In the non-antioxidant 'panel,' no significant associations were observed for any of the micronutrients examined. Thus, this study does not support the hypothesis that diets high in antioxidant micronutrients reduce the risk of *incident* knee OA. On the other hand, the data suggest that some of these micronutrients, vitamin C in particular, may reduce the risk of *progression* of OA among those who already have some radiographic changes (Table 9.18).

If antioxidants are, indeed, protective for individuals with OA, we are left with questions about why the effect appears to be confined to those with existing radiographic changes. One possible explanation relates to differences in the intra-articular environment of normal and OA knees. For example, several pathologic mechanisms, including raised intra-articular pressure,[7] low grade inflammation,[38] and increased metabolic activity[6] increase the opportunity for oxidative damage in an osteoarthritic knee. Therefore, antioxidants could play a greater role in preventing the progression, rather than the incidence, of structural damage that might result from a variety of non-metabolic insults, such as joint trauma.[40]

Table 9.18 Epidemiological studies of nutritional factors in OA

Reference	Nutritional factor studied	Outcome variables	Results
37	Dietary intake of antioxidants: (vitamin C, vitamin E, β-carotene)	Knee OA, incidence and progression	Vitamin C appeared to protect against OA progression (but not incidence)
44	Dietary intake and serum level of vitamin D	Knee OA, incidence and progression	Vitamin D appeared to protect against OA progression (but not incidence)
42	Serum level of vitamin D	Hip OA, incidence and progression	Vitamin D appeared to protect against incidence of hip OA

Another important observation in this study was that the effect of vitamin C was stronger and more consistent than the effects of β-carotene and vitamin E. Relatively little is known about the tissue distribution and bio-availability of antioxidant molecules within joints. For example, it is not clear whether lipophilic molecules(such as vitamin E or β-carotene) are available at sites of cartilage damage. If lipophilic molecules gain only limited access to tissue compartments at which damage is manifest, hydrophilic antioxidants (such as vitamin C) may be the only agents in this class that are likely to benefit the disorder. An alternative explanation is that the protective effects of vitamin C relate to its role in the biosynthesis of cartilage collagen fibrils and proteoglycan molecules, rather than to its antioxidant properties.

Clinical trials

Benefit from vitamin E therapy has been suggested by the results of several small clinical trials, the most rigorous of which was an industry-sponsored 6-week double-blind placebo-controlled trial of 400 mg alpha-tocophorol (vitamin E) in 56 patients with OA.[39] Those treated with vitamin E experienced greater improvement in every efficacy measure, including pain at rest (69 per cent better with vitamin E vs 34 per cent better with placebo, $p < 0.05$), pain on movement (62 per cent better with vitamin E vs 27 per cent with placebo, $p < 0.01$) and use of analgesics (52 per cent less on vitamin E; 24 per cent less on placebo, $p < 0.01$). The rapid response in symptoms observed in this study is unlikely to have been due to an effect of vitamin E on structural changes in the osteoarthritic joint in this disorder, and suggests the beneficial effect might result from some metabolic action, such as inhibition of arachidonic acid metabolism. On the other hand, a more recent, independently-funded, 6-month double-blind study in which 77 patients with knee OA were assigned randomly to receive vitamin E, 500 IU/day, or placebo, found no benefit of vitamin E over the placebo for pain, stiffness, or function.[40]

Selenium has also been tested in a clinical trial as a therapy for OA symptoms. Hill and Bird conducted a six-month double-blind placebo-controlled study of Selenium-ACE, a proprietary nutritional supplement in the United Kingdom, among thirty patients with OA of various joints.[41] The 'active' treatment contained, on average, 144 μg of selenium and unspecified quantities of vitamins A, C, and E. In fact, the 'placebo' also contained 2.9 μg of selenium. Pain and stiffness scores remained similar for the two groups at all time points, leading the authors to conclude that their data did not provide evidence of efficacy for selenium-ACE in relieving OA symptoms.

Studies of vitamin D

In a separate investigation we tested the association of vitamin D status on the *incidence* and *progression* of knee OA among the cohort of participants in the Framingham OA Cohort Study described above.[44] The methodology for this investigation was essentially identical to that in the study of antioxidant micronutrient intake in OA,[37] except that the analysis was confined to a subset of 550 individuals who participated in the dietary assessment and also provided serum for assay of 25-hydroxy vitamin D. Dietary intake of vitamin D and serum 25-hydroxy vitamin D levels were modestly correlated in this sample ($r = 0.24$), and, as in our study of the association of vitamin C to OA,[37] were unrelated to *incident* disease. Risk of *progression*, however, increased three-fold among participants in the middle and lower tertiles for vitamin D dietary intake (odds ratio for lowest vs. highest tertile = 4.0, 95 per cent, CI = 1.4–11.6) and vitamin D serum level (OR = 2.9, 95 per cent, CI = 1.0–8.2). Low serum vitamin D level also predicted cartilage loss, as assessed by loss of joint space (OR = 2.3, 95 per cent, CI = 0.9–5.5) and osteophyte growth (OR = 3.1, 95 per cent, CI = 1.3–7.5). We concluded that low serum level, and low dietary intake, of vitamin D were each associated with a highly significant increase in the risk of *progression* of knee OA (Table 9.18).

Lane *et al.*[42] subsequently examined the relationship of serum 25-and 1,25-hydroxy vitamin D to the development of radiographic hip OA among Caucasian women more than 65 years old who were participating in the Study of Osteoporotic Fractures. They measured serum vitamin D levels in 237 subjects, randomly selected from 6051 women who had pelvic radiographs taken at the baseline examination and again after 8 years of follow-up. Radiographs were graded with a scoring system based on individual radiographic features of OA, and cases were defined using three proxy definitions of incident hip OA: (1) a summary grade requiring definite osteophytosis or joint-space narrowing, with at least one other feature, (2) development of definite joint-space narrowing, (3) development of definite osteophytosis. *Change* in summated individual radiographic features (IRF) scores and *change* in minimal joint-space width was analyzed as continuous measures. Multivariate analyses were adjusted for age, clinic, weight at age 50, and health status.

Individuals in the lowest tertile for serum 25-hydroxy vitamin D level were at significantly increased risk for incident hip OA based on joint-space narrowing, but the association was weaker when the summary grade was used, and no association was observed when the osteophyte definition was used. In the analyses treating these variables as continuous measures, low vitamin D level was associated with loss of joint-space width ($p = 0.02$), and increase in summated IRF score ($p = 0.06$). An increased risk for incident joint-space narrowing among those in the middle tertile for 25-hydroxy vitamin D level was also apparent, but did not reach statistical significance. These findings are consistent with the possibility that vitamin D has a protective effect with respect to loss of cartilage, but not with respect to the development of osteophytes (Table 9.18).

Thus, two independent epidemiological studies have demonstrated an inverse association between vitamin D status and risk for OA. Both of these studies used a prospective design and included relatively robust measures of vitamin D status. The observations of Lane *et al.*[42] are of considerable importance because of their remarkable similarity to the findings for knee OA in the Framingham Study.[43] Furthermore, they suggest that vitamin D may protect against incident OA, at least at the hip. Taken together, these studies provide the most compelling evidence for the role of any nutritional factor in the development of OA. In view of their observational nature, however, clinical trials are required to confirm the possibility that vitamin D might play a role in the secondary prevention of OA and, if the results are positive, to determine the optimal way to promote the use of vitamin D supplements for OA, given the potential for toxicity.[44]

Folic acid and cobalamin

Based on observational studies that showed rises in osteocalcin and alkaline phosphatase in vitamin B12 deficient patients, following treatment with Cobalamin,[45] Flynn *et al.* conjectured that folic acid and cobalamin might influence the course of OA through effects on osteoblast metabolism and bone.[46] They performed a two-month double-blind randomized three-arm cross-over clinical trial of 6400 μg folate versus 6400 μg folate with 20 μg cyanocobalamin versus placebo among 30 individuals with symptomatic hand OA. Participants were assessed for tender joints, grip strength, symptoms, and analgesic use. In their analyses, the authors stratified the participants according to their baseline grip strength. Some benefits were found among some strata for certain measures of grip strength and tender joints favoring the folate /cyanocobalamin arm. Few differences, however, were noted in pain scores, global assessments, or analgesic use, suggesting that this intervention had limited, if any, efficacy.

In fact, the influence of dietary intake of folate was also tested also in the Framingham Osteoarthritis study, where it was used as a non-antioxidant 'control' micronutrient.[37] That investigation found no convincing effect of dietary folate intake on either incidence or progression of knee OA.

Selenium and iodine: studies of Kashin-Beck disease

Kashin-Beck disease is an osteoarthropathy of children and adolescents that occurs in geographic areas of China in which deficiencies of both selenium and iodine are endemic. Strong epidemiological evidence supports the environmental nature of this disease.[47] Although the clinical and radiological characteristics of Kashin-Beck disease differ from OA, its existence raises the possibility that environmental factors also play a role in the occurrence of this disorder.

Selenium deficiency, in conjunction with pro-oxidative products of organic matter in drinking water, and contamination of grain by fungi have been proposed as environmental causes of Kashin-Beck disease. The efficacy of selenium supplementation in preventing the disorder, however, is controversial. Because selenium is an integral component of iodothyronine deiodinase and of glutathione peroxidase, Moreno-Reyes et al.[48] studied iodine and selenium metabolism in 11 villages in Tibet in which Kashin-Beck disease was endemic, and in one village in which it was not. They found iodine deficiency to be the main determinant of Kashin-Beck disease in these villages, although it should be noted that selenium levels were very low in all the subgroups examined. In an accompanying editorial, Utiger[47] inferred that Kashin-Beck disease probably results from a combination of deficiencies of both of these elements, and speculated that growth plate cartilage is both dependent on locally produced triiodothyronine and is sensitive to oxidative damage.

It should be noted that there is little, if any, evidence to suggest that Kashin-Beck disease has any similarities with OA. Furthermore, the single published clinical trial of supplemental selenium (Selenium-ACE) in the treatment of symptoms associated with OA did not demonstrate efficacy for this product.[41]

Summary

Although little attention has been paid to this field, many biological mechanisms exist by which micronutrients can hypothetically influence OA. These relate to their antioxidant and anti-inflammatory properties, effects on bone, and role in cartilage metabolism. Vitamin C, for example, is an antioxidant and a co-factor in biosynthesis of articular cartilage collagen and proteoglycan. Vitamin C supplementation has been shown to reduce the severity of incident OA in animal models. Consistent with these observations, higher intake of dietary vitamin C in humans was found to be associated with a reduction in the risk of progression of knee OA. Adequate levels of vitamin D are critical to bone health and may modify the response of subchondral bone to cartilage damage. This has not been studied in animal models, but observational cohort studies in humans have shown an association between higher serum levels of 25-hydroxy-vitamin D and slower OA radiographic progression of the hip and knee. 'Protective' effects have also been demonstrated for β-carotene, but are less consistent than those found for Vitamins C and D. Vitamin E has also been tested in clinical trials, with inconsistent results. Clinical trials of selenium, cyanocobalamin

and folate have failed to show convincing evidence of the efficacy of these compounds in treatment of OA symptoms.

Currently, a role for vitamins C and D in slowing the progression of OA seems more plausible than one for the other vitamins and micronutrients discussed above. Further studies are needed to replicate the published observations, however, and to test the efficacy of dietary supplementation in prospective randomized controlled trials. The data are insufficient to permit a recommendation that therapeutic doses of vitamins C or D be prescribed for the prevention or treatment of OA.

Key points

1. Despite enormous public interest in the relationship between diet and arthritis, few scientific studies have tested the relationship between nutritional factors and OA.

2. Dietary micronutrients have the potential to influence pathophysiologic processes in OA through antioxidant effects and their participation in metabolic and inflammatory pathways.

3. Clinical trials of vitamin E and other micronutrient supplements often have included only small numbers of subjects, and have had generated negative or inconsistent results.

4. A study of the relationship of dietary antioxidant micronutrient intake to knee OA among the Framingham cohort suggested that vitamin C had a protective effect with respect to radiographic progression of knee OA.

5. Two observational studies of vitamin D status (dietary intake and serum levels) have suggested the protective effects of adequate levels of vitamin D with respect to radiographic progression of knee and incident hip OA.

6. Although definitive conclusions from future research are awaited, it seems appropriate to advise people with OA to follow general public health recommendations by increasing their daily consumption of fruits and vegetables and optimizing their vitamin D status (the current RDA for vitamin D is 800 IU). The data are insufficient to permit a therapeutic dose of vitamins C or D to be prescribed for either the prevention or treatment of OA.

References

(An asterisk denotes recommended reading.)

1. **Frei, B.** (1994). Reactive oxygen species and antioxidant vitamins: mechanisms of action. *Am J Med* **97**(Suppl. 3A):5S–13S.

2. **Jacques, P.F., Chylack, L.T., and Taylor, A.** (1994). Relationships between natural antioxidants and cataract formation. In B. Frei (ed.), *Natural Antioxidants in Human Health and Disease*. San Diego: Academic Press, pp. 515–33.

3. **Gaziano, J.M.** (1994). Antioxidant vitamins and coronary artery disease risk. *Am J Med* **97**(Suppl. 3A):18S–21S.

4. **Hennekens, C.H.** (1994). Antioxidant vitamins and cancer. *Am J Med* **97**(Suppl. 3A):2S–4S.

5. **Boveris, A., Oshino, N., and Chance, B.** (1972). The cellular production of hydrogen peroxide. *Biochem J* **128**:617–30.

6. **Blake, D.R., Unsworth, J., Outhwaite, J.M.,** *et al.* (1989). Hypoxic-reperfusion injury in the inflamed human. *Lancet* **11**:290–3.

7. **Ames, B.N., Shigenaga, M.K., and Hagen, T.M.** (1993). Oxidants, antioxidants and the degenerative diseases of aging. *Proc Natl Acad Sci USA* **90**:7915–22.

8. **Henrotin, Y., Deby-Dupont, G., Deby, C., Debruin, M., Lamy, M., and Franchimont, P.** (1993). Production of active oxygen species by isolated human chondrocytes. *Br J Rheumatol* **32**.

9. **Rathakrishnan, C., Tiku, K., Raghavan, A., and Tiku, M.L.** (1992). Release of oxygen radicals by articular chondrocytes: A study of luminol-dependent

chemoluminescence and hydrogen peroxide secretion. *J Bone Miner Res* **7**:1139–48.

10. **Briviba, K. and Seis, H.** (1994). Non-enzymatic antioxidant defense systems. In: B. Frei (ed.), *Natural Antioxidants in Human Health and Disease.* San Diego: Academic Press, pp. 107–128.

11. **Hankinson, S.E., Stampfer, M.J., Seddon, J.M.,** *et al.* (1992). Nutrient intake and cataract extraction in women: a prospective study. *BMJ* **305**(6849):335–9.

12. **Peterkofsky, B.** (1991). Ascorbate requirement for hydroxylation and secretion of procollagen: relationship to inhibition of collagen synthesis in scurvy. *AM J Clin Nutr* **54**:1135S–40S.

13. **Spanheimer, R.G., Bird, T.A., and Peterkofsky, B.** (1986). Regulation of collagen synthesis and mRNA levels in articular cartilage of scorbutic guinea pigs. *Arch Biochem Biophys* **246**:33–41.

14. **Houglum, K.P., Brenner, D.A., and Chijkier, M.** (1991). Ascorbic acid stimulation of collagen biosynthesis independent of hydroxylation. *Am J Clin Nutr* **54**:1141S–3S.

15. **Schwartz, E.R. and Adamy, L.** (1997). Effect of ascorbic acid on arylsulfatase activities and sulfated proteoglycan metabolism in chondrocyte cultures. *J Clin Invest* **60**.

16. **Sandell, L.J. and Daniel, L.C.** (1988). Effects of ascorbic acid on collagen mRNA levels in short-term chondrocyte cultures. *Connect Tiss Res* **17**:11–22.

17. **Peterkofsky, B., Palka, J., Wilson, S., Takeda, K., and Shah, V.** (1991). Elevated activity of low molecular weight insulin-like growth factor binding proteins in sera of vitamin C deficient and fasted guinea pigs. *Endocrinol* **128**:1769–79.

18. **Bhalla, A.K., Wojno, W.C., and Goldring, M.B.** (1987). Human articular chondrocytes acquire AU-,25(OH)2 vitamin D-3 receptors. *Biochim Biophy Acta* **931**:26–32.

19. **Radin, E.L., Paul, I.L., and Tolkoff, M.J.** (1970). Subchondral changes in patients with early degenerative joint disease. *Arthritis Rheum* **13**:400–5.

20. **Layton, M.V., Golstein, S.A., Goulet, R.W., Feldkamp, L.A., Kubinski, D.J., and Bole, G.G.** (1988). Examination of subchondral bone architecture in experimental osteoarthritis by microscopic computed axial tomography. *Arthritis Rheum* **31**.

21. **Milgram, J.W.** (1983). Morphological alterations of the subchondral bone in advanced degenerative arthritis. *Clin Orthop Rel Res* **173**:293–312.

22. **Kellgren, J.H. and Lawrence, J.S.** (1962). *The Epidemiology of Chronic Rheumatism: Atlas of Standard Radiographs.* Oxford, UK: Blackwell Scientific.

23. **Anonymous.** (1976). Cartilage and bone in osteoarthrosis. *Brit Med J* **2**:4–5.

24. **Dequecker, J., Mokassa, L., and Aerssens, J.** (1995). Bone density and osteoarthritis. *J Rheumatol* **22**(Suppl. 43):98–100.

25. **Dedrick, D.K., Goldstein, S.A., Brandt, K.D., O'Connor, B.L., Goulet, R.W., and Albrecht, M.** (1993). A longitudinal study of subchondral plate and trabecular bone in cruciate-deficient dogs with osteoarthritis followed up for 54 months. *Arthritis Rheum* **36**:1460–7.

26. **Radin, E.L. and Rose, R.M.** (1986). Role of subchondral bone in the initiation and progression of cartilage damage. *Clin Orthop Rel Res* **213**:34–40.

27. **Pottenger, L.A., Philips, F.M., and Draganich, L.F.** (1990). The effect of marginal osteophytes on reduction of varus–valgus instability in osteoarthritis knees. *Arthritis Rheum* **33**.

28. **Smythe, S.A.** (1987). Osteoarthritis, insulin and bone density. *J Rheumatol* **14**(Suppl.):91–3.

29. **Zhang, Y., Hannan, M., Chaisson, C., McAlindon, T., Evans, S., and Felson, D.** (1997). Low bone mineral density (BMD) increases the risk of progressive knee osteoarthritis (OA) in women. *Arthritis Rheum* **40**:1798.

30. **Dieppe, P., Cushnaghan, J., Young, P., and Kirwan, J.** (1993). Prediction of the progression of joint space narrowing in osteoarthritis of the knee by bone scintigraphy. *Ann Rheum Dis* **52**:557–63.

31. **Kiel, D.P.** Vitamin D, calcium and bone: descriptive epidemiology. (1995). In: I.H. Rosenberg (ed.), *Nutritional Assessment of Elderly Populations: Measurement and Function.* New York: Raven, pp. 277–90.

32. **Pangamala, R.V. and Cornwell, D.G.** (1982). The effects of vitamin E on arachidonic acid metabolism. *Ann NY Acad Sci.*

33. **Felson, D.T.** (1995). Weight and osteoarthritis. *J Rheumatol* **22**(Suppl. 43): 7–9.

34. **Sokoloff, L. and Mickelsen, O.** (1965). Dietary fat supplements, body weight and osteoarthritis in DBA/2JN mice. *J Nutr* **85**:117–21.

35. **Schwartz, E.R., Leveille, C., and Oh, W.H.** (1981). Experimentally induced osteoarthritis in guinea pigs: effect of surgical procedure and dietary intake of vitamin C. *Lab Animal Sci* **31**:683–7.

36. **Meacock, S.C.R., Bodmer, J.L., and Billingham, M.E.J.** (1990). Experimental OA in guinea pigs. *J Exp Path* **71**:279–93.

37. *McAlindon, T.E., Jacques, P., Zhang, Y., Hannan, M.T., Aliabadi, P., Weissman, B., Rush, D., Levy, D., and Felson, D.T.** (1996). Do antioxidant micronutrients protect against the development and progression of knee osteoarthritis? *Arthritis Rheum* **39**(4):648–56.
    This observational study, based on the Framingham Knee OA Study cohort, tested the possibility that dietary intake of antioxidant micronutrients (vitamins A, C, and E) reduces the incidence and progression of knee OA. The results suggest a protective effect of vitamin C with respect to the progression of knee OA.

38. **Schumacher, Jr., H.R.,** (1995). Synovial inflammation, crystals and osteoarthritis. *J Rheumatol* **22**(Suppl. 43):101–3.

39. **Blankenhorn, G.** (1986). Clinical efficacy of spondyvit (vitamin E) in activated arthroses. A multicenter, placebo-controlled, double-blind study. *Z Orthop* **124**:340–3.

40. **Brand, C., Snaddon, J., Bailey, M., and Cicuttini, F.** (2001). Vitamin E is ineffective for symptomatic relief of knee osteoarthritis: a six month double blind, randomised, placebo controlled study. *Ann Rheum Dis* **60**(10):946–9.

41. **Hill, J. and Bird, H.A.** (1990). Failure of selenium-ace to improve osteoarthritis. *Br J Rheumatol* **29**(3):211–3.

42. *Lane, N.E., Gore, L.R., Cummings, S.R.,* *et al.* (1999). Serum vitamin D levels and incident changes of radiographic hip osteoarthritis: a longitudinal study. Study of Osteoporotic Fractures Research Group. *Arthritis Rheum* **42**(5):854–60.
    This observational study tested the relationship between vitamin D status and hip OA. The results suggest a protective effect of vitamin D with respect to incident hip OA.

43. *McAlindon, T.E., Felson, D.T., Zhang, Y.,* *et al.* Relation of dietary intake and serum levels of vitamin D to progression of osteoarthritis of the knee among participants in the Framingham Study. (1996) *Ann Intern Med* **125**(5):353–9.
    This observational study, based on the Framingham Knee OA Study cohort, tested the possibility that vitamin D reduces the incidence and progression of knee OA. The results suggest a protective effect of vitamin D on the progression of knee OA.

44. **Koutkia, P., Chen, T.C., and Holick, M.F.** (2001). Vitamin D intoxication associated with an over-the-counter supplement. *N Engl J Med* **345**(1):66–7.

45. **Carmel, R., Lau, K.H., Baylink, D.J., Saxena, S., and Singer, F.R.** (1998). Cobalamin and osteoblast-specific proteins. *N Engl J Med* **319**(2):70–5.

46. **Flynn, M.A., Irvin, W., and Krause, G.** (1994). The effect of folate and cobalamin on osteoarthritic hands. *J Am Coll Nutr* **13**(4):351–6.

47. **Utiger, R.D.** (1998). Kashin-Beck disease—expanding the spectrum of iodine-deficiency disorders. *N Engl J Med* **339**(16):1156–8.

48. **Moreno-Reyes, R., Suetens, C., Mathieu, F.,** *et al.* (1998). Kashin-Beck osteoarthropathy in rural Tibet in relation to selenium and iodine status [see comments]. *N Engl J Med* **339**(16):1112–20.

9.11 Physical therapy

9.11.1 Exercise for the patient with osteoarthritis

Marian A. Minor

Physical disability and poor health often accompany OA. This decline, which intensifies, as people grow older, is a complex phenomenon influenced by pain, lower extremity impairments, poor physical fitness, obesity and co-morbidity, as well as OA severity. In addition to functional losses, low levels of daily physical activity and exercise are common problems, and OA often becomes a risk factor for inactivity-related diseases. There is mounting evidence that exercise can modify a number of the factors associated with disability and enhance health status and quality of life.[1-3] There is also information to indicate that particular types of exercises and joint motion may improve circulation and metabolism within the joint.[4,5]

Practitioners, aware of the benefits of exercise and risks of inactivity, often encourage patients to 'exercise' but do not provide specific information to facilitate adoption or maintenance. This chapter describes the problems created by inactivity in OA, reviews the rationale and evidence for specific types of exercise, and presents exercise recommendations appropriate in hip and knee OA.

Inactivity, de-conditioning and disability in OA

In the United States of America, OA is the most common form of arthritis, and the most common cause of physical disability and dependency.[6] Hip and knee OA account for more trouble walking, getting in and out of a chair, climbing stairs, performing self-care, household tasks, shopping, and doing errands, in persons over 65 than any other disease.[7] People with OA report significant losses in home and community activities; spend more time in sedentary activities such as sleeping and watching television, and require more time to complete tasks that they still perform. Among those with moderate to severe knee OA, marked changes in gait, joint loading, strength and range of motion have been demonstrated in both the affected and the non-affected extremity, with changes at the hip and ankle as well as the knee.[8] In elderly persons, the risk for physical disability attributable to hip and knee OA is as great as that of cardiovascular disease and greater than any other medical condition.[9]

Secondary inactivity-related conditions also arise in the presence of OA. People over 45, report arthritis as a major reason for limiting physical activity.[10] Those with arthritis tend to be physically inactive and cardiovascularly de-conditioned.[11,12] People who are inactive are at twice the risk for death, compared to those who are moderately active.[13]

Thus, the full impact of OA encompasses pain, impairments in strength and flexibility ranging far beyond the affected joint, altered biomechanics, asymmetrical gait, physical disability, loss of independence, cardiovascular

de-conditioning, and increased risk for a number of inactivity-related diseases, particularly cardiovascular disease. OA-related disability is influenced by a variety of factors. A number of these factors can be modified with exercise: flexibility, strength, cardiovascular fitness, energy expenditure, endurance, pain, and obesity.

The relationship between exercise and OA

Historically, vigorous physical activity—even weight bearing—was proscribed for a person with joint pathology. Today, we understand the deleterious effects of prolonged inactivity and the benefits of regular exercise for people with OA. We are also learning more about the relationship of exercise to the onset and progression of OA, and the effects of various types of exercise on joints.

Does exercise cause arthritis?

A number of studies have investigated the incidence of hip or knee OA related to sports, physical activity, and other factors, such as body weight, occupation, and prior joint injury. Cheng and colleagues[14] categorized over 15 000 individuals in terms of level of physical activity, gender, and age. For both men and women, running more than 20 miles per week and greater weight were the only factors significantly related to OA. In other studies, prior joint injury, participation in sports for more than 10 years, female gender, high levels of physical activity, and increased body weight increased the risk for hip or knee OA.[15-17] Spector *et al.*[18] reported that former elite female athletes were at increased risk for both hip and knee OA. There also have been attempts to study the relative contribution of specific sports to OA. Cooper *et al.*[19] found differences among various sports with respect to the risk for hip OA (Table 9.19). For women, tennis and swimming resulted in the highest risk; for men, golf presented the greatest risk. Currently, we do not have enough sport-specific information to direct

Table 9.19 Sport-specific risk for hip OA (Ref. 19). Odds ratios (95% confidence interval), adjusted for body mass index, hip injury, and Heberden's nodes

Sport	Men	Women
Tennis	1.0 (0.6–2.0)	1.9 (1.3–2.8)
Swimming	1.2 (0.7–1.9)	1.8 (1.2–2.7)
Soccer	1.1 (0.7–1.6)	Not reported
Cricket	0.9 (0.5–1.5)	0.5 (0.1–2.6)
Golf	1.5 (0.8–2.9)	1.2 (0.5–2.6)
Any sport	1.0 (0.5–1.9)	1.3 (0.9–1.7)

Modified from Ref. 19.

people toward or away from specific sports. For example, it is puzzling that swimming was associated with increased hip OA in women, and that soccer and tennis were less risky than golf for men. Overall, it appears that moderate exercise is not a risk factor for OA.

There are, however, activity-related recommendations that may reduce the risk of hip and knee OA:

- maintain proper body weight[20]
- exercise and participate in sports in moderation[14,18]
- reduce the occurrence of sport-related joint injury[16,19]
- minimize occupational tasks such as heavy lifting and excessive knee bending and squatting[17]

Exercise, joint health, and disease progression of OA

There are continuing questions about the effects of exercise on a joint already affected by OA. A number of research reports challenge previous assumptions that rest promotes healing and exercise damages OA joints. Joint immobilization leads to articular cartilage atrophy[21] and weakening of the peri-articular muscles and ligaments, whereas regular joint motion and intermittent weight bearing are beneficial to both cartilage[21,22] and muscle.

Dynamic exercise, both resisted and non-resisted, may promote joint health. Cycling and walking increased synovial circulation in effused knees.[4] At faster speeds (160° per second), cycling and resistance exercise resulted in improved oxygen partial pressure in the joint, whereas isometric exercise and slow movement (60° per second) did not produce the same benefit.[5] A study of synovial fluid from OA knees found a decrease in the levels of interleukin-1 β (IL-1 β), a cytokine that mediates the degradation of articular cartilage, in subjects who participated in a walking and strengthening exercise program in comparison with a non-exercising control group.[23]

The type of exercise performed determines the physiologic and metabolic responses. Although dynamic exercise improved synovial blood flow in subjects with knee joint effusions, prolonged isometric contraction of the quadriceps and extreme knee flexion decreased synovial blood flow.[4] The assumption that isometric exercise is safer for an arthritic joint than dynamic exercise has been called into question by a series of studies using an instrumented femoral head prosthesis. These studies showed that rapid and/or maximal isometric contraction of the gluteal muscles increased hip joint contact pressure more than walking or cycling.[24] In a study of patients with knee OA, in which synovial fluid was analyzed before and after 12 weeks of quadriceps strengthening exercise and low intensity walking, no adverse effects were noted on articular cartilage metabolism, as reflected by changes in concentrations of glycosaminoglycans and of chondroitin sulphate epitopes 3B3 and 7D4.[25] Some weight-bearing activities increase joint loading and may need to be modified if they increase joint pain or other joint symptoms. For example, stair descent and ascent, one-legged stance, and carrying loads greater than 10 per cent of body weight may significantly increase loading of the hip.[24,26] Squatting, climbing, and walking at faster speeds, particularly in the presence of obesity or lower extremity malalignment, increases biomechanical stress at the knee.[27,28]

In summary, current evidence supports the safety of moderate, weight-bearing, dynamic exercise with respect to both the joint and general health. Too often, people with hip or knee arthritis are cautioned against *all* weight-bearing activities, such as walking, running, dancing, and stair climbing. However, many people with hip or knee involvement do not need to avoid these activities.

Exercise as a preventive and rehabilitative intervention

Range of motion, strengthening, and aerobic exercises improve health and function in people with OA. In a systematic review of conditioning exercise in subjects with hip or knee OA, Van Baar *et al.* examined the results of 11

randomized controlled trials.[3] Although the measured outcomes varied, most studies measured pain, self-reported disability, and walking performance. Positive results were reported for each measure with effect sizes varying from small to large. The rationale for, and evidence supporting the benefit of, the three major modes of conditioning exercise and a consideration of specific exercise for patients with OA are presented below.

Range of motion/flexibility

Knee and hip OA are associated consistently with decreased range of motion of all joints in both lower limbs.[8,29] Decreased hip motion is associated with pain, loss of function, limitations in physical activity, decreased walking speed, decreased stride length, and increased energy expenditure.[29–31] Loss of knee extension reduces walking efficiency, and limited knee flexion interferes with using stairs or transferring to a toilet or bathtub.[32] In addition to these functional problems, inadequate joint motion is harmful to the joint itself.

For adequate nutrition and balanced catabolic and anabolic activity, articular cartilage requires regular joint motion with compression and decompression.[22,33] Prolonged immobilization and inadequate joint loading result in cartilage atrophy.[21] Additionally, inactivity results in loss of flexibility and decreased compliance of the joint capsule, ligaments, and synovium. Compliance in these structures is associated with a decrease in the peak impact load on the joint.[34]

Daily exercise that includes a full active range of motion and periods of weight bearing and non-weight bearing is the optimal prescription for maintenance of joint health. Some people may benefit from an individually designed flexibility program that takes into account joint pathology and impairments. For many, general flexibility may be maintained in accordance with the American College of Sports Medicine (ACSM) and Centers for Disease Control and Prevention (CDC) recommendations for adults[35] (Table 9.20). It is important to remember that OA in a single joint commonly leads to decreased motion and loss of flexibility in adjacent and contralateral joints. Therefore, comprehensive exercise recommendations should address general needs for range of motion and flexibility.

Aerobic exercise

Inactivity is as dangerous as smoking, obesity, and an elevated cholesterol level in increasing the likelihood of coronary artery disease, atherosclerosis, hypertension, diabetes, and some types of cancer.[36] Cardiovascular de-conditioning and an increased risk of such diseases are common in people with lower extremity OA.[11,12] There is no question that regular physical activity improves health for people of all ages, and that increasing physical activity improves health at any age. In a sample of nearly 10 000 men over 40 years of age who were followed for 5 years, becoming fit reduced the mortality risk by 44 per cent. A one-minute increase in the duration of treadmill test time over the study period decreased the risk of cardiovascular death by 8.6 years.[13] Aerobic exercise, which requires repetitive, rhythmic motion and activation of the major muscle groups, improves general health, physical fitness, function and quality of life for people with OA.[3,23,37–39] Evidence is mounting that dynamic exercise also has a positive effect on joint health.[4,5,23]

Numerous controlled trials have reported positive results of aerobic exercise (walking, cycling, water exercise) for people with hip or knee OA.

Table 9.20 Recommendations for musculoskeletal flexibility

Mode:	Gentle static stretching
Frequency:	Minimum 2–3 days/week
Intensity:	Stretch to a position of mild tension/discomfort
Duration:	Hold position for 10–30 seconds
Repetitions:	3–4 repetitions for each stretch

Source: Taken from Ref. 35.

Outcomes include improved cardiovascular fitness, improved function, and walking performance, and decreased disability, pain, and depression. Study samples included subjects from 40–85 years who were recruited from community and clinical sites. Exercise periods varied from 4–12 weeks and included supervised and home programs. Follow up periods were as long as one year. Some studies used initial periods of physical therapist-directed exercise (strengthening, flexibility, balance, coordination, locomotion) in either individualized or small group programs. Results from these aerobic and conditioning programs indicate that a variety of interventions, both weight bearing and partial weight bearing, are well-tolerated and lead to improvements in fitness, function, and health status.

Muscle strengthening exercise

Lower extremity strength is related to disability in people with hip and knee OA.[29,40] Static and dynamic strength deficits as great as 60 per cent are common. In a comprehensive cross-sectional study of determinants of pain and disability among subjects with hip and knee OA, van Baar[29] reported significant and clinically important strength deficits in all motions at the hip and knee, irrespective of the disease site. In this study, kinesiologic variables were more closely and consistently related to pain and disability than radiographic severity.

In knee OA, quadriceps weakness results from neuromuscular inhibition[41] that occurs in the presence of pain and effusion, and from disuse atrophy that results from inactivity. There is also some evidence that quadriceps weakness may precede OA and be a disease risk factor.[42] It is not clear if knee OA results in diminished quadriceps muscle mass. Studies have reported both decreased[43] and increased[42] quadriceps muscle mass in women with knee OA.

In addition to the importance of strength for function, muscle is a major shock absorber for joints. An adequately conditioned muscle mass and the ability to generate force quickly attenuate impact loads. The necessary components—muscle mass, contractile velocity, force production, endurance for repetitive motions, and motor skill—are often compromised by joint pathology, pain, and inactivity. A comprehensive exercise program designed to improve strength, endurance, and motor control includes strength training, functional exercises, and balance activities. Functional exercises are activities such as partial-squats (deep knee bending may cause discomfort), arising from and sitting in a chair, and stepping up and down on one or two steps. Functional exercises encompass both concentric (muscle shortens during torque production) and eccentric (muscle lengthens during torque production) muscle training. For example, the partial squat exercise trains the quadriceps concentrically as the quadriceps contracts and shortens to extend the knee and raise the body. Eccentric training occurs as the knee bends while the quadriceps lengthens but maintains tension to control the speed and amount of knee bending. Muscle training can be designed to reduce impairment, improve function, and protect joints from abnormal stresses and excessive loading.

Recent controlled trials of strength training in OA have focused primarily on knee OA.[41,44–46] Subjects, ranged in age from 34–85 years, came from community and clinical settings, and had symptoms for 3–80 months. The exercise interventions were diverse in content, intensity, and frequency. Most contained isometric and dynamic exercise, a variety of modes of external resistance (i.e., elastic bands, isokinetic dynamometer), and some included functional exercises (i.e., stepping, squats). Frequency of exercise ranged from twice weekly to daily. Interventions were taught and carried out in supervised sessions, home programs, or a combination. Study periods varied from 8 weeks to 18 months.

Results included increased knee strength, decreased pain, and improvement in function. Of the three studies that provided physiologic information, two reported improvement in voluntary muscle activation (a decrease in muscle inhibition) after the exercise period.[41,45] One study reported less energy expenditure for self-paced walking.[46] Strengthening programs that addressed multiple joints (hips, knees, and ankles) and functional training reported significant improvements in balance, gait, and independence as well as strength.[38,41,45,46]

Exercise recommendations

The challenge for the person with OA is to find and maintain safe and effective exercise routines. People with OA are a heterogeneous population, ranging widely in age, morbidity, impairments, functional goals, and interests. People with severe involvement may require individualized therapy and support to become more active. On the other hand, many people are interested in, and capable of exercising more vigorously to improve physical fitness. Others may not be able to exercise for the duration or intensity recommended for improving fitness and will benefit from recommendations and support to increase daily physical activity.

Physical activity for health

General health depends upon adequate levels of regular physical activity. The levels of physical activity necessary to improve and maintain general health are less intense than those required to improve physical fitness in an already active person. Guidelines for improving health are couched in terms of regular physical activity to reduce health risks, rather than targeted exercise to train a specific component of physical fitness. The recommendations for health are whole body, dynamic activity performed at low to moderate intensity on most days of the week, accumulating 30 minutes of moderate physical activity each exercise day[36] (Table 9.21). Activity accumulated in three 10-minute bouts appears to provide the same health benefits as a continuous 30-minute session. People for whom 10 minutes is too much, can start with 1 or 2 minutes of walking, knowing that the goal is 10 minutes. This is good news for people with arthritis or other limitations who may be unable to exercise for a longer duration or with greater intensity. This also is important information for health care providers who now can recommend safe and effective activity to improve health and prevent unnecessary disability for almost everyone.

Exercise for cardiovascular and musculoskeletal fitness

Most of the OA exercise studies reported to date have set exercise goals in accordance with the parameters of intensity, duration, and frequency recommended for cardiovascular and muscular fitness by the ACSM, CDC, and the US Surgeon General.[35,36] Guidelines for improving physical fitness, both cardiovascular and musculoskeletal, recommend continuous exercise bouts at moderate levels of intensity[35] (Table 9.22). These recommendations can be exercise goals for many people with hip or knee OA; however, initial exercise may need to be at lower levels of intensity and duration, and increased as tolerated.

Walking for exercise with OA

Walking is a safe, effective, and accessible form of aerobic exercise for people with OA. Studies have shown that free speed walking produces a minimal increase in hip joint contact pressures, much less than that generated by maximal isometric contraction or one-legged standing.[24] Studies of

Table 9.21 Physical activity recommendations for health

Activity:	Daily activity (walking, yard work, etc.)
Frequency:	Most days of the week
Intensity:	Moderate; 55–70% of age-predicted maximal heart rate; RPE 2–4
Duration:	Accumulate at least 30 minutes of activity (e.g., three 10-minute bouts)

RPE, Rating of perceived exertion (scale 0–10).
Source: Taken from Ref. 36.

Table 9.22 Recommendations for physical fitness

Cardiovascular fitness

Mode:	Rhythmic, aerobic exercise (walking, jogging, cycling, swimming, etc.)
Frequency:	3–5 days/week
Intensity:	70–85% age-predicted maximal heart rate; RPE 4–5
Duration:	20–30 minutes continuous

Muscular fitness

Mode:	Dynamic, resistance exercise for major muscle groups
Frequency:	2–3 days/week on alternate days
Volume:	8–10 exercises; resistance adequate to induce moderate, volitional fatigue after 8–12 repetitions. If the subject is more than 50–60 years of age or frail, or the primary goal is to improve endurance, choose a level of resistance that will produce moderate fatigue after 10–15 repetitions.

RPE, Rating of perceived exertion (scale 0–10).

Source: Taken from Ref. 35.

patients with a knee effusion have shown that synovial blood flow increases with dynamic exercise, such as walking and cycling.[4]

Lightweight athletic shoes with variable lacing, hindfoot control, a midsole of shock-absorbing materials, and a continuous sole offer support and shock-attenuating properties. Adding an insole of viscoelastic materials increases shock absorption.[47] In subjects without joint involvement, viscoelastic insoles were shown to decrease the shock measured at the proximal tibia by 42 per cent in subjects walking 4 km (2.4 miles) per hour. Such insoles range in price from $20–30 and are available in stores that sell athletic shoes. For some people with OA, mild control of pronation and shock absorption provided by commercially available shoes and insoles may decrease knee and hip discomfort associated with walking; others may require the greater biomechanical correction afforded by semi-rigid or rigid orthoses. This type of correction requires professional services (physical therapist, orthotist) for evaluation and fitting of customized devices. Costs can vary from $100–400 and are rarely covered by insurance or managed care plans.

Faster walking speeds increase biomechanical stress on the knee joint. In normal knees, this is not harmful, and walking or running does not damage the joint. However, in the presence of malalignment, joint instability, or diminished proprioception, increasing walking speeds may increase joint forces. Among patients with medial tibiofemoral compartment OA, increased walking speed was associated with increased loading of the medial compartment.[27]

Exercise stress testing

Current guidelines state that men younger than age 40 and women younger than 50 who are asymptomatic and have no more than one cardiovascular risk factor can begin a moderate intensity exercise program with medical clearance, and do not require physician-supervised cardiovascular stress testing.[48] Table 9.23 contains the guidelines, a list of cardiovascular risk factors and definitions of moderate and intense exercise. On the other hand, initiation of a *vigorous* exercise program does merit exercise stress testing in sedentary men older than 40 and women older than 50.

Novice exercisers should understand the risks imposed by vigorous, rather than moderate intensity exercise, and learn methods to monitor and regulate exercise intensity. Heart rate, as a percentage of maximal, is often suggested as a guide; however, many people have trouble taking their own pulse. A rating of perceived exertion (RPE) or a simple talk test may be more useful for self-monitoring. The RPE scale (0, no exertion; 10, extremely strong exertion) is a valid method to assess exercise intensity or exertion. A level of 2–5 encompasses low to moderate intensity exercise. The talk test

Table 9.23 Guidelines for exercise stress testing

Perform supervised exercise stress test for

♦ Apparently healthy: men ≥40 years; women ≥50 years, for vigorous exercise only

♦ Persons at risk* with no symptoms: all ages, for vigorous exercise only

♦ Persons at risk* with symptoms and disease: all ages, for moderate or vigorous exercise

♦ There is no requirement to perform maximal or diagnostic exercise stress testing for healthy or asymptomatic people prior to aerobic exercise of only moderate intensity

* See below

Persons at Risk have two or more of the following Risk Factors for Cardiovascular Disease

♦ Hypertension (blood pressure ≥160/90 mm Hg)

♦ Serum cholesterol ≥240 mg/dL (6.2 mmol/L)

♦ Cigarette smoking

♦ Diabetes mellitus

♦ Family history of cardiovascular disease

Definitions of exercise intensity are as follows

Moderate: well within the subject's current capacity; sustainable comfortably for 60 minutes; non-competitive activity. 50–75% of MHR = RPE 3–5

Vigorous: substantial challenge; fatigue within 20 minutes; >75% of MHR = RPE >5

RPE, rating of perceived exertion (0–10);
MHR, age-predicted maximal heart rate

Source: Taken from Ref. 47.

is based on the fact that moderate intensity exercise does not cause shortness of breath in individuals with normal pulmonary function. Being able to carry on a normal conversation, talk in complete sentences, or recite a poem while exercising indicate that the effort is no more than moderate.

Considerations in prescribing an exercise program

Disease severity/joint alignment

The severity of OA may affect individual response to exercise. In a study of patients with knee OA, Fransen and colleagues[49] reported that participants with a smaller medial compartment joint-space width (implying loss of articular cartilage) did not respond as well to the exercise intervention as did those with greater joint-space width. It has been noted that genu varus may increase loading of the medial compartment of the knee during walking, and that loading increases with faster walking speeds.[27,28] It is not known whether the increased loading of the medial compartment is harmful, or if changes in lower extremity alignment by use of orthoses (heel wedges, semi-rigid or rigid insoles, or knee braces) will reduce the loading in a meaningful way (see Chapter 7.2.5). People with impairments due to hip or knee OA expend more energy in walking a given distance than those without joint involvement.[11,31,46] This increased energy expenditure may result in early onset fatigue and diminished neuromuscular control. Fig. 9.12 depicts increased energy expenditure and cost of self-paced

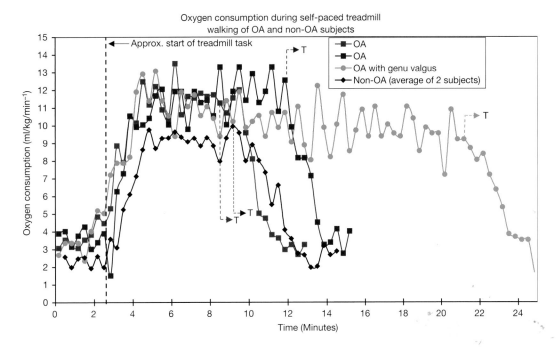

Fig. 9.12 Oxygen consumption during a 0.25 mile (0.15 km) self-paced treadmill walk by 4 age- and gender-matched subjects (two with knee OA, two without OA) and one subject with knee OA who had marked bilateral genu valgus. Respiratory gases were collected and measured with a portable analyzer and software package (MedicalGraphics VO2000). Values for the non-OA subjects were nearly identical and are presented as an average. Energy expenditure (oxygen consumption in ml/kg/min^{-1}) is displayed on the *y* axis. Time (minutes) of the treadmill walking is displayed on the *x* axis. 'T' denotes termination of treadmill walking for each subject. Data are shown for 2 minutes of recovery after cessation of treadmill walking. Energy cost of the task is comprised of the energy expenditure and the time taken to complete the task. OA subjects demonstrated greater energy expenditure and energy cost than the non-OA subjects.

Source: Taken from Stratman, J. Minor M: Oxygen consumption during daily tasks: Preliminary study of the effects of knee osteoarthritis (OA). *International Conference on Health Promotion and Disability Prevention in Rheumatic Disease: Evidence for Exercise and Physical Activity*, St. Louis, MO, 2002.

walking of women with knee OA compared to age-matched peers without knee OA.[50]

Exercise recommendations for people with severe disease should:

- include an assessment of their biomechanical needs
- set initial exercise levels well within current capacity
- monitor for pain and aggravation of symptoms
- modify the exercise, if necessary.

When impairments such as pain, weakness, limited motion, or joint instability interfere with increasing physical activity, referral to a physical and/or occupational therapist is warranted. The therapist can assess the patient and develop a treatment plan that includes education, home exercise, and joint protection as needed. Four to 12 outpatient visits are available through most health care plans in the United States of America and can be used for the initial visit and for periodic review and revision of the plan as the patient progresses to a self-directed exercise or activity program.

Pain

Pain is the major symptom of OA and a common reason for people to limit physical activity. However, the mechanisms of pain in OA are not well understood. There is relatively little correlation between the radiographic severity of OA and the severity of joint pain. Furthermore, little information is available regarding the course of joint pain as a person with OA begins to exercise. Specific recommendations for exercise in the presence of pain do not exist. Studies have indicated that strengthening regimens reduce joint pain in subjects with knee OA, and that compliance with these programs is good. It might be suggested that muscle-conditioning programs be implemented before aerobic exercise. However, many people with symptomatic hip or knee OA tolerate walking for aerobic exercise and can walk vigorously and frequently enough to improve cardiovascular fitness without increasing their symptoms or their requirement for analgesics. The best recommendations that can be made at this time are to:

- begin each session with exercises for flexibility and musculoskeletal and cardiovascular warm-up (gentle stretching, low intensity calisthenics, 2–5 minutes of slow paced walking or cycling with no resistance)
- exercise within a pain-free range and avoid postures or activities that increase pain or cause joint swelling
- supply biomechanical support by using foot orthoses, if needed, and selecting shock attenuating footwear.

The exercise program should be designed and self-monitored to avoid immediate pain as well as delayed onset muscle soreness. Pain is not necessary to achieve benefit and is a major reason for exercise non-compliance.

Age

Age is not a contraindication to conditioning exercise—the usual guidelines apply in the elderly. In a study of people between the ages of 68–85, approximately 50 per cent of who reported physician-diagnosed mild to moderate OA; 6 months of resistance and/or aerobic exercise resulted in gains in strength and endurance and no increase in pain or reported joint symptoms. Joint symptoms and exercise-related injuries were infrequent and similar in those with and without OA.[51] Although the presence of impairments that may affect balance or increase fracture risk need to be considered in the exercise recommendation, there is good evidence that older people, even with joint involvement, can learn to exercise vigorously and enjoy improved health and fitness.

Obesity

Being overweight is a risk factor in knee OA (see Chapter 2). Losing weight is associated with both reduced symptoms of knee OA and a decreased risk for developing the disease.[20] Although little information exists about obesity, joint effects, and exercise, general knowledge can be applied to this situation. Carrying extra weight adds stress to hip and knee with walking, running, climbing and descending stairs. Biomechanical studies indicate that carrying a load greater than 10 per cent of body weight increases stress on the hip and knee.[24] However, people who need to reduce must include regular aerobic exercise in their weight loss program. Caloric balance and weight control require regular physical activity. Therefore, adequate physical activity and exercise are essential, albeit challenging, for obese people with painful joints. Moderately paced walking, bicycling, and water exercise, have demonstrated safety and efficacy as exercise modalities for people with hip or knee OA, and are appropriate for those who are overweight.

Summary

OA-related disability and poor health are closely related to musculoskeletal and cardiovascular deficits. Many of the determinants of disability and poor health are potentially preventable or reducible through regular physical activity and exercise. Appropriate exercise, performed regularly, may reduce pain, increase mobility, strengthen muscle, improve neuromuscular function, improve cardiovascular health, reduce the fatigue generated by performance of daily tasks, and help manage weight. The current recommendations for regular physical activity and exercise have been proposed by the ACSM, CDC, and the US Surgeon General. Promotion of adequate levels of exercise and habitual physical activity for all people, including people with arthritis, has become a public health priority. The majority of exercise studies in OA have based exercise protocols upon these published recommendations for cardiovascular and muscular fitness (Table 9.22). These exercise recommendations may be used as goals for most people with OA, with consideration of other activity-limiting conditions. For some people, the level of exercise necessary to improve fitness may not be feasible. In these instances, it is appropriate to direct efforts toward achieving recommended levels of physical activity for health (Table 9.21).

Key points

1. OA is a major reason for physical inactivity and cardiovascular and muscular de-conditioning.

2. OA in one hip or knee is associated with gait disturbance and decreased strength and range of motion of all other lower extremity joints.

3. Walking and cycling at moderate intensity are safe and effective methods to improve cardiovascular fitness for many people with hip and knee OA.

4. Lower extremity strength training improves function and endurance and decreases pain in subjects with knee OA.

5. Accumulation of 30 minutes of moderate physical activity on most days of the week confers significant health benefits even to people who are not able to exercise at conditioning levels.

Acknowledgement

I wish to thank Joshua Stratman, BHS, SPT, for his assistance in the preparation of this manuscript. Work on this chapter was supported in part by US Department of Education, National Institute on Disability and Rehabilitation Research under special project number H133B980022.

References

(An asterisk denotes recommended reading.)

1. *Felson, D.T., Lawrence, R.C., Hochberg, M.C., McAlilndon, T., Dieppe, P.A., Minor, M.A., Blair, S.N., Berman, B.M., Fries, J.F., Weinberger, M., Lorig, K.R., Jacobs, J.J., and Goldberg, V. (2000). NIH Conference. Osteoarthritis: New insights. Part 2: Treatment approaches. *Ann Int Med* **133**(9):726–37.
   This edited summary of a scientific conference, 'Stepping Away from OA,' held at the National Institutes of Health in 1999, presents a multidisciplinary perspective to the management of OA.

2. Minor, M.A. (1999). Exercise in the treatment of osteoarthritis. In K.D. Brandt (ed.), *Rheumatology Clinics of North America*. Philadelphia: W.B. Saunders, **25**(2):397–415.

3. *van Baar, M.E., Assendelft, W.J.J, Dekker, J., Oostenforp, R.A.B., and Bijlsma, J.W.J. (1999). Effectiveness of exercise therapy in patients with osteoarthritis of the hip or knee. *Arthritis Rheum* **42**:1361–89.
   This is a systematic review of experimental studies of aerobic and strengthening exercise in patients with hip and knee OA.

4. *James, M.J., Cleland, L.G., Gaffney, R.D., Proudman, S.M., and Chatterton, B.E. (1994). Effect of exercise on 99Tc-DTPA clearance from knees with effusions. *J Rheumatol* **21**:501–4.
   This study investigates synovial blood flow in knees of patients with rheumatoid arthritis or OA and demonstrates specific physiologic effects of different modes of exercise and weight bearing.

5. Miltner, O., Scheider, U., Graf, J., and Neithard, F.U. (1997). Influence of isokinetic and ergometric exercises on oxygen partial pressure measurement in the human knee joint. In Nemoto and LaManna (eds), *Oxygen Transport to Tissue XVIII*. New York: Plenum Press, pp. 183–9.

6. Felson, David, T., MD, MPH, Lawrence, Reva, C., MPH Dieppe, Paul, A. MD and Hirsch, Rosemarie, MD, MPH *et al.* (2000). Osteoarthritis: New Insights: Part 1: The Disease and Its Risk Factors. [NIH Conference] *Ann Int Med* **133**(7):635–46.

7. Ettinger, Jr., W.H. (1998). Physical activity, arthritis and disability in older people. *Clin Ger Med* **12**:633–40.

8. Messier, S.P., Loeser, R.F., Hoover, J.L., Semble, E.L., and Wise, C.M. (1992). Osteoarthritis of the knee: Effects on gait, strength and flexibility. *Arch Phys Med Rehab* **73**:29–36.

9. Guccione, A.A., Felson, D.T., Anderson, J.J., Anthony, J.M., Zhang, Y., and Wilson, P.W. (1994). The effects of specific medical conditions on functional limitations of elders in the Framingham Study. *Am J Public Health* **84**:351–8.

10. Yelin, E. (1992). Arthritis. The cumulative impact of a common chronic condition. *Arthritis Rheum* **35**:489–97.

11. Minor, M.A., Hewett, J., Webel, R., Dreisinger, T., and Kay, D. Exercise tolerance and disease related measures in persons with rheumatoid arthritis and osteoarthritis. *J Rheumatol* **15**(6): 905–11.

12. Philbin, E.F., Groff, G.D., Ries, M.D., and Miller, T.E. (1995). Cardiovascular fitness and health in patients with end-stage osteoarthritis. *Arthritis Rheum* **38**:799–805.

13. Blair, S.N., Kohl, H.W., Barlow, C.E., Paffenbarger, R.S., Gibbons, L.W., and Macera, C.A. (1995). Changes in physical fitness and all-cause mortality. A prospective study of healthy and unhealthy men. *JAMA* **273**:1093–8.

14. Cheng, Y., Macera, C.A., Davis, D.R., Ainsworth, B.E., Troped, P.J., and Blair, S.N. (2000). Physical activity and self-reported, physician-diagnosed osteoarthritis: Is physical activity a risk factor? *J Clin Epi* **53**(3):315–22.

15. Felson, D.T., Zhang, Y., Hannan, M., Naimark, A., Weissman, B., Aliabadi, P., and Levy. (1997). Risk factors for incident radiographic knee osteoarthritis in the elderly. *Arthritis Rheum* **40**:728–33.

16. Cooper, C., Snow, S., McAlindon, T.E., Stuart, B., Coggon, D., and Dieppe, P.A. (2000). Risk factors for the incidence and progression of radiographic knee osteoarthritis. *Arthritis Rheum* **43**(5):995–1000.

17. Coggon, D., Croft, P., Kellingray, S., Barrett, D., McLaren, M., and Cooper, C. (2000). Occupational physical activities and osteoarthritis of the knee. *Arthritis Rheum* **43**(7):1443–9.

18. Spector, T.D., Harris, P.A., Hart, D.J., Cicuttini, F.M., Nandra, D., Etherington, J., Wolman, R.L., and Doyle, D.V. (1996). Risk of osteoarthritis associated with long-term weight-bearing sports. *Arthritis Rheum* **39**(6): 988–96.

19. Cooper, C., Inskip, H., Croft, P., Campbell, L., Smith, G., McLaren, M., and Coggon, D. (1998). Individual risk factors for hip osteoarthritis: Obesity, hip injury and physical activity. *Am J Epi* 147(6):516–22.

20. Felson, D.T. and Chaisson, C.E. (1997). Understanding the relationship between body weight and osteoarthritis. *Baillière's Clin Rheumatol* 11:671–81.

21. Palmoski, M.J., Colyer, R.A., and Brandt, K.D. (1980). Joint motion in the absence of normal loading does not maintain normal articular cartilage. *Arthritis Rheum* 23:325–34.

22. Houlbrooke, K., Vause, K., and Merrilees, M.J. (1990). Effects of movement and weightbearing on the glycosaminoglycan content of sheep articular cartilage. *Aus J Physiother* 3:88–91.

23. Messier, S.P., Loeser, R.F., Mitchell, M.N., Valle, G., Morgan, T.P., Rejeski, W.J., and Ettinger, W.H. (2000). Exercise and weight loss in obese older adults with knee osteoarthritis: A preliminary study. *J Am Geriat Soc* 48:1062–72.

24. *Tackson, S.J., Krebs, D.E., and Harris, B.A. (1997). Acetabular pressures during hip arthritis exercises. *Arthritis Care Res* 10:308–319.

   This paper is one of a series of reports based on information obtained with an instrumented femoral head prosthesis that relayed data about hip joint pressures during various types of exercise and activities. The important effect of muscle contraction on joint forces is shown.

25. Bautch, J.C., Clayton, M.K., Chu, Q., and Johnson, K.A. (2000). Synovial fluid chondroitin sulphate epitopes 3B3 and 7D4 and glycosaminoglycan in human knee osteoarthritis after exercise. *Ann Rheum Dis* 59:887–91.

26. Neumann, D.A. (1989). Biomechanical analysis of selected principles of hip joint protection. *Arthritis Care Res* 2:146–155.

27. Schnitzer, T.J., Poppovich, J.M., Andersson, G.B.J., and Andriacchi, T.P. (1993). Effect of piroxicam on gait in patients with osteoarthritis of the knee. *Arthritis Rheum* 36:1207–13.

28. Sharma, L., Hurwitz, D.E., Thonar, E.J., Sum, J.A., Lenz, M.E., Dunlop, D.D., et al. (1998). Knee adduction moment, serum hyaluronan level, and disease severity in medial tibiofemoral osteoarthritis. *Arthritis Rheum* 41:1233–40.

29. van Baar, M.E., Dekker, J., Lemmens, J.A., Oostendorp, R.A., and Bijlsma, J.W. (1998). Pain and disability in patients with osteoarthritis of hip or knee: the relationship with articular, kinesiological, and psychological characteristics. *J Rheumatol* 25:125–33.

30. Steultjens, M.P., Dekker, J., vanBaar, M.E., Oostendorp, R.A., and Bijlsma, J.W. (2000). Range of joint motion and disability in patients with osteoarthritis of the knee or hip. *Rheumatology* 39:955–61.

31. Waters, R.L., Perry, J., Conaty, P., Lunsford, B., and O'Meara, P. (1987). The energy cost of walking with arthritis of the hip and knee. *Clin Orthop* 214:278–84.

32. Badley, E.M., Wagstaff, S., and Wood, P.H.N. (1984). Measures of functional ability (disability) in arthritis in relation to impairment of range of joint movement. *Ann Rheum Dis* 43:563–9.

33. Buckwalter, J.A. (1995). Osteoarthritis and articular cartilage use, disuse, and abuse: Experimental studies. *J Rheumatol* (Suppl. 43) 22:13–15.

34. Radin, E.L. and Paul, I.L. (1970). Does cartilage compliance reduce skeletal impact loads? The relative force-attenuating properties of articular cartilage, synovial fluid, periarticular soft tissues and bone. *Arthritis Rheum* 13:139–44.

35. Pate, R.R., Pratt, M., and Blair, S.N., et al. (1995). Physical activity and public health. A recommendation from the Centers for Disease Control and Prevention and the American College of Sports Medicine. *JAMA* 273:402–7.

36. *U.S. Department of Health and Human Services: Physical Activity and Health: A Report of the Surgeon General, 1996. Available at: http://www.cdc.gov/nccdphp/sgr/sgr.htm (Accessed March 13, 2001).

   This US Surgeon General Report, the first since the report on smoking, provides an indepth review of the dangers of inactivity and the benefits of physical activity in the general population and in populations with a chronic disease. Recommendations are provided.

37. Minor, M.A., Hewett, J.E., Webel, R.R., Anderson, S.K., and Kay, D.R. (1989). Efficacy of physical conditioning exercise in patients with rheumatoid arthritis or osteoarthritis. *Arthritis Rheum* 32:1397–1405.

38. Ettinger, W.H., Burns, R., Messier, S.P., et al. (1997). A randomized trial comparing aerobic exercise and resistance exercise with a health education program in older adults with knee osteoarthritis. *JAMA* 277:25–31.

39. VanBaar, M.E., Dekker, J., Oostendorp, R., Bijl, D., Voorn, T.B., Lemmens, J.A.M., and Bijlsma, W.J. (1998). The effectiveness of exercise therapy in patients with osteoarthritis of the hip or knee: A randomized clinical trial. *J Rheumatol* 25:2432–9.

40. McAlindon, T.E., Cooper, C., Kirwan, J.R., and Dieppe, P.A. (1993). Determinants of disability in osteoarthritis of the knee. *Ann Rheum Dis* 52:258–62.

41. *Hurley, M.V. and Scott, D.L. (1998). Improvements in quadriceps sensorimotor function and disability of patients with knee osteoarthritis following a clinically practicable exercise regime. *Br J Rheumatol* 37:1181–87.

   This report describes the exercise methods used in a successful muscle-conditioning program for patients with knee OA. The exercise protocol and a number of outcome measures are also presented in detail.

42. Slemenda, C., Brandt, K.D., Heilman, K., et al. (1997). Quadriceps weakness and osteoarthritis of the knee. *Ann Intern Med* 127:97–104.

43. Toda, Y., Segal, N., Toda, T., Kato, A., and Toda, F. (2000). A decline in lower extremity lean body mass per body weight is characteristic of women with early phase osteoarthritis of the knee. *J Rheumatol* 27:2449–54.

44. Maurer, B.T., Stern, A.G., Kinossian, B., Cook, K.D., and Schumacher, H.R. (1999). Osteoarthritis of the knee: Isokinetic quadriceps exercise versus an educational intervention. *Arch Phys Med Rehabil* 80:1293–9.

45. O'Reilly, S., Muir, K., and Doherty, M. (1999). Effectiveness of a home exercise on pain and disability from osteoarthritis of the knee: A randomized controlled trial. *Ann Rheum Dis* 58:15–19.

46. Petrella, R.J. and Bartha, C. (2000). Home based exercise therapy for older persons with knee osteoarthritis: a randomized clinical trail. *J Rheumatol* 27:2215–21.

47. Voloshin, D. and Wosk, J. (1981). Influence of artificial shock absorbers on human gait. *Clin Ortho Rel Res* 160:52–6.

48. Gordon, N.F., Kohl, H.W., Scott, C.B., Gibbons, L.W., and Blair, S.N. (1992). Reassessment of the guidelines for exercise testing. *Sports Med* 13:293–302.

49. Fransen, M., Crosbie, J., and Edmonds, J. (2000). Physical therapy is effective for patients with osteoarthritis of the knee: a randomized controlled clinical trial. *J Rheumatol* 28:156–64.

50. Stratman, J. and Minor, M. Oxygen consumption during daily tasks: Preliminary study of the effects of knee osteoarthritis (OA). *International Conference on Health Promotion and Disability Prevention in Rheumatic Disease: Evidence for Exercise and Physical Activity*, St. Louis, MO, 2002.

51. Coleman, E.A., Buchner, D.M., Cress, M.E., Chan, B.K.S., and deLateur, B.J.: The relationship of joint symptoms with exercise performance in older adults. *J Am Geriat Soc* 44:14–21, 1996.

9.11.2 Other physical therapies

Nicola Walsh and Michael Hurley

The aims of treatment for non-pharmacological interventions in OA are similar to those for pharmacological management—to control pain, reduce joint stiffness, limit joint damage, and improve function and health-related quality of life, with the least amount of adverse detrimental effects.

Several of the more commonly administered physical therapies aim to initiate pain relief, either via the 'pain gate' concept or the release of endogenous opioids.[1] However, pain relief in itself may not necessarily lead to spontaneous improvement in strength or function, as patients may still refrain from activities they believe will cause pain or further joint damage. Consequently, the interventions described below are rarely given individually, but are usually combined with advice, education, and exercise as a complete package of care.

The quality and quantity of research into physical therapy interventions is broad. Exercise, education, and self-management are well researched and are shown to be the most successful non-pharmacological interventions. The physical therapy modalities described in this chapter are generally less researched. Most of the studies that have been published are methodologically poor, therefore the benefits and efficacy of these modalities are equivocal.

Acupuncture

With mounting scepticism and disillusionment in pharmacological and traditional physical means of pain relief, the use of alternative or complementary therapies is becoming increasingly prevalent. Acupuncture is one of the most popular interventions. A recent survey of acupuncturists in the United Kingdom, reported that around 50 per cent of their applied treatments were for axial or peripheral OA.[2] Interest and acceptance are such that acupuncture is becoming increasingly utilized within healthcare systems.

It is claimed that the analgesic effect of acupuncture is obtained through neuro-humoral mechanisms—mechanical stimulation of high threshold A-δ fibres initiating production of opioid derivatives, including endorphins.[3] Other theories claim bio-electromagnetic factors acting via 'meridians' or 'energy channels' run through the body, and that 'normal' energy flow may be altered with pathological change.[4] It is suggested that acupuncture needling alters electrical activity around these 'energy channels' with subsequent homeostatic changes. All these theories are contentious and tenuous and have little research support.

Acupuncture is widely used for chronic pain conditions, including headaches, low back pain and a variety of visceral disorders. However, systematic reviews suggest the evidence regarding efficacy is inconclusive, with no probable increased benefits when compared to waiting list controls or sham treatments,[5] and studies with the most rigorous methodology demonstrate no improvement in pain following acupuncture.[5]

A recent systematic review of acupuncture in axial and peripheral OA reported very conflicting results, but found no evidence to suggest that acupuncture evoked a better response than sham needling (acupuncture at non-specific points).[6] A systematic review specifically examining acupuncture for knee OA also failed to conclusively support its use, although there was some evidence to suggest that acupuncture elicits more pain relief than sham needling.[7]

The inconclusive findings of acupuncture studies highlight the methodological problems inherent in this intervention. The popularity, widespread use, negligible side effects and possible benefits, however, suggest that acupuncture warrants further investigation. Consideration should be given to the propriety of sham needling as an appropriate control intervention, since non-specific needling may induce therapeutic effects.[6] Appropriate dose and extent of treatment also requires further investigation.

Electrotherapy

Electrotherapeutic modalities are widely used in physiotherapy departments to decrease pain associated with OA. Popular treatments include ultrasound, interferential therapy, electromagnetic energy, laser, and transcutaneous electrical nerve stimulation.[8] The proposed physiological effects of these modalities include deep heating, increased blood flow, reduced muscle-spasm, promotion of inflammatory response, and pain relief.[9] However, despite ubiquitous use of electrotherapy in the treatment of OA and other musculoskeletal disorders, there is a paucity of evidence demonstrating they are beneficial.

Ultrasound (US) is probably the most commonly used electrotherapy modality, especially for hip, knee, and vertebral OA. It is claimed that the therapeutic effects are derived from sound wave absorption, which alters cell function, vascularity, and collagen extensibility, resulting in a pro-inflammatory effect.[10] However, there are very few trials examining the efficacy of US for OA and those published, to date, are generally methodologically flawed, or demonstrate no beneficial effect.[11] A meta-analysis of US in other musculoskeletal conditions concluded that it has no role in the relief of pain.[11]

Transcutaneous electrical nerve stimulation (TENS) receives widespread use in many acute and chronic pain conditions. The main theoretical rationale for pain relief is that electrical stimulation of large diameter neural fibres 'closes the pain gate'. Alternatively, counter-irritant stimulation may facilitate release of endogenous opioid substances.[1] TENS has been subject to more rigorous testing of its efficacy than most other electrotherapy and non-pharmacological interventions, allowing a recent Cochrane Review regarding knee OA to conclude that TENS can effect pain relief when used at high frequency or strong burst mode for more than four weeks.[12] Although most studies are performed on knee OA, there is no reason to believe that these analgesic effects would not also be produced in other affected joints. Additionally, as the modality produces only occasional side effects of mild skin irritation at the electrode site, and can be applied by the patient, it is both a clinical and cost effective intervention.

Interferential therapy (IFT) is a means of delivering low-frequency stimulation, resulting from the interference between two medium frequency currents.[9] Physiological effects of this treatment modality differ according to the level of stimulation and type of nerves fibres that are stimulated. Stimulation of motor nerves leads to muscle contraction and as a result increases circulation in the area. This is of limited use in OA where active exercise is of proven benefit, so external stimulation is an unnecessary, time-consuming intervention. Sensory nerve stimulation is also theoretically possible, facilitating opioid production and 'closing the pain-gate'.[1] However, despite the theoretical basis of IFT, there is no evidence for its benefit in stimulating healing, and only limited evidence supporting analgesic effects.[9] Considering the similar therapeutic effects to TENS—a proven modality—it would seem prudent to use the latter for OA treatment.

Electromagnetic energy fields have been used in a variety of orthopaedic and musculoskeletal conditions with varied success. Pulsed or continuous delivery results in tissue heating and subsequent increased circulation of the treated area. Cell membrane potentials may also be effected although this theory remains contentious.[13] Studies utilizing this modality are relatively few. One pilot study suggested that pulsed treatment relieved pain in subjects with hand and knee OA,[14] but verification in larger, methodologically sound trials has not been forthcoming.

Low-level laser therapy (LLLT) has evolved as a therapeutic intervention for OA over the last decade. Therapeutic doses are used that are too low to induce thermal effects within the tissues and the physiological benefits are thought to derive from photochemical reactions at cellular level, which produce an anti-inflammatory effect.[15] Determining efficacy is difficult, as studies have used a wide diversity of laser class, dosage, and site of application. A recent review failed to conclude whether LLLT was beneficial in the treatment of OA due to this heterogeneity of application.[16] Further well-designed studies are necessary to determine whether with optimal treatment, prescription of this modality is a beneficial intervention for OA.

There are many laboratory-based studies that demonstrate the physiological effects of *electrotherapy* modalities that should theoretically produce therapeutic effects. Unfortunately, in general, clinical trials have failed to support these findings, noting little or no therapeutic benefits. It has been claimed that such an inability to replicate laboratory findings may be due to inappropriate timing, dosage, and modality when used clinically.[9] Until clinical trials replicate laboratory findings, electrotherapy cannot be considered an efficacious, cost-effective, evidence-based intervention for OA. However, it should be noted that patients generally like electrotherapy treatments and the considerable placebo effects could be used to enhance other aspects of a treatment package.

Balneotherapy

Balneotherapy (hydrotherapy or spa therapy) is one of the oldest recorded treatments for rheumatic conditions. It utilizes buoyancy—the assistant and resistant properties offered by water- in combination with the purported 'healing' effects of warm, mineral rich waters. The aim is to relieve muscle spasm, increase joint range of motion and muscle strength, with subsequent improvement in function.[17]

Spa Therapy is normally delivered on a 2–3 week residential basis at spa resorts (primarily in Europe or the Middle East) and consists of daily thermal bathing, exercise sessions, mudpacks, and jet massage.[18] Patients may also have their drugs and diet reviewed. Understandably, this is a popular and often effective treatment for patients. The period of respite care in a relaxing environment, with the patient removed from domestic and vocational pressures, has obvious physical and psychological benefits. This may account for the reported benefits of this type of intervention. The holistic nature of spa treatment makes it impossible to determine whether the regime is itself the beneficial aspect, or whether individual aspects have therapeutic effects.

Hydrotherapy consisting of exercise in a heated pool is also popular with patients, and has been reported to be effective in relieving pain, improving joint range of motion, and patient function and quality of life.[19,20] Due to demand and limited resources however, treatments are normally of short duration with little possibility of follow-up treatment.

Trials report that patients with a variety of rheumatic conditions benefit from balneotherapy, with reductions in pain and muscle spasm, and accompanying improvements in functional activities.[20,21] Unfortunately, these trials are generally methodologically flawed, and the dearth of high-quality studies in this area precludes confirmation of the benefits of balneotherapy. At present it is an expensive intervention based on poor scientific evidence.

Further, quality studies are necessary for comparing the benefits of hydrotherapy with spa therapy, as well as the specific interventions associated with holistic spa treatments. Until the effectiveness of balneotherapy is proven to exceed the benefits of land-based exercise and other treatment modalities, and long-term benefits of treatment are established, economic burdens are likely to exclude it from many healthcare agendas.[22]

Orthoses

The use of orthoses in the management of OA is becoming increasingly widespread as biomechanical implications of the disease become more apparent. Supports, braces, and corrective devices may assist in relieving pain and improving function of affected joints. Orthoses are used primarily for the weight-bearing joints' particularly the knees that are commonly affected by OA, for the relief of pain whilst walking and standing. Consequently most research regarding orthotic interventions focuses on such devices, however, orthoses may also be applied in hand/wrist OA and axial spondylosis.

They are used to attenuate vertical forces applied to the skeleton at heel-strike; realign unstable or structurally deficient joints with amelioration or restoration of normal force distribution; improve proprioception; and improve stability and patient perception of instability.[23,24]

The knee is the joint most readily treated by supportive sleeves, correction braces, and lateral heel wedges. *Lateral heel wedging* can help decrease pain in medial compartment OA,[25] presumably by correcting and improving varus deformity by encouraging a valgus position, thus reducing the pressure on the medial aspect of the joint line. However, long-term benefits of these devices have yet to be established.

Neoprene sleeves and valgus correction braces are also used in knee OA (Fig. 9.13). Compliance with these devices is a problem, however, as they are bulky and awkward for elderly patients to apply. These devices purportedly reduce knee adduction moments that have been implicated in the development and progression of OA,[23] although other studies suggest that neoprene fails to alter adduction alignment.[27] Neoprene sleeves are more likely to have an effect on joint proprioception than knee alignment. The fabric structure is not strong enough to reposition the joint, but the increased pressure and cutaneous stimulation may possibly enhance patient joint position sense.[27] A study comparing neoprene sleeves and valgus bracing used in conjunction with medical therapy and medical therapy alone, noted an increase in function and decrease in pain for the orthotic intervention group,[26] also that valgus braces were probably more effective.

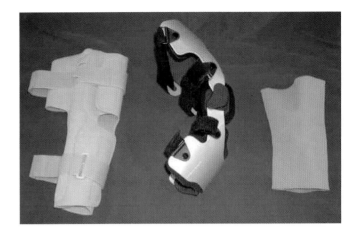

Fig. 9.13 Braces and supports for knee osteoarthritis.

The hip joint does not lend itself readily to orthotic intervention, although heel lifts have been used with modest effects on pain relief.[28] Orthotic intervention for low back pain remains questionable since clinical trials are generally of poor quality. There is limited evidence to suggest that lumbar supports are more beneficial than no treatment, but there is considerable uncertainty regarding their efficacy compared to other treatments for low back pain.[29]

Wrist and hand supports are also used to improve function in activities of daily living, by maintaining an appropriate, pain free position. Although these are readily supplied, no evaluation of their efficacy is available.

Further controlled studies are necessary to conclude whether these devices are efficacious interventions. Research particularly needs to take into account long-term patient compliance. Previous work suggests that compliance even with small devices is poor in the longer-term, so it is likely that patients will discard more cumbersome appliances.

Walking aids

Sticks and crutches are supplied to reduce the stress applied to weight-bearing joints and to improve patient stability during ambulation. Unfortunately, walking aids are not always popular with patients, who perceive them as being for the elderly and infirm. They can also be impractical and cumbersome when performing other functional activities. Recent years have seen improvements in the design of walking aids, with greater attention to the ergonomic requirements of the devices. Contemporary aids are lighter, and protect wrist and hand joints more effectively through moulded handgrips (Fig. 9.14).

Historically, patients have been encouraged to use walking aids on the contralateral side to the problematic joint, thus encouraging improved weight distribution, and an energy efficient gait pattern.[30] A recent study confirmed this is an appropriate method for patients with hip OA, producing a mechanically advantageous long lever arm, which reduces the deleterious effects of body weight on the affected hip. For knee patients walking aids function as a vertical load-sharing implement and cannot effect forces in the frontal plane. Therefore patients may use a walking aid in either hand with equal effect, although due to movement of the centre of gravity use in the contralateral hand may be more energy efficient especially for older patients.[30] However, the benefits of walking aids on patient function have received little investigation, so it is not possible to determine clinical effectiveness.[31]

Thermotherapy

Superficial heat or cold have been used for many years for the relief of pain in a variety of musculo-skeletal disorders. Heat applied through hot water

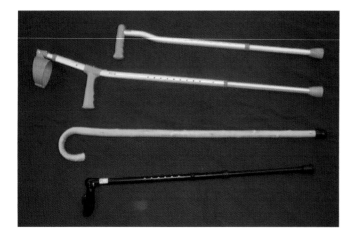

Fig. 9.14 A selection of walking aids. The appropriate height for the handle of a walking aid is determined by measuring the distance from the ulnar styloid to the ground, while standing.

bottles or various heated packs, relieves pain presumably due to stimulation of afferent nerve fibres that 'close the pain gate', improved local circulation, increased collagen extensibility, reduced muscle spasm, and improved range of motion.[32] Similarly, cold therapy applied through ice packs or baths may relieve pain via the 'pain-gate' mechanism, reduced peripheral nerve excitability, and reduction in joint effusions and oedema.[32]

There are few studies of thermotherapy in OA, but a recent review of thermotherapy in rheumatoid arthritis patients noted that it was safe, easily administered, and preferred by patients to no treatment at all.[33] Although there is a lack of direct evidence supporting thermotherapy for OA, it appears to be a simple, cost-effective, means of assisting pain control, and therefore is an appropriate tool in patient self-management regimes.

Mobilization and manipulation

Physiotherapists, osteopaths and chiropractors, to reduce joint pain and stiffness, and increase range of motion, use these manual techniques. *Manipulation* consists of high velocity thrusting movements and is popular with patients who often gain short-term benefit.[34,35] However, the population suitable for this treatment is relatively small, and only trained practitioners should perform manipulations. Ill-considered manipulation, particularly in the cervical area, can be dangerous and potentially fatal.[34]

Mobilizations generally consist of small oscillatory accessory joint movements, administered to either the peripheral or axial skeleton. Similar to manipulations, their aim is to relieve pain and increase range of motion. There has been very little evaluation of these techniques, but the studies that have been performed suggest minimal efficacy in relieving pain and in improving range of movement and function.[34]

Manual therapies tend to require a course of treatment, so are generally time consuming. Despite this and the lack of evidence, it is still commonly used in outpatient departments in conjunction with other modalities such as electrotherapy and exercise. Further work is necessary to determine the efficacy of these interventions especially at different stages of disease progression, as there is a possibility that benefits will differ accordingly.[36]

T'ai Chi

T'ai Chi is an ancient Chinese form of exercise, integrating controlled movements with relaxation. The regime is thought to maintain flexibility and mobility, enhance stability, and improve an individual's sense of well-being.[37] A recent pilot study of T'ai Chi in OA noted improvements in functional mobility, self-efficacy, and quality of life after a 12-week course.[38]

Despite some methodological problems associated with this study, and a paucity of supporting literature, T'ai Chi would appear to be an appropriate intervention for OA patients. The combination of exercise (which is known to be effective) with stress relief and relaxation (also considered an appropriate means of symptom control) encourages a holistic approach to patient management.

Contemporary treatment programmes need to integrate physical activity with an understanding of the psychological aspects of OA if patients are going to benefit from, and adhere to changes in lifestyle in the longer-term.

Massage

Patients frequently report that rubbing or massaging a joint temporarily relieves pain, probably because the mechanical stimulus excites large diameter nerve fibres closing the pain gate.[1] The additional application of topical agents, either pharmacological or homeopathic, may enhance the benefits of massage.

There are no trials comparing the effects of massage with sham treatments in OA. However, one back pain study reported that massage was no better than manipulation, but was inferior to TENS, in relieving pain.[39] The innate reaction to rub a painful joint and the reported subjective benefits mean that massage is likely to be used by patients and encouraged by practitioners.

Patellar taping

Patellar taping in conjunction with localized exercise has been used for the treatment of anterior knee pain with reported analgesic effects.[40,41] Pain is thought to arise from abnormal patella alignment within the trochlea groove, with subsequent alterations in activation of the vastus medialis obliquus (VMO), and vastus lateralis muscles. Taping the patello-femoral joint is considered to encourage realignment of the patella through inhibition of the vastus lateralis and to unload painful structures, whilst promoting localized exercise to maintain normal joint mechanics in the long-term.[42] The proposed rationale for pain relief is that taping holds the patella in a correctly aligned position, allowing improved timing and magnitude of vastii contraction.[43] However, the ability of the external cutaneous tape to maintain this alignment with repeated contraction is questionable.[44] An alternative explanation is that taping enhances motor activation through cutaneous stimulation and proprioceptive feedback, although this mechanism has been refuted since placebo taping fails to effect a motor response.[45]

One pilot study found that short-term taping did decrease pain in patients with patello-femoral OA.[46] However, repetition on a larger scale failed to support these initial findings.[47] The ambiguous evidence in support of taping, in addition to the proven pain relieving effects of active exercise alone, suggests that tape is of limited benefit in the management of OA.

Summary

Non-pharmacological interventions that relieve pain and improve function are considered essential in the management of OA. Exercise and self-management programmes provide the cornerstone to this approach as they are proven, efficacious modalities. Unfortunately, the variety of physical interventions used to support these approaches is either grossly under-researched or is methodologically flawed, limiting the inferences that can be drawn from published work. There is some evidence that certain modalities are efficacious (e.g. TENS, thermotherapy). Other modalities are widely used despite inconclusive research findings (e.g. US, acupuncture, manual therapy). Further, well-designed clinical trials are necessary to establish the suitability of these interventions.

Establishing clinical effectiveness of non-pharmacological modalities is complex, and careful consideration of methodology is essential if research findings are to be replicated in clinical practice. The interventions described in this chapter are rarely delivered in isolation, but are integrated with other pharmacological and non-pharmacological approaches that collectively influence the patient's pain and function. Future research agendas should consider the effects of complex 'packages of healthcare', the typical manner in which they are delivered, and the patients they are administered to. This approach will increase the likelihood of achieving clinical and cost effectiveness and improve patient satisfaction and outcome.

Key points

1. There is reasonable evidence that TENS, thermotherapy and orthoses provide short-term pain relief in the treatment of OA, but little evidence supporting the efficacy of many widely used physical therapy modalities.

2. The ubiquitous use of these modalities in the treatment of this prevalent condition has significant, though largely unevaluated cost consequences.

3. Many physical therapy treatments are popular with patients, and have considerable placebo effects, which may be utilized by therapists when delivering a package of care.

4. These modalities require evaluation of their efficacy, clinical, and cost effectiveness.

5. Traditional research methodologies may be too restrictive in evaluating the benefits of these treatments that are delivered as a complex 'package of healthcare'.

Further reading

Campbell, M., Fitzpatrick, R., Haines, *et al.* (2000). Framework for design and evaluation of complex interventions to improve health. *Br Medic J* **321**:694–6.

Hurley, M. and Walsh, N. (2001). Physical, functional and other non-pharmacological interventions for Osteoarthritis. *Baillieres Clin Rheumatol* **15**(4):569–81.

References

(An asterisk denotes recommended reading.)

1. Melzack, R. and Wall, P. (1965). Pain mechanisms: a new theory. *Science* **150**:971–9.

2. Wadlow, G. and Peringer, E. (1996). Retrospective survey of patients of practitioners of traditional Chinese acupuncture in the UK. *Complementary Therap Medic* **4**:1–7.

3. Sims, J. (1997). The mechanism of acupuncture analgesia: a review. *Complementary Therap Medic* **5**:102–11.

4. Darras, J-C., de Vernejoul, P., and Albarede, P. (1992). Nuclear medicine and acupuncture: a study of the migration of radioactive tracers after injection at acupoints. *Am J Acupuncture* **20**:245–55.

5. Ezzo, J., Berman, B., Hadhazy, V., Jadad, A., Lao, L., and Singh, B. (2000). Is acupuncture effective for the treatment of chronic pain? A systematic review. *Pain* **86**:217–25.

6. *Ernst, E. (1997). Acupuncture as a symptomatic treatment of osteoarthritis: a systematic review. *Scand J Rheumatol* **26**:444–7.

   This paper highlights the contradictory evidence for acupuncture in pain relief. Methodological flaws are outlined, and the necessity for future research to clarify the benefits of this modality are discussed.

7. Ezzo, J., Hadhazy, V., Birch, S., Lao, L., Kaplan, G., Hochberg, M., and Berman, B. (2001). Acupuncture for Osteoarthritis of the Knee. *Arthritis Rheum* **44**:819–25.

8. Pope, G. (1995). A survey of the electrotherapeutic modalities: ownership and use in the NHS in England. *Physiotherapy* **81**:82–91.

9. Watson, T. (2000). The role of electrotherapy in contemporary physiotherapy practice. *Manual Therapy* **5**:132–41.

10. Maxwell, L. (1992). Therapeutic ultrasound; its effects on the cellular and molecular mechanisms of inflammation and repair. *Physiotherapy* **78**:921–6.

11. van der Windt, D., van der Heijden, G., van der Berg, S., ter Riet, G., de Winter, A., and Bouter, L. (1999). Ultrasound therapy for musculoskeletal disorders: a systematic review. *Pain* **81**:257–71.

12. *Osiri, M., Welch, V., Brosseau, L., *et al.* (2001). Transcutaneous electrical nerve stimulation for knee osteoarthritis (A Cochrane Review). *Cochrane Library* **2**.

    A comprehensive systematic review demonstrating efficacy of high rate/short burst TENS in relieving pain and stiffness. Further methodologically sound research is required to conclude the benefits of this treatment.

13. Goodman, R. and Henderson, A. (1991). Transcription and translation in cells exposed to extremely low frequency electromagnetic fields. *Bioelectrochem Bioenergetics* **25**:335–55.

14. Trock, D., Bollet, A., Dyer, R., Fielding, L., Miner, W., and Markoll, R. (1993). A double blind trial of the clinical effects of pulsed electromagnetic fields in osteoarthritis. *J Rheumatol* **20**:456–60.

15. Baxter, G. (1996). Low intensity laser therapy. In S. Kitchen and S. Bazin (eds), *Clayton's Electrotherapy* (10th ed.). London: WB Saunders, pp. 154–78.

16. Brosseau, L., Welch, V., Wells, G., *et al.* (2001). Low level laser therapy (Class I, II and III) for treating Osteoarthritis (A Cochrane Review). *The Cochrane Library* **2**.

17. McNeal, R. (1990). Aquatic therapy for patients with rheumatic disease. *Rheum Dis Clin North Am* **16**:915–29.

18. Romain, F. (2000). Magnitude and duration of the effects of two spa therapy courses on knee and hip osteoarthritis: an open prospective study in 51 consecutive patients. *Joint Bone Spine* **67**:296–304.

19. Hall, J., Skevington, S., Maddsion, P., Chapman, K. (1996). A randomised and controlled trial of hydrotherapy in rheumatoid arthritis. *Arthritis Care Res* **9**:206–15.

20. Verhagen, A., de Vet, H., de Bie, R., Kessels, A., Boers, M., and Knipschild, P. (1997). Taking baths: The efficacy of balneotherapy in patients with arthritis. A systematic review. *J Rheumatol* **24**:1964–71.

21. *Verhagen, A., de Vet, H., de Bie, R., Kessels, A., Boers, M., and Knipschild, P. (2001). Balneotherapy for rheumatoid arthritis and osteoarthritis (A Cochrane Review). *The Cochrane Library* **3**.

    A systematic review reporting patient-perceived benefits of treatment. However, trials were methodologically flawed, and heterogeneity of protocol prevents evidence-based conclusions of efficacy to be established to date.

22. Patrick, D., Ramsey, S., Spencer, A., Kinne, S., Belza, B., and Topolski, T. (2001). Economic evaluation of aquatic exercise for persons with osteoarthritis. *Medic Care* **39**:413–24.

23. Sharma, L., Song, J., Felson, D., Cahue, S., Shamiyeh, E., and Dunlop, D. (2001). The role of knee alignment in disease progression and functional decline in knee osteoarthritis. *JAMA* **286**:188–95.

24. Draper, E., Cable, J., Sanchez-Ballester, J., Hunt, N., Robinson, J., and Strachan, R. (2000). Improvement in function after valgus bracing of the knee. An analysis of gait symmetry. *J Bone Joint Surg* **82**(B):1001–5.

25. Crenshaw, S., Pollo, F., and Calton, E. (2000). Effects of Lateral-Wedged Insoles on Kinetics at the Knee. *Clin Orthop Rel Res* **375**:185–92.

26. Kirkley, A., Webster-Bogaert, S., Litchfield, R., *et al.* (1999). The effect of bracing on varus gonarthrosis. *J Bone Joint Surg* **81**(A):539–48.

27. Hewett, T., Noyes, F., Barber-Westin, S., and Heckmen, T. (1998). Decrease in knee joint pain and increase in function in patients with medial compartment arthrosis: a prospective analysis of valgus bracing. *Orthopaedics* **21**:131–8.

28. Oshawa, S. and Veno, R. (1997). Heel lifting as a conservative therapy for osteoarthritis of the hip: based on the rationale of Pauwels' intertrochanteric osteotomy. *Prosthetics Orthotics Int* **21**:153–8.

29. van Tulder, M., Jelleman, P., van Poppel, M., Nachemson, A., and Bouter, L. (2001). Lumbar supports for prevention and treatment of back pain (A Cochrane Review). *The Cochrane Library* **1**.

30. Mendelson, S., Milgron, C., Finestone, A., *et al.* (1998). Effect of cane use on tibial strain and strain rates. *Am J Phys Medic Rehab* **11**:333–8.

31. Rogers, J.C. and Holm, M.B. (1992). Assistive technology device use in patients with rheumatic diseases: a literature review. *Am J Occupational Therapy* 46:120–7.

32. Collins, K. (1996). Thermal Effects. In S. Kitchen and S. Bazin (eds), *Clayton's Electrotherapy*, (10th ed.). London: WB Saunders, pp. 93–109.

33. *Welch, V., Brosseau, L., Shea, B., McGowan, J., Wells, G., and Tugwell, P. (2001). Thermotherapy for treating rheumatoid Arthritis (A Cochrane Review). *The Cochrane Library* 2.
     A systematic review noting patient preference for thermotherapy, but no evidence to suggest disease modifying effects. No harmful effects were reported.

34. Hurwitz, E., Aker, P., Adams, A., Meeker, W., and Shakelle, P. (1996). Manipulation and mobilisation of the cervical spine. A systematic review of the literature. *Spine* 21:1746–60.

35. Meade, T., Dyer, S., Browne, W., Townsend, J., and Frank, A. (1990). Low back pain of mechanical origin: randomised comparison of chiropractic and hospital outpatient treatment. *Br Med J* 300:1431–7.

36. Maitland, G. (1991). *Peripheral Manipulation* (2nd ed.). Oxford: Butterworth-Heinemann, Oxford.

37. Da-hong, Z. (1992). Preventive geriatrics: An overview from traditional Chinese medicine. *Am J Chinese Medic* 10:32–9.

38. Hartman, C., Manos, T., Winter, C., Hartman, D., Li, B., and Smith, J. (2000). Effects of T'ai Chi Training on Function and Quality of Life Indicators in Older Adults with Osteoarthritis. *J Am Geriat Soc* 48:1553–9.

39. Furlan, A., Brosseau, L., Welch, V., and Wong, J. (2000). Massage for low back pain (A Cochrane Review). *The Cochrane Library* 4.

40. Herrington, L. and Payton, C. (1997). Effects of corrective taping of the patella on patients with patellofemoral pain. *Physiotherapy* 83:566–72.

41. Handfield, T. and Kramer, J. (2000). Effect of McConnell taping on perceived pain and knee extensor torques during isokinetic exercise performed by patients with patellofemoral pain syndrome. *Physiotherapy Canada* 50:39–44.

42. Crossley, K., Cowan, S., Bennell, K., and McConnell, J. (2000). Patellar taping: is clinical success supported by scientific evidence? *Manual Therapy* 5:142–50.

43. McConnell, J. (1996). Management of patellofemoral problems. *Manual Therapy* 1:60–6.

44. Cerny, K. (1995). Vastus medialis oblique/vastus lateralis muscle activity ratios for selected exercises in persons with and without patellofemoral pain syndrome. *Physical Therapy* 75:672–83.

45. Ernst, G., Kawaguchi, J., and Saliba, E. (1999). Effect of patellar taping on knee kinetics of patients with patellofemoral pain syndrome. *J Orthop Sports Phys Ther* 29:661–7.

46. Cushnaghan, J., McCarthy, C., and Dieppe, P. (1994). Taping the patellar medially; a new treatment for osteoarthritis of the knee joint? *Br Med J* 308:753–5.

47. Quilty, B., Tucker, M., and Dieppe, P. (1998). Patello-femoral joint disease disability, quadriceps Dysfunction and response to physiotherapy. NHS national Research and Development Programme, Physical and Complex Disabilities, Report No. PCD/A1/123.

9.12 Occupational therapy for the patient with osteoarthritis

Jeanne L. Melvin

Occupational therapists are concerned with what occupies a person's time and hands and with how to help the patient regain functional independence with those activities. This concern with function has led many occupational therapists to specialize in treating the hand and upper extremity. Because painful OA of the hand joints is such a common problem, this chapter will focus on the conservative management of hand OA and on how the occupational therapist can help patients with OA—particularly of the hand joints, but also of other joints—improve their functional ability.

The occupational therapist must assess functional performance in the person with OA in order to teach the patient how to manage their disease by eliminating factors that may exacerbate the disease; by reducing pain, stiffness, and inflammation; maintaining range of motion (ROM); maintaining or increasing muscle strength; restoring muscle balance; reducing stress on the involved joints, and maintaining or increasing functional independence, including participation in avocational activities (Table 9.24).

These goals are achieved through education of the patient in principles of joint protection, training in ergonomics and education in body mechanics and posture; education in energy conservation and management of fatigue; therapeutic exercise; splinting; use of thermal modalities; training in behavioral management of pain and symptoms; training in alternative methods for accomplishing a task (adaptive methods), and use of assistive devices, for example, a dressing stick or enlarged handles[1,2] (Table 9.25). Assessment of the home and the work site by the therapist may be required. In addition, in some countries, occupational therapists may be involved in the fabrication of foot orthotics and shoe adaptations.

Hand involvement in OA

Previously, hand OA was typically described as affecting the interphalangeal joints (IPJs) and trapeziometacarpal joint (TMJ) of the thumb, that is, the first carpometacarpal joint (CMCJ)[3] (Fig. 9.15). (In the remainder of this chapter the CMCJ of the thumb will be referred to as the TMJ, because this terminology is gaining increased usage and, in the case of the thumb base, is more specific. The term, CMCJ, will be used to refer only to the CMCJs of the other digits.) Although these are the joints that tend to be the most symptomatic in people with hand OA, osteophytes can occur also at the metacarpophalangeal joints (MCPJs), where they may contribute to triggering of flexor tendons, and OA of the carpal joints can limit motion and cause pain.[4,5] The pattern of OA joint involvement in women is similar to that in men, but women are more likely than men to have more severe involvement of the hand joints and more likely to have generalized OA.[6–8]

In a multidisciplinary study in which occupational therapists assessed 77 patients who had been referred because of problems with hand OA,[5] 39 per cent of the patients had complaints related to tendon involvement, including crepitus (32 per cent), triggering (12 per cent), and locking (4 per cent). Wrist ROM was limited in all planes: 60 per cent of the 77 patients were limited in wrist flexion, 44 in extension, 49 in ulnar deviation, and 32 in radial deviation.

People with hand OA may be asymptomatic or may experience the following problems: aching in the joints with exposure to cold or changes in weather (considered to be a response to changes in barometric pressure); joint pain, particularly with use; joint swelling due to synovitis; secondary muscle aching, spasm; muscle weakness, due to disuse or reflex inhibition of muscle contraction; joint tenderness; stiffness with static positioning ('gelling'); limited joint mobility; joint and/or tendon crepitus; and tendon triggering.[7–9] The most likely causes of joint stiffness include low-grade inflammation, effusion, synovial thickening, muscle shortening, and fibromyalgia.[1]

Pain associated with hand OA

Articular cartilage degeneration and osteophytosis may cause mild stiffness or decreased ROM in patients with OA, but are generally painless. Even in the absence of swelling, redness, or warmth, hand pain may be associated

Table 9.24 Therapeutic goals in occupational therapy for patients with OA

- Elimination of aggravating factors
- Reduction of pain, stiffness, and inflammation
- Maintenance or improvement, of range of motion (ROM)
- Maintenance or improvement, of muscle strength
- Restoration of muscle balance
- Reduction of stress on the involved joints
- Maintenance or improvement in functional independence, including participation in avocational activities

Table 9.25 Approaches used to achieve the goals of occupational therapy in patients with OA

- Education of the patient in principles of joint protection
- Improvement, ergonomics, through education in body mechanics and posture
- Education in energy conservation and management of fatigue
- Therapeutic exercise for upper extremities
- Splinting
- Use of thermal modalities
- Training in alternative methods for accomplishing a task (adaptive methods)
- Behavioral management of pain and symptoms
- Use of assistive devices, for example, a dressing stick or enlarged handles

with low-grade inflammation. Even mild joint effusions can cause disability.[10] Pain can also result from impingement or stretching of the joint capsule over a sharp osteophyte. In the spine and lower extremities, weight bearing on thin articular cartilage can transmit pressure to sensory nerves in subchondral bone; in the hand joints, this may be of minimal importance. However, lateral pinch generates compression forces on the TMJ that are 12 times greater than those at the tip of the thumb and index finger.[11] In a TMJ in which the articular cartilage has been lost, this stress can increase pressures in the subchondral bone. Other factors that have been identified as sources of joint pain in OA, especially in weight-bearing joints, include periostitis at sites of bony remodeling, periarticular muscle spasm, and bone angina resulting from decreased blood flow and elevated intraosseous pressure.[12] In many patients, OA pain is amplified by fibromyalgia, depression, anxiety, or poor sleep.[8,13] When that is the case, management of the OA pain can be facilitated by reducing the intensity of the amplifier.[14,15]

Anticipation of hand pain during functional activities can result in muscle guarding that extends up the entire extremity into the neck. It is important to address this problem because women with inflammatory digital OA tend to have concomitant OA of the cervical spine. About one-third of the patients referred to this author for splinting for thumb OA have cervical muscle tension or pain that began after the development of their hand pain and appears to be related to muscle guarding of the limb to protect the thumb. In addition to protective hand splints, such patients need education in conscious measures to relax the extremity during functional activities. (See discussion below on patient education.)

Generalized ligamentous laxity, with consequent joint hypermobility, albeit within the range of normal, is found in a substantial proportion of normal people. Recent studies suggest that hypermobility, especially in the TMJ, may result in capsular and ligamentous strain that is a source of joint pain, promotes uneven cartilage wear, and may ultimately be a cause of OA.[16]

Specific joint and tendon involvement

Several types of deformity may result from hand OA[7–9,17,18]

- bony enlargement of the joint (Fig. 9.16)
- angulation deformity of the IPJ, related to asymmetric cartilage degeneration or asymmetric osteophytosis (Fig. 9.16)
- mallet finger deformity, resulting from attrition of the distal attachment of the extensor communis tendon over a dorsal osteophyte (Fig. 9.17)

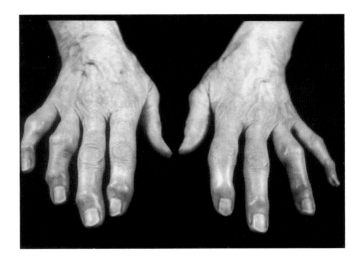

Fig. 9.16 Classic primary OA, with bony enlargement of the DIPJs (Heberden's nodes) and PIPJs (Bouchard's nodes). Acute inflammation of the DIPJs and angulation deformity of the right middle and ring finger DIPJs are apparent.

Source: Reprinted from the Clinical Slide Collection on the Rheumatic Diseases, © 1991. Used with the permission of the American College of Rheumatology.

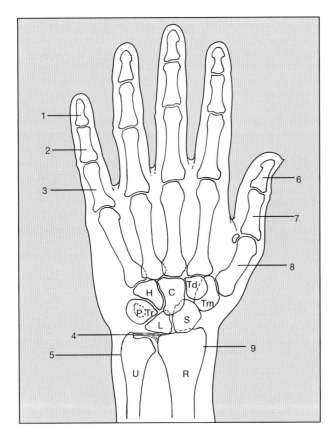

Fig. 9.15 Bones of the hand and wrist: (1) distal phalanx; (2) middle phalanx; (3) proximal phalanx; (4) triangular fibrocartilage; (5) ulnar styloid; (6) distal phalanx of thumb; (7) proximal phalanx of the thumb; (8) metacarpal; (9) radial styloid; (H) hamate; (C) capitate; (Td) trapezoid; (Tm) trapezium; (S) scaphoid (also called navicular); (L) lunate; (Tr) triquetrum; (P) pisiform; (U) ulna; (R) radius.

Source: Taken from Ref. 3. The trapeziometacarpal joint (TMJ) is also commonly referred to as the 1st carpometacarpal joint (CMC).

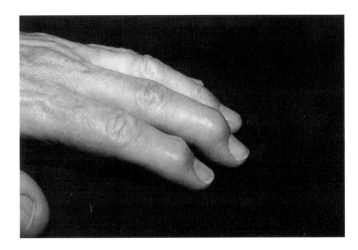

Fig. 9.17 Mallet finger deformity. The middle finger DIPJ is fixed in flexion. At this stage it may be difficult to tell if the extensor tendon is ruptured or the deformity is due to an osteophyte.

- a classic thumb deformity consisting of TMJ adduction, MCPJ hyperextension (or lateral deviation), and IPJ (Fig. 9.18) flexion
- enlargement and subluxation of the TMJ, producing characteristic 'squaring' of the joint (Fig. 9.19)
- loss of flexion of the involved digit due to volar osteophytosis, or loss of extension due to dorsal osteophytosis.

Generally, if these deformities are painless, no treatment is indicated. However, education in adaptive methods and provision of assistive devices to reduce disability may be helpful for patients with loss of joint motion (Table 9.24).

Distal and proximal interphalangeal joints

In the hand, osteophytes at the distal interphalangeal joints (DIPJs) are named in honor of a famous Welsh physician and are referred to as Heberden's nodes; at the proximal interphalangeal joints (PIPJs), they are named after a famous French physician and referred to as Bouchard's nodes (Fig. 9.16). Osteophytes at these joints are diagnostic of OA. The result is a lumpy, unevenly deformed joint. Mucoid cysts are more common in the DIPJs than in the PIPJs, and often evolve into osteophytes.[19] The considerable magnitude of the shear forces acting on these joints contributes to the predominance of DIPJ involvement.[20,21]

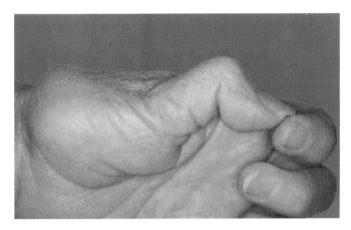

Fig. 9.18 Classic thumb deformity, with adduction of the TMJ, hyperextension of the MCPJ and flexion of the IPJ.

Source: The figure was provided by James Strickland, MD.

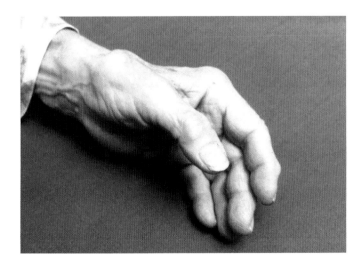

Fig. 9.19 OA of the TMJ, resulting in classical 'squaring' of the joint.

Source: The figure was provided by Kenneth Brandt, MD.

Thumb joints

OA can affect all of the joints of the thumb, but is most common in the TMJ.[7,17,20] Symptoms include pain or aching around the base of the thumb that may radiate down the digit or up the forearm and is usually most intense during pinch. OA of the TMJ may mimic de Quervain's tenosynovitis (see section below on evaluation). Tenderness over the TMJ and stiffness of the TMJ upon awakening from sleep or after a period of inactivity are common. If inflammation is severe, swelling, warmth, and redness may be present. Inflammation of the TMJ often occurs from overuse or repetitive strain and may be apparent in the absence of radiographic evidence of OA. With progression of the disease, the TMJ subluxes and contracture of the thumb adductor muscles occurs, reducing the ability to press the palm completely flat on a table or to fully spread the thumb web space. This creates difficulty in grasping large objects and encourages hyperextension or lateral deviation of the MCPJ and flexion of the IPJ (Fig. 9.18).

The articular surfaces of the TMJ are incongruous and are stabilized by the surrounding ligaments and the intracapsular palmar beak ligament (sometimes referred to as the anterior or volar oblique ligament), which originates from the trapezium and attaches to the articular margin of the metacarpal beak (or prominence) (Fig. 9.20). The beak ligament is a major static stabilizer of the TMJ, especially in the presence of joint hypermobility, and its attrition from functional strain parallels the progressive degeneration of the palmar articular surface of the TMJ. The beak ligament has been found to be nonfunctional in end-stage OA of the TMJ.[22,23]

Bony hypertrophy around the margins of the TMJ contributes to subluxation, which is evidenced by a characteristic squared appearance[23] (Fig. 9.19). A diagnosis of TMJ OA may be made on the basis of the squared appearance, presence of a positive grind test (see section below on evaluation) or the radiograph findings. Repetitive pinch, grasp, and twisting activities, and nonprehensile application of force with the heel of the hand,

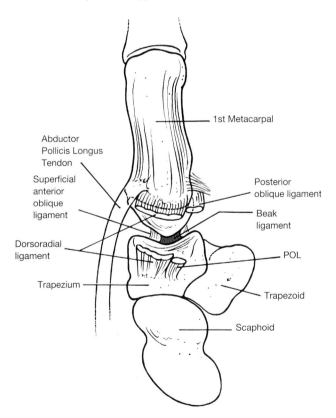

Fig. 9.20 The beak ligament of the TMJ (also called the anterior or volar oblique ligament), shown in red, is an important stabilizer of the TMJ. POL = posterior oblique ligament.

Source: The figure was provided by James Strickland, MD.

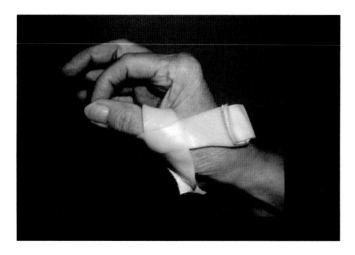

Fig. 9.21 Immobilization splint, designed by the author,[17] to prevent flexion, extension, and deviation of the MCPJ of the thumb. This splint is very effective in treating synovitis and instability of the 1st MCPJ. IPJ inflammation can be aggravated by this splint, however, and is a contraindication to the use of this splint.

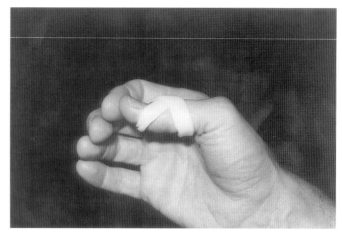

Fig. 9.22 A figure-8 splint for instability or pain in the thumb IPJ. Use of this splint will increase flexion forces on the MCPJ.

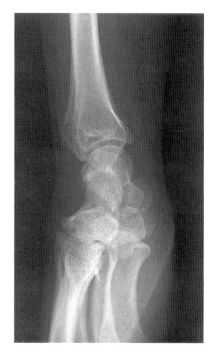

Fig. 9.23 The carpe bossu (carpal boss). Note the osteophytosis on the dorsum of the capitate and base of the metacarpal bone. This may be apparent clinically as bony swelling at this site.

Source: The figure was provided by Kenneth Buckwalter, MD.

for example, stapling papers or manually squeezing oranges aggravates symptoms of TMJ arthritis.

Pain and inflammation in the TMJ due to use can occur in adults at any age, but OA of this joint tends to occur in women over 40 years of age who have joint laxity and, often, a shallow dorsal radial facet on the trapezium.[16,27] A painful thumb can limit activities: a severely painful thumb can reduce hand function by nearly 50 per cent.

OA can also affect any of the other three trapezial joints (pantrapezial or scaphoid-trapezium-trapezoid (STT) arthritis) (Fig. 9.15). Clinically, this presents as pain over the affected joint(s) during wrist motion. Often, point tenderness, decreased grip and pinch strength, and loss of wrist motion are apparent.[24] Pantrapezial arthritis may occur with the TMJ as the only symptomatic joint. In a review of 200 hand radiographs of patients referred for surgery for OA of the TMJ, Swanson *et al.*[25] found OA in 100 per cent of the TMJs, 86 per cent of the trapezial-2nd MCPJ, 35 per cent of the trapezial-trapezoid joints, and 45 per cent of the scaphotrapezial joints (STJ). In another study of elderly female patients, the presence of severe OA of the STJ identified those with calcium pyrophosphate crystal deposition disease (CPPD) with a sensitivity of 83 per cent and specificity of 73 per cent, even when other signs of CPPD in the hand were absent.[26]

Inflammation of the small sesamoid bones (sesamoiditis) over the volar aspect of the thumb MCPJ is common in older women with OA and is often triggered by gripping a hard surface for a prolonged period. It is believed that sesamoiditis results from traumatic microtears in the perisesamoid tendon and/or sesamoid-metacarpal articulation.[28] Acute point tenderness is usually present over the sesamoid bones on the volar aspect of the thumb MCPJ; signs of tenosynovitis of the flexor pollicis longus, with which sesamoiditis may be confused, are usually absent. Splinting the thumb MCPJ (Fig. 9.21) for 2–3 weeks, and application of cold four times a day, is usually very effective in resolving the symptoms.

The thumb IPJ can become enlarged and stiff in a flexed position, or enlarged and unstable. Instability is disabling, making surgical arthrodesis the treatment of choice. For those who are not surgical candidates, a figure-8 splint can provide functional stability (Fig. 9.22). As with triggering of the IPJs of the other digits, thumb IPJ triggering is treated with a splint to decrease IP flexion, which reduces irritation and results in decrease in thickening of the flexor tendon sheath or in the size of the nodule catching on the transverse annular ligament on the volar aspect of the sheath. Triggering of the thumb IPJ is common, often occurs in conjunction with sesamoiditis, and necessitates a MCPJ splint that is elongated to block IPJ flexion.

Wrist and carpometacarpal joints

OA of the wrist (radiocarpal joint) is generally secondary to other diseases, for example, intercarpal instability, Kienböck's disease (osteonecrosis of the lunate), scaphoid nonunion, malunited fractures or CPPD disease. Scapholunate instability, with collapse or rotary subluxation of the scaphoid, is a precursor of OA.[29] Untreated Kienböck's disease progresses to pancarpal arthritis.[30]

OA of the second or third CMCJ results in osteophytosis of the involved joint at the dorsal base of the second or third metacarpal and the distal dorsal lip of the trapezoid or capitate, producing a firm prominence, the carpe bossu (carpal boss), proximal to the insertion of the radial wrist extensors[20,31] (Fig. 9.23). Patients report the gradual development of a firm, tender mass. The overlying wrist extensor tendons can become

Table 9.26 Assessment of the OA hand

- pain (at rest, during ROM, and during function)
- stiffness
- tenderness during palpation
- swelling and inflammation
- tendon pain, triggering, crepitus, and lag
- strength testing
- ROM active, passive, and lag
- grind test
- Finkelstein test
- function and disability
- current self-management strategies

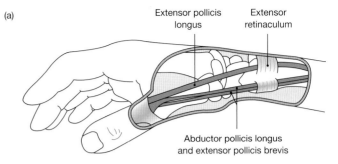

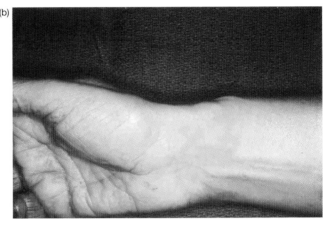

Fig. 9.24 The tenosynovitis of de Quervain. (a) Diagram of underlying anatomy. Note that the tendon sheaths of the extensor pollicis brevis and abductor pollicis longus run distal to the styloid process of the radius and the TMJ. (b) Note the swelling immediately proximal to the radial styloid, reflecting inflammation of the sheaths of the above tendons.

Source: (a) Reproduced with permission from Shipley, M. 1985. *Pocket Picture Guides to Clinical Medicine. Rheumatic Diseases.* Baltimore, MD: Williams & Wilkins, pp.1–93.
(b) The photograph was provided by Alex Mih, MD.

inflamed with manual activity. This condition occurs most commonly in men in their third decade and is often misdiagnosed as a ganglion. Conservative management includes splinting and use of anti-inflammatory medications.[20,32]

Evaluation of the hand with OA

Evaluation of the OA hand should include assessment of all of the features listed in Table 9.26. A 'hard-end feel' at the end of the range in the affected joins indicates that motion is limited by osteophytes. If a difference exists between active and passive ROM (ROM lag), the cause (e.g., muscle weakness, triggering, swelling, tenosynovitis) should be ascertained and treated.

Because of the similarities of pain patterns, the main differential diagnosis for TMJ OA is de Quervain's tenosynovitis (inflammation of the first dorsal wrist compartment containing the extensor pollicis brevis and abductor pollicis longus tendons) (Fig. 9.24). Two assessments can help distinguish these two conditions[17]:

- The 'grind test' (metacarpal compression and rotation), which is a specific test for localizing pain and/or crepitus to the TMJ.
- The Finkelstein test (full thumb flexion and wrist ulnar deviation) (Fig. 9.25), which is specific for localizing pain in the first dorsal tendon compartment.
- Treatment of these two conditions differs. OA of the TMJ requires a hand-based splint that blocks adduction; de Quervain's tenosynovitis requires a forearm-based, radial gutter splint that block tendon motion, but permits TMJ adduction.

Treatment by the occupational therapist of pain, stiffness, and inflammation in the OA hand

In a study of hand OA in the elderly by Moratz *et al.*,[5] disability was more often associated with pain than with limited motion or reduced strength. This finding is supported by clinical experience and other studies. The focus of hand therapy for OA is to maintain function through the reduction of pain, inflammation, and stiffness, and to help the patient adapt or compensate for loss of ROM. The main approaches to symptom reduction are the use of analgesics/nonsteroidal anti-inflammatory drugs (NSAIDs), splinting, thermal modalities, elastic gloves, and use of joint protection techniques. Corticosteroid injections may be indicated for acute joint inflammation. Steroid injections are more effective when combined with splint immobilization.

Splinting

If a DIPJ becomes so painful that it interferes with hand function, a rigid, custom-molded, thermoplastic cylindrical orthosis or tri-point splint that blocks flexion (made from 1/16 in. thermoplastic splinting material) can reduce pain, improve overall hand function, and reduce muscular guarding by allowing the patient to use the hand without fear of pain or trauma (Fig. 9.26).

For the PIPJ, rigid immobilization can be employed for severe pain but, generally, is not an acceptable option for the patient because it limits hand function. Furthermore, it can result in shortening of the collateral ligaments, limiting mobility of the PIPJ.

Results of two studies[32,33] have indicated that approximately 80 per cent of patients with TMJ disease who were referred for surgery found that splinting provided sufficient symptomatic relief so that they did not require operation. The first study[32] evaluated a short opponens (hand-based, permitting wrist motion) splint and the second, a long opponens (forearm based, restricting wrist motion) splint. Both splints included a C-bar over the web space to stabilize the thumb in abduction and prevent adduction and other motion[33] of the TMJ. A short opponens splint, permitting wrist motion, has greater patient acceptance and appears to be as effective as a long opponens splint that restricts the wrist and creates additional limitations.

For OA of the TMJ, the author recommends a custom-fitted, thermoplastic, immobilization splint that provides a C-bar to stabilize the TMJ in abduction but permits full mobility of the thumb IPJ and wrist (Fig. 9.27). This splint was evaluated with a protocol requiring continuous use for 2–3 weeks and then, once the patient became pain-free for as long as 3 hours

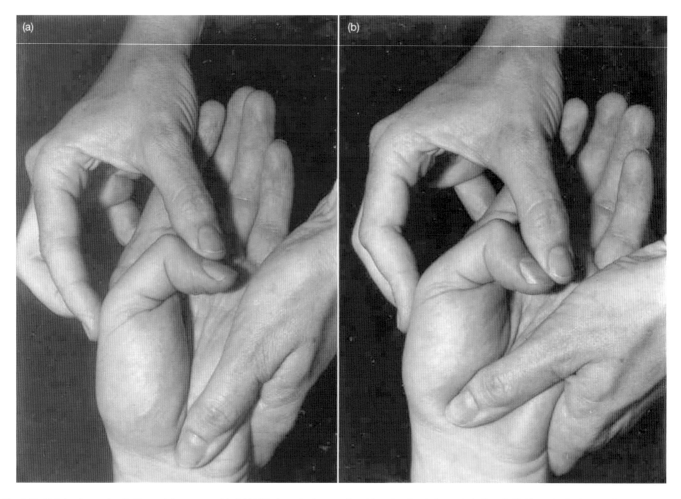

Fig. 9.25 Finkelstein test for de Quervain's tenosynovitis. (a) With the wrist in neutral position, the thumb is passively flexed. (b) The wrist is then gently deviated in the ulnar direction while the thumb is held in flexion to fully stretch the extensor pollicis brevis and abductor pollicis longus tendons. The test is positive if the patient experiences sharp pain over the radial styloid, indicating inflammation in the first dorsal wrist compartment.

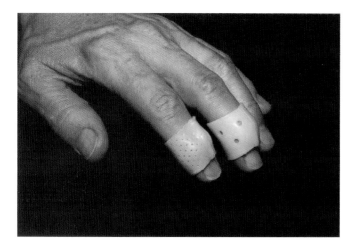

Fig. 9.26 DIPJ immobilization splints made of 1/16 in. Aquaplast™. One is pre-perforated and the other has been perforated manually. Use of a simple cylinder splint can decrease nocturnal joint pain and reduce joint pain and trauma during the day. Patients consider this an effective self-management tool.

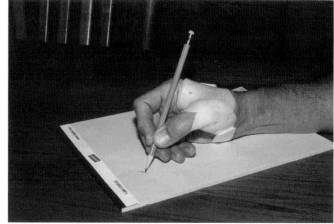

Fig. 9.27 TMJ-MCPJ stabilization splint, designed by the author, to stabilize the TMJ in the neutral resting position and provide maximal immobilization without restricting the wrist. The MCPJ is included only to provide attachment of the C-bar over the web space, to prevent TMJ adduction.

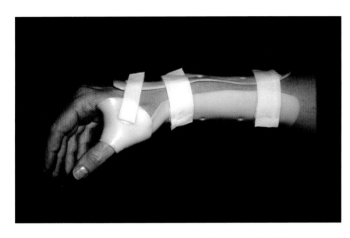

Fig. 9.28 Full circumferential wrist-thumb immobilization splint, fabricated from 1/16 in. Aquaplast™, for scaphoid-trapezial-trapezoid (i.e., STT, pantrapezial) OA (3).

without it, using it only during stressful activities. In a three-month follow-up study of 35 patients using this type of splint, 80 per cent complied with instructions, 17 per cent were pain-free after treatment, while another 68 per cent reported significant reduction in pain. Seven of 23 patients were able to reduce their dose of NSAID or discontinue NSAID use. Seventy-one per cent continued to use the orthosis to reduce pain during specific activities.[34] Sixty per cent reported that the orthotic allowed them to stop worrying about their thumb (which reduces muscle guarding). The ideal outcome is to eliminate pain and inflammation for 3 months to reduce the sensitivity of the joint capsule, permitting the patient to tolerate moderate stress without an increase in symptoms.[35]

Several commercially available TMJ splints do not include a C-bar over the web space. However, any orthotic without a C-bar will permit adduction of the thumb at the TMJ and may not sufficiently immobilize the TMJ to adequately treat inflammation in that joint. Pantrapezial OA requires a splint that immobilizes the wrist as well as the TMJ (Fig. 9.28). Patients with wrist or hand pain often develop subconscious muscle guarding to protect the joint and require education in methods to relax the extremity when they wear the splint, because guarding can reduce the effectiveness of the splint.[35]

Thermal modalities

Most people with OA cringe at the idea of applying cold to their hands because warmth feels better. Generally, those with acute synovitis of the TMJ are the most receptive to use of cold modalities. Cold seems to work best when acute inflammation is present. Cold should be used only if it results in improvement in ROM or a decrease in pain or swelling.

The prime focus of therapy for OA should be effective daily self-management *at home*. This goal is best accomplished by using thermal modalities that can be readily replicated at home, for example, hand exercises may be performed in a sink filled with warm water or shoulder and neck exercises in the shower.

Treatment of joint stiffness

For stiffness of PIPJs or DIPJs, some soft splint options are available. Self-adhesive tape, such as Coban™, can be used because it restricts motion slightly and reminds the patient to be cautious with use of the joint. However, the tape gets dirty easily. Another option (especially at night) is to wrap an inch-wide strip of plastic food wrap (4 in. long) firmly, but not tightly, around the joint. This material will self-adhere and keep the joint warm, increasing the patient's comfort.

If stiffness limits functional ability in the morning, the overnight use of Futuro Thermoelastic Gloves® or Isotoner® gloves (inverted to avoid pressure from seams) may be helpful.[36] Because hand OA is usually bilateral, patients can use the glove on one hand and employ the other hand as a control, permitting them to ascertain whether the treatment actually works.

Garfinkel *et al.*[37] demonstrated that a yoga regimen combined with patient education for 10 weekly sessions reduced stiffness, pain, and tenderness, and improved ROM in hand joints of patients with symptomatic OA. In comparison, control subjects, showed no significant improvement.

Patient education: philosophy of self-management

Many patients believe they have two options: 'to give in to their arthritis' or 'to suffer through their pain.' They need to be taught that joint inflammation can be aggravated by activities that cause pain and that performing activities painlessly may help assure a measure of 'joint protection.' Although many sports enthusiasts believe 'No pain, no gain,' this is not the correct approach to treatment of patients with arthritis, in which the *greatest gain results from no pain*. Pain causes muscle spasm, increasing stress on the joint. If it is persistent, pain may lead to muscle contracture. Hence, it is important that patients exercise and use their joints in performance of their daily activities in a pain-free fashion.

It is helpful to teach patients to pay attention to their pain. Whenever an activity causes joint pain, the patient should try to ascertain the cause of the pain to determine what changes can be made to permit the activity to be performed painlessly.[38] It is important that therapists and physicians teach patients how to problem-solve, that is, to find ways to reduce joint pain during activity, rather than merely giving them a list of generic 'do's and don'ts.' Occupational therapists can teach patients the basic principles of joint care and adapting or altering activity to reduce stress on the OA joint. It is useful to have the patient make a list of those daily activities that cause pain and of their solutions for reducing that pain. The list can then be reviewed with the therapist. Involving spouses and caregivers in adapting the home or fabricating simple assistive devices, such as a dressing stick or thickened handles, has the benefit of allowing them to make a direct, meaningful contribution in reducing the patient's pain and disability.

Self-management training is an educational process, and the philosophy of empowering patients to manage their arthritis/illness and their health that began as a series of classes within a public health model is now being integrated within physical and occupational therapy clinics.[39]

Management of OA based on principles of joint protection

Cordery originated the concept of joint protection training as a therapeutic intervention for patients with rheumatoid arthritis (RA) in 1965.[40] Since that time it has been used for patients with RA in clinics throughout the Western world. Although these principles were loosely applied also to OA over the years, in 1998, Cordery adapted and defined them for OA, in general,[2] and, later, for OA of the hand, in particular.[41] Schreuer *et al.*[42] found that women with hand OA had less pain and were able to perform activities in less time after they have been trained in principles of joint protection and use of adaptive equipment. These principles, in fact, provide a philosophy of care for the person with OA.

Increase muscle strength and physical fitness

Muscle strength is needed to maintain ROM, and should be assessed routinely and improved, if necessary. Strengthening exercises need to be performed in a pain-free manner,[43] because pain inhibits the strength of muscle contraction, this often requires isometric exercise[44] or water exercise (aqua or pool therapy), which has proved to be one of the most effective means of exercise for people with OA.[45]

Aerobic exercise can effectively reduce OA pain[46] (see Chapter 9.11.1). Fitness exercise improves stamina, reduces stress and depression, and improves sleep,[13] all of which can help reduce pain and symptoms of OA.

Maintain ROM

Joint motion promotes healthy cartilage and muscles. Behavioral pain management techniques, medications, and, splinting for hand OA, can play an important role in maintaining ROM. To reduce pain, many patients avoid use of the involved joint, but this promotes stiffness and may lead to contracture and loss of motion. Loss of ROM in one joint will alter the loading of adjacent joints.

Reduce excessive loading on joints

Osteophytes develop at sites at which the greatest stresses are generated.[4] Muscle contraction produces considerable force on the joints; reducing the strength required to perform an activity will reduce loading of the joint.[47] This may be accomplished by a variety of techniques; for the hands, use of enlarged handles, nonslip surfaces, and stabilizing devices (e.g., to hold bowls or prevent sauce pans from moving), can reduce the grip strength needed to stabilize the item. The load on an OA joint can also be reduced by using lighter objects and employing wheels and ambulation aids[48] and by eliminating some activities, such as stair climbing and single-leg standing (e.g., while getting into and out of a bathtub) (see Table 9.24 for other suggestions). Peak dynamic load can be attenuated by using shock absorbers, such as rubber mats on which to stand, viscoelastic shoe inserts, and shock-absorbing athletic shoes designed for running (rather than for walking).[2] Strong muscles improve joint efficiency and reduce the load on weight-bearing joints.[49]

Avoid joint pain during activities

Joint pain in patients with hand OA is usually related to weight bearing on damaged articular cartilage, pressure on nerves caused by osteophytes, and inflammation. Pain can lead to protective muscle spasm that will restrict joint ROM. Pain during use of an involved joint causes uncoordinated function, which can lead to abnormal distribution of stress on the joint. Any activity or posture that causes pain should be avoided. Muscle strengthening, stabilizing orthoses, assistive devices, and modification of activities, can reduce joint pain in patients with OA.

Balance activity and rest

People with OA do not exhibit fatigue as a result of a systemic disease, as do persons with inflammatory joint diseases, such as RA. The person with OA, however, may be biomechanically inefficient and require higher energy expenditure than normal for everyday tasks, such as walking, and may be physically deconditioned (see Chapter 9.11.1). Rest breaks reduce repetitive stress on joints. People with hand joint OA who perform repetitive hand activities in a static posture, such as at a desk or computer, should utilize the upper extremity and hand stretches to relieve muscle tension in the hands. Because tired muscles cannot control loading of the joint or act effectively as shock absorbers, they cannot fully protect the joint.[2] Stretching, strengthening exercises, and rest breaks can reduce muscle fatigue.

Avoid maintaining joint positions for prolonged periods of time

People with OA are prone to 'gelling' or stiffness and discomfort after periods of inactivity. Muscles tire quickly in static positions and are then less

Table 9.27 Interventions for common limitations due to OA in joints of the hand and other sites

Limitation	Treatment
1. Severe morning stiffness	Thermoelastic gloves at night; active ROM in warm water; gentle stretching exercises at bedtime
2. Loss of full grip due to decreased finger ROM	Enlarged or nonslip handles on equipment and devices
3. Inability to hold objects because of joint pain	Instruction in joint protection techniques; enlarged handles; adaptive methods; education on optimal treatment for inflammation
4. Inability to fully extend fingers and use palmar hand surface	Assistive devices for specific activities
5. Inability to apply pinch because of TMJ or pantrapezial joint pain	MCP-TM splint to restrict TM joint motion during activities; pantrapezial arthritis also requires immobilization of the wrist
6. Inability to hold objects because of thumb metacarpal adduction contracture (the most common thumb deformity)	Reduced thickness of handles to accommodate diminished web space
7. Inability to apply pinch because of thumb IPJ, MCPJ, or TMJ instability	Thumb orthosis to stabilize IPJ alone, MCPJ alone, or combined MCP-TMJ or TM-MCP-IPJs
8. Cervical pain and decreased ROM (evaluate for nerve root compression and decreased hand strength)	Training in joint protection principles; assistive devices; soft collar for positioning (not immobilization)
9. Shoulder pain: decreased UE dressing and bathing	Adaptive methods and assistive devices
10. Back pain: decreased toilet, tub, and low seat transfer, and more difficult lower extremity dressing/bathing	Assistive devices to don pants, shoes, socks, tie shoe laces and remove shoes; transfer bars, bathing aids, adapted seats
11. Spinal arthritis with progressive deformity	Home evaluation of chairs, bed, and posture during leisure activities and sleep, deep breathing for spinal mobility, fitness and posture exercise
12. Decreased hip flexion: decreased LE dressing, toilet, or low seat transfer	Assistive devices to don pants, shoes, socks, tie shoe laces; raised toilet seats
13. Decreased hip abduction: decreased perineal care	Adaptive bathing and toileting devices, raise chairs for leisure sitting
14. Decreased knee flexion or knee pain; more difficult lower extremity dressing and low seat transfer	Assistive devices to don pants, shoes, and socks and to tie shoe laces; walker adaptations if necessary
15. First MTPJ pain/stiffness; limiting ambulation endurance	Foot orthoses with metatarsal bar, lightweight shoes with cushioned rocker soles
16. Decreased ambulation and coordination, risk of falling	Home safety evaluation, education and adaptation

ROM, range of motion; TMJ, trapeziometacarpal joint; MCPJ, metacarpophalangeal joint; IPJ, interphalangeal joint; UE, upper extremity; LE, lower extremity; MTPJ, metatarsophalangeal joint.
Source: Taken from Ref. 50.

effective in supporting the joints. Instructing the patient to put the involved limb through its ROM every 15–20 minutes may minimize stiffness and facilitate muscle function.

Compensation for limited joint mobility: assistive devices and adaptive methods

People with OA may have limited ROM or joint contractures, with or without joint pain. As indicated above, assistive devices or adaptive methods to reduce stress on the joint are therapeutic interventions for pain and inflammation. For example, for the patient with limited back or hip mobility who cannot reach his feet to don socks, a sock donner or dressing stick may be recommended to improve function. For people with limited finger flexion, function can be improved by building up handles so that force can be exerted within the available ROM. Patients with an adduction contracture of the thumb or a narrow web space may require handles to be narrowed to fit their limited web space.

Patients often require instruction in how the use of levers can reduce stress. For example, enlarging the head of a car key permits greater leverage in turning on the ignition. Lengthening a faucet handle makes turning the faucet easier. Patients must be warned, however, that the reverse effect can also occur; for example, lifting an item with a long lever, such as a $2\frac{1}{2}$ footlong reacher, increases the impact of the lifted weight on the joints of the hand. Table 9.27 provides examples of some common adaptive devices and interventions that are helpful for joint protection and improvement of function of people with OA.[50]

Summary

Many people with hand joint OA are asymptomatic. Usually, it is the onset of pain that impairs function that leads the person with OA to seek medical attention. The primary purpose of management is to control the pain and inflammation and maintain optimal ROM, and in the early stages of the disease, to return the patient to a state of painless OA. These goals are more readily achieved in patients with hand OA than in those with OA of other joints because weight-bearing forces are less of a factor in the hand than, for example, in joints of the spine or lower extremity. The guidelines for protection of OA joints in the hand, cited herein, provide a comprehensive approach to optimizing joint function and reducing load on the joint. Successful management of symptomatic OA requires a broad approach to improving joint physiology through self-management training that includes ROM exercise, cardiovascular fitness exercise, weight control, nutrition, stress management, and the reduction of factors that can amplify joint pain, such as poor sleep, depression, anxiety, fatigue, and deconditioning.

Key points

1. Severe thumb pain can limit hand function by nearly 50 per cent.

2. Hand pain elicits muscular guarding throughout the upper extremity and can aggravate cervical OA.

3. Custom-made thermoplastic thumb splints can be very effective for resolving the symptoms of OA in the basal thumb joint, and often eliminate the need for surgery.

4. Patients with limited joint mobility and decreased functional ability, whether painful or painless, should be evaluated by an occupational therapist and should receive advice and training in the use of assistive devices and adaptive methods to improve function and protect the arthritic joint.

References

(An asterisk denotes recommended reading.)

1. Bland, J.H., Melvin, J.L., and Hasson, S. (2000). Osteoarthritis. In: J.L. Melvin, K.M. Ferrell (eds). *Rheumatologic Rehabilitation Series, Volume II, Adult Rheumatic Diseases*. Bethesda, MD: American Occupational Therapy Association, pp. 81–124.

2. *Cordery, J.C. and Rocchi, M. (1998). Joint Protection and Fatigue Management. In: J.L. Melvin, G. Jensen (eds). *Rheumatologic Rehabilitation Series, Volume 1 Assessment and Management*, Bethesda, MD: American Occupational Therapy Association, pp. 311–16.
   This paper provides a rationale for training patients with arthritis in principles of joint protection.

3. Melvin, J.L. (1989). *Rheumatic Disease in the Adult and Child* (3rd ed.). Philadelphia: FA Davis, pp. 1–607.

4. Buckland-Wright, J.C., Macfarlane, D.G., and Lynch, J.A. (1991). Osteophytes in the osteoarthritic hand: their incidence, size, distribution, and progression. *Ann Rheum Dis* **50**:627–30.

5. Moratz, V., Muncie, Jr., H.L., and Miranda-Walsh, H. (1986). Occupational management in the multidisciplinary assessment and management of osteoarthritis. *Clin Ther* **9**(Suppl. B):24–9.

6. Chaisson, C.E., Zhang, Y., Sharma, L., Kannel, W., and Felson, D.T. (1999). Grip strength and the risk of developing radiographic hand osteoarthritis: results from the Framingham Study. *Arthritis Rheum* **42**:33–8.

7. *Burkholder, J.F. (2000). Osteoarthritis of the hand: a modifiable disease. *J Hand Ther* **13**:79–89.
   This current article provides an excellent description of occupational therapy for patients with hand OA.

8. Dieppe, P. (1994). Osteoarthritis: clinical features and diagnostic problems. In: J.H. Klippel, P. Dieppe (eds). *Rheumatology*. St Louis: Mosby Yearbook, pp. 7.4.1–16.

9. Bland, J.H. and Stulberg, S.D. (1985). Osteoarthritis: pathology and clinical patterns. In: W.M. Kelley, E.D. Harris, S. Ruddy, C.B. Sledge (eds). *Textbook of Rheumatology (2nd ed.)*. Philadelphia: WB Saunders, pp. 1471–90.

10. Bland, J.H. (2000). Pathophysiology of cartilage and joint structures in rheumatic disease. In: J.L. Melvin, K.M. Ferrell (eds). *Rheumatologic Rehabilitation Series, Volume II, Adult Rheumatic Diseases*. Bethesda, MD: American Occupational Therapy Association, pp. 21–34.

11. Cooney, W. and Chao, E. (1977). Biomechanical analysis of static forces in the thumb during hand function. *J Bone Joint Surg* **59**(A):27.

12. Altman, R.D. and Dean, D. (1989). Pain in Osteoarthritis. Introduction and Overview. *Sem Arthritis Rheum* **18**(4 Suppl. 2):1–4.

13. Moldofsky, H., Lue, F.A., and Saskin, P. (1987). Sleep and morning pain in primary osteoarthritis. *J Rheumatol* **14**:124–8.

14. Russell, I.J., Melvin, J.L., and Siegel, M. (2000). Fibromyalgia Syndrome. In: J.L. Melvin, K.M. Ferrell (eds). *Rheumatologic Rehabilitation Series, Volume II, Adult Rheumatic Diseases*, Bethesda, MD: American Occupational Therapy Association, pp. 121–60.

15. *Melvin, J.L. (1996). *Fibromyalgia syndrome: Getting Healthy*. Bethesda: American Occupational Therapy Association, pp. 27–46.
   This 51 page book for patients emphasizes a wellness-based, self-management approach to recovery from fibromyalgia. It contains specific guidelines for progressive exercise and nutrition to improve energy, and sleep and stress management.

16. Jonsson, H. and Valtysdottir, S.T. (1995). Hypermobility features in patients with hand osteoarthritis. *Osteoarthritis Cart* **3**:1–5.

17. Melvin, J.L. (2002). Osteoarthritis of the hand: conservative and postoperative therapy. In: E.J. Mackin, A.D. Callahan, A.L. Osterman, T.M. Skirven, L.H. Schneider (eds). Hunter-Makin-Callahan *Rehabilitation of the Hand and Upper Extremity* (5th ed.). St. Louis: Mosby.

18. Swanson, A.B. and de Groot-Swanson, G. (1985). Osteoarthritis in the hand. *Clin Rheum Dis* **11**:393–420.

19. Kleinert, H.E., Kutz, J.E., Fishman, J.H., and McCraw, L.H. (1972). Etiology and treatment of the so-called mucous cyst of the finger. *J Bone Joint Surg* **54**(A):1455–58.

20. Siegel, D.B., Gelberman, R.H., and Smith, R. (1992). Osteoarthritis of the hand and wrist. In: R.W. Moskowitz, D.S. Howell, V.M. Goldberg, H. Mankin (eds). *Osteoarthritis: Diagnosis and Medical-Surgical Management* (2nd ed.). Philadelphia: WB Saunders, pp. 547–58.

21. Culver, J.E. and Fleegler, E.J. (1987). Osteoarthritis of the distal interphalangeal joint. *Hand Clin* **3**:385–403.

22. Moulton, M.J., Parentis, M.A., Kelly, M.J., Jacobs, C., Naidu, S.H., and Pellegrini, Jr., V.D. (2001). Influence of metacarpophalangeal joint position on basal joint-loading in the thumb. *J Bone Joint Surg Am* **83**(A):709–16.

23. Pellegrini, Jr., V.D. (1996). The basal articulations of the thumb: pain, instability and osteoarthritis. In: C.A. Peimer (ed.). *Surgery of the Hand and Upper Extremity.* New York: McGraw-Hill, pp. 1019–42.

24. Crosby, E.B., Linscheid, R.L., and Dobyns, J.H. (1978). Scaphotrapezial trapezoidal arthrosis. *J Hand Surg* **3**:223–34.

25. Swanson, A.B. and de Groot-Swanson, G. (1976). Disabling osteoarthritis in the hand and its treatment. In *Symposium on Osteoarthritis.* St Louis: CV Mosby, pp. 196–232.

26. Stucki, G., Hardegger, D., Bohni, U., and Michel, B.A. (1999). Degeneration of the scaphoid-trapezium joint: a useful finding to differentiate calcium pyrophosphate deposition disease from osteoarthritis. *Clin Rheumatol* **18**:232–7.

27. Dray, G.J. and Jablon, M. (1987). Clinical and radiologic features of primary osteoarthritis of the hand. *Hand Clin* **3**:351–69.

28. Parks, B.J. and Hamlin, C. (1986). Chronic sesamoiditis of the thumb: pathomechanics and treatment. *J Hand Surg Am* **11**:237–40.

29. Watson, H.K. and Ballet, F.L. (1984). The SLAC wrist: Scapholunate advanced collapse pattern of degenerative arthritis. *J Hand Surg* **9**(A): 358–65.

30. Lichtman, D.M., Alexander, A.H., Mack, G.R., and Gunther, S.F. (1982). Kienböck's disease: Update on silicone replacement arthroplasty. *J Hand Surg* **7**(A):343–7.

31. Cuono, C.B. and Watson, H.K. (1979). The carpal boss: surgical treatment and etiologic considerations. *Plast Reconstr Surg* **63**:88–93.

32. Swigart, C.R., Eaton, R.G., Glickel, S.Z., and Johnson, C. (1999). Splinting in the treatment of arthritis of the first carpometacarpal joint. *J Hand Surg Am* **24**:86–91.

33. Dell, P.C., Brushart, T.M., and Smith, R.J. (1978). Treatment of trapeziometacarpal arthritis: results of resection arthroplasty. *J Hand Surg* **3**:243–9.

34. Melvin, J.L. and Carlson-Rioux, J. (1989). Orthotic Treatment for Osteoarthritis of the Thumb Carpometacarpal Joint: Evaluation of Efficacy and Compliance (abstract). *Arthritis Care Res* **2**:S10.

35. Melvin, J.L. (In preparation). Splinting treatment for arthritis of the hand. In J.L. Melvin, E.A. Nalebuff (eds). *The Hand in Rheumatic Disease-Evaluation, Therapy and Surgery.*

36. McKnight, P.T. and Kwoh, C.K. (1992). Randomized, controlled trial of compression gloves in rheumatoid arthritis. *Arthritis Care Res* **5**:223–7.

37. Garfinkel, M.S., Schumacher, H.R., Hsain, A., Levy, M., and Reshetar, R.A. (1994). Evaluation of a yoga based regimen for treatment of osteoarthritis of the hands. *J Rheumatol* **21**:2341–3.

38. *Melvin, J.L. (1995). *Osteoarthritis: Caring for Your Hands.* Bethesda, MD: American Occupational Therapy Association, pp. 14–17.
    This inexpensive booklet, that may be given to the patient by the therapist, contains useful information about comprehensive home programs for patients with specific hand problems. It contains a space for the therapist to provide patient-specific recommendations for exercise, joint protection, and splinting.

39. Boutaugh, M.L. and Brady, T. (1998). Patient Education for Self-Management. In: J.L. Melvin, G. Jensen (eds). *Rheumatologic Rehabilitation Series, Volume 1 Assessment and Management.* Bethesda, MD: American Occupational Therapy Association, pp. 219–58.

40. Cordery, J. (1965). Joint protection: a responsibility of the occupational therapist. *Am J Occup Ther* **19**:285–94.

41. Cordery, J. (In preparation). Joint protection for arthritis of the hand. In: J.L. Melvin, E.A. Nalebuff (eds). *The Hand in Rheumatic Disease: Evaluation, Therapy and Surgery.*

42. Schreuer, N., Palmon, O., and Nahir, A.M. (1994). An occupational therapy group workshop for patients with osteoarthritis of the hands. *Work* **4**:147–50.

43. Melvin, J.L. (In preparation). Therapeutic exercise and thermal modalities in the management of the hand with arthritis. In: J.L. Melvin, E.A. Nalebuff (eds). *The Hand in Rheumatic Disease-Evaluation, Therapy and Surgery.*

44. *Lockard, M.A. (2000). Exercise for the patient with upper quadrant osteoarthritis. *J Hand Ther* **13**(2):175–83.
    This paper is a good source of information on exercise for patients with OA of upper extremity joints.

45. Suomi, R. and Lindauer, S. (1997). Effectiveness of the Arthritis Foundation Aquatic Program on strength and range of motion in women with arthritis. *J Aging Phys Activity* **5**:341–51.

46. Minor, M., Hewett, J., Webel, R., Anderson, S., and Kay, D. (1989). Efficacy of physical conditioning exercise in rheumatoid arthritis and osteoarthritis. *Arthritis Rheum* **32**:1396–405.

47. Radin, E.L. (1987). Osteoarthritis: What is known about prevention. *Clin Orthop* **222**:60–5.

48. Neumann, D.A. and Hase, A.D. (1994). An electromyographic analysis of the hip abductors during load carriage: Implications for hip joint protection. *J Orthop Sports Phys Ther* **19**:296–304.

49. Radin, E.L, Paul, I.L., and Rose, R.M. (1975). The mechanical aspects of osteoarthrosis. *Bull Rheum Dis* **26**:862–5.

50. Melvin, J.L. (2000). Self-care strategies for persons with arthritis and connective tissue diseases. In: C. Christiansen (ed.) *Ways of Living: Self-care Strategies for Special Needs* (2nd ed.). Bethesda, MD: American Occupational Therapy Association, pp. 145.

9.13 Patient education

Julie Barlow and Kate Lorig

There are several features of OA that pose considerable challenges for both patients and physicians. First, the chronic nature of OA means that management of the condition spans a third or more of the total lifetime of the patient. Second, pain is a major feature, from the point of view of the patient. Third, medical and surgical interventions are, at best, only partially ameliorative. Finally, both physicians and patients often subscribe to the widespread belief that OA is an inevitable consequence of old age and that little can be done for it. Indeed, patients are often told, 'You will have to learn to live with it.' They are seldom taught 'how to live with it.' The operative word, however, is 'learn.' Patient education is an important aspect of treatment for all people with OA and, for many, it is the most important intervention.

This chapter will discuss OA patient education from three perspectives: (1) what the patient wants and needs; (2) what is known about the effectiveness of various forms of patient education; and (3) how physicians can integrate patient education into clinical practice.

The patient's perspective

The usual role of the physician is to diagnose and then, based on scientific knowledge of anatomy, physiology, pharmacology, and so on, to suggest a treatment plan. The unique role of the physician is as holder and applier of scientific knowledge.

Many patients, on the other hand, are not particularly interested in scientific knowledge, except as it applies to helping them get on with their lives. For them, a disease is just that: a 'dis-ease.' Unfortunately, patients are often educated as though they were health professionals. They are taught about the physiological causes of their disease and instructed to follow prescribed medical or exercise routines. These instructions sometimes have little to do with the disease as experienced by the patient.

The onset of a chronic disease, such as OA, has been described as a 'biographical disruption,' thus indicating the adverse impact that a chronic disease can have on a person's life.[1] In a large qualitative study, Corbin and Strauss[2] identified three major ways in which the lives of patients with chronic conditions were disrupted. First, patients had to conform to a new set of medical issues. That is, they had to take medicine, exercise in new ways, visit physicians, and carry out other activities necessitated by their disease. Second, they had to accommodate changes in their life roles. For example, they had to change the patterns of their work, family, social, and recreational lives. Sometimes, these accommodations were small, such as asking for help in opening jars, and, sometimes, very large, such as moving to be closer to relatives. Finally, people with chronic conditions have an altered and often uncertain future.

The findings of Corbin and Strauss have been verified in both qualitative and quantitative studies of people with OA. Disruption, lack of certainty, and a changed sense of identity combined with multiple losses (e.g. loss of valued activities due to physical limitations, a reduced social network, loss of independence) can lead to emotional reactions such as depression, frustration, or anger. For example, it has been estimated that 20–40 per cent of people with arthritis are clinically depressed, and that depression is similar in OA and rheumatic arthritis (RA) patients.[3] An interview-based exploration of personal models of OA[4] showed that the 61 older people (mean age 72, SD 7.8) believed their condition to be fairly serious and chronic, although amenable to control by one or more treatments recommended by their health care practitioner. Not surprisingly, patients who viewed their condition as more serious made greater use of medical services and self-management activities, and had a poorer quality of life. Pain was viewed as the major symptom of OA and was used by patients to assess 'seriousness.' A study of 86 people with knee OA (mean age 61) adds support for this finding,[5] showing that disability, instability of the knee joint, and anxiety about knee OA were also sources of distress for many. Interestingly, although 41 of the sample had not tried education or advice, educational interventions were cited as a priority for research.

Community samples of OA patients identified pain, activity problems, and depression as their major concerns. When rheumatologists were asked about the concerns of patients, they gave similar responses, but rated them to be less important than did patients.[6] Despite the major role played by pain from the patient's perspective, pain does not always correlate with the extent of OA when assessed radiographically.[7] This situation demonstrates how potential discrepancies between patient and provider perspectives can emerge. Table 9.28 suggests some ways in which patients and health care providers differ in how they view OA.

Other studies have found that the beliefs of arthritis patients and their physicians differ. For example, physicians believe that their patients are much more compliant than they actually are.[8] They also believe that their patients know less about their disease and use non-traditional therapists more than is the reality.[6] A final set of studies has shown that patients find physicians their most credible source of information.[9] Unfortunately, many physicians do not feel that they are effective in educating their patients.

In summary, patients and their physicians have similar, but not concordant, concerns and beliefs. To the extent that concerns and beliefs are similar, communication and education are possible. One of the first rules in establishing good patient/physician communication is for the physician to solicit, and then act on, the concerns of the patient. Specific techniques for doing this are discussed later. Pain and disability are the two greatest concerns of OA patients—concerns that should be addressed by patient

Table 9.28 How views of patients and providers differ

Views of the provider	Views of the patient
Anatomy and physiology	Why do I feel bad?
Behaviors to maintain or improve health	Behaviors to solve problems
Facts about disease	Beliefs about disease
Skills to perform health behaviors	Skills to maintain a 'normal' life
Frustration about non-compliance	Frustration about living with disease
Fear of malpractice	Fear about the future

Table 9.29 Key issues for people with OA

Concerns of people with OA:

♦ Pain

♦ Fatigue

♦ Disability

♦ Psychological consequences of OA

♦ Social consequences of OA

The level of concern does *not* always correlate with objective disease assessment criteria (e.g. X-rays).

---

education programs. In an excellent review of the biobehavioral mechanisms of these symptoms in OA patients,[7] Dekker *et al.* concluded that 'pain and disability are associated with degeneration of cartilage and bone (articular level) with muscle weakness, limitation in joint motion (kinesiological level), limitation with anxiety coping styles, attention focus on symptoms, and possibly depression (psychological level)'. (See Table 9.29.)

What we know about OA patient education

The growing interest in patient education as a valuable tool in rheumatological disease management has been matched by a burgeoning of published studies. Whilst the majority pertains to people with RA, there is an increasing interest in provision of education for people with OA. Overall, the somewhat limited literature suggests that OA patient education can increase the practice of healthy behaviors, improve health status, and decrease health care utilization.

Definition of terms

Before discussing specific programs and their outcomes, some definitions are necessary. 'Patient education' is any set of planned educational activities designed to help patients change behaviors, health status, or health care utilization. While it is true that most patient education programs also alter the knowledge that patients have, this is not the ultimate aim. Changes in knowledge are necessary, but not sufficient, to bring about changes in behaviors or health status; if all that was necessary was having the correct knowledge, there would be few overweight patients and most would exercise appropriately and be compliant with medication taking. In short, good patient education combines the giving of knowledge with skills development, problem solving, and motivational activities.

Patients' are people with diagnosed disease. When health professionals see these people in a clinical setting, they are patients. Most of the time, however, they are people living in the community who happen to have OA.

'Health status,' for the purpose of this chapter, refers to health from the perspective of the patient. For people with OA, this means disability, pain, fatigue, and psychological distress (e.g. depression). Health status does not refer to X-ray findings or joint space. While these physiological states of disease may relate to patient symptoms, by themselves they are usually not important to patients. Of greater import, is the impact that changes in these disease states have on the patient's life.

Two other terms which merit discussion are 'coping' and 'self-management.' These terms are often incorrectly used as synonyms. Coping is the response to a negative stimulus and is usually short term. In contrast, self-management entails a wide range of skills such as planning, problem solving, and using consultants, and is long term. Consider for example, that businesses advertize for managers, not copers. For patients with long-term chronic conditions such as OA, self-management becomes the key ingredient in successful patient education.

Examples of OA patient education with a specific focus

Having examined some of the important concepts, we will now turn to what is known about OA patient education. Many studies have focused on determining the effectiveness of a specific therapy and modality such as cognitive pain management, or, exercise. One very small study ($n = 8$) focused on weight management.[10] Following a 17-week group intervention, all participants reached their expected weight loss (5–20 pounds). Given the importance of avoiding obesity in OA, it is surprising that weight control has not attracted more attention in its own right. However, diet or nutrition does often feature in multi-component interventions.

Relaxation or cognitive pain management is widely thought to be helpful for people with arthritis. One of the most popular cognitive techniques is progressive muscle relaxation, which teaches patients to tense and relax muscles in a systematic manner.[11] Other cognitive techniques include visualization or guided imagery, distraction or thinking of something other than pain, and various forms of meditation. For a short overview of cognitive pain management techniques see *The Arthritis Helpbook*.[12] While there have been a number of studies evaluating these modalities with non-OA patients, there have been few parallel studies focusing on OA. Investigators have demonstrated that cognitive pain management techniques, are useful in decreasing pain, and, sometimes, depression, for RA and AS patients.[13–16]

The results of studies using relaxation with OA patients have been somewhat mixed. Laborde and Powers randomized 160 people with OA into five groups.[17] Group one received an informational brochure, group two received instructions in joint protection, group three received relaxation training plus the brochure, group four received all three interventions, and group five received no intervention. Participants receiving relaxation training (when compared to controls) demonstrated significant reduction in pain ($p < 0.005$). In a study of 222 hip and knee surgery patients (73 per cent OA), Daltroy *et al.* used four interventions: informational classes, Benson's relaxation training, both of these interventions combined, and no intervention. They found no main effects for length of hospital stay, post-operative pain, anxiety, or medication usage.[18]

Calfas *et al.* studied 40 OA patients.[19] The intervention group participants were taught cognitive pain management techniques, while control participants received lectures from health professionals. As in the Daltroy study, there were no main effects, although both groups demonstrated decreases in depression and improvements in physical functioning. Finally, Keefe *et al.*[20] found that cognitive behavioral techniques were more effective than didactic arthritis education and standard care in reducing pain and psychological distress among people with OA.

Several conclusions can be drawn from these few studies. First, for some OA patients, cognitive pain management techniques may be useful. However, when used as the only behavioral modality, or when combined only with didactic material, these techniques do not appear to be very powerful. Use of cognitive techniques is usually new to patients with OA and, like all other new behaviors, these techniques need practicing before effects can occur. Moreover, such techniques need to be maintained in order to afford continued benefits, thus, greater emphasis should be placed on long-term practice.

Another behavior taught in most arthritis patient education programs is that of exercise. In the past, it was believed that arthritis patients needed to be careful when exercising; the fear was that they would 'wear out their joints.' In the past fifteen years, we have learned the importance of a full conditioning program for people with OA, and educational interventions focusing on exercise are proliferating. Minor *et al.*, have conducted a series of important studies on this subject. Twenty-four OA and RA patients were randomized to a physical conditioning program including aerobic exercise (walking or swimming) or a range of motion exercise program. Compared to the range of motion group, the aerobic group demonstrated improvements in walking time, morning stiffness, pain, and grip strength.[21] In a second study, 40 RA and 80 OA patients were randomized to an aerobic walking group program, a group aerobic aquatic program, or a range of motion group. The aerobic groups, compared to the range of motion group, improved significantly in aerobic capacity, endurance, physical activity, anxiety, and depression.[22]

Allegrante et al.[23] developed a walking program for people with knee OA, based on a synthesis of theoretical and empirical precepts. A randomized, controlled study ($n = 102$) compared the eight-week program with weekly phone calls about activities of daily living.[24] Immediately following the program, walking group participants had significantly decreased their disability and increased the six-minute walk distance. There were no changes in joint involvement, suggesting that there were no adverse effects from the walking program. However, at 12-month follow-up, there were no differences between the groups[25] and initial gains in physical activity and walking had returned to baseline values among the intervention group. It should be noted that the follow-up sample was much reduced (i.e. 29 and 23 of the original intervention and control groups). Nonetheless, the importance of sustaining changes in behavior after the end of educational interventions was highlighted.

Examples of multi-component OA patient education

The above discussion suggests that patient education interventions aimed at specific strategies can be helpful in reducing pain, disability, and weight, and increasing exercise activity, at least in the short term. Next, we will combine the teaching of several behavioral strategies (see Table 9.30).

The most widely delivered multi-component program is the six-week Arthritis Self-Management Program (ASMP).[26] This program is taught in the community by teams of trained lay leaders who conduct two-hour weekly group sessions with 10–15 people (75 per cent with OA). The ASMP has been successfully adapted and tested among Spanish-speaking participants.[27] The following are the major findings from a series of studies conducted in the United States of America:

1. In four-month randomized trails, ASMP participants, when compared to wait list controls, experienced increased physical activity, increased use of cognitive pain management techniques, and decreased pain.[26]

2. Reinforcement after one year did not add to the effect; both reinforced and non-reinforced groups retained most of the initial gains two years after the original course.[28]

3. Participants that were followed for four years continued to demonstrate decreased pain; they also decreased their arthritis-related visits to physicians.[29]

4. The mechanisms by which the ASMP affects pain appear to be much more psychological than behavioral. The program enhances self-efficacy of participants, increasing their confidence that they can do something about specific disease-related problems. The changes in self-efficacy are significantly associated with changes in pain. There are no significant associations between changes in pain and changes in behaviors (exercise and the use of cognitive pain management techniques).[30]

A series of studies conducted on the ASMP in the UK (>50 per cent OA), including a randomized controlled trial, report similar findings in terms of increased arthritis self-efficacy, greater use of self-management behaviors (e.g. exercise, diet), better communication with physicians and improved psychological well being (e.g. less depressed and more increased positive mood).[31–33] There was no difference in outcomes between people with RA or OA. In contrast to US findings, there was no change in visits to general

Table 9.30 Common elements of multi-component programs

The program takes place in small groups
The program is carried out over several weeks
The program is highly participatory
The program includes structured practice and feedback
The program is geared to the concerns of the patients

practitioners (GP) at 4 months, although a decrease in visits among the intervention group was noted at 12 months.

The ASMP is now sponsored and/or organized by national voluntary arthritis organizations (Arthritis Foundation, Arthritis Society, Arthritis Care) in the United States of America, Australia, Canada, and Great Britain, respectively.

Another series of studies was conducted by Goeppinger et al. with 450 subjects (72 per cent OA) living in rural areas. Participants were randomized to a small group self-management program similar to the ASMP, a home-study program with the same content, or a wait list control group.[34] At four months, both intervention groups demonstrated improvements in knowledge, self-care behaviors, perceived helplessness and pain, when compared to controls; these improvements were sustained for one year.[35] There were no significant changes in depression or function, nor were there differences between the two intervention groups—both interventions had high (82 per cent) retention rates and high acceptability to the participants. When the control group participants were allowed to choose, half chose the small group and half the home-study interventions.[36] This finding illustrates that group programs are not the ideal format of education for everyone; some people prefer individualized programs based on home study.

Bill Harvey et al. utilized a quasi-experimental pre-test post-test design to study 76 inner-city (mostly African-American) low literacy participants with OA, who attended a 10-hour group intervention.[37] Trained lay leaders taught the classes. Results included increased knowledge, exercise, use of assistive devices, and improved attitude ($p < 0.05$ function).

Collectively, these studies suggest that group or individualized, multi-component interventions that are based on issues of salience to patients can have a positive influence on quality of life. The interventions were all community-based and utilized non-health professionals as instructors; they appeared useful for a wide stratum of people with OA—urban and rural, people with little education, university graduates, and people of different races. Two studies have investigated the use of lay instructors compared to instruction given by health professionals.[38,39] In both studies, outcomes for participants taught by professionals were the same as those taught by lay people.

Examples of different delivery systems of OA patient education

Several studies have examined other patient education delivery systems. Nineteen women age >50, with knee OA, were randomized to individualized 15–30 minute sessions or a small group, one-hour session.[40] A nurse-physician team taught both interventions. There were no differences in outcomes between groups, both groups improved in knee flexion, knee extension, and pain. There were no changes in weight, mobility, physical activity, anxiety, or depression. The failure of this study to change behaviors suggests the need for education to be carried out in several sessions over time.

Goeppinger et al. conducted a dissemination study of a home-study arthritis education program combined with the availability of a community advisor. Participants improved in behaviors, helplessness, pain, and depression.[41] When this study was repeated without advisors, no beneficial effects were noted (personal communication).

The importance of personalization was also demonstrated by Weinberger et al.[42] Four hundred and thirty-nine OA patients (70 per cent Black, 88 per cent female) in a general medicine practice were randomized to receive monthly phone calls, attend the clinic, or to receive both monthly phone calls and attend the clinic. There were no significant clinic-by-phone interactions. Those contacted by phone had less disability and pain than those not receiving phone calls. The benefits accrued by those in receipt of phone calls have to be balanced against the increased contact time and the associated increased cost of providing and training interviewers. Nonetheless, the value of regular discussion about OA and its management is highlighted.

Finally, three studies have utilized computers for patient education. Seventy-two OA patients from small-town senior centers used a computer

Table 9.31 Tentative conclusions from the reviewed studies

Patient education is most effective when several behaviors are taught

Patient education should be based on the concerns and problems of the patient

Patient education should be interactive and personalized

If tutors are well trained; professional qualifications do not appear to give any advantage

Many methods of patient education are effective: small group, proactive telephone, home study, and computerized formats

The most effective programs are carried out over a period of time (e.g. weeks, months)

Focusing on self-management skills and behaviors appears to be more effective than acquisition of knowledge or compliance to a set of prescribed behaviors

to access eight OA lessons, totaling less than three hours. Significant pre-post increases were reported in knowledge, exercise, rest, and use of heat; no differences were reported in locus of control or pain.[43] OA patients belonging to a large health maintenance organization (HMO) filled out questionnaires about their arthritis.[44] Utilizing a computer program, the questionnaires were analyzed, and participants received highly personalized letter responses with self-management suggestions; they also received a book about arthritis self-management and an audio relaxation tape. Every three months they repeated the questionnaire and received a response showing progress or problems since the previous questionnaire. At six months, study participants who completed the program, when compared to controls, reported less pain, greater mobility, and greater sense of control over their symptoms. There were also trends towards less health care utilization. A similar mail-delivered program was investigated in a randomized, controlled trial by Fries *et al.*[45] among a mixed group of arthritis patients, including some with OA. The mail-delivered program comprised individualized, computer-generated advice, the ASMP, and the *Arthritis Helpbook*. At 6 months, intervention participants had decreased pain, improved joint count, increased self-efficacy, increased exercise, and were making fewer visits to physicians. (See Table 9.31.)

Patient education in clinical practice

The following are suggestions for integrating patient education into clinical practice; most of these suggestions require little or no extra time:

1. Frame teaching to match the concerns and expectations of the patient. For example, if patients are concerned about pain, suggest that exercise will help reduce pain by strengthening muscles. Also, reassure patients that they will not 'wear out' their joints and that they will not make their arthritis worse by exercising. In reality, the reverse is true. Tell them that they will make their arthritis worse by not exercising.

2. Be specific—do not just suggest that a patient walk more. Find out what they can do now and suggest that they do this, four times a week, adding a further 10 per cent a week until they can exercise for 20–30 minutes.

3. Tell patients what you want them to do. If you do not tell a patient to walk, practice relaxation, or loose weight, they will not do it. Many times patients tell us that they are not doing things because their doctor never told them to.

4. Inform patients of the purposes and expected effects of medications. Also, tell them when to expect effects. Patients usually think that they are taking medications, in order to help them to feel better. They should be told that sometimes medications do not make them feel better, rather they prevent symptoms from becoming worse, or they slow the progression of the disease. Another patient expectation is that medications will make them feel better in a short period of time, usually

hours, or at most, a day. When this does not happen they stop taking the medication. By knowing what to expect, and when to expect it, there is greater compliance with medication taking.[46]

5. It is probably easier for patients to add new behaviors than to eliminate established ones. For example, starting an exercise program is easier for most patients than changing eating habits.[47]

6. Ask patients to tell you how they are going to integrate your suggestion into their lives. For example, ask them when they are going to take their medicine or do their exercises. Do not let them repeat your exact words; rather, get them to think about how they will do things. In this way, you can often identify and discuss problems before they occur.

7. Use a combination of educational strategies; this can be done in any setting. Have literature for your patients, tell them what you want them to do, have videotapes of exercise programs that they can borrow, and teach your office staff to reinforce what is taught. In this way your patients will not get mixed messages.

8. Involve your office staff—patients learn a great deal from the receptionist and other staff in the office or practice. Be sure that everyone is giving the same messages to patients.

9. Refer—in a short visit you cannot possibly do all the necessary teaching. Many patients will never find their way to patient education courses, exercise classes, or voluntary arthritis organizations without your suggestion. Most patients, especially new patients and those not previously referred, should not leave your office without some sort of a referral. To make referrals easier, have referral prescription pads made up at any copy shop. They should contain the names of books, tapes, and organizations, which you have found helpful. In addition, they should contain phone numbers. All you have to do is check-off what you what the patient to do.

   Another time saving way of doing referrals is to have a bulletin board in the waiting area; across the top it can say 'Things your doctor suggests.' Have someone on your staff assigned to keep the board updated with new information about classes, support groups, new literature and tapes, and local arthritis organizations.

10. Monitor progress—make note what you asked patients to do, so that next time you see them you can ask about the arthritis class, or exercise program, or whatever. This personalizes the visit and shows the patient you are truly interested: it also gives you direct feedback on the programs to which you are referring.

In summary, patient education can be one of the most important interventions for OA. It is true that this is a disease that patients 'have to learn to live with': the operative work is 'learn.' The job of good clinical practice is to assist patients with the process of learning, thus enabling them to establish a satisfactory quality of life.

Key points

1. Education is a key aspect of treatment for people with OA.

2. The literature on OA suggests patient education can increase the practice of healthy behaviors (e.g. exercise, diet), improve aspects of health status (e.g. mood), and decrease health care utilization.

3. Change in knowledge is necessary *but* is rarely sufficient to bring about lasting changes in behaviors or health status.

4. Ability to self-manage is a key ingredient in effective patient education.

5. Patient education does not always impact on OA pain: rather the person's perceived ability to manage life with OA is enhanced (i.e. pain is a less dominant feature of the participant's life).

6. Long-term maintenance of behavior change is essential.

7. Effective education can be group or individualized, single- or multi-component, so long as participants perceive the content as salient.

References

(An asterisk denotes recommended reading.)

1. Bury, M. (1991). The sociology of chronic illness: a review of research and prospects. *Sociol Health Illness* **13**:451–68.

2. Corbin, J.M. and Strauss, A. (1988). *Unending work and care: managing chronic illness at home.* San Franciso: Jossey-Bass.

3. Hawley, D.J. and Wolfe, F. (1993). Depression is not more common in rheumatoid arthritis: a 10-year longitudinal study of 6153 patients with rheumatic disease. *J Rheumatol* **20**:2025–31.

4. Hampson, S.E., Glasgow, R.E., and Zeiss, A.M. (1994). Personal models of osteoarthritis and their relation to self-management activities and quality of life. *J Behav Med* **17**:143–58.

5. Tallon, D., Chard, J., and Dieppe, P. (2000). Exploring the priorities of patient with osteoarthritis of the knee. *Arthritis Care Res* **13**:312–19.

6. Lorig, K., Cox, T., Cuevas, Y., Kraines, R.G., and Britton, M.C. (1984). Converging and diverging beliefs about arthritis: Caucasian patients, Spanish-speaking patients and physicians. *J Rheumatol* **11**(1):76–9.

7. Dekker, J., Bot, B., Van der Woude, L.H.C., and Bijlsma, J.W.J. (1992). Pain and disability in osteoarthritis: a review of biobehavioral mechanisms. *J Behav Med* **15**(2):189–213.

8. Allegrante, J.P., Peterson, M.G.E., Kovar, P.A., and Gordon, K.A. (1990). Beliefs held by physicians and patients regarding compliance with treatment and educational needs in arthritis and musculoskeletal diseases. In *Proceedings of 25th Annual Meeting: Arthritis Health Professions Ass in Seattle*, WA, S204.

9. Hanumappa, S., Murphy, B.N., and Schumacher, H.R. (1988). Patient sources of information about treatment of arthritis. In *23rd Annual Meeting: Arthritis Health Professions Ass in Houston*, TX, S162.

10. Templeton, C.L., Petty, B.J., and Harter, J.L. (1978). Weight control—a group approach for arthritis clients. *J Nutritional Educ* **10**:33–5.

11. Jacobson, E. (1938). *Progressive relaxation.* Chicago: University of Chicago Press.

12. Lorig, K. and Fries, J. (1995). *The Arthritis Helpbook.* Reading: Addison-Wesley, pp. 191–206.

13. Basler, H.D. and Rehfisch, H.P. (1991). Cognitive-behavioral therapy in patients with ankylosing spondylitis in a German self-help organization. *J Psychosom Res* **35**:345–54.

14. Bradley, L.A., Young, L.D., Anderson, K.O., Turner, R.A., Agudelo, C.A., McDaniel, L.K., Pisko, E.J., Semble, E.L., and Morgan, T.M. (1987). Effects of psychological therapy on pain behaviour of rheumatoid arthritis patients: treatment outcome and six-month follow-up. *Arthritis Rheum* **30**:1105–14.

15. Parker, J.C., Frank, R.G., Beck, N.C., Finan, M., Walker, S., Hewett, J.E., Broster, C., Smarr, K., Smith, E., and Kay, D. (1988). Pain management in rheumatoid arthritis patients: a cognitive behavioral approach. *Arthritis Rheum* **31**:593–601.

16. Radojevic, V., Nicassio, P.M., and Weisman, M.H. (1992). Behavioral intervention with and without family support for rheumatoid arthritis. *Behav Therapy* **23**(1):13–30.

17. Laborde, J.M. and Powers, M.J. (1983). Evaluation of educational interventions for osteoarthritis. *Multiple Linear Regression Viewpoints* **12**:12–37.

18. Daltroy, L., Morlino, C., and Liang, M. (1989). Preoperative education for total hip and knee replacement patients. In *24th Annual Meeting: Arthritis Health Professions Association in Cincinnati*, OH, S193.

19. Calfas, K.J., Kaplan, R.M., and Ingram, R.E. (1992). One-year evaluation of cognitive-behavioral intervention in osteoarthritis. *Arthritis Care Res* **5**(4):202–9.

20. Keefe, F.J., Caldwell, D.S., Williams, D.A., Gil, K.M., Mitchell, D., *et al.* (1990). Pain coping and training in the management of osteoarthritic knee pain: a comparative study. *Behav Therapy* **21**:49–62.

21. Minor, M.A., Hewett, J.E., and Kay, D.R. (1986). Monitoring for harmful effects of physical conditioning exercise (PCE) with arthritis patients. *Arthritis Rheum* **29**:S144.

22. Minor, M.A., Hewett, J.E., Webel, R.R., Anderson, S.K., and Kay, D.R. (1989). Efficacy of physical conditioning exercise in patients with rheumatoid arthritis and osteoarthritis. *Arthritis Rheum* **23**(11):1396–405.

23. *Allegrante, J.P., Kovar, P.A., MacKenzie, C.R., Peterson, M.G.E., and Gutin, B. (1993). A walking education program for patients with osteoarthritis of the knee: theory and intervention strategies. *Health Educ Quarterly* **20**: 63–81.
    An excellent description of program development drawing on empirical and theoretical literature.

24. Kovar, P.A., Allegrante, J.P., MacKenzie, C.R., Peterson, M.G.E., and Gutin, B. (1992). Supervised fitness walking in patients with osteoarthritis of the knee: a randomized, controlled trial. *Ann Intern Med* **116**:529–34.

25. Sullivan, T., Allegrante, J.P., Peterson, M.G.E, Kovar, P.A., and MacKenzie, C.R. (1998). One-year follow-up of patients with osteoarthritis of the knee who participated in a program of supervised fitness walking and supportive patient education. *Arthritis Care Res* **11**:228–33.

26. Lorig, K. and Holman, H.R. (1993). Arthritis self-management studies: a twelve year review. *Health Educ Quarterly* **20**:17–28.
    A useful summary of the development and evaluation of the most widely used, community based arthritis self-management program.

27. Lorig, K., Gonzalez, V.M., and Ritter, P. (1999). Community-based Spanish language arthritis education program: a randomized trial. *Medical Care* **37**:957–63.

28. Lorig, K. and Holman, H. (1989). Long-term outcomes of an arthritis self-management study: effects of reinforcement efforts. *Soc Sci Med* **29**:221–4.

29. Lorig, K., Mazonson, P., and Holman, H. (1993). Evidence suggesting that health education for self-management in patients with chronic arthritis has sustained health benefits while reducing health care costs. *Arthritis Rheum* **36**(4):439–46.

30. Lorig, K., Seleznick, M., Lubeck, D., Ung, E., Chastain, R., and Holman, H.R. (1989). The beneficial outcomes of the arthritis self-management course are inadequately explained by behavior change. *Arthritis Rheum* **32**(1):91–5.

31. Barlow, J.H., Turner, A., and Wright, C.C. (2000). A Randomized Controlled Study of the Arthritis Self Management Program in the UK. *Health Educ Res: Theory Practice* **15**:665–80.

32. Barlow, J.H., Williams, B., and Wright, C. (1999). 'Instilling the strength to fight the pain and get on with life': learning to become an arthritis self-manager through an adult education program. *Health Educ Res: Theory Practice* **14**:533–44.

33. Barlow, J.H., Williams, R.G., and Wright, C. (1997). Improving arthritis self-management in older adults: 'just what the doctor didn't order'. *Br J Health Psychol* **2**:175–85.

34. Goeppinger, J., Brunk, S.E., Arthur, M.W., and Reidesel, S. (1987). The effectiveness of community-based arthritis self-care programs. *Arthritis Rheum* **30**:S194.

35. Goeppinger, J., Arthur, M.W., Baglioni, A.J., Brunk, S.E., and Hawdon, J.E. (1988). Effectiveness of arthritis self-care education: a longitudinal perspective. In *23rd Annual Meeting: Arthritis Health Professions Association in Houston*, TX, S155.

36. Goeppinger, J., Arthur, M.W., Baglioni, A.J., Brank, S.E., and Brunner, C.M. (1989). A re-examination of the effectiveness of self-care education for persons with arthritis. *Arthritis Rheum* **32**:706–16.

37. Bill-Harvey, D., Rippy, R., Abeles, M., Donald, M.J., Dawning, D., Ingemito, F., *et al.* (1989). Outcome of an osteoarthritis education program for low-literacy patients taught by indigenous instructors. *Patient Educ Counsel* **13**:133–42.

38. Lorig, K., Feigenbaum, P., Regan, C., Ung, E., and Holman, H.R. (1986). A comparison of lay-taught and professional-taught arthritis self-management courses. *J Rheumatol* **13**(4):763–7.

39. Cohen, J.L., Sauter, R., DeVellis, R.F., and DeVellis, B.M. (1986). Evaluation of arthritis self-management courses led by lay persons and by professionals. *Arthritis Rheum* **29**:388–93.

40. Doyle, T.H. and Granda, J.L. (1982). Influence of two management approaches on the health status of women with osteoarthritis. *Arthritis Rheum* **25**:S153.

41. Goeppinger, J., Macnee, C., Anderson, M.K., Boutaugh, M., and Stewart, K. (1995). From research to practice: the effects of jointly sponsored dissemination of an arthritis self-care nursing intervention. *Applied Nursing Res* **8**(3):106–13.

42. Weinberger, M., Tierney, W.M., Booker, P., and Katz, B. (1989). Can the provision of information to patients with osteoarthritis improve functional status. *Arthritis Rheum* **23**(12):1577–83.

43. Rippey, R.M., Bill, D., Abels, M., Day, J., Downing, D.S., Pfeiffer, C.A., *et al.* (1987). Computer-based patient education for older persons with osteoarthritis. *Arthritis Rheum* **30**(8):932–5.

44. Gale, F.M., Kirk, J.C., and Davis, R. (1994). Patient education and self-management: randomized study of effects on health status of a mail-delivered program. *Arthritis Rheum* **37**(9):S197.

45. Fries, J.F., Carey, C., and McShane, D.J. (1997). Patient education in arthritis: randomized controlled trial of a mail delivered program. *J Rheumatol* **27**:1378–83.

46. Daltroy, L.H., Katz, J.N., and Liang, M.H. (1992). Doctor-patient communications and adherence to arthritis treatments. *Arthritis Care Res* **5**:S19.

47. Mullen, P.D., Simons-Morton, D.G., Ramirez, G., *et al.* (1993). A meta-analysis of studies evaluating patient education for three groups of preventive behaviors. In *Prevention '93 in St. Louis*, MO.

9.14 Social support

Steven A. Mazzuca and Morris Weinberger

The relationship between the pathophysiology of OA and clinical outcomes of pain and functional impairment is complex.[1] Only 30–40 per cent of subjects with radiographic evidence of OA report significant joint pain.[2,3] While pain and function are related to the presence and radiographic severity of OA, persons with comparable radiographic changes experience markedly different levels of joint pain and dysfunction.[4,5] In his chapter on the reasons that patients with OA hurt (Chapter 7.3.2), Dr. Hadler asserts that persons with joint pain *decide* to become patients— who then acquire a diagnosis of OA if radiographs of the joint show appropriate changes— not because the experience of musculoskeletal pain is new, but because they have come to perceive that the quality or severity of their pain and related dysfunction have outstripped their capacity to cope effectively with it. Among the factors that influence one's capacity to cope with, and counteract, the effects of joint pain is social support. This chapter describes social support as a potential moderator and/or mediator of joint pain and functional impairment in OA. It summarizes research evidence concerning the capacity of social support to enhance the effectiveness of therapeutic interventions in OA, describes some practical methods, based on previous research, for assessing and utilizing social support in practice and offers some guidelines for monitoring and minimizing the burden of support of the patient by family members and friends.

Overview of social support

For decades, social scientists have hypothesized that, persons who are exposed to stressful life events (for example, death of a loved one, divorce, marriage, childbirth, onset of a chronic or life-threatening illness) experience worse health outcomes than those who avoid major stressors. However, the strength of the observed correlations between exposure to stressful life events and health parameters is only modest. This consistent observation has led social scientists to explore factors that may influence the stress–health relationship. One of the factors that has been examined as a potential explanatory factor is variation between patients in the amount or nature of social support available to them.

What is social support?

Social support is generally defined as the gratification of basic social needs through interactions with others.[6] Within the context of health, social support refers to processes by which interpersonal relationships promote physical, social, and emotional well being.[7] Like many terms used by social scientists, 'social support' has come to be used commonly in other research disciplines and by the general public. This is a double-edged sword, however. While common usage of the term assures a broad appreciation of its importance, the popularity of the term also makes communication of precise operational definitions of social support and, therefore, implications of research findings, more difficult.

Two theoretical approaches to social support are popular today among social scientists. The *social network approach* emphasizes the quantifiable, structural characteristics of support systems.[8,9] This approach assumes that factors such as the size of a social network and the frequency with which members contact one another are critical. All social ties, which an individual possesses, are assumed to be both accessible and supportive. An alternative conceptualization represents a *functional approach* to understanding support systems.[10,11] This approach emphasizes discrete types of support and the degree to which each type of basic social need is fulfilled by one or more persons. As such, this latter approach makes qualitative distinctions among the types of support from which a person may benefit. For patients with chronic medical conditions, supportive functions include:[12]

1. *Esteem support* to promote feelings of self-esteem, belonging, and acceptance, despite difficulties or personal faults (also known as emotional support);

2. *Informational support* to assure understanding of the medical condition and an accurate appraisal of prognosis and the risks and benefits of treatment options;

3. *Instrumental support* in the form of financial and other tangible assistive services (e.g., help with transportation and other activities of daily living);

4. *Social companionship*, which, while lacking the emotional aspects of esteem support, may provide beneficial sources of distraction from worries and promote positive affect.

Social network and functional approaches are not antithetical. They may provide different, but complementary, information.[13] Social networks reflect support that is potentially available (that is, the totality of the social resources from which persons may draw), while functionally defined support better represents the resources actually used in response to specific stressors.

How does social support operate to maintain health?

Two causal models are currently used by social science researchers attempting to explain how social support influences health (Fig. 9.29). The *additive* or *main-effects model* posits that social support is beneficial, regardless of the stress level of a person.[14–16] Within this theoretical perspective, it is generally hypothesized that, by providing individuals with an overall sense of well-being and a recognition of self-worth, a supportive social network prevents, or directly counterbalances, the negative effects of stressors—thereby affording a measure of protection against poor health outcomes.

In contrast, the *buffering model* (Fig. 9.29) asserts that social support influences health only when a stressor is present.[12,17,18] Accordingly, when an individual is exposed to a potential stressor, sources of functional support can be tapped to attenuate the perceived threat to well-being and/or to mount effective emotional and behavioral coping responses to counteract any negative health-related sequelae. However, the buffering model maintains that, in the absence of stress, social support does not affect health.

Who can provide social support?

Regardless of how social support is defined or how it operates to maintain health (as a prophylaxis against stress, in general, or as a buffer against

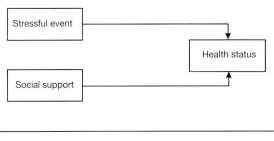

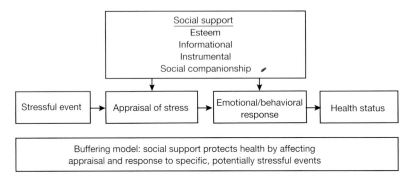

Fig. 9.29 Alternative theoretical models of the effects of social support on health status.

specific stressors), a further distinction between the sources of social support is important.

Social scientists differentiate between primary and secondary social groups. *Primary social groups* are composed of persons involved in personal, intimate, and non-specialized relationships (e.g., families). While primary group members often develop close, intimate, and enduring relationships with each other, primary relationships are not always loving or supportive. Primary group members need not live in close physical proximity, but periodic interaction is necessary to maintain primary group status.

In contrast, members of *secondary social groups* relate to one other in the context of limited, specific roles (e.g, as coworkers). In secondary groups, members have few emotional bonds and ties are impersonal; relationships are task-oriented and members associate to achieve specific, practical goals; interactions are more superficial and utilitarian than in primary groups.

Adapting these definitions, potential *primary sources of social support* are generally considered to be the family of the patient and close friends. Persons capable of functioning as primary sources of social support usually comprise a limited group of individuals with whom the patient shares deeply personal, often intimate, relationships. The support offered by primary sources is non-specialized; that is, primary sources can perform a variety of emotional, informational, tangible, and social functions. In contrast, *secondary sources of social support* are usually a larger group of less intimate acquaintances who can offer context-specific, but nevertheless valuable, support (e.g., health care professionals, members of peer-support groups). Notably, through repeated contact over time, secondary sources of social support can evolve into primary sources.

Research on social support in arthritis

To date, research on the effects of social support on outcomes in arthritis has been dominated by investigations of patients with rheumatoid arthritis (RA). Even though patients with RA and OA differ with respect to clinical, therapeutic, and demographic characteristics, to the extent that patients

with either disease must cope with stressful life events, joint pain, and the prospect of progressive dysfunction, several conclusions about social support and RA may generalize to patients with OA:

1. In numerous observational studies (both cross-sectional and longitudinal) comparing patients with differing levels of social support, patients with higher levels of support also reported more effective coping strategies,[19] greater psychological adjustment to illness,[20] greater self-esteem,[21] fewer depressive symptoms,[22–24] and higher levels of life satisfaction.[25]

2. The participation of family and friends (primary sources of social support) in cognitive-behavioral therapy for arthritis patients can enhance the capacity of such interventions to reduce the psychological impact of arthritis[26] and prolong initial therapeutic response to treatment.[27]

3. Instruction of patients on how to communicate their needs for support to family members can increase compliance[28] and a sense of control over pain.[29]

4. The beneficial effects of social support are more consistently seen in psychological and behavioral outcomes than in changes in pain and functional impairment.[7]

Observational studies in osteoarthritis

A limited number of observational studies of social support in OA have been published, the results of which are consistent with several of the above generalizations from studies of RA. Summers *et al.*[30] demonstrated that psychological variables are stronger correlates of joint pain in patients with hip and knee OA than are objective (radiographic) indicators of disease severity. While social support *per se* was not among the psychological variables included in that study, the variables that were included (depression, anxiety, coping style) are all related to social support.

In a longitudinal study of 193 patients with OA, Weinberger *et al.*[31] found that patients' satisfaction with their social support was more strongly related to the presence of identifiable sources of their functional support than to the size, or level of activity, of their overall social network. However, neither functional nor structural aspects of social support were found to buffer the effects of stressors on health outcomes over an interval of six months.

This investigation was followed by a larger study ($n = 439$) of the direct benefits of social support in OA.[32] In this study, low self-esteem was associated with joint pain, physical disability, and psychological disability. In addition, physical disability was related to a lack of tangible support, and the absence of a sense of belonging was inversely related to psychological health. These relationships were independent of the effects of stress, that is, the data were consistent with a direct main effect (rather than a buffering effect) of social support on health.

Prospective intervention studies targeted at patients with OA indicate a clearly positive role for social support in explaining health outcomes. In two such studies, social support was shown to be a factor in the long-term response of OA patients to treatment. Calfas et al.[33] evaluated a cognitive-behavioral modification intervention designed to teach OA patients to become more aware of the thoughts, beliefs, and actions engendered by their joint pain; to avoid overestimating the threat represented by that pain; to believe they can cope effectively; and to adapt their behaviors to control pain and maintain function. While only immediate post-intervention improvements in quality of life could be attributed to the intervention, structural social support and mobility at baseline were the only significant (inverse) predictors of depressive symptoms 12 months after intervention.

Using a different form of non-pharmacological treatment of arthritis, Minor et al.[34] showed that aerobic walking and aquatic exercise programs (three 60-minute sessions per week for 12 weeks) had significant positive effects on physical and emotional function in patients with OA or RA. In a secondary analysis of self-directed maintenance of the exercise routines by the subjects, the investigators determined that the perceived support of friends for continued exercise was a significant predictor of exercise behavior 9 months after completion of the study intervention;[35] by 18 months, social support was no longer a direct predictor of self-directed behavior. However, at that point, prior exercise behavior (to which social support had contributed) became a significant determinant.

Social support as a non-pharmacological intervention in osteoarthritis

The literature contains several controlled evaluations of educational interventions for patients with OA, in which elements of the design of the intervention were intended to facilitate support of patients by family members, friends, or peers. While the discrete effects of such elements cannot be teased out of the overall results, their support-engendering potential is noteworthy, nevertheless.

The most widely documented model for arthritis patient education is the Arthritis Self-Management Program (ASMP) designed and tested by Lorig and colleagues at Stanford University.[36,37] Now disseminated in the United States of America, Canada, Australia, and New Zealand, the basic paradigm for the ASMP is a series of 6 two-hour sessions that combine conventional topics of patient education (e.g., disease processes, exercise, side effects of drugs) with cognitive-behavioral techniques (e.g., relaxation exercises, contracting for explicit changes in self-management behaviors). Participation of family members is encouraged, but the discrete effects of such participation have not been documented. Participants are led through a communication exercise in which they learn to elicit support from family and friends. Most notable is the fact that the ASMP is designed to be led by an autonomous lay person who is also an arthritis patient. Formative evaluation data from early trials of the ASMP showed greater knowledge gains among participants in sessions led by health professionals, but greater implementation of self-care behaviors (e.g, relaxation techniques) in sessions with lay leaders.[38]

Kovar et al.[39] published a trial in which the intervention (supervised walking and patient education for patients with symptomatic knee OA) included social support from secondary sources. The authors designed the 8-week intervention (three 90-minute sessions per week) to include both

supportive encouragement by the intervention facilitator (a physical therapist) and peer interactions during educational and walking sessions.[40] In comparison with subjects in an attention-control group, patients participating in the walking/education program exhibited significant improvements in walking capacity, functional status, and joint pain.[39]

Interventions designed to improve social support

More direct evidence for the beneficial effects of social support can be found in a series of reports by Weinberger et al.[41–43] In an early study of social support in OA, subjects (193 patients with knee and/or hip OA) were telephoned bi-weekly for 6 months by a research assistant, to document current stressors, social support, and arthritis outcomes.[31] An uncontrolled (and unexpected) observation in this study was that social support and functional status parameters both improved significantly over the 6 months.[41] This observation led to the hypothesis that periodic communication between lay personnel and patients, about the status of their OA, could serve a beneficial, supportive function.

The hypothesis was tested directly in a randomized controlled trial of various strategies for achieving periodic communication between trained lay personnel and OA patients for the purpose of reviewing the health of the subject.[42] Contacts were structured to assure a uniform set of inquiries concerning medications (compliance, adequacy of supply); joint pain; presence of gastrointestinal symptoms; status of acute symptoms due to comorbid conditions (e.g., hypertension, diabetes, cardiac or pulmonary disease); recall of the next scheduled outpatient visit; barriers to keeping clinic appointments; and recall of an 'after-hours' telephone number at which healthcare providers could be reached. Two formats for delivery of the intervention were studied: a monthly telephone call and an in-person interview at each scheduled clinic visit, immediately prior to seeing the physician. Four hundred thirty-nine patients with OA were assigned randomly to one of four treatment conditions: telephone intervention, in-clinic intervention, both telephone and in-clinic intervention, or neither (a pure control group).

After one year of contacts and informational support under their assigned conditions, subjects in the groups receiving monthly telephone calls exhibited significant improvement in joint pain and physical function. In contrast, the in-clinic intervention was not beneficial and, in fact, had an adverse effect on physical health.[42] Several possible explanations may be offered for this observation. Perhaps most importantly, the clinic may be a poor setting in which to deliver such interventions. When patients have an appointment with their physician, the busy clinical environment and thoughts about the primary purpose of the visit may undermine efforts to provide support. In contrast, telephone calls were made at times convenient for the patient—if the patient was busy or feeling ill, interviewers were instructed to call back at a more convenient time.

It is especially noteworthy that the effects of the telephone intervention were strongest among those patients who were maintained on a stable medical regimen throughout the study.[43] The magnitude of experimental effects on pain and physical function (65 and 53 per cent of the respective pooled standard deviations) for this subsample of subjects was more than twice that found in the study as a whole. Effects of this size compare favorably to the results of open-label trials of non-steroidal anti-inflammatory drugs.[44]

More recently, two other models of social support intervention have been evaluated in patients with OA. Keefe et al.[45] evaluated the effects of participation by spouses of patients with knee OA in coping skills training (CST). Eighty-eight OA patients with persistent knee pain were randomly assigned to 1 of 3 conditions: (1) CST for OA pain with both patient and spouse in attendance, (2) a conventional CST intervention with no spousal involvement, or (3) an arthritis education spousal support (AE-SS) control group. All treatment was carried out in 10 weekly, 2-hour group sessions. The results indicated that after completion of treatment, patients whose spouses participated with them in CST had significantly lower levels of pain, psychological disability and pain behavior, and higher scores on measures of coping attempts, marital adjustment, and self-efficacy, than patients in the AE-SS control condition. Compared to the control group, patients who participated alone in CST (without spouse involvement) had significantly higher post-treatment levels of self-efficacy and marital adjustment. However, levels of pain and psychological disability in the CST group improved only marginally, compared to the controls.

In addition, Cronan et al.[46,47] examined the effects of social support and educational interventions designed to promote appropriate usage of health care resources in a health maintenance organization (HMO) by patients with OA. Both interventions, alone and in combination, were evaluated with respect to health care costs over three years, in comparison with those generated by a control (no intervention) group. The social support intervention consisted of 10 weekly group sessions of two hours duration, followed by 10 monthly sessions. The sessions consisted of unstructured group discussion and were designed to foster empathy, cohesiveness, participation and sharing of information, and coping techniques among group members. While there were no significant changes in health status in treatment or control groups between baseline and annual post-intervention assessments,[47] health care costs in the groups receiving either or both interventions were lower, on average, than those in the control group by $1279/participant/year over 3 years.[48] Implementation of the social support intervention was less expensive than implementation of either the educational or combined interventions. However, attrition in the social support group was greater than in the education group.

Social support in clinical practice

Assessment of social support

To our knowledge, currently available instruments for the measurement of quantitative and functional aspects of social support have not been validated for 'real-world' clinical use. Nevertheless, the basic definitions and causal assumptions about the interrelatedness of social support and well-being provide an adequate framework within which social support can be assessed briefly, as a part of the patient history, by asking the following questions:

- Are you married?
- Are there other family members or friends with whom you keep close contact?
- To whom do you talk when something is bothering you?
- Whose advice do you trust for information about your health?
- On whom do you count when you need help doing something?
- What do you do socially for recreation or relaxation?

Structural issues of social support include the marital status of the patient and the number and roles of persons other than a spouse (e.g., friends, and other family members) with whom the patient maintains close or frequent contact. Membership in a church congregation or in social organizations may be suggestive of the types of supportive environments and activities available to the patient. As an added measure, questions about specific supportive functions (that is, emotional, tangible, informational, companionship) may identify areas of need that are currently unmet.

Enhancement of social support in care of the patient with OA

With the exception of the social support interventions designed by Weinberger et al.[42] and Keefe et al.,[45] specific protocols or guidelines for addressing social support in clinical practice have not been subjected to controlled evaluation among patients with OA. Nevertheless, published evidence of the effects of social support in OA care,[31–33,35] and general social support dynamics implicit in previous intervention studies in RA[26–29] and OA,[38,39] offer a firm basis for a systematic approach to addressing social support in clinical practice. Elements of that approach can be listed as follows:

1. Include the primary support-giver (usually the spouse) in discussions regarding prognosis, self-care recommendations, and drug and side effects;

2. Have the support-giver accompany the patient to self-care education programs;

3. Monitor the continued functionality of the relationship between patient and support-giver;

4. Encourage the support-giver to maintain social ties outside the relationship/marriage;

5. Consider specific functional requirements of the patient for assistance by community service organizations with respect to transportation, nutrition, and other activities;

6. Between office visits, implement periodic (e.g., monthly) telephone calls from office staff to monitor the patient's health status and effects and side effects of therapy, and to reinforce self-care;

7. Be alert to the need for peer support or a mental health professional for the support-giver during times of high stress.

When the social history of a patient reveals a primary relationship with an individual who is committed to the general well being of that patient, every effort should be made to permit that individual to fulfill his or her role as a primary support-giver. With the permission of the patient, the person primarily entrusted with a supportive role should be present during any discussions between physician and patient in which information regarding prognosis, self-care recommendations, expected effects of treatment, and side effects of medications is provided. To the extent that primary support-givers are able to participate in the clinical encounter, the information that is shared will enable them to anticipate the stresses the patient will endure and to adapt existing support schemes to accommodate the new demands of drug therapy, exercise regimens, and adherence to principles of joint protection. Most free standing programs of arthritis self-care education (e.g., the ASMP) permit, but do not require, attendance of 'significant others.' Patients enrolling in such programs should be encouraged to attend with their primary support-giver.

Research on the interrelationships among patients with RA and their family members has revealed several pitfalls in the mustering of social support which, on face value, bear mention in the context of care for OA. Either by their own limitations, or because of temporary and uncontrollable circumstances, primary support-givers cannot always be counted upon to be unfailing sources of help and encouragement. Among the real or perceived behaviors of family and friends that can, at times, be detrimental to the well being of the patient are the trivialization of symptoms, pessimistic comments, and over-solicitousness.[20] For some patients, social support may be helpful only as a buffer against stress (e.g., a flare of disease activity); as the stress subsides, the otherwise supportive actions of others can be perceived as threats to the sense of autonomy and self-esteem of the patient.[48] The clinician should assess, periodically, the functionality of relationships between OA patients and family members or other support-givers to identify early on changes that may compromise the patient's ability to cope with OA. If current arrangements for specific supportive functions (e.g., tangible support, social companionship) cannot be repaired and maintained, alternative sources of functional support need to be considered (see below).

The clinician who utilizes social support in practice must recognize that support-givers pay an emotional cost to fulfill their roles. This is a particular concern when support-givers are elderly and have their own array of medical conditions, or when children of elderly adults with OA have obligations to their own families. In such cases, the support-givers themselves are subject to stress. Interviewing the spouses of patients with RA, Revenson and Majerovitz[49] found that support-givers often feel burdened and are hesitant to reveal the stress of their role to their spouse (that is, the patient). Many support-givers find they can be more helpful to their spouse if they maintain and nurture social ties outside the marriage. Also, with the help of support groups or mental health professionals, about a third of the spouses of patients with RA learn to cope with the prolonged burden of their roles.[49]

Physicians and their staff should consider themselves the chief source of *informational support* for all patients (and their support-givers) coping with OA. This responsibility extends beyond the disclosure of essential information required during routine office visits to enable patients to make informed choices about their treatment. As demonstrated by Weinberger *et al.*,[42] periodic contact by telephone for the purpose of assessing the health status of the patient and reinforcing self-care can have dramatic, beneficial effects on the physical and psychological well-being of patients with OA—over and above routine clinical contact.

The responsibility of the clinician also entails making patients and their care givers aware of community service organizations specializing in *instrumental support*, in the forms of transportation, nutrition, personal hygiene, and other domestic needs of the elderly and infirm. While health care professionals strive to provide a degree of *emotional support* to all patients, this need may be greatest for elderly OA patients who, because of widowhood or the death of close friends, may have no primary source of social support. Older OA patients may have support-givers who are themselves elderly or burdened by other commitments (e.g., the child of a patient with OA may also be a parent). In such cases, clinicians can facilitate access to secondary sources of support. For example, many community hospitals maintain mutual support groups for patients with specific diseases and their family members. Such opportunities are available also through local volunteer health organizations, such as the Arthritis Foundation. Many local churches include multi-functional service to the elderly among their missions.

Finally, the Internet represents a vast resource permitting interaction among people with a common interest. Between December 1998 and August 2000, the percentage of American households with Internet access rose from 26.2–41.5 per cent—a 58% increase in less than 2 years.[50] Most volunteer health organizations (and many doctors' offices) have web sites. In addition to providing extensive patient information on OA, the Arthritis Foundation web site also contains a series of 'message boards' on which people with a common interest (e.g., coping skills, women and arthritis, surgery) can post questions and comments and receive feedback from others.[51] While accessibility of the Internet in minority households and among the elderly has lagged somewhat, relative to that in other segments of the population, experts project that penetration of the Internet into all segments of our society will continue to grow for the foreseeable future.[50] Therefore, the ability to provide sound advice about informational or other supportive resources on the Internet will become increasingly important as more patients go online.

Summary

Social support is the gratification of basic social needs through interactions with others. A large and active network of persons providing social support to an individual can counteract the effects of daily stress on the patient's sense of general well being. In addition, when a patient is faced with a specific stressor (e.g., an exacerbation of joint pain), specific types of functional support (i.e., emotional, informational, tangible, social companionship) can help the patient maintain an accurate perspective when appraising the new threat to well-being and mount effective coping responses. The size of a patient's social network and availability of specific types of functional support are easily obtainable in the patient's history. Involvement of key individuals who have insight into the stresses faced by the patient and the patient's typical response to stress may improve the ability of the patient to cope effectively with chronic pain and dysfunction. The evidence clearly supports the proposition that provision of informational support and interim monitoring of patient progress (e.g., by a brief telephone call) results in improved patient outcomes.

Key points

1. A large and active network of persons providing social support to an individual can counteract the effects of daily stress on the individual's sense of general well being.

2. When a patient is faced with a specific stressor (e.g., an exacerbation of joint pain) the accurate appraisal of the new threat to well being and the implementation of effective coping responses can be facilitated by provision of appropriate functional support (i.e., emotional, informational, instrumental, social companionship).

3. Information relevant to the characterization of a patient's social network and the availability of specific types of functional support is easily obtainable in the patient's history.

4. Involvement of key individuals who have insight into the stresses faced by the patient and into the patient's typical response to stress may improve the ability of the patient to cope effectively with chronic pain and dysfunction.

5. Informational support from health professionals and interim monitoring of patient progress results in improved patient outcomes.

Acknowledgment

Supported in part by grants from the National Institutes of Health (AR20582, AR43348, AR43370).

References

(An asterisk denotes recommended reading.)

1. Hadler, N.M. (1992). Knee pain is the malady—not osteoarthritis. *Ann Intern Med* **116**:598–9.

2. Lawrence, J.S., Bremner, J.M., and Bier, F. (1966). Osteoarthrosis, prevalence in the population and relationship between symptoms and X-ray changes. *Ann Rheum Dis* **25**:1–24.

3. Cobbs, S., Merchant, W.R., and Rubin, T. (1957). The relationship of symptoms to osteoarthritis. *J Chron Dis* **5**:197–204.

4. Davis, M.A., Ettinger, W.H., Neuhaus, J.M., and Mallon, K.P. (1991). Knee osteoarthritis and physical functioning: evidence from the NHANES I Epidemiologic Followup Study. *J Rheumatol* **18**:591–8.

5. Davis, M.A., Ettinger, W.H., Neuhaus, J.M., Barclay, J.D., and Segal, M.R. (1992). Correlates of knee pain among US adults with and without radiographic knee osteoarthritis. *J Rheumatol* **19**:1943–9.

6. Kaplan, B.H., Cassel, J.C., and Gore, S. (1977). Social support and health. *Medical Care* **15**:47–58.

7. Lanza, A.F. and Revenson, T.A. (1993). Social support interventions for rheumatoid arthritis patients: the cart before the horse? *Health Edu Q* **20**:97–117.

8. Berkman, L.F. and Syme, L. (1979). Social networks, host resistance, and mortality: a nine-year follow-up study of Alameda County residents. *Am J Epidemiol* **109**:186–204.

9. Mitchell, R.E. and Trickett, E.J. (1980). Social networks as mediators of social support: an analysis of the effects and determinants of social networks. *Com Mental Health J* **16**:27–44.

10. Sarason, I.G., Levine, H.M., Basham, R.B., and Sarason, B.R. (1983). Assessing social support: the social support questionnaire. *J Personality Social Psychol* **44**:127–39.

11. Porritt, D. (1979). Social support in crisis: quantity or quality. *Soc Sci Med* **13**(A):715–21.

12. *Cohen, S. and Willis, T.A. (1985). Stress, social support, and the buffering hypothesis. *Psychol Bull* **98**:310–57.
    This review of the literature on social support presents evidence for alternative theoretical models of the mechanism of action of social support in promoting health.

13. Pearlin, L.I. (1989). The sociological study of stress. *J Health Social Behav* **30**:241–56.

14. Blazer, D. (1982). Social support and mortality in an elderly community population. *Am J Epidemiol* **115**:684–94.

15. Norris, F.H. and Murrell, S.A. (1984). Protective function of resources related to life events, global stress, and depression in older adults. *J Health Soc Behav* **25**:424–37.

16. Williams, A.W., Ware, J.E., and Donald, C.A. (1981). A model of mental health, life events, and social support applicable to general populations. *J Health Soc Behav* **22**:324–36.

17. Dean, A. and Lin, N. (1977). The stress-buffering role of social support: problems and prospects for systematic investigation. *J Nerve Mental Disord* **165**:403–17.

18. Dohrenwend, B.S. and Dohrenwend, B.P. (1978). Some issues in research on stressful life events. *J Nerve Mental Disord* **168**:7–15.

19. Manne, S.L. and Zautra, A.J. (1989). Spouse criticism and support: their association with coping and psychological adjustment among women with rheumatoid arthritis. *J Personality Soc Psychol* **56**:608–17.

20. Affleck, G., Pfeiffer, C., Tennen, H., and Fifield, J. (1988). Social support and psychological adjustment to rheumatoid arthritis. *Soc Sci Med* **27**:71–7.

21. Fitzpatrick, R., Newman, S., Lamb, R., and Shipley, M. (1988). Social relationships and psychological well-being in rheumatoid arthritis. *Soc Sci Med* **27**:399–403.

22. Brown, G.K., Wallston, K.A., and Nicassio, P.M. (1989). Social support and depression in rheumatoid arthritis: a one-year prospective study. *J Appl Soc Psychol* **19**:1164–81.

23. Fitzpatrick, R., and Newman, S., Archer, R., and Shipley, M. (1991). Social support, disability and depression: a longitudinal study of rheumatoid arthritis. *Soc Sci Med* **33**:605–11.

24. Goodenow, C., Reisine, S.T., and Grady, K.E. (1990). Quality of social support and associated social and psychological functioning in women with rheumatoid arthritis. *Health Psychol* **9**:266–84.

25. Smith, C.A., Dobbins, C.J., and Wallston, K.A. (1991). The mediational role of perceived competence in psychological adjustment to rheumatoid arthritis. *J Appl Soc Psychol* **21**:1218–47.

26. Bradley, L.A., Young, L.D., and Anderson, K.O., *et al.* (1987). Effects of psychological therapy on pain behavior of rheumatoid arthritis patients. *Arthritis Rheum* **30**:1105–14.

27. Radojevic, V., Nicassio, P.M., and Weisman, M.H. (1992). Behavioral intervention with and without family support for rheumatoid arthritis. *Behav Ther* **23**:13–30.

28. DeVellis, B.M., Blalock, S.J., Hahn, P.M., DeVellis, R.F., and Hochbaum, G.M. (1988). Evaluation of a problem-solving intervention for patients with arthritis. *Patient Edu Couns* **11**:29–42.

29. Parker, J.C., Frank, R.G., Beck, N.C., *et al.* (1988). Pain management in rheumatoid arthritis patients: a cognitive-behavioral approach. *Arthritis Rheum* **31**:593–601.

30. Summers, M.N., Haley, W.E., Reveille, J.D., and Alarcon, G.S. (1988). Radiographic assessment and psychological variables as predictors of pain and function in osteoarthritis of the knee or hip. *Arthritis Rheum* **31**:204–9.

31. Weinberger, M., Hiner, S.L., and Tierney, W.M. (1987). Assessing social support in elderly adults. *Soc Sci Med* **25**:1049–55.

32. Weinberger, M., Tierney, W.M., Booher, P., and Hiner, S.L. (1990). Social support, stress and functional status in patients with osteoarthritis. *Soc Sci Med* **30**:503–8.

33. Calfas, K.J., Kaplan, R.M., and Ingram, R.E. (1992). One-year evaluation of cognitive-behavioral intervention in osteoarthritis. *Arthritis Care Res* **5**:202–9.

34. Minor, M.A., Hewett, J.E., Webel, R.R., Anderson, S.K., and Kay, D.R. (1989). Efficacy of physical conditioning exercise in patients with rheumatoid arthritis or osteoarthritis. *Arthritis Rheum* **32**:1396–405.

35. Minor, M.A. and Brown, J.D. (1993). Exercise maintenance of persons with arthritis after participation in a class experience. *Health Edu Q* **20**:83–95.

36. Lorig, K., Lubeck, D., Kraines, R.G., Seleznick, M., and Holman, H.R. (1985). Outcomes of self-help education for patients with arthritis. *Arthritis Rheum* **28**:680–5.

37. Lorig, K. and Holman, H.R. (1989). Long-term outcomes of an arthritis self-management study: effects of reinforcement efforts. *Soc Sci Med* **29**:221–4.

38. Lorig, K., Feigenbaum, P., Regan, C., Ung, E., Chastain, R.L., and Holman, H.R. (1986). Comparison of lay-taught and professional-taught arthritis self-management courses. *J Rheumatol* **13**:763–7.

39. *Kovar, P.A., Allegrante, J.P., MacKenzie, C.R., Peterson, M.G.E., Gutin, B., and Charlson, M.E. (1992). Supervised fitness walking in patients with osteoarthritis of the knee. *Ann Intern Med* **116**:529–34.

   This study illustrates how the social support derived from participation in a group exercise program may contribute to improved health outcomes in patients with OA.

40. Allegrante, J.P., Kovar, P.A., MacKenzie, C.R., Peterson, M.G.E., and Gutin, B. (1993). A walking education program for patients with osteoarthritis of the knee: theory and intervention strategies. *Health Edu Q* **20**:63–81.

41. Weinberger, M., Hiner, S.L., and Tierney, W.M. (1986). Improving functional status in osteoarthritis: the effect of social support. *Soc Sci Med* **23**:899–904.

42. *Weinberger, M., Tierney, W.M., Booher, P., and Katz, B.P. (1989). Can provision of information to patients with osteoarthritis improve functional status? A randomized, controlled trial. *Arthritis Rheum* **32**:1577–83.

   This is the first published randomized controlled trial of a social support intervention in OA. The results of this study have been highly influential in the development of guidelines for management of OA.

43. *René, J., Weinberger, M., Mazzuca, S.A., Brandt, K.D., and Katz, B.P. (1992). Monthly telephone contacts with lay personnel reduce join pain in patients with knee osteoarthritis maintained on stable medical management. *Arthritis Rheum* **35**:511–15.

   This secondary analysis of data from the original article by Weinberger and colleagues (above) provides evidence that the beneficial effects of social support are direct and not mediated (or confounded) by changes in other aspects of OA management, such as changes in NSAID treatment.

44. Anderson, J.J., Firschein, H.E., and Meenan, R.F. (1989). Sensitivity of a health status measure to short-term clinical changes in arthritis. *Arthritis Rheum* **32**:844–50.

45. *Keefe, F.J., Caldwell, D.S., Baucom, D., *et al.* (1996). Spouse-assisted coping skills training in the management of osteoarthritic knee pain. *Arthritis Care Res* **9**:279–91.

   This study illustrates how involvement of the patient's spouse in promoting effective coping strategies can improve patient outcomes.

46. Cronan, T.A., Groessl, E., and Kaplan, R.M. (1997). The effects of social support and education interventions on health care costs. *Arthritis Care Res* **10**:99–110.

47. Cronan, T.A., Hay, M., Groessl, E., Bigatti, S., Gallagher, R., and Tomita, M. (1998). The effects of social support and education on health care costs after three years. *Arthritis Care Res* **11**:326–34.

48. Cohen, S. (1988). Psychological models of the role of social support in the etiology of physical disease. *Health Psychol* **7**:269–97.

49. Revenson, T.A. and Majerovitz, S.D. (1990). Spouse's support provision to chronically ill patients. *J Soc Personal Relationships* **7**:575–86.

50. U.S. Department of Commerce. National Telecommunications and Information Administration. Falling through the net: toward digital inclusion. Available at: http://www.ntia.doc.gov/ntiahome/fttn00/contents00.html

51. Arthritis Foundation. Communities. Available at: http://www.arthritis.org/communities/default.asp

9.15 Depression in osteoarthritis

Dennis C. Ang and Kurt Kroenke

As the population ages, OA and depression are becoming increasingly common concerns for primary care physicians. Pain and decreased mobility, two important symptoms of OA, can lead to changes in psychological status and social functioning. Due to the unidimensional focus on the biomedical model of OA, many physicians evaluate and treat only the physical illness and fail to diagnose concomitant depression. Many patients with depression selectively focus on the somatic components of their depressive syndrome and minimize or even deny affective and cognitive symptoms. When depression occurs in patients with OA, its recognition and treatment are particularly important for good outcomes. This chapter discusses the complex interaction between symptoms of OA and depression, and suggests interventions to improve the diagnostic and therapeutic acumen of the primary care physicians.

Depression in general medical patients

Medical conditions are associated with an increased risk of depressive symptoms and disorders, particularly when the illness is chronic. Among outpatients in general medicine clinics, most studies have found the prevalence of active depression to be approximately 5–10 per cent,[1,2] with one report noting a 20 per cent prevalence among those who utilized health care extensively.[3] Depressed patients make more office visits and more telephone calls to their physicians, undergo more tests and evaluations, take more medications, and are more likely to be hospitalized for medical disorders than patients who are not.[4] The individual and societal burdens of depression are enormous in terms of: their economic costs (over $40 billion annually in the United States of America); disability days; and their pervasive effects on physical, mental and social well being.[5,6]

Overall, the primary care physician may fail to make the diagnosis of depression in at least 50 per cent of cases.[7] Underdetection also occurs in patients with OA; in a study of 200 consecutive patients with OA of the hip or knee, general practitioners significantly underestimated functional disability, anxiety, and depression in 50–70 per cent.[8] Given the propensity for the depressed patient to present with physical complaints, recognition of depression in the patient with chronic diseases remains a challenge.

A variety of instruments have been developed to facilitate identification of affective disorders. The 21-item Beck Depression Inventory, 20-item Zung Self-Assessment Depression Scale and 20-item Center for Epidemiologic Studies Depression Screen have been used widely to screen for depression.[9] Although much effort has gone into the development of these efficient and reliable standardized symptom-report measures, they are not intended for use as diagnostic instruments for case identification, but are measures of the severity of depressive symptoms. High scores require confirmation of a diagnosis of depression by additional inquiry about the presence of criteria of major depression[10] (Table 9.32). Five or more of the symptoms enumerated in Table 9.32, including depressed mood or loss of interest or pleasure, are required to make a diagnosis of *major depression*. Patients with fewer symptoms, but a history of such symptoms for more than at least 2 years, are classified as having *dysthymia*, a chronic form of depression. Those with depressed mood (anhedonia) and at least two other

DSM-IV depressive symptoms, but not a chronic history (2 or more years), are classified as having *minor depression*.

The PHQ-9 (Fig. 9.30) is a nine-item depression scale from the newly validated Patient Health Questionnaire based on the DSM-IV criteria for the diagnoses of depressive disorders. In addition to its utility as a diagnostic instrument, the PHQ-9 may be used to assess the severity of depressive symptoms. Cutpoints of 5, 10, 15, and 20 represent mild, moderate, moderately severe, and severe depression, respectively.[11] Alternatively, a single sensitive screening question, 'Have you been bothered by feeling down or depressed?' may be used to identify depressive states.[12] Patients who answer affirmatively can then be questioned about additional features for major depression.

Depressive symptoms that do not meet the criteria for major depression are sometimes characterized as subthreshold depression and are more prevalent than major depression. Subthreshold depression is associated with as much or more impairment in social and occupational functioning than major depression[13] and may explain some of the variations in pain reported by individuals with OA.

Primary care providers tend to attribute subthreshold depressive symptoms to coexisting medical disorders and are less likely to treat these symptoms than major depression.[14] Untreated subthreshold depression can amplify somatic symptoms and disability in the chronically ill patient. Among those with OA, evaluation of depressive symptoms is further complicated by the overlap between symptoms attributable to OA (e.g., pain) and those attributable to depression (e.g., diminished interest in activities because of pain). This makes it even more important for physicians caring for such patients to understand how to best identify those patients needing treatment for subclinical depression.

It is generally reasonable to provide psychosocial support initially to ameliorate depressive symptoms and distress even when these do not meet the diagnostic criteria for major depression. Subthreshold depression on should be viewed as an important area for intervention, especially in conditions such as OA, whose symptoms are partly influenced by the psychological state of the patient. Understanding the complex interaction between mood and symptom reporting in OA may be important in predicting the response to therapy and determining the patient's adherence to treatment, thereby improving the effectiveness of treatment.

The physical illness–depression relationship

The relationship between chronic physical conditions and psychological distress is not well understood. Several alternative theories have been proposed to explain the association and the effects of a chronic physical disorder on a person's psychological state.[15] The roles of life stresses, resource deprivation, and the contribution of pain are briefly described below.

Limitations in physical and social functioning due to illness are thought to result in low self-esteem.[16] Generally, people place great value on being able to master important aspects of their lives. The experience of inescapable

Table 9.32 Criteria for a major depressive episode*

1. Five (or more) of the following symptoms have been present during the same two-week period and represent a change from previous functioning; at least one of the symptoms is either (1) depressed mood or (2) loss of interest or pleasure.

   (1) Depressed mood most of the day, nearly every day, as indicated by either subjective report (e.g. feels sad or empty) or observation made by others (e.g. appears tearful).

   (2) Markedly diminished interest or pleasure in all, or almost all, activities most of the day, nearly every day (as indicated by either subjective account or observation made by others).

   (3) Significant weight loss when not dieting or weight gain (e.g. a change of more than 5 per cent of body weight in a month), or decrease or increase in appetite nearly everyday.

   (4) Insomnia or hypersomnia nearly every day.

   (5) Psychomotor agitation or retardation nearly every day (observable by others, not merely subjective feelings of restlessness or being slowed down).

   (6) Fatigue or loss of energy nearly every day.

   (7) Feeling of worthlessness, or excessive or inappropriate guilt (which may be delusional), nearly every day (not merely self-reproach or guilt about being sick).

   (8) Diminished ability to think or concentrate or indecisiveness, nearly everyday (either by subjective account or as observed by others).

   (9) Recurrent thoughts of death (not just fear of dying), recurrent suicidal ideation without a specific plan, or a suicide attempt or a specific plan for committing suicide.

2. The symptoms do not meet the criteria for a manic-depressive episode.

3. The symptoms cause clinically significant distress or impairment in social, occupational, or other important areas of functioning.

4. Symptoms are not due to the effects of a substance (e.g. a drug of abuse, a medication) or a general medical condition such as hypothyroidism.

5. In the case of the loss of a loved one, symptoms that persist for longer than two months or are characterized by marked functional impairment, morbid preoccupation with worthlessness, suicidal ideation, psychotic symptoms, or psychomotor retardation may represent major depressive episode, but in less severe or prolonged cases, the symptoms may simply be bereavement.

Source: Taken from Ref. 10.

Over the last 2 weeks, how often have you been bothered by any of the following problems?

	Not at all	Several days	More than half the days	Nearly every day
1. Little interest or pleasure in doing things................	0	1	2	3
2. Feeling down, depressed, or hopeless................….…	0	1	2	3
3. Trouble falling or staying asleep, or sleeping too much..……....…..….	0	1	2	3
4. Feeling tired or having little energy......…......…....…	0	1	2	3
5. Poor appetite or overeating..................…........………	0	1	2	3
6. Feeling bad about yourself—or that you are a failure or have let yourself or your family down......	0	1	2	3
7. Trouble concentrating on things, such as reading the newspaper or watching television………....….	0	1	2	3
8. Moving or speaking so slowly that other people could have noticed? Or the opposite—being so fidgety or restless that you have been moving around a lot more than usual.............….………….	0	1	2	3
9. Thoughts that you would be better off dead or of hurting yourself in some way....….................….	0	1	2	3

(*For office coding: Total Score* _____ = _____ + _____ + _____)

If you checked off any problems, how difficult have these problems made it for you to do your work, take care of things at home, or get along with other people?

Not difficult at all	Somewhat difficult	Very difficult	Extremely difficult
☐	☐	☐	☐

Fig. 9.30 Primary Care Evaluation of Mental Disorders Patient Health Questionnaire (PRIME-MD PHQ). The PHQ was developed by Drs. Robert L. Spitzer, Janet B.W. Williams, Kurt Kroenke, and colleagues. For research information, contact Dr. Spitzer at rls8@columbia.edu. PRIME-MD® is a trademark of Pfizer Inc. Copyright© 1999 Pfizer Inc. All rights reserved. Reproduced with permission.

and undesirable events, unaltered by effort to overcome disability, may result in helplessness. Elderly people are likely to have some age-related comorbidity, and pain and functional impairment resulting from OA may be perceived as an additional burden to the normal demands of daily living. Functional restrictions imposed by OA give rise to helplessness, which may predispose to anxiety and depression.[17]

Social resources are affected when the chronically ill person withdraws from the supportive social interactions necessary to maintain his psychological well being. It has been shown that persons who experience negative life events report lower levels of perceived support.[18] The favorable influence of social support on depressive symptoms of patients with OA and rheumatoid arthritis (RA) has been reported previously.[19]

Also, persistent pain may substantially mediate the relationship between chronic physical illness and depression, as indicated in a study of patients with RA. Chronic pain is strongly related to depression.[20]

OA and psychological variables

OA is a prototypical example of a chronic disorder that is highly prevalent and a major cause of functional impairment among the elderly.[21] Pain and disability are its major symptoms. Although several studies have indicated a relationship between the presence of OA, as judged by radiographic measures, and the occurrence of clinical symptoms,[22,23] many patients report pain and functional impairment in daily activities far in excess of the levels suggested by objective medical evaluation.[24] Symptoms of OA are believed to be associated not only with the degeneration of cartilage and bone, muscle weakness and limitations in joint motion, but also with psychological factors,[25] which are likely to influence the perception of pain and the degree of functional impairment experienced by patients with OA.

Depression, anxiety, and OA

Depressive and anxiety disorders are prevalent in subjects with musculoskeletal symptoms in the general population[26] and primary care practice,[27] and are even more prevalent among patients with musculoskeletal symptoms who are referred to rheumatologists.[28] Among persons with a variety of chronic diseases, depression and anxiety were most common among those with OA, whereas those with diabetes and heart disease appeared to be the least psychologically distressed.[29] Other studies have suggested that various chronic medical illnesses are associated with a similarly elevated risk of depression.[30] The association between OA and depression has been confirmed in both clinic and community samples.[31,32]

Maisiak[33] found that patients with OA were three times as likely as nonarthritic people to have a depressed mood, while those with rheumatoid arthritis were only about twice as likely as nonarthritic patients to be depressed. Hawley and Wolfe noted definite depression (as defined by a score ≥23 on the Center for Epidemiological Studies Depression Scale) in 17 per cent of patients with hip or knee OA[34]—nearly twice the prevalence found in general medical patients by Coulehan et al.[35] O'Reilly[36] found that depression was strongly associated with the level of disability in subjects with OA. Except among subjects with OA at the highest level of educational attainment, depression was a better predictor than pain or disability of who would be under the care of a physician.[37]

Among outpatients with knee OA, Salaffi et al.[38] found that the severity of joint pain correlated significantly with depression and anxiety. Self-reported disability in patients with symptomatic knee OA is shown as being strongly related to anxiety, even after controlling for pain severity and body mass index.[39] These findings suggest a significant impact of depression and anxiety on the severity of pain and functional impairment of persons who seek care for OA.

Catastrophizing, hypochondriasis, and life stresses

Catastrophizing has been defined as an individual's tendency to focus on and exaggerate the threat value of painful stimuli and to negatively evaluate one's ability to deal with pain.[40] Catastrophizing bears a direct relationship to depression and chronic pain.[41] A catastrophizing reaction to pain may strengthen the patient's tendency to avoid pain-related activities, thereby enhancing muscle weakness which then may mediate the association between psychological processes (anxiety and avoidance) and symptoms of OA (pain and disability).[42]

Lichtenberg et al.[43] found hypochondriasis scores in the Minnesota Multiphasic Personality Inventory were strongly predictive of pain severity among patients with knee OA. Furthermore, there is some evidence that 'daily hassles' (repetitive chronic irritations, such as troubles with family life or work, excessive noise, frustrations with living conditions) are linked to the severity of joint pain in patients with knee OA.[44]

Social support and coping resources

The impact of stress due to chronic diseases is influenced by social support and personal coping resources. Poor coping strategies are a significant predictor of pain, health status, and depression in patients with knee OA.[41] Older persons with high levels of personal coping resources are less depressed than older persons with low levels.[45] Hopman-Rock et al.[46] concluded that seeking social support as a coping style is a more important predictor of quality of life than either the chronicity of pain or physical disability among those with chronic, episodic, or sporadic pain in the hip or knee. Among individuals with severe arthritis, personal coping resources explained 28 per cent of the variance of depressive symptoms as reported in a longitudinal study of aging in Amsterdam.[18]

A population-based sample of older persons revealed that having many close social relationships, the presence of a partner, feelings of mastery, and high self-esteem had direct, favorable effects on measures of depression among patients with self-reported arthritis (OA and RA).[18] In contrast, helplessness appeared to be an important factor in determining self-reported pain severity in knee OA.[47] On the other hand, mastery, having many diffuse social relationships, and receiving emotional support seem to mitigate the influence of arthritis on depressive symptoms.[18]

Psycho-educational interventions for depression in OA

Nonpharmacologic measures are as important as—and often more important than—drug treatment for OA. Although they are useful for treatment of OA pain, analgesics and anti-inflammatory drugs fail to deal with concomitant depression and anxiety, two important symptom-modifying factors in patients with OA. Psycho-educational interventions encompass both traditional educational or teaching activities and psychological interventions. The two most common examples are self-management (SM) programs and cognitive behavioral therapy (CBT).

SM programs are broadly focused, rather than concentrating on the disease, and provide a combination of disease-related information and assistance in learning and adapting new activities and skills. Using group interaction and mutual support, participants discuss and plan how to implement new behaviors. Programs may be led by lay persons and may include topics such as general information about arthritis, accomplishment of goals, energy-saving techniques, time management, and problem solving. Reports of such programs indicate a trend toward improvement in measures of pain,[48] depression, and anxiety[49] at the completion of the program. Lorig et al.[50] evaluated the effectiveness of a multi-component arthritis SM program which included disease-specific education, design of individualized exercise and relaxation programs, provision of information about the appropriate use of damaged joints, and methods for solving problems that arose from OA. The intervention produced significant and sustained benefits beyond those seen with conventional therapy (e.g., analgesics and NSAIDs).

Most psychological interventions used in management of OA incorporate a combination of cognitive and behavioral strategies. CBT is more narrowly focused and emphasizes control of pain and acquisition of new skills, such as cognitive restructuring and diversion. Evaluation by Keefe et al.[49] of a 10-week CBT intervention designed to improve pain coping skills of patients with knee OA indicated that such training was more effective in reducing pain, anxiety, and depression than participation in an arthritis education group. Furthermore, those who continued to apply these new skills experienced significantly lower levels of anxiety and depression 6 months later, than patients who discontinued using the new learned pain coping skills.[51] However, the initial gains in pain relief with CBT had dissipated by 12 months after the intervention, suggesting that booster interventions may be necessary.

Keefe et al.[52] evaluated the effects of a spouse-assisted CBT training on pain, psychological disability, and physical disability, by using the Arthritis Impact Measurement Scales (AIMS). After treatment, patients in the spouse-assisted CBT group exhibited significantly lower levels of pain, anxiety, and depression than those in the control group, which received education-spousal support. These benefits persisted for as long as one year and appeared to be mediated by improvements in marital adjustment and self-efficacy.[53]

Pharmacological interventions

Treatment of subthreshold depression with drugs is controversial, because few data exist from clinical trials to provide guidance in the management of patients with this level of depression. A comparison of paroxetine, 20–40 mg/d, with maprotiline, 100–150 mg/d, in patients with subthreshold depression indicated that both agents had good antidepressant properties and were comparably effective.[54] Minaprine, an antidepressant not available in the United States of America, provided greater 'global improvement' than placebo.[55] The structure of minaprine is different from that of conventional tricyclic antidepressant drugs. Results of preclinical studies suggest that minaprine facilitates serotonergic and dopaminergic neurotransmission by both presynaptic and postsynaptic effects.[56] However, the exact neuronal sites on which minaprine exerts its effects are unknown, and it does not affect noradrenergic neurotransmission.

A meta-analysis of newer pharmacological therapies for clinical depression in adults concluded that the efficacy of selective serotonin reuptake inhibitors (SSRIs, e.g., paroxetine, sertraline, fluoxetine) was comparable to that of first- and second-generation tricyclic antidepressants (e.g., amitriptyline, nortriptyline, respectively).[57] A trial comparing paroxetine to amitriptyline for treatment of depression in patients with RA shows no differences in efficacy,[58] although paroxetine was better tolerated than amitriptyline.

The adverse effects commonly seen with SSRIs include nausea, headache, insomnia, and diarrhea; those that are common with tricyclics are dry mouth, constipation, dizziness, blurred vision, tremors, and urinary retention. The anticholinergic effects and orthostatic hypotension that plague many elderly patients taking tricyclics make SSRIs the first line therapy for depression. Table 9.33 lists the classes of antidepressants and their doses.[59]

Practical recommendations

The authors suggest the following general diagnostic and therapeutic approach to depression in patients with OA:

1. Depression screening should be performed for OA patients with significant pain and functional impairment that are out of proportion to the objective findings. The 9-item Patient Health Questionnaire can be used as a diagnostic instrument and a measure of severity of depressive symptoms (Fig. 9.30).

2. Patients with mild depression should be encouraged to participate in mutual support groups to learn more about their pain and OA, in general. By attending support groups, they will learn energy saving techniques and problem solving skills, which will improve their ability to cope with their illness.

3. Psychosocial support provided through regular telephone contact with an office nurse can help promote self-care.

4. If depression is more than mild, antidepressant medications should be considered in addition to supportive therapy. Patients initiating antidepressant therapy should be followed up within the first 1–2 weeks with an office visit or telephone call. This first contact is important for assessing compliance and evaluating side effects, rather than for establishing efficacy (which is often gradual over the first 4 weeks of

Table 9.33 Antidepressant medications

Drug	Starting dose	Maximum dose	Comments
SSRIs			
Sertraline (Zoloft®)	12.5 mg/d	50–75 mg/d	First line therapy; start with a low dose which may then be increased
Fluoxetine (Prozac®)	10 mg 3 times/wk	20 mg/d	
Paroxetine (Paxil®)	5 mg/d	20 mg/d	
Citalopram (Celexa®)	10 mg/d	20–40 mg/d	
Tricyclics			
Desipramine (Norpramine®)	25 mg/d	100 mg/d	Second line therapy; useful for severely depressed patients for whom SSRI therapy has not provided adequate improvement
Nortriptyline (Pamelor®)	10 mg/d	50 mg/d	Nortriptyline has fewer anticholinergic side effects and is less sedating than amitriptyline
Amitriptyline (Elavil®)	10 mg/d	100 mg/d	
Others			
Bupropion (Wellbutrin®)	75 mg/d	150 mg bid (am and afternoon)	CNS stimulant effect may be useful for depressed patients with low energy level
Mirtazapine (Remeron®)	15 mg/d	45 mg/d	Useful for patients with concomitant sleep problems
Nefazodone (Serzone®)	50 mg bid	150 mg bid	Useful for patients with depression with features of anxiety
Venlafaxine (Effexor®)	25 mg bid	100–150 mg bid	Second line therapy (may cause elevation of blood pressure)

SSRI, selective serotonin reuptake inhibitor.

Source: Taken from Ref. 58, with permission.

treatment). Patients should be informed that early side effects often improve or resolve with continued use of the drug. Three contacts in the first 12 weeks are recommended for depressed patients beginning on medication. In patients who do not improve substantially within the first 6 weeks, the dose of the medication should be increased. If the patient is still significantly depressed after an additional 6 weeks, an alternative medication should be prescribed.

5. Referral to a mental health specialist is warranted for patients who continue to have substantial depression after 12 weeks. Indications for immediate referral of the depressed patient include suicidal ideation, bipolar disorder, and psychotic symptoms. Patients who have a good response to antidepressants should continue on the drug for at least 4–9 months after remission is achieved. For those with two or more recurrences of major depression, chronic maintenance treatment with an antidepressant may be warranted.

Conclusion

Even in the absence of a diagnosable depressive disorder, the presence of depressive symptoms places people with OA at risk for adverse functional outcomes. Primary care physicians are in a unique position to address issues relevant to the patient's psychological well being and should be alert to the manifestations of depression in patients with OA. Single questions about mood are quite sensitive in screening for depression, and a brief questionnaire can be used to gauge severity and monitor the response to treatment. Psychological treatment and antidepressant medication are effective and may improve pain and function in patients with OA.

Summary

The prevalence of major depression has been estimated to be 5–10 per cent; three times as many people may have significant subclinical depressive symptoms. Primary care physicians miss the diagnosis in at least half of the cases. Underrecognition is due, in part, to inadequate time to obtain a history of depressive symptoms and the prominence of somatic complaints as the main manifestation of depression in patients with comorbid medical illnesses. In patients with OA, the overlap of symptoms attributable to arthritis, such as musculoskeletal pain, and those attributable to depression makes the diagnosis far more complicated. Psychological variables exert a huge influence on the perception of pain and degree of functional impairment experienced by patients with OA. Changes in functional status and heightened pain awareness in patients with OA may signify the onset of depression. Use of simple screening questionnaires by the primary care physician can help considerably with recognition of depression. It is reasonable to provide psychosocial support to ameliorate mild depressive symptoms in patients with OA. Use of antidepressants is indicated for those with moderate to severe depression. Referral to a mental health specialist is warranted for those who continue to have substantial residual depressive symptoms.

Key points

1. As depression increases pain and pain-related disability, as well as global impairment in other domains of health-related quality of life, untreated subthreshold depression can amplify somatic symptoms and disability in OA.

2. Symptoms of OA are associated not only with the degeneration of cartilage and bone, muscle weakness, and limitation in joint motion, but also with depression and anxiety.

3. Arthritis self-management programs that deal with improving self-efficacy, energy-saving techniques, and problem solving, using

group interaction and mutual support formats, can reduce the severity of depressive symptoms and joint pain.

4. A trial of an antidepressant is reasonable for patients with OA who have major depression, dysthymia, persistent minor depression, or subthreshold depression.

References

1. Borus, J.F., Howes, M.J., Devins, N.P., Rosenberg, R., and Livingston, W.W. (1988). Primary health care providers' recognition and diagnosis of mental disorders in their patients. *Gen Hosp Psychiatry* **10**:317–21.

2. Perez-Stable, E.J., Miranda, J., Munoz, R.F., and Yu-Wen, Y. (1990). Depression in medical outpatients: underrecognition and misdiagnosis. *Arch Intern Med* **150**:1083–8.

3. Pearson, S.T., Katzelnick, D.J., Simon, G.E., Manning, W.G., Helstad, C.P., and Henk, H.J. (1999). Depression among high utilizers of medical care. *J Gen Intern Med* **14**:461–8.

4. Katon, W., Berg, A.O., Robins, A.J., and Risse, S. (1986). Depression: medical utilization and somatization. *West J Med* **144**:564–8.

5. Simon, G.E., Von Korff, M., and Barlow, W. (1995). Health care costs of primary care patients with recognized depression. *Arch Gen Psychiatry* **52**:850–6.

6. Spitzer, R.L., Korenke, K., Linzer, M., Hahn, S.R., Williams, J.B., deGruy, F.V. 3rd, *et al.* (1995). Health related quality of life in primary care patients with mental disorders. Results from the PRIME-MD 1000 study. *JAMA* **274**: 1511–7.

7. Ormel, J., Van der Brink, W., Koeter, M.W.J., *et al.* (1990). Recognition, management and outcome of psychological disorders in primary care: a naturalistic follow-up study. *Psychol Med* **20**:909–23.

8. Memel, D.S., Kirwan, J.R., Sharp, D.J., and Hehir, M. (2000). General practitioners miss disability and anxiety as well as depression in their patients with osteoarthritis. *Br J Gen Practice* **50**:645–8.

9. Mulrow, C.D., Williams, J.W., Gerety, M.B., *et al.* (1995). Case finding instruments for depression in primary care settings. *Ann Intern Med* **122**:913–21.

10. Diagnostic and statistical manual of mental disorders (4th ed.). (1994). Washington DC: American Psychiatric Association, p. 327.

11. Kroenke, K., Spitzer, R.L., and Williams, J.B.W. (2001). The PHQ-9. Validity of a brief depression severity measure. *J Gen Intern Med* **16**:606–13.

12. Kroenke, K. (2001). Depression screening is not enough. *Ann Intern Med* **134**:418–20.

13. Johnson, J., Weissman, M.M., and Klerman, G.L. (1992). Service utilization and social morbidity associated with depressive symptoms in the community. *JAMA* **267**:1478–83.

14. Coulehan, J.L., Schulberg, H.C., Block, M.R., Janosky, J.E., and Arena, V.C. (1990). Depressive symptomatology and medical co-morbidity in primary care clinic. *Intern J Psychiatr Med* **20**(4):335–47.

15. Vilhjalmsson, R. (1998). Direct and indirect effects of chronic physical conditions on depression: A preliminary investigation. *Soc Sci Med* **47**(5): 603–11.

16. Blake, R.L. (1991). Social stressors, social supports and self-esteem as predictors of morbidity in adults with chronic lung disease. *Family Pract Res J* **11**:65–74.

17. Ozment, J.M. and Lester, D. (1998). Helplessness and depression. *Psychol Rep* **82**(2):434.

18. Procidano, M.E. and Heller, K. (1983). Measures of perceived social support from friends and from family: Three validation studies. *Am J Community Psychol* **II**:1–24.

19. *Penninx, B.W., Tilburg, T.V., Deeg, D.J., Kriegsman, D.M., Boeke, J.P., and Eijk, J.T. (1997). Direct and buffer effects of social support and personal coping resources in individuals with arthritis. *Soc Sci Med* **44**(3):393–402.

    This study provides evidence of the benefits of social support and of personal coping resources on depressive symptoms in a community-based sample of older persons with OA and RA.

20. Brown, G.K. (1990). A causal analysis of chronic pain and depression. *J Abnormal Psychol* **99**:127–37.

21. Wood, P.H.N. (1976). Osteoarthritis in the community. *Clin Rheum Dis* 2:495–507.

22. Lethbirdge-Cejku, M., Scott, W.W., Jr., Reichle, R., *et al.* (1995). Association of radiographic features of osteoarthritis of the knee with knee pain: data from the Baltimore Longitudinal Study of Aging. *Arthritis Care Res* 8:182–8.

23. Hochberg, M.C., Lawrence, R.C., Everett, D.P., and Cornoni-Huntley, J. (1989). Epidemiological associations of pain in osteoarthritis of the knee. *Semin Arthritis Rheum* 18(Suppl. 2):4–9.

24. Bole, G.G. (1985). Osteoarthritis, Rheumatology, and Immunology. A.S. Cohen and J.C. Bennett (eds). New York: Grune & Stratton, pp. 332–41.

25. *Dekker, J., Boot, B., van der Woude, L.H., and Bijlsma, J.W.J. (1992). Pain and Disability in Osteoarthritis: A Review of Biobehavioral Mechanisms. *J Behav Med* 15(2):189–213.
   An excellent review of the biobehavioral mechanisms of pain and disability in OA.

26. Kroenke, K. and Price, R.K. (1993). Symptoms in the community: prevalence, classification and psychiatric comorbidity. *Arch Intern Med* 153:2474–80.

27. Kroenke, K., Spitzer, R.L., Williams, J.B.W., Linzer, M., Hahn, S.R., deGruy, F.V., and Brody, D. (1994). Physical symptoms in primary care: predictors of psychiatric disorders and functional impairment. *Arch Fam Med* 3:774–9.

28. O'Malley, P.G., Jackson, J.L., Kroenke, K., Yoon, I.K., Hornstein, E., and Dennis, G.L. (1998). The value of screening for psychiatric disorders in rheumatology referrals. *Arch Intern Med* 158:2357–62.

29. Penninx, B.W., Beekman, A.T., Ormel, J., Kriegsman, D.M., Boeke, J.P., Van Eijk, J.T., and Deeg, D.J. (1996). Psychological status among elderly people with chronic diseases: does type of disease play a part? *J Psychosom Res* 40(5):521–34.

30. DeVellis, B.M. (1993). Depression in the rheumatic diseases. *Ballieres Clin Rheumatol* 7:241–7.

31. Wells, K.B., Golding, J.M., and Burnam, M.A. (1989). Affective, substance abuse and anxiety disorders in persons with arthritis, diabetes, heart disease, high blood pressure or chronic lung conditions. *Gen Hosp Psychiatry* 11:320–7.

32. Stewart, A.L., Greenfield, S., Hays, R.D., Wells, K., Rogers, W.H., Berry, S., McGlynn, E.A., and Ware, J.E. (1989). Functional status and well being of patients with chronic conditions: results from the medical outcomes study. *JAMA* 262:907–13.

33. Maisiak, R. (1990). Arthritis and the risk of depression: An epidemiological case control study. *Arthritis Care Res Abstr* 3:C36.

34. Hawley, D.J. and Wolfe, F. (1993). Depression is not more common in rheumatoid arthritis: a 10 year longitudinal study of 6153 patients with rheumatic disease. *J Rheumatol* 20:2025–31.

35. Coulehan, J.L., Schulberg, H.C., Block, M.R., Janosky, J.E., and Arena, V.C. (1990). Depressive symptomatology and medical co-morbidity in a primary care clinic. *Intern J Psychiatr Med* 20(4):335–47.

36. O'Reilly, S.C., Jones, A., Muir, K.R., and Doherty, M. (1998). Quadriceps weakness in knee OA: The effect on pain and disability. *Ann Rheum Dis* 57:588–94.

37. *Dexter, P. and Brandt, K. (1994). Distribution and predictors of depressive symptoms in osteoarthritis. *J Rheumatol* 21:279–86.
   This cross-sectional study of community living persons highlights the importance of assessing depression in persons who seek care for OA.

38. Salaffi, F., Cavalieri, F., Nolli, M., and Ferraccioli, G. (1996). Analysis of disability in knee osteoarthritis. Relationship with age and psychological variables but not with radiographic score. *J Rheumatol* 23:1037–44.

39. *Creamer, P.M., Lethbridge-Cejku, and Hochberg, M.C. (2000). Factors associated with functional impairment in symptomatic knee osteoarthritis. *Rheumatology* 39:490–6.
   Helplessness is an important determinant of disability in patients with symptomatic knee OA and predisposes to depression. This study provides further support for interventions targeting helplessness and anxiety in patients with OA.

40. Sullivan, M.J.L., Bishop, S., and Pivik, J. (1995). The pain catastrophizing scale: development and validation. *Psychol Assess* 7:524–32.

41. Geisser, M.E., Robinson, M.E., Keefe, F.J., and Weiner, M.L. (1994). Catastrophizing, depression and the sensory, affective and evaluative aspects of chronic pain. *Pain* 59(1):79–83.

42. Dekker, J., Tola, P., Auftemkampe, G., and Winckers, M. (1993). Negative affect, pain and disability in osteoarthritis patients: the mediating role of muscle weakness. *Behav Res Ther* 31:203–6.

43. Lichtenberg, P.A., Skehan, M.W., and Swensen, C.H. (1984). The role of personality, recent life stress and arthritic severity in predicting pain. *J Psychosom Res* 28:231–6.

44. Lichtenberg, P.A., Swensen, C.H., and Skehan, M.W. (1986). Further investigation of the role of personality, lifestyle and arthritic severity in predicting pain. *J Psychosomatic Res* 30:327–37.

45. Roberts, B.L., Dunkle, R., and Haug, M. (1994). Physical, psychological and social resources as moderators of the relationships of stress to mental health of the very old. *J Gerontol Soc Sci* 49:35–43.

46. Hopman-Rock, M., Kraaimaat, F.W., and Bijlsma, J.W. (1997). Quality of life in elderly subjects with pain in the hip or knee. *Qual Life Res* 6(1):67–76.

47. Creamer, P., Lethbridge-Cejku, M., and Hochberg, M.C. (1999). Determinants of pain severity in knee osteoarthritis: effect of demographic and psychosocial variables using 3 pain measures. *J Rheumatol* 26:1785–92.

48. Kovar, P.A., Allegrante, J.P., MacKenzie, R., *et al.* (1992). Supervised fitness walking in patients with osteoarthritis of the knee. *Ann Intern Med* 116:529–34.

49. Keefe, F.J., Caldwell, D.S., Williams, D.A., *et al.* (1990). Pain coping skills training in the management of osteoarthritic knee pain: a comparative study. *Behav Therapy* 21:49–62.

50. Lorig, K.R., Mazonson, P.D., and Holman, H.R. (1993). Evidence suggesting that health education for self-management in patients with chronic arthritis has sustained health benefits while reducing health care costs. *Arthritis Rheum* 36(4):439–46.

51. Keefe, F.J., Caldwell, D.S., Williams, D.A., Gil, K.M., Mitchell, D., Robertson, C., *et al.* (1990). Pain coping skills training in the management of osteoarthritic knee pain II: Follow-up results. *Behavior Therapy* 21: 435–47.

52. Keefe, F.J., Caldwell, D.S., Baucom, D., Salley, A., Robinson, E., Timmons, K., Beaupre, P., Weisberg, J., and Helms, M. (1996). Spouse-assisted coping skills training in the management of osteoarthritic knee pain. *Arthritis Care Res* 9(4):279–91.

53. Keefe, F.J., Caldwell, D.S., Baucom, D., Salley, A., Robinson, E., Timmons, K., Beaupre, P., and Helms, M. (1999). Spouse assisted coping skills training in the management of knee pain in osteoarthritis: long term followup results. *Arthritis Care Res* 12(2):101–11.

54. Szegedi, A., Wetzel, H., Angersbach, D., Dunbar, G.C., Schwarze, H., Philipp, M., and Benkert, O. (May 1997). A double blind study comparing paroxetine and maprotiline in depressed outpatients. *Pharmacopsychiatry* 30(3):97–105.

55. Parnetti, L., Sommacal, S., Morselli, L.A., and Senin, U. (1993). Multicentre controlled randomized double-blind placebo study of minaprine in elderly patients suffering from prolonged depressive reaction. *Drug Invest* 6:181–8.

56. Biziere, K., Worms, P., Kan, J.P., Mandel, P., Garattini, S., and Roncucci, R. (1985). Minaprine, a new drug with antidepressant properties. *Drugs Under Exp Clin Res* 11(12):831–40.

57. *Williams, J.W., Mulrow, C., Cynthia, D., Chiquette, E., Noel, P.H., Aguilar, C., and Cornell, J. (2000). A systematic review of newer pharmacotherapies for depression in adults: evidence report summary: clinical guideline, Part 2. *Ann Intern Med* 132(9):743–56.
   This excellent review of new and old pharmacotherapies for depression is useful for primary care physicians confronted with the choice of drug therapy for depressed patients.

58. Bird, H. and Broggini, M. (2000). Paroxetine versus amitriptyline for treatment of depression associated with rheumatoid arthritis: a randomized double blind parallel group study. *J Rheumatol* 27:2791–7.

59. Koenig, H.G. (1999). Late-life depression: How to treat patients with comorbid chronic illness. *Geriatrics* 54(5):56–61.

9.16 Coping strategies for the patient with osteoarthritis

Francis J. Keefe, Ann Aspnes, David S. Caldwell, and Susmita Kashikar-Zuck

Patients with OA vary greatly in their abilities to cope with the disease.[1] Consider two patients both of whom have very similar levels of OA of the hips. The first patient, a 70-year old man, reports having severe hip pain, is discouraged, spends most of his time in a wheelchair, and is increasingly dependent upon his family. The second patient, a 72-year old woman, reports having minimal to moderate pain, is optimistic about the future, walks daily, and is very active socially. In order to explain such variations in adjustment, biobehavioral scientists are increasingly turning their attention to coping processes in patients with OA. Over the past 10 years a number of research studies have examined coping in OA patients and investigated whether training in coping skills can reduce pain and psychological disability.

This chapter provides an overview of recent studies in the OA coping literature. The chapter is divided into four sections. The first section presents a biopsychosocial model of coping in OA and contrasts it with the more traditional biomedical models of OA. The second section focuses on methods for assessing coping in OA. The third section describes coping skills training and arthritis education interventions used to enhance coping efforts of OA patients. The fourth section highlights a number of important future directions for work in this area.

Conceptual background

OA is typically assessed and treated on the basis of a biomedical or disease model. This model, depicted in Fig. 9.31, focuses on impairment as the primary cause of pain and disability. Impairment in the form of cartilage destruction and changes in bone surfaces can range from minimal to severe. According to the biomedical model, patients with severe impairment can be expected to have more severe pain and higher levels of disability than patients with minimal impairment. Treatments based on this model are designed to correct or minimize the effects of underlying impairments. Thus, a surgical joint replacement might be used to treat a patient with very advanced disease. Alternatively, medical treatments in the form of non-steroidal anti-inflammatory agents might be used to treat a patient with moderate disease and significant swelling.

The biomedical model has several problems. First, the relationship between the degree of impairment and the amount of pain and disability is not uniform. Some patients with advanced disease report less pain than patients with minimal disease. Second, patients who receive the same medical or surgical treatment often show very different outcomes. For example, two patients with very similar demographic and medical profiles may show quite different outcomes following a knee replacement surgery.

The biopsychosocial model of OA is depicted in Fig. 9.32. The major tenet of this model is that to understand pain and disability in OA, one needs to not only be concerned about impairment, but also about psychological and social factors. This model differs in several ways from the biomedical model. First, it highlights the important role that coping and appraisal play in determining adjustment to OA. Coping refers to the efforts that patients make to deal with or minimize the effects of their disease. Coping strategies might include, for example, relaxing, pacing activities, or intentionally calming oneself when upset or feeling pain. Coping strategies that are adopted and

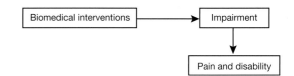

Fig. 9.31 The biomedical model

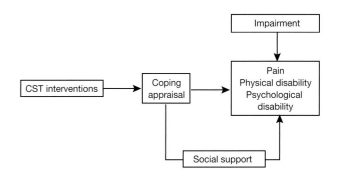

Fig. 9.32 The biopsychosocial model.

used over a long time period can have a significant impact on pain and disability. Appraisal refers to the way in which a patient views their situation and their own ability to cope effectively with it. Second, the biopsychosocial model takes a broader view of disability and considers not only pain and disability, but also psychological disability due to depression, anger, frustration, or guilt. Finally, this model considers the social context of OA. Patients who receive support from a spouse or family members may cope much more effectively with OA.

Assessing coping in OA patients

Researchers have taken two basic approaches to the assessment of coping in OA patients. The first approach involves assessing general coping skills and the second involves assessing pain-specific coping skills.

Assessing general coping skills

Conceptual background

Folkman and Lazarus[2] proposed a general model of stress and coping that has been used to analyze coping in many medical conditions, including OA. According to this model, the relationship between a stressful event (e.g. having arthritis) and health outcomes (e.g. pain and disability) is mediated by two factors: coping strategies and appraisal. Coping strategies are a person's efforts to reduce, manage, or deal with stress. Appraisal refers to a person's perceptions of their situation as being potentially threatening/harmful (primary appraisal) and their perceptions about their own ability to cope effectively (secondary appraisal).

A major tenet of Lazarus and Folkman's[2] stress and coping model is that the particular coping strategies used by the person are likely to have important consequences for their adjustment. For example, an individual with OA who uses planned problem solving as a coping strategy (e.g. seeking out educational information about their disease in an active fashion) is very likely to have less pain and disability than a patient who uses escape-avoidance strategies to deal with their disease (e.g. simply wishing their condition would go away). According to this model, how an individual appraises their arthritis is a very important determinant of adjustment. The OA patient who anticipates a high level of pain and dysfunction and doubts their own ability to cope may become much more disabled by their disease.

To measure general coping efforts used by OA patients, researchers have used three questionnaire instruments. These instruments are somewhat similar in that they are based on the same general coping model, but also have notable differences.

The Ways of Coping Scale (WOC)

The WOC[3] is the most general measure of coping that has been used to assess coping in OA patients. This is a 66-item questionnaire that asks respondents to describe the most stressful event they have experienced in the past month and then to indicate on a 4-point scale (0, not used, 3, used a great deal) how often they have used different strategies to cope with the event. The WOC has eight subscales, each of which assesses a distinct coping strategy. These strategies include confrontive coping, distancing, self-control, seeking social support, accepting responsibility, escape-avoidance, planned problem-solving, and positive reappraisal. Sample items for each of the WOC subscales are presented in Table 9.34. Research has shown that the WOC is internally reliable, and alpha coefficients for the subscales generally fail in the moderately high range (i.e. from 0.61 to 0.79).[3]

A recent study by Burke and Flaherty[4] used the WOC to assess coping in a sample of elderly women with OA. The study found that the most frequently employed strategy was self-control, for example keeping feelings to one's self. Other commonly used strategies included positive reappraisal and distancing. Correlational analyses revealed that there was a significant negative relationship between the use of escape-avoidance strategies and health status. That is, women who reported that they cope with arthritis by engaging in wishful thinking and hoping were much more likely to have poor physical health and psychological functioning.

The WOC has the advantages of being theoretically based, having wide applicability, and good reliability. The WOC was initially developed for use in stress research, and has only recently been extended to arthritis populations. Further research is needed to determine whether this very general coping instrument is likely to be useful in understanding pain and disability in OA patients.

The Jalowiec Coping Scale (JCS)

The JCS[5] is also based on Folkman and Lazarus' model of stress and coping, but was specifically designed to be applicable to medical populations. The JCS is a self-report instrument that consists of 40 items designed to measure coping strategies derived from the Folkman and Lazarus model. Patients are asked to rate each item on a 5-point scale (1–5, never to almost always) to indicate how often they use that strategy.

Jalowiec[5] conducted a study to identify the underlying factor structure of the JCS. Subjects included patients having a variety of medical conditions (e.g. cardiac patients, arthritis patients, pulmonary patients, and cancer patients) as well as nonpatients (e.g. relatives of patients, nurses, and graduate students.). A factor analysis of patients' responses on the JCS identified three factors that accounted for a significant proportion of variance in questionnaire responses. The three factors were: (1) confrontive coping (e.g. thinking through solutions), (2) palliative coping (e.g. accepting one's situation), and (3) emotive coping (e.g. getting nervous/angry). The factors were found to be highly reliable showing evidence of good internal consistency (alphas ranging from 0.70 to 0.85) and test-retest reliability (test-retest coefficients ranging from 0.78 to 0.91).

Downe-Wambolt[6] used the JCS to study coping in a sample of women having OA. This study found that the most frequently used coping strategies were palliative strategies such as accepting the situation and being resigned to one's fate. The next most frequently used coping strategies were confrontive strategies, such as thinking through solutions and maintaining control over the situation. Data analysis revealed that the overall level of coping as assessed by total scores on the JCS was related to life satisfaction. Women who reported high levels of coping were found to have much higher levels of life satisfaction than those reporting low levels of coping.[6]

The JCS appears to be a reliable instrument that has the advantage of being specifically designed for use with medical populations. Available evidence suggests that there is a relationship between the frequency of coping, as assessed by the JCS, and life satisfaction in OA patients.

The Arthritis Appraisal and Ways of Coping Scale (AAWOC)

The AAWOC is an arthritis-specific coping questionnaire based on Lazarus and Folkman's stress and coping model.[7] In developing the AAWOC Regan et al.[7] modified items from the WOC to make them more relevant to arthritis patients. For example, two WOC items ('changed something so that things would turn out all right' and 'bargained or compromised to get something positive from the situation') were changed because in these patients having arthritis is a given fact that cannot be changed, bargained, or compromised with. These two items, thus, were combined to form the AAWOC item 'modified my plans or activity to get something positive from the situation.' The AAWOC also included items from the Catastrophizing subscale from the Coping Strategies Questionnaire,[8] a pain-specific coping measure we will discuss below. The AAWOC differs from the WOC and JCS in that it not only assesses coping strategies, but also appraisal. On the AAWOC, there are items that assess primary appraisal (threat/harm/loss) and secondary appraisal (self efficacy).

Regan et al.[7] carried out a factor analysis of the AAWOC and identified five coping factors. The coping factors included: dependency, adapting, distancing, anger-withdrawal, and expanding thoughts and actions. Table 9.35 lists sample items for each of the factors. The AAWOC has been found to

Table 9.34 Subscales of the WOC and sample items

Subscale	Sample item
Confrontive coping	Stood my ground and fought for what I wanted
Distancing about it	Made light of the situation; refused to think too much about it
Self-controlling	I tried to keep my feelings to myself
Seeking social support	Talked to someone to find out more about the situation
Accepting responsibility	Criticized or lectured myself
Escape-avoidance	Wished that the situation would go away or somehow be over
Planned problem-solving	I knew what had to be done so I doubled my efforts to make it work
Positive reappraisal	Changed or grew as a person in a good way

Table 9.35 Coping subscales of the AAWOC and sample items

Subscale	Sample item
Dependency	Talked to someone who could do something
Adapting	Did something to help myself relax
Anger-withdrawal	Took it out on other people
Distancing	Refused to think about it too much
Expanding thought and action	Thought about a person I admire and used that as a role model

have acceptable reliability. Test–retest reliability for each of the factors ranged from 0.45 to 0.82 and internal consistency reliabilities ranged from 0.64 to 0.81. The internal consistency estimate for the items measuring appraisal was also found to be good: primary appraisal scale alpha = 0.83, as were the estimates for internal consistency for the secondary appraisal items, alphas = 0.75 to 0.90.

Regan *et al.*[7] have presented evidence supporting the construct validity of the AAWOC. Arthritis patients scoring high on items measuring fear of harm or threat (primary appraisal) and low on items measuring perceived self-efficacy (secondary appraisal) had higher levels of pain and depression. Patients' scores on the coping factors were also found to relate to adjustment. Individuals who scored high on the dependency factor had higher levels of pain and depression and lower activity levels. Individuals scoring high on the anger-withdrawal factor had higher levels of depression and lower activity levels.

To summarize, the AAWOC is a theoretically based instrument that shows reasonably good psychometric properties. In addition, it has the advantage of being specifically applicable to arthritis patients. Scores on the AAWOC are shown as being related to pain, depression, and activity level in OA patients.

Comment

The general measures of coping in OA research are based on Lazarus and Folkman's model of stress. The AAWOC was specifically developed for use with arthritis populations and research has provided support for its reliability and validity. Of the general coping measures currently available, the AAWOC appears to be the instrument of choice for use with OA patients.

Assessing pain-specific coping strategies

Conceptual background

OA patients consider pain to be the most common and difficult problem they have to contend with.[9] Not surprisingly, a major focus in coping research has been on understanding the use of strategies patients specifically employ to cope with pain. Pain coping strategies have been defined as the cognitive and behavioral methods patients use to tolerate, deal with, or minimize their pain.[8] These strategies might include distraction, calming self-statements, or changing activity level. In a chronic disease such as OA these strategies can have a substantial impact on pain and function. Patients who develop and apply adaptive strategies over long time periods may have much less pain and lower levels of disability. Those patients, however, who develop and apply maladaptive strategies may be much more disabled by their pain.

Assessment of pain coping strategies

The most commonly used method of assessing pain coping strategies in arthritis patients is the Coping Strategies Questionnaire (CSQ).[8] This 44-item instrument measures the frequency of use and perceived effectiveness of a variety of cognitive–behavioral pain coping strategies. The CSQ contains seven subscales, each of which measures a different cognitive or behavioral strategy. Table 9.36 lists the subscales along with sample items. Questionnaire respondents rate each item indicating how frequently they use that strategy when they feel pain. The item ratings are made using a 7-point scale (0, never; 3, sometimes; and 6, always). The last two items of the questionnaire asks subjects to provide two ratings of the overall effectiveness of the pain coping strategies: (1) how much their strategies allow them to control pain (0, no control; 3, some control; and 6, complete control), and (2) how much their strategies allow them to decrease pain (0, cannot decrease it at all; 3, can decrease it somewhat; and 6, can decrease it completely).

Table 9.37 summarizes data for each of the CSQ subscales gathered from a sample of 51 patients having OA of the knees.[1] As can be seen, these patients varied in the frequency of coping strategies. Patients reported frequent use of coping self-statements, praying, and hoping and rarely reported the use of catastrophizing and reinterpreting pain strategies. Patients rated the perceived effectiveness of their pain coping strategies in controlling and decreasing pain in the moderate range (2.96–3.56).

To assess the internal reliability of the CSQ, Cronbach alpha coefficients were computed for each subscale. As displayed in Table 9.37, these coefficients were in the 0.78 to 0.89 range indicating that this measure has good degree internal consistency.

Table 9.36 Coping Strategy Questionnaire: subscales and sample items

Subscale	Sample item
Diverting attention	I try to think of something pleasant
Reinterpreting pain sensations	I don't think of it as pain but rather as a dull or warm feeling
Coping self-statements	I tell myself I can overcome the pain
Ignoring pain sensations	I don't think about the pain
Catastrophizing	It is terrible and I feel it is never going to get any better
Praying and hoping	I pray to God it won't last long
Increasing activity level	I leave the house and do something, such as going to the movies or shopping

Table 9.37 Coping Strategies Questionnaire statistical data

Subscale	Item rating			Factor loading	
	α^*	M	SD	1	2
Factor 1: Coping attempts					
Diverting attention	0.84	2.55	1.56	0.83	−0.05
Reinterpreting pain sensations	0.89	1.18	1.50	0.78	0.15
Coping self-statements	0.82	4.06	1.36	0.75	0.03
Ignoring pain sensations	0.78	2.40	1.41	0.70	0.34
Praying and hoping	0.80	3.41	1.52	0.67	−0.44
Increasing activity level	0.78	2.89	1.45	0.79	−0.08
Factor 2: Self-control and rational thinking					
Catastrophizing	0.74	1.29	1.15	0.37	−0.63
Ability to control pain	—	3.56	1.13	0.30	0.71
Ability to decrease pain	—	2.96	1.12	0.06	0.76

* Cronbach's (1970) alpha. Alpha coefficients were based on $n = 52$ (including 1 subject who was missing data on other measures).

Source: Reprinted from Keefe, F.J., Caldwell, D.S., Queen, K.T., Gil, K.M., Martinez, S., Crisson, J.E., Ogden, W., and Nunley, J. 1987. Pain coping strategies in osteoarthritis patients. *J Consult Clin Psychol* **55**:208–12. Reprinted with the permission of the author. © 1987, American Psychological Association.

Factor analysis of CSQ responses revealed two factors accounting for 60 per cent of the variance in questionnaire responses. The subscales and factor loadings for each of these factors are shown in Table 9.37. Patients scoring high on the first factor, Coping Attempts, are active copers in that they report frequent use of a wide variety of strategies including diverting attention, reinterpreting pain, coping self-statements, ignoring pain sensations, praying and hoping, and increasing activity level. Patients scoring high on the second factor, Pain Control and Rational Thinking, report they are effective in decreasing and controlling pain and also avoid overly negative thinking (catastrophizing) when having pain. Interestingly, these same two factors with nearly identical factor loadings have been identified by Parker et al.[10] in a study of pain coping strategies used by rheumatoid arthritis (RA) patients.

Several studies of pain coping have been conducted with patients having OA of the knees. Our initial study,[1] for example, found that patients scoring high on the Pain Control and Rational Thinking factor had significantly lower levels of pain, physical disability, psychological disability, and overall psychological distress than patients scoring low on this factor. In a second study,[11] high scores on Pain Control and Rational Thinking were also related to functional impairment. Patients scoring high on this factor took less time to make transfers from standing to sitting and standing to reclining position. They also walked a 5-meter course more rapidly and reported on the Arthritis Impact Measurement Scales that they had higher levels of dexterity, mobility, and household activities. These findings regarding coping are particularly impressive, because they were obtained after controlling for demographic variables (age, sex) and medical status variables (X-ray evidence of disease, obesity status, financial disability/workers compensation status) believed to explain pain and disability in this population.

Further evidence for the validity of pain coping strategies in understanding pain and disability has come from treatment outcome studies. For example, research has shown that changes in scores on the Pain Control and Rational Thinking factor of the CSQ are related to short- and long-term outcomes of pain coping skills training in OA patients.[12,13] Patients who showed increases on the Pain Control and Rational Thinking factor were more likely to show immediate improvements in physical disability.[1] Patients who showed increases on this factor during treatment also were found to have lower levels of pain, physical disability, and pain behavior at six months follow-up.[11]

The Pain Coping Inventory

The Pain Coping Inventory[14] has recently been used in a study of coping in patients having pain due to osteoarthritis of the hip or knee.[15] This study used the PCI to assess: (1) passive coping—as measured by the PCI-resting scale that assesses the tendency to cope with pain by avoiding physical activity, and (2) active coping as measured by the PCI-pain transformation scale (e.g. pretending the pain is not there) and the PCI-lowering demands scale (e.g. working at a slower pace). Coping was assessed at baseline and patients were followed for 36 weeks. Data analyses examined the degree to which baseline coping predicted subsequent disability and pain. In patients having OA of the knee, high scores on the resting scale predicted much higher levels of disability and high scores on the pain transformation scale predicted much higher levels of pain. Interestingly, in patients with OA of the hip, no significant relationship was found between coping styles and pain and disability. This finding may have been due to the small numbers of OA hip patients included in the study. Also, the authors noted that the hip patients were less obese, had less pain at baseline, and had had pain for a shorter period of time. This suggests that the hip OA patients may have been more physically fit and less likely to show a relationship between resting and pain and disability. In any event, these findings suggest that the PCI may be useful in assessing coping in OA patients. Additional research using this measure, particularly comparing patients having OA of the knees and hips, appears to be warranted.

Daily Coping Inventory[16]

All of the coping measures discussed thus far ask patients, at a single point in time, to report retrospectively on how they cope with arthritis or arthritis pain. The DCI has the advantage of assessing coping at a specific point close to the actual occurrence of the event. Real-time reporting reduces the problems associated with recall. Repeated administrations of the DCI can also detect individual variation in the use of coping techniques.

Affleck et al.[17] adapted the DCI for chronic pain patients. This version has seven items on different coping strategies. Patients answer 'yes' or 'no' as to whether they used a particular category of coping during the day. These categories include: (1) direct action, 'did something specific to try to reduce the pain;' (2) relaxation, 'did something to help me relax;' (3) distraction, 'diverted attention from the pain by thinking about other things or engaging in some activity;' (4) redefinition, 'tried to see the pain in a different light that made it seem more bearable;' (5) emotional venting, 'expressed emotions to reduce my anxiety, frustration, or tension about the pain;' (6) spiritual support, 'sought spiritual support or comfort concerning my pain;' and (7) emotional/social support, 'sought emotional support from loved ones, friends, or professionals concerning my pain.'

A recent study used the DCI to examine the effects of type of arthritis (OA vs RA) and gender on daily pain, mood, and coping.[18] A sample of 71 persons with OA and 76 persons with RA completed daily diary questionnaire booklets for 30 days. Included in the diary booklet was the DCI, a daily joint pain assessment, and a daily mood assessment. Data analyses revealed that RA patients reported higher levels of daily pain and that women, regardless of the type of arthritis, reported more pain than men. Women, regardless of disease, were more likely to use emotion-focused coping than men were. Men were much more likely than women to report increased negative mood after a more painful day. Interestingly, emotion-focused coping seemed to help OA patients in that their pain improved after a day in which they used more emotion-focused coping. RA patients showed the opposite pattern, that is, an increase in pain after a day in which they used more emotion-focused coping. This study demonstrates the utility of the DCI in analyzing the effects of gender and disease on coping. Future studies should take advantage of computer advances in daily recording methods and the use of the DCI. Patients could, for example, enter their diary recording directly into a handheld computer for instantaneous reporting. The data would then be available for a researcher or clinician to download and analyze.

Comment

Research suggests that a focus on specific pain coping strategies may be useful in understanding pain and functional disability in OA patients. The CSQ has been used in a number of studies conducted in our lab and is now being used in several ongoing studies by other investigators. Available evidence provides support for the reliability and validity of this instrument in assessing pain-specific coping strategies in OA patients. The DCI has only recently been investigated as a daily pain coping measure in OA patients, but appears to have promise.

Coping skills training for OA patients

Over the past 10 years, behavioral researchers have developed and refined protocols that teach arthritis patients how to cope with their disease.[12,19] To illustrate the methods used in these protocols, a brief description of a pain coping skills training intervention for OA is detailed below.[12] Readers interested in a more detailed description are referred to a recent chapter by Keefe, Beaupre, and Gil[20] or can contact us by email (keefe003@mc.duke.edu) to ask for an electronic version of our detailed treatment manual. The present description includes a discussion of the general treatment format, treatment rationale, and specific coping skills training methods. Research studies that have tested the efficacy of coping skills interventions for OA patients are also presented.

General format

This pain coping skills training intervention is carried out in group sessions consisting of 6–9 patients. The sessions are held weekly for 10 weeks and last 90 minutes. Two therapists serve as group leaders: a psychologist having a background in cognitive–behavioral approaches to pain management, and a nurse having experience in educational interventions. Each session involves the presentation of didactic material on pain coping, followed by a discussion of the material, and guided practice with the skills learned.

The small group format is an ideal one for training in pain coping skills. It provides patients with exposure to other individuals who have similar problems and concerns about their arthritis. The group setting is also small enough that each patient has an opportunity to talk and to get individual attention from the therapists. Finally, the group setting provides opportunities for patients to learn from each other. Patients who are experiencing success in the use of newly learned pain coping skills often serve as effective models for other patients in the group.

Treatment rationale

The treatment rationale is introduced early in the group sessions and is designed to help patients reconceptualize their pain and to understand that they have a role to play in coping with their disease. The rationale has three basic elements: (1) presentation of an adaptational model, (2) discussion of the gate control theory, and (3) description of skills training.

The adaptational model used in the treatment rationale focuses on patients' adjustment to their disease. Patients are asked to identify changes in their life that have occurred as a result of having OA and pain symptoms. Specifically they are asked about changes in three areas of adjustment: (1) daily activities (e.g. ability to work, carry out household chores, participate in recreational activities), (2) thoughts (e.g. thoughts about self, others, and the future), and (3) feelings (e.g. anxiety, anger, or depression). Several points are highlighted in the discussion. These include the fact that: (a) the changes identified are common and shared by most of the patients, (b) the patterns of adjustment have usually developed gradually over the course of time, and (c) that the changes in adjustment can, in turn, influence arthritis pain (e.g. feeling discouraged is often associated with increased pain). Patients are told that training in coping skills can provide a new and more effective alternative to learned patterns of adjustment.

The second element of the rationale consists of a simplified presentation of the gate control theory of pain.[21] The discussion begins with a brief description of traditional pain theories that highlights some of the problems of these theories such as the failure to explain the absence of pain following injury (e.g. in battlefield and sports injuries), the poor correlation between amount of tissue damage and amount of perceived pain, and the failure to account for psychological and behavioral factors that can influence pain. The gate control theory is then presented as an alternative to traditional pain theories. This theory highlights the fact that pain is a complex experience and that the patient's own cognitive and behavioral responses can influence pain. Patients are asked to identify specific thoughts, feelings, and behaviors that they have found influence their own pain. Coping skills are then introduced as techniques for altering cognitive and behavioral responses to pain and thereby enhancing pain control.

The third component of the rationale is designed to help patients understand that learning how to cope with arthritis is a skill. Like any skill, practice is important. Patients are given the opportunity to practice each coping skill in the group setting and the therapists provide feedback and guidance on performance. At the end of each session, the patients are also given explicit instructions about how to practice at home and their compliance with these instructions is monitored at the start of the next group session. Obstacles to regular practice are pinpointed in the group sessions and problem solving is used to identify innovative ways to overcome these obstacles.

Specific skills training

The coping skills training protocol is designed to increase patients' sense of control over pain and to reduce the use of catastrophizing variables that have been related to pain in OA patients.

Controlling pain through attention diversion

To help patients control and decrease pain more effectively, they are provided with systematic training in three attention diversion techniques: progressive relaxation training, imagery, and distraction methods. Progressive relaxation training[22] consists of slowly tensing and relaxing major muscle groups starting with those in the feet and legs and progressing to those in the face, scalp, and neck. The therapists initially demonstrate the relaxation exercises and then use a relaxation tape to guide patients through the relaxation process. Patients are asked to listen to the relaxation tape at least twice daily. Imagery is introduced as a way to heighten relaxation and enhance pain control. Patients are asked to focus on a pleasant image (e.g. relaxing at the beach or by a mountain lake or stream) and to try to involve each of their senses in the imagery. They are encouraged to use pleasant imagery at the end of each relaxation session and whenever they are feeling increased pain. The distraction techniques help patients alter thought patterns during episodes of increased pain. One distraction method involves counting backwards slowly from 100–1. Another technique involves focusing on distracting features of the physical environment such as a pleasant picture on the wall or a photo of a loved one. To help patients become more aware of the pain reducing effects of distraction, they are asked to record their pain level before and after practice and note any differences in pain that occur.

Controlling pain by changing activity patterns

Patients are trained in two activity-based coping skills for controlling pain: activity–rest cycling and pleasant activity scheduling. Activity–rest cycling is designed to help patients better pace their activities over the day.[23] Many OA patients overdo daily activities such as shopping or yard work and push themselves until they reach the point of pain tolerance before stopping and allowing themselves to rest. In activity–rest cycling, patients learn to break up activities they tend to overdo into periods of moderate activity followed by limited rest. A patient who reports having severe knee pain after hours of yard work, for example, might be taught to break up the yard work into 30-minute periods of work followed by 10 minutes of rest. The activity–rest cycle works best when it is repeated frequently. To encourage repetition of the cycle patients are asked to keep track of the number of activity–rest cycles they complete each week. As patients become accustomed to the cycle, the amount of time spent in the activity phase of the cycle can be increased and the amount of time spent in the rest phase decreased.

Pleasant activity scheduling[24] is a second activity-based coping skill that helps patients manage pain better. Many patients with moderate or severe arthritis pain have reduced their involvement in pleasant activities and tend to live very restricted and unrewarding lifestyles. As a result, they have few distractions from pain and often feel discouraged and depressed. To counter this behavioral pattern, patients are encouraged to identify a range of pleasant activities they might enjoy doing. A list of 20–30 activities is typically developed and patients are asked to select activity goals from this list on a weekly basis. Different goals are set each week and patients' attainment of these goals is systematically monitored in the group. Many patients report reductions in pain and improvements in mood when they are involved in pleasant activities.

Spouse-assisted pain coping skills

Previous research has shown that RA patients with supportive spouses are more likely to use active coping styles, while patients whose spouses are highly critical use more maladaptive coping styles and show worse psychological adjustment.[25] Influenced by these findings, a coping skills training protocol has been developed for OA patients and their spouses.[26] Couples attend group sessions that include pain coping skills training in the gate control theory of pain, distraction, activity–rest cycling, and pleasant activity scheduling. In addition, the patients and their spouses are trained in couple skills, such as communication, behavioral rehearsal, and mutual goal setting. Spouses can help the patients learn and maintain the use of pain coping strategies.

Research on coping skills interventions for OA patients

One controlled study has tested the efficacy of coping skills training for OA patients.[12,13] Ninety-nine patients having OA of the knees were randomly assigned to one of three interventions: pain coping skills training, arthritis education, or a standard care control condition. Patients in the pain coping skills training condition received an intervention identical to that described above: that is, 10 weekly, 90-minute sessions focused on enhancing pain coping skills. Patients in the arthritis education intervention attended 10 weekly, 90-minute group sessions that used a lecture–discussion format to present basic information on the diagnosis and treatment of OA. Patients in the standard care condition continued with their routine care. Data analysis revealed that patients in the pain coping skills training condition had significantly lower levels of pain and psychological disability than patients in the arthritis education or standard care condition. At 6-months follow-up, patients in the pain coping skills training condition had significantly lower levels of psychological and physical disability than patients in the arthritis education condition, and marginally lower levels of psychological and physical disability than patients in the standard care condition. Correlational analyses showed that changes in coping were related to treatment outcome. Patients in the pain coping skills training condition who showed increases in scores on the Pain Control and Rational Thinking (PCRT) factor of the Coping Strategies Questionnaire had significantly lower levels of pain, physical disability, psychological disability, and pain behavior at long-term follow-up.

Calfas et al.[27] have also conducted a study comparing the efficacy of a cognitive–behavioral coping skills training intervention and a traditional educational intervention for patients having OA. This study found that both the coping skills training group and the educational group had significant improvements in depression and short-term (6 months) improvements in physical and psychological functioning. There was a borderline ($p < 0.07$) tendency for the coping skills training group to show improvement relative to the education group when comparing outcomes before and after treatment. At 1-year follow-up, however, these group differences were not apparent. These findings suggest that both educational and coping skills training interventions may have benefits for OA patients, but that patients may have difficulty maintaining their treatment gains.

One approach to enhancing the short- and long-term effects of a coping skills training intervention is to combine it with an educational program designed to increase patients knowledge about their disease. Lorig and her colleagues[28] were the first to investigate the efficacy of a combined coping skills training and arthritis education intervention for OA patients. Their protocol, called the Arthritis Self-Management Program, systematically taught patients about their disease and also provided training in relaxation, exercise, and a variety of cognitive self-management strategies. Training was carried out in group sessions of 10–15 patients that met weekly for two hours for six weeks. Each group was led by two lay leaders who had been trained in the program. Outcome data have demonstrated that this program is effective in reducing pain and improving knowledge about arthritis in a heterogeneous population of arthritis patients, 75 per cent of whom had OA.[28,29] A 4-year follow-up of the Arthritis Self-Management Program has shown that patients were able to maintain their gains in pain relief and that they also showed a highly significant reduction in physician office visits.[30] The program appears to be cost-effective in that the savings in terms of medical care substantially outweighed the costs of the program. In fact, Lorig et al.[30] estimated that if only 1 per cent of individuals with OA in the United States of America participated in the program the net savings over four years would be $14 500 000.

One study was conducted to examine the efficacy of spouse-assisted coping skills training.[26,31] Patients were assigned to one of three treatment groups: (1) spouse-assisted pain coping skills training, (2) conventional coping skills training without spouses, or (3) arthritis eduction with spouses. Patients who completed the spouse-assisted pain coping skills training protocol showed less psychological disability and lower pain ratings than patients in the other treatment conditions. They also had better marital adjustment scores and self-efficacy ratings than those patients who participated in the arthritis education with their spouses. At a 12-month follow-up, overall self-efficacy was still highest in patients who completed the spouse-assisted coping skills training. Those patients whose self-efficacy ratings increased upon completion of the spouse-assisted coping skills training were more likely to report less pain, psychological disability, and physical disability at the 12-month follow-up. Results suggest promise in involving partners in future coping skills interventions for patients with OA.

Taken together, the results of recent treatment outcome studies suggest that coping skills training or combined coping skills training and arthritis education interventions can reduce pain and improve the psychological functioning of patients with OA.

Future directions

Recent studies suggest that a focus on coping is important in understanding pain and disability in patients having OA. The results of these studies have potentially important implications for future assessment and treatment efforts.

One area of future research possibilities is in gender differences in coping methods. A study of 72 male and 96 female patients with OA examined coping differences.[32] Female patients reported greater levels of pain and physical disability. Under observation, women with OA also showed more pain behavior than men. Analysis found that these results were mediated by catastrophizing, a maladaptive coping style that exaggerates the negative impact of pain and one's inability to cope with pain. Future research might test interventions targeted to reduce catastrophizing in women as a function of gender-specific coping skills training. Research on other gender differences in coping styles might yield more information on individual coping styles.

Coping skills training may have different success depending on an individual readiness to adapt to new coping strategies. Another research direction might consider Prochaska and DiClemente's stages of change model.[33] This model posits that individuals differ in how able and willing they are to make lifestyle changes. Prochaska and DiClemente identified five stages of change: (1) precontemplation, (2) contemplation, (3) preparation, (4) unprepared action, and (5) prepared maintenance. In a recent study, distinct clusters were identified that fell into these five stages using cluster analysis of stages of change ratings from a sample of 103 patients with RA and 72 patients with OA.[34] Interventions could be developed to move patients from one stage to the other to maximize the benefits of coping skills training.

Recent studies of emotional disclosure (where a person is asked to talk about stressful life experiences either alone or with the help of a clinician) have reported significant health benefits.[35–37] These studies found that subjects who participated in emotional disclosure reported health problems less frequently than those who did not. In the study by Esterling,[35] the immune systems of patients who completed emotional disclosure also showed increased functioning. A study currently being conducted in our lab is testing the efficacy of private emotional disclosure and clinician-assisted emotional disclosure in reducing pain, psychological disability, and physical disability in patients with RA. Emotional disclosure should be explored as a means to pain reduction and improved coping in OA patients.

In terms of assessment, clinicians working with populations of OA patients need to be more aware of how individual patients cope with their disease. Patients who report their coping strategies are ineffective and who tend to worry and focus excessively on the negative aspects of pain may be at risk for increased pain and disability. To identify these patients, clinicians may wish to gather baseline data on coping using questionnaire instruments such as the CSQ or AAWOC. Individuals who are having difficulty coping could be referred for coping skills training interventions that may prevent the development of maladaptive behavioral and cognitive responses to OA. Periodic assessments of coping may also be useful in tracking patients' progress over the course of treatment. Our clinical observations suggest that patients who have a good response to medical or surgical treatments for OA, for example, often show an increase in the use and perceived effectiveness of their own cognitive and behavioral coping skills.

In terms of treatment, there are a number of important future directions. First, coping skills training and related educational interventions need to be more fully integrated into the management of OA. One obstacle has been the costs involved in having psychologists or highly skilled mental health professionals conduct such treatments. Studies by Lorig et al.,[28,29] however, suggest that nurse educators and lay individuals can deliver these interventions in a cost-effective manner. Innovative computer-based formats for coping skills training are also being developed and evaluated and are likely to significantly reduce the costs of this intervention.

Second, methods for enhancing the long-term efficacy of coping skills training interventions need to be developed. The relapse prevention model developed by Marlatt and Gordon[38] can serve as a theoretical foundation to guide therapists interested in enhancing the maintenance of coping skills training interventions in arthritis patients.[39] This model maintains that relapse is a process and that patients can learn to analyze and to cope with specific episodes of relapse. Arthritis patients, for example, can be trained to recognize early warning signs of a setback or relapse and then to apply coping skills in a timely fashion. Through behavioral rehearsal arthritis patients can also learn strategies for dealing with major setbacks or relapse episodes. Finally, by training arthritis patients in self-monitoring and self-reinforcement skills one can potentially maintain a much more frequent use of coping skills.

Conclusions

The coping perspective has much to offer clinicians working with OA patients. Research findings gathered over the past 15 years suggest that an analysis of coping can not only help in understanding pain and disability, but that it can also be useful in symptom management. By extending the coping perspective even more fully into clinical practice, one may be able to significantly reduce the pain and suffering experienced by OA patients.

Key points for clinical practice 1

1. There is growing evidence that pain coping strategies (as assessed using the Coping Strategies Questionnaire) is related to pain and disability in patients with arthritis.

2. Interestingly, the effects of patients pain coping are evident even after controlling for the effects of demographic variables and medical status variables.

Key points for clinical practice 2

1. Systematic training in nonpharmacological pain control techniques can reduce pain and disability.

2. Training typically focuses on two sets of techniques: (a) those designed to control pain through attention diversion (relaxation, imagery, distraction methods) and (b) those designed to control pain by changing activity patterns (activity–rest cycling and pleasant activity scheduling).

3. Recent evidence indicates that involving spouses in pain coping skills training may be helpful in patients having OA.

4. Spouse-involvement in coping skills training appears to be more effective than spouse involvement in an informational/support intervention.

References

(An asterisk denotes recommended reading.)

1. Keefe, F.J., Caldwell, D.S., Queen, K.T., Gil, K.M., Marinez, S., Crisson, J.E., Ogden, W., and Numley, J. (1987). Pain coping strategies in osteoarthritis patients. *J Consul Clin Psychol* **55**:208–12.

2. Lazarus, R.S. and Folkman, S. (1984). *Stress, appraisal and coping.* New York: Springer.

3. Folkman, S., Lazarus, R.S., Dunkel-Schetter, C., DeLongis, A., and Gruen, R. (1986). The dynamics of a stressful encounter: cognitive appraisal, coping and encounter outcomes. *J Pers Soc Psychol* **50**:992–1003.

4. Burke, M. and Flaherty, M.J. (1993). Coping strategies and health status of elderly arthritic women. *J Adv Nurs* **18**:7–13.

5. Jalowiec, A. (1988). Confirmatory factor analysis of the Jalowiec Coping Scale. In C.F. Waltz and O.L. Strickland, *Measuring Client Outcomes.* New York: Springer, pp. 287–308.

6. Downe-Wambolt, B. (1991). Stress, emotions and coping: a study of elderly women with OA. *J Adv Nurs* **16**:1328–35.

7. Regan, C.A., Lorig, K., and Thorensen, C.E. (1988). Arthritis appraisal and ways of coping: scale development. *Arthritis Care Res* **1**:139–50.

8. Rosenstiel, A.R. and Keefe, F.J. (1983). The use of coping strategies in chronic low back pain patients: Relationship to patient characteristics and current adjustment. *Pain* **17**:33–40.

9. Kazis, L.E., Meenan, R.F., and Anderson, J. (1983). Pain in the rheumatic diseases: Investigations of a key health status component. *Arthritis Rheum* **4**:10–13.

10. Parker, J.C., Frank, R.G., Beck, N.C., Smarr, K.L., Phillips, L.R., Smith, E.I., Anderson, S.K., and Walker, S.E. (1988). Pain management in rheumatoid arthritis patients: A cognitive-behavioral approach. *Arthritis Rheum* **29**:1456–66.

11. Keefe, F.J., Caldwell, D.S., Queen, K.T., Gil, K.M., Martinez, S., Crisson, J.E., Ogden, W., and Nunley, J. (1987). Osteoarthritic knee pain: A behavioral analysis. *J Consul Clin Psychol* **55**:208–12.

12. Keefe, F.J., Caldwell, D.S., Williams, D.A., Gil, K.M., Mitchell, D., Robertson, D., Robertson, C., Martinez, S., Nunley, J., Beckham, J.C., and Helms, M. (1990). Pain coping skills training in the management of osteoarthritic knee pain: A comparative study. *Behavior Therapy* **21**:49–62.

13. Keefe, F.J., Caldwell, D.S., Williams, D.A., Gil, K.M., Mitchell, D., Robertson, C., Martinez, S., Nunley, J., Beckham, J.C., Crisson, J.E., and Helms, M. (1990). Pain coping skills training in the management of osteoarthritic knee pain: Follow-up results. *Behavior Therapy* **21**:435–48.

14. Kraaimaatt, F.W. and van Schevikhoven, R.E.O. (1984) *Inventarisatielijst Pijngedrag (Pain Coping Inventory).*

15. Hopman-Rock, M., Kraaimaatt, F.W., Odding, E., and Bijlsma, J.W.J. (1998). Coping with pain in the hip or knee in relation to physical disability in community-living elderly people. *Arthritis Care Res* **11**:588–602.

16. Stone, A.A. and Neale, J. (1984). The effects of 'severe' daily events on mood. *J Pers Soc Psychol* **46**:137–44.

17. Affleck, G., Urrows, S., Tennen, H., and Higgins, P. (1992). Daily coping with pain from rheumatoid arthritis: patterns and correlates. *Pain* **51**:221–9.

18. Affleck, G., Tennen, H., Keefe, F.J., Lefebvre, J.C., Kashikar-Zuck, S., Wright, K., Starr, K., and Caldwell, D.S. (1999). Everyday life with osteoarthritis or rheumatoid arthritis: independent effects of disease and gender on daily pain, mood, and coping. *Pain* **83**:601–9.

19. Bradley, L.A., Young, L.D., Anderson, K.O., Turner, R.A., Agudelo, C.A., McDaniel, L.K., Pisko, E.J., Semble, E.L., and Morgan, T.M. (1987). Effects of psychological therapy on pain behavior of rheumatoid arthritis patients: Treatment outcome and six month follow-up. *Arthritis Rheum* **30**:1105–14.

20. *Keefe, F.J., Beaupre, P.M., and Gil, K.M. (1996). Group therapy for patients with chronic pain. In R.J. Turk and R.J. Gatchel, *Psychological Approaches for Pain Management: A Practitioner's Handbook.* New York: Guilford Press. pp. 254–82.
   This chapter provides a very detailed and practical guide to conducting cognitive-behavioral coping skills training groups for patients having pain.

21. Melzack, R. and Wall, P. (1965). Pain mechanisms: A new theory. *Science* **50**:971–9.

22. Bernstein, D.A. and Borkovec, T.D. (1973) *Progressive relaxation training: A manual for the helping professions.*

23. Gil, K.M., Ross, S.L., and Keefe, F.J. (1988). Behavioral treatment of chronic pain: Four pain management protocols. In: R.D. France and K.R. Krishnan, *Chronic Pain.* New York: American Psychiatric Press, pp. 376–413.

24. Lewinsohn, P.M. (1975). The behavioral study and treatment of depression. In: M. Hersen, R.M. Eisler, and P.M. Miller, *Progress in Behavior Modification: Volume 1.* New York: Academic Press, pp. 19–65.

25. Manne, S.L. and Zautra, A.J. (1990). Couples coping with chronic illness: Women with rheumatoid arthritis and their healthy husbands. *J Behav Med* **13**:327–42.

26. Keefe, F.J., Caldwell, D.S., Baucom, D., Salley, A., Robinson, E., Timmons, K., Beaupre, T., Weisberg, J., and Helms, M. (1996). Spouse-assisted coping skills training in the management of osteoarthritic knee pain. *Arthritis Care Res* **9**:279–91.

27. Calfas, K.J., Kaplan, R.M., and Ingram, R. (1992). One-year evaluation of cognitive-behavioral intervention in osteoarthritis. *Arthritis Care Res* **5**:202–9.

28. Lorig, K., Laurin, J., and Holman, H.R. (1984). Arthritis self-management: a study of the effectiveness of patient education in the elderly. *Gerontologist* **24**:455–62.

29. Lorig, K., Lubeck, D.P., Kraines, R.G., Seleznick, M., and Holman, H.R. (1985). Outcomes of self-help education for patients with arthritis. *Arthritis Rheum* **28**:680–5.

30. Lorig, K.R., Mazonson, P.D., and Holman, H.R. (1993). Evidence suggesting that health education for self-management in patients with chronic arthritis has sustained health benefits while reducing health care costs. *Arthritis Rheum* **36**:439–46.

31. *Keefe, F.J., Caldwell, D.S., Baucom, D., Salley, A., Robinson, E., Timmons, K., Beaupre, P.M., Weisberg, J., and Helms, M. (1999). Spouse-assisted coping skills training in the management of knee pain in osteoarthritis: Long-term follow-up results. *Arthritis Care Res* **12**:101–11.

    This paper presents one of the few controlled studies of a couples-based approach to pain management training.

32. Keefe, F.J., Lefebvre, J.C., Egert, J.R., Affleck, G., Sullivan, M.J., and Caldwell, D.S. (2000). The relationship of gender to pain, pain behavior, and disability in osteoarthritis patients: The role of catastrophizing. *Pain* **87**:325–34.

33. *Prochaska, J.O. and DiClemente, C.C. (1998) Towards a comprehensive, transtheoretical model of change: states of change and addictive behaviors. In: W.R. Miller and N. Heather, *Applied Clinical Psychology* (2nd ed.). *Treating Addictive Behavior*. New York: Plenum Press, pp. 3–24.

    This is an excellent overview of a comprehensive theory that can be used to understand issues of maintenance and relapse in patients having a variety of health conditions.

34. Keefe, F.J., Lefebvre, J.C., Kerns, R.D., Rosenberg, R., Beaupre, P.M., Prochaska, J., Prochaska, J.O., and Caldwell, D.S. (2000). Understanding the adoption of arthritis self-management: stages of change profiles among arthritis patients. *Pain* **87**:303–13.

35. Esterling, B.A., Antoni, M.H., Fletcher, M.A., Marguilies, S., and Schniederman, N. (1994). Emotional disclosure through writing of speaking modulates latent EpsteinBarr Virus antibody titers. *J Consul Clin Psychol* **62**:130–40.

36. Greenberg, M.A., Wortman, C.B., and Stone, A.A. (1996). Emotional expression and physical health: Revising traumatic memories or fostering self-regulation? *J Pers Soc Psychol* **71**:588–602.

37. *Pennebaker, J.W. (1992). Putting stress into words: The impact of writing on psychological absentee and self-reported emotional well being measures. *Am J Health Promotion* **6**:280–7.

    This paper highlights recent findings supporting the benefits of emotional disclosure interventions.

38. Marlatt, G.A. and Gordon, J.R. (1985) *Relapse Prevention*. New York: Guildford.

39. Keefe, F.J. and Van Horn, Y. (1993). Cognitive-behavioral treatment of rheumatoid arthritis pain: Maintaining treatment gains. *Arthritis Care Res* **6**:213–22.

9.17 Irrigation of the osteoarthritic joint

John D. Bradley

Irrigation of a joint (JI) has been widely referred to as joint lavage. Lavage means 'the washing out of an organ,' whereas irrigate has multiple meanings, including 'to wash out or flush with water or other fluid' and 'to refresh by watering.' As a treatment for OA, JI theoretically could be beneficial by virtue of the removal of particulate debris from the joint space (e.g., loose bodies of cartilage and bone, calcium crystals). In addition, it might have 'refreshing' effects on joint tissues, particularly the articular cartilage and synovium, or by mobilizing phlogistic materials (e.g., degradative enzymes, cytokines) from the tissues, altering cellular behavior through the change it produces in the extracellular environment. Finally, JI could be efficacious by reducing the temperature of the joint or distension of the joint capsule.

Regardless of the mechanism, clinical benefits associated with JI were reported in 1934 in patients undergoing arthroscopy.[1] With the development of surgical interventions performed via arthroscopy, the benefits of the JI, relative to those of the surgery itself, have been debated. Only recently has the importance of the placebo effect of JI been appreciated and assessed. In contrast to the enthusiastic appraisal of JI expressed in the 1995 guidelines[2] for management of OA published by the American College of Rheumatology Subcommittee on OA Guidelines, the revision of these guidelines, published in 2000,[3] contained a considerably more conservative endorsement.[4] However, the recently published European League Against Rheumatism recommendations for the management of knee OA continue to support JI as an effective treatment.[4]

Possible mechanisms underlying the beneficial effect of JI

Cartilage fragments of varying size and soluble cartilage matrix proteins, presumably released as a result of disruption of the articular cartilage surface, may be found in OA synovial fluid.[5,6] These particulate fragments and soluble matrix molecules can be phagocytized by synovial macrophages,[7] inciting an inflammatory response.[8] JI would remove these fragments, thereby reducing the inflammatory response. Clinical improvement may correlate with the mass of the fragments removed by the irrigation procedure.[9] Removal of calcium-containing crystals from the joint space and tissues might also be important.[10] Such crystals have been demonstrated in the early phases of OA in animal models,[11] and their prevalence in human OA may be insufficiently appreciated because of the poor sensitivity and specificity of routine light microscopic techniques and standard radiographs.[12] Deposits of calcium crystals have been found in a substantial proportion of OA knees evaluated by arthroscopy, and their detection (and removal) may correlate with the clinical response to arthroscopic irrigation.[13,14] In addition to reducing the pain associated with OA, reduction of synovial inflammation may diminish the impact on the articular cartilage of cytokines, matrix metalloproteinases, and toxic oxygen radicals.[15] A 'disease-modifying' effect of JI has not been demonstrated, however.

Clinical trials

Numerous reports of JI have been published, describing a variety of techniques for performance of the procedure. Many represent uncontrolled observations. While generally enthusiastic about the results,[16–18] some investigators have noted that the response to JI was inversely related to the severity of radiographic changes of OA.[16] The following discussion will focus on randomized, controlled trials of JI.

JI was evaluated by Dawes et al. in 20 subjects randomized to receive either a 10 ml injection of saline (the placebo group) after aspiration of the knee or 2 L continuous irrigation with saline through 14 gauge needles placed into the superolateral and medial aspects of the knee.[19] In both treatment groups, evaluation 12 weeks later showed similar reductions in overall, rest, and night pain, in comparison with the baseline values, with differences between the groups slightly favoring the placebo. Technical limitations of this study included possible 'streaming' of the irrigation fluid from the inflow to the outflow port, which might have reduced the effectiveness of irrigation, and the failure to employ intra-articular anesthesia, resulting in pain during and immediately after the procedure. Furthermore, neither the subjects nor the investigator who performed the assessments were effectively blinded to the identity of the treatment.

The tidal irrigation (TI) method of JI was compared to conservative medical management in a single-blinded (blinded physician-assessor) trial reported by Ike et al.[20] The subjects were at least 21 years old; had Kellgren and Lawrence[21] grade I–III radiographic changes of OA; had had an inadequate response to intra-articular corticosteroids, physical therapy, NSAIDs, and analgesics; and had persistent knee pain on motion or at rest. During a two-week 'stabilization period,' all subjects were instructed in a medical management approach that included instruction in isometric exercise and joint protection principles, and modification of their NSAID/analgesic regimen. Subjects were then randomized to receive TI or not.

The TI procedure involved intra-articular instillation of 50 mL of 0.25 per cent bupivicaine, placement of a 14 gauge needle into a single superolateral port, aspiration of the knee, and sequential instillation and withdrawal of fresh 20–80 mL aliquots of sterile saline until 1 L of saline had been passed through the knee. Follow-up evaluations were performed weekly for one month, and then monthly for two additional months. Outcome measures included function tests, such as the times required to walk 50 feet and to ascend and to descend 4 steps, and measurement of pain associated with each of these activities on a 100 mm visual analog scale (VAS).

The initial protocol called for enrolment of 120 subjects, but because an interim analysis revealed statistically significant differences favoring TI, only 77 subjects were enrolled. Fifty-seven completed the study. Eight of the 10 medical management subjects and 2 of the 10 TI subjects who withdrew did so because of inadequate symptom control. TI was statistically superior to medical management alone in improving pain after walking and after ascending steps; maximum reported pain; frequency of knee stiffness; physician-assessed knee tenderness; and global efficacy, as judged by both the physician and the subject. These differences were apparent at the first follow-up assessment and persisted throughout the 12 weeks. The authors recognized that some of the apparent benefit might have been attributable to a placebo effect, but noted '… any potential participant who had first been informed of the distension-irrigation mechanics of tidal knee irrigation would readily distinguish any sham procedure we might devise as being quite different from true tidal knee irrigation and thus could never be truly blinded to the treatment being performed.'

TI performed in a fashion similar to that in the above study[20] was compared to arthroscopic surgery in a single-blinded (blinded physician-assessor) randomized study reported by Chang et al.,[22] which involved a similar subject population. Notably, fewer than half of the subjects reported being able to walk more than 4 blocks at the time of enrolment; about half were using an assistive device for walking; and the mean 50-foot walk time was 15 seconds (about twice the normal). Notably, of the more than 200 subjects who, at screening, appeared to be eligible to participate in this study, over half experienced sufficient improvement with conservative medical management prior to randomization to make TI or arthroscopy unnecessary. Of the 18 randomized to receive arthroscopy, 3 did not undergo the procedure. Each of the remaining 15 subjects underwent some form of surgical intervention during arthroscopy: 8 underwent surgical repair of the medial meniscus and 7 of the lateral meniscus. Improvement was defined as reduction of at least one point on a 10-point Arthritis Impact Measurement Scales (AIMS)[23] pain scale; an increase of at least 1 cm on a 10 cm VAS for 'overall well-being' assessed by the subject; and reduction of at least one point on a 4-point physician's global disease severity scale.

Arthroscopy and, particularly, repair of the meniscus, was associated with improvement in AIMS pain and physical activity, well-being, and knee tenderness at 3 and 12 months, compared to the baseline values. The 14 subjects in the TI control group showed significant improvement, relative to baseline, only in AIMS pain at 12 months. Only two significant between-group differences (knee tenderness and the physician's global assessment) were found, both of which favored arthroscopy. Neither group showed improvement in range of motion, swelling, AIMS physical functioning or social activity, or in the 50-foot walk time. Interestingly, the radiographic grade of OA (the study was restricted to subjects with Kellgren and Lawrence grade I–III changes) was not predictive of outcome, and signs and symptoms of meniscus damage did not predict the pathology identified at arthroscopy. The degree of cartilage damage, as assessed by arthroscopy, and AIMS depression and anxiety scores correlated with the severity of knee pain. The authors recognized that the subjects' assessments were likely affected by '… the very strong and highly probable surgical placebo effect.'

Using a Latin square design, Ravaud et al.[24] evaluated the effects of JI and intra-articular corticosteroid injection on symptoms in 98 subjects with knee OA. About half of the subjects in the JI and non-JI groups were randomized to receive an intra-articular corticosteroid injection, while the others received an intra-articular injection of saline. The JI procedure was single-blinded (using a blinded physician assessor) but the placebo-controlled corticosteroid injection was double-blinded. Under local anesthesia with lidocaine, two 14 gauge cannulae were placed in the suprapatellar areas, medially and laterally, of the JI subjects. One liter of saline flowed from the medial to the lateral port, with intermittent interruption of flow and manipulation of the knee to facilitate filling, lavage, and drainage. Clinical assessments were completed at baseline and 1, 4, 12, and 24 weeks after the procedure(s), and included the subject's assessment of pain in the treated knee over the past week and of their global status, and their score on the Lequesne algofunctional index.[25] 'Response' was defined as a 30 per cent reduction in VAS pain, relative to baseline. Use of NSAIDs and analgesics was permitted during the study, but these medications were discontinued shortly before each assessment.

All of the subjects had baseline VAS knee pain ≥ 40 mm and Kellgren and Lawrence grade II–IV radiographic changes; about half had evidence of a knee effusion. Two-thirds had bilateral knee involvement and one-third had severe (grade IV) radiographic changes. Randomization yielded comparable groups except that knee pain in the JI plus intra-articular corticosteroid group was significantly lower at baseline than in the other groups. Five subjects did not receive their assigned treatment and 4 incorrectly received JI. A greater proportion of subjects in the placebo group than in

the intra-articular steroid group were lost to follow-up, mostly because of inefficacy of treatment.

Intra-articular corticosteroid injection significantly improved knee pain, global status, and Lequesne index scores only at weeks 1 and 4, whereas the JI group reported improvement in pain at weeks 4, 12, and 24, and in global status at weeks 4 and 12. While the authors concluded that the effects were 'additive,' the only benefit of intra-articular corticosteroid injection in combination with JI was an improvement in the 'early' response, that is, at weeks 1 and 4. The authors noted: 'We also cannot discount the possibility that the joint lavage effect was due only to a powerful placebo effect' and commented that '…joint lavage would be easily distinguished from any other (intra-articular) procedure.'

In a simplified study design, Bradley et al.[26] performed a randomized, double-blinded evaluation of TI; using a modification of the method described by Ike[17] and Chang.[19] Notably, in contrast to other studies of TI, this study included a sham irrigation (SI) control group. In all subjects, the skin and joint capsule were anesthetized with 1 per cent lidocaine and 0.25 per cent bupivicaine. A small sample of synovial fluid was aspirated (when possible) prior to intra-articular injection of 20 mL of bupivicaine. Subjects were prevented from viewing the blinded portion of SI or TI by the positioning of a drape, but were able to view the supply bag of saline at the edge of the drape. A closed system of tubing, stopcocks, a 50 mL syringe, and an empty waste bag was assembled for each subject. The identity of the treatment to be given was kept in a sealed envelope, which was opened by the procedurist immediately before treatment was given.

For TI subjects, a 14 gauge cannula was placed in the knee joint through a lateral suprapatellar port; for SI subjects, the cannula was placed in the anesthetized subcutaneous tissue abutting, but not penetrating, the joint capsule. While TI proceeded with 20–30 'exchanges' of saline (30–50 mL each), for SI, the saline was drawn into the syringe and 3–5 mL per 'exchange' was infiltrated into the pericapsular subcutaneous tissue over a period of time comparable to that required for actual injection into and aspiration of fluid from, the knee joint for TI; the remainder of the saline was expelled directly into the waste bag. In both treatment groups, the knee was maintained in relaxed extension, and the anterior knee was massaged periodically. The time required for the entire procedure was 45–60 minutes. Upon completion of the procedure, the procedurist left the room and the blinded assessor, who was not aware of which treatment had been given, asked the subject to guess the identity of their treatment (SI or TI) and to express their level of certainty about their guess.

The primary outcome measure was the change from baseline in the Western Ontario-McMaster Universities OA Index (WOMAC)[27] pain score, using an intent-to-treat analysis. Joint tenderness and swelling, 50-foot walk time, and the investigator's global assessment were recorded. Subjects also completed the WOMAC physical functioning and stiffness scales and the Quality of Well-Being scale. Assessments were made at baseline and 3, 6, and 12 months after the procedure.

The 180 subjects in the study met the ACR clinical criteria for OA, had current knee pain, and were ambulatory without assistance. Randomization was stratified according to the severity of X-ray scores; most subjects had Kellgren and Lawrence grade II–III changes. The SI and TI groups were comparable with respect to age; sex; race; marital status; duration of knee symptoms and the frequency of bilateral knee symptoms. However, the SI group had significantly higher (worse) WOMAC pain and physical functioning scores at baseline.

Subjects were allowed to take NSAIDs during the study, but only about 10 per cent of each study group did so. Acetaminophen was provided as a 'rescue analgesic,' but mean daily consumption was only 1 g per day in both groups and changed little over the course of the study.

About 90 per cent of subjects in both the TI and SI group guessed they had received TI, and nearly one-fourth of subjects in both groups were 'absolutely certain.' Over half of the minority who guessed they had received SI were 'not certain.'

Outcomes data were available for over 97 per cent of subjects in each group at each time point (Table 9.38). Two TI subjects did not receive TI because of technical difficulties; 5 subjects in each group received an

Table 9.38 Outcomes of JI and SI in patients with knee OA

Variable	Enrollment (week 1)		Baseline (week 0)		12 Weeks		24 Weeks		52 Weeks	
	Sham	TI	Sham	TI	Sham	TI	Sham	TI	Sham	TI
N	91	89	91	89	91	87	89	87	89	88
Difficulty with knee over past week?										
(assessed by subjects)										
None	0	1	2	2	17	21	13	18	15	16
Mild	17	23	17	26	34	32	31	32	26	34
Moderate	38	39	40	41	25	24	30	24	27	26
Severe	23	23	24	16	12	4	11	11	16	9
Extreme	13	3	8	3	2	6	4	1	4	1
Tenderness, mean ± SD (range, 0–3)	0.76 ± 0.72	0.55 ± 0.58	0.63 ± 0.57	0.53 ± 0.55	0.46 ± 0.64	0.43 ± 0.68	0.56 ± 0.64	0.49 ± 0.61	0.52 ± 0.68	0.59 ± 0.74
Swelling, mean ± SD (range, 0–3)	0.69 ± 0.68	0.56 ± 0.71	0.58 ± 0.62	0.64 ± 0.71	0.37 ± 0.55	0.48 ± 0.71	0.34 ± 0.52	0.3 ± 0.53	0.33 ± 0.56	0.3 ± 0.49
50 Foot walk time, seconds, mean ± SD	11.9 ± 4.1	10.7 ± 3.5	11.2 ± 3.4	10.6 ± 3.4	10.6 ± 2.5	10.2 ± 3.4	10.5 ± 2.5	10.2 ± 3.2	10.8 ± 3.2	10.1 ± 3.2
WOMAC pain score, mean ± SD (range, 5–25)	14.5 ± 3.9	13.5 ± 3.9	14.5 ± 3.8	13.2 ± 3.9	11.2 ± 4.3	10.4 ± 4.2	11.8 ± 4.7	11.1 ± 3.9	11.9 ± 4.6	10.4 ± 3.9
WOMAC function score, mean ± SD (range, 17–85)	50.2 ± 13.8	47 ± 12.6	51.5 ± 14.1	45.4 ± 12.4	40.7 ± 14.5	37.9 ± 14.6	42.8 ± 14.3	38.9 ± 3.9	41.9 ± 14.7	37.9 ± 13.5

JI, joint irrigation; SD, standard deviation.

Differences between the group that received TI and the group that received SI were not statistically significant at any time point.

The data shown with respect to difficulty with knee over past week represent the number of subjects.

Source: Taken from Ref. 26.

intra-articular corticosteroid injection during the course of follow-up. After adjustment for baseline scores, no differences between TI and SI were apparent for any of the outcomes. Both groups showed about 20 per cent improvement in WOMAC pain and physical functioning. Furthermore, neither demographic nor radiographic features, the presence of a synovial effusion at the time of treatment, synovial fluid leukocyte count, nor the presence of crystals in the synovial fluid were predictors of improvement. The authors concluded that the benefit of TI is largely attributable to a placebo effect. *Post hoc* administration of questionnaires addressing depression, self-efficacy, and ability to cope with pain showed that positive and active pain coping strategies were associated with greater degrees of benefit, regardless of which treatment was given.[28]

A three-arm randomized comparison of arthroscopic debridement, arthroscopic irrigation, and sham arthroscopy in the treatment of knee OA has been recently reported in an abstract by Moseley *et al.*[29] All subjects were sedated in the operating room and received soft tissue anesthesia with bupivicaine. Multiple skin incisions were then made, consistent with the performance of arthroscopy, but the sham group received no articular puncture or instrumentation. Arthroscopic surgery included chondroplasty and meniscectomy, as appropriate. Arthroscopic irrigation involved a minimum of 10 L of saline, which was flushed continuously through separate inflow and outflow ports. The physician assessor was blinded to the procedure employed. Clinical assessments were performed at baseline, 2 and 6 weeks, and 3, 12, 18, and 24 months, and included measures of pain, function, and satisfaction. Sixty subjects were randomized to each treatment arm. Baseline characteristics, including age, sex, race, radiographic severity of OA, physical and mental health, were similar among the treatment groups.

All treatments resulted in reduction of joint pain at 6, 12, and 24 months, but the sham group reported less pain and greater functional improvement 2 weeks post-operatively than the two arthroscopy groups. All three groups showed functional improvement at 6, 12, and 24 months. Satisfaction and

function, as assessed by physical performance, did not vary significantly among the treatment groups. Neither radiographic severity nor evidence of ligament laxity predicted outcomes. Consistent with the findings of Bradley *et al.*,[26] the authors stated: 'The results of this study suggest the improvement is due to the placebo effect. Patients undergoing placebo arthroscopy experienced improvement in pain and function and satisfaction with surgery similar to their arthroscopic lavage and debridement cohorts.'

A smaller study by Caracuel *et al.*[30] also reported recently in an abstract, compared the effectiveness of a series of 5 weekly intra-articular hyaluronate (HA) injections, JI, and JI plus HA in 37 subjects with Kellgren and Lawrence grade II knee OA. 'Cold sterile 0.9 per cent saline' was used as the irrigant. The Lequesne index and VAS pain and global status were used as the outcome measures, but only the global status data was reported in the abstract. At the end of one month (at which time the HA subjects received their last injection), improvement in global status was nearly twice as great among JI subjects as in the HA group, but the combination of HA injection and JI was not significantly better than JI alone. Blinding was not described and, unfortunately, no placebo HA group was employed. Outcomes, therefore, were susceptible to subjects' expectations and to an unmeasured placebo effect. It is possible that the efficacy of JI in this study may have been attributable, at least in part, to its novelty and, perhaps, to specific aspects of the treatment experience, for example, cooling of the joint.

Several abstracts[13,31–33] have been published reporting the findings of a multicenter, prospective, randomized comparison of low-volume (250 mL) and high-volume (3 L) arthroscopic irrigation as treatment for 'early knee OA.' The two treatment groups were comparable with respect to demographic features and arthroscopically assessed intra-articular damage and inflammation. Assessments were performed at baseline, 1, and 3 months, and included the WOMAC and a physician global assessment. Physician assessors and subjects were reportedly blinded to the treatment assignment, but the mechanism of subject blinding and the success of blinding were not described.

Table 9.39 Controlled studies of JI as treatment for knee OA

Authors/references	Treatments compared	Number of subjects	Blinding	Difference between treatments with respect to pain	Difference between treatments with respect to function
Dawes et al.[19]	2 L continuous JI vs 10 mL IA saline	20	BA	No	No
Ike et al.[20]	1 L tidal JI vs medical management	77	BA	Favored JI	No
Chang et al.[22]	1 L tidal JI vs arthroscopy	29	BA	Favored arthroscopy	No
Ravaud et al.[24]	1 L interrupted JI, with or without IA steroid or IA placebo	98	BA for JI steroid for DB	Favored JI +/− steroid over placebo	Favored JI +/− steroid over placebo
Brion et al.[33]	250 mL vs 3 L arthroscopic irrigation	90	BA	Favored 3 L	No
Bradley et al.[26]	1 L tidal JI vs sham JI	180	DB, BA	No	No
Moseley et al.[29]	10 L arthroscopic irrigation vs 10 L arthroscopic debridement vs sham arthroscopy	180	DB, BA	No	No

JI, joint irrigation; IA, intra-articular; BA, blinded assessor; DB, double blinded.

Both treatment groups showed improvement in comparison with their baseline status, but the high-volume JI group experienced greater improvement at 3 months than the low-volume JI group.[31] Counterintuitively, lower intra-articular inflammation scores at baseline were associated with greater improvement. A subsequent subset analysis indicated that the presence of crystalline material was not associated with arthroscopic evidence of intra-articular damage or inflammation but predicted greater improvement with JI, regardless of the volume of irrigating fluid employed.[13] An algorithm utilizing clinical assessment of morning stiffness, joint line tenderness, and night pain has been proposed to correlate with arthroscopic evidence of crystalline deposits[32] and, therefore, might be predictive of benefit from JI, but this has not been tested.

In an analysis that included 90 subjects, the change in total WOMAC score for the low-volume JI subjects was not significantly different from that for the high-volume JI subjects at 12 months, but the WOMAC pain scale and a VAS pain assessment favored high-volume JI. Notably, the magnitude of pain relief resulting from these procedures was relatively small, that is, ≤ 21 per cent of the scale of the measurement instrument (WOMAC or VAS).[33]

Summary

Variable improvement has been observed following JI used as a treatment for knee OA. The duration of clinical improvement may exceed 12 months. Predictors of response have been difficult to identify. Radiographic severity of OA and X-ray evidence of chondrocalcinosis, the presence of synovial fluid crystals, and even the severity of articular cartilage damage and synovial inflammation, as determined arthroscopically, do not predict the response to JI. Nonetheless, and perhaps because of its heightened sensitivity in comparison with radiography and light microscopic evaluation of the presence of synovial fluid crystals, arthroscopic visualization of crystalline deposits may be predictive of an enhanced response to JI. The volume and specific characteristics of the irrigation fluid and the method of delivery and removal of the fluid may be important determinants of the efficacy of JI, but the superiority of one particular JI technique over any other has not been demonstrated.

Although the procedure seems safe, JI, performed either through a needle or with arthroscopic visualization, has not proved superior to sham procedures in a broad range of patients with knee OA. Placebo effects are particularly prominent with invasive interventions. Needle puncture placebos have greater impact than oral placebos[34,35] and, the more elaborate the procedure, the greater the potential for a placebo effect.[36] Objective improvement can be achieved as a result of placebo effect, as has been demonstrated in a sham-controlled study of lymphoplasmapheresis in patients with rheumatoid arthritis.[37]

Conclusion

There is a plausible rationale for use of JI in the symptomatic treatment of patients with knee OA. Uncontrolled data support the efficacy of this procedure, but results of controlled clinical trials have yielded variable results (Table 9.39). Recent sham-controlled studies indicate that the placebo effect may account for most, if not all, of the benefit which patients derive from this procedure.

While there are clearly practical and ethical issues related to performance of placebo-controlled trials, particularly for interventional procedures,[38] results of recent sham-controlled studies of JI demonstrate the necessity of including such control groups in the evaluation of this procedure.

Key points

1. Removal of joint debris, including crystalline deposits, is a logical objective of JI.

2. Needle irrigation is simple and reasonably safe; however, the optimal technique for this procedure is unknown.

3. The clinical benefit of JI is variable; predictors of benefit are uncertain.

4. Sham-controlled studies indicate that the symptomatic benefit of JI is attributable to a placebo effect.

References

(An asterisk denotes recommended reading.)

1. **Burman, M.S., Finkelstein, F.H., and Mayer, L.** (1934). Arthroscopy of the knee joint. *J Bone Joint Surg* **16**:255–68.

2. **Hochberg, M.C., Altman, R.D., Brandt, K.D.,** *et al.* (1995). Guidelines for the medical management of osteoarthritis. Part II: OA of the knee. *Arthritis Rheum* **38**:1541–6.

3. American College of Rheumatology Subcommittee on Osteoarthritis Guidelines (2000). Recommendations for the medical management of OA of the hip and knee: 2000 Update. *Arthritis Rheum* **43**:1905–15.

4. **Pendleton, A., Arden, N., Dougados M.,** *et al.* (2000). EULAR recommendations for the management of knee OA: report of a task force of the Standing Committee for International Clinical Studies Including Therapeutic Trials (ESCISIT). *Ann Rheum Dis* **59**:936–44.

5. **Evans, C.H., Mears, D.C., and Stanititski, C.L.** (1982). Ferrographic analysis of wear in human joints. Evaluation by comparison with arthroscopic examination of symptomatic knees. *J Bone Joint Surg Br* **64**(B):572–8.

6. Cheung, H.S., Ryan, L.M., Kozin, F., and McCarty, D.J. (1980). Identification of collagen subtypes in synovial fluid segments from arthritic patients. *Am J Med* **68**:73–9.

7. Myers, S.L., Flusser, D., Brandt, K.D., and Heck, D.A. (1992). Prevalence of cartilage shards in synovium and their association with synovitis in early and endstage OA. *J Rheumatol* **19**:1247–51.

8. Boniface, R.J., Cain, P.R., and Evans, C.H. (1988). Articular responses to purified cartilage proteoglycans. *Arthritis Rheum* **31**:258–66.

9. Ranginwala, M.A., Michalska, M., and Block, J.A. (1995). Pain improvement and quantity of articular debris after arthroscopy for OA of the knee. *Arthritis Rheum* **38**(Suppl.):240.

10. Concoff, A.L. and Kalunian, K.C. (1999). What is the relation between crystal and OA? *Curr Opin Rheumatol* **11**:436–40.

11. Schumacher, H.R., Rubinow, A., Rothfuss, S., *et al.* (1994). Apatite crystal clumps in synovial fluid are an early finding in canine OA. *Arthritis Rheum* **37**(Suppl.):346.

12. Kurian, J., Butler, J., Daft, L., Carrera, G., and Derfus, B. (1999). The high prevalence of pathologic calcium crystals in pre-operative joints. *Arthritis Rheum* **42**(Suppl.):145.

13. Kalunian, K., Singh, R., Klashman, D., Myers, S., Ike, R., Skovron, M.L., and Moreland, L. (1996). Crystalline material in early OA predicts outcome after arthroscopic irrigation. *Arthritis Rheum* **39**(Suppl.):173.

14. O'Connor, R.L. (1973). The arthroscope in the management of crystal-induced synovitis of the knee. *J Bone Joint Surg Am* **55**(A):1443–9.

15. *Ryan, L.M. and Cheung, H.S. (1999). The role of crystals in OA. *Rheum Dis Clinic NA* **25**:257–67.

   This is an exceptionally detailed description of the pathophysiologic significance of articular crystals in the development and progression of OA.

16. Ike, R.W., Arnold, W.J., Simon, C., and Eisenberg, G.M. (1987). Tidal knee irrigation as an intervention for chronic knee pain due to OA of the knee. *Arthritis Rheum* **30**(Suppl.):17.

17. Mohr, B.W., Danao, T., Gragg, L.A., and Segal, A.M. (1991). Tidal knee lavage for OA and rheumatoid arthritis: long-term results. *Arthritis Rheum* **34**(Suppl.):85.

18. Edelson, R., Burks, R.T., and Bloebaum, R.D. (1995). Short-term effects of knee washout for OA. *Am J Sports Med* **23**:345–9.

19. Dawes, P.T., Kirlew, C., and Haslock, I. (1987). Saline washout for knee OA: results of a controlled study. *Clin Rheumatol* **6**:61–3.

20. *Ike, R.W., Arnold, W.J., Rothschild, E.W., Shaw, H.L., the Tidal irrigation Cooperating Group. (1992). Tidal irrigation versus conservative medical management in patients with OA of the knee: a prospective randomized study. *J Rheumatol* **19**:772–9.

   This clear and thoughtful description of a seminal controlled study of tidal irrigation identifies and discusses key issues in the assessment of this treatment modality.

21. Kellgren, J.H. and Lawrence, J.S. (1957). Radiographical assessment of osteo-arthrosis. *Ann Rheum Dis* **16**:494–501.

22. *Chang, R.W., Falconer, J., Stulberg, S.D., Arnold, W.J., Mannheim, L.M., and Dyer, A.R. (1993). A randomized controlled trial of arthroscopic surgery versus closed-needle joint lavage for patients with OA of the knee. *Arthritis Rheum* **36**:289–96.

   This is a provocative comparison of low-cost, low-risk tidal irrigation and high-cost, higher-risk arthroscopy as treatments for knee OA.

23. Meenan, R.F., Gertman, P.M., and Mason, J.H. (1980). Measuring health status in arthritis: the Arthritis Impact Measurement Scales. *Arthritis Rheum* **23**:146–52.

24. *Ravaud, P., Moulinier, L., Giraudeau, B., *et al.* (1999). Effects of joint lavage and steroid injection in patients with OA of the knee. Results of a multicenter, randomized, controlled trial. *Arthritis Rheum* **42**:475–82.

   This is a well-designed study evaluating the additive value of intra-articular corticosteroids and joint irrigation that illustrates the difficulties in performing blinded trials of invasive procedures.

25. Lequesne, M.G. and Samson, M. (1991). Indices of severity in OA for weight bearing joints. *J Rheumatol* **18**:16–18.

26. *Bradley, J.D., Heilman, D.K., Katz, B.P., G'Sell, P., Wallick, J.A., and Brandt, K.D. (2002). Tidal irrigation as treatment for knee osteoarthritis: a sham-controlled, randomized, double-blinded evaluation. *Arthritis Rheum* **46**:100–8.

   This paper describes an adequately powered, successfully blinded, sham-controlled evaluation of tidal irrigation as a treatment for knee OA, which demonstrates that sham/placebo was as effective as the 'active' treatment.

27. Bellamy, N., Buchanan, W.W., Goldsmith, C.H., Campbell, J., and Stitt, L.W. (1988). Validation study of WOMAC: a health status instrument for measuring clinically important patient relevant outcomes to antirheumatic drug therapy in patients with OA of the hip or knee. *J Rheumatol* **15**:1833–40.

28. Bradley, J.D., Heilman, D.K., and G'Sell, P. (2000). Do psychological factors 'predict' response to tidal lavage (TL) and sham lavage (SL) in knee OA (KOA)? *Arthritis Rheum* **43**(Suppl.):337.

29. Moseley, B., Wray, N., Kuykendal, D., and Petersen, N. (2001). Arthroscopic treatment of OA of the knee: A prospective, randomized, placebo-controlled trial. *Trans Orthop Res Soc* **26**:662.

30. Caracuel, M.A., Munoz-Villanueva, M.C., Escudero, A., *et al.* (2001). Effects of joint lavage and hyaluronic acid infiltration in patients with OA of the knee. *Ann Rheum Dis* **60**(Suppl. 1):228–9.

31. Kalunian, K., Klashman, D., Singh, R., *et al.* (1995). Office-based arthroscopy in early OA of the knee: preliminary results of a multi-center study of the effects of visually guided irrigation on outcome. *Arthritis Rheum* **38**(Suppl.):240.

32. Concoff, A., Singh, R., Klashman, D., *et al.* (1997). A clinical algorithm for identifying occult crystalline disease in patients with knee OA. *Arthritis Rheum* **40**(Suppl.):239.

33. Brion, P.H., Moreland, L.W., Myers, S.L., *et al.* (2000). Visually-guided irrigation in patients with early knee OA: A multi-center randomized, controlled trial. *Arthritis Rheum* **43**(Suppl.):338.

34. Lasagna, L. (1955). Placebos. *Sci Am* **193**:68–71.

35. Traut, E.F. and Passarelli, E.W. (1956). Study in the controlled therapy of degenerative arthritis. *Arch Intern Med* **98**:181–6.

36. Kaptchuk, T.J., Goldman, P., Stone, D.A., and Stason, W.B. (2000). Do medical devices have enhanced placebo effects? *J Clin Epidemiol* **53**:786–92.

37. Wallace, D.J., Goldfinger, D., Lowe, C., Nichols, S., Weiner, J., Brachman, M., and Klinenberg, J.R. (1982). A double-blind, controlled study of lymphoplasmapheresis versus sham apheresis in rheumatoid arthritis. *N Engl J Med* **306**:1406–10.

38. Macklin, R. (1999). The ethical problems with sham surgery in clinical research. *N Engl J Med* **341**:992–6.

9.18 Surgical approaches to preserving and restoring articular cartilage

Joseph A. Buckwalter and L. Stefan Lohmander

Most patients and many physicians consider joint replacement as the only surgical option for the treatment of OA joints, yet procedures that preserve or restore articular cartilage instead of resecting and replacing it with synthetic materials or fusing the involved joint make up an important part of the spectrum of treatments available to patients with degenerative joints. These procedures can decrease pain and improve joint function for selected patients. This patient group includes younger patients with localized loss or early articular cartilage degeneration, especially those individuals with normal joint alignment, good joint stability, muscle strength, and a functional range of motion.[1,2] For these individuals maintaining or restoring synovial joint structure and function may make possible a high level of physical activity and delay or eliminate the need for joint replacement or fusion. Further improvements in the methods of preserving and restoring articular cartilage can expand the role of these operations to include treatment of older individuals with early degenerative disease and even individuals with advanced joint degeneration.

Procedures performed with the intent of preserving or restoring articular cartilage surfaces include joint debridement with shaving of fibrillated cartilage, and perforation of subchondral bone to stimulate formation of a new articular surface. Osteotomy, resection arthroplasty, and resection of localized regions of degenerated articular cartilage followed by implantation of periosteal, perichondrial, and osteochondral autografts and allografts to create a new articular surface, also belong to this category of treatment.[1–3] Differences in joint anatomy, size, and function as well as technical limitations, have restricted application of these procedures to selected joints. Surgeons have used joint debridement and resection or penetration of subchondral bone most commonly for treatment of OA of the knee and less frequently for the elbow, shoulder, hip, ankle, and other joints. Osteotomies have been used for the treatment of OA of the knee and hip, while resection arthroplasties appear to be most effective for treatment of OA involving the first metatarsophalangeal joint, the carpometacarpal joint of the thumb, and less in other joints. Periosteal, perichondrial, and osteochondral grafts have been used in a variety of joints including the knee, hip, and hand joints.

Experimental procedures now being developed to preserve or restore articular surfaces include implantation of growth factors, chondrocytes, and mesenchymal stem cells with synthetic matrices or combinations of growth factors, cells, and matrices.[1,3] Although the effectiveness of these procedures has not yet been demonstrated in treating osteoarthritic joints, experimental studies suggest they have the potential to improve current procedures performed with the intent of restoring articular cartilage.

Joint debridement

Joint debridement usually includes joint irrigation, resecting cartilage flaps, and removing loose cartilaginous, osteochondral, and meniscal fragments. In some instances it includes shaving regions of severely degenerated meniscal and articular cartilage surfaces, resecting synovium and removing osteophytes (cheilectomy).[1] Although surgeons have debrided osteoarthritic joints for more than 50 years by arthrotomy[4,5] or by arthroscopy,[3,6–16] and recommended the procedure for selected patients, the efficacy of debridement to alter the course of OA, or durably relieve pain or improve joint function, has not been established by blinded prospective long-term controlled, randomized studies.

The lack of such studies makes critical evaluation of the effects of different procedures involved in joint debridement especially important in making treatment decisions for individual patients. Removal of chondral flaps, free cartilage, and osteochondral and meniscal fragments that cause mechanical disturbances of joint function has been reported to improve function and decrease symptoms.[13,17] In addition, since intra-articular osteochondral fragments can cause synovitis and excoriation of articular cartilage,[18] removing free tissue fragments may slow progression of joint damage. The potential benefits of other debridement procedures are less clear. The available evidence does not support routine synovectomy and removal of osteophytes, but these procedures may still have specific indications. For example, resection of osteophytes either as an isolated procedure or combined with other debridement procedures can decrease pain and improve motion in selected patients with OA of the elbow, ankle, and first metatarsophalangeal joints.[19–23]

Despite widespread clinical use, shaving or debriding fibrillated articular cartilage and menisci remains controversial. Although careful removal of fibrillated tissue can leave a smoother articular surface, published reports of animal experiments and clinical studies do not demonstrate beneficial effects of this procedure. Shaving normal animal articular cartilage did not stimulate regeneration of an articular surface,[24,25] and in one experiment the remaining cartilage degenerated following shaving.[24] Fibrillated human osteoarthritic cartilage may respond differently to debridement, but clinical studies indicate that shaving is not likely to restore an articular surface. In one group of patients, shaving fibrillated patellar cartilage during arthrotomy produced unpredictable outcomes.[26,27] Only 25 per cent of the patients had satisfactory results, and the investigator concluded that the procedure is disappointing and ineffective. Examination of five patellar articular surfaces from patients treated by shaving did not show cartilage regeneration,[28] and arthroscopic shaving of fibrillated human femoral articular cartilage did not restore a smooth articular surface and may have increased fibrillation and chondrocyte necrosis.[29]

Despite the lack of evidence for beneficial effects of debridement on joint structure and function, other than correcting mechanical disturbances of joint function due to free or displaced tissue fragments, and questions concerning its clinical efficacy,[30] many clinical series indicate that joint debridement decreases pain.[1] The symptomatic improvement could result from a placebo effect.[14] Experimental injection of cartilage particles and even purified cartilage proteoglycans may, in animals, lead to synovial inflammation, joint effusion, increased degradative enzyme activity and cartilage friability, pitting, and discoloration.[31,32] Although the effect of cartilage and meniscal particles on the progression of OA in humans has not been demonstrated, observations from experimental studies combined with the clinical observation that joint irrigation may temporarily decrease pain in osteoarthritic joints[30,33] suggest that removal of tissue debris and joint irrigation could improve symptoms by decreasing a source of synovial irritation.

Penetration of subchondral bone

Debridement of a joint may be combined with penetration of subchondral bone to stimulate formation of a new articular surface. In regions with full thickness loss or advanced degeneration of articular cartilage, penetration of the exposed subchondral bone disrupts subchondral blood vessels leading to formation of a fibrin clot over the bone surface.[3,34,35] If the surface is protected from excessive loading, undifferentiated mesenchymal cells can migrate into the clot, proliferate, and differentiate into cells with the morphologic features of chondrocytes.[36] In many instances they form a fibrocartilage-like repair tissue over the bone surface.[37,38]

A variety of methods have been developed to penetrate subchondral bone to stimulate formation of a new cartilaginous surface including resection of sclerotic subchondral bone, drilling through the subchondral bone, abrasion of the articular surface and making multiple small diameter defects with an awl or similar instrument, a technique referred to as 'microfracture'.[1] It is not clear which method of penetrating subchondral bone produces the best new articular surface, and differences in patient selection and technique among surgeons using the same method may be responsible for variations in results, making it difficult to compare techniques. However, comparison of bone abrasion with subchondral drilling for treatment of an experimental chondral defect in rabbits showed that while neither treatment predictably restored the articular surface, drilling appeared to produce better long-term results than abrasion.[39] This observation fits well with experimental work showing that tissue that grows up through multiple drill holes that pass from the articular surface into vascularized bone will spread over exposed subchondral bone between holes and form a fibrocartilage-like articular surface.[40] It also suggests that small diameter holes that leave the bone intact between defects lead to the formation of more stable repair tissue than abraded bone surfaces.[39] Many reports suggest a decrease in symptoms following recovery from the procedure.[4,5,41–44]

Development of arthroscopic surgery has decreased the morbidity associated with joint debridement and drilling or abrasion of subchondral bone. Arthroscopic abrasion of chondral and osteochondral lesions in osteoarthritic joints with a motorized burr can decrease symptoms.[7,11,13,37,38] Typically, a superficial layer of subchondral bone, 1–3 mm thick, is removed to expose subchondral bone blood vessels. Following surgery, the resulting fibrin clot and immature repair tissue is protected from excessive loading, but early controlled joint motion is encouraged.

Examination of joint surfaces following arthroscopic abrasion has shown that in many individuals it results in formation of tissue that varies in composition from dense fibrous tissue with little or no type II collagen, to hyaline cartilage-like tissue with predominantly type II collagen.[37,38] In some patients this tissue persists for years. Some of the variability in the clinical results of this procedure may result from the variability in the extent and quality of the repair tissue. However, no studies have documented a relationship between the extent and type of repair tissue and the symptomatic or functional results.

Prospective randomized controlled trials of arthroscopic abrasion treatment of osteoarthritic joints have not been reported, but several authors have reviewed series of patients and found that these procedures can decrease the symptoms of OA of the knee. In general, 60–80 per cent good or excellent results have been reported at 12 months after surgery, with decrease in pain and stiffness.[11,16,37,38,45] The probability of a satisfactory outcome appears to decrease with the increasing severity of OA.[11] Other investigators have noted less good results, with 40–50 per cent early failures and only 12 per cent of the patients with no symptoms at two years after surgery.[7,38]

Although an increase in radiographic joint-space following subchondral abrasion presumably indicates formation of a new articular surface, the development of this new surface does not necessarily result in symptomatic improvement.[37,38] Thus, about half of 59 patients treated with abrasion arthroplasty had evidence of increased radiographic joint-space two years after treatment, but one-third of these individuals either had no symptomatic improvement or more severe symptoms.[8,9]

These observations suggest that formation of a new articular surface following penetration of subchondral bone does not necessarily relieve pain. This lack of predictable benefit may result from variability among patients in the severity of the degenerative changes, joint alignment, patterns of joint use, age, perception of pain, pre-operative expectations or other factors. It may also result from the inability of the newly formed tissue to replicate the properties of articular cartilage. Examination of the tissue that forms over the articular surface following penetration of subchondral bone shows that it lacks the structure, composition, mechanical properties, and in most instances the durability of articular cartilage.[3,34,35,40] For these reasons, even though it covers the subchondral bone, it may fail to distribute loads across the articular surface in a way that avoids pain with joint loading and further degeneration of the joint.[1,3]

Despite the evidence that penetration of subchondral bone stimulates formation of fibrocartilaginous repair tissue and reports of symptomatic improvement in several series of patients,[16,38,45] the clinical value of this approach remains uncertain. One investigator concluded that while joint debridement can improve symptoms in many patients, abrasion or drilling of subchondral bone does not benefit patients with OA of the knee and may increase symptoms.[8] The short periods of follow-up, lack of well-defined evaluations of outcomes, lack of randomized controlled trials, and the possibility for a significant placebo effect[14] or an improvement in symptoms due to joint irrigation alone[30,33] make it very difficult to define the indications for penetration of subchondral bone to stimulate formation of a new articular surface.

Osteotomies

Treatment of an osteoarthritic joint with an osteotomy consists of cutting the bone adjacent to the involved joint and then stabilizing the cut bone surfaces in a new position, thereby changing the alignment and the resulting load of the joint surfaces. Joint debridement may be combined with osteotomy,[46] but this approach is not widely used. Osteotomies are planned to decrease loads on the most severely damaged regions of the joint surface, to bring regions of the joint surface that have remaining articular cartilage into opposition with regions that lack articular cartilage or correct joint malalignment, which may be contributing to symptoms and joint dysfunction (Fig. 9.33). Most hip and knee osteotomies performed to treat OA alter joint alignment in the coronal plane (varus and valgus osteotomies). However, some hip osteotomies are designed to change joint alignment in the sagittal plane (flexion and extension osteotomies), or alter the relationship of the joint surfaces by rotation of the femoral head relative to the acetabulum (rotational osteotomies). The optimal planes and degrees of joint realignment for specific OA joints have not been defined. Nonetheless, clinical experience shows that osteotomies of the hip and knee can decrease symptoms and stimulate formation of a new articular surface.[1] However, the mechanisms of symptomatic improvement and formation of new articular surfaces remain poorly understood. The decreased pain may result from decreasing stresses on regions of the articular surface with the most advanced cartilage degeneration, decreasing intraosseous pressure or formation of a new articular surface.[1]

Most clinical studies have shown that osteotomies lead to improvement in the radiographic signs of joint damage, including resolution of subchondral cysts, decreased subchondral bone density, and increased radiographic joint-space. This latter change may result either from the altered relationship between the articular surfaces or the formation of a new articular surface. Osteotomies may thus alter joint alignment to separate previously opposed joint surfaces or they may rotate a cartilage covered articular surface into opposition with a surface consisting of exposed bone, thus creating a radiographically visible cartilage space where prior to the osteotomy bone opposed bone. In one series of 757 osteotomies performed to treat OA of the hip, the radiographic joint-space increased immediately following the procedure in approximately one-third of the patients.[47] In these patients the increased joint-space presumably resulted from alterations in the relationships between the joint surfaces. In another third of the patients

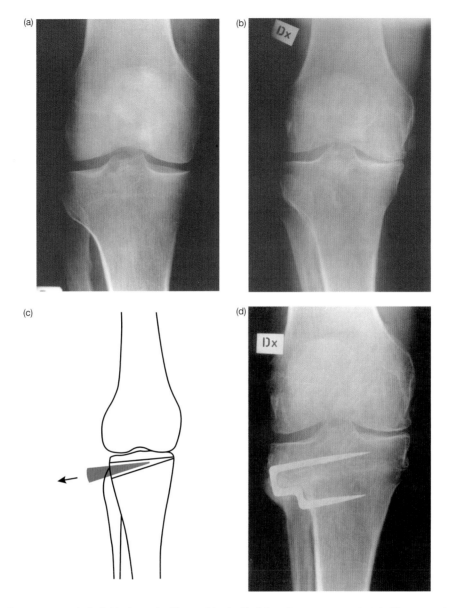

Fig. 9.33 (a) X-ray film (standing anteroposterior) of right knee of a 44-year old male. Medial meniscectomy approximately 10 years ago. Intermittent knee pain when walking, with some functional limitations. No radiological signs of OA, but borderline narrowing of medial joint-space is seen. (b) X-ray film of same patient 13 years later, age 57. Now, persistent knee pain on walking, resting and sometimes night pain with significant functional limitations. Medial osteophytes and loss of medial joint-space can be seen. Osteoarthritis clinically and radiologically. (c) High tibial osteotomy of right knee performed at age 57. Lateral bone wedge was removed to decrease load in the medial compartment. (d) X-ray film of same knee performed two years later, at age 59. The osteotomy is healed. There is an apparent increase in medial joint-space. There was an improvement in walking distance, and a significant decrease in pain.

the radiographic joint-space increased during the next 18 months, and these individuals had better clinical results. This suggests that over 18 months these patients may have developed a new articular surface in some areas of the joint as a result of the altered loading. Evidence that hip osteotomies stimulate formation of fibrocartilage-like tissue over articular surfaces that previously consisted of exposed bone supports this suggestion.[48,49]

Reports of the treatment of knee OA with osteotomies also describe increased radiographic joint-space accompanied by decreased subchondral sclerosis, and in some people formation of a new fibrocartilage articular surface.[1] One group of investigators biopsied the articular cartilage of the medial femoral condyle at the time of osteotomy, and then again at two years after osteotomy in 19 patients with degenerative disease of the medial side of the knee joint.[50] The biopsies showed formation of a new fibrocartilage articular surface in nine patients, no change in eight patients, and

deterioration of the articular surface in two patients. Radiographic examination showed that six knees had improved, 11 had remained unchanged, and two had deteriorated. There was, however, no correlation between the histological score, the radiographic appearance, the postoperative varus-valgus angle, or the clinical results. A similar study of 14 patients found proliferation of new fibrocartilage on the tibial condyle in eight patients and on the medial femoral condyle in nine patients, two years following osteotomy.[51] No correlation was found between regeneration of an articular surface and clinical outcome.

Long-term follow-up of patients treated with osteotomies for hip and knee OA show that the clinical results deteriorate with time.[47,52] At one year following surgery 70 per cent of 103 hips treated by intertrochanteric osteotomy had a good result, at five years 51 per cent had a good result, and at ten years only 30 per cent of the hips still showed a beneficial effect of the osteotomy.[53] Several studies of knee osteotomy for OA also report deterioration with time, with between 15 and 57 per cent of patients reporting useful knee function at 9–15 years after osteotomy.[52,54,55] Variables that appear to adversely affect the results of a knee osteotomy include advanced patient age, obesity, severe joint degeneration, joint instability, limited joint motion, operative over correction or under correction, and post operative loss of correction.[52,54–56] However, many patients who appear to be optimal candidates for osteotomy and who have a good initial surgical outcome, tend to develop recurrent pain and evidence of advancing OA with time.

Several studies report, however, that the results of osteotomies can be improved through better technique and patient selection.[57,58] Evaluation of pre-operative joint mechanics may also lead to improved results. Surgeons generally use radiographs that demonstrate joint alignment, subchondral bone density, and cartilage space to plan osteotomies that will redistribute articular surface loading. They base this practice on the assumption that static joint alignment can be used to predict dynamic loading in a joint. However, one group of investigators studied patients with varus gonarthrosis using gait analysis and found that the patients could be separated into two groups: those with high adduction moments at the knee and those with low adduction moments.[59,60] The two groups did not differ in preoperative knee score, initial knee alignment, post-operative knee alignment, age or weight; but those with high pre-operative adduction moments had only 50 per cent good or excellent results at an average of 3.2 years following osteotomy, compared with 100 per cent good or excellent results for patients with low pre-operative adduction moments.[59] With increasing time the results for both groups deteriorated, but the patients with low pre-operative adduction moments maintained better clinical results.[60]

At present, the overall clinical results of hip and knee osteotomies vary more than those of joint replacement, and the relationships between the degree of alteration of joint loading, type of osteotomy, quality and extent of articular surface repair, radiographic changes, and clinical outcome remain unclear. Given the available information, identifying the patients most likely to benefit from osteotomy, planning the optimal osteotomy for a specific joint, and predicting the outcome of the procedure for an individual patient are difficult. However, investigations by Odenbring suggest that advances in osteotomies through improved selection of patients, pre-operative planning, and surgical techniques have the potential to provide better and longer lasting results than unicompartmental arthroplasty in the young and physically active patient.[57,58,61] However, this remains to be proven in a controlled, randomized trial.

Disadvantages of the commonly used 'bone wedge removal' osteotomies are loss of correction during healing, and a long period of fixation in a cast during healing of the osteotomy. A recently introduced method of callus distraction osteotomy attempts to improve on these disadvantages. Here, pins are drilled into the bone on each side of a single cut osteotomy, and an external frame attached (Fig. 9.34). The frame is then slowly adjusted (by the patient) over the course of several weeks to months. During this time, the resulting defect is filled by callus and bone. When the correct angular correction is reached, the frame is locked in place until the defect is completely healed. The patient is allowed full weight bearing during the treatment. Early results are encouraging, but longer follow-up of large patient series is needed to confirm the value of this technique.[62–65]

Resection arthroplasty

Resection of an osteoarthritic joint surface followed by joint motion results in the formation of connective tissue and fibrocartilage over the surfaces of the resected bone.[1,3,34] In addition to motion, some distraction, or at least limited loading, of the new joint facilitates formation of articular surfaces, whereas immobilization and compression may lead to a bony or fibrous union. The articulations that result from resection arthroplasty generally lack stability and may be painful, but in selected patients and joints they can provide acceptable function.

Resection arthroplasty is most successful in joints that do not require a high degree of stability and where shortening due to resection of bone does not prevent near normal function. One of the most commonly performed

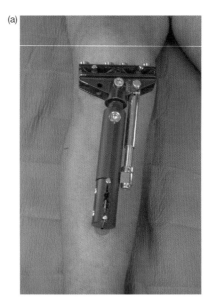

(a)

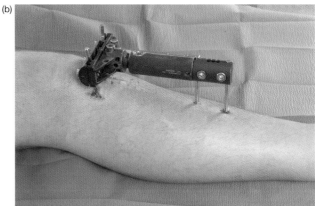

(b)

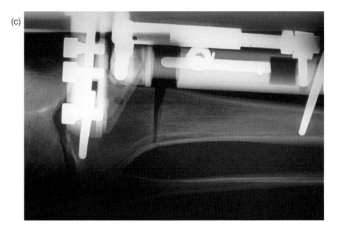

(c)

Fig. 9.34 (a), (b), and (c) Callus distraction osteotomy (hemicallotasis) of right knee, with external fixation was applied. The external fixator was gradually adjusted until planned correction with medial opening wedge was obtained. Osteotomy callus tissue was allowed to heal and the fixator was removed. Full weight bearing and activity was allowed during treatment.

Source: Illustrations kindly provided by S. Toksvig-Larsen, G. Magyar, and A. W-Dahl, Lund University Hospital.

resection arthroplasties, the Keller arthroplasty (performed to treat hallux valgus deformity and OA of the first metatarsophalangeal joint) consists of resecting damaged articular cartilage along with 30–50 per cent of the proximal portion of the proximal phalanx of the great toe.[66,67] Several weeks following surgery most patients begin active motion of the joint and proceed to develop satisfactory motion usually with minimal discomfort. The reasons for the relatively good clinical outcomes of these procedures have not been fully explored. Possibly the limited loading and early motion at the resection site allows formation of a new articular surface on the resected bone end. The limited loading of the newly formed articular surface may also prevent degeneration of this tissue and decrease the probability of pain from motion.

Fibrous or fibrocartilage-like articular surfaces also form after resection arthroplasty of the hip or knee. These procedures are most commonly performed in an attempt to save some joint function following a failed total joint arthroplasty or to treat joint infections that cannot be controlled by other means. Generally, the instability of the joint and in some instances limb shortening and pain compromise function.[68,69]

Soft tissue grafts

Treatment of osteoarthritic joints by soft tissue grafts usually involves debriding the joint and interposing soft tissue grafts consisting of fascia, muscle, tendon, periosteum, or perichondrium between debrided or resected articular surfaces.[3] The potential benefits of soft tissue grafts relative to resection arthroplasty or penetration of subchondral bone include introduction of a new cell population along with an organic matrix, a decrease in the probability of ankylosis before a new articular surface can form, and some protection of the graft or host cells from excessive loading. The success of soft tissue arthroplasty depends not only on the severity of the joint abnormalities and the type of graft, but also on post-operative motion to facilitate generation of a new articular surface.

Soft tissue interposition arthroplasties have been used most frequently to treat osteoarthritic joints of the upper extremity; in particular, tendon or fascia arthroplasty treatment of OA of the thumb carpometacarpal joint.[70] This procedure has been found to provide acceptable relief of symptoms in a high proportion of the patients and to retain some joint motion.

Fascial arthroplasty has been used for other joints of the upper extremity including the elbow. In selected young patients with post-traumatic OA of the elbow, some surgeons have used soft tissue interposition arthroplasty as an alternative to total joint arthroplasty. The functional results of elbow soft tissue arthroplasty for OA have varied among patient groups, with between 56 and 80 per cent good results at 1–4 years after surgery.[71,72]

Animal experiments and clinical experience show that perichondrial and periosteal grafts can replace lost or degenerated regions of articular cartilage.[1] These grafts have the potential advantage of containing cells with the capacity to differentiate into chondrocytes and synthesize a cartilaginous matrix. In an early study, Engkvist and Johansson treated 26 patients with painful stiff small joints with rib perichondrial arthroplasty.[73] Some individuals had improved motion and decreased pain, but a roughly equal number were not improved. Subsequent reports suggested that patient age was directly related to the results.[74] In metacarpophalangeal joint arthroplasties 100 per cent of the patients in their twenties and 75 per cent of the patients in their thirties had good results. In proximal interphalangeal joint arthroplasties 75 per cent of the patients in their teens and 66 per cent of the patients in their twenties had good results. None of the patients older than 40 years had a good result with either type of arthroplasty. The authors concluded that perichondrial arthroplasty could be used for treatment of post-traumatic OA of the metacarpophalangeal joint and proximal interphalangeal joints of the hand in young patients. Perichondrial grafts have also been used to replace lost or damaged cartilage in the knee.[75]

The clinical observation that perichondrial grafts produced the best results in younger patients agrees with the concept that age may adversely affect the ability of undifferentiated cells or chondrocytes to form an articular surface, or that with age the population of cells that can form an articular surface declines.[76] The age-related differences in the ability of cells to form a new articular surface may also help explain some of the variability in the results of other procedures including osteotomies or procedures that penetrate subchondral bone. That is, younger people may have greater potential to produce a more effective articular surface when all other factors are equal.

Cartilage grafts

Compared with soft tissue grafts, cartilage or meniscal grafts have the advantage of more closely resembling the structure and composition of articular cartilage and have the potential for transplantation of viable chondrocytes. Experimental work using meniscal[77] and sternal cartilage[78] autografts has shown promising results. Because of their greater availability and because they can be prepared in any size, osteochondral allografts have been used more frequently to replace damaged segments of articular surfaces.

Clinical experience with fresh allografts show that they can restore an articular surface and provide good results in many patients with damaged joint surfaces.[79–81] Results have been considerably less encouraging in patients with OA. Frozen osteochondral allografts may produce results that compare favorably with fresh allografts for the treatment of localized defects of the distal femoral articular surface.[82] Use of frozen allografts makes it possible to perform the surgical reconstructions electively and allows time for more extensive testing of the donors for possible viral and bacterial infections.

More recent developments in this area include the use of autogenous osteochondral grafts taken from non load-bearing areas of the knee joint, and transferred to areas of cartilage damage in the same knee, so-called mosaicplasty.[83]

In summary, these studies show that osteochondral allografts can provide at least temporary improvement in symptoms and function for selected patients with isolated regions of damaged articular cartilage. The results indicate that in selected patients restoring localized regions of an articular surface can at least temporarily improve joint function.

Experimental treatments

Experimental surgical methods of restoring articular cartilage include implantation of growth factors, cells, and artificial matrices. In animal experiments, these approaches have resulted in the formation of new articular surfaces following creation of an acute cartilage or cartilage and subchondral bone defect in normal joints.[2] When interpreting these studies it is important to recognize that methods which stimulate articular cartilage formation in a normal animal joint will not necessarily lead to similar success in an adult damaged or osteoarthritic human joint.

Growth factors influence a variety of cell activities including cell proliferation, migration, matrix synthesis, and differentiation. Many of these factors have been shown to affect chondrocyte metabolism and chondrogenesis.[1] Bone matrix contains a variety of these molecules including Transforming Growth Factor Betas, Insulin-like Growth Factors, Bone Morphogenic Proteins, Platelet Derived Growth Factors and others. In addition, mesenchymal cells, endothelial cells, and platelets produce many of these factors. Thus, osteochondral injuries and exposure of bone due to loss of articular cartilage may locally release agents that affect the formation of cartilage repair tissue. They probably have an important role in the formation of new articular surfaces after currently used surgical procedures for this purpose.

Local treatment of chondral or osteochondral defects with these factors has the potential to stimulate restoration of an articular surface superior to that formed after penetration of subchondral bone alone, especially in joints with normal alignment and range of motion and with limited regions of cartilage damage. A recent experimental study of the treatment of partial thickness cartilage defects with timed release of TGF-Beta showed that this growth factor can stimulate cartilage repair.[84] Despite the early promise of this approach, the wide variety of growth factors, their multiple effects, the interactions among them, the possibility that the responsiveness of cells to growth factors may decline with age[76,85] and the limited understanding of their effects in osteoarthritic joints make it difficult to develop a simple strategy for using these agents to treat patients with OA. However, development of growth factor based treatments for early cartilage damage in younger people appears more promising.

The limited ability of host cells to restore articular surfaces[3] has led investigators to seek methods of transplanting cells that can form cartilage into chondral and osteochondral defects. Experimental work has shown that both chondrocytes and undifferentiated mesenchymal cells placed in articular cartilage defects survive and produce a new cartilage matrix.[76] About 80 per cent of rabbit osteochondral defects treated with allograft articular chondrocytes embedded in collagen gels healed within twenty-four weeks.[86] Other investigators have reported similar results with chondrocyte transplantation in experimental models.[87–89] Cultured mesenchymal stem cells also appear to be able to repair large osteochondral defects;[90] within two weeks of transplantation they differentiate into chondrocytes and begin to produce a new articular surface.

In addition to these animal experiments with cell transplants, the use of autologous chondrocyte transplants for treatment of localized cartilage defects of the femoral condyle or patella in 23 patients has been reported.[91] The investigators harvested chondrocytes from the patients, cultured the cells for 14–21 days, and then injected them into the area of the defect and covered them with a flap of periosteum. At two or more years following chondrocyte transplantation 14 of 16 patients with condylar defects and 2 of 7 patients with patellar defects had good or excellent clinical results. Biopsies of the defect sites showed hyaline-like cartilage in 11 of 15 femoral and one of seven patellar defects. A subsequent longer-term follow-up of 7 years of 61 patients treated with the same method provides supportive results with regard to tissue quality of the transplants, and duration of the beneficial clinical effect.[92] These results indicate that chondrocyte transplantation combined with a periosteal graft can promote restoration of an articular surface in humans, but further work and larger patient series are needed to assess the function and durability of the new tissue and determine if it improves joint function and delays or prevents joint degeneration, and if this approach will be beneficial in OA joints. We still lack controlled, randomized comparisons with alternative methods for treating the same conditions.

Treatment of chondral defects with growth factors or cell transplants requires a method of delivering and in most instances at least temporarily stabilizing the growth factors or cells in the defect. For these reasons, the success of these approaches often depends on an artificial matrix. In addition, artificial matrices may allow, and in some instances stimulate ingrowth of host cells, matrix formation, and binding of new cells and matrix to host tissue. Combined with materials currently used to fabricate artificial joints they have the potential to improve the fixation of the artificial joints. Implants formed from a variety of biologic and non-biologic materials including treated cartilage and bone matrices, collagens, collagens and hyaluronan, fibrin, carbon fiber, hydroxyapatite, porous polylactic acid, polytetrafluoroethylene, polyester, and other synthetic polymers facilitate restoration of an articular surface.[76] However, lack of studies that directly compare different types of artificial matrices makes it difficult to evaluate their relative merits. For example, in animal experiments collagen gels have proven to be an effective way of implanting chondrocytes and mesenchymal stem cells,[1] and fibrin has been used to implant and allow timed release of a growth factor.[84] Treatment of osteochondral defects in rats and rabbits with carbon fiber pads resulted in restoration of a smooth articular surface consisting of firm fibrous tissue that filled the pads.[93] Use of the same approach to treat osteochondral defects of the knee in humans produced a satisfactory result in 77 per cent of 47 patients evaluated clinically and arthroscopically three years after surgery.[93]

No blinded, controlled, and randomized trials have yet been published that compare the patient-relevant outcomes of different methods of regeneration or repair of the injured joint cartilage: abrasion, microfracture, soft tissue grafts, osteochondral grafts, chondrocyte transplantation, or natural history. The clinical series published up to this date have generally contained small numbers of patients with variable forms and locations of joint damage, and the outcome measures used to report the results have too rarely been standardized, validated, or patient-relevant.[94] It may thus be that the results reported are associated with significant patient, examiner, and publishing bias. The specific indications for, and the value of these methods remain to be defined.

Conclusions

Current surgical treatments that attempt to preserve or restore articular cartilage include joint debridement, penetration of subchondral bone, osteotomy and replacement of lost or damaged articular cartilage with soft tissue or cartilage grafts. Unfortunately, the efficacy of these procedures has not been demonstrated by prospective, controlled randomized studies, and the basic mechanisms by which they may relieve pain and improve function remain poorly understood. Generally, these procedures produce less predictable results than joint replacement, and their efficacy as measured by relief of symptoms and improved function varies among joints, patients, and procedures. Debridement of osteoarthritic joints may provide limited symptomatic relief in some patients, but prospective randomized controlled clinical studies are needed to define the indications and optimal techniques for this approach. The same is true of the multiple methods of stimulating formation of a new articular surface by penetration of subchondral bone. In selected patients, an osteotomy will decrease pain, but more work is needed to refine the indications and improve the technique. In particular, we need to learn more about how altering loads on the articular surfaces and subchondral bone affects joint pain and regeneration or preservation of articular cartilage, develop better methods of assessing the static and dynamic loads on articular surfaces and determine how osteotomies alter these loads. Resection arthroplasties and soft tissue interposition arthroplasties can be effective in a limited number of joints, but the resulting instability, shortening, and in some instances, pain, make these procedures inappropriate for many joints and patients.

Osteochondral allografts can replace limited regions of articular degenerated cartilage, but they have less value in joints with more extensive changes. Promising experimental methods of stimulating formation of a new joint surface include growth factors, cell transplants, and artificial matrices. Thus far, none of these approaches has been shown to regenerate a tissue in the osteoarthritic joint that duplicates the structure, composition, mechanical properties, and durability of articular cartilage, nor have these methods been compared in controlled clinical trials to other approaches to stimulating formation of a new articular surface in localized chondral defects.

It is unlikely that any one of these methodologies will be generally successful in the treatment of OA. Instead, the available clinical and experimental evidence indicates that future optimal surgical methods of preserving and restoring articular surfaces will begin with a detailed analysis of the structural and functional abnormalities of the involved joint, and the patient's expectations for future joint use. Based on this analysis the surgeon will develop a treatment plan that potentially combines correction of mechanical abnormalities (including malalignment, instability, and intra-articular causes of mechanical dysfunction), debridement that may or may not include limited penetration of subchondral bone and applications of growth factors or implants that may consist of a synthetic matrix that incorporates cells or growth factors, followed by a post-operative course of controlled loading and motion.

Key points

1. Surgical methods that attempt to preserve or restore joint cartilage include debridement, penetration of subchondral bone, osteotomy, transplantation of soft tissue, osteochondral grafts or chondrocytes, or implantation of artificial matrices.

2. Several of these methods have shown promise, with evidence of generation of new joint tissue, and relief of symptoms, providing some 'proof-of-principle.'

3. However small the patient series are, results appear to deteriorate with time, and the specific indications for individual methods remain uncertain.

4. None of the techniques, perhaps with the exception of osteotomy, has shown a durable effect in OA.

5. We lack randomized, controlled trials that compare the benefits and risks of the different techniques with the natural history of the condition.

6. Published results to date may thus be associated with significant patient, investigator, and publication bias.

References

(An asterisk denotes recommended reading.)

1. **Buckwalter, J.A. and Lohmander, S.** (1994). Operative treatment of osteoarthrosis: Current practice and future development. *J Bone Joint Surg* **76A**:1405–18.

2. **Buckwalter, J.A., Mow, V.C., and Ratcliffe, A.** (1994). Restoration of injured or degenerated articular surfaces. *J Am Acad Ortho Surg* **2**:192–201.

3. **Buckwalter, J.A. and Mow, V.C.** (1992). Cartilage repair in osteoarthritis. In: R.W. Moskowitz *et al.* (eds), *Osteoarthritis: Diagnosis and Medical/Surgical Management.* Philadelphia: Saunders, pp. 71–107.

4. **Haggart, G.E.** (1940). The surgical treatment of degenerative arthritis of the knee joint. *J Bone Joint Surg* **22**:717–29.

5. **Magnuson, P.B.** (1941). Joint debridement: surgical treatment of degenerative arthritis. *Surg Gynecol Obstet* **73**:1–9.

6. **Aichroth, P.M., Patel, D.V., and Moyes, S.T.** (1991). A prospective review of arthroscopic debridement for degenerative joint disease of the knee. *Int Orthop* **15**:351–5.

7. **Baumgaertner, M.R., Cannon, W.D., Vittori, J.M., Schmidt, E.S., and Maurer, R.C.** (1990). Arthroscopic debridement of the arthritic knee. *Clin Orthop Rel Res* **253**:197–202.

8. **Bert, J.M.** (1993). Role of abrasion arthroplasty and debridement in the management of osteoarthritis of the knee. *Rheum Dis Clin NA* **19**(3):725–39.

9. **Bert, J.M. and Maschka, K.** (1989). The arthroscopic treatment of unicompartmental gonarthrosis. *J Arthroscopy* **5**:25.

10. **Dandy, D.J.** (1991). Arthroscopic debridement of the knee for osteoarthritis. *J Bone Joint Surg* **73**(B):877–8.

11. **Ewing, J.W.** (1990). Arthroscopic treatment of degenerative meniscal lesions and early degenerative arthritis of the knee (chap. 9). In: J.W. Ewing (ed.), *Articular Cartilage and Knee Joint Function. Basic Science and Arthroscopy.* New York: Raven Press, pp. 137–45.

12. **Jackson, R.W., Silver, R., and Marans, R.** (1986). The arthroscopic treatment of degenerative joint disease. *J Arthroscopy* **2**:114.

13. **Johnson, L.L.** (1980). *Diagnostic and Surgical Arthroscopy.* St. Louis: CV Mosby.

14. **Moseley, J.B., Wray, N.P., Kuykendall, D., Willis, K. and Landon, G.C.** (1994). Arthroscopic treatment of osteoarthritis of the knee: a prospective, randomized, placebo-controlled trial: results of a pilot study. In *American Academy of Orthopaedic Surgeons 61st Annual Meeting.* New Orleans, LA: American Academy of Orthopaedic Surgeons.

15. **Rand, J.A.** (1991). Role of arthroscopy in osteoarthritis of the knee. *J Arthroscopy* **7**:358

16. **Sprague, N.F.** (1981). Arthroscopic debridement for degenerative knee joint disease. *Clin Orthop* **160**:118–23.

17. **Hubbard, M.J.S.** (1987). Arthroscopic surgery for chondral flaps in the knee. *J Bone Joint Surg* **69B**:794–6.

18. **Huber, M.J., Schmotzer, W.B., Riebold, T.W., Watrous, B.J., Synder, S.P., and Scott, E.A.** (1992). Fate and effect of autogenous osteochondral fragments implanted in the middle carpal joint of horses. *Am J Vet Res* **53**:1579–88.

19. **Geldwert, J.J., Rock, G.D., McGrath, M.P., and Mancuso, J.E.** (1992). Cheilectomy: still a useful technique for grade I and grade II hallux limitus/rigidus. *J Foot Surg* **31**:154–9.

20. **Hawkins, R.B.** (1988). Arthroscopic treatment of sports-related anterior osteophytes in the ankle. *Foot Ankle* **9**:87–90.

21. **Mann, R.A. and Clanton, T.O.** (1988). Hallux rigidus: treatment by cheilectomy. *J Bone Joint Surg* **70A**:400–06.

22. **Morrey, B.F.** (1992). Primary degenerative arthritis of the elbow. Treatment by ulnohumeral arthroplasty. *J Bone Joint Surg* **74B**:409–13.

23. **Tsuge, K. and Mizuseki, T.** (1994). Debridement arthroplasty for advanced primary osteoarthritis of the elbow. Results of a new technique in 29 elbows. *J Bone Joint Surg* **76B**:641–6.

24. **Kim, H.K.W., Moran, M.E., and Salter, R.B.** (1991). The potential for regeneration of articular cartilage in defects created by chondral shaving and subchondral abrasion. *J Bone Joint Surg* **73A**:1301–15.

25. **Mitchell, N. and Shepard, N.** (1987). Effect of patellar shaving in the rabbit. *J Orthop Res* **5**:388–92.

26. **Bentley, G.** (1980). Chondromalacia patellae. *J Bone Joint Surg* **52A**:221–32.

27. **Bentley, G. and Dowd, G.** (1984). Current concepts of etiology and treatment of chondromalacia patellae. *Clin Orthop* **189**:209–28.

28. **Milgram, J.W.** (1985). Injury to articular cartilage joint surfaces. I. Chondral injury produced by patellar shaving: a histopathologic study of human tissue specimens. *Clin Orthop Rel Res* **192**:168–73.

29. **Schmid, A. and Schmid, F.** (1987). Results after cartilage shaving studied by electron microscopy. *Am J Sports Med* **15**:386–7.

30. **Gibson, J.N.A., Whit, M.D., Chapman, V.M., and Strachan, R.K.** (1992). Arthroscopic lavage and debridement for osteoarthritis of the knee. *J Bone Joint Surg* **74B**:534–7.

31. **Boniface, R.J., Cain, P.R. and Evans, C.H.** (1988). Articular response to purified cartilage proteoglycans. *Arthritis Rheum* **31**:258–66.

32. **Evans, C.H., Mazzocchi, R.A., Nelson, D.D., and Rubash, H.E.** (1984). Experimental arthritis induced by intra-articular injection of allogenic cartilaginous particles into rabbit knees. *Arthritis Rheum* **27**:200–15.

33. **Livesley, P.J., Doherty, M., Needoff, M., and Moulton, A.** (1991). Arthroscopic lavage of osteoarthritic knees. *J Bone Joint Surg* **73B**:922–6.

34. **Buckwalter, J.A. and Cruess, R.** (1991). Healing of musculoskeletal tissues. In: C.A. Rockwood and D. Green (eds), *Fractures.* Philadelphia, PA: Lippincott.

35. **Buckwalter, J.A., Rosenberg, L.C., and Hunziker, E.B.** (1990). Articular cartilage: composition structure, response to injury and methods of facilitating repair. In: J.W., Ewing (ed.), *Articular Cartilage and Knee Joint Function: Basic Science and Arthroscopy,* New York: Raven Press, pp. 19–56.

36. **Shapiro, F., Koide, S., and Glimcher, M.J.** (1993). Cell origin and differentiation in the repair of full-thickness defects of articular cartilage. *J Bone Joint Surg* **75A**:532–53.

37. **Johnson, L.L.** (1986). Arthroscopic abrasion arthroplasty. Historical and pathologic perspective: Present status. *Arthroscopy* **2**:54–9.

38. **Johnson, L.L.** (1990). The sclerotic lesion: Pathology and the clinical response to arthroscopic abrasion arthroplasty. (chap. 22). In: J.W., Ewing (ed.), *Articular Cartilage and Knee Joint Function. Basic Science and Arthroscopy,* New York: Raven Press, pp. 319–33.

39. **Fenkel, S.R., Menche, D.S., Blair, B., Watnik, N.F., Toolan, B.C., and Pitman, M.I.** (1994). A comparison of abrasion burr arthroplasty and subchondral drilling in the treatment of full-thickness cartilage lesions in the rabbit. *Trans Orthop Res Soc* **19**:483.

40. **Mitchell, N. and Shepard, N.** (1976). The resurfacing of adult rabbit articular cartilage by multiple perforations through the subchondral bone. *J Bone Joint Surg* **58A**:230–3.

41. **Bentley, G.** (1978). The surgical treatment of chondromalacia patellae. *J Bone Joint Surg* **60B**:74–81.

42. **Insall, J.** (1974). The Pridie debridement operation for osteoarthritis of the knee. *Clin Orthop* **101**:61–7.

43. **Ficat, R.P., Ficat, C., Gedeon, P.K., and Toussaint, J.B.** (1979). Spongialization: A new treatment for diseased patellae. *Clin Orthop* **144**:74–83.

44. **Childers, J.C. and Ellwood, S.C.** (1979). Partial chondrectomy and subchondral bone drilling for chondromalacia. *Clin Orthop* **144**:114–20.

45. **Friedman, M.J., Berasi, D.O., Fox, J.M., Pizzo, W.D., Snyder, S.J., and Ferkel, R.D.** (1984). Preliminary results with abrasion arthroplasty in the osteoarthritic knee. *Clin Orthop* **182**:200–0.

46. **Ha'eri, G.B. and Wiley, A.M.** (1980). High tibial osteotomy combined with joint debridement: a long-term study of results. *Clin Orthop* 151:153–9.

47. **Weisl, H.** (1980). Intertrochanteric osteotomy for osteoarthritis. A long-term follow-up. *J Bone Joint Surg* **62B**:37–42.

48. **Beyers, P.D.** (1974). The effect of high femoral osteotomy on osteoarthritis of the hip. *J Bone Joint Surg* **56B**:279–90.

49. Itoman, M., Yamamoto, M., Yonemoto, K., Sekiguchi, M., and Kai, H. (1992). Histological examination of surface repair tissue after successful osteotomy for osteoarthritis of the hip. *Int Orthop Germany* **16**:118–21.

50. Bergenudd, H., Johnell, O., Redlund-Johnell, I., and Lohmander, L.S. (1992). The articular cartilage after osteotomy for medial gonarthrosis: biopsies after 2 years in 19 cases. *Acta Orthop Scand* **63**(4):413–16.

51. Odenbring, S., Egund, N., Lindstrand, A., Lohmander, L.S., and Willén, H. (1992). Cartilage regeneration after proximal tibial osteotomy for medial gonarthrosis. *Clin Orthop Rel Res* **277**:210–16.

52. Insall, J.N., Joseph, D.M., and Msika, C. (1984). High tibial osteotomy for varus gonarthrosis. A long-term follow-up study. *J Bone Joint Surg* **66A**:1040–8.

53. Reigstad, A. and Gronmark, T. (1984). Osteoarthritis of the hip treated by intertrochanteric osteotomy. A long-term follow up. *J Bone Joint Surg* **66A**:1–6.

54. Berman, A.T., Bosco, S.J., Kirshner, S., and Avolio, A. (1991). Factors influencing long-term results in high tibial osteotomy. *Clin Orthop* **272**:192–8.

55. Matthews, L.S., Goldstein, S.A., Malvitz T.A., Katz, B.P., and Kaufer, H. (1988). Proximal tibial osteotomy. Factors that influence the duration of satisfactory function. *Clin Orthop* **229**:193–200.

56. Coventry, M.B., Ilstrup, D.M., and Wallrichs, S.L. (1993). Proximal tibial osteotomy. A critical long-term study of eighty-seven cases. *J Bone Joint Surg* **75A**:196–201.

57. Dell, P.C. and Muniz, R.B. (1987). Interposition arthroplasty of the trapeziometacarpal joint for osteoarthritis. *Clin Orthop Rel Res* **220**:27–34.

58. Odenbring, S., Egund, N., Lindstrand, A., and Tjornstrand, B. (1989). A guide instrument for high tibial osteotomy. *Acta Orthop Scand* **60**:449–51.

59. Prodromos, C.C., Andriacchi, T.P., and Galante, J.O. (1985). A relationship between gait and clinical changes following high tibial osteotomy. *J Bone Joint Surg* **67A**:1188–94.

60. *Wang, J-W., Kuo, K.N., Andriacchi, T.P., and Galante, J.O. (1990). The influence of walking mechanics and time on the results of proximal tibial osteotomy. *J Bone Joint Surg* **72A**:905–09.

    Identifies the importance of gait mechanics for the outcome of tibial osteotomy for knee OA.

61. Odenbring, S., Tjornstrand, B., Egund, N., et al. (1989). Function after tibial osteotomy for medial gonarthrosis below aged 50 years. *Acta Orthop Scand* **60**:527–31.

62. Magyar, G., Toksvig-Larsen, S., and Lindstrand, A. (1999). Hemicallotasis open-wedge osteotomy for osteoarthritis of the knee. Complications in 308 operations. *J Bone Joint Surg Br* **81**(3):449–51.

63. Magyar, G., Ahl, T.L., Vibe, P., Toksvig-Larsen, S., and Lindstrand, A. (1999). Open-wedge osteotomy by hemicallotasis or the closed-wedge technique for osteoarthritis of the knee. A randomised study of 50 operations. *J Bone Joint Surg Br* **81**(3):444–8.

64. Magyar, G., Toksvig-Larsen, S., and Lindstrand, A., (1999). Changes in osseous correction after proximal tibial osteotomy: Radiostereometry of closed- and open-wedge osteotomy in 33 patients. *Acta Orthop Scand* **70**(5):473–7.

65. Magyar, G., Toksvig-Larsen, S., and Lindstrand, A., (1998). Open wedge tibial osteotomy by callus distraction in gonarthrosis. Operative technique and early results in 36 patients. *Acta Orthop Scand* **69**(2):147–51.

66. Richardson, E.G. (1987). The foot in adolescents and adults. In: A.H. Crenshaw (ed.), *Campbell's Operative Orthopaedics*. St Louis: CV Mosby, pp. 829–988.

67. Sherman, K.P., Douglas, D.L., and Benson, D.A. (1984). Keller's arthroplasty: Is distraction useful? *J Bone Joint Surg* **66B**:765–9.

68. Falahee, M.H., Matthews, L.S., and Kaufer, H. (1987). Resection arthroplasty as a salvage procedure for a knee with infection after a total arthroplasty. *J Bone Joint Surg* **69A**:1013–21.

69. Lettin, A.W.F., Neil, N.J., Citron, N.D., and August, A. (1990). Excision arthroplasty for infected constrained total knee replacements. *J Bone and Joint Surg* **72B**:220–4.

70. *Odenbring, S., Egund, N., Knutson, K., Lindstrand, A., and Larsen, S.T. (1990). Revision after osteotomy for gonarthrosis. A 10–19 year follow-up of 314 cases. *Acta Orthop Scand* **61**:128–30.

    A long-term follow-up of tibial osteotomy for OA that identifies important risk factors for poor outcome of this procedure.

71. Shahriaree, H., Sajadi, K., Silver, C.M., and Sheikholeslamzadeh, S. (1987). Excisional arthroplasty of the elbow. *J Bone Joint Surg* **61A**:922–7.

72. Knight, R.A. and Zandt, I.L.V. (1952). Arthroplasty of the elbow. *J Bone Joint Surg* **34A**:610–18.

73. Engkvist, O. and Johansson, S.H. (1980). Perichondrial arthroplasty: a clinical study in twenty-six patients. *Scand J Plast Reconstr Surg* **14**:71–87.

74. Seradge, H., Kutz, J.A., Kleinert, H.E., Lister G.D., Wolff, T.W., and Atasoy., E. (1984). Perichondrial resurfacing arthroplasty in the hand. *J Hand Surg* **9A**:880–6.

75. Homminga, G.N., Bulstra, S.K., Bouwmeester, P.M., and Linden, A.J.V.D. (1990). Perichondrial grafting for cartilage lesions of the knee. *J Bone Joint Surg* **72** B:1003–7.

76. Buckwalter, J.A., Woo, SL-Y., Goldberg, V.M., et al. (1993). Soft tissue aging and musculoskeletal function. *J Bone Joint Surg* **75A**:1533–48.

77. Kusayama, T., Tomatsu, T., Akasaka, O., and Imai, N. (1991). Autogenous meniscus grafts in articular cartilage defects—an experimental study. *Tokai J Exp Clin Med* **16**:145–51.

78. Vachon, A.M., McIlwraith, C.W., Powers B.E., McFadden, P.R., and Amiel, D. (1992). Morphologic and biochemical study of sternal cartilage autografts for resurfacing induced osteochondral defects in horses. *Am J Vet Res* **53**:1038–47.

79. Locht, R.C., Gross, A.E., and Langer, F. (1984). Late osteochondral allograft resurfacing for tibial plateau fractures. *J Bone Joint Surg* **66A**:328–35.

80. Meyers, M.H., Akeson, W., and Convery, F.R. (1989). Resurfacing the knee with fresh osteochondral allograft. *J Bone Joint Surg* **71A**:704–13.

81. Gross, A.E., Beaver, R.J., and Mohammed, M.N. (1992). Fresh small fragment osteochondral allografts used for posttraumatic defects in the knee joint. In: G.A.M., Finerman, and F.R. Noyes (eds), *Biology and Biomechanics of the Traumatized Synovial Joint: The Knee as a Model*. Rosemont, IL: American Academy of Orthopaedic Surgeons, pp. 123–41.

82. Flynn, J.M., Springfield, D.S., and Mankin, H.J. (1994). Osteoarticular allografts to treat distal femoral osteonecrosis. *Clin Orthop Rel Res* **303**:38–43.

83. Hangody, L., Feczko, P., Bartha, L., Bodo, G., and Kish, G. (2001). Mosaicplasty for the treatment of articular defects of the knee and ankle. *Clin Orthop* **391** (Suppl.):S328–36.

84. Hunziker, E.B. and Rosenberg. R. (1994). Induction of repair partial thickness articular cartilage lesions by timed release of TGF-Beta. *Trans Orthop Res Soc* **19**:236.

85. Pfeilschifter, J., Diel, I., Brunotte, K., Naumann, A., and Ziegler, R. (1993). Mitogenic responsiveness of human bone cells in vitro to hormones and growth factors decreases with age. *J Bone Miner Res* **8**:707–17.

86. Wakitani, S., Kimura, T., Hirooka, A., et al. (1989). Repair of rabbit articular surfaces with allograft chondrocytes embedded in collagen gel. *J Bone Joint Surg* **71B**:74–80.

87. Itay, S., Abramovici, A., Ysipovitch, Z., and Nevo, Z. (1988). Correction of defects in articular cartilage by implants of cultures of embryonic chondrocytes. *Trans Orthop Res Soc* **13**:112.

88. Noguchi, T., Oka, M., Fujino, M., Neo, M., and Yamamuro, T. (1994). Repair of osteochondral defects with grafts of cultured chondrocytes. Comparison of allografts and isografts. *Clin Orthop Rel Res* **302**:251–8.

89. Robinson, D., Halperin, N., and Nevo, Z. (1990). Regenerating hyaline cartilage in articular defects of old chickens using implants of embryonal chick chondrocytes embedded in a new natural delivery substance. *Calcif Tissue Int* **46**:246–53.

90. Wakitani, S., Goto, T., Mansour, J.M., Goldberg, V.M., and Caplan, A.I. (1994). Mesenchymal stem cell-based repair of a large articular cartilage and bone defect. *Trans Orthop Res Soc* **19**:481.

91. Brittberg, M., Lindahl, A., Nilsson, A., Ohlsson, C., Isaksson, O., and Peterson, L. (1994). Treatment of deep cartilage defects in the knee with autologous chondrocyte transplantation. *N Engl J Med* **331**:889–95.

92. *Peterson, L., Brittberg, M., Kiviranta, I., Lundgren, Åkerlund, E., and Lindahl, A. (2002). Autologous chondrocyte transplantation. Biomechanics and long-term durability. *Am J Sports Med* **30**:2–12.

    A long-term follow-up of 61 patients treated with chondrocyte transplantation.

93. Muckle, D.S. and Minns, R.J. (1990). Biological response to woven carbon fiber pads in the knee: A clinical and experimental study. *J Bone and Joint Surg* **72B**:60–2.

94. *Lohmander, L.S. (1998). Cell-based cartilage repair—Do we need it, can we do it, is it good, can we prove it? *Curr Opin Orthop* **9**(6):38–42.

    A critical discussion of the current state-of-the-art for chondrocyte transplantation.

9.19 Arthroplasty and its complications

Kaj Knutson

Arthroplasty is the reconstruction, by natural modification or artificial replacement, of a diseased, damaged, or ankylosed joint. This chapter deals with endoprosthetic joint replacement arthroplasty.

Clinical picture

Joint degeneration in OA is slow and gradual. The OA joint may be painful on weight bearing when radiographs show only a reduced thickness of the joint cartilage. However, some patients have asymptomatic joint degeneration. The degenerative process goes on to complete loss of cartilage and rebuilding of the subchondral bone. Finally, the joint is painful even at rest. The time from the onset of OA on radiographs to the onset of pain or to the complete loss of cartilage varies considerably between patients and between joints.

In hinge-like joints, such as the knee, one part of the joint often takes more load than the other with an asymmetric progress of the degeneration. As a result, a varus or valgus malalignment follows which increases the uneven load distribution. The end result is a severely malaligned joint, with subluxation of the condyles. However, pain reduces joint mobility, which, together with sclerosis of the loaded parts of the condyles, osteophytes, and fibrosis of the joint capsule, stops the process at some advanced level. Sometimes the joint spontaneously ankyloses.

Historical review

One hundred years ago, attempts were made to treat diseased joints with endoprosthetic replacement. Péan designed a rubber ball to replace the humeral head, and Gluck an ivory hinge for the knee, which were implanted in patients with tuberculous joints. The initial failures were due to unsuitable materials and surgical technique, as well as to a lack of antisepsis and proper indications. A search for implant materials for fracture treatment and joint replacement continued, and by the middle of the century, stainless steel, cobalt-chromium alloy, and acrylics were found to be suitable. The first successes came with a stainless steel, reinforced acrylic hinged knee prosthesis, introduced by Walldius in 1953. The Walldius knee was further developed into a cobalt-chromium hinge that was universally accepted; it relied on fibrous encapsulation of its stems in the femoral and tibial shafts. Young and Shiers independently made similar designs.

Parallel with this development, attempts were made to treat arthritic joints with materials interposed between the joint surfaces. The idea was to prevent the degenerated surfaces from making direct contact, thus reducing pain and the progression of attrition and malalignment. Autogenous materials, such as fascia lata and split-thickness skin grafts, were used, but also pig-bladder and synthetic materials have been tried. In weight-bearing joints, the materials were too soft, or they evoked a serious foreign-body reaction. However, autogenous materials in the joints of the upper extremity still have their use in modern orthopaedic surgery in rheumatoid patients. In the 1950s, inert metal alloys were successfully introduced as hemiprostheses, replacing one of a pair of degenerated articular surfaces,

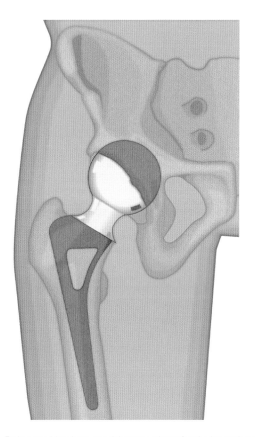

Fig. 9.35 Early monobloc (one piece) hemiprosthesis for the hip with a metal head articulating against acetabulum. This concept is still in use for the elderly with a cervical hip fracture where the acetabular cartilage is intact.

for example, the Smith–Petersen hip cup and the MacIntosh tibial inlay. Femoral head-replacing prostheses were also introduced (Fig. 9.35).

Evolution of hip prostheses

The Charnley low-friction arthroplasty

An important breakthrough came with the work of Charnley.[1] He realized that a hip hemiarthroplasty, with a metal head articulating against subchondral bone in the acetabulum, would never achieve the low friction of a normal joint; high friction caused the implants to loosen by putting stress on the boundaries between the bone and the implant. Others, such as McKee, had tried metal-against-metal hip implants with screw fixation, but Charnley found that the friction was still too high and the fixation inadequate. From a chemist in the field of dental surgery, Charnley had learnt

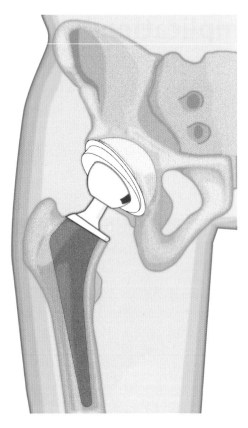

Fig. 9.36 Modern cemented hip prosthesis with a smooth stem, a modular 28-mm head and a HDPE cup; a design based on the low-friction arthroplasty of Charnley. The use of a collar at the neck of the stem is optional.

about self-curing acrylic resin that could be used for implant fixation: a powder of polymethyl methacrylate was mixed with fluid methyl methacrylate, giving a doughy cement that could be used to fill the gap between the stem of a hip prosthesis and the femoral shaft. The cement cured in 15 minutes, with some heat generation. Once cured, the substance was inert and strong enough to keep the femoral component fixed to the bone. Charnley also looked for other materials to use as an articulating surface against the prosthesis. Low friction was first achieved with an acetabular cup of polytetrafluoroethylene (PTFE) and was improved by gradual reduction of the head diameter from 42 to 22 mm. Despite low friction the PTFE wore rapidly and the wear particles evoked a strong foreign-body reaction—another cup material was needed. High-density polyethylene (HDPE) combined inertness with low friction and low wear rate. In 1962, Charnley's low-friction arthroplasty (LFA) was finalized with a set of orthopaedic instruments and a strict surgical routine for the procedure. Although the procedure was a success, Charnley continued to refine the operation. The components were redesigned to improve cement pressurization during insertion, which also improved cement interlocking with the intramedullary cancellous bone. He also introduced drill holes in acetabulum, lavage systems and brushes for cleaning the cancellous surfaces and the technique of plugging the distal femoral canal with a bone-block to further improve fixation. Hundreds of similar all-cemented designs have since been introduced on the market (Fig. 9.36).

Prevention of deep infection

Another important step in making the LFA a safe procedure was the development of an ultraclean environment for the operation. Charnley assumed that the seven per cent deep infection rate in the early years was due to intraoperative contamination. Operating in a small tent-like enclosure in

the operating room, with a vertical flow of filtered air, reduced the number of infective particles to two per cent. Further reduction was achieved with body gowns of new impermeable materials, a helmet with glass visor, body exhaust systems, and double gloves. After ten years' development the infection rate was less than one-tenth of the original rate. Today, further reduction of the infection rate has been achieved with prophylactic antibiotics given during surgery or added to the bone cement for slow release locally.

Improvement in cementing technique

The load of an implant is carried to the bone through shearing forces in the cement. This load is high, and methods have been employed to increase the strength of the cement and, thus, prevent it from deforming and cracking. The traditional mixing of cement in a bowl led to air entrapment causing porous and weakened cement. Low viscosity cement was easier to mix, and centrifugation after mixing reduced the number of large voids, while micro-porosity was the same. Mixing in thin air (so-called partial vacuum) has been shown to improve further the fatigue properties of cement and is nowadays commonly used. The cement is mixed in a cartridge and then injected and pressurized using a cement gun.

The cement monomer is toxic, the curing process generates high temperatures which may cause heat necrosis of the bone, and the cement is brittle, and more so with age. Once the cement is loose, it wears down and generates cement particles that can induce an inflammatory process, which increases bone resorption and promotes further loosening of the implant. Concern about heat necrosis during the cement-curing process has led to the development of new types of cement with lower heat generation. However, in vivo measurements of interfacial temperatures have not supported the validity of this concern in arthroplasty. At least one of the new low-heat generating cements had to be withdrawn because of poor mechanical properties.[2] As an alternative, biological fixation methods, with direct bone-to-implant contact, were investigated.

Cementless cup fixation

The HDPE cup was reinforced with a metal outer shell in an attempt to better redistribute the load and to minimize deformation through creep of the plastic material. The metallic shell was supplied with an outer thread to allow cementless fixation by screwing the cup into the acetabular cavity. However, the screw cup had only the inadequate area of the edge of the threads in contact with bone, and results were inferior. Instead, a layer of porous coating was added to the metal shell to combine instant macrolocking with later microlocking through bone ingrowth.[3] Concern was expressed that the cup failed to make bone contact centrally, thus preventing bone ingrowth, which cannot span millimetre-wide gaps. Conventional screws inserted through holes in the metal shell were introduced. The thickness of the metal shell had to be increased to harbour the screw heads, thus reducing the thickness of the plastic parts to an unsafe level, with increased plastic deformation and wear as a result. Because of the screw holes, only a fraction of the plastic shell was actually supported by the metal shell. The latest step is a solid metal shell with a smooth inner surface that makes full contact with the plastic part. These porous-coated cups rely on under-reamed acetabulae and a peripheral pressfit for fixation. This latter type of acetabular implant has proved to be as reliable as cemented HDPE cups (Fig. 9.37).

Cementless stem fixation

Porous coating for biological fixation is also used in the femoral shaft.[4] The technique requires a large number of sizes to allow optimal filling of the medullary cavity for an initial, stable press-fit (Fig. 9.38). Initial stability is essential to bone ingrowth and as little as $150\,\mu$ of micromotion has been found to prevent it. The natural variability in the shape of the proximal femur makes it impossible to obtain more than isolated areas with good bone-to-prosthesis contact.

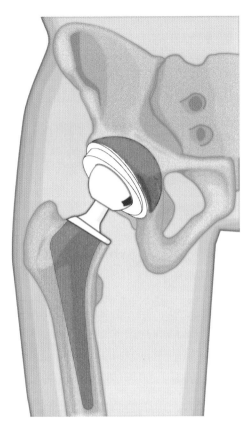

Fig. 9.37 Hybrid hip prosthesis with a conventional cemented femoral stem and a metal backed porous coated cementless HDPE cup fixed to the acetabulum by initial press-fit and later bone ingrowth.

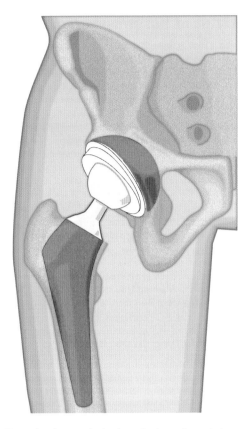

Fig. 9.38 Cementless hip prosthesis where the femoral stem is large enough to give press-fit fixation against the cortical bone for bone ingrowth into a porous surface. The same applies to the cup. The head is ceramic made of aluminum oxide or zirconium oxide for wear reduction. The HDPE cup-liner can be replaced by one with a ceramic articulating surface.

The shafts of uncemented femoral components are considerably stiffer than the femoral cortex. This has been pointed out as a possible explanation of the common problem of mid-thigh pain during the first postoperative year. Attempts have been made to improve the elasticity match of the femoral component by weakening the distal end. This can be done with slots or hollow implants, a thinner stem with an outer sleeve, and by using titanium alloy components. However, more flexible implants have more interfacial motion and less ingrowth in porous surfaces. As is often seen, the solution to one problem causes another.[5]

Bioactive coatings

In later years, great interest has been focused on bioactive coatings to create an active bond between the implant and the bone bed. The coating most often used is made of hydroxyapatite. The bioactive coating improves early fixation, but does not replace the need for porous coating or press-fit design. Its effect is probably short lasting, and the coating may resorb or become yet another source of particles that may interfere with the articulation, thus creating more wear.

Wear[6]

Concern about wear has led to improvement in the surface quality of the femoral heads and the use of ceramic heads (Fig. 9.38). Ceramic cups have been designed for the same reason. Also the polyethylene cup material has been modified with higher density, increased intermolecular cross-linkage, and storage in inert gases to prevent oxidative degradation. A renewed interest in metal-against-metal articulation has also started. Modern production techniques make it possible to produce perfectly matching pairs with minimal wear. Modern metal-to-plastic implants have a wear rate of 0.1–0.2 mm per year; ceramic and all-metal articulations are more than ten times better. The friction in all-metal articulations is the same as in the LFA, and the high friction found by Charnley has since been ascribed to his having evaluated a poorly designed copy of the McKee–Farrar prosthesis.

The Scandinavian national arthroplasty registers

In 1975, the Swedish Orthopaedic Society initiated a prospective nationwide study of knee arthroplasty.[7–9] It was followed by a national hip arthroplasty study in 1979.[10] The Norwegian and Finnish counterparts have started similar registers.[11–14] The registers use the unique social security numbers to keep track of all patients. Individual patient mortality has been checked against national census registers. Data are regularly analysed by actuarial methods to calculate the cumulated risk of revision for various groups of patients, implants, and surgical techniques. The results provide a better calculation of risks than reports from highly specialized units and are part of an ongoing quality control of joint replacement procedures. The registers have shown some underperforming designs, but also that the modern conventional cemented implants have been a safe choice.

The registers focus on revision, but not all revisions are equal and clinical performance is not taken into account. Another problem is that results are so good that differences become obvious only after prolonged observation times, when the implants have already been replaced by newer models. Nonetheless, these large-scale studies have given information that could not have been collected in any other way, and they were never meant to replace detailed studies in smaller units. Selected data from the registers have also been used to analyse uncommon conditions, complications, and revision techniques.

Currently used hip prostheses

In Europe, sales statistics show that total hip arthroplasties are more often carried out with cemented femoral stems than without, while cemented and uncemented cups are equally common. In Scandinavian countries, the usual procedure is a cemented total hip replacement with a cobalt-chromium-molybdenum or stainless steel femoral component articulating against a HDPE acetabular cup. The four most common types in Sweden were Charnley, Lubinus SP, Exeter polished, and Scan Hip. Head sizes varied between 22 and 28 mm. Use of a cement-restricting plug, lavage, cleaning of the bone bed, and cement pressurization of vacuum-mixed cement with a gun was standard practice and affected the revision rate, according to the Swedish Total Hip Arthroplasty Register.[10] The same source shows a cumulative revision rate of 0.6 per cent for infection at ten years. This infection rate was influenced by the use of ultraclean air filtration and of gentamicin-containing bone cement, but not by the use of body-exhaust gowns. The ten-year revision rate for loosening was just above ten per cent; it was higher in men and in younger patients. Modern implants differed little. The limited experience of uncemented implants has so far not encouraged its continued use. These findings have been supported by the Norwegian Arthroplasty Register, in which uncemented implants had twice as high a risk of revision as the cemented implants, and even more among younger patients.[13]

Evolution of knee prostheses

It was soon realized that the low-friction technique, with HDPE-against-metal components fixed with bone cement, was also the solution for knee arthroplasty. The interposition implants were developed into surface replacements, with a HDPE tibial component and a metal runner on the femoral condyle, as in the knee prostheses developed by Gunston, Marmor, and Buchholz. These implants were suitable for single-compartment degeneration (Fig. 9.39). For generalized degeneration, it was easier to use interconnected parts (Geomedic) or true bicondylar implants, for example, the Freeman–Swanson knee. Later, the patellar articulation was included and the implants became tricompartmental or 'total knees' (Fig. 9.40).

Hinged implants were more anatomically redesigned, as in the French GUEPAR prosthesis, and soon included HDPE bearings to avoid direct metal-to-metal connections as in the St. Georg hinged prosthesis. Hybrid solutions were created, either as rotating hinges or stabilized prostheses with more than single-axis mobility. The latter had loose interference connections between the tibial and femoral parts, restricting varus and valgus mobility, and a forced roll-back of the femoral component on the tibia through a cam axis or similar design. Most of these implants were fixed with bone cement.

Improvements in surgical technique

The initial clinical experience of knee arthroplasty was rewarding, with good mobility, stability, and pain relief. However, the failure rate was higher than for contemporary hip arthroplasties. Large implants were easy to use because they replaced both the degenerated joint surfaces and the accompanying stabilizing structures. The positioning of the implants relative to the bony parts was simplified by using long intramedullary stems. Despite the rigid fixation, these implants had a high failure rate because of loosening and deep infection.[7] During the 1980s, large implants were replaced by smaller ones, as more was learned about soft tissue techniques with ligament release procedures to correct deformities. The surface replacement prostheses were supplied with increasingly complex guide instruments to ensure proper alignment of the leg, position of the implant, and soft tissue balance. Surface replacement prostheses rely on the support of the condylar cancellous bone for fixation, and the same cement injection technique as in hip arthroplasty was used.

Improvement of fixation

Further attempts were made to improve prosthetic fixation. In particular, the tibial component constituted a problem because of its basically flat

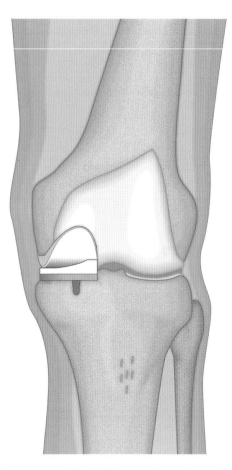

Fig. 9.39 Unicompartmental (medial) knee prosthesis with a metal femoral component and a metal backed HDPE tibial component for use in single compartment OA.

design; the first polyethylene tibial components covered only a part of the resected tibial condyle. They were anchored to the cement and bone bed by a textured surface or by small dovetail-shaped pegs. Development of better fixation was a gradual process, starting with better coverage by using more sizes, short intracondylar stems, integrated metal reinforcement, or a metal base plate with stems, pegs, or screws. Parallel to this, attempts were made to reduce the stresses transmitted through the tibial component. Initially, the femoral and tibial parts were highly congruent, allowing only single-axis rotation. Thus, the rotation of the lower leg around its longitudinal axis was restricted by the implant, causing high stresses on the fixation. By redesigning the articulate surfaces into a flat tibial contact area, these stresses were instead transmitted through the soft tissues. However, in solving one problem another problem was created; articulating a curved femoral component on a flat tibial component meant a very high stress level at the point of contact, resulting in an increased wear rate.

Cementless fixation

Biological fixation methods with direct bone-to-implant contact have also been investigated in knee arthroplasty. Initial macroscopic fixation is a prerequisite for microscopic fixation, where bone grows on the surface of the implant. The former was achieved through a press-fit design, with additional screw fixation, and the latter through a porous coating of the implant. The first design to be clinically used was the PCA total knee by Hungerford and Kenna, which had a porous layer of chrome-cobalt beads sintered to the metal parts. Others followed, using titanium alloy components having a porous wire mesh fixed to the substrate by diffusion bonding. Porous titanium surfaces were also created by plasma-spraying metal on a cold metal

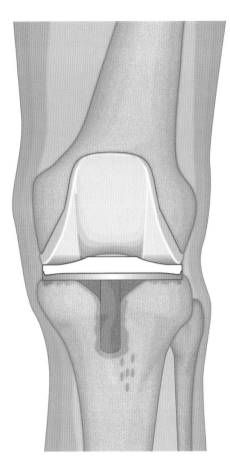

Fig. 9.40 Symmetrical total (tricompartmental) knee prosthesis with a cemented metal tibial tray, which holds a modular HDPE articulating surface. Soft tissue tension can be adjusted by changing the thickness of the plastic component. Patella (not shown) can also be fitted with a HDPE surface.

substrate. Again, it seemed that a problem was solved, but instead new problems were created. The sintering process changed the properties of the substrate metal, making it more vulnerable to metal fatigue; beads came off and tibial trays broke. Also, little, if any, bone ingrowth has been found at the examination of postmortem retrieved tibial components. Furthermore, the porous structure greatly enlarged the surface, causing increased risk of metal ion leakage into the surrounding tissues. Although the alloys were inert, the isolated ions were not.

Micromotion

Computer-assisted radiostereometric analysis (RSA) of tibial component migration can detect very small changes in the prosthetic position over time.[15] Collected data have indicated that most implants migrate for up to one year after insertion, but then they stabilize;[16] a small subset migrated more and continued to migrate. Cases that were eventually revised for loosening all belonged to the continuously migrating group. Thus, the loosening process was gradual and started shortly after implantation. The pattern was the same, whether the interface material was bone cement, polyethylene, or metal. Less migration was seen when a water-cooled saw-blade was used to cut bone, instead of cutting with a conventional heat-generating blade.[17] Proper alignment of the leg also reduced migration.

RSA has also been used to record the inducible displacement of the tibial component when the replaced knee is physiologically loaded. The observed micromotion occurs at a level that inhibits bone ingrowth in porous surfaces. However, stems and screws have a stabilizing effect, which reduces interfacial motion.

RSA indicates that the early findings govern the final outcome of the arthroplasty, influenced by prosthetic design, surgical technique, fixation and position of implants, alignment, and bone quality. The interface in stable implants has been shown to be mainly dense fibrocartilage. Unstable implants have a softer, fibrous tissue encapsulation permeable to polyethylene wear particles. These, and other wear particles induce an inflammatory reaction capable of inducing bone resorption (osteolysis), making failure more likely.[18]

Currently used knee prostheses

Early single-compartment OA of the knee can be treated with unicondylar implants. The original designs have been modified but still have femoral onlay parts with pegs for fixation. On the tibial side they have HDPE parts with a flat top. They can be used with or without a metal backing, and they rely on bone cement for fixation. Some recently introduced designs have femoral components that are fixed to the femoral condyle after bone resection. The tibial part is often metal backed (Fig. 9.39), sometimes with screw fixation. Guide instruments are used to make accurate cuts. These implants are available with or without porous coating, for cemented or cementless fixation. The fraction of knee arthroplasties for OA performed with unicondylar implants varies from country to country.[19] In Sweden it is high; approximately one-fifth.[9]

Advanced or generalized OA of the knee is, nowadays, treated with tricompartmental (total) knee prostheses (Fig. 9.40). Most of them are cobalt-chromium-molybdenum alloy implants with an anatomic-shaped femoral component. Both smooth and porous-coated femoral implants are used, and cementless fixation is regarded as safe. The tibial component is usually modular, with a cemented metal tray that gains additional stability from a short central stem or from pegs. The HDPE part is usually fixed to the tray with a snap-fit. Modularity is increasingly popular, and several implants can be fitted with stem extension and wedges to fill the gap between the implant and the worn-down tibial condyle. Attempts are being made to reduce the high-contact stresses inherent in knee prosthesis with a flat tibial component and a rounded femoral component. By changing the tibial component to a more 'dished' shape, a higher degree of congruence is achieved with larger contact area. The most radical design has a fully congruent HDPE component, which has a second articulation on its lower surface against the flat and polished top of the metal tray. By separating the articulation for flexion from that of axial rotation, these discal knees combine a large contact area with low shear forces and wear (Fig. 9.41).

In total knees, a HDPE patellar component can be fitted. It usually has the shape of a small button and is cemented against the resected joint surface of the patella. Metal backing is avoided because of the thin implant that may wear through causing metal to scratch against metal. The need for patellar replacement is debated.[20]

Stabilized implants with a forced roll-back of femur on tibia have limited use in primary knee arthroplasty, the exception being patellectomized knees, and knees with severe insufficiency of the posterior cruciate ligament.

In Sweden the most common unicompartmental knee is the Endo Link, and the most common total knees are AGC, Freeman–Samuelson, and PFC, while in Norway the discal LCS knee is mostly used. In Europe, sales statistics show that three-quarter of the tibial components are cemented, whereas cementless femoral fixation is slightly more common than cemented.

Ankle arthroplasty

Symptomatic OA of the ankle is rare and often secondary to deformity, joint instability, ankle fractures, or vascular necrosis of the talus. The condition is painful; cartilage reduction and osteophyte formation lead to early loss of motion. The most common surgical treatment is ankle fusion through an anterior approach or lateral with malleolar osteotomy; oblique screws are inserted through the joint for fixation.[21]

In sedentary OA patients aged over 60, without instability, deformity, or neuropathic disorders, but with normal vascular status, a joint replacement arthroplasty may be considered. A variety of implants have been designed, most of them having a metal talar dome and an HDPE tibial insert, having more or less constrained articulation. Cement fixation was commonly used. A few porous-coated designs intended for biological fixation have more recently been introduced. These implants are discal and have a lower congruent talar articulation and an upper flat tibial articulation that eliminates shear forces (Fig. 9.42).

Ankle replacement arthroplasty is still being investigated. The original two-part designs had a low-success rate that deteriorated with time, whereas the discal designs are more promising. However, reports are few and short-term.[21,22]

Foot arthroplasties

OA of the subtalar joints and the first metatarsophalangeal joints has been experimentally treated with joint replacement arthroplasty. The most extensive attempt has used silicone rubber interposition in the first metatarsophalangeal joint. Safe alternative methods, such as arthrodesis, osteotomy, and resection arthroplasty, have completely replaced these experimental methods.[23]

Shoulder arthroplasty

OA of the shoulder follows the same pattern as OA of other joints: the cartilage is reduced in the loaded areas, and the periphery of the humeral head and glenoid is enlarged with osteophytes; usually, the rotator cuff remains intact or mildly degenerated. Fibrosis of the joint capsule restricts mobility, but this restriction is compensated by the thoracoscapular mobility. OA of the shoulder is not the main indication for shoulder arthroplasty, a procedure constituting one per cent of all large joint arthroplasties. The implants used today are all similar unconstrained designs derived from the original Neer design, but with a modular, anatomically-sized head fixed with a taper to a humeral stem (Fig. 9.43); an HDPE glenoid surface replacement component is optional. The approach is anterior, through the deltopectoral groove. Only the subscapularis tendon is divided and then the joint dislocated to obtain access. At closure, the tendon can be lengthened to improve joint mobility (since this tendon is often shortened in OA). Prosthetic components are press-fit or cemented. A simple metal cup fixed to the surface of the head has been designed for hemiarthroplasty—its usefulness in OA has not been established.

Little has been reported concerning the clinical outcome of shoulder hemiarthroplasty—pain relief is incomplete, and mobility depends on the condition of the rotator cuff and the shoulder muscles. A glenoid component seems to increase pain relief, at least for as long as it remains fixed. Failure of this component, however, is quite common.

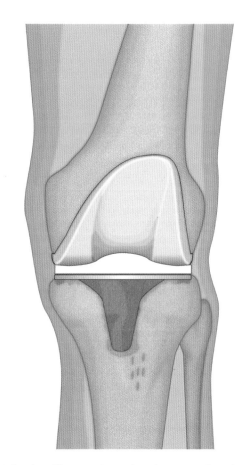

Fig. 9.41 Discal total knee prosthesis where the upper surface of the fully congruent HDPE component allows flexion-extension only, while the lower surface allows axial rotation. The femoral component is asymmetrical (left/right) to better mimic the original anatomy of the femoral condyle.

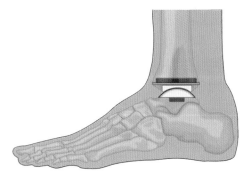

Fig. 9.42 Discal ankle prosthesis with a congruent distal talar articulation for flexion-extension and a flat upper tibial articulation that eliminates shear forces.

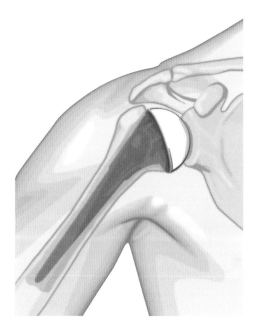

Fig. 9.43 Shoulder prosthesis with a cemented humoral stem and modular head that can be chosen (diameter/thickness) to fit the anatomy. A small glenoid HDPE articular surface can also be fitted.

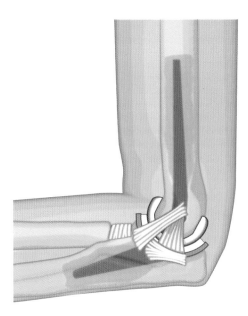

Fig. 9.44 Elbow prosthesis with cemented stems and a HDPE articular surface fixed to the ulnar component.

Elbow arthroplasty

The elbow is a hinge-like joint and the first attempts to replace it were performed using hinged prostheses. Because of the high failure rate, with loosening due to overload of the bone-cement interface, the hinge was abandoned. Today, constrained surface replacement implants with short stems, such as the capitellocondylar and Kudo implants, are used when possible (Fig. 9.44). In severely destroyed joints, 'sloppy' hinged prostheses may be used; they allow some axial rotation along the shafts, which reduces the interfacial stress. The approach is either posterior through the triceps tendon or lateral, with detachment of the radial collateral ligament. OA of the elbow is a rare condition and more than 95 per cent of all elbow arthroplasties are performed for other indications.

Arthroplasties of the hand

OA of the fingers affects both the proximal and distal joints. The initially painful arthritis and joint degeneration eventually cause stiff, slightly deformed, but stable joints that need not be treated with implants, although such are available for rheumatoid arthritis.

The commonest OA affliction of the hand is found in the saddle-shaped trapeziometacarpal (TMC) joint of the thumb. Every fourth woman will develop some joint degeneration and as many as one in twenty will be a candidate for surgery.[24] Often the loss of cartilage is combined with subluxation of TMC joint, and the end-stage is pantrapezial OA with fixed adduction contracture.

Surgical treatment of TMC OA includes partial or total excision of the trapezium with ligament reconstruction and interposition of tendinous structures or a silicone rubber implant. The implant can be designed to replace the base of the first metacarpal or the trapezium. Cemented ball-and-socket prostheses, like miniature hip prostheses, are also being evaluated in the TMC joint.[24]

Primary OA of the wrist is rare and in many cases unilateral. Although silicone rubber interposition devices and cemented or porous-coated ball-and-socket prostheses have been designed for use in rheumatoid arthritis, they are seldom used in OA. Arthrodesis of the wrist permanently relieves pain and improves finger function, but at the expense of motion—this affects daily living activities. Partial wrist fusion and proximal row carpectomy are alternatives in localized, often secondary, OA of the wrist joints.[25]

Arthroplasty complications

General complications

The prevalence of symptomatic OA increases with the age of the patient, as also the risks of general complications due to major surgery. Improvements in risk assessment and anesthesiological technique have made it possible to offer arthroplasty even to the very old. Early reports on hip arthroplasty have dealt mainly with surgical risk aspects and early clinical outcome. These reports indicate that the immediate mortality rate was 0.5–2 per cent, mainly because of cardiac problems and pulmonary embolism. One type of pulmonary embolism was seen during pressurization of cement in the femoral shaft. It has been suggested that thromboplastic products are pushed out into the venous circulation in the cancellous bone by the cement. Changes in surgical technique with the introduction of lavage, brushing, and retrograde cement-filling of the shaft have eliminated this risk of intraoperative *mors subita*. With modern hip arthroplasty technique and hypotensive epidural anesthesia, Sharrock et al.[17] have reported 0.1 per cent mortality at the Hospital for Special Surgery in New York.

The risk of deep-vein thrombosis has been reported to be 10–70 per cent, and pulmonary embolism 1–4 per cent. Half of the thrombi were proximal and sometimes asymptomatic, and these were associated with pulmonary embolism. Deep-vein thrombosis, even when treated, is associated with later deep-venous insufficiency. Many methods have been introduced to reduce these figures: by using an epidural instead of general anesthesia, the risk was reduced to less than half. Mechanical methods, such as leg elevation, graduated elastic compression stockings, foot compression pumps, and early ambulation all contribute. The main improvement came with pharmacological prophylaxis. Dextran, heparin, dihydroergotamine, antithrombin III, and warfarin/dicumarol have been successfully used. Today, the low molecular weight heparins are favoured because of simple administration (once daily), and good prophylactic effect with negligible pulmonary embolism and few bleeding complications. Similarly good results, that is, 11 per cent deep-vein thromboses and 1 per cent pulmonary embolisms, have been reported using hypotensive epidural anesthesia combined with aspirin.[17]

Urinary retention is a common problem seen in one-third of the patients undergoing hip arthroplasty. Indwelling catheters are used to prevent retention and to monitor kidney function, but they increase the risk of urinary tract infection.

Rare general complications include paralytic intestinal obstruction, gastrointestinal bleeding, kidney dysfunction, cardiac failure, arrhythmia and infarction, pulmonary infection, stroke, and postoperative confusion and psychosis. The best prevention against these complications is a properly selected, well-informed, well-nourished, well-monitored patient, with blood loss replaced and pain-free. The importance of being pain-free has recently led to changes in the postoperative routines, including continued epidural analgesia, personally adjusted doses, and even self-administration of morphine.

Local complications in hip arthroplasty

Intraoperative complications

The surgical procedure of hip arthroplasty is quite safe, but some intraoperative complications remain. The hip is close to both vessels and nerves; accidental damage to these structures has been reported (neural damage in 0–3 per cent[26]). Especially when arthroplasty is combined with lengthening of the hip, distension of the sciatic nerve may cause injury.

The preparation of the bone beds has been reported to cause fractures of the greater trochanter, the shaft, and acetabulum, particularly when uncemented press-fit prostheses are used (shaft fractures in 2–20 per cent[27]). If not dislocated, they usually heal uneventfully. The orientation of the implants must be reasonably correct to allow a normal range of motion and stability. Malpositioned components may cause impingement, early loosening, and dislocation. Failure to anchor the components properly may result in the patient having a prosthesis that is loose from the beginning. One serious intraoperative complication is bacterial contamination of the joint.

Early postoperative complications

Early local postoperative complications include delayed wound healing, deep infection, dislocation, avulsion of the greater trochanter, or pseudarthrosis of a trochanteric osteotomy. Dislocation has been reported in 0.5–5 per cent. The joint can usually be reduced and the problem may resolve as a pseudocapsule develops around it. Dislocation is associated with prior surgery of the hip, use of a posterior approach, and malaligned components, but not with head size, leg, or neck length, or nursing instructions.[28] Trochanteric problems are reported with the same frequency and to these should be added the formation of heterotopic bone seen in every other patient. When pronounced, it may seriously reduce mobility.

Late postoperative complications

Late local complications include loosening of implants, delayed infection, osteolysis, periprosthetic fractures, implant wear, and breakage. Wear has so far been unavoidable, but it causes no problems during the first ten postoperative years. Severe wear of the cup may result in instability and dislocation of the joint. More serious is the bone loss caused by osteolysis triggered by wear particles; this asymptomatically reduces the bone stock later needed for revision.

Loosening

Loosening of components is the indication for 80 per cent of the hip revisions; using survival statistics, the risk is approximately 10 per cent at 10 years and is higher in men and in younger patients. Modern cemented implants differ little from one another. Most steps in modern cementation technique have an impact on prosthetic survival. In half of the revisions, both components are exchanged and, overall, more stems than cups. Standard revision usually means the recementation of new, sometimes larger components. Components designed for revision, with a prolonged stem to create anchorage below the previous implant, are used in cases with severe bone loss. Various oddly shaped acetabular cups have been designed to fit and fill various defects.

An alternative method to compensate for severe bone loss is to fill the femoral shaft with morselized cancellous bone grafts from donors. Donated bone consists of heads from previous hip arthroplasties, temporarily stored in a bone bank at $-80\,°C$ until tests show that it is safe to use for reconstruction. A cavity is created centrally in the shaft with impaction instruments and a conventional implant is cemented into the cavity. Cortical defects are covered with stainless steel mesh, fixed with wires. After some years, the impaction-grafted shafts show a normalized cortex, but the central core of dead donor bone remains dead. Early results are promising, but long-term results are lacking. Acetabular bone defects can be treated in the same manner.

Deep infection

Deep infection is a serious complication. Three types are encountered: early and delayed postoperative, and late hematogenous, that is, bacterial seeding from some other focus, such as urinary tract, gall bladder, lungs, or dental abscess. The former are regarded as intraoperative contaminations. Typically, the patient is not pain-free, the erythrocyte sedimentation rate remains elevated, and, sometimes, low-grade fever is noted. Wound healing may be disturbed or a fistula may develop. Radiographic examination usually shows rapid loosening of the components that is indistinguishable from aseptic loosening. Osteolysis and perforation of the cortex are subsequently seen. The clinical condition can range from no signs of infection to life-threatening septic shock.

A broad spectrum of microorganisms has been isolated from infected hip arthroplasties; staphylococci are seen in half of the cases, with more

Staphylococcus epidermidis than *Staphylococcus aureus* infections. The latter was the most common infective organism in the early days of hip arthroplasty, and the change in bacteriologic findings may be due to modern antimicrobial prophylaxis. Some bacteria are glycocalyx-forming, and this protects them from the effects of antibiotics and body defence mechanisms.

Surgical treatment of deep infection, without removal of the implants, can occasionally be effective in cases with well-fixed components. Antibiotics alone can only slow down the destructive process, but this may be the only alternative in elderly persons with medical contraindications to surgery. For the majority, the only safe method is removal of the implant. A controversial question is whether, and if so, when to reimplant a new prosthesis. Leaving the patient without a hip joint—the Girdlestone procedure—causes leg shortening, severe limp, and often pain, and is therefore usually avoided. Buchholz has a long experience of one-stage revision, that is, immediate reimplantation of a new prosthesis using bone cement loaded with gentamicin or other appropriate antibiotics. Other investigators have waited months to years before reimplantation, that is, a two-stage revision. Modern two-stage techniques include extraction of the prosthesis, a 6-week period with chains of gentamicin-containing cement beads inserted in the bone defects and antibiotic treatment on the basis of the cultures, and then reimplantation of a new prosthesis. Alternatively a prosthesis-shaped spacer of gentamicin-loaded acrylic cement can be used during the interim period. The overall success rate is in the range of 75–95 per cent.

Local complications in knee arthroplasty

Wound healing disturbances

The knee may have undergone surgery before arthroplasty. This increases the risk of conflicting skin incisions with healing disturbances. Overdistension of the capsular sutures due to oversized implants may cause capsular dehiscence. The end result may be wound rupture and skin necrosis, and a high risk of deep infection. An exposed implant must be promptly covered and a gastrocnemic muscle-flap can be turned over the anterior part of the joint to save the patient from serious consequences. Wound-healing problems are more common, and more often associated with deep infection when large and complex implants are used.

Patellar problems

Correct articulation of patella is a prerequisite for knee function. Medial capsular dehiscence, a tight lateral patellar retinaculum, malposition of components, unbalanced ligaments, and deformed patella are some reasons for patellar subluxation and dislocation, which make the knee weak and unreliable. All of the causes of patellar dislocation can be corrected, but the results of revision are unpredictable. In patients with an unresurfaced patella, pain is not uncommon but it usually resolves with time. Resurfacing the patella is not without problems. The component is thin and wears quickly because of a small contact area; deformation of the component causes loosening; and the anchoring holes make the patella weaker, increasing the risk of fatigue fracture. Lateral release to improve patellar tracking may render the patella avascular, which causes flattening and fragmentation of patella. Overall, six per cent of all revisions are made due to patellar problems including secondary resurfacing of the patella.[20]

Instability

During total knee arthroplasty, the mechanical axis is restored, that is, the knee is so aligned that it is placed on the axis joining the hip with the ankle. Specially designed instruments are used to achieve correct bone cuts; soft tissues around the knee must then be released to balance ligament tensions. Failure to do so may cause instability and even complete dislocation of the joint. Seven per cent of all revisions are due to instability and 15 per cent due to other mechanical reasons.[10] For revision of unstable knees, implants with more or less inherent stability are available. Some reports indicate that unbalanced tension may accelerate loosening of the implant, and the same is found when the mechanical axis is not corrected. Ligament insufficiency is a minor problem. If muscle control is good, or if the knee is protected in a brace, the ligament spontaneously adapts within a few months.

Loosening

Loosening of components, mainly the tibial, is the indication in half of all revisions. In total knee arthroplasty, the cumulative risk of revision for loosening is three per cent at 10 years. This risk has constantly been reduced by improvements in instrumentation, prosthetic design, and cementation technique; as for unicompartmental implants the risk is twice as high, with less improvement over time. The best revision results are achieved if a new total knee implant is used with exchange of all components. If bone loss is minor, a primary type of implant is used, or else a thicker long-stem revision type is advocated. Modular systems have spacers that can be fitted on any of the prosthetic contact areas to compensate for bone loss. Central bone defects after loose stems can be reconstructed with bank bone in the same way as hips, but experience of this is limited.

Deep infection

Deep infection occurs after intraoperative contamination, primarily or after secondary procedures, and in the form of hematogenous seeding from distant foci, most commonly leg ulcers. Early or hematogenous septic arthritis can be treated with conventional therapy, that is, debridement and lavage. Delayed or late infection may occur as chronic arthritis, with fibrosis and joint contracture. Eventually the implants become loose. Late infection can also occur as an abscess or a fistula. Usually, the bone–cement interface is also infected, and revision is needed. The infection may occasionally be necrotizing, toxic, and life threatening; in such a case, prompt removal of the implant or even amputation may be necessary.

The cumulative risk of revision for deep infection is below 1 per cent at 10 years. Half of the revisions are performed as one- or two-stage exchange arthroplasties, and the remainder as knee fusions. The eradication rate after exchange arthroplasty is 75–95 per cent, regardless of the staging technique. However, the clinical success rate is lower; residual pain and restricted mobility are common. An attempt to preserve leg length by use of a cement spacer in the void after the removed implant is an attractive possibility in two-stage revision, but it has not been shown to improve mobility. Deep infection in combination with large implants, severe bone loss, a disrupted extensor mechanism, or soft tissue damage, is not suitable for exchange arthroplasty. Attempts have been made using resection arthroplasty, that is, leaving the joint empty; the results have been discouraging because of instability, pain, and persistent deep infection. More reliable results have been achieved with knee fusion; a modified two-stage technique is used. The empty knee is fixed with a stable external fixator, plates, or an intramedullary rod, and gentamicin-containing cement beads are inserted and combined with appropriate antibiotic treatment. After six weeks, the beads are removed and at the same time an autogenous cancellous bone graft is placed around the joint. Healing can be expected in 90 per cent, but it may take 4–8 months; failed fusion can be treated with another attempt.

Local complications in ankle arthroplasty

The complication rate after ankle arthroplasty is high. Delayed wound healing has been reported in 40 per cent and deep infection in 3–5 per cent. In one report, radiolucent zones were seen in 88 per cent after one year, and loosening of almost all components after six years. More typical results show that one-fourth of the components have loosened after five years; the talar component is most often involved. Impingement, malleolar fracture, subluxation, and dislocation are also reported. Serious complications are treated with ankle fusion or exchange arthroplasty.

Local complications in shoulder arthroplasty

Complications occurred in 11 per cent of a mixed material, using the Neer prosthesis; other similar designs produced the same complication rate. The most frequent complication, one-third of patients, is impingement with the acromion, rotator cuff tears, and tuberosity problems, followed by instability. The loosening, seen in a few per cent, mainly affects the glenoid component. In a compilation of 13 reports with various durations of follow-up, half of the glenoid components had a radiolucent zone, and 2–10 per cent shift in position, indicating that loosening might be imminent or underestimated. In one six-year follow-up of Neer arthroplasties, many of the humeral components showed a shift in position, although the clinical results continued to be excellent.

Other rare complications include intra- or postoperative periprosthetic fractures, intraoperative nerve injury, notably of the axillary nerve, and deep infection. Pain is sometimes reported in otherwise successful shoulder arthroplasties; one reason for this is OA pain from the acromioclavicular joint.

Loose glenoid components can be exchanged, if bone stock so permits, by temporarily removing the modular humeral head. In half the revisions, the glenoid component is permanently removed and a bone graft is placed in the defect. Instability can be treated with a new larger head or soft-tissue repair; infection is treated with component removal. In hemiarthroplasty, glenoid attrition and medialization of the head weaken the joint and make it painful. Secondary glenoid replacement is sometimes possible, but a similar effect can be achieved by replacing the head by a bipolar type, where the inside of the outer head articulates against a smaller humeral head.

Local complications in elbow arthroplasty

Most reports on elbow arthroplasty are based on materials with a majority of rheumatoid cases. The most common complications with modern surface replacements are ulnar nerve palsy in 20–40 per cent and instability or dislocation in 10 per cent. Wound-healing disturbances are not uncommon and deep infection is seen in a few per cent; implant loosening is a less common problem than infection. The overall revision rate is estimated at 5 per cent after five years with the best designs; hinged prostheses with a 'sloppy' or similar rotation are used for revision. Infected cases are, as a rule, treated with resection arthroplasty; fusion is not an alternative because of the limited usefulness of a stiff elbow.

Local complications in silicone rubber arthroplasties

Silicone rubber has been used extensively as an interpositional implant, with good early results. Some loss of motion is common when the implant bridges from one shaft, over the joint, to the next cortical shaft. Although the material is soft and pliable, fatigue fracture of the implant is a common finding after some years. The fracture may pass unnoticed, but may lead to malalignment, instability, and dislocation. The implant may also fret against the hard cortical shafts causing the production of wear particles. These are not so biocompatible as the bulk material, and severe synovitis and cyst formation have been noted in the adjacent bones. Concern regarding this reaction has limited the use of silicone implants in joints where other options are available.

Key points

1. Surgical treatment for osteoarthritic joint degeneration include debridement, joint resection, interposition arthroplasty, osteotomy, and endoprosthetic joint replacement.

2. Endoprosthetic joint replacement of the hip and knee is nowadays a common, safe, and successful procedure. It is still commonly based on Charnley's 40-year old low-friction arthroplasty where a polyethylene cup articulated against a polish metal head. These parts were fixed to bone using bone cement, an acrylic polymer.

3. Improvements in design and technique have reduced the failure rate but still revision surgery has to be performed for loosening, wear, and infection.

4. Loosening is prevented by injection of pore free cement under pressure in a dry bone bed.

5. Loosening is also prevented by use of cementless fixation where bone grows into a porous surface with bioactive coating.

6. Wear in the hip is decreased by use of modified polyethylene or by replacing it with a metal-on-metal or ceramic articulation.

7. Wear in the knee is decreased by the use of a discal polyethylene part, which increases the contact area.

8. Infection is prevented by performing the operation in an ultraclean theatre.

9. Infection is also prevented by giving antibiotic prophylaxis.

10. Future development will be directed towards solutions for other joints and for simple and safe revision procedures.

References

(An asterisk denotes recommended reading.)

1. *Waugh, W. (1990). John Charnley. The man and the hip. London: Springer-Verlag.

    A good overview of the importance of Charnley's work and the difficulties he had to overcome in creating the modern hip arthroplasty.

2. Linder, L. (1995). Boneloc®—the Christiansen experience revisited. Acta Orthop Scand 66:205–6.

3. Yahiro, M.A., Gantenberg, J.B., Nelson, R., Lu, H.T.C., and Mishra, N.K. (1995). Comparison of the results of cemented, porous-ingrowth, and threaded acetabular cup fixation. A meta-analysis of the orthopaedic literature. J Arthroplasty 10:339–50.

4. Rothman, R.C. and Cohn, J.C. (1990). Cemented versus cementless total hip arthroplasty: a critical review. Clin Orthop Rel Res 254:153–69.

5. *Huiskes, R. (1993). Failed innovation in total hip replacement. Diagnosis and proposals for a cure. Acta Orthop Scand 64:699–716.

    Shows the complex interaction between commerce and science and its effect on the evolution of hip replacements.

6. Selvik, G. (1974). Roentgen stereophotogrammetry. A method for the study of kinematics of the skeletal system. Thesis, University of Lund, Sweden. Reprinted 1989 in Acta Orthop Scand 60 (Suppl. 232).

7. Knutson, K., Lindstrand, L., and Lidgren, L. (1986). Survival of knee arthroplasties. A nation-wide multicentre investigation of 8000 cases. J Bone Joint Surg Br 68(B):795–803.

8. Knutson, K., Lewold, S., Robertsson, O., and Lidgren, L. (1994). The Swedish knee arthroplasty register. A nation-wide study of 30 003 knees 1976–92. Acta Orthop Scand 65:375–86.

9. Robertsson, O., Knutson, K., Lewold, S., and Lidgren, L. (2001). The Swedish Knee Arthroplasty Register 1975–1997. An update with special emphasis on 41 223 knees operated on in 1988–97. Acta Orthop Scand 72:503–13.

10. Malchau, H., Herberts, P., and Ahnfelt, L. (1993). Prognosis of total hip replacement in Sweden: follow-up of 92 675 operations performed 1978–90. Acta Orthop Scand 64:497–506.

11. Espehaug, B., Havelin, L.I., Engesæter, L.B., Vollset, S.E., and Langeland, N. (1995). Early revision among 12 179 hip prostheses. A comparison of 10 different brands reported to the Norwegian Arthroplasty Register, 1987–93. Acta Orthop Scand 66:487–93.

12. Havelin, L.I., Espehaug, B., Vollset, S.E., Engesæter, L.B., and Langeland, N. (1993). The Norwegian arthroplasty register: a survey of 17 444 hip replacements 1987–90. Acta Orthop Scand 64:245–51.

13. Havelin, L.I., Espehaug, B., Vollset, S.E., and Engesæter, L.B. (1994). Early failures among 14 009 cemented and 1326 uncemented prostheses for primary coxarthrosis: the Norwegian Arthroplasty Register, 1987–92. Acta Orthop Scand 65:1–6.

14. Havelin, L.I., Vollset, S.E., and Engesæter, L.B. (1995). Revision for aseptic loosening of uncemented cups in 4352 primary total hip prostheses: a report from the Arthroplasty Register. Acta Orthop Scand 66:494–500.

15. Sharrock, N.E., Cazan, M.G., Hargett M.J.L., Williams-Russo, P., and Wilson Jr., P.D. (1995). Changes in mortality after hip and knee arthroplasty over a ten-year period. Anesth Analg 80:242–8.

16. *Ryd, L., Albrektsson, B.E.J., Carlsson, L., Dansgård, F., Herberts, P., Lindstrand, A., et al. (1995). Roentgen stereophotogrammetric analysis as a predictor of mechanical loosening of knee prostheses. J Bone Joint Surg Br 77:377–83.

    RSA is an important research tool to demonstrate early prosthetic migration. Its real value lies in its ability to predict failure, as shown in this study.

17. Toksvig-Larsen, S., Ryd, L., and Lindstrand, A. (1990). An internally cooled saw-blade for bone cuts: lower temperatures in 30 knee arthroplasties. Acta Orthop Scand 61:321–3.

18. Oparaugo, P.C., Clarke, I.C., Malchau, H., and Herberts, P. (2001). Correlation of wear debris-induced osteolysis and revision with volumetric wear-rates of polyethylene: a survey of 8 reports in the literature. Acta Orthop Scand 72:22–8.

19. Grelsamer, R.P. (1995). Current concepts review. Unicompartmental osteoarthrosis of the knee. J Bone Joint Surg Am 77(A):278–92.

20. *Rand, J.A. (1994). Current concepts review. The patellofemoral joint in total knee arthroplasty. J Bone Joint Surg Am 76(A):612–20.

    Many of the design changes in modern knee prostheses are based on fashion more than on science.

21. Goodman, S. and Lidgren, L. (1992). Polyethylene wear in knee arthroplasty. Acta Orthop Scand 63:358–64.

22. Johnson, K.A. (1991). Ankle replacement arthroplasty. In B.M. Morrey (ed.), Joint replacement arthroplasty. Rochester: Churchill Livingstone, pp. 1173–82.

23. Campbell II, D.C. (1991). Arthroplasty of the metatarsophalangeal joint. In B.M. Morrey (ed.), Joint replacement arthroplasty. Rochester: Churchill Livingstone, pp. 1183–92.

24. Cooney, W.P. (1991). Arthroplasty of the thumb axis. In B.M. Morrey (ed.), Joint replacement arthroplasty. Rochester: Churchill Livingstone, pp. 173–94.

25. Wood, M.B. (1991). Alternative reconstructive procedures. In B.M. Morrey (ed.), Joint replacement arthroplasty. Rochester: Churchill Livingstone, pp. 271–35.

26. Wasielewski, R.C., Crossett, L.S., and Rubash, H.E. (1992). Neural and vascular injury in total hip arthroplasty. Orthop Clin North Am 23:219–35.

27. Kavanagh, B.F. (1992). Femoral shaft fractures associated with total hip arthroplasty. Orthop Clin North Am 23:249–457.

28. Morrey, B.F. (1992). Instability after total hip arthroplasty. Orthop Clin North Am 23:237–48.

9.20 Weight loss and osteoarthritis

Kenneth R Muir and Jonathan Webber

The prevalence and incidence of knee OA is strongly associated with weight. For the hip joint and the hand the true relationships are less clear.

For the knee, subjects with a Body Mass Index (BMI) of ≥ 30 have a much higher rate of OA than those who are overweight (BMI >25 and <30).[1] Weight by the mid-late thirties predicts the risk of subsequent radiographic knee OA better than current weight, suggesting that obesity is a cause rather than an effect of knee OA.[2]

Since obesity is a potentially preventable risk factor, weight loss may be an important strategy in reducing the burden of both current and future knee OA.[3] The difficulty of achieving successful and meaningful weight loss has previously limited intervention studies based on weight reduction. Studies in which weight loss has been achieved, however, have indicated subsequent improvement in the symptoms of those with knee OA.[4–6] Indeed, it has been estimated that between a quarter and a half of all knee OA may be prevented by eliminating obesity.[7]

Weight, BMI, and osteoarthritis

Accurate measurement of body fat is rarely feasible in clinical practice. In order to assess the degree of obesity, that is a measure of weight for height, the BMI is widely used. BMI is calculated as the weight (in kg) divided by the height (in metres) squared (Wt/Ht^2). A healthy BMI for white Caucasian populations lies in the range $18.5–25\,kg\,m^{-2}$, where the risk of ill health and premature mortality is minimized. Above a BMI of $25\,kg\,m^{-2}$ there is a progressive increase in the risk of many diseases, including type 2 diabetes and hypertension. Overweight represents a BMI in the range $25–30\,kg\,m^{-2}$, obesity a BMI above $30\,kg\,m^{-2}$, and morbid obesity a BMI above $40\,kg\,m^{-2}$.

For the knee a high BMI, or being overweight relative to normal or light weight for a given age group has been shown to associate with structural OA.[8–13] Furthermore, being overweight also associates with knee pain and lower limb disability.[14] Prospective studies that have allowed investigation of the temporal relationship between obesity and knee pain have shown that excess relative weight precedes the development of the condition and therefore is likely to be contributory to the causation of OA.[2] Obesity is more strongly associated with bilateral than unilateral OA, and obese patients report more symptoms for a given level of radiographic structural change.[2]

For the hip, a relationship between being overweight and radiographic changes of OA has been observed in some but not all studies.[8,11,13,15,16] Furthermore, data showing a clear temporal relationship between excess weight that precedes the onset of the condition and hip OA and thus indicates a causal pathway are less clear-cut than for the knee.

Significantly, such data that are available for the hand are also equivocal.[15,17]

Mechanistic considerations

The way in which weight can influence OA is an important consideration when planning options for intervention.

Body fat distribution has a major influence on the relationship between obesity and most obesity-related comorbidities. For example, intra-abdominal (visceral) fat is more closely linked to type 2 diabetes and cardiovascular disease than is subcutaneous fat.[18] For a given BMI, type 2 diabetes and cardiovascular disease are greater in men than women. This is mainly explained by a greater preponderance of visceral fat in men. However, when it comes to OA of weight-bearing joints, the relationship between obesity and pain does not appear to be much influenced by indices of body fat distribution.[10,19] In most studies BMI is the best predictor of knee OA.[20] Thus, the epidemiological evidence points to the mechanical effects of obesity being critical.

However, the story may be somewhat more complex than the simple biomechanical one would suggest. Some studies have found an association between hand OA and obesity.[15] This, together with the observations that excess weight seems to be a stronger risk factor for women rather than men, has allowed speculation of metabolic or hormonal effects as a possible mechanistic explanation. Humoral factors produced by adipose tissue (of which there are many, including oestrogen and tumour necrosis factor) may also be important. Following menopause the main site of oestrogen production in a woman is the peripheral fat. The higher rates of OA in older women together with the observation of oestrogen receptors on chondrocytes has therefore suggested a role for this hormone in the condition. Increased adipose tissue-produced oestrogen is also proposed to account for the observed raised prevalence of breast and other cancers in obese women.[21]

One recent interventional study[22] lends credence to the hypothesis that adipose tissue-derived substances may have an important role to play in OA. Loss of body fat (as assessed by bioelectrical impedance analysis) in obese patients in a weight loss programme was more closely linked to symptomatic relief from knee OA than was change in body weight.[23] This implies that humoral factors produced by adipose tissue may be more important than mechanical effects of weight *per se*. It is unclear, however, from this study what the differential effects of weight loss and a physical activity programme were on knee OA symptoms.

An alternative explanation, however, is that reduced quadriceps strength relative to body weight is greater in women than in men.[23] Such an observation, together with the more substantial and consistently observed effects of excess weight on the knee joint, suggest that a biomechanical mechanism is perhaps more directly suggested. Sharma *et al.*[24] have investigated further the relationship of BMI to knee OA severity with varus and valgus malalignment and observed that the effects of weight were much greater in varus knees. Such observations would again be consistent with a mechanical/loading explanation as varus alignment transmits greater forces across the knee joint. These results, if confirmed, would also suggest that the therapeutic effects of weight loss would be most effective in those with varus knee alignment.

Does weight loss improve osteoarthritis symptoms?

Whilst the effects of weight loss on other obesity-related comorbidities has been the subject of much research,[25,26] there is a relative paucity of data

Table 9.40 Benefits seen from a 10% weight loss[30]

Comorbidity	Improvement seen with weight loss
Diabetes	50% fall in fasting glucose
Hypertension	10–20 mmHg fall
Cholesterol	10% fall
Asthma[31]	9% increase in FVC and FEV_1
Knee osteoarthritis	50% reduction in new knee OA[23]
	Significant knee pain reduction and improved functional status[24] (12–15% weight loss)

examining the consequences of weight loss on OA. In patients with morbid obesity (BMI > 40 kg m^{-2}) who underwent gastroplasty for weight loss, moderate surgical weight loss (<27 kg) was as effective as much greater weight loss (>45 kg) in improving lower back, knee, ankle, and foot pain.[27]

Other studies have suggested that weight loss may reduce the symptoms and disability of knee and hip OA. Older women who had lost about 5 kg during a 10-year period had a 50 per cent reduction in the development of new symptomatic knee OA.[28]

So far there are scant data available from randomized trials assessing weight loss as an intervention for OA. Data that are available are from relatively small trials using short-term outcomes. They do, however, support the proposition that if weight loss can be achieved then symptomatic relief will follow.

In a trial of acupuncture and electrotherapy in a Chinese population, Huang et al.[6] demonstrated significant relief in symptoms from knee OA in patients who achieved reasonable weight loss. Shafshak also demonstrated that significant weight loss could be achieved in obese patients with knee OA using a mixed intervention that included electroacupuncture.[29] Messier et al.[5] in a preliminary study of exercise and weight loss in obese older American adults with knee OA, showed that weight loss could be achieved in these patients and that pain scores were lower in the weight loss group. However, the results did not reach statistical significance, though this may have reflected limited power given the small sample size.

More recently Huang and colleagues studied overweight and obese Chinese patients (n = 126) with bilateral knee OA defined by the Altman classification.[6] Significant pain relief was obtained in those subjects who were able to lose weight by a combination of acupuncture, dietary counselling, and an aerobic exercise programme, but only in those subjects who lost more than 15 per cent of their initial weight. This threshold for the benefits of weight loss is greater than that seen for the effects of weight loss on many other parameters (Table 9.40). It is clear, for example, that weight loss of 5–10 per cent is associated with marked improvements in diabetes control and blood pressure.[30] One other important finding of the Huang study[6] was that those who had less severe knee OA benefited the most from weight loss. This supports the supposition that initiatives based around weight loss should be an early management strategy in OA patients.

Strategies for weight loss

All of the evidence reviewed above, although based on small studies, suggests that weight loss in overweight and obese patients is a useful treatment for knee OA and possibly also for OA affecting other weight-bearing joints. It should also be considered as a primary preventative strategy for knee OA. Weight loss is undoubtedly of benefit for most other obesity-related comorbidities.[26]

The missing piece of the jigsaw is how to help patients achieve and maintain enough weight loss to improve their symptoms. Much of the literature on weight loss in obese patients has been very pessimistic and there is a widespread perception that hardly anyone succeeds in maintaining significant weight loss. However, this perception may be wrong. Up to 20 per cent of patients may achieve and maintain a 10 per cent or more weight loss over

a 4-year period.[32] The US National Weight Control Registry provides information on many individuals who have been very successful at long-term weight loss maintenance. Whilst strategies used by patients to achieve initial weight loss vary, those who maintain weight loss are characterized by the following:

- eating a diet low in fat and high in carbohydrate,
- frequent self-monitoring, and
- undertaking regular physical activity.

Once patients have maintained a weight loss for 2–5 years the chances of longer-term success greatly increase.[32]

Opportunities

There is increasing recognition that obesity is a chronic condition that deserves to be taken seriously and not dismissed as a non-medical problem that the patient should sort out for oneself. Recent estimates of the costs of obesity to society[33] have served to emphasize that ignoring the problem is not the answer.

Evidence for effective strategies for weight loss is growing. No single approach is likely to be successful, and it is the combination of dietary counselling, physical activity, and behavioural approaches that are required as the core of any programme. Whether or not there are additional benefits on OA of increased physical activity,[5] there is clear evidence that adding in activity is important in long-term weight loss maintenance.[34]

Alongside these approaches there are likely to be more effective drugs available for longer-term use in the near future.[35] None of these drugs is likely to be a panacea for obesity, but they are likely to increase the number of patients able to achieve and maintain a medically useful weight loss. There is potential to link the prescribing of these drugs to continued attendance at either individual or group sessions for weight management education and support.

Until now knee pain and OA have not been included as end-points in pharmaceutical studies with the currently available drugs (orlistat and sibutramine). Their limited license (1–2 years therapy at present) necessitates further long-term trials with OA-related end-points in addition to effects on other comorbidities. At present cessation of drug treatment is followed by weight regain in most cases. Comparisons of the effectiveness of these agents needs to be made with the natural history of untreated obesity (progressive weight gain).[36] Within the last 20 years the prevalence of adult obesity has tripled in the UK from around 6–7 per cent to around 20 per cent.[37] This rapid increase in obesity is due to a combination of more sedentary lifestyles and changed eating patterns (in particular increased snacking and fat consumption).[38] Currently the average adult in the UK puts on about 10–15 kg in weight from the ages of 20–65. Clearly strategies to effectively manage obesity must take this background into account.

Orlistat (Xenical®) is a pancreatic lipase inhibitor that blocks the digestion and hence absorption of about 30 per cent of dietary fat. In clinical trials, orlistat, at 120 mg three times a day with meals has been associated with about 10 per cent weight loss at one year in comparison with about 6 per cent for placebo.[39] The UK license for this drug only allows its prescription if patients are able to lose 2.5 kg by dietary and lifestyle changes in the month prior to commencing therapy. Orlistat should only be continued beyond 3 months if the patient has lost greater than 5 per cent of their weight at this time. About 40 per cent of patients who achieved this 3-month weight loss in trials lost 10 per cent of their weight after 12 months therapy.[39] The predictable side effects of orlistat are confined to the gut and include fatty stools and diarrhoea. These side effects are minimized if the patient is able to follow a low-fat diet.

Sibutramine (Reductil®) is a centrally acting agent that appears to enhance satiety by its actions to inhibit serotonin (5-HT) and noradrenaline reuptake in the hypothalamus and other brain regions. In human trials most weight loss with sibutramine appears to be due to reduced food intake, although in rodent studies increased energy expenditure is also of importance. At a dose of 15 mg once daily, sibutramine therapy is associated with about 7–9 per cent weight loss after 6 months with a 4–5 kg weight loss greater than placebo at 12 months.[40] Most side effects of sibutramine are mild (dry mouth, insomnia, constipation), but its central sympathomimetic effects lead to increases in heart rate and blood pressure that can be significant in some patients. These side effects mean that sibutramine is contraindicated in those with coronary artery disease, heart failure, and uncontrolled hypertension, and that pulse and blood pressure should be measured at fortnightly intervals for the first three months of therapy.

For those with morbid obesity, obesity surgery (bariatric surgery), either gastric restriction or bypass procedures, is likely to dramatically improve symptoms and function related to OA of weight-bearing joints.[41] Bariatric surgery may also result in sufficient weight loss for patients to become eligible for joint replacement surgery, even if their symptoms remain significant after such weight loss.[42] Finally, the increased rate of perioperative complications seen in obese patients undergoing total knee arthroplasties[43] is likely to be reduced with effective preoperative weight loss.

Conclusion

Being overweight is a causal and potentially modifiable risk factor for knee OA in particular. The difficulties in achieving significant and lasting weight loss in overweight/obese patients remain, but new approaches offer good potential. Long-term large trials are currently underway. Weight loss also offers health benefits for a number of other common diseases that often co-associate with large joint OA.

Key points

1. High Body Mass Index is a strong causal risk factor for knee OA and possibly also a risk factor for OA of the hip and hand.

2. Reduction in weight has been shown to alleviate the symptoms of knee OA in short-term trials.

3. The difficulties of achieving and maintaining weight loss dictate that further data are required from larger long-term trials to fully evaluate the potential of this intervention.

References

(An asterisk denotes recommend reading.)

1. Felson, D.T. (1995). Weight and osteoarthritis. *J Rheumatol* **22**:7–9.

2. *Felson, D.T., Anderson, J.J., Naimark, A., *et al.* (1998). Obesity and knee osteoarthritis. *Ann Intern Med* **109**:18–24.
   Data concerning the temporal relationship of excess weight preceding the OA thus confirming the potential for therapeutic intervention.

3. *Nevitt, M.C. and Lane, N. (1999). Body weight and osteoarthritis. *Am J Med* **107**(6):632–3.
   Short but clear overview of the relationship of markers of weight and OA.

4. Williams, R.A. and Foulsham, B.M. (1981). Weight reduction in osteoarthritis using phentermine. *Practitioner* **2**:225–31.

5. *Messier, S.P., Loeser, R.F., Mitchell, M.N., Valle, G., Morgan, T.P., Rejeski, W.J., *et al.* (2000). Exercise and weight loss in obese older adults with knee osteoarthritis: a preliminary study. *J Am Geriatr Soc* **48**(9):1062–72.
   Early data which shows the short-term potential of weight loss as an adjunct therapy to exercise in older OA patients.

6. Huang, M-H., Chen, C-H., Chen, T-W., Weng, M-C., Wang, W-T., and Wang, Y-L. (2000). The effects of weight reduction on the rehabilitation of patients with knee osteoarthritis and obesity. *Arthritis Care Res* **13**(6):398–405.

7. Felson, D.T. and Zhang, Y. (1998). An update on the Epidemiology of knee and hip osteoarthritis with a view to prevention. *Arthritis Rheum* **41**:1343–55.

8. Gelber, A.C., Hochberg, M.C., Mead, L.A., Wang, N.Y., Wigley, F.M., and Klag, M.J. (1999). Body mass index in young men and the risk of subsequent knee and hip osteoarthritis. *Am J Med* **107**(6):542–8.

9. White-O'Connor, B., Sobal, J., and Munci, H.L. Jr. (1989). Dietary habits, weight history, and vitamin supplement use in elderly osteoarthritis patients. *J Am Dietetic Assoc* **89**(3):378–82.

10. Hochberg, M.C., Lethbridge-Cejku, M., Scott, W.W. Jr., Reichle, R., Plato, C.C., and Tobin, J.D. (1995). The association of body weight, body fatness and body fat distribution with osteoarthritis of the knee: data from the Baltimore Longitudinal Study of Aging. *J Rheumatol* **22**(3):488–93.

11. Felson, D.T. and Chaisson, C.E. (1997). Understanding the relationship between body weight and osteoarthritis. *Baillieres Clin Rheumatol* **11**(4): 671–81.

12. Cicuttini, F.M., Baker, J.R., and Spector, T.D. (1996). The association of obesity with osteoarthritis of the hand and knee in women: a twin study. *J Rheumatol* **23**(7):1221–6.

13. Felson, D.T. (1996). Weight and osteoarthritis. *Am J Clin Nutr* **63**(3 Suppl.): 430S–432S.

14. Jordan, J.M., Luta, G., Renner, J.B., Linder, G.F., Dragomir, A., Hochberg, M.C., and Fryer, J.G. (1996). Self-reported functional status in osteoarthritis of the knee in a rural southern community: the role of sociodemographic factors, obesity, and knee pain. *Arthritis Care Res* **9**(4): 273–8.

15. Oliveria, S.A., Felson, D.T., Cirillo, P.A., Reed, J.I., and Walker, A.M. (1999). Body weight, body mass index, and incident symptomatic osteoarthritis of the hand, hip, and knee. *Epidemiology* **10**(2):161–6.

16. Sturmer, T., Gunther, K.P., and Brenner, H. (2000). Obesity, overweight and patterns of osteoarthritis: the Ulm Osteoarthritis Study. *J Clin Epidemiol* **53**(3):307–13.

17. Vingard, E., Alfredsson, L., and Malchau, H. (1997). Lifestyle factors and hip arthrosis. A case reference study of body mass index, smoking and hormone therapy in 503 Swedish women. *Acta Orthop Scand* **68**(3):216–20.

18. Knight, T.M., Smith, Z., Whittles, A., Sahota, P., Lockton, J.A., Hogg, G., *et al.* (1992). Insulin resistance, diabetes, and risk markers for ischaemic heart disease in Asian men and non-Asian men in Bradford. *Br Heart J* **67**:343–50.

19. Hart, D.J. and Spector, T.D. (1993). The relationship of obesity, fat distribution and osteoarthritis in women in the general population: the Chingford Study. *J Rheumatol* **20**(2):331–5.

20. Coggon, D., Reading, I., Croft, P., McLaren, M., Barrett, D., and Cooper, C. (2001). Knee osteoarthritis and obesity. *Int J Obes Relat Metab Disord* **25**(5):622–7.

21. Hulka, B., Liu, E., and Lininger, R. (1994). Steroid hormones and risk of breast cancer. *Cancer* **74**:1111–4.

22. Toda, Y., Toda, T., Takemura, S., Wada, T., Morimoto, T., and Ogawa, R. (1998). Change in body fat, but not body weight or metabolic correlates of obesity, is related to symptomatic relief of obese patients with knee osteoarthritis after a weight control program. *J Rheumatol* **25**:2181–86.

23. Slemenda, C., Heilman, D.K., Brandt, K.D., Katz, B.P., Mazzuca, S.A., Braunstein, E.M., and Byrd, D. (1998). Reduced quadriceps strength relative to body weight: a risk factor for knee osteoarthritis in Women? *Arthritis Rheum* **41**(11):1951–59.

24. Sharma, L., Lou, C., Cahue, S., and Dunlop, D. (2000). The mechanism of the effect of obesity in knee osteoarthritis: the mediating role of malalignment. *Arthritis Rheum* **43**(3):568–75.

25. Wing, R.R., Koeske, R., Epstein, L.H., Nowalk, M.P., Gooding, W., and Becker, D. (1987). Long-term effects of modest weight loss in type II diabetic patients. *Arch Intern Med* **147**:1749–53.

26. Oster, G., Thompson, D., Edelsberg, J., Bird, A.P., and Colditz, G.A. (1999). Lifetime health and economic benefits of weight loss among obese persons. *Am J Public Health* **89**(10):1536–42.

27. McGoey, B.V., Deitel, M., Saplys, R.J., and Kliman, M.E. (1990). Effect of weight loss on musculoskeletal pain in the morbidly obese. *J Bone Joint Surg Br* **72**(2):322–3.

28. Felson, D.T., Zhang, Y., Anthony, J.M., Naimark, A., and Anderson, J.J. (1992). Weight loss reduces the risk for symptomatic knee osteoarthritis in women. The Framingham Study. *Ann Intern Med* **116**(7):535–9.

29. Shafshak, T.S. (1995). Electroacupuncture and exercise in body weight reduction and their application in rehabilitating patients with knee osteoarthritis. *Am J Chinese Med* **23**(1):15–25.

30. *Goldstein, D.J. (1992). Beneficial health effects of modest weight loss. *Int J Obesity* **16**:397–415.
    Key review highlighting the health benefits of modest weight loss and clearly showing that normalisation of body weight is not necessary for these benefits.

31. Stenius-Aarniala, B., Poussa, T., Kvarnstrom, J., Gronlund, E-L., Ylikahri, M., and Mustajoki, P. (2000). Immediate and long term effects of weight reduction in obese people with asthma: randomised controlled study. *Br Med J* **320**:827–32.

32. Wing, R.R. and Hill, J.O. (2001). Successful weight loss maintenance. *Ann Rev Nutr* **21**:323–41.

33. National Audit Office. (2001). *Tackling Obesity in England*. HC 220. London: The Stationary Office.

34. Fogelholm, M., Kukkonen-Harjula, K., Nenonen, A., and Pasanen, M. (2000). Effects of walking training on weight maintenance after a very-low-energy diet in premenopausal obese women: a randomized controlled trial. *Arch Intern Med* **160**(14):2177–84.

35. Mertens, I.L. and Van Gaal, L.F. (2000). Promising new approaches to the management of obesity. *Drugs* **60**(1):1–9.

36. Rossner, S. (1992). Factors determining the long-term outcome of obesity treatment. In: Bjornzorp, P., Brodoff, B.N. (eds), *Obesity*. Philadelphia: JB Lippincott, pp. 712–9.

37. Prescott-Clarke, P. and Primatesta, P. (1999). *Health Survey for England 1997*:HMSO.

38. Prentice, A.M. and Jebb, S.A. (1995). Obesity in Britain: Gluttony or Sloth? *Br Med J* **311**:437–9.

39. Sjostrom, L., Rissanen, A., Andersen, T., Boldrin, M., Golay, A., Koppeschaar, H.P.F., *et al.* (1998). Randomised placebo-controlled trial od orlistat for weight loss and prevention of weight regain in obese patients. *Lancet* **352**:167–73.

40. James, W.P.T., Astrup, A., Finer, N., Hilsted, J., Kopelman, P., Rossner, S., *et al.* (2000). Effect of sibutramine on weight maintenance after weight loss: a randomised trial. *Lancet* **356**:2119–25.

41. Albrecht, R.J. and Pories, W.J. (1999). Surgical intervention for the severely obese. *Baillieres Best Pract Res Clin Endocrinol Metab* **13**(1):149–72.

42. Parvizi, J., Trousdale, R.T., and Sarr, M.G. (2000). Total joint arthroplasty in patients surgically treated for morbid obesity. *J Arthroplasty* **15**(8):1003–8.

43. Winiarsky, R., Barth, P., and Lotke, P. (1998). Total knee arthroplasty in morbidly obese patients. *J Bone Joint Surg* **80A**(12):1770–4.

9.21 Patient adherence

Alison Carr

Estimates of adherence to treatment in OA range from 50–95 per cent, but these are probably overestimates as many derive from clinical trials. Identifying patients who are non-adherent is problematic because of the complexity of factors determining adherence. Traditionally, the assumption has been that adherence is directly related to the patient's understanding and recall of information about their disease and treatment, and most early interventions to promote adherence focused on increasing patients' understanding and knowledge. It is now clear that this view is over-simplistic and that patients come to the consultation with specific beliefs and expectations about illness and treatment that they use to interpret the information they receive and to evaluate the effectiveness of treatment. Non-adherence takes many forms (taking a reduced dose, taking an increased dose, missing doses, changing the frequency of doses, having medication 'breaks', stopping the intervention), which make it difficult to measure accurately, and both the patients and clinicians frequently underestimate it. More effective methods for assessing and promoting adherence are based around increasing clinicians' understanding of those factors influencing adherence and enabling patients and clinicians to share and negotiate treatment decisions.

What is adherence?

Adherence describes the extent to which patients follow a prescribed treatment regimen or life style advice that is the result of an agreed, informed decision made by the patient and clinician working in partnership. It was developed to replace the concept of compliance, which has been criticized for being paternalistic; implying that non-compliance is deviant behaviour and the consequent ineffectiveness of the intervention, the patient's fault.

Many types of non-adherence have been described, most of which represent partial or incomplete adherence. Non-adherence to medication, for example, may include: receiving a prescription but not having it made up at the pharmacy; taking an incorrect dose (higher or lower than recommended); taking medication at the wrong times; forgetting doses of medication or increasing the frequency of doses; and stopping the treatment too soon.[1] Most studies and clinical trials use arbitrary definitions of adherence based on missed doses without any understanding of the reasons for non-adherence, what level of adherence is required to achieve treatment efficacy or how adherence is related to treatment outcome. Some studies, for example, have found improved outcome in adherent compared with non-adherent patients regardless of whether they were taking active treatment or placebo, suggesting that the relationship between adherence and outcome is not straightforward. Moreover, clinicians' definitions of adherence may differ significantly from those of patients. Qualitative research suggests that patients with arthritis do not consider adherence, as defined by clinicians, to be an issue and do not describe themselves as non-adherent even when they are not adhering to their prescribed medication regimens.[2]

These issues: the lack of a clear, agreed definition of adherence; the disparity between clinicians' and patients' conceptualization of adherence; the limited understanding of those factors influencing adherence; and the many types of adherence, have significantly hampered attempts to measure and promote adherence in clinical practice.

How common is non-adherence?

Estimates across all diseases suggest that at least 38 per cent of patients do not follow short-term medication treatment plans and 30–70 per cent do not adhere to medication regimens for long-term treatment.[1,3,4] Non-adherence to lifestyle modifications such as diet or exercise is even higher with more than 75 per cent of patients unable or unwilling to follow advice.[5] In a chronic disease such as rheumatoid arthritis, adherence behaviour appears to be consistent over time in around 60 per cent of patients (36 per cent are consistently adherent and 24 per cent consistently non-adherent).[6]

In OA, estimates for non-adherence to non-steroidal anti-inflammatory drugs derived from research are in the range 5–40 per cent, suggesting generally high adherence to medication within the context of clinical trials. Clinical trials of non-pharmacological interventions in OA report similar levels of non-adherence; around 30 per cent for home exercise.[7] In primary care, patient self-reported estimates of non-adherence to OA medication are around 40 per cent.[8]

The consequences of non-adherence

Although a direct link between adherence and clinical outcome has not been established in many conditions, the potential individual and societal costs of non-adherence are considerable.[9] Non-adherence to some medication (such as in diabetes, hypertension or organ transplantation) could result in serious morbidity or mortality.[10] In other conditions, it may lead to unnecessary investigations or changes to more aggressive treatment. In OA, non-adherence to analgesia (and therefore ineffective pain control) may result in treatment with NSAIDs and the associated risk of serious side effects.

Little data are available on the consequences of full adherence for outcome and side-effect profile. Most research has examined the factors influencing adherence as a means of influencing and promoting it, on the assumption that adherence will benefit the patient. This assumption may be incorrect. For many treatments, it is not clear whether full adherence results in better outcome or a worse side-effect profile.

What factors influence adherence?

Although non-adherence is very common across all treatments and disease groups, repeated studies have failed to identify stable characteristics that identify non-adherent patients. This is partly because non-adherence is often undetected, even by very experienced clinicians,[11] but predominantly because it reflects the complex interaction of many different factors from the quality of the relationship between patient and clinician to patients' personal beliefs about illness and treatment.

Patient characteristics

Most studies have failed to find any association between adherence and age, gender, intelligence, or education,[3] although in one longitudinal study of RA patients, older, female patients and more disabled patients were more likely to be adherent to treatment.[6] Existing evidence in OA suggests that adherence is independent of age, gender, or disease severity.[12]

Adherence is influenced by certain psychological and personality factors. Patients who are depressed are three times as likely to be non-adherent to all medical regimens as non-depressed patients;[13] conscientious patients are more likely to be adherent than those who are not conscientious;[14] and adherence is most likely when patients' preferred style of coping with illness is most congruent with the contextual features or demands of the medical regimen.[15]

Patients' knowledge and understanding of treatment

A large body of research has attempted to explain non-adherence in terms of the patient's failure to understand or to remember instructions, or their inability to realize the importance of treatment.[16] Parallel studies have called for better patient education[17] or an improvement in clinicians' communication skills[18] as a means of improving adherence. However, the implicit assumption that patients who have a better understanding of their disease and treatment are more likely to adhere to treatment is oversimplistic. Non-adherence is as frequent in life saving treatments as in mild, symptom-modifying treatments,[19] and rates of non-adherence are just as high amongst health professionals as amongst patients.[20]

There is ample evidence that many doctors in secondary care give patients detailed information about diagnosis, treatment, and possible outcomes. There is also evidence that patients retain 17–60 per cent of this information immediately post consultation.[21] However, remembering the information does not necessarily mean that it will be acted upon.[22] More recent research suggests that patients remember information that has meaning or importance for them but that their interpretation of the information may differ from that of the doctor. Patients evaluate information about diagnosis and treatment in the context of their pre-existing beliefs about their illness, and either reinterpret this information so that it is compatible with their beliefs or reject it completely if it cannot be accommodated within their beliefs.[23]

Lack of awareness of patients' interpretation of information can result in inaccurate assumptions about patient knowledge and behaviour. These misunderstandings can be associated with non-adherence. One study of patients in primary care identified fourteen categories of misunderstanding between the doctor and patient, all of which were associated with actual or potential adverse outcomes such as non-adherence.[24] In some cases, these misunderstandings arose from actions taken by the patient to preserve the relationship with the doctor (e.g., medication is taken even though not understood, because of the fear that further treatment will be withheld).

The doctor–patient relationship

Whilst it is estimated that around 40 per cent of any clinician's patients will not follow their treatment recommendations,[25] there are particular aspects of the doctor–patient relationship that can influence adherence. The quality of the emotional relationship between doctor and patient, for example, has been associated with adherence. Adherence is improved when: doctors are emotionally supportive, providing encouragement and reassurance; and when the patient is treated as an equal partner. It is compromised when: there is unresolved tension in the consultation; where the doctor fails to answer the patient's questions; when the doctor expresses anger, anxiety, or other negative emotions; and when a passive doctor is consulted by an active patient.[26]

The treatment regimen

Studies have consistently supported the intuitive assumption that adherence is related to the complexity of the treatment regimen. Patients with OA are more likely to adhere to treatment prescribed as once or twice daily doses because that is their preferred pattern of medication use.[27] Adherence is higher to treatment regimens that can be easily accommodated within the patient's daily routine[1] and lifestyle interventions that build on pre-existing behaviour (e.g., exercise interventions in patients who exercised regularly before treatment).[28]

Patients' perceptions of risk

Fear of side effects is frequently cited as a reason for non-adherence; around 60 per cent of patients with RA report fear of side effects as an influence on their decisions to alter drug dosage or frequency.[1] In OA, 59 per cent of patients have significant concerns about the potential effects of their OA treatment that outweigh their perception of how necessary the medication is in managing their arthritis (Mitchell, Horne, Cooper, and Carr, 2001, unpublished data). Where perceived necessity of the treatment is outweighed by concerns about its risks, adherence is low.[29]

Patients' perceptions of risk do not always reflect medical perceptions. This is probably because medical understanding of risk is based on data from groups and couched in the language of statistical risk, whereas patients' understanding is based on observation, personal experience, and discussion in personal networks and the public arena. They weigh the risks and benefits of treatment in the context of what outcomes and risks are important to them. For example, in relation to analgesia, which is associated with fears about addiction and tolerance (the belief that their bodies will become used to the medication), patients with RA and OA are willing to suffer significant levels of pain to avoid these risks.[1,30]

There is also evidence that the evaluation of risk is influenced by the principle of discounting. That is, risks are more likely to be taken if they correspond to immediate symptomatic benefit than if they prevent some future adverse event or produce some longer-term benefit. Whilst this appears to be the case in RA,[1] it is less clear that discounting is of any value in OA where most medication is prescribed for symptomatic benefit. Qualitative data from patients with OA suggests that, rather than seeking immediate pain relief, patients will delay the use of analgesics and NSAIDs because of their fear of tolerance and their belief that they may be even more in need of treatment in later disease.[30]

Beliefs and expectations about illness and treatment

There is increasing evidence that patients' understanding and beliefs about the causes and nature of their illness may differ significantly from the biomedical model used by clinicians. These sets of beliefs are constructed on the basis of: patients' previous experience of illness; their general understanding of biology; the cultural meaning of symptoms and disease; their everyday roles and responsibilities; information from other doctors, popular literature and the media; advice from family and friends; and the social acceptability of their symptoms. Reported beliefs about the causes of RA include: heredity, occupation, stress, the environment, physical trauma, auto-immunity and personal behaviour[31,32] and there is some evidence that patients' beliefs about the causes of OA are very similar (Mitchell, Horne, Cooper, and Carr, 2001, unpublished data).

In addition to beliefs about the causes and consequences of illness, patients hold specific beliefs and expectations about treatment that are closely related to their illness beliefs. Beliefs about treatment in OA are comprised of general beliefs about the necessity, usefulness, and potential harm of all medical treatments and specific beliefs about treatment for OA. These beliefs in turn influence patients' expectations of treatment and the ways in which they evaluate its efficacy.[1]

Recent studies suggest that illness and treatment beliefs can predict and influence patients' health behaviour, adherence, and outcome.[23,29,33] Treatment beliefs have been shown to influence adherence to medication in asthma, renal and cardiac disease, and cancer;[29] attendance at cardiac rehabilitation;[34] and adoption of lifestyle changes following myocardial infarction.[35]

Illness and treatment beliefs can influence adherence in a number of ways.

Through the interpretation of symptoms

Patients who do not interpret their symptoms as evidence of disease or ill health are unlikely to seek medical help and less likely to adhere to treatment regimens if they do seek medical help, than those for whom symptoms are manifestations of disease. Most patients with arthritis initially attribute their symptoms to stress rather than illness, or normalize them in the context of ageing or activities in a way that represents prevailing societal and cultural beliefs.[36] A study of elderly people in the same US city found cultural differences in the causal attributions for OA between white non-hispanic and black Americans, with white non-hispanic Americans more likely than black Americans to normalize OA as part of ageing. More than one-third of black Americans, compared with 8 per cent of white non-hispanic Americans, attributed OA to working in cold, wet conditions.[37] Cultural differences in the perception and attribution of OA symptoms have also been reported in UK patients (Mitchell, Horne, Cooper, and Carr, 2001, unpublished data). In this population, Caucasian patients perceived more symptoms that they attributed to OA than non-Caucasian patients. They also reported more treatment-related symptoms than non-Caucasian patients.

Similarly, patients who attribute their symptoms to a disease other than that with which they have been diagnosed (e.g., attributing joint pain to cancer rather than OA), are unlikely to take medication for a disease that they do not believe they have.

Through fears about the potential harm of treatment

Fears about the risk of addiction and tolerance to any medication are common across all diseases and have been associated with non-adherence.[1] Patients with OA express fears of addiction, tolerance, and side effects with conventional analgesic drugs such as paracetamol that had led some to delay the use of analgesics for the later stages of the disease when they feared they might need them more.[30] There is a suggestion that patients balance these fears against their perceived necessity for the treatment in managing the condition[29] and make decisions about adherence accordingly. Some of the non-adherence to analgesia in OA may be explained by the fact that in general, patients with OA do not perceive analgesics as very necessary in managing their OA, but have high levels of concern about analgesic addiction, tolerance, and side effects (Mitchell, Horne, Cooper, and Carr, 2001, unpublished data).

Other treatment beliefs that have been associated with non-adherence include the belief that medication should only be taken when the person feels ill and that the body needs a rest from medicines from time to time.[1]

Through unrealistic expectations of treatment

Patients and clinicians may have unrealistically high or unnecessarily low expectations of treatment. Expectations of complete and immediate symptomatic relief and a return to full physical functioning have been reported in relation to glucosamine sulphate and joint replacement surgery in OA.[30,38] Conversely, the expectation that nothing can be done for OA has been reported by around 25 per cent of elderly people in the United States of America.[37]

The specific link between expectations and adherence in OA has not yet been established, although it is the subject of current research in a number of centres, but there is evidence from some qualitative research in RA that patients allow themselves a 'trial of treatment' during which they evaluate the effectiveness of treatment against their expectations.[1] This suggests that patients who have unrealistically high expectations are likely to abandon treatment that fails to match those expectations. Patients with very low expectations of treatment may be less likely to take the risk of experiencing side effects for a treatment that is unlikely to work.

As with illness beliefs, there are cultural differences in expectations of treatment. Non-Caucasian patients in the United Kingdom are more likely than Caucasian patients to expect that treatment will be effective

in controlling their OA (Mitchell, Horne, Cooper, and Carr, 2001, unpublished data).

Assessing adherence

Despite the fact that non-adherence is as common as adherence, it is frequently undetected.[11] Even in patients whom physicians know well, the sensitivity of clinical judgement for detecting non-adherence is only 10 per cent.[39] Clinical judgement as the sole method of measuring adherence is therefore very unreliable and likely to yield highly inaccurate assessments. A variety of other methods from biological markers to patient self-report are available, some of which are only suitable for research. Identifying a method for assessing adherence that is valid, accurate, ethical, and practical remains the greatest challenge in adherence research.

Direct measures of adherence

Biological and physiological measures

Biological methods involve measuring blood levels or urinary excretion of medication or, for specific exercise-related interventions, measuring muscle strength and proprioception against a standardized protocol. They are considered the most objective methods of assessing adherence but have a number of serious limitations. Genetic differences in the absorption, excretion, and metabolism of drugs; the intermittent timing of assessments (usually only at the consultation); ethical issues around privacy and autonomy; and the cost of tests mean that, at best, biological methods provide an estimation of adherence for a period around the time of the assessment (not necessarily for the whole treatment period) that is only practical for use in research situations.

Direct observation of adherence

Direct observation of physical therapy interventions or medication taking have similar practical, cost, and ethical limitations as biological methods and will overestimate likely adherence to the same interventions when used in clinical practice where direct observation is not possible.

Indirect measures of adherence

Electronic medication dispensers

A variety of electronic medication dispensers are available that record the opening of a medication bottle or removal of a tablet or capsule from a packet. Some are combined with alarms that remind patients when to take medication. Their main drawback is that they can only give indirect estimations of adherence because they give no information about whether or how the medication was actually taken or by whom.

Uptake of prescriptions and pill counts

Checking whether a prescription has been dispensed or a repeat prescription ordered can give an indication of adherence but, as with electronic dispensers, gives no information about whether the medication has been taken according to the prescribed regimen, or by the person for whom it was prescribed. Similarly, returned pill counts give no information about how or by whom the medication has been taken or how many tablets have been lost or thrown away.

Patient self-report

Self-reported adherence through questionnaires or by direct questioning in consultation is the most widely used method in clinical practice. Estimates of adherence vary significantly depending upon the method used and the way it is administered. For example, questionnaires completed in the consulting room will give higher estimates of adherence than structured interviews conducted in the patient's home by independent researchers. Similarly, judgemental or leading questions from the clinician will result in overestimates of adherence compared with non-judgemental, or information-intensive approaches. The information-intensive approach[11] involves asking the patient what medications they are taking, in what dose and how often and whether they have experienced any side effects. It has been recommended as a strategy for assessing and promoting adherence in routine clinical practice.[40] Non-judgemental approaches include prefacing questions about medication use with general statements such as 'People often have difficulty taking their medication for one reason or another'.[41]

However well-designed the method, there is evidence that patients overestimate the actual rate of adherence by up to 19 per cent[42] and this should be taken into account when using any self-report measure. Nevertheless, a meta-analysis of self-report measures of adherence suggests they are valid and reliable methods for use in clinical practice, with a sensitivity of 55 per cent and specificity of 87 per cent for detecting non-adherence.[41] Comparisons of self-report with other methods of estimating adherence suggest it may be more accurate than most other methods.[42]

Clinical clues

Sequences of clinical clues that can be used to identify patients who are not adhering to treatment have been devised for use in clinical practice.[41] They suggest that non-adherence should be considered in: patients who do not attend appointments; patients in whom there is a loss of responsiveness to a previously adequate dose of treatment; patients who do not respond to what is usually an adequate dose of treatment; or patients who do not exhibit usual or common side effects of treatment (such as increased urinary frequency with diuretic use).

Whilst these are useful indicators of possible non-adherence, they are not pathognomic of non-adherence. Although non-adherence in patients who do not attend their clinic appointments is around 95 per cent, non-adherence in patients who do attend is still around 40 per cent.[43] Similarly, response to therapy and the occurrence of common side effects are related to many factors other than adherence, with which there is only a weak correlation for most treatments.[42]

Combining clinical clues with other methods of measuring adherence can produce more accurate estimates. For example, combining self-reported non-adherence with lack of response to therapy had a sensitivity of 83 per cent and specificity of 66 per cent for non-adherence.[44]

How to promote adherence

Although there is evidence that some interventions can improve adherence, few lead to any improvement in outcome.[9] Those that do improve adherence are complex interventions involving a combination of several methods such as information, counselling, medication reminders or prompts, self-monitoring, and family therapy. These complex interventions are probably addressing intentional non-adherence (reducing the dose, having treatment breaks, or stopping the course of treatment early) as well as unintentional non-adherence (forgetting doses, or failing to understand the treatment regimen), thus accounting for their effectiveness.

Most interventions to promote adherence have focused on increasing patient understanding and knowledge of their disease and treatment through written information and educational interventions, and improving doctor–patient communication in the consultation through standardized consultation schedules or interviews.

Increasing patient knowledge and understanding

Well-written, well-designed information about what the treatment is, when and how to take it, and what to do if a dose is missed or if side-effects are experienced can significantly improve patient knowledge (although not necessarily adherence) and is most effective when the information is individualized or personalized.[45] One way of individualizing information in a way that improves knowledge, satisfaction, and adherence[46] is through the use of reminder charts. These enable treatment regimens to be tailored to patients' daily routines and clearly place daily medications in the context of four daily anchors that are stable and relevant to the patient (such as work or mealtimes).

Table 9.41 The knowledge gap in adherence

1. The link between adherence and clinical outcome has not been established for many treatments so it is not clear that full adherence will always be beneficial.

2. All current measures of adherence are either: subject to significant measurement error or reporting bias; expensive; unethical; or act as adherence interventions. Appropriate, accurate tools for research and clinical practice are urgently needed.

3. Traditional interventions for promoting adherence are largely unsuccessful. More innovative methods, based on the factors determining adherence should be developed and evaluated.

4. Because most interventions have been unsuccessful, it is not clear whether it is possible to 'cure' adherence or whether improving adherence requires constant or repeated interventions.

Verbal reinforcement of written information increases its effectiveness by indicating to the patient that the clinician feels the information is important and relevant; providing the opportunity to check patient understanding and interpretation; and increasing patients' uptake and recall.[45]

Written information has the advantage of being available as a constant resource for the patient and their partner, family and friends, all of whom have a role in adherence. Alternative media (such as audio or video tapes, interactive computer programs, mind maps, and the telephone) should be available for patients with impaired sight and those who have reading difficulties, and translations are necessary for non-English speaking patients. Interactive computer programs have demonstrated improved adherence, increased knowledge, and more realistic treatment expectations in patients with OA.[47] (Table 9.41 summarizes the knowledge gap in adherence.)

Improving doctor–patient communication in the consultation

Patients' illness and treatment beliefs play an important role in determining adherence to treatment but are rarely elicited within the clinical consultation. This is largely because most clinicians assume that patients will adhere if they understand and remember medical information about their disease and treatment, and are unaware that patients may reinterpret and reject this information if it cannot be accommodated within their beliefs. Proposed strategies for improving communication within the consultation are based on an understanding of the role of patients' beliefs and include: eliciting patients' beliefs about illness and treatment; identifying their expectations of treatment and negotiating realistic treatment goals.[48,49] Standardized protocols to promote adherence in the clinical consultation have been devised[17,50] and are given in Table 9.42. Whilst their effectiveness in promoting adherence in OA has not been evaluated, they are based on robust evidence about what influences adherence and how doctor–patient communication can be improved.

Conclusion

Non-adherence to treatment is as common as adherence but is frequently undetected or under-estimated by clinicians. The factors influencing adherence are complex and go beyond a simple understanding or recall of information to include personality, mood, and beliefs about illness and treatment. Many methods for assessing adherence are either subject to significant measurement error or are unsuitable for clinical practice. Similarly, interventions to promote adherence are largely unsuccessful, probably because they fail to address patients' beliefs and expectations. However, improving communication in the clinical consultation to enable patients' beliefs and expectations and the ways in which they take medication to be elicited, may not only result in more accurate assessments of adherence but

Table 9.42 Structured protocols for assessing and promoting adherence in clinical practice

Steps	Method	
	Daltroy[50]	Roter and Hall[40]
1	Elicit patient's concerns	Assess patient's knowledge, beliefs and expectations about treatments
2	Discuss concerns	Discuss misunderstanding and misinformation
3	Doctor and patient share their illness beliefs	Clearly describe treatment plans and goals
4	Doctor and patient share their treatment goals	Discuss patient's concerns about treatment plan including ability to adhere
5	Treatment goals agreed	Negotiate and agree treatment plan with patient
6	Doctor and patient share treatment beliefs	Check understanding of treatment goals and plan by asking patient to repeat in their own words
7	Potential barriers to adherence are identified	At follow-up check adherence
8	Plans made to overcome these	
9	Doctor provides written information annotated with individual patient details/concerns	

will also improve understanding about the barriers to adherence and thereby provide the basis for effective interventions to promote adherence. These methods require extensive evaluation in patients with OA. However, promoting adherence will only be of benefit if it improves clinical outcome and it is by no means clear that this would be the case. Increased adherence might just as easily be associated with a worse side-effect profile. Establishing the relationship between adherence and outcome should be the next step in adherence research in OA.

Key points for clinical practice

1. Non-adherence is very common and is frequently under-estimated by clinicians and patients.

2. Non-adherence is rarely due solely to lack of understanding or poor recall of information.

3. The reasons for non-adherence are complex and include patients' beliefs and expectations about their illness and treatment that might be very different from clinicians' beliefs.

4. Adherence should be routinely assessed in all patients by asking them what medications they are taking, how they are taking them, and whether they have had any problems.

5. Non-adherence should be considered when: the patient is failing to respond to a treatment that previously worked; the patient does not respond to a treatment that generally has a good response in this condition; there are clear indications that the patient might have difficulty adhering (e.g. the treatment regimen is too difficult to follow, the patient is depressed or anxious about treatment, the patient's partner or relatives do not agree with treatment).

6. Explore possible barriers to adherence by eliciting patients' beliefs about their illness and treatment.

7. Giving information alone, without eliciting patients' beliefs will not significantly improve adherence.

Selected further reading

Myers, L.B. and Midence, K. eds (1998). *Adherence to Treatment in Medical Conditions*. Amsterdam: Harwood Academic Publishers.

References

(An asterisk denotes recommended reading.)

1. *Donovan, J.C.L. and Blake, D.R. (1992). Patient non-compliance: deviance or reasoned decision-making. *Soc Sci Med* **34**:507–13.
   This paper significantly advances understanding of adherence from the patient's perspective, highlighting that what clinicians perceive as non-adherence is seen by patients as completely logical, understandable behaviour. It is a landmark paper in the compliance/adherence literature.

2. Donovan, J.L. (1995). Patient decision making: the missing ingredient in compliance research. *Int J Tech Ass Health Care* **11**:443–55.

3. DiMatteo, M.R. (1994). Enhancing patient adherence to medical recommendations. *JAMA* **271**:79.

4. Conrad, P. (1985). The meaning of medications: another look at compliance. *Soc Sci Med* **20**:29–37.

5. Brownwell, K.D., Marlatt, G.A., Lichtenstein, E., and Wilson, G.T. (1986). Understanding and preventing relapse. *Am Psychol* **41**:765–82.

6. Viller, F., Guillemin, F., Briancon, S., Moum, T., Suurmeijer, T., and van den Heuvel, W. (1999). Compliance to drug treatment of patients with rheumatoid arthritis: a 3 year longitudinal study. *J Rheumatol* **26**:2114–22.

7. O'Reilly, Muir, K.R., and Doherty, M. (1999). Effectiveness of home exercise on pain and disability from osteoarthritis of the knee: a randomised controlled trial. *Ann Rheum Dis* **58**:15–19.

8. Weinberger, M., Tierney, W.M., and Booher, P. (1989). Common problems experienced by adults with osteoarthritis. *Arthritis Care Res* **2**:94–100.

9. *Haynes, R.B., Montague, P., Oliver, T., McKibbon, K.A., Brouwers, M.C., and Kanani, R. (2001). Interventions for helping patients to follow prescriptions for medications. *The Cochrane Database of Systematic Reviews*, Issue 2, The Cochrane Collaboration.
   This is the most recent systematic review of interventions to promote adherence. It discusses the limitations of existing studies and interventions and highlights the lack of evidence for a link between adherence and outcome.

10. Irvine, *et al.* (1999). *Psychosomatic Med* **61**:566–75.

11. *Steele, D.J., Jackson, T.C., and Gutmann, M.C. (1990). Have you been taking your pills? The adherence monitoring sequence in the medical interview. *J Fam Pract* **30**:294–9.
   This paper describes a method for assessing and promoting adherence in routine clinical practice.

12. Rejeski, W.J., Brawley, L.R., Ettinger, W., Morgan, T., and Thompson, C. (1997). Compliance to exercise therapy in older participants with knee osteoarthritis: implications for treating disability. *Med Sci Sports Exercise* **29**:977–85.

13. DiMatteo, M.R., Lepper, H.S., and Croghan, T.W. (2000). Depression is a risk factor for noncompliance with medical treatment: meta-analysis of the effects of anxiety and depression on patient adherence. *Arch Int Med* **160**:2101–7.

14. Christensen, A.J. and Smith, T.W. (1995). Personality and patient adherence: correlates of the five-factor model in renal dialysis. *J Behav Med* **18**:305–13.

15. Christensen, A.J. (2000). Patient-by-treatment context interaction in chronic disease: conceptual framework for the study of patient adherence. *Psychosom Med* **62**:435–43.

16. DiMatteo, M.R. (1994). Enhancing patient adherence to medical recommendations. *JAMA* **271**:79–83.

17. Roter, D.L. and Hall, J.A. (1994). Strategies for enhancing patient adherence to medical recommendations. *JAMA* **271**:80–1.

18. Bartlett, E.E., Grayson, M., Barker, R., Levine, D.M., Golden, A., and Libber, S. (1984). The effects of physician communication skills on patient satisfaction, recall and adherence. *J Chron Dis* **37**:755–64.

19. **Krall, R.L.** (1991). Interaction of compliance and patient safety. In: J.A. Cramer and B. Spilker (eds), *Patient Compliance in Medical Practice and Clinical Trials*. New York: Raven Press.

20. **Morse, E.V., Simon, P.M., and Balson, P.M.** (1993). Using experiential training to enhance health professionals' awareness of patient compliance issues. *Acad Med* **68**:693–7.

21. **Anderson, J.L., Dodman, S., Kopelman, M., and Fleming, A.** (1979). Patient information recall in a rheumatology clinic. *Rheum Rehab* **18**:18–22.

22. **Tuckett, D.A., Boulton, M., and Olson, C.** (1985). A new approach to the measurement of patients' understanding of what they are told in medical consultations. *J Health Soc Behav* **26**:27–38.

23. **Donovan, J.L., Blake, D.R., and Fleming, W.G.** (1989). The patient is not a blank sheet: lay beliefs and their relevance to patient education. *Br J Rheumatol* **28**:58–61.

24. **Britten, N., Stevenson, F.A., Barry, C.A., Barber, N., and Bradley, C.P.** (2000). Misunderstandings in prescribing decisions in general practice: qualitative study. *Br Med J* **320**:484–8.

25. **Epstein, L.H. and Cluss, P.A.** (1982). A behavioural medicine perspective on adherence to long-term medical regimens. *J Consult Clin Psychol* **50**:950–71.

26. **Hall, J.A., Roter, D.L., and Katz, N.R.** (1988). Correlates of provider behaviour: a meta-analysis. *Med Care* **26**:657–75.

27. **Punchak, S., Goodyer, L.I., and Miskelly, F.** (2000). Use of an electronic monitoring aid to investigate the medication pattern of analgesics and non-steroidal anti-inflammatory drugs prescribed for Osteoarthritis. *Rheumatology* **39**:448–9.

28. **Daltroy, L.H., Robb-Nicholson, C., Iversen, M.D., Wright, E.A., and Liang, M.H.** (1995). Effectiveness of minimally supervised home aerobic training in patients with systemic rheumatic disease. *Br J Rheumatol* **34**:1064–9.

29. *****Horne, R. and Weinman, J.** (1999). Patients' beliefs about prescribed medicines and their role in adherence to treatment in chronic physical illness. *J Psychosom Res* **47**:555–67.

   This paper provides evidence for the relationship between patients' beliefs about illness and treatment and their adherence to treatment. John Weinman and Rob Horne are at the forefront of research in this area.

30. **Carr, A.J., Hughes, R.A., and Stowers, K.** (2000). What influences placebo response to a complementary therapy, glucosamine sulphate? *Arthritis Rheum* **43**:S223.

31. **Williams, G.H.** (1986). Lay beliefs about the causes of rheumatoid arthritis: their implications for rehabilitation. *Int Rehab Med* **8**:65–8.

32. **Affleck, G., Pfeiffer, C., Tennen, H., and Fifield, J.** (1987). Attributional processes in rheumatoid arthritis patients. *Arthritis Rheum* **30**(8):927–31.

33. **Scharloo, M. and Kaptein, A.A.** (1997). Measurements of illness perceptions in patients with chronic somatic illness: a review. In: K.J. Petrie and J.A. Weinman (eds), *Perceptions of Health and Illness*. Amsterdam: Harewood Academic Publishers.

34. **Cooper, A., Weinman, J., and Jackson, G.** (1999). Illness perceptions as predictors of rehabilitation attendance in patients with coronary heart disease. *Heart* **82**:234–6.

35. **Weinman, J., Petrie, K.J., and Sharpe, N.** (2000). Causal attributions in patients and spouses following a heart attack and subsequent lifestyle changes. *Br J Health Psychol* **5**:263–73.

36. **Sakalys, J.A.** (1997). Illness behaviour in rheumatoid arthritis. *Arthritis Care Res* **10**:229–37.

37. **Goodwin, J.S., Black, S.A., and Satish, S.** (1999). Aging versus disease: the opinions of older black, Hispanic and non-hispanic white Americans about the causes and treatment of common medical conditions. *J Am Ger Soc* **47**:973–9.

38. **Woolhead, G.M., Carr, A.J., Wilkinson, M., Bannister, G.C., and Ackroyd, C.E.** (1996). Expectations of treatment and its outcome in patients awaiting joint replacement surgery and general orthopaedic outpatient referrals. *Arthritis Rheum* **39**:S174.

39. **Gilbert, J.R., Evans, C.E., Haynes, R.B., and Tugwell, P.** (1980). Predicting compliance with a regimen of digoxin therapy in family practice. *Can Med Assoc J* **123**:119–22.

40. **Roter, D.L. and Hall, J.A.** (1994). Strategies for enhancing patient adherence to medical recommendations. *JAMA* **27**(1):80.

41. **Stephenson, B.J., Rowe, B.H., Haynes, R.B., Macharia, W.M., and Leon, G.** (1993). Is this patient taking the treatment as prescribed? *JAMA* **269**(21):2779–81.

42. **Haynes, R.B., Taylor, D.W., Sackett, D.L., Gibson, E.S., Bernholz, C., and Mukherjee, J.** (1980). Can simple clinical measurements detect patient non-compliance? *Hypertension* **2**:757–64.

43. **Richardson, J.L., Skilton, D.R., Krailo, M., and Levine, A.M.** (1990). The effect of compliance with treatment on survival among patients with haematologic malignancies. *J Clin Oncol* **8**:356–64.

44. **Inui, T.S., Carter, W.B., and Pecoraro, R.E.** (1981). Screening for noncompliance among patients with hypertension: is self-report the best available measure? *Med Care* **19**:1061–64.

45. **Raynor, D.K.** (1998). The influence of written information on patient knowledge and adherence to treatment. In L. Myers and K. Midence (eds), *Adherence to Treatment in Medical Conditions*. London: Harwood, pp. 83–111.

46. **Sandler, D.A., Mitchell, J.R.A., Fellows, A., and Garner, S.T.** (1989). Is an information booklet for patients at a teaching hospital useful and helpful? *Br Med J* **298**:1511–13.

47. **Edworthy, S.M. and Devins, G.M.** (1999). Improving medication adherence through patient education distinguishing between appropriate and inappropriate utilization. *J Rheumatol* **26**(8):1647–9.

48. **Horne, R.** (1999). Patients' beliefs about treatment: the hidden determinant of treatment outcome? *J Psychosom Res* **47**:491–5.

49. *****Carr, A.J. and Donovan, J.L.** (1998). Why doctors and patients disagree. *Br J Rheumatol* **37**:1–6.

   This review article pulls together all the existing evidence from medical, social, and anthropological research that provides some explanation for the misunderstandings that can arise between clinicians and patients and suggests clinical methods to improve communication.

50. **Daltroy, L.H.** (1993). Doctor patient communication in rheumatological disorders. *Balliere's Clin Rheumatol* **7**:221–39.

10 Outcome assessment in osteoarthritis: a guide for research and clinical practice

Heike A. Bischoff, Ewa M. Roos, and Matthew H. Liang

The basic goals in managing OA are to reduce symptoms (pain, stiffness, instability), and to maintain and improve function. This chapter will focus on patient-derived measures, which add an important dimension to the assessment of OA. Objective findings of structural or physiological joint abnormality are frequently discordant with the patient's experience of symptoms. Mapping patient-based assessments to objective measures is a major challenge of research. Correlating these findings is also necessary to understand the clinical relevance of objective findings.

Introduction

To evaluate whether a treatment is working, one needs to assess whether the patient is getting better or worse in a disease where early symptoms are subtle and unfold over years. In advanced disease, where significant structural damage has occurred, the assessment of pain in weight-bearing joints is confounded by the fact that patients adapt to pain by giving up activities to spare themselves of symptoms. These self-imposed limitations may further aggravate the problem by accelerating physical deconditioning. Functional ability, especially among older individuals, may not solely be joint related, but influenced by comorbid conditions, manifestations of frailty (i.e., falls, decreased balance, impaired vision, and hearing), and psychosocial factors such as depression. Comprehensive assessment should include these non-joint related determinants of function.[1,2] At the other end of the age spectrum, younger patients with early OA may have less severe symptoms but a higher functional demand. Special assessment is required to capture this.

Definitions

Impairment, disability, and handicap refer to the major impacts of illness on individuals.[3] *Impairment* is the 'objective' loss or abnormality of psychological, physiological, or anatomical structure or function, and signifies a pathological state. In OA, measures of impairment include the radiographic assessment of cartilage thickness and examination findings of joint deformity and reduced range of motion.

Impairment can result in *disability* or restricted ability, or inability to perform normal activities. Disability can affect behavior, communication, personal care, locomotion, dexterity, and activities of daily living. Disability or function cannot be captured by a single standard measure because at any given time it is the result of three factors: capacity, will, and need. Capacity is the physical and mental potential to do something; will includes personality factors such as drive and motivation; and need is the requirement to perform certain functions dictated by the environment. In clinical practice, function is improved or maintained by manipulating or enhancing capacity, will, or need. *Handicap* is the disadvantage for an individual that limits fulfillment of normal functions. Handicaps include work, ability, social integration, and economic self-sufficiency. Questionnaires developed to evaluate health status or quality of life measure a multi-attribute state that includes physical, emotional, and social functioning.

In 2000, a new classification, the ICIDH-2, was suggested by the WHO (www.who.int/icidh). This classification introduces a new 'health' instead of an 'illness' perspective and recognizes interactions between the components. Most outcome measures discussed in this chapter were developed prior to the ICIDH-2. Carr, who suggests that the psychosocial impact of OA may have been underestimated,[4] has highlighted the value of going beyond disability to measure handicap in OA.

Symptoms of OA and reported functional difficulties should be considered within the experience of the patient. There is a view that the report of the patient is subjective and less important or, less objective, than hard clinical findings. However, in the last three decades clinical research has produced a number of sophisticated questionnaires with excellent psychometric properties to measure pain, well-being, and functional limitations (physical, emotional, or social), and their metric properties match and in some cases perform better than traditional objective measures of disease impairment.

Validity, reliability, and *sensitivity* to change are the basic psychometric attributes that describe the performance of quantitative measures (Table 10.1). Studies show that patient-derived data are valid, reliable, and as sensitive or more sensitive to change than traditional radiographic measures or physical findings in musculoskeletal diseases.[5–7] We review these assessment methods and indicate how they can be practically incorporated in patient care.

Table 10.1 Validity, reliability, and sensitivity to change

Psychometric attributes	Meaning
Validity	Capacity to measure what the instrument purports to measure.
Four types of validity	Face validity: experienced individuals judge an instrument to measure the domain of interest (for instance, joint pain).
Content validity	Extent to which a measure is able to comprehensively evaluate the domain of interest (e.g., all joint symptoms).
Construct validity	Measures obtained with an instrument are consistent with hypothetical constructs (or concepts) related to the domain of interest (e.g., physical disability resulting from rheumatic diseases).
Criterion validity	Assessment by comparing the instrument to a 'gold standard' (such as, a pathognomonic finding or a biopsy).
Reliability (reproducibility)	Intra-rater reliability refers to whether the same rater at two different time points (i.e., one week apart) comes up with the same result when the phenomenon measured has not changed.
	Inter-rater reliability refers to whether two different raters come up with the same result. The instrument is considered reliable if the measurements show little random error.
Sensitivity	Capacity to detect any changes.
Responsiveness	The ability to detect a clinically meaningful change.

Patient self-assessment

Patient self-assessment techniques are simple and readily accepted by patients. The information is provided by the patient and generally collected by questionnaire, either self-administered or administered by an interviewer. Ratable domains include joint symptoms, and emotional, physical, and social functioning.

Neither function nor a change in a function is an absolute state. It is relative to an individual's experience, goals, expectations, and physical ability. Investigators have sought ways to recognize this and to improve responsiveness by a number of approaches that might be termed individualized or patient-specific subject assessment.

Instruments that take patients preferences into account can be generic like the Patient-Specific Functional Scale,[8,9] or disease-specific like the Patient-Specific Index.[10,11] The major advantage of these instruments is the high responsiveness for the individual. The Patient-Specific Functional Scale is easy to use, does not require a computer, and can be used in settings such as a physical therapy practice, where a variety of conditions are treated. Another approach is to ask the respondent to identify the areas of most importance to them, to rate their importance, and then using multivariate statistical techniques to estimate the weight that the individual attributes to each factor.[12]

A technique first used to evaluate behavioral interventions—goal-attainment scaling—has attractive features for measuring change from an individual's perspective and mirrors what happens normally in the negotiation between a patient and a health care provider.[13] With this method subjects are asked to name, or select from a list, their priority areas or problem areas and then after an intervention, to state whether these areas have improved and to what extent.

Another way of obtaining individual outcome data is to ask the subject and/or a proxy whether or not a change has occurred ('transition question'),[14] how large is the change,[15] how important or relevant is the change,[16] and how satisfied they are with the resultant change.[17] The judgment of any or all of these could be done by the patient or by an independent rater and the data suggests that these will not necessarily be the same. If patients are asked about a meaningful change, the framing of the question(s) and the timing of when the questions should be asked in relationship to the intervention need careful consideration because the extent of recall bias is unknown. An independent judge could be a health care professional uninvolved with the subject's care or a caretaker such as a family or significant other when the subject is unreliable. A related construct such as satisfaction with the change, a change that allows resumption of normal work, or a change that requires assistance are also possibilities. These questions could be used in both group and individual applications.

Using item response theory and computerized testing a respondent could be presented with items from a large battery of questions that are more 'difficult' or 'easier' than one already answered, to quickly triangulate their position on a scale where items are equally spaced in terms of difficulty across the entire range scale ('equi-discriminating'). With equal differences between item difficulty across the range of the scale, when respondents move a particular number of points, one can be relatively sure that he has moved the same distance on some true scale of difficulty.

A problem for all methods is that the perception of change in a state, such as functional status, derives its significance and meaning in comparison to the starting state as much as any other referent. Studies suggest that perceived change of physical and sensory states may be a power function.[18] For instance, persons who start at a low level of function on a scale and change a relatively small distance along the dimension may perceive the change as clinically significant. However, persons starting with a much higher physical function may view the same size change as a trivial improvement, and would need a much larger change to judge it as clinically significant. Thus, even with equi-discriminating scales, the responsiveness of these scales still provokes the question of whether or not the same amount of change in an underlying dimension is clinically significant at all levels or a function of the level at which one starts.

Results of health assessment questionnaires are generally reported as aggregates or summations of the weighted or unweighted items. In contrast, a signal measurement strategy identifies one or more 'target' joints or symptoms from an inventory that the patient identifies as areas in which potential improvement would have personal importance. This customizes the evaluation process to the individual and improves the efficiency of the measure by concentrating on items with the highest potential for response. This strategy reduced response variation in patients with OA undergoing total hip or knee joint-replacement surgery[19] and in a clinical trial comparing two NSAIDs.[20]

The signal measurement strategy may be problematic, however, because different individuals may chose different signals and the stability of patient choices has not been demonstrated over time. Other problems include the possibility of overlooking relevant or clinically important changes in items not chosen as signals, the tendency of patients to choose the functional items that are most severely affected and possibly less responsive, and the added time needed to negotiate preferences.

We believe that transition questions should be part of the assessment battery to capture the patient's view. Their use raises a number of methodological questions, such as:

1. How should the global assessment of change be framed?

2. Should the valuation rate importance or satisfaction with a clinical state? We believe satisfaction is a different construct, equally important, and separately ratable even when no change has occurred.

3. How should the assessment be posed to minimize response biases and maximize reliability? Response bias and unreliable responses threaten the validity of using such measures in resource allocation decisions.

Evaluating importance will address the conceptually unsatisfactory task of generalizing weights or utilities from normal populations to the ill individual. If patient-oriented instruments are to find a role in patient care, the importance of any change needs to be assessed and the individual should assess it. Valid, responsive instruments in groups of subjects may not be so in individuals. Sensitivity is a statistical property of measures, whereas responsiveness is a measure of its importance and thus an individual judgment worthy of separate evaluation. For measures of function and quality of life, responsiveness should be based on the subject's valuation of the magnitude of change and its importance. For measures of impairment or disease activity the physician is the best judge.

Pain rating and pain scales

As pain perception is a subjective experience it is conceptually most appropriate to be assessed by patients themselves. The major tools used to evaluate pain include verbal transition scales (VTS), verbal rating scales (VRS) or Likert scales, numerical rating scales (NRS), and visual analog scales (VAS). The VTS has the respondent estimate whether the pain has been stable or has changed over a period of time (better or worse). With the VRS, the respondent is asked to quantify his or her pain, ranging, for example, from total absence (no pain) to extreme pain, with a number of intermediate levels (mild, moderate, severe). The NRS has the respondent assign a number from an ordinal scale, usually ranging from 0 to 10 (no pain to extreme pain), or from 0 to 100 (no pain to extreme pain), rather than endorsing an adjective. The VAS is typically a 10 cm line marked 'least' at one end 'most' at the other end on which the patient marks their level of pain, and the distance from this point to the origin of the line is recorded. All of these techniques show changes when an intervention is effective.

As a general principle, more reproducible information is obtained by framing the question in a specific and consistent manner, such as specifying the period of time and whether one is interested in the worst pain or average pain during that period.[21] Irrespective of the period covered by the questions, however, people seem to weigh the most pain experience disproportionally and/or remember their current discomfort.

Verbal transition, verbal rating, and numerical rating scales are the most practical, and most patients find them easy to use. A number summarizes the VRS and NRS, and the VAS[22] offers the theoretical advantages of a continuous pain score. However, some patients cannot complete a VAS or NRS. The addition of adjectives (mild, moderate, severe) along the line can improve comprehension, but individuals may circle or check these anchors instead of marking the line. This phenomenon, which is more frequent when a vertical scale is used, technically converts the VAS into a verbal rating scale equivalent and results in significant loss of sensitivity.[23]

Pain scales that require the respondent to endorse a facial expression that corresponds to their affective state are useful in evaluating pain in children,[24] or across different languages.[25] However, faces scales cannot be completed over the telephone and their validity in OA has not been studied.

Pain questionnaires

The McGill pain questionnaire,[26] based on an inventory of 78 adjectives, is an attempt to describe pain as a multidimensional process with sensory, emotional, social, and behavioral inputs. It also exists in a shorter version[27] but has received only limited application in OA research.

The Knee Pain Scale, a self-administered 12-item questionnaire, was developed in an OA population to evaluate the intensity and frequency of knee pain in transfer and ambulation.[28] This valid and reliable scale, if it proves to be responsive, may become a valuable tool for pain assessment in clinical trials.

Symptoms other than pain

Joint stiffness (early morning after awakening, or after a period of inactivity) is frequently reported in clinical trials. The duration of morning stiffness can be a reliable measure when assessed by experienced interviewers[29] and after standardization of the question.[30] In clinical trials, morning stiffness, measured either by VRS or VAS, is generally responsive to active therapy.[31] Other patient-reported symptoms of OA include swelling, decreased range of motion, grinding, and instability.[32]

Physical function

The demands on physical function vary with age and physical activity level. Most outcome measures in OA are validated in elderly populations and reflect the physical function needed for their daily life. However, it is estimated that more than 5 per cent of individuals aged 35–54 have radiographic signs of knee OA and many of these may have previously sustained a knee injury, not uncommonly in sports, and have a higher than average physical activity level. Therefore in subjects with post-traumatic knee OA, regardless of whether they are younger or older than 50 years, it may be more relevant to assess limitations in more demanding activities such as kneeling, squatting, running, jumping, and pivoting than physical activities required for daily living.[32] To evaluate physical function or change in physical function it is necessary to evaluate the subject with an age-appropriate instrument that reflects the functional demands or expectations of that age group.

Health status or quality of life instruments

A variety of self-administered or interviewer-assisted instruments have been applied to the study of OA. Measures developed for general populations are referred to as *generic*, while others, distinguished as *disease-* or *joint-specific*, refer to OA specific instruments or involve specific joints involved with OA.

Generic instruments

Generic health status questionnaires that have been applied to OA populations include the Sickness Impact Profile[33] (SIP), the Nottingham Health Profile[34,35] (NHP), and the Medical Outcome Study (MOS) Short Form-36 (SF-36)[36] (Table 10.2). All have excellent psychometric properties in general populations and have been tested for reliability and validity, at least to some extent, in orthopedic surgery patients or populations with OA.[35,37–39]

The SIP[33] has 138 yes–no questions that take approximately 30 minutes to complete unaided or with an interviewer. Individual items are weighted and aggregated to provide scores for seven dimensions: physical (ambulation, mobility, body care, movement), psychological (communication, social interaction, emotional behavior, alertness behavior), sleep and rest, eating, work, home management, and recreational activities. The SIP has proven to be responsive in the evaluation of joint arthroplasty.[5,40,41] However, in a study of patients undergoing total hip replacement for OA or rheumatoid arthritis the SF-36 was more sensitive to change than the SIP.[42]

The NHP[43] is a 38-item self-administered questionnaire that can be completed in approximately 10 minutes. It was designed for population surveys to measure mobility, pain, emotion, energy level, sleep, and social isolation. The instrument has been validated in OA[35] and used in a study of total hip arthroplasty.[44] The NHP may not be sensitive enough, however, to assess small improvements in individuals with either mild or very severe OA.

Table 10.2 Overview of joint-, disease-specific and generic instruments used for OA patients

Instruments	No. of questions	No. of domains	Time to complete	Measurement level			Administration method		Assesses measurement levels in separate scores
				Impairment	Disability	Handicap	Patient administered	Observer administered	
Disease and joint specific									
HRQ	15	1	10	λ	λ		λ		
THAOEQ	15			λ	λ	λ			
Lequesne Indices	10 knee	1	10	λ	λ			λ	
	10 hip								
WOMAC	24	3	5	λ	λ		λ		λ
KOOS	42	5	10	λ	λ	λ	λ		λ
Oxford	12	1	5	λ	λ		λ		
Generic									
SIP	138	7	30	λ	λ	λ	λ	λ	λ
NHP	38	6	10	λ	λ	λ	λ		λ
SF-36	36	8	10	λ	λ		λ		λ

The SF-36,[36] the most widely used health status measure, is a self-administered questionnaire with excellent psychometric properties that takes less than 10 minutes to complete.[39] It has been modified for use in multiple languages. In evaluating outcome of hip joint arthroplasty[44] the SF-36 performs as well as the SIP and a short version of the AIMS.[45] A shorter version (SF-12) is available. It has not been studied in patients with OA *per se* but appears equally sensitive to change as the Physical Component Summary Scores of the SF-36 in patients with low back pain.[46]

Joint-specific instruments

Instruments to rate single joints have been developed to evaluate outcomes of joint surgery.[47,48] Until recently, these instruments were not standardized, untested for reliability and validity, and based on arbitrary anthropometric criteria or on the assessment of the surgeon. However, the Harris Hip Score has recently been shown to be valid and reliable and can be used by a physician or a physiotherapist to evaluate outcome of total hip replacement.[49] The Hip Rating Questionnaire (HRQ), developed to assess total hip replacement, is another of the few instruments that has been tested for validity, reliability, and responsiveness.[50,51] It takes approximately 10 minutes to answer the 15 questions that probe the overall impact of the arthritis, walking ability, and performance in daily life activities.

The Total Hip Arthroplasty Outcome Evaluation Questionnaire is based on a consensus recommendation of the American Academy of Orthopedic Surgeons (AAOS), the HIP Society, and the Société Internationale de Chirurgie Orthopédique et de Traumatologie (SICOT).[52] The baseline (15 questions) and postoperative forms (13 questions) include items on pain, level of activity, ADL, walking capacity, gait, patient satisfaction, expectations, and reasons for choosing the operation. The instrument is valid and reliable but its responsiveness has not been assessed.[52]

Disease- and joint-specific instruments

The Lequesne Indices of Severity for Osteoarthritis of the Hip and the Knee[53] and the Western Ontario and McMaster Universities Osteoarthritis Index (WOMAC)[54] have had wide use (Table 10.2). The Lequesne Indices have one 10-item scale for the knee and one 10-item scale for the hip. Trained individuals can administer these in 5–10 minutes. Both scales rate pain or discomfort, stiffness, performance on activities of daily living, and the need for assistive devices in maximum walking capacity. In the hip scale an additional question addresses arthritis-related sexual dysfunction in sexually active women. The knee and the hip indices are reliable[53,55] and responsive in clinical trials.[53,56,57]

The WOMAC Osteoarthritis Index[54] is a 24-item questionnaire focusing on pain, stiffness, and functional limitation related to knee and/or hip OA. The WOMAC is available in two versions, one using verbal rating scales and another using VAS; both can be completed in less than five minutes. The WOMAC has been extensively tested for validity, reliability, and responsiveness,[57,58] translated into several languages, and used as the main outcome in evaluations of pharmacological,[57,58] surgical,[40,59] and acupuncture therapy trials.[60]

The Lequesne Indices had similar sensitivity to change as the Doyle[61] and the WOMAC indices in a trial comparing meclofenate to diclofenac sodium for OA of the knee.[58] Both instruments are recommended for long-term OA research studies.[62] However, the Lequesne Indices have disadvantages. Some items are not clearly described. The time period covered is not stated. There is no clear 'breakpoint' within categories of 'walking distance' and interviewer training is required. In a study comparing the psychometric properties of the self-reported Lequesne and the WOMAC in patients having total hip replacement, it was concluded that the self-reported Lequesne should be used with caution until additional testing of its metric properties and validity has been performed.[63]

Knee injury and Osteoarthritis Outcome Score

The Knee Injury and OA Outcome Score (KOOS) was developed for short- and long-term follow-up studies of knee injury that often results in knee OA.[64] It is a 42-item, self-administered questionnaire based on the WOMAC 3.0, therefore WOMAC scores can be derived from it. The measure has five subscales: Pain, Symptoms, Activities of Daily Living, Sport and Recreation Function, and knee-related Quality of Life. The KOOS has been validated for patients aged 15–80 with knee injury and OA.[32,65] Because of high sensitivity and high responsiveness over time the two KOOS subscales for sport/recreation function and knee-related quality of life can be added to the WOMAC in younger or physically more active patients.[66] The KOOS has been used as the main outcome measure for evaluating short- and long-term effects of knee surgery and physiotherapy[66,67] and is recommended for use in cartilage repair trials.[68]

Oxford Hip/Knee Score

Ten years after the WOMAC, a new 12-item instrument designed for patients undergoing hip or knee arthroplasty was published and found practical, reliable, valid, and sensitive.[69] However, concerns about the clarity, coverage, and content validity of the score have been raised, possibly resulting from too few and thus complex questions.[70] The major reason for substituting the currently recommended WOMAC with a new instrument would be higher responsiveness, which might allow fewer patients but similar study power in clinical trials. No comparison of responsiveness between the Oxford Scale and WOMAC has been published.

Semi-objective assessments

Semi-objective assessments combine patient-report and the assessment by the physician of the subject's report. These include analgesic/antiinflammatory medication consumption, joint counts, and performance testing.

Consumption of medications

Although quantification of the use of medications for OA could reflect how much discomfort a patient experiences this approach has limitations. Many patients with OA reduce their level of medication use after a few years, even if symptoms persist.[71] Potential explanations for this include the natural evolution of the disease (maximal OA symptoms generally occur in the first few years[72]), limitation of joint use to reduce symptoms, adaptation to pain, drug side effects and their limited efficacy.

Physical examination

Few physical examination findings of OA have been tested for their reliability and sensitivity to change over time.[29,73]

Performance tests

Timed walk

Timed walking capacity measures lower-limb function.[74] The measure is obtained by calculating the time a patient needs to walk a predetermined distance (e.g., 20 or 50 meters) as fast as possible. The validity of timed walking capacity in OA has been demonstrated.[75] Timed walking capacity has been shown to improve in trials evaluating pharmacological, rehabilitation, and surgical interventions for knee OA[37,13]. Walking time is therefore included in recommendations for long-term OA trials.[53] In practice it is important to standardize the instructions and the type and amount of encouragement given. We find that a female assessor, as against a male assessor, may encourage a male subject to walk faster!!

Muscle strength

Muscle strength testing has infrequently been used in the evaluation of OA,[76,77] even though its measurement is reliable, valid, and responsive. In an elderly population, muscle strength of the lower limb was a better predictor of walking velocity than joint pain;[78] quadriceps muscle strength was a stronger predictor of functional impairment than the radiological severity of knee OA.[79]

Longitudinal data suggest that muscle weakness may be a risk factor for development of knee OA,[80] though further evaluation of the same cohort revealed no differences in quadriceps strength between patients with radiographically stable OA and those with radiographically progressive OA.[81] Interestingly, no significant differences were found between progressive and non-progressive groups with respect to baseline WOMAC pain and changes in WOMAC pain over time.

Functional Assessment System (FAS)

The FAS consists of 20 items divided into 5 groups: hip impairment (range of motion measured by goniometer), knee impairment (range of motion measured by goniometer), physical disability (performance tests), social disability, and pain. Social disability and pain are assessed by observer-administered questions. The FAS is validated for total hip and knee replacement patients.[82] However, in a follow-up study after total hip replacement, self-administered questionnaires like the WOMAC and SF-36 were more responsive measures of pain and function than range of motion, performance tests, and observer-administered questions (FAS).[37]

Objective methods

Objective measures include physical findings from direct or indirect evaluation of the joint. Our discussion is limited to physical examination methods since other methods, such as imaging, arthroscopy, and biochemical markers are covered elsewhere.

Joint count

The Doyle Index[61] was adapted for OA populations from the Ritchie Index[83] for use in rheumatoid arthritis. It is a standardized examination protocol of 48 OA target joints. The examiner records the number of joints in which pain or tenderness is produced under firm digital pressure or movement. Each joint is scored on a 4-point scale (0, no tenderness; 1, patient complained of pain; 2, patient complained of pain and winced; 3, patient complained of pain, winced, and withdrew the joint). The index has been tested for reliability, validity, and sensitivity to change,[61] and has been used in OA trials.[58,84] The index seems best suited to generalized OA, and a joint count is recommended for the long-term evaluation of a drug with disease modification properties in OA.[46]

Physical examination

In a comparison of swelling, crepitus, tenderness, and instability in subjects with OA of the knee only, bony tenderness and tibio-femoral crepitus showed moderate to good intra-rater and inter-rater reliability.[85] Not surprisingly, the reproducibility of joint count, range of motion measures, and bony swelling assessment can be improved by training and standardization of the procedures.[30]

Joint circumference

Measurement of joint circumference or bony *swelling* or *enlargement* is one of the most reliable physical signs of OA,[85] as confirmed in a cross-sectional study.[86] The validity of this method for cross-sectional studies is, however, questionable because of variation in joint shape and size. Joint circumference may be suitable for longitudinal assessment, but the rate of change is not known and it is unlikely to be sensitive.

Range of motion

The techniques that have been tested show important variations inter- and intra-rater reliability.[87] The general findings can be summarized as follows: (1) measurements of passive motion are generally greater than those for active motion; (2) intra-rater reliability is better than inter-rater reliability; (3) reliability can be substantially improved with proper training and standardization of the examination;[30] (4) range of motion is a responsive

outcome following hip arthroplasty;[37] and (5) warming-up exercises, before measurements, may affect the results.[88]

Methodologic considerations

The factors that influence a patient's report or perception of their function and health status have been little studied. What has been documented suggests sources of both random and systematic bias. Factors that influence reporting include the time of the day when questions are asked;[89] the season;[90,91] the learning effect from previous experience with a questionnaire; and possibly the effects of warming-up.[92] Mental health influence reports of physical functioning in patients after total hip replacement.[2]

Informing the patients of their previous answers influences their response, and may be condition specific. When a pain VAS was used in patients with rheumatic conditions with and without giving their previous answers, the majority of patients overestimated their previous pain score 2 weeks afterwards.[93] However, in a trial of NSAIDs for hip and knee OA Bellamy et al.[94] were not able to reduce response variation when the baseline WOMAC was given to patients before the follow-up WOMAC was completed.

Floor and ceiling effects

Health status instruments are sometimes insensitive to change in individuals who score near the extreme values for a scale. The *floor effect* refers to an inability to measure improvement in individuals already at the minimal disability score, and the *ceiling effect* refers to the inability to measure deterioration in individuals at the worst possible score.[95]

Which instrument to choose?

The choice of which instrument to use depends on which joints are under study (some instruments being joint-specific), the purpose of the study, the responsiveness of the instrument, and practical considerations such as the need for an interviewer and the time required to complete the questionnaire.

Because of their narrow focus, joint- or disease-specific instruments may be more pertinent and more sensitive to change in studies assessing specific joints. However, because of their broader coverage, generic instruments may detect complications, side effects, or unintended consequences. Generic instruments are also particularly valuable in studies of resource allocation or health policy because they permit comparison of the impact of the disease or therapy across a variety of medical conditions.[39] For studies of OA, the inclusion of both a disease-specific and a generic instrument has been suggested.[39,62]

Lessons learned from research relevant to the practice setting

An international task force has proposed guidelines for long-term clinical trials to evaluate potential disease modifying drugs in OA.[62] Such guidelines are also relevant to the practitioner who is evaluating whether a patient is getting better or worse (Table 10.3). Restrictions in time and available resources, however, may limit the application of these guidelines to the practice setting.

Table 10.4 summarizes a suggested comprehensive, practical assessment of OA. The approach follows a step-wise progression, starting with open-ended screening questions and utilizing principles of good questionnaire construction. These questions rapidly establish the priorities of the patient and assess whether the condition has changed. If deterioration has occurred the questions progress to more detailed systematic review, especially in the complicated elderly, reticent, stoic, or unreliable historian. Observation of the gait of the patient and the ability to transfer from a chair to the examination table will help to confirm reported problems. For the reliable patient who is stable and doing well, the examination adds little. However, when

Table 10.3 Recommended outcome assessment for evaluating therapy for OA[67]

	Symptomatic slow-acting drugs*	Disease-modifying drugs**
Measures	(5 to 8 of the following)	(One of the following)
	1. Pain scale	Assessment of the cartilage status and rate of change by serial:
	2. Algofunctional indices:	1. Radiography (joint space narrowing)
	(a) Lequesne Index	2. Fiberoptic arthroscopy
	or	3. Other techniques:
	(b) WOMAC 3	(a) CT-scan
	3. Medication consumption:	(b) MRI
	(a) Analgesics	(c) Ultrasonography
	(b) NSAIDs	
	4. Physical examination:	
	(a) Doyle Index (original or adaptations)	
	(b) Articular mobility	
	5. Timed performances:	
	(a) Walk 20 or 50 meters	
	(b) Go up and down a standard flight of stairs	
	6. Global judgment of effectiveness:	
	(a) From the patient	
	(b) From the physician	
	7. Quality of life scale	
Duration	3–12 months	Therapeutic trial‡—2–4 years
		Prophylactic trial§—many years

* Drugs that are neither rapidly acting analgesics nor non-steroidal, anti-inflammatory agents nor chondroprotective, but have a slow onset of action and are alleged to improve OA symptoms.

** Drugs that may prevent, retard, or reverse cartilage lesions in humans.

‡ Aimed at slowing or reversing the OA articular changes.

§ Aimed at preventing the development of OA change (in selected high-risk populations).

Table 10.4 Clinical assessment of OA patients (every 6–12 months)

Parameters	Assessment
Global rating	Verbal transition scale (VRS)
	Are you better, same, or worse?
Pain	Numerical rating scale (NRS)
	Over the last month, how much discomfort have you had on a scale of 1–5 (5, the most)?
	Have you had:
	(1) Pain at rest?
	(2) Pain with any weight bearing?
	(3) Pain at night?
Function	What is the most difficult thing for you to do on a regular day?
Examination	Range of motion and effect of mobilization on pain
	Functional testing, if necessary (see Table 10.5)
Therapy	Analgesics
	NSAIDs
	Joint aspirations
	Intra-articular steroids

NRS, numeric rating scale; VRS, verbal rating scale.

there has been a change in reported problems, development of new problems, or change in medication use and activity, the assessment will provide insight into potential management strategies. When severe discomfort is reported, knowing what critical functions are disturbed, such as sleep or weight bearing, permits more sensitive grading of the pain.

The physical examination will identify coexisting peri-articular soft tissue lesions (e.g., trochanteric or anserine bursitis) that may respond to local therapy. Biomechanical factors such as leg length discrepancies, contractures, valgus or varus deformities that may cause ligament strain, can be managed with orthotics. Muscle strength testing can identify a therapeutic target. Finally, whether mobilizing the joint induces discomfort may be used as a clue for unreported functional limitation. For the unreliable historian, simple performance tests may quickly identify potential functional problems and the joints that may be involved (Table 10.5).

With the current state of therapy, radiographic imaging may have a place in assessing structural change, but has little value in the routine monitoring of patients because of its poor correlation with symptoms and function. Radiographs are most useful when surgery is contemplated, when there has been a major change in symptoms or physical findings, or when another diagnosis is under consideration.

General principles

The development of valid, reliable, patient-centered questionnaires have taught us how to pose more useful and quantitative questions for the

Table 10.5 Screening for functional disability in patients with OA

Task	Musculoskeletal areas tested	Function
Touch fingers to palmar crease*	Finger small joints (F)	Grip
Touch index finger pad to thumb pad	Thumb (AB, O) and thumb opponens muscle (S)	Grip and pinch
Place palm of hand to contralateral	Wrist (F) and Trochantershoulder (AD)	Hygiene (perineal and back care)
Touch 1st MCP joint to top of head	Shoulder (AB, F, ER) and elbow (F)	Hygiene (face, neck, hair, oral), feeding, and dressing
Touch waist in back	Shoulder (IR)	Dressing and low back care
Touch tip of shoe	Back, hip, and knee (F) and elbow (E)	Dressing of lower extremities
Arise from chair without using hands†	Hip girdle and quadriceps rectus femoris (S)	Transfer ability
Stand unassisted	Hip, knee, and ankle (F, E) and quadriceps femoris muscle (S)	Standing
Step over a 6-inch block	Hip, knee, and ankle (F, E) and Hip girdle (S)	Stairs
Gait	Hip, knee, ankle, and small joints of feet (F, E), hip girdle and quadriceps femoris muscle (S)	Walking

AB, abduction; ER, external rotation; F, flexion; E, extension; AD, adduction; IR, Internal rotation; O, opposition; S, strength.

* If abnormal, test grip strength; lateral pinch strength is the last to diminish.

† If abnormal, test ability to get up from bed.

Source: Adapted from Liang et al.,[74] with permission.

day-to-day monitoring of the patient with OA. The minimal history should include questions that are:

1. comprehensible—stated in the simplest language;

2. consistent—framed in a way to ensure reproducible replies (having the same anchors, time of reference and response categories);

3. mutually exclusive—minimal overlap with one another;

4. sensitive to change—respond to the range of severity.

Functional diagnosis

It is important to recognize that functional decline from OA may be hastened by chronic and acute illnesses. Many individuals decline slowly, accommodate the decline in function, and accept it. Unfortunately, by the time function has declined effective intervention may prove more difficult. Regular functional evaluation is particularly useful in this regard. Function is an important end point to be measured in a standardized, quantitative manner. A measurement of improvement, such as a timed walk is more sensitive to actual change than self-reported function, whereas the self-report reflects the patient's perception of their ability best. Two approaches are useful to screen for functional problems: (1) the one-second drill asks the patient what single function is the most difficult for him or her to perform during the day, and how difficult it is on a scale of 1 to 5; (2) the 10-second drill permits patients to express how they are affected by the condition, communicate which activity is the most difficult, compare their condition to baseline, and determine their priority for treatment. Questioning in the 10-second drill might take the following course:

1. How does your condition affect you?

2. What is the most: (a) difficult thing for you to do in an average day? (b) important thing for us to work on?

3. What can you not do: (a) that you were able to do? (b) that you need or would like to do?

4. Are you able to sleep through the night?

In patients with polyarticular OA, or when the patient is a poor observer or cognitively impaired, a systematic inventory of activities of daily living (ADL) such as ambulation, dressing, eating, personal hygiene, transfers, and toileting should be obtained (ADEPTT is a mnemonic). Disease-specific[54] or joint-specific[50] instruments might be administered while the

patient is waiting to be seen. To be most helpful, the physician should incorporate these ratings into his assessment to obtain additional details on the problem areas.

Functional testing

A useful method of evaluating function in elderly, sick, cognitively impaired, or unreliable subjects is performance testing.[96] One performance test that can be done rapidly in the office, to screen for potential problems, has the patient imitate the assessor in maneuvers that test musculoskeletal areas (Table 10.4). If there is asymmetry between sides, or if the patient is unable to perform these maneuvers because of pain or mechanical restrictions, limitations in certain self-care areas probably exist. The 'GALS' screen[97] is a validated screen of musculoskeletal abnormality that shows a good correlation (Spearman correlation: 0.31–0.70) with disability related to ADL.[98]

In following functional ability, adoption of a single-signal function can help the evaluator and the physician to focus on relevant problems. However, because function is multi-determinant, interrelated factors (e.g., mental health, social, and economic environment, comorbid conditions, vocational status, frailty) impact on function. When function is not proportional to objective evidence, these factors should be explored.

Key points

How to evaluate symptomatic OA?

1. Evaluate pain, function, and quality of life.

2. Use patient self-assesment.

3. Use questionnaire validated for OA and age group/functional demands.

References

(An asterisk denotes recommended reading.)

1. *Greenfield, S., Apolone, G., McNeil, B.J., and Cleary, P.D. (1993). The importance of co-existent disase in the occurrence of postoperative complications and one-year recovery in patients undergoing total hip replacement. *Med Care* **31**:141–54.

Comprehensive assessment should include non-joint related determinants of function, such as mental health, comorbid conditions, and indicators of frailty among older patients.

2. Bischoff, H.A., Lingard, E.A., Losina, E., Roos, E.M., Phillips, C.B., Mahomed, N.N., Baron, J.A., Barrett, J., and Katz, J.N. (2001). The role of non-hip-related factors associated with poor functional outcome 3 Years After Total Hip Replacement (Abstract). *Arthritis Rheum* **44**(suppl):S184.

3. Liang, M.H. and Jette, A.M. (1981). Measuring functional ability in chronic arthritis: a critical review. *Arthritis Rheum* **24**:80–6.

4. Carr, A.J. (1999). Beyond disability: measuring the social and personal consquences of osteoarthritis. *Osteoarthritis Cart* **7**:230–8.

5. Liang, M.H., Larson, M.G., Cullen, K.E., and Schwartz, J.A. (1985). Comparative measurement efficiency and sensitivity of five health status instruments for arthritis research. *Arthritis Rheum* **28**:542–7.

6. Ryd, L., Kärrholm, J., and Ahlvin, P. (1997). Knee scoring systems in gonarthrosis. Evaluation of interobserver variability and the envelope of bias. *Acta Orthop Scand* **68**(1):41–5.

7. Sun, Y., Sturmer, T., Gunther, K., and Brenner, H. (1997). Reliability and validity of clinical outcome measurements of osteoarthritis of the hip and knee—a review of the literature. *Clin Rheumatol* **16**(2):185–98.

8. Chatman, A.B., Hyams, S.P., Neel, J.M., Stratford, P.W., Schomberg, A., and Stabler, M. (1997). The patient-specific functional scale: measurement properties in patients with knee dysfunction. *Phys Ther* **88**(8):820–9.

9. Westaway, M.D., Stratford, P.W., and Binkley, J.M. (1998). The Patient-specific functional scale: Validation of its use in persons with neck dysfunction. *J Orthop Sports Phys Ther* **27**(5):331–8.

10. Wright, J., Rudicel, S., and Feinstein, A. (1994). Ask patients what they want. Evaluation of individual complaints before total hip replacement. *J Bone Joint Surg Br* **76B**(2):229–34.

11. Wright, J.G. and Young, N.L. (1997). The patient-specific index: asking patients what they want. *J Bone Joint Surg Am* **79A**(7):974–83.

12. O'Boyle, C.A., McGee, H., Hickey, A., O'Malley, K., and Joyce, C.R. (1992). Individual quality of life in patients undergoing Hip Replacement. *Lancet* **339**:1088–91.

13. *Liang, M.H., Partridge, A.J., Larson, M.G., Gall, V., and Taylor, J. (1984). Evaluation of Comprehensive Rehabilitation Services for Elderly Homebound Patients with Arthritis and Orthopedic Disability. *Arthritis Rheum* **27**:258–66.

Goal-attainment scaling has attractive features for measuring change from an individuals perspective. Subjects are asked to name, or select from a list, their priority areas or problem areas and then after an intervention, to state whether these areas have improved and to what extent.

14. Pincus, T., Summey, J.A., Soraci, S.A., Jr, Wallston, K.A., and Hummon, N.P. (1983). Assessment of patient satisfaction in activities of daily living using a modified Stanford Health Assessment Questionnaire. *Arthritis Rheum* **26**:1346–53.

15. Meenan, R.F., Mason, J.H., Anderson, J.J., Guccione, A.A., and Kazis, L.E. (1992). AIMS2. The content and properties of a revised and expanded Arthritis Impact Measurement Scales Health Status Questionnaire. *Arthritis Rheum* **35**:1–10.

16. Larson, C. (1963). Rating scale for hip disabilities. *Clin Orthop* **31**:85–93.

17. Harris, W.H. (1969). Traumatic arthritis of the hip after dislocation and acetabular fractures: treatment by mold arthroplasty. An end result study using a new method of result evaluation. *J Bone Joint Surg Am* **51A**:737–55.

18. Nunnally, J.C. and Bernstein, I.H. (1994). *Psychometric Theory* (3rd ed.). New York: McGraw-Hill.

19. Bellamy, N., Buchanan, W.W., Goldsmith, C.H., Campbell, J., and Duku, E. (1990). Signal measurement strategies: are they feasible and do they offer any advantage in outcome measurement in osteoarthritis? *Arthritis Rheum* **33**:739–45.

20. Barr, S., Bellamy, N., Buchanan, W.W., Chalmers, A., Ford, P.M., Kean, W.F., et al. (1994). A comparative study of signal versus aggregate methods of outcome measurement based on the WOMAC Osteoarthritis Index. *J Rheumatol* **21**:2106–12.

21. Williams, R.C. (1988). Toward a set of reliable and valid measures for chronic pain assessment and outcome research. *Pain* **35**:239–51.

22. Huskisson, E.C. (1974). Measurement of pain. *Lancet* **2**:1127–31.

23. Scott, J. and Huskisson, E.C. (1976). Graphic representation of pain. *Pain* **2**:175–84.

24. Bieri, D., Reeve, R.A., Champion, G.D., Addicoat, L., and Ziegler, J.B. (1990). The Faces Pain Scale for the self-assessment of the severity of pain experienced by children: development, initial validation, and preliminary investigation for ratio scale properties. *Pain* **41**:139–50.

25. Lorish, C.D. and Maisiak, R. (1986). The Face Scale: a brief, nonverbal method for assessing patient mood. *Arthritis Rheum* **29**:906–9.

26. Melzack, R. (1975). The McGill pain questionnaire: major properties and scoring methods. *Pain* **1**:277–99.

27. Melzack, R. (1987). The short-form McGill Pain Questionnaire. *Pain* **30**:191–7.

28. Rejeski, W.J., Ettinger, W.H. Jr, Shumaker, S., Heuser, M.D., James, P., Monu, J., et al. (1995). The evaluation of pain in patients with knee osteoarthritis: the knee pain scale. *J Rheumatol* **22**:1124–9.

29. Jones, A., Hopkinson, N., Pattrick, M., Berman, P., and Doherty, M. (1992). Evaluation of a method for clinically assessing osteoarthritis of the knee. *Ann Rheum Dis* **51**:243–5.

30. Bellamy, N., Carette, S., Ford, P.M., Kean, W.F., le Riche, N.G., Lussier, A., et al. (1992). Osteoarthritis antirheumatic drug trials. I: Effects of standardization procedures on observer dependent outcome measures. *J Rheumatol* **19**:436–43.

31. Bellamy, N. and Buchanan, W.W. (1984). Outcome measurement in osteoarthritis clinical trials: the case for standardization. *Clin Rheumatol* **3**:293–303.

32. Roos, E.M., Roos, H.P., and Lohmander, L.S. (1999). WOMAC Osteoarthritis Index—additional dimensions for use in post-traumatic osteoarthritis of the knee. *Osteoarthritis Cart* **7**(2):216–21.

33. Bergner, M., Bobbitt, R.A., Pollard, W.E., Martin, D.P., and Gilson, B.S. (1976). The Sickness Impact Profile: validation of a health status measure. *Med Care* **14**:57–67.

34. McDowell, I.W., Martini, C.J., and Waugh, W. (1978). A method for self-assessment of disability before and after hip replacement operations. *Br Med J* **2**:857–9.

35. Hunt, S.M., McKenna, S.P., and Williams, J. (1981). Reliability of a population survey tool for measuring perceived health problems: a study of patients with osteoarthrosis. *J Epidemiol Community Health* **35**:297–300.

36. *Ware, J.E., Jr and Sherbourne, C.D. (1992). The MOS 36-item short-form health survey (SF-36). A conceptual framework and item selection. *Med Care* **30**:473–83.

SF-36 is the most widely used generic outcome measure. Norms are available for multiple countries (www.sf-36.com).

37. Nilsdotter, A.K., Roos, E.M., Westerlund, J.P., Roos, H.P., and Lohmander, L.S. (2001). Comparative responsiveness of measures of pain and function after total hip replacement. *Arthritis Rheum* **45**(3):258–62.

38. Summers, M.N., Haley, W.E., Reveille, J.D., and Alarcon, G.S. (1988). Radiographic assessment and psychologic variables as predictors of pain and functional impairment in osteoarthritis of the knee or hip. *Arthritis Rheum* **31**:204–9.

39. Bombardier, C., Melfi, C.A., Paul, J., Green, R., Hawker, G., Wright, J., et al. (1995). Comparison of a generic and a disease-specific measure of pain and physical function after knee replacement surgery. *Med Care* **33**:AS131–44.

40. Laupacis, A., Bourne, R., Rorabeck, C., Feeny, D., Wong, C., Tugwell, P., et al. (1993). The effect of elective total hip replacement on health-related quality of life. *J Bone Joint Surg Am* **75A**:1619–26.

41. Liang, M.H., Fossel, A.H., and Larson, M.G. (1990). Comparisons of five health status instruments for orthopedic evaluation. *Med Care* **28**:632–42.

42. Stucki, G., Liang, M.H., Phillips, C., and Katz, J.N. (1995). The Short Form-36 is preferable to the SIP as a generic health status measure in patients undergoing elective total hip arthroplasty. *Arthritis Care Res* **8**(3):174–81.

43. Wiklund, I. and Romanus, B. (1991). A comparison of quality of life before and after arthroplasty in patients who had arthrosis of the hip joint. *J Bone Joint Surg Am* **73A**:765–9.

44. Katz, J.N., Larson, M.G., Phillips, C.B., Fossel, A.H., and Liang, M.H. (1992). Comparative measurement sensitivity of short and longer health status instruments. *Med Care* **30**:917–25.

45. Wallston, K.A., Brown, G.K., Stein, M.J., and Dobbins, C.J. (1989). Comparing the short and long versions of the Arthritis Impact Measurement Scales. *J Rheumatol* **16**:1105–9.

46. Riddle, D.L., Lee, K.T., and Stratford, P.W. (2001). Use of sf-36 and sf-12 health status measures a quantitative comparison for groups versus individual patients. *Med Care* **39**(8):867–78.

47. Larson, C. (1963). Rating scale for hip disabilities. *Clin Orthop* **31**:85–93.

48. Harris, W.H. (1969). Traumatic arthritis of the hip after dislocation and acetabular fractures: treatment by mold arthroplasty. An end result study using a new method of result evaluation. *J Bone Joint Surg Am* **51A**:737–55.

49. Söderman, P. and Malchau, H. (2001). Is the Harris Hip Score System useful to study the outcome of total hip replacement? *Clin Orthop* **384**:189–97.

50. Johanson, N.A., Charlson, M.E., Szatrowski, T.P., and Ranawat, C.S. (1992). A self-administered hip-rating questionnaire for the assessment of outcome after total hip replacement. *J Bone Joint Surg Am* **74A**:587–97.

51. Mancuso, C.A. and Charlson, M.E. (1995). Does recollection error threaten the validity of cross-sectional studies of effectiveness? *Med Care* **33**:AS77–88.

52. Katz, J.N., Phillips, C.B., Poss, R., Harrast, J.J., Fossel, A.H., Liang, M.H., et al. (1995). The validity and reliability of a total hip arthroplasty outcome evaluation questionnaire. *J Bone Joint Surg* **77A**:1528–34.

53. Lequesne, M.G., Mery, C., Samson, M., and Gerard, P. (1987). Indexes of severity for osteoarthritis of the hip and knee. Validation—value in comparison with other assessment tests. *Scand J Rheumatol* (Suppl. 65):85–9.

54. *Bellamy, N., Buchanan, W.W., Goldsmith, C.H., Campbell, J., and Stitt, L.W. (1988). Validation study of WOMAC: a health status instrument for measuring clinically important patient relevant outcomes to antirheumatic drug therapy in patients with osteoarthritis of the hip or knee. *J Rheumatol* **15**:1833–40.

    The WOMAC is the best validated, and now most widely used knee/hip OA-specific instrument with domains of pain, stiffness, and lower limb function.

55. Pavelka, K., Gatterova, J., Pelitskova, Z., Svarcova, Z., Fencl, F., Urbanova, Z., et al. (1992). Correlation between knee roentgenogram changes and clinical symptoms in osteoarthritis. *Rev Rhum Mal Osteoartic* **59**:553–9.

56. Mazieres, B., Masquelier, A.M., and Capron, M.H. (1991). A French controlled multicenter study of intraarticular orgotein versus intraarticular corticosteroids in the treatment of knee osteoarthritis: a one-year follow up. *J Rheumatol* (Suppl. 27):134–7.

57. Bellamy, N., Bensen, W.G., Ford, P.M., Huang, S.H., and Lang, J.Y. (1992). Double-blind randomized controlled trial of flurbiprofen-SR (ANSAID-SR) and diclofenac sodium-SR (Voltaren-SR) in the treatment of osteoarthritis. *Clin Invest Med* **15**:427–33.

58. Bellamy, N., Kean, W.F., Buchanan, W.W., Gerecz-Simon, E., and Campbell, J. (1992). Double blind randomized controlled trial of sodium meclofenamate (Meclomen) and diclofenac sodium (Voltaren): post validation reapplication of the WOMAC Osteoarthritis Index. *J Rheumatol* **19**: 153–9.

59. Bellamy, N., Buchanan, W.W., Goldsmith, C.H., Campbell, J., and Stitt, L. (1988). Validation study of WOMAC: a health status instrument for measuring clinically important patient relevant outcomes following total hip or knee arthroplasty in osteoarthritis. *J Orthop Rheumatol* **1**:95–108.

60. Takeda, W. and Wessel, J. (1994). Acupuncture for the treatment of pain of osteoarthritic knees. *Arthritis Care Res* **7**:118–22.

61. Doyle, D.V., Dieppe, P.A., Scott, J., and Huskisson, E.C. (1981). An articular index for the assessment of osteoarthritis. *Ann Rheum Dis* **40**:75–8.

62. Lequesne, M., Brandt, K.D., Bellamy, N., Moskowitz, R., Menkes, C.J., Pelletier, J.P., et al. (1994). Guidelines for testing slow acting drugs in osteoarthritis. *J Rheumatol* **21**(Suppl. 41):65–71.

63. Stucki, G., Sangha, O., Stucki, S., et al. (1998). Comparison of the WOMAC (Western Ontario and McMaster Universities) osteoarthritis index and a self-report format of the self-administered Lequesne-Algofunctional index in patients with knee and hip osteoarthritis. *Osteoarthritis Cart* **6**(2):79–86.

64. *Roos, E.M. KOOS homepage. In: www.koos.nu

    The KOOS includes the WOMAC and assesses symptoms, function, and quality of life in younger or physically more active patients with knee injury and OA.

65. Roos, E.M., Roos, P.H., Lohmander, L.S., Ekdahl, C., and Beynnon, B.D. (1998). Knee injury and Osteoarthritis Outcome Score (KOOS)—Development of a self-administered outcome measure. *J Orthop Sports Phys Ther* **78**(2): 88–96.

66. Englund, M., Roos, E.M., Roos, H.P., and Lohmander, L.S. (2001). Patient-relevant outcomes fourteen years after meniscectomy: influence of type of tear and size of resection. *Rheumatology* **40**:631–9.

67. Roos, E.M., Roos, H.P., Ryd, L., and Lohmander, L.S. (2001). Substantial disability 3 months after meniscectomy: a prospective study of patient-relevant outcomes. *Arthroscopy* **16**(6):619–26.

68. Mandelbaum, B.R., Romanelli, D.A., and Knapp, T.P. (2000). Articular cartilage repair: assessment and classification. *Operative Techniques Sports Med* **8**(2):90–7.

69. Dawson, J., Fitzpatrick, R., Murray, D., and Carr, A. (1998). Questionnaire on the perceptions of patients about total knee replacement. *J Bone Joint Surg Br* **80B**(1):63–9.

70. McMurray, R., Heaton, J., Sloper, P., and Nettleton, S. (1999). Measurement of patient perceptions of pain and disability in relation to total hip replacement: the place of the Oxford hip score in the mixed methods. *Qual Health Care* **8**(4):228–33.

71. Lequesne, M., Dougados, M., Abiteboul, M., Bontoux, D., Bouvenot, G., Dreiser, R.L., et al. (1990). How to evaluate the long-term course of osteoarthritis. Tests for trials of fundamental treatments (spine excluded). *Rev Rhum Mal Osteoartic* **57**:24S–31S.

72. Auquier, L., Paolaggi, J.B., Cohen de Lara, A., Siaud, J.R., Limon, J., Emery, J.P., et al. (1979). Long term evolution of pain in a series of 273 coxarthrosis patients. *Rev Rhum Mal Osteoartic* **46**:153–62.

73. Cushnaghan, J., Cooper, C., Dieppe, P., Kirwan, J., McAlindon, T., and McCrae, F. (1990). Clinical assessment of osteoarthritis of the knee. *Ann Rheum Dis* **49**:768–70.

74. Spiegel, J.S., Paulus, H.E., Ward, N.B., Spiegel, T.M., Leake, B., and Kane, R.L. (1987). What are we measuring? An examination of walk time and grip strength. *J Rheumatol* **14**:80–6.

75. Marks, R. (1994). Reliability and validity of self-paced walking time measures for knee osteoarthritis. *Arthritis Care Res* **7**:50–3.

76. Fisher, N.M., Gresham, G.E., Abrams, M., Hicks, J., Horrigan, D., and Pendergast, D.R. (1993). Quantitative effects of physical therapy on muscular and functional performance in subjects with osteoarthritis of the knees. *Arch Phys Med Rehabil* **74**:840–7.

77. Hochberg, M.C., Lethbridge-Cejku, M., Plato, C.C., Wigley, F.M., and Tobin, J.D. (1991). Factors associated with osteoarthritis of the hand in males: data from the Baltimore Longitudinal Study of Aging. *Am J Epidemiol* **134**:1121–7.

78. Chang, R.W., Dunlop, D., Gibbs, J., and Hughes, S. (1995). The determinants of walking velocity in the elderly. An evaluation using regression trees. *Arthritis Rheum* **38**:343–50.

79. McAlindon, T.E., Cooper, C., Kirwan, J.R., and Dieppe, P.A. (1993). Determinants of disability in osteoarthritis of the knee. *Ann Rheum Dis* **52**:258–62.

80. Slemenda, C., Heilman, D.K., Brandt, K.D., Katz, B.P., Mazzuca, S.A., Braunstein, E.M., and Byrd, D. (1998). Reduced quadriceps strength relative to body weight: a risk factor for knee osteoarthritis in women? *Arthritis Rheum* **41**(11):1951–9.

81. Brandt, K.D., Heilman, D.K., Slemenda, C., Katz, B.P., Mazzuca, S.A., Braunstein, E.M., and Byrd, D. (1999). Quadriceps strength in women with radiographically progressive osteoarthritis of the knee and those with stable radiographic changes. *J Rheumatol* **26**:2431–7.

82. Öberg, U., Öberg, B., and Öberg, T. (1994). Validity and reliability of a new assessment of lower-extremity function. *Phys Ther* **74**:861–71.

83. Ritchie, D.M., Boyle, J.A., Mclnnes, J.M., Jasani, M.K., Dalakos, T.G., Grieveson, P., et al. (1968). Clinical studies with an articular index for the assessment of joint tenderness in patients with rheumatoid arthritis. *Q J Med* **37**:393–406.

84. Buckland-Wright, J.C., Macfarlane, D.G., Lynch, J.A., and Jasani, M.K. (1995). Quantitative microfocal radiography detects changes in OA knee joint space width in patients in placebo controlled trial of NSAID therapy. *J Rheumatol* **22**:937–43.

85. Cushnaghan, J., Cooper, C., Dieppe, P., Kirwan, J., McAlindon, T., and McCrae, F. (1990). Clinical assessment of osteoarthritis of the knee. *Ann Rheum Dis* **49**:768–70.

86. Theiler, R., Stucki, G., Schütz, R., Hofer, H., Seifert, B., Tyndall, A., *et al.* (1996). Parametric and nonparametric measures in the assessment of knee and hip osteoarthritis: interobserver reliability and correlation with radiology. *Osteoarthritis Cart* **4**:35–42.

87. Bellamy, N. (1993). Mechanical and electromechanical devices. In *Musculoskeletal Clinical Metrology*. Dodrecht: Kluwer Academic Publishers, pp. 117–34.

88. Roberts, W.N., Liang, M.H., Pallozzi, L.M., and Daltroy, L.H. (1988). Effects of warming up on reliability of anthropometric techniques in ankylosing spondylitis. *Arthritis Rheum* **31**:549–52.

89. Bellamy, N., Sothern, R.B., and Campbell, J. (1990). Rhythmic variations in pain perception in osteoarthritis of the knee. *J Rheumatol* **17**:364–72.

90. Hawley, D.J. and Wolfe, F. (1994). Effect of light and season on pain and depression in subjects with rheumatic disorders. *Pain* **59**:227–34.

91. Harris, C.M. (1984). Seasonal variations in depression and osteoarthritis. *J R Coll Gen Pract* **34**:436–9.

92. Spiegel, J.S., Paulus, H.E., Ward, N.B., Spiegel, T.M., Leake, B., and Kane, R.L. (1987). What are we measuring? An examination of walk time and grip strength. *J Rheumatol* **14**:80–6.

93. Marks, R. (1994). Reliability and validity of self-paced walking time measures for knee Osteoarthritis. *Arthritis Care Res* **7**:50–3.

94. Bellamy, N., Goldsmith, C.H., and Buchanan, W.W. (1991). Prior score availability: Observations using the WOMAC osteoarthritis Index (Letter). *Br J Rheumatol* **30**:150–1.

95. Stucki, G., Stucki, S., Bruhlmann, P., and Michel, B.A. (1995). Ceiling effects of the Health Assessment Questionnaire and its modified version in some ambulatory rheumatoid arthritis patients. *Ann Rheum Dis* **54**:461–5.

96. Liang, M.H., Gall, V., Partridge, A.J., and Eaton, H. (1983). Management of functional disability in homebound patients. *J Fam Practice* **17**:429–35.

97. Doherty, M., Dacre, J., Dieppe, P., and Snaith, M. (1992). The 'GALS' locomotor screen. *Ann Rheum Dis* **51**:1165–9.

98. Plant, M.J., Linton, S., Dodd, E., Jones, P.W., and Dawes, P.T. (1993). The GALS locomotor screen and disability. *Ann Rheum Dis* **52**:886–90.

11

Prospects for pharmacological modification of joint breakdown in osteoarthritis

11.1 Pharmacological modification of joint breakdown in OA: Do we need it, can we do it, can we prove it, is it good?

Kenneth Brandt, Michael Doherty, and L. Stefan Lohmander

The currently available treatments for OA focus on decreasing pain and improving function, with varying degrees of success. When this fails, destroyed joints can be replaced by arthroplasty, often with good long-term outcome. However, we still lack reliable means of intervening in the disease process of OA in order to stop or slow down the gradual destruction of articular cartilage and other joint tissues, which is a hallmark of this disease. We could thus summarize the current situation as in Table 11.1(a) and (b) below, while the solutions outlined in (c) and (d) still largely elude us. The chapters within this section focus on item (c), while previous sections of this book deal with the other points.

Do we need pharmacological modification of joint breakdown in OA?

The few long-term studies available on the natural history of OA suggest that many patients with mild or moderate OA actually do not progress much in their disease, but remain on the same level of pain and function for years, or even in some cases improve.[1–3] It is argued that for these patients pharmacological prevention of joint breakdown is not a relevant treatment choice.[4,5] This large group of patients with mild or moderate, non-progressive (or only very slowly progressive) disease might thus be better served by greater attention to, and research on items (a) and (e) than items (c) and (d) in the list above.

On the other hand, there is enough progressive OA around to generate a yearly rate per 100 000 individuals (within the most relevant group aged between 60 and 80) of some 300–500 hip replacements for OA in the Scandinavian countries.[6] This translates into some 10 000 hips replaced for OA per year in Sweden, with a population of about 9 million. Higher and lower rates are reported from other areas, and to this number should be added the rate of knee replacements for OA, which may approach that for hips in many countries.

In addition, several studies have highlighted the high risk of severe OA at a young age following joint injuries.[7–9] These young patients with OA, often in their thirties and forties, present a significant challenge. They have high expectations of physical activity and ability to work, while the orthopedic surgeon is often reluctant to replace their failed joint due to the

significantly increased risk of implant wear, loosening, and reoperation in these young patients (Buckwalter and Lohmander, Chapter 9.18; Knutson, Chapter 9.19).

These facts provide a rationale for treatments that would stop or slow joint destruction in OA, and provide patient-relevant benefit for the patients with progressive OA.

Can we do it?

Chapter 11.2.1 deals with the biological aspects of disease modification in OA. The author provides some evidence that pharmacological modification of joint breakdown in OA is a reality in animal models. The advantages and limitations of these animal models are further explored in Chapter 11.3. In Chapter 11.1.2, Kenneth Brandt discusses the clinical perspectives of disease modification in OA, and describes some early results from human clinical trials, which suggest that pharmacological modification of joint destruction in OA may be possible. However, the experience also suggests that most of the agents tested so far have been either ineffective or associated with significant side effects, or both. OA is a chronic but not life-threatening disease. The acceptance level for side effects of disease modifying pharmacological treatment of OA will likely be low.

Can we prove it?

A major problem facing the introduction of any disease modifying OA therapy is the lack of reliable and convenient outcome measures to document changes in joint structure, function, or metabolism resulting from the treatment. It may even be argued that until such measures are developed, it will be difficult to prove the efficacy of even the most promising drug candidate.

A comparison with the development of new osteoporosis treatment is instructive. For this disease, a reliable and convenient outcome measure in the form of bone density was available early on, and subsequently supplemented with systemic biomarkers of bone turn over measured in urine and blood. These measures could in turn be related to a clinically relevant and measurable outcome: fracture. Finally, agents were available early on that could be used to probe validity of these measures in animal models.

In OA the indirect measurement of joint cartilage thickness by plain radiography is still being standardized, and its relationship with a clinically relevant outcome is yet unproven in the context of the clinical trial (Chapters 11.4.1 and 11.4.2). Magnetic resonance imaging shows considerable promise as an alternative or complementary method to monitor the structure of cartilage and other joint tissues, but is equally not validated in regard to its relationship with clinical or other measures of outcome (Chapter 11.4.3). Other measures such as arthroscopy, ultrasonography, or mechanical probing of cartilage quality also remain to be validated (Chapters 11.4.4, 11.4.5 and 11.4.6). Biomarkers for OA are being developed and show promise, but for lack of an agent with proven disease-modifying effect, it remains difficult to validate biomarkers for OA as outcome measures (Chapter 11.4.7).

Table 11.1 Treating OA now and in the future, we need to:

a) Treat the pain, improve the function

b) Replace the joint that is lost

c) Detect cartilage loss before it is too severe and prevent further loss

d) Help grow back lost cartilage

e) Better understand low-cost, low-tech solutions to a very common health problem

Is it good (for the patient)?

With today's technology it is a challenge, but not impossible, to show a structure-modifying effect of a pharmacological agent for OA. Some consensus has been reached on clinical trial methodology to evaluate structure modification, as described by Nicholas Bellamy in Chapter 12. However, it remains to be proven that structure modification, such as slowing or reversal of joint structural change in OA, actually translates into a relevant and measurable patient benefit, and with which delay if any. Such benefit could be improvement as determined by patient-relevant outcome questionnaires, health-related quality of life, and/or a delay of need for joint replacement.

References

1. Sahlström, A., Johnell, O., and Redlund-Johnell, I. (1993). The natural course of arthrosis of the knee. *Acta Orthop Scand* **63**(Suppl. 248):57.

2. Dieppe, P.A., Cushnaghan, J., and Shepstone, L. (1997). The Bristol 'OA500' Study: progression of osteoarthritis (OA) over 3 years and the relationship between clinical and radiographic changes at the knee joint. *Osteoarthritis Cart* **5**:87–97.

3. Dieppe, P., Cushnaghan, J., Tucker, M., Browning, S., and Shepstone, L. (2000). The Bristol 'OA500 study': progression and impact of the disease after 8 years. *Osteoarthritis Cart* **8**:63–8.

4. Dieppe, P. (1999). Osteoarthritis: time to shift the paradigm: this includes distinguishing between severe disease and common minor disability. *Br Med J* **318**:1299–300.

5. Chard, J.A., Tallon, D., and Dieppe, P.A. (2000). Epidemiology of research into interventions for the treatment of OA of the knee joint. *Ann Rheum Dis* **59**:414–8.

6. Ingvarsson, T., Hägglund, G., Jónsson Jr., H., and Lohmander, L.S. (1999). Incidence of total hip replacement for primary osteoarthrosis in Iceland 1982–1996. *Acta Orthop Scand* **70**:229–33.

7. Lohmander, L.S. and Roos, H. (1994). Knee ligament injury, surgery and osteoarthrosis. Truth or consequences? *Acta Orthop Scand* **65**:605–9.

8. Roos, H., Laurén, M., Adalberth, T., Roos, E.M., Jonsson, K., and Lohmander, L.S. (1998). Knee osteoarthritis after meniscectomy: prevalence of radiographic changes after twenty-one years, compared with matched controls. *Arthritis Rheum* **41**:687–93.

9. Englund, M., Roos, E.M., Roos, H.P., and Lohmander, L.S. (2001). Patient-relevant outcomes fourteen years after meniscectomy. Influence of type of meniscal tear and size of resection. *Rheumatology* **40**:631–9.

11.2 Disease modifying osteoarthritis drugs (DMOADs)

11.2.1 The biological perspective

Peter Ghosh

Structure modifying OA drugs (SMOADs) have been defined as agents that reverse, retard, or stabilize the underlying pathology of OA, thereby slowing its progression and possibly providing symptomatic relief in the long term. While the 'structures' considered in this definition include articular cartilage and subchondral bone, these tissues are not of uniform composition and undergo continuous adaptation and remodeling throughout the development of OA. These circumstances render the evaluation of putative SMOADs extremely difficult since loss of tissue integrity in one part of a joint may be accompanied by a compensatory biosynthetic response in another, resulting in overall structural changes, which may appear to be beneficial. This is particularly evident in the early stages of OA, which is probably the most amenable to therapeutic intervention. In human subjects, unlike animal models, direct tissue analysis is not generally possible and imaging techniques are used to assess changes in cartilage and bone in OA joints. Joint-space narrowing, as determined radiographically, is currently used to follow cartilage loss in OA and has been employed to assess the effects of drugs on OA progression. However, this approach has been shown to be open to many systematic errors and stringent precautions must be employed to ensure reproducible and meaningful measurements. Magnetic resonance imaging allows joint soft tissues, including cartilage, to be visualized and this technique in combination with contrast agents holds promise as a potential means of following proteoglycan and collagen changes in cartilage and determining the ability of SMOADs to preserve these matrix components. Although no drug has yet been shown to qualify as a SMOAD, studies with animal models of OA indicate that such agents do exist and with the evolution of validated non-invasive means for their assessment in human subjects it is likely that they will be available in the not too distant future.

While the concept of disease or structural modification in OA by therapeutic agents has been recognized for over 50 years, it was not until the early 1990s that committees were established to clarify definitions and standardize methodological approaches for their evaluation and the registration of such agents.[1,2]

SMOADs were considered to fall broadly into two categories: (1) those agents which slowed, arrested, or reversed structural changes in OA joints while concomitantly relieving the symptoms of the disease, and (2) drugs that achieved the same as (1) but provided no improvement in symptoms in the short term. For SMOADs corresponding to (2), symptomatic improvement was expected to occur in the long term and it was considered that other drugs, such as analgesics or nonsteroidal anti-inflammatory drugs (NSAIDs), would probably have to be used to supplement this class of SMOADs in the intervening period.

Irrespective of the time course of action, both categories required identification of a 'structural' component within the OA joint, which faithfully represents the status of the disease at a particular phase of its development and which would be amenable to modification by a therapeutic agent. If such structural biomarkers could be identified it was then assumed that these would allow the relative effects of a drug or placebo treatments, which were administered to a suitable number of patients, to be evaluated over a period of time, which was long enough for the structural component to change sufficiently for it to be accurately measured and permit differentiation between the respective treatments.

Fundamental to this approach is the identification of those structural features of OA that are amenable to observation using currently available noninvasive methodologies and which were meaningful in terms of our understanding of the pathology of the disease. In this chapter we attempt to address these issues, but since at the time of writing no drug has yet been approved by the FDA for classification as a SMOAD we are compelled to illustrate much of the discussion with studies using animal models whose joint tissues have been sampled at various stages of OA progression and where the effects of putative SMOADs have been evaluated at the molecular level using validated techniques.

Structural changes associated with disease progression in OA

As described more fully elsewhere in this book, OA is a disorder of multifactorial etiology that generally has a long and variable period of asymptomatic development that affects the composition and structure of all tissues of the joint including articular cartilage (AC), bone, ligaments, synovium, and synovial fluid. In the late stages of OA the pathology is characterized by substantial degradation and loss of AC accompanied by subchondral bone necrosis, remodelling, and synovial inflammation. However, since the functions of the respective components of the joint are integrated and failure of one will inevitably lead to molecular and cellular changes in the others, it is important to appreciate that a SMOAD that may appear to produce a measurable change at one site in an OA joint may in fact be exerting its pharmacological effects elsewhere. For example, a SMOAD that has no direct effects on cartilage metabolism may still mitigate its loss by decreasing the levels of cytokines released by synoviocytes, which promote catabolic proteinase production by chondrocytes.

Although the cellular and biochemical events that are responsible for such interrelated tissue changes in OA joints are comprehensively reviewed elsewhere (see Chapter 7) we include here a brief account of the main structural and functional features of AC and subchondral bone, as these tissues, by definition, are target sites for SMOADs. In addition we highlight some of the difficulties and concerns that may be encountered in using these joint tissues as structural/disease biomarkers of OA because of the limitations in the techniques that can monitor the complex temporal and regional changes that may coexist within these joints during the initiation and progression of this disease.

Articular cartilage

The primary function of AC is to transmit and disperse mechanical stresses imposed across joints during load bearing and to facilitate, with the assistance of synovial fluid, low-friction articulation. These important functions of AC are made possible by its unique composition and structure. In simple terms, AC may be considered as a anisotropic biomaterial composed of a three-dimensional network of type II collagen fibrils that are inflated by underhydrated proteoglycan (PG) aggregates (aggrecans). The living element of AC is the chondrocyte that senses and responds to changes in its environment by synthesizing an extracellular matrix necessary to sustain cartilage function throughout the animal's lifetime. Articular cartilage, like bone, obeys Wolff's Law in that the resident chondrocytes respond to the mechanical stresses placed upon them by synthesizing a matrix that is the most capable of dispersing the applied stresses.[3] However, this adaptive response may be modified by extrinsic factors, such as cell senescence or hormonal changes as occurs following the female menopause or during synovial inflammation when cytokines, free radicals, and proteinase may diffuse into cartilage and modify chondrocyte metabolism. It is apparent therefore, that AC may fail, as occurs in OA, when the chondrocyte is unable to maintain an extracellular matrix capable of resisting the loads applied to it during normal weight-bearing functions.

Experiments undertaken in the author's laboratories over several years using an ovine model of OA, have provided valuable insights into the adaptive response of AC chondrocytes to alterations to mechanical stresses, the nature of which are commonly associated with the initiation and progression of human OA. In this model, both hindlimbs of aged ewes are subjected to lateral meniscectomy and two weeks after surgery animals are allowed normal weight-bearing exercise. Age matched nonoperated ewes maintained under the same conditions are used as controls. At necropsy, six months post meniscectomy, knee joints from all animals are dissected and the tibial plateaux divided into 26 zones as shown by the grid pattern in Fig. 11.1(b). Each zone is then subjected to histological, biochemical, and biomechanical, microanalysis.[4] On the lateral tibia plateaux of the meniscectomized joints the classical pathological hallmarks of early OA were clearly evident (Fig. 11.1(a)), with focal AC lesions almost down to the bone (zones 2 and 6 in Fig. 11.1(b)) and prominent osteophytes at the outer margin of the joint, particularly posteriorly (zones 9 and 13 in Fig. 11.1). Topographical microanalysis of the composition of AC over the surface of the lateral tibial plateaux showed that the sulfated glycosaminoglycans (a marker of PGs) (Fig. 11.2) were depleted from the lesion and adjacent zones, and this loss was accompanied by an increase in water content and AC thickness (Fig. 11.2). By contrast, the PG content of AC located along the outer lateral margin of the OA joints was elevated and cartilage was thicker, relative to the same regions of nonoperated control joints (Fig. 11.2). Although the AC of the medial compartment of the operated joints appeared macroscopically normal (Fig. 11.1) microanalysis for S-GAGs revealed an overall increase and redistribution of this component, such that the highest amounts present were now located towards the outer regions of this compartment (zones 20, 21, and 23 in Fig. 11.2). In the nonoperated control group these regional cartilage S-GAG concentrations correlated with AC thickness ($R = 0.86$). However, this correlation was lost following meniscectomy ($R = 0.18$). Determination of the effective shear modulus (ESM) (G') for each of the 26 zones shown in Fig. 11.1 using a micro dynamic indentor[5] (Fig. 11.2) demonstrated a marked change in G' in both the medial and lateral compartments of the operated joints. In the meniscectomized compartment there was an overall decline in ESM, but in the posterior half of the outer margins on the medial side (zones 24 and 26) it increased. The correlation between S-GAG and ESM, which prior to meniscectomy was reasonable ($R = -0.81$), was also lost following establishment of OA ($R = 0.01$). Analysis of collagen birefringence using picrosirius

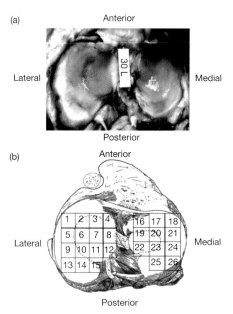

Fig. 11.1 (a) Photograph of the tibial plateau from an aged ewe, six months following lateral meniscectomy to induce OA. Note the cartilage lesion and formation of large osteophytes along the rim of the lateral compartment. The medial compartment appears macroscopically normal. (b) Grid pattern used for topographical biomechanical and biochemical analysis of articular cartilage of the tibial plateaux from OA and nonoperated control animals. The broken lines represent the normal position of the menisci.

red-stained coronal histological sections cut across the lesion area (zones 5, 6, 7, 8) indicated disruption of the alignment and/or assembly of collagen fibres at the surface and deep regions of lateral AC.

What do these findings tell us with respect to the structural changes that take place in AC of OA joints? Firstly, they show that degradation of AC in one compartment of a joint is associated with a spectrum of AC matrix changes throughout the rest of the joint. Secondly, while the AC adjacent to the focal lesion or in another compartment may appear macroscopically normal or even 'better' than normal AC, as judged by measurements of its thickness or PG content, it may still be biomechanically inadequate. Thirdly, these animal experiments suggest that collagen fibril integrity and/or assembly, particularly in the superficial zone of AC may be a more useful marker of early AC structural change in OA than its thickness or PG content. Similar conclusions have been reached by other investigators using AC from canine models[6–8] and human AC obtained at autopsy or following joint replacement surgery.[9–11]

Given that a disturbance in joint mechanics, as occurs in OA subjects, is accompanied by both catabolic and anabolic changes in cartilage, the question arises, whether it is logical to use joint-space narrowing (JSN), which is considered to correlate with AC loss as a marker of disease progression. The problem is compounded by the difficulty of obtaining a satisfactory radiograph of the knee over the long periods required to detect joint-space changes in OA.[12] Failure to reproducibly position the patient in the X-ray beam at each visit can introduce errors in image magnification and measurement of joint-space width, due to malalignment of the beam axis with the surface of the tibial plateaux.[12] Problems in assessing JSN may also arise because of the inability of X-rays to identify injuries and degenerative changes in joint soft tissues such as the menisci and ligaments. Since these weight-bearing structures also serve to reduce contact between the AC surfaces, their extrusion or failure can lead to a reduction in the radiologically determined joint width without loss of AC.[13,14] These and other issues related to the radiological assessment of joints are discussed in detail elsewhere (see Appendix 4).

On the basis of the above considerations, it is clear that the use of conventional X-ray imaging technology to study structural changes in OA joints is fraught with many problems, yet this technique is still considered

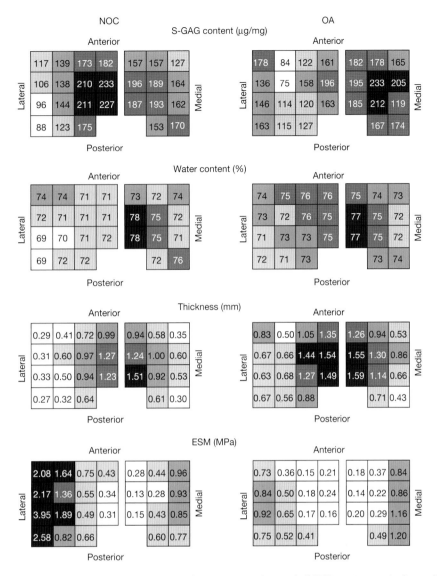

Fig. 11.2 Topographical analysis of articular cartilages on the tibial plateaux from nonoperated controls (NOC), meniscectomized ewes (OA) for sulfated glycosaminoglycans (S-GAG), water content, thickness, and effective shear moduli (ESM), using the zones shown in Fig. 11.1. The numbers shown in each zone represent the mean of six animals in each group and the dark shading corresponds to the highest values and light to the lowest. Note the marked changes in all parameters in both the lateral and medial compartments, six months following induction of OA.

to be the 'gold standard' by many. Moreover, it has and will continue to be used as a method of demonstrating disease modification in OA as illustrated by a recent double-blind clinical study, which reported that OA patients who consumed 1.5 grams of glucosamine sulphate a day for three years only lost −0.06 mm of joint space in the medial compartment of their knees, while a matched placebo group showed a −0.31 mm reduction leading the authors to suggest that this compound was a SMOAD.[15]

Magnetic resonance imaging (MRI) has been proposed as an alternative methodology for identifying early joint changes in OA. Validated methods for quantitating cartilage volume, PG, or water content in cadaveric or post surgical AC specimens have been described[16–19] thereby confirming the potential of this technique. However, the low resolution and sensitivity of currently available commercial instruments has so far limited the use of this technique for the evaluation of SMOADs in patients. In addition, the ability of MRI to detect cartilage changes in OA must also be examined in the light of the compensatory response of AC to the alterations in mechanical stresses introduced across joints during the initiation and progression of the disease, as highlighted in our animal studies. While MRI does have the distinct advantage of

allowing meniscal extrusion and other soft tissue changes, which are known to influence JSN, to be detected,[13] the use of this technique to identify small topographical variations in the PGs and abnormalities in collagen assembly in AC still lies within the realms of developmental research. Nevertheless, this research has shown that MRI combined with contrast agents such as Gd-$(DTPA)^{2-}$ or other instrument modifications is capable of detecting changes in tissue PGs and collagens at the molecular level.

The subchondral bone and intraosseous circulation in OA

Radiological, anatomical, and histological studies have confirmed that calcified cartilage (CC) and the adjacent subchondral bone of OA joints all undergo structural modification during the development of OA. These subchondral changes may even take place before macroscopic signs of degeneration are evident in AC.[20,21]

Typical subchondral bone changes in OA joints are illustrated in Figs 11.3 and 11.4, which again were derived from studies using our ovine OA model induced by lateral meniscectomy. In those regions of the joint subjected to high focal stresses and below the AC lesion zone (Fig. 11.3), the cortical plate is seen to be thickened (subchondral sclerosis), while in the cancellous bone the fatty marrow spaces between trabeculae are increased.

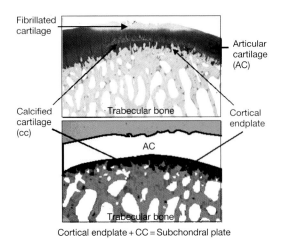

Fig. 11.3 Photomicrograph of a Toluidine-blue stained histological section of the lesion and adjacent region of a femoral condyle from a laterally meniscectomized ewe (top) and a line drawing of this region (bottom) showing the noncalcified articular cartilage (AC), calcified cartilage (CC), cortical endplate and trabecular (cancellous) bone. The subchondral bone plate (SCP) is considered as the CC + cortical endplate. Note the thickened subchondral bone beneath the AC lesion area.

As is evident from these figures and noted in studies of human subchondral bone,[22] microinjuries and fragmentation of trabeculae occur in OA joints. These cortical and cancellous bone changes are invariably accompanied by the advancement of the CC mineralization front (tide mark) into the AC, and this latter response is considered to be one of the main reasons for cartilage thinning in OA joints.[22–24] The extent and nature of the metabolic response of the subchondral bone and its vascular tissues to the altered mechanical stresses introduced by OA, may be further modified by the interactions of resident cells with circulating factors, such as cytokines, prostanoids, free radicals, hormones, vitamins, growth factors, and with some drugs. The subchondral bone response to the nitric oxide free radical donor, glyceryl trinitrate (GTN), in a group of meniscectomized sheep who were administered the drug for six months is an example of this[25] and the results are shown in Fig. 11.4. As can be readily seen, GTN increased the subchondral bone plate thickness not only in the meniscectomized lateral compartment but also on the medial side when it corrected the loss induced by OA in the outer region of the femoral condyle. These bone-preserving effects of GTN appeared to be mediated by the known ability of nitric oxide radicals to inhibit osteoclastic bone resorption[26] and were consistent with the clinical use of this agent to increase bone mineral density (BMD) in postmenopausal women.[27] The thickened subchondral bone plate in joints of the GTN-treated animals would be expected to reduce the shock absorbing qualities of the subchondral bone, thereby increasing the stresses borne by the overlaying AC and thus contributing to its degradation. In a parallel study on the AC from these animals, this appeared to be the case.[28] Other bone antiresorptive drugs such as bisphosphonates are also under investigation as potential SMOADs.[29,30] In the Myers et al. study,[30] an ACL deficient canine OA model was used and although the bisphosphonate reduced bone turnover in the unstable knees it did not diminish cartilage loss or osteophyte formation. Oestrogen replacement therapy (ERT) in post menopausal women has been shown to slow the progression of their OA as determined by conventional radiographic measurement of JSN.[31] In a

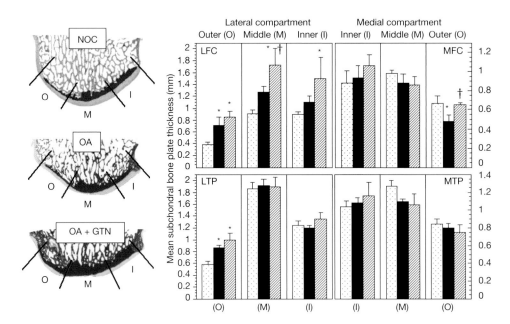

Fig. 11.4 Left-hand side, representative photomicrograph of Masson trichrome stained histological sections of lateral femoral condyles from nonoperated controls (NOC), laterally meniscectomized (OA) animals and OA animals treated for six months with the nitric oxide donor, glyceryl trinitrate (GTN). Right-hand side, using sections from six animals in each group the mean (± SEM) subchondral bone plate (SCP) thickness of the inner (I), middle (M), and outer (O) regions of the medial (M) and lateral (L) femoral condyles (FC) and tibial plateaux (TP) were determined using computer-assisted analysis of digitized images. Significant increases in SCP thickness occurred in all zones (inner, middle, and outer) of the lateral compartment in OA joints and this was elevated further by GTN treatment. In the outer zone of the MFC, GTN treatment restored SCP thickness to NOC values ▨ = NOC, ■ = OA, ▨ = OA + GTN.

*Significantly different from NOC ($p < 0.05$).

†OA + GTN significantly different from OA ($p < 0.05$).

group of ovariectomized ewes subjected to meniscectomy to induce OA, ERT not only maintained BMD but preserved the levels of PGs in their AC.[32] Similarly, the interleukin-1 inhibitor, Diacerhein, was found to partially protect AC as well as reduce subchondral plate thickness but not osteophyte formation.[33] In contrast, calcium pentosan polysulfate (CaPPS), administered orally to OA sheep for six months mitigated vascular invasion of the CC and reduced osteophyte formation at the margin of the tibial plateaux (see Fig. 11.5). Other studies with the same model showed that CaPPS maintained AC integrity as well as its biomechanical properties, in regions adjacent to the OA lesions.[34,35]

Structural modification in OA by therapeutic agents, as exemplified by the few experimental studies cited here, could therefore include drugs that normalize subchondral bone turnover or reduce osteophyte formation in those regions of OA joints subjected to high focal stresses. Moreover, these adaptive bone changes in OA joints are more readily monitored and quantitated by existing imaging techniques, such as microfocal radiography, high-resolution computer tomography, and bone scintigraphy.

Angiogenesis and vascular invasion of the calcified cartilage occurs contemporaneously with subchondral plate remodelling in weight-bearing areas of OA joints; the vessels originating in the trabecular bone. The numbers of these vessels crossing the cortical plate and calcified cartilage normally decreases with ageing, but in OA femoral and humeral heads the numbers increase[36] and may provide a major route for solute exchange

with AC.[22] Venous congestion and elevated intraosseous pressure in the subchondral vasculature of OA joints has been proposed as an important cause of joint pain in patients with primary disease.[37–40] Histological studies of OA femoral heads have revealed that the marrow spaces of the cancellous bone become engorged with lipid, cholesterol, and fibrin deposits.[40–42] Venous stasis and hypertension arising from the subchondral thrombosis accompanied by variable bone necrosis can be a relatively early histological event in OA and may be present before cartilage degeneration is evident.[43] As the disease progresses, bone necrosis becomes more widespread, particularly in and adjacent to the eburnated bone and the distal areas of femoral heads.[37,40,41] In a study of 25 heads of femur removed at the time of total joint replacement surgery for OA, 16 showed widespread loss of osteocyte viability and bone death, leading these investigators to suggest that OA of the hip was strongly associated with episodic osteocyte death, which may have existed for many years prior to the appearance of clinical symptoms.[44] Haematological studies of blood from many patients with generalized OA have demonstrated the existence of a hypercoagulable and/or hypofibrinolytic state. This may predispose such patients to thrombosis and vascular dysfunctions, particularly at compromised sites such as in the subchondral vasculature of OA joints.[40–42] It has been proposed that certain blood coagulation and fibrinolytic factors might be employed as surrogate markers of OA.[42]

From the above discussion it may be deduced that agents, which possess the ability to mobilize thrombi and lipids within the subchondral vascular of OA joints, may qualify as both disease- and symptom-modifying OA drugs. Potent anticoagulant activity in itself would be undesirable, as the potential risk of gastrointestinal bleeding in older patients, who may have been chronic users of NSAIDs, would outweigh any benefits that might be obtained by improving their subchondral blood circulation. However, agents with low anticoagulant activity but high fibrinolytic, lipolytic, and antiinflammatory activities might be acceptable candidates. One class of drugs, the pentosan polysulphates (PPS), which have been studied for more than 40 years as thromboprophylactics, would appear to meet this criteria.[45] In human and veterinary clinical studies undertaken with CaPPS and NaPPS, improvement in OA symptoms was accompanied by normalization of fibrinolytic and lipolytic parameters in patients' blood for up to four weeks post treatment.[45] Furthermore, recent laboratory research has shown that CaPPS protected AC by reducing aggrecanase activity[46] and upregulating the production of tissue inhibitor of matrix metalloproteinases-3 (TIMP-3) by chondrocytes and synovial cells.[47] These haematological and chondroprotective activities of CaPPS may account for its ability to reduce osteophyte formation and subchondral angiogenesis in the sheep OA model (Fig. 11.5).

Conclusion

The biological changes that take place in all OA joint tissues are extremely diverse and vary with the cause and the phase of the disease. In the early and mid stages it is common to find regions of cartilage and subchondral bone where catabolic processes are proceeding, adjacent to tissues undergoing predominantly hypermetabolic changes. Structural changes in OA and its modification by drugs must take into consideration the adaptable nature of joint connective tissues and accommodate such dynamic complexities into methods of assessment. Unfortunately the noninvasive methods currently available for detecting structural changes in OA joints are not capable of achieving this. For these reasons, the demonstration of disease or structural modification in OA by therapeutic agents is presently based on studies using animal models. While these models cannot truly simulate the diverse time dependent, hormonal, and genetic events, which take place in human OA, they have allowed direct topographic sampling and detailed analysis of joint tissues collected during the early, middle, and late stages of OA. The pool of knowledge generated by these animal studies has allowed potential biomarkers for human OA research to be identified and has spawned new strategies for treatment. If disease modification in OA is to become a reality, the limitations of present methods of assessing structural changes in joint

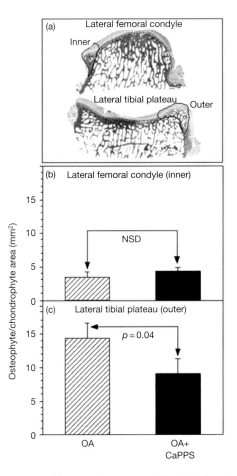

Fig. 11.5 Representative Masson trichrome-stained histological sections of the lateral femoral condyle and lateral tibial plateau from an OA sheep joint showing osteophyte development at the inner and outer margins (a). In OA animals ($n = 6$) treated orally with 20 mg/kg CaPPS each week, osteophyte size (as determined by computer assisted analysis of digital images) in the lateral condyle remained unaffected by treatment (b) but was reduced in the lateral tibial plateaux (c).

tissues must be resolved and the complexities of the OA disease process recognized.

Key points

1. Structural modifying OA drugs (SMOADs) are defined as agents that slow, arrest, or reverse those structural changes that take place in OA joints, which reflect its underlying pathology.

2. This pathology exists primarily in cartilage, fibrocartilage (menisci), subchondral bone and in other joint tissues, such as synovial fluid and synovium. However, noninvasive methods that are capable of demonstrating structural or molecular changes in these tissues are still undergoing development and validation.

3. On the other hand, studies using animal models that permit joint tissue to be analyzed using well established analytical procedures have provided valuable insights into the structural changes that take place in OA during initiation and early progression of the disease. Furthermore, such studies have allowed putative SMOADs to be identified.

4. While X-ray imaging is presently the gold standard for assessing structural modification in OA, the inability of this technique to show joint soft tissue changes directly, is a distinct disadvantage.

5. MRI, in contrast to X-ray imaging, is capable of capturing and storing data from both hard and soft joint tissues of OA joints and will allow some of the changes, which occur in their extracellular matrices to be quantitated. This technique, therefore, offers considerable potential as a method of demonstrating pharmacological modification of joint breakdown in OA.

References

(An asterisk denotes recommended reading.)

1. Dougados, M., Devogelaer, J.P., Annefeldt, M., *et al*. (1996). Recommendations for the registration of drugs used in the treatment of osteoarthritis. *Ann Rheum Dis* **55**:552–7.

2. *Altman, R., Brandt, K., Hochberg, M., *et al*. (1996). Design and conduct of clinical trials in patients with osteoarthritis: Recommendations from a task force of the Osteoarthritis Research Society. *Osteoarthritis Cart* **4**:217–43.

    This report records the recommendations of a task force convened to examine therapeutic management in OA. The report provides definitions for the classes of drugs to be used and presents guidelines for their clinical assessment.

3. Helminen, H.J., Hyttinen, M.M., Lammi, M.J., *et al*. (2000). Regular joint loading in youth assists in the establishment and strengthening of the collagen network of articular cartilage and contributes to the prevention of osteoarthrosis later in life: A hypothesis. *J Bone Miner Metabol* **18**:245–57.

4. Appleyard, R., Burkhardt, D., Ghosh, P., *et al*. (2002). Topographical relationships between cartilage biochemical and dynamic biomechanical properties in an ovine model of osteoarthritis. *Osteoarthritis Cart (submitted for publication)*.

5. Appleyard, R.C., Swain, M.V., Khanna, S., and Murrell, G.A.C. (2001). The accuracy and reliability of a novel hand-held dynamic indentation probe for analysing articular cartilage. *Phys Med Biol* **46**:1–10.

6. Setton, L.A., Mow, V.C., and Howell, D.S. (1995). Mechanical behavior of articular cartilage in shear is altered by transection of the anterior cruciate ligament. *J Orthop Res* **13**:473–82.

7. LeRoux, M.A., Arokoski, J., Vail, T.P., *et al*. (2000). Simultaneous changes in the mechanical properties, quantitative collagen organization, and proteoglycan concentration of articular cartilage following canine meniscectomy. *J Orthop Res* **18**:383–92.

8. Jurvelin, J.S., Arokoski, J.P., Hunziker, E.B., and Helminen, H.J. (2000). Topographic variation of the elastic properties of articular cartilage in the canine joint. *J Biomech* **33**:669–75.

9. Bader, D.L., Kempson, G.E., Egan, J., Gilbey, W., and Barrett, A.J. (1992). The effects of selective matrix degradation on the short-term compressive properties of adult human articular cartilage. *Biochim Biophys Acta* **1116**:147–54.

10. Obeid, E.M.H., Adams, M.A., and Newman, J.H. (1994). Mechanical properties of articular cartilage in knees with unicompartmental osteoarthritis. *J Bone Joint Surg Br* **76B**:315–9.

11. Franz, T., Hasler, E.M., Hagg, R., Weiler, C., Jakob, R.P., and Mainil-Varlet, P. (2001). *In situ* compressive stiffness, biochemical composition, and structural integrity of articular cartilage of the human knee joint. *Osteoarthritis Cart* **9**:582–92.

12. *Mazzuca, S.A., Brandt, K.D., and Katz, B.P. (1997). Is conventional radiography suitable for evaluation of a disease-modifying drug in patients with knee osteoarthritis? *Osteoarthritis Cart* **5**:217–26.

    This paper draws our attention to the limitations associated with the use of conventional radiology for determining joint-space narrowing in OA and questions its use to evaluate structural modifying OA drugs in a clinical setting.

13. Adams, J.G., McAlindon, T., Dimasi, M., Carey, J., and Eustace, S. (1999). Contribution of meniscal extrusion and cartilage loss to joint-space narrowing in osteoarthritis. *Clin Radiol* **54**:502–6.

14. Fife, R.S., Brandt, K.D., Braunstein, E.M., *et al*. (1991). Relationship between arthroscopic evidence of cartilage damage and radiographic evidence of joint space narrowing in early osteoarthritis of the knee. *Arthritis Rheum* **34**:377–82.

15. Reginster, J.Y., Deroisy, R., Rovati, L.C., *et al*. (2001). Long-term effects of glucosamine sulphate on osteoarthritis progression: A randomised, placebo-controlled clinical trial. *Lancet* **357**:251–6.

16. Bashir, A., Gray, M.L., and Burstein, D. (1996). Gd-DTPA^{2-} as a measure of cartilage degradation. *Magn Reson Med* **36**:665–73.

17. Bashir, A., Gray, M.L., Hartke, J., and Burstein, D. (1999). Nondestructive imaging of human cartilage glycosaminoglycan concentration by MRI. *Magn Reson Med* **41**:857–65.

18. *Burstein, D., Bashir, A., and Gray, M.L. (2000). MRI techniques in early stages of cartilage disease. *Invest Radiol* **35**:622–38.

    This article provides an excellent review of the potential of MRI to evaluate cartilage and other soft tissue changes in OA joints.

19. Eckstein, F., Reiser, M., Englmeier, K-H., and Putz, R. (2001). *In vivo* morphometry and functional analysis of human articular cartilage with quantitative magnetic resonance imaging—from image to data, from data to theory. *Anat Embryol* **203**:147–73.

20. Bailey, A.J. and Mansell, J.P. (1997). Do subchondral bone changes exacerbate or precede articular cartilage destruction in osteoarthritis of the elderly? *Gerontology* **43**:296–304.

21. Carlson, C.S., Loeser, R.F., Jayo, M.J., Weaver, D.S., Adams, M.R., and Jerome, C.P. (1994). Osteoarthritis in cynomolgus macaques: A primate model of naturally occurring disease. *J Orthop Res* **12**:331–9.

22. *Imhof, H., Sulzbacher, I., Grampp, S., Czerny, C., Youssefzadeh, S., and Kainberger, F. (2000). Subchondral bone and cartilage disease: A rediscovered functional unit. *Invest Radiol* **35**:581–8.

    This article provides a comprehensive review of the close interplay between cartilage and subchondral bone in OA.

23. Hulth, A. (1993). Does osteoarthrosis depend on growth of the mineralized layer of cartilage. *Clin Orthop* **287**:19–24.

24. Oegema, T.R., Jr., Carpenter, R.J., Hofmeister, F., and Thompson, R.C. (1997). The interaction of the zone of calcified cartilage and subchondral bone in osteoarthritis. *Microsc Res Tech* **37**:324–32.

25. Cake, M.A., Read, R.A., Hwa, S-Y., and Ghosh, P. Glyceryl trinitrate increases subchondral bone thickness and density in an ovine meniscectomy model of osteoarthritis. *Osteoarthritis Cart (submitted for publication)*.

26. Ralston, S.H., Ho, L.P., Helfrich, M.H., Grabowski, P.S., Johnstone, P.W., and Benjamin, N. (1995). Nitric oxide: A cytokine induced regulator of bone resorption. *J Bone Miner Res* **10**:1040–9.

27. Jamal, S.A., Browner, W.S., Bauer, D.C., and Cummings, S.R. (1998). Intermittent use of nitrates increase bone mineral density: The study of osteoporotic fractures. *J Bone Miner Res* **13**:1755–9.

28. Cake, M. (2001). PhD *Thesis*. Murdoch University, WA, Australia.

29. Cocco, R., Tofi, C., Fioravanti, A., *et al*. (1999). Effects of clodronate on synovial fluid levels of some inflammatory mediators, after intra-articular

administration to patients with synovitis secondary to knee osteoarthritis. *Boll Soc Ital Biol Sper* **75**:71–6.

30. Myers, S.L., Brandt, K.D., Burr, D.B., O'Connor, B.L., and Albrecht, M. (1999). Effects of a bisphosphonate on bone histomorphometry and dynamics in the canine cruciate deficiency model of osteoarthritis. *J Rheumatol* **26**:2645–53.

31. Felson, D.T. and Nevitt, M.C. (1999). Estrogen and osteoarthritis: How do we explain conflicting study results? *Prev Med* **28**:445–8.

32. Parker, D., Smith, S.M., Hwa, S-Y., Smith, M.M., and Ghosh, P. (2000). Estrogen replacement therapy mitigates the loss of joint cartilage proteoglycans and bone mineral density induced by ovariectomy and osteoarthritis. *Osteoarthritis Cart* **8**(suppl 8): 546.

33. Hwa, S-Y., Burkhardt, D., Little, C., and Ghosh, P. (2001). The effects of orally administered Diacerein on cartilage and subchondral bone in an ovine model of osteoarthritis. *J Rheumatol* **28**:825–34.

34. Appleyard, R., Swain, M., and Ghosh, P. (2000). Modification of the dynamic shear modulus and phase lag properties of tibial plateau articular cartilage in an ovine model of osteoarthritis by oral administration of calcium pentosan polysulfate. *Trans Orthop Res Soc Meeting* 320.

35. Hwa, S-Y., Smith, M.M., Sambrook, P., and Ghosh, P. The protective effects of calcium pentosan polysulfate on calcified cartilage integrity in the medial compartment of joints of an ovine model of osteoarthritis. *Osteoarthritis Cart (submitted for publication).*

36. Lane, L.B., Villacin, A., and Bullough, P.G. (1977). The vascularity and remodelling of subchondral bone and calcified cartilage in adult human femoral and humeral heads. *J Bone Joint Surg Br* **59B**:272–8.

37. Arnoldi, C.C. (1994). Vascular aspects of degenerative joint disorders. *Acta Orthop Scand* **65**:1–82.

38. *Kiaer, T. (1987). The intraosseous circulation and pathogenesis of osteoarthritis. *Med Sci Res* **15**:759–63.

    This review provides an excellent introduction to the pathological events that occur in the subchondral bone and vasculature of OA joints.

39. Arnoldi, C.C., Lemberg, R.K., and Linderholm, H. (1975). Intraosseous hypertension and pain in the knee. *J Bone Joint Surg Br* **57B**:360–3.

40. *Bullough, P.G. and DiCarlo, E.F. (1990). Subchondral avascular necrosis— a common cause of arthritis. *Ann Rheum Dis* **49**:412–20.

    This report draws our attention to the abnormalities that exist in the subchondral vasculature of many OA joints.

41. Cheras, P.A., Freemont, A.J., and Sikorski, J.M. (1993). Intraosseous thrombosis in ischemic necrosis of bone and osteoarthritis. *Osteoarthritis Cart* **1**:291–32.

42. Cheras, P.A., Whitaker, A.N., Blackwell, E.A., Sinton, T.J., Chapman, M.D., and Peacock, K.A. (1997). Hypercoagulability and hypofibrinolysis in primary osteoarthritis. *Clin Orthop* **334**:57–67.

43. Levin, D., Norman, D., Zinman, C., Misselevich, I., Reis, D.N., and Boss, J.H. (1999). Osteoarthritis-like disorder in rats with vascular deprivation-induced necrosis of the femoral head. *Pathol Res Pract* **195**:637–47.

44. Wong, S.Y.P., Evans, R.A., Needs, C., Dunstan, C.R., Hills, E., and Garvan, J. (1987). The pathogenesis of osteoarthritis of the hip—evidence for primary osteocyte death. *Clin Orthop* **214**:305–12.

45. Ghosh, P. (1999). The pathobiology of osteoarthritis and the rationale for the use of pentosan polysulfate for its treatment. *Sem Arthritis Rheum* **28**:211–67.

46. *Munteanu, S.E., Ilic, M.Z., and Handley, C.J. (2000). Calcium pentosan polysulphate inhibits the catabolism of aggrecan in articular cartilage explant cultures. *Arthritis Rheum* **43**:2211–8.

    Since aggrecanase is responsible for the turnover of proteoglycans in normal and OA cartilage, its inhibition could provide a means of slowing disease progression. This report demonstrates that CaPPS was capable of inhibiting aggrecanase and reducing proteoglycan loss from cartilage at concentrations readily achievable in vivo.

47. Takizawa, M., Ohuchi, E., Yamanaka, H., *et al.* (2000). Production of tissue inhibitor of metalloproteinases 3 is selectively enhanced by calcium pentosan polysulfate in human rheumatoid synovial fibroblasts. *Arthritis Rheum* **43**:812–20.

11.2.2 The clinical perspective

Kenneth D. Brandt

Definition of DMOADs and rationale for their use

Although the pathologic hallmark of OA is a progressive loss of articular cartilage over the habitually loaded areas of the diarthrodial joint, it is clear that not only the cartilage, but *all* of the tissues of the joint are affected in OA: the subchondral bone, synovium, capsule, ligaments, periarticular muscle, and sensory neurons whose endings lie within these tissues (see Chapter 5). Abnormalities in any of these tissues may be of etiologic importance in the condition that is recognized clinically as OA.

Although in most cases the pathologic changes of OA are asymptomatic, because of the sheer prevalence of OA, the prevalence of significant joint pain and disability in even a minority of those with pathologic changes results in enormous medicoeconomic and socioeconomic burdens (see Chapters 3 and 9.14). Until recently, pharmacological therapy for OA was aimed exclusively at symptom relief and has been based mainly on the use of acetaminophen and other analgesics and nonsteroidal anti-inflammatory drugs (NSAIDs). However, as greater understanding of the pathogenetic mechanisms in OA has accrued, interest has burgeoned in the development of new classes of drugs that are not primarily analgesics or anti-inflammatory agents but whose mechanism of action is directed at the inhibition of catabolic processes or stimulation of anabolic processes in the OA joint. These agents were initially called 'chondroprotective drugs', but because of the recognition that the pathologic changes of OA are much more extensive than those in cartilage alone, more recently they have been designated Disease-Modifying OA Drugs, DMOADs,[1] or Structure-Modifying OA Drugs, SMOADs.[2] For the most part, these agents have been designed to act upon pathogenetic mechanisms in articular cartilage; to a lesser extent, they have been directed at processes in subchondral bone.

The ability of articular cartilage to withstand—in most cases, for a lifetime—repeated loading and motion is attributable to the properties of the extracellular matrix produced by its chondrocytes. As described in Chapters 7.2.1.1 and 7.2.1.4, these properties depend on interactions between the fibrillar and nonfibrillar components of the matrix. The fibrillar components of articular cartilage are types II, IX, and XI collagen. The nonfibrillar components include aggrecan, the dominant high molecular weight proteoglycan; smaller proteoglycans, such as decorin and biglycan; and a variety of other noncollagenous proteins, such as cartilage oligomeric matrix protein (COMP). It is likely that all of these components are important for the normal function of articular cartilage; in a number of cases, mutations in the genes responsible for their synthesis have been shown to result in joint damage indistinguishable from that of OA. (see Chapter 4.2).

In normal articular cartilage a balance exists between matrix synthesis and degradation. OA is characterized by increased degradation and inadequate synthesis of matrix, resulting in cartilage destruction (although, at least until the very late stages of the disease, synthesis of proteoglycans, collagens, and other matrix molecules is increased, presumably reflecting repair activity by the chondrocytes).

Matrix metalloproteinases (MMPs)

Matrix metalloproteinases, zinc-dependent proteinases with a common domain structure, are the principal matrix-degrading enzymes of the extracellular matrix of articular cartilage. More than 20 MMPs have been identified (see tables 1–4, Chapter 7.2.1.2). On the basis of their structure and substrates specificities, they can be subdivided into collagenases, gelatinases,

Table 11.2 Properties of the tissue inhibitors of matrix metalloproteinases (TIMPs)

Property	TIMP-1	TIMP-2	TIMP-3	TIMP-4
MMPs inhibited	All, except for most MT-MMPs	All	All	MMP-1, -2, -3, -7, -9
Molecular mass	20.6 kDa	21.5 kDa	21.6 kDa	22.3 kDa
Expression	Inducible	Constitutive	Inducible	—
Expressed in cartilage	Yes	Yes	Yes	—
Binding to pro-MMPs	MMP-9	MMP-2	MMP-2, -9	MMP-2

MT-MMP, membrane type MMP.

Source: Taken from Bigg, H.F. and Rowan, A.D. 2001. *Curr Opin Pharma* **1**:314–20.[3]

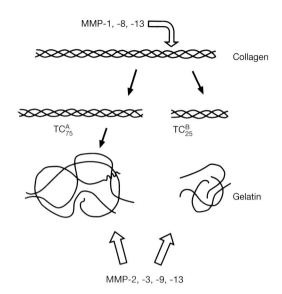

Fig. 11.6 Cleavage of the triple helix of collagen by MMP. Collagenases cleave triple-helical collagen into two fragments (TC^A and TC^B) at a specific site, three-fourths the length of the molecule downstream from the aminoterminus. The cleaved collagen undergoes denaturation, and other MMPs are able to degrade the polypeptides.

Source: Taken from Ref. 6.

stromelysins, membrane-type MMPs (MT-MMPs) and others. Acting in concert, they can degrade all of the components of articular cartilage. Control of MMP activity in cartilage occurs at a variety of levels, including regulating of gene expression, activation of the secreted proenzymes, and inhibition of the active enzymes by endogenous inhibitors, such as the Tissue Inhibitors of Metalloproteinases (TIMPs), a family of inhibitors that form irreversible one-to-one complexes with the MMPs[3,4] (Table 11.2). Theoretically, therapeutic intervention may be targeted at each of these loci.

Native fibrillar collagen types I, II, and III are degraded by MMP-1, -8, and -13. More recently, it has been shown that MMP-2 and -14 are also capable of degrading native fibrillar collagen.[4,5] All of these collagenolytic enzymes are synthesized by the chondrocytes in human OA cartilage. In each case, cleavage of the collagen fibril occurs at a specific site, approximately three-fourths of the distance from the amino terminus in all 3 chains of the triple helix. At physiologic temperature (e.g., *in vivo*) the cleaved helix unwinds and the ends are subject to further degradation by collagenolytic enzymes and other proteinases[6] (Fig. 11.6). MMP-13 appears to be the predominant collagenase involved in degradation of the articular cartilage matrix in OA, although MMP-2, -8, and -14 may also be involved.[4,7] When the local balance between active MMPs and their inhibitors is altered so that the active enzymes are present in excess, cartilage destruction may occur. Broadly speaking, the objective in developing DMOADs that aim at therapeutic inhibition of MMP(s) is to restore the stoichiometry by decreasing the level of active enzyme and/or increasing the level of inhibitors.

As an alternative to inhibition of degradation of the collagen network in articular cartilage, direct inhibition of cartilage proteoglycan loss also represents a reasonable therapeutic target for a DMOAD. Some concern has been expressed, however, that the increased proteoglycan synthesis in OA may represent a normal physiologic response to tissue damage, and that inhibition of this 'repair response' may be undesirable. Although it was originally believed as being mediated by MMPs, proteoglycan loss in OA has now been shown to be due chiefly to 'aggrecanases', members of the ADAM (a disintegrin and metalloproteinase) family of enzymes. Two aggrecanases have been identified[8,9] and it is likely that more exist.

Cytokines

Because ADAM-17 is involved in the processing of pro-tumor necrosis factor-α (pro-TNF-α) it is known also as TNF-α-converting enzyme (TACE).[10] TNFα can stimulate its own production through autocrine and paracrine mechanisms, and can also induce chondrocytes and synovial cells to generate other cytokines, proteases, and prostaglandin E$_2$ (PGE$_2$). The ADAMs can be inhibited by synthetic MMP inhibitors, but are generally unaffected by the TIMPs, although TIMP-3 is an effective inhibitor of TACE[11] and of ADAMTS-4 and -5 (aggrecanase-1 and -2, respectively).[12]

The proinflammatory cytokine, interleukin-1β (IL-1β), appears to play a more important role than TNF-α in destruction of the cartilage matrix in OA.[13,14] Like TNFα, IL-1β can stimulate its own production through autocrine and paracrine mechanisms and can induce synthesis by articular cartilage and synovium of other cytokines, proteases, including the MMPs; and PE G$_2$. Like TNF, IL-1β is synthesized as a precursor but is released into the extracellular matrix in an active form. IL-1β-converting enzymes (ICE), also called caspase-1, located in the plasma membrane, are responsible for generating the mature form of IL-1β.[15] Levels of ICE have been shown to be upregulated in articular cartilage and synovium from patients with OA.[16] Thus, pharmacological inhibition of ICE and TACE represent potential targets for DMOAD. The results of a recent clinical trial of diacerein, an anthraquinone derivative that appears to inhibit the synthesis and activity of IL-1 in patients with hip OA, are discussed below.

Activation of cells by IL-1 occurs through association of the cytokine with a specific cell-surface receptor, IL-1R. Two such receptors have been identified, IL-1R type I and in-IR type II.[17] The type I receptor has a slightly higher affinity for IL-1β than for IL-1α and is responsible for signal transduction. The number of type I IL-1R on OA chondrocytes is increased, rendering them more sensitive than normal chondrocytes to stimulation by IL-1β.[18] This results in up-regulation of the gene expression of a number of catabolic factors, including MMPs, which mediate cartilage destruction.

IL-1R is shed from the chondrocyte surface and may exist in the extracellular matrix and synovial fluid as a soluble IL-1 receptor (sIL-1R). Because its ligand-binding capacity is preserved, sIL-1R may function as a physiologic inhibitor of IL-1 and thereby regulate the activation of IL-1R on the cell surface. In addition, IL-1 receptor antagonist (IL-1Ra) a competitive inhibitor of IL-1R, can block a number of the catabolic pathways that are activated by IL-1, including chondrocyte synthesis of collagenase, PGE$_2$, and nitric oxide, all of which may lead to degradation of the extracellular matrix.[19,20] Although IL-1Ra levels in OA are higher than normal, they are far below that which would be needed to inhibit the markedly increased levels of IL-1β that are present.

Inhibition of signaling pathways involved in cytokine synthesis

The P38 mitogen-activated protein (MAP) kinase pathway and the nuclear factor, κB (NF-κB), are significantly involved in the synthesis of inflammatory cytokines and MMPs that are up-regulated in OA.[19] Compounds that inhibit P38 MAP kinase can block the production of some proinflammatory cytokines, such as IL-1β and TNFα[21] (Fig. 11.7), and have been designated cytokine-suppressive anti-inflammatory drugs (CSAIDs). Such agents have been shown to inhibit production of nitric oxide (NO) by OA cartilage from humans[22] and to have efficacy in animal models of inflammatory arthritis.[23] Inhibitors of NF-κB, therefore, have been considered as potential therapeutic agents for OA. In the collagen-induced arthritis model, when activation of NF-κB was inhibited by *in vivo* transfection of decoy oligodeoxynucleotides, reduction in the expression of IL-1β and TNFα in synovium and reduction in the severity of bone and cartilage damage were noted.[24] No clinical trials of inhibitors of MAP kinase or NF-κB have been undertaken in patients with OA, however.

Chapter 7.4.1 provides an excellent review of the cytokines, growth factors, and enzymes in synovium of OA joints that are likely to play an important role in various aspects of the pathology of OA, such as osteophyte formation, sclerosis of subchondral bone, and breakdown of the articular cartilage.

Synthetic MMP inhibitors

With the hope that they would be useful as DMOADs, synthetic MMP inhibitors have been designed that mimic the *in vivo* effects of TIMPs in blocking MMP activity. Initially, such inhibitors were designed to mimic part of the peptide sequence that surrounds the collagen cleavage site in interstitial collagenase,[25] permitting the inhibitor to fit tightly within the active site of the enzyme. The zinc atom in the active site of the collagenase molecule was then chelated through a zinc-binding group, such as an hydroxamate, carboxylate, aminocarboxylate, sulfhydryl, or phosphoric acid derivative.[26] Because of the effectiveness of hydroxamates as a zinc

chelator, most synthetic MMP inhibitors have been hydroxamates, but other ligands have been developed. Although the earlier compounds exhibited poor oral availability, more recently developed inhibitors exhibit good absorption from the gastrointestinal tract. Clinical trials of these agents have generally been conducted in patients with cancer, rather than OA, but the studies have nonetheless been helpful in disclosing a number of side effects that might mitigate the effectiveness of these drugs in treatment of patients with OA (see below). Recent reviews by Mengshol *et al.*[6] and by Pelletier *et al.*[27] provide excellent discussions of the rationale for use of MMP inhibitors in treatment of patients with OA.

The availability of crystal structures of the catalytic sites of a number of the MMPs has permitted the design of inhibitors that have selectivity for different members of the MMP family (Fig. 11.8). Compounds have been developed that exhibit enhanced inhibitory activity against MMPs whose tertiary structure includes a 'deep pocket' in the active site (such as gelatinase A, gelatinase B, and stromelysin-1), with much less activity against interstitial collagenase and matrilysin.[28] Thus, inhibitors with greater *selectivity* for gelatinase or collagenase have been developed, but *specificity* for only a single MMP has not been achieved[29] (Table 11.3).

Because MMPs are involved in normal physiologic processes whose inhibition might result in excessive deposition of extracellular matrix, the use of specific inhibitors, rather than of agents with broad MMP inhibition may be advantageous. It is not known, however, *which* MMP(s) should be inhibited in treatment of OA, although a wide variety of evidence suggests that collagenase inhibition might be useful. On the other hand, numerous redundancies exist in the activities of the MMPs in articular cartilage, and inhibition of one MMP may lead to compensation by others with similar substrate specificity.

Clinical trials of MMP inhibitors in humans with OA

Table 11.4 provides a list of MMP inhibitors that have been studied in clinical trials in humans, as published in the year 2000.[26] Although BAY-12-9566 showed promise in animal models of arthritis[30] and a small, small, short-term clinical trial suggested it was effective also in patients with OA,[31] a major large-scale phase III clinical trial was halted because of a report of increased tumor growth and decreased survival in patients with small cell carcinoma of the lung who were treated with this agent.[32] Lack of efficacy of Ro 32-3555 led to discontinuation by the manufacturers of their MMP inhibitor program in rheumatoid arthritis and also of an early-phase OA program for the compound, RS-130-830. Doxycycline, which was shown to have activity against collagenase and gelatinase *in vitro*[33] and efficacy in a canine model of OA *in vivo*,[34] is the only 'MMP inhibitor' (see below) currently being studied in a randomized placebo-controlled trial in patients with OA.

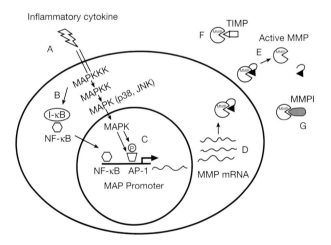

Fig. 11.7 Targets of MMP inhibition. The letters denote key regulatory steps in MMP gene regulation targeted by current and possible future therapies. A, Inflammatory cytokine receptor binding. B, Receptor activation, signaling pathway activation. C, MMP transcription. D, MMP mRNA stability and translation. E, Proteolytic cleavage and activation of MMPs. F, Tissue inhibitor of metalloproteinases (TIMP) protein binding and active site inhibition. G, Synthetic MMP inhibitors (MMPi). Inhibition of MMP gene expression can occur at steps A–D. MAPK, mitogen-activated protein kinase; JNK, c-Jun N-terminal kinase; NF-κB, nuclear factor κB; IκB, inhibitor of nuclear factor κB; AP-1, activator protein 1.

Source: Taken from Ref. 6.

Table 11.3 Inhibitory profiles of selected MMP inhibitors

Inhibitor* (assay)	MMP-1	MMP-2	MMP-3	MMP-7	MMP-9
Marimastat (IC$_{50}$)	5	6	200	20	3
CGS 27023A (K$_1$)	33	20	43	—	8
Prinomastat (K$_1$)	8	0.08	0.27	54	0.26
Solimastar (IC$_{50}$)	10	80	30	5	70
BAY 12-9566 (K$_1$)	>5000	11	134	—	301
Ro 32-3555 (K$_1$)	3	154	527	—	59
BMS-275291 (IC$_{50}$)	25	41	157	—	25
RS-130.830 (K$_1$)	590	0.22	9	1200	0.58

* Because assay conditions vary, the values shown provide only approximate comparisons.

Source: Taken from Brown, P.D. 2000. *Exp Opin Invest Drugs* **9**:2167–77.[26]

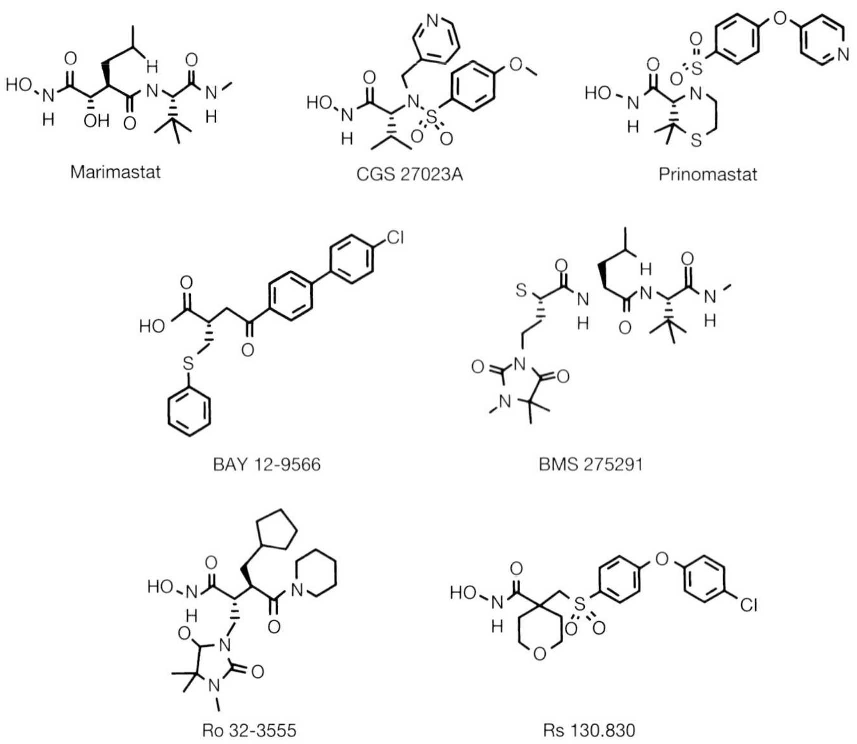

Marimastat

CGS 27023A

Prinomastat

BAY 12-9566

BMS 275291

Ro 32-3555

Rs 130.830

Fig. 11.8 Structures of some MMP inhibitors.

Source: Taken from Ref. 26.

Table 11.4 MMP inhibitors tested in clinical trials in humans

Compound	Company	Indication	Status of Trial
Prinomastat	Agouron/Pfizer	Cancer	Phase III
		Macular degeneration	Phase II
BAY 12-9566	Bayer	Cancer and OA	Suspended
Marimastat	BritishBiotech/ Schering-Plough	Cancer	Phase III
CGS 27023A	Novartis	Cancer	Suspended
RMS 275291	Celltech/Bristol- Myers Squibb	Cancer	Phase II
Metastat	CollaGenex	Cancer	Phase I
Neovastat	Aeterna	Cancer	Phases III
Ro 32-3555	Roche	Rheumatoid arthritis	Suspended
RS-130.830	Roche	OA	Suspended

Source: From Brown, P.D. 2000. *Exp Opin Invest Drugs* **9**:2167–77.[26]

Musculoskeletal syndrome in patients treated with MMP inhibitors

Notably, clinical use of MMP inhibitors has been associated with soft tissue rheumatism syndromes, such as musculoskeletal pain, Dupuytren's contracture (Fig. 11.9), and frozen shoulder. These adverse effects were first reported in studies with marimastat, the first synthetic MMP inhibitor developed for clinical use,[35] which was assessed in cancer trials but not in patients with arthritis. However, Ro-31-9790 produced similar musculoskeletal problems, leading to termination of its evaluation as an arthritis

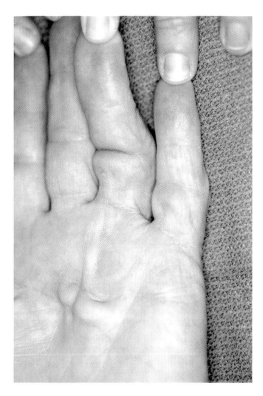

Fig. 11.9 Dupuytren's contracture, such as the soft tissue changes, has been noted following treatment with MMP inhibitors, such as marimastat. Note the cords, pits, and contractures.

Source: Figure kindly provided by Alex Mih, MD.

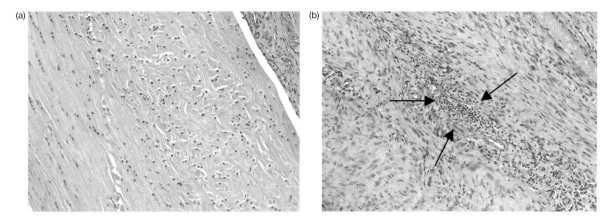

Fig. 11.10 (a) Joint capsule from a control animal, showing scattered, condensed fibroblast nuclei in a dense collagen matrix. (b) Joint capsule from a marimastat-treated animal, showing a marked increase in fibroblast cellularity and nuclear size, with perivascular aggregates of lymphocytes (arrows). Magnification ×200 for both photos.

Figures kindly provided by Drs. V. Baragi and H. Welgus.

treatment.[36] In contrast, these musculoskeletal complaints do not appear to be associated with RO-32-3555, BAY-12-9566, or doxycycline.

Although no tissue has been available for study from humans who developed a musculoskeletal syndrome during treatment with an MMP inhibitor, histopathological studies in animals have revealed an intense fibroplastic proliferation in the synovium[37] (Fig. 11.10). The underlying mechanism is obscure. However, the histopathology is similar to that observed in the murine knee joint in the presence of increased levels of transforming growth factor-β (TGF-β),[38] raising the possibility that the MMP inhibitor blocked degradation of TGF-β within the joint (although no measurements of TGF-β levels were reported).

These musculoskeletal problems in patients treated with MMP inhibitors may be due to inhibition of constitutive MMPs required in normal physiology. If so, they may argue for the use of MMPs with greater specificity, rather than nonselective MMP inhibitors. More information is needed in this area. Regardless of the cause, if the drug is effective in treatment of cancer, such adverse effects might be acceptable; however, their occurrence is likely to be viewed differently in patients with OA, that is, a risk-benefit ratio that might be acceptable in patients with cancer may be unacceptable in patients with OA.

The doxycycline knee OA clinical trial

The clinical trial of doxycycline in patients currently in progress, funded by the National Institutes of Health, is based on *in vitro* observations that showed that this drug inhibited collagenase and gelatinase in a concentration-dependent fashion[33] and *in vivo* studies that showed it was effective in animal models of OA when administered prophylactically[34] or therapeutically[35] and that, in reasonable doses, it inhibited levels of total and active collagenase and gelatinase in extracts of OA cartilage.[39]

The mechanism of action underlying the beneficial effects of doxycycline in animal models of OA is unclear. In comparison with MMP inhibitors developed recently by industry, doxycycline is only a relatively weak chelator of divalent cations, such as zinc and calcium. On the other hand, although chelation of zinc might account for the decreased levels of *active* enzyme seen in extracts of OA cartilage from animals and humans treated with doxycycline, it cannot account for the reduction in levels of *total* gelatinase and *total* collagenase in the extracts. The latter observation, however, may be explained by the fact that the presence of doxycycline during activation of latent pro-MMPs results in autocatalysis of the molecule to low molecular weight, enzymatically inactive fragments.[40] Furthermore, Amin *et al.*[41] have shown that doxycycline reduces the level of message for inducible nitric oxide synthase (iNOS) by chondrocytes. This may be

relevant because NO is present in markedly increased quantities in OA cartilage and stimulates production of MMPs by the chondrocytes.[42]

Administration of the selective iNOS inhibitor, N-iminoethyl-L-lysine, at an early stage of the disease in a canine cruciate-deficiency model of OA was shown recently to reduce the severity of chondropathy, in association with reduction in the activities of MMPs in the cartilage, and IL-1β in the synovium, and the extent of chondrocyte apoptosis.[43] These data raise the possibility that selective inhibitors of iNOS, which are currently being evaluated as symptomatic therapy for OA in the hope that they will be accompanied by less GI toxicity than nonsteroidal anti-inflammatory drugs, may also exhibit DMOAD activity.

The clinical trial of doxycycline that is in progress will be completed in November, 2002. In this study, 432 women with primary knee OA have been randomized to placebo or to doxycycline, 100 mg/bid. The subjects 45–64 years of age, in the upper tertile of the population with respect to their body mass index, have evidence of unilateral knee OA in conventional standing anteroposterior radiographs. These selection criteria were employed on the basis of epidemiological evidence that the uninvolved knee in such subjects is at high risk for developing OA over the next two years.[44] Hence, it was considered that such subjects afforded an opportunity to examine the effects of doxycycline treatment on both the *progression* of radiographic changes of OA in the knee that was involved at baseline and the *incidence* of OA in the uninvolved contralateral knee. Subsequent studies, however, have shown that the radiographically normal knee, in fact, often exhibits structural changes of OA in the patellofemoral or lateral view, or an increase in uptake of a bone-seeking isotope on scintigraphy, relative to age- and sex-matched nonarthritic controls.[45] Therefore, this study will not provide information on the ability of doxycycline to prevent incident OA, but should provide an indication of whether doxycycline exhibits DMOAD activity in patients at a relatively early radiographic stage of knee OA and/or with moderately advanced radiographic changes.

Intra-articular hyaluronan injection

An arthroscopic study has suggested that intra-articular injections of hyaluronan (HA) may exhibit DMOAD activity.[46] Patients with knee OA were treated with weekly injections of an intra-articular HA formulation for three consecutive weeks every three months (a total of 12 injections over the year), or with conventional measures without intra-articular injection. Based on arthroscopic observations at baseline and again one year later, the authors concluded that HA treatment slowed the progression of chondropathy. However, only 36 patients were studied; the level of chondropathy at baseline was less severe in the HA group than in those treated conventionally, and the proportion of patients who required an NSAID for management of symptoms during the study was twice as great in the control group as in the HA group.

Although arthroscopy is a useful tool for evaluation of pathology of the meniscus and intra-articular ligaments and assessment of the joint surface, it is less useful for detecting anatomic or biochemical changes in the OA joint and has not been shown to be an accurate, sensitive, reproducible, and validated outcome measure for evaluation of chondropathy in OA. Cartilage thickness and the mechanical quality of the cartilage cannot be assessed by arthroscopy unless a striking loss of cartilage has occurred. Although probing the cartilage may provide some useful information about the resilience of the tissue, the probe assesses changes in only a small area of the cartilage and cannot simulate the effects of load bearing (see Chapter 9.8).

Glucosamine

Similarly, although a recent report[47] has suggested that, in comparison with placebo, treatment with glucosamine sulfate, 1500 mg/d, reduced the rate of joint-space narrowing in standing knee radiographs, concern has been expressed about the suitability of the radiographic methods employed in that study to discern true cartilage loss (i.e., joint-space narrowing greater than that which could be explained by random measurement error alone) and the possibility that the concomitant decrease in knee pain experienced by subjects in the glucosamine arm could have affected positioning of the knee on serial radiographic examinations (see Chapter 11.4.2). Similar results have been reported in an abstract by Pavelka et al.,[48] and raise similar concerns.

A multi-center clinical trial of glucosamine/chondroitin sulfate in patients with knee OA, supported by the National Institutes of Health, is currently in progress in subjects with knee OA. The experimental design includes 5 treatment arms: glucosamine, 1500 mg/d; chondroitin sulfate, 1200 mg/d; glucosamine and chondroitin sulfate, in the above doses; celecoxib, 200 mg/d; and placebo. Some 318 patients will be enrolled in each treatment arm to evaluate the effects of the above therapies on symptoms; in addition, half of the patients in each arm will undergo knee radiography at baseline, 1 and 2 years later, in an attempt to ascertain whether any of the above treatments exhibits DMOAD activity. It is expected that this study will be completed in 2004.

The ECHODIAH study

All of the clinical trials described above employed the OA knee as the target joint. It is notable, therefore, that a 3-year placebo-controlled trial in patients with hip OA, the Evaluation of the Chondromodulating Effect of Diacerein in OA of the Hip (the ECHODIAH Study)[49] has recently been reported in which the authors concluded that diacerein, a derivative of the anthraquinone, rhein, exhibited DMOAD activity. Diacerein has been shown to inhibit the production and activity of IL-1 and secretion of MMPs,[50] but, in contrast to cyclooxygenases inhibitors, to have no effect on synthesis of prostaglandins. In animal models of OA, treatment with diacerein has been reported to prevent, or reduce the severity of, joint damage.[51–53] In clinical trials in patients with hip or knee OA, this agent has been shown to be superior to placebo in reducing pain and improving function.

In the ECHODIAH study,[49] approximately 500 patients were randomized to receive either diacerein or placebo over a 3-year treatment period. The dropout rate was about 40 per cent, due chiefly to loose stools in the diacerein arm and lack of efficacy in the placebo arm. Nonetheless, in both the intent-to-treat and completor analyses, a significantly smaller percentage of patients in the diacerein group than in the placebo group exhibited at least 0.5 mm of joint-space narrowing—a magnitude of joint-space loss here greater than that which can be accounted for by random measurement error. Furthermore, among those subjects who completed 3 years of

treatment, the mean rate of joint-space narrowing was significantly lower with diacerein than with placebo. Although this study failed to demonstrate a beneficial effect of diacerein on symptoms, washout periods that were scheduled prior to clinic visits for subjects who were taking concomitant analgesics/ NSAIDs were not rigorously observed, perhaps precluding demonstration of an effect of diacerein on symptoms as seen in other studies.[54,55]

Bone as a target for DMOAD therapy in OA

Although the bulk of the work on DMOAD development to date has focused on pathogenetic mechanisms in articular cartilage, a clinical trial of the bisphosphonate, ricedronate, has recently been initiated in patients with knee OA. This study, which should be completed by the summer of 2003, involves 4 treatment arms (placebo; ricedronate 5 mg or 15 mg daily; or a single weekly dose of ricedronate), with approximately 300 patients per arm, is based upon demonstration of clinical efficacy of ricedronate in a guinea pig model of OA,[2] evidence that increased formation and resorption of bone in the OA joint can be inhibited by treatment with bisphosphonates,[56] and the suggestion in a scintigraphic study[57] that uptake of a bone-seeking isotope may be associated with progression of knee OA (see Chapter 11.4.5).

As indicated in Chapter 7.2.2.1, pharmacological agents that suppress bone turnover remodeling could have beneficial effects in OA by preserving the bony architecture. Treatment with bisphosphonates, agents that inhibit oseoclast activity and hence the activation of new remodeling sites in bone, will result in an increase in density of the subchondral plate. If, however, as has been suggested by some investigators, increased density of the subchondral bone may drive the progression of OA, drugs that reduce bone turnover could, in fact, be detrimental in OA. Furthermore, by reducing the rate of bone turnover, bisphosphonates could theoretically prevent the alterations in the geometry of the bone ends that represent an adaptation to alterations in local mechanical stresses in OA.

In preclinical studies we found that administration of a bisphosphonate to dogs in which OA had been induced by anterior cruciate ligament transection reduced the rates of bone resorption and bone formation, but did not have a significant effect on the severity of articular cartilage damage.[56] Indeed, treatment was associated with a decrease in the proteoglycan concentration of the cartilage, suggesting the possibility that it inhibited repair activity by the chondrocytes and resulted in a cartilage that was softer and less able to tolerate mechanical stress than OA cartilage from untreated animals, although biomechanical testing of the cartilage was not performed. In contrast to these results, intra-articular injection of another bisphosphonate, etidronate, was found to reduce the severity of pathologic changes in the canine cruciate-deficiency model.[58]

Finally, with respect to the likelihood that a DMOAD targeted at bone will have a beneficial effect in OA, it should be borne in mind that changes in articular cartilage in some cases of secondary OA (such as in OA occurring after an osteochondral fracture or in patients with Paget's disease of bone) may be the consequence of primary alterations in the bony architecture of the joint, in primary (idiopathic) OA the changes in the bony architecture of the joint are secondary and represent an attempt to adapt to alterations in stress on the joint (see Chapter 7.2.2.1). It is theoretically possible that inhibition of this adaptive response could, over the long run, aggravate the joint pathology in OA. For this reason, the results of the clinical trial of ricedronate described above should provide important information about the role of bone in OA.

Limitations of outcome measures for evaluating DMOADs

Limitations that exist in the outcome measures available today for the evaluation of a putative DMOAD deserve emphasis. Chapter 11.4.2 documents the limitations of knee radiography in such studies; neither magnetic resonance imaging nor chondroscopy have been validated for this purpose nor have biochemical or immunochemical measurements of the concentration of 'marker' molecules in body fluids been shown to have predictive value as a surrogate for OA progression (see Chapter 11.4.7).

Participants in a recent workshop that addressed the suitability of various radiological/radiographic methods for the evaluation of a putative DMOAD in a study with a 'reasonable' sample size and 'reasonable' duration of treatment (i.e., ≤3 years) concluded that *none* of the existing protocols met that objective.[59] They emphasized, however, that analyses of film archives from recent studies supported by industry and by government that have utilized fluoroscopically-assisted and nonfluoroscopically-assisted imaging techniques can provide important information about the rate and variability of joint-space narrowing (JSN, a surrogate for articular carilage loss) in subjects with knee OA. Such data, which could be generated very rapidly, would be of great benefit in making an accurate judgment about the longitudinal performance of such protocols with respect to their sensitivity to JSN and variability in measurement of JSN. The availability of this information would be of great help in determining whether *any* of these protocols is suitable for use in a randomized control trial of a DMOAD.

Therefore, despite the important advances in our understanding of the pathogenetic mechanisms underlying tissue damage in the OA joint and the availability of pharmacological agents that may modify those pathogenetic processes, the unreliability of outcome measures available for use in clinical trials of DMOADs that would involve a reasonable number of patients and/or reasonable duration of treatment continues to inhibit significantly progress in DMOAD development.

Is a DMOAD effect clinically important?

The clinical significance of the DMOAD effect demonstrated in the ECHODIAH study (see above) is unclear. Nearly 20 per cent of subjects in the placebo group and 14.5 per cent in the diacerein group underwent hip replacement surgery during the study, a difference that was not statistically significant. It is unclear whether slowing the rate of progression of cartilage damage in OA pharmacologically will be accompanied by clinically meaningful benefit.

Among patients with OA, the relationship between the severity of symptoms and the severity of radiographic changes of OA is poor. In a longitudinal study by Ledingham *et al.*[60] of 350 subjects with knee OA, neither the severity of knee pain nor change in knee pain severity predicted loss of joint space, although radiographic severity of OA at baseline was associated with an increase in joint pain during the study. Dougados *et al.*[61] noted that change in disability over a one-year period among subjects who exhibited joint-space loss in routine knee radiographs was no different from that in subjects who did not develop joint-space loss. Similarly, no significant relationship was noted between joint-space loss and an increase in joint pain. In another study, Massardo *et al.*[62] noted a lack of correlation between joint pain, disability, and radiographic severity of knee OA, although that study involved only 31 subjects. However, in a long-term study of 400 patients with knee OA, Dieppe *et al.*[63] found no correlation between the progression of X-ray changes and the progression of joint pain or disability. It should not be assumed a priori, therefore, that a pharmacological agent exhibiting DMOAD activity in humans will have a favorable impact on *clinically important* outcomes, such as joint pain, function, disability, and the need for joint replacement surgery.

Although it is possible that the poor correlation that has been noted between radiographic progression and clinical progression is due to the lack of precision of plain radiography in evaluating structural change, the origin of joint pain in patients with knee OA is multifactorial and may relate to factors such as anxiety, depression, quadriceps strength, and the patient's coping skills—changes that do not have radiographic correlates (see Chapter 7.3.2).

Remember, OA is a disease of all of the tissues in the diarthrodial joint, not only of cartilage and bone

It must be remembered that OA is a disease of an organ (i.e., the diarthrodial joint) and not only of the specific tissue(s) that DMOADs have been designed to affect (e.g., articular cartilage, subchondral bone). It is possible therefore, that the benefit of pharmacological inhibition of degradative enzyme activity in articular cartilage may not be apparent in patients in whom the local mechanical environment is so mechanically disadvantageous to the cartilage as to overwhelm the effects of the drug. To date, none of the clinical trials of DMOADs that have been initiated in humans has taken such variables into account. In future studies it may be advisable to stratify subjects at entry into the study on the basis of, e.g., their quadriceps strength, degree of varus/valgus instability, or level of proprioceptive acuity. Support for this concept is provided by the observation in dogs in which OA was produced by transection of the anterior cruciate ligament, that diacerein did not exhibit DMOAD activity if sensory input from the unstable extremity had been significantly reduced prior to the creation of joint instability,[64] whereas a significant DMOAD effect was apparent in the unstable knee of neurologically intact dogs.[39]

Key points

1. Based on an increase in our understanding of pathogenetic mechanisms underlying damage to tissue of the OA joint, pharmacological agents have been developed whose main mechanism of action is aimed at inhibition of matrix-degrading enzymes, such as collagenase, gelatinase, or stromelysin; or inhibition of cytokines, such as TNF-α or interleukin-1β, or of signaling pathways involved in the synthesis of such cytokines.

2. Clinical trials of such agents, chiefly matrix metalloproteinase inhibitors, have generally been conducted in patients with cancer, rather than with OA. Except for a trial of doxycycline in subjects with knee OA, a randomized clinical trial of which is currently in progress, other trials of MMP inhibitors have been halted because of a lack of efficacy or appearance of adverse effects.

3. Although it has been claimed that intra-articular injections of hyaluronan and oral treatment with glucosamine sulfate reduce the progression of cartilage damage in OA joints, better evidence for both of these claims is required.

4. In a recent clinical trial of diacerein, in humans with hip OA, although the dropout rate was about 40 per cent, the results suggested that the drug significantly reduced the rate of cartilage loss, as judged by radiographic joint-space narrowing.

5. A significant impediment to the development of structure-modifying drugs for OA is the unreliability of outcome measures suitable for use in clinical trials involving a reasonable number of patients and/or a reasonable duration of treatment.

6. Finally, even if drug is shown to slow the progression of cartilage damage in OA, it should not be assumed a priori that it will have a favorable impact on clinically important outcomes, such as joint pain or function.

References

(An asterisk denotes recommended reading.)

1. **Lequesne, M., Brandt, K., Bellamy, N.**, *et al.* (1994). Guidelines for testing slow-acting and disease-modifying drugs in osteoarthritis. (published correction appears in *J Rheumatol* (1994). 21:2395) *J Rheumatol* **41**(Suppl.):65–73.

2. **Beary, J.F.** (2001). Joint structure modification in osteoarthritis: development of SMOAD drugs. *Curr Rheumatol Rep* **3**:1–7.

3. Bigg, H.E. and Rowan, A.D. (2001). The inhibition of metalloproteinases as a therapeutic target in rheumatoid arthritis and osteoarthritis. *Curr Opin Pharmacol* **1**:314–20.

4. Woessner, J.F., Jr. and Nagase, H. (2000). *Matrix Metalloproteinases and TIMPs.* Oxford: Oxford University Press, pp. 1–238.

5. Konttinen, Y.T., Ceponis, A., Takagi, M., *et al.* (1998). New collagenolytic enzymes cascade identified at the pannus—hard tissue junction in rheumatoid arthritis: destruction from above. *Matrix Biol* **17**:585–601.

6. *Mengshol, J.A., Mix, K.S., and Brinckerhoff, C.E. (2002). Matrix metalloproteinases as therapeutic targets in arthritic diseases. *Arthritis Rheum* **46**:13–20.

   An excellent discussion of the rationale for the use of matrix metalloproteinase inhibitors in treatment of patients with OA.

7. Ohuchi, E., Imai, K., Fujii, Y., Sato, H., Seiki, M., and Okada, Y. (1997). Membrane type 1 matrix metalloproteinase digests interstitial collagens and other extracellular matrix macromolecules. *J Biol Chem* **272**:2446–51.

8. Tortorella, M.D., Burn, T.C., Pratta, M.A., *et al.* (1999). Purification and cloning of aggrecanase-1: a member of the ADAMTS family of proteins. *Science* **284**:1664–66.

9. Abbaszade, I., Liu, R.Q., Yang, F., *et al.* (1999). Cloning and characterization of ADAMTS11, an aggrecanase from the ADAMTS family. *J Biol Chem* **274**:23443–50.

10. Black, R.A., Rauch, C.T., Kozlosky, C.J., *et al.* (1997). A metalloproteinase disintegrin that releases tumour-necrosis factor-a from cells. *Nature* **385**:729–35.

11. Armour, A., Siocombe, P.M., Webster, A., *et al.* (1998). TNF-α converting enzyme (TACE) is inhibited by TIMP-3. *FEBS Lett* **435**:39–44.

12. Kashiwagi, M., Tortorella, M., Nagase, H., and Brew, K. (2001). TIMP-3 is a potent inhibitor of aggrecanase 1 (ADAM-TS4) and aggrecanase 2 (ADAM-TS5). *J Biol Chem* **276**(16):12501–4.

13. Caron, J.P., Fernandes, J.C., Martel-Pelletier, J., *et al.* (1996). Chondroprotective effect of intraarticular injections of interleukin-1 receptor antagonist in experimental osteoarthritis: suppression of collagenase-1 expression. *Arthritis Rheum* **39**:1535–44.

14. Van de Loo, F.A.J., Joosten, L.A.B., van Lent, P.L.E.M., Arntz, O.J., and van den Berg, W.B. (1995). Role of interleukin-1, tumor necrosis factor α, and interleukin-6 in cartilage proteoglycan metabolism and destruction: effect of in situ blocking in murine antigen- and zymosan-induced arthritis. *Arthritis Rheum* **38**:164–72.

15. Kronheim, S.R., Mumma, A., Greenstreet, T., *et al.* (1992). Purification of interleukin-1 beta converting enzyme, the protease that cleaves the interleukin-1 beta precursor. *Arch Biochem Biophys* **296**:698–703.

16. Saha, N., Moldovan, F., Tardif, G., Pelletier, J.-P., Cloutier, J.-M., and Martel-Pelletier, J. (1999). Interleukin-1β-converting enzyme/caspase-1 in human osteoarthritic tissues: localization and role in the maturation of interleukin-1β and interleukin-18. *Arthritis Rheum* **42**:1577–87.

17. Slack, J., McMahan, C.J., Waugh, S., *et al.* (1993). Independent binding of interleukin-1 alpha and interleukin-1 beta to type I and type II interleukin-1 receptors. *J Biol Chem* **268**:2513–24.

18. Sadouk, M., Pelletier, J.P., Tardif, G., Kiansa, K., Cloutier, J.M., and Martel-Pelletier, J. (1995). Human synovial fibroblasts coexpress interleukin-1 receptor type I and type II mRNA: the increased level of the interleukin-1 receptor in osteoarthritic cells is related to an increased level of the type I receptor. *Lab Invest* **73**:347–55.

19. Martel-Pelletier, J., di Battista, J.A., and Lajeunesse, D. (1999). Biochemical factors in joint articular tissue degradation in osteoarthritis. In J.Y. Reginster, J.P. Pelletier, J. Martel-Pelletier, and Y. Henrotin (eds), *Osteoarthritis: Clinical and Experimental Aspects.* Berlin: Springer-Verlag, pp. 156–87.

20. Martel-Pelletier, J., Alaaeddine, N., and Pelletier, J.P. (1999). Cytokines and their role in the pathophysiology of osteoarthritis. *Front Biosci* **4**:D694–703.

21. Young, P., McDonnell, P., Dunnington, D., Hand, A., Laydon, J., and Lee, J. (1993). Pyridinyl imidazoles inhibit IL-1 and TNF production at the protein level. *Agents Actions* **39**(Spec. No.):C67–9.

22. Martel-Pelletier, J., Mineau, F., Jovanovic, D., Di Battista, J.A., and Pelletier, J.-P. (1999). Mitogen-activated protein kinase and nuclear factor κB together regulate interleukin-17-induced nitric oxide production in human osteoarthritic chondrocytes: possible role of trans-activating factor

mitogen-activated protein kinase-activated protein kinase (MAPKAPK). *Arthritis Rheum* **42**:2399–409.

23. Badger, A.M., Griswold, D.E., Kapadia, R., *et al.* (2000). Disease-modifying activity of SB 242235, a selective inhibitor of p38 mitogen-activated protein kinase, in rat adjuvant-induced arthritis. *Arthritis Rheum* **43**:175–83.

24. Tomita, T., Takeuchi, E., Tomita, N., *et al.* (1999). Suppressed severity of collagen-induced arthritis by in vivo transfection of nuclear factor κB decoy oligodeoxynucleotides as gene therapy. *Arthritis Rheum* **42**:2532–42.

25. Grams, F., Crimmin, M., Hinnes, L., *et al.* (1995). Structure determination and analysis of human neutrophil collagenase complexed with hydroxamate inhibitor. *Eur J Cell Biol* **34**:14012–20.

26. Brown, P.D. (2000). Ongoing trials with matrix metalloproteinase inhibitors. *Exp Opin Invest Drugs* **9**:2167–77.

27. *Pelletier, J.P., Martel-Pelletier, J., and Abramson, S.B. (2001). Osteoarthritis, an inflammatory disease. Potential implication for the selection of new therapeutic targets. *Arthritis Rheum* **44**:1237–47.

   An excellent discussion for the rationale of the use of matrix metalloproteinase inhibitors in treatment of patients with OA.

28. Betz, M., Huxley, P., Davies, S.J., *et al.* (1997). 1.8-Å crystal structure of the catalytic domain of human neutrophil collagenase (matrix metalloproteinse-8) complexed with a peptidomimetic hydroxamate primed-side inhibitor with a distinct selectivity profile. *Eur J Biochem* **247**(1):356–63.

29. Whittaker, M., Floyd, C.D., Brown, P., and Gearing, A.J.H. (1999). Design and therapeutic application of matrix metalloproteinase inhibitors. *Chem Rev* **99**:2735–76.

30. Chau, T., Jolly, G., Plym, M.J., *et al.* (1998). Inhibition of articular cartilage degradation in dog and guinea pig models of osteoarthritis by the stromelysin inhibitor, BAY 12-9566 (abstract). *Arthritis Rheum* **41**(Suppl.):S300.

31. Leff, R.L. (1999). Clinical trials of a stromelysin inhibitor. *Ann NY Acad Sci* **878**:201–7.

32. Hughes, S. (1999). Bayer drug casts shadow over MMP inhibitors in cancer. Scrip No 2477, Oct 1 1999, p. 20.

33. Yu, L.P., Smith, G.N., Hasty, K.A., and Brandt, K.D. (1991). Doxycycline inhibits Type XI collagenolytic activity of extracts from human osteoarthritic cartilage and of gelatinase. *J Rheumatol* **18**:1450–2.

34. Yu, L.P., Smith, G.N., Brandt, K.D., *et al.* (1992). Reduction of the severity of canine osteoarthritis by prophylactic treatment with oral doxycycline. *Arthritis Rheum* **35**:1150–9.

35. *Hutchinson, J.W., Tierney, G.M., Parsons, S.L., and Davis, T.R.C. (1998). Dupuytren's disease and frozen shoulder induced by treatment with matrix metalloproteinase inhibitor. *J Bone Joint Surg Br* **80B**:907–8.

   This paper describes the musculoskeletal syndrome associated with use of matrix metalloproteinase inhibitors.

36. Bigg, H.F. and Rowan, A.D. (2001). The inhibition of metalloproteinases as a therapeutic target in rheumatoid arthritis and osteoarthritis. *Curr Opin Pharma* **1**:314–20.

37. Renkiewicz, R., Qiu, L., Lesch, C. *et al.* (Submitted). Broad-spectrum matrix metalloproteinase inhibitor marimastat–induced musculoskeletal side effects in rats.

38. Bakker, A.C., van de Loo, F.A., van Beuningen, H.M., *et al.* (2001). Overexpression of active TGF-beta-1 in the murine knee joint: evidence for synovial-layer-dependent chondro-ostephyte formation. *Osteoarthritis Cart* **9**:128–36.

39. Smith, G., Jr., Yu, L., Jr., Brandt, K., and Capello, W. (1998). Oral administration of doxycycline reduces collagenase and gelatinase activities in extracts of human osteoarthritic cartilage. *J Rheumatol* **25**:532–5.

40. Smith, G.N., Jr., Brandt, K.D., and Hasty, K.A. (1996). Activation of recombinant human neutrophil procollagenase in the presence of doxycycline results in fragmentation of the enzyme and loss of enzyme activity. *Arthritis Rheum* **39**:235–44.

41. Amin, A.R., Attur, M.G., Thakker, G.D., *et al.* (1996). A novel mechanism of action of tetracyclines: effects on nitric oxide synthases. *Proc Natl Acad Sci USA* **93**:14014–19.

42. Lotz, M. (1999). The role of nitric oxide in articular cartilage damage. In: K.D. Brandt (ed.), *Osteoarthritis.* Philadelphia: WB Saunders Company, pp. 269–82.

43. Pelletier, J-P., Javonovic, D.V., Lascau-Coman, V., *et al.* (2000). Selective inhibition in inducible nitric oxide synthase reduces progression of experimental osteoarthritis in vivo: possible link with the reduction of chondrocyte apoptosis and caspase 3 level. *Arthritis Rheum* **43**:1290–9.

44. Hart, D.J., Doyle, D.V., and Spector, T.D. (1999). Incidence and risk factors for radiographic knee osteoarthritis in middle-aged women: the Chingford Study. *Arthritis Rheum* **42**:17–24.

45. Mazzuca, S., Brandt, K., Schauwecker, D., *et al.* (2000). The utility of scintigraphy in explaining x-ray changes and symptoms of knee osteoarthritis. *Trans Orthop Res Soc* **25**:234.

46. Listrat, V., Ayral, X., Patarnello, F., *et al.* (1997). Arthrocopic evaluation of potential structure modifying activity of hyaluronan (Hyalgan) in osteoarthritis of the knee. *Osteoarthritis Cart* **5**:153–60.

47. Reginster, J.Y., Deroisy, R., Rovati, L.C., *et al.* (2001). Long-term effects of glucosamine sulphate on osteoarthritis progression: a randomised, placebo-controlled clinical trial. *Lancet* **357**(9252):251–6.

48. Pavelka, K., Gatterova, J., Olejarova, M., *et al.* (2000). A long-term, randomized, placebo controlled, confirmatory trial on the effects of glucosamine sulfate on knee osteoarthritis progression. *Osteoarthritis Cart* **8**(Suppl.):S6–7.

49. Dougados, M., Nguyen, M., Berdah, L., Mazieres, B., Vignon, E., and Lequesne, M. (for the ECHODIAH Investigators Study Group). (2001). Evaluation of the structure-modifying effects of diacerhein in hip osteoarthritis. *Arthritis Rheum* **44**:2539–47.

50. Boittin, M., Redini, F., Loyau, G., and Pujol, J.P. (1993). Matrix deposition and collagenase release in cultures of rabbit articular chondrocytes exposed to diacethylrhein. *Osteoarthritis Cart* **1**:39–40.14.

51. Bendele, A.M., Bendele, R.A., Hulman, J.F., and Swann, B.P. (1996). Beneficial effects of treatment with diacerhein in guinea pigs with osteoarthritis. *Rev Prat* **46**:35–9.

52. Mazieres, B. (1997). Diacerhein in a post-contusive model of osteoarthritis: structural results with 'prophylactic' and 'curative' regimens (abstract). *Osteoarthritis Cart* **5**(Suppl. A):73.

53. Smith, G.N., Myers, S.L., Brandt, K.D., Mickler, E.A., and Albrecht, M.E. (1999). Diacerhein treatment reduces the severity of osteoarthritis in the canine cruciate-deficiency model of osteoarthritis. *Arthritis Rheum* **42**:545–54.

54. Nguyen, M., Dougados, M., Berdah, L., and Amor, B. (1994). Diacerhein in the treatment of osteoarthritis of the hip. *Arthritis Rheum* **37**:529–36.

55. Pelletier, J.P., Yaron, M., Haraoui, B., *et al.* (2000). Efficacy and safety of diacerhein in osteoarthritis of the knee: a double-blind placebo-controlled trial. *Arthritis Rheum* **43**:2339–48.

56. Myers, S.L., Brandt, K.D., Burr, D.B., O'Connor, B.L., and Albrecht, M. (1999). Effects of a bisphosphonate on bone histomorphometry and dynamics in the canine cruciate-deficiency model of osteoarthritis. *J Rheumatol* **26**:2645–53.

57. Dieppe, P., Cushnaghan, J., Young, P., and Kirwan, J. (1993). Prediction of the progression of joint space narrowing in osteoarthritis of the knee by bone scintigraphy. *Ann Rheum Dis* **52**:557–63.

58. Howell, D.S., Altman, R.D., Pelletier, J.-P., Martel-Pelletier, J., and Dean, D.D. (1995). Disease-modifying antirheumatic drugs: current status of their application in animal models of osteoarthritis. In: K.E. Kuettner, and V.E. Goldberg (eds). *Osteoarthritic Disorders* Chicago: American Academy of Orthopedic Surgeons, pp. 365–77.

59. *Brandt, K.D., Mazzuca, S.A., Conrozier, T., *et al.* (2002). *Which is the best radiologic/radiographic protocol for a clinical trial of a structure-modifying drug in patients with knee osteoarthritis?* Proceedings of January 17–18, 2002 Workshop in Toussus-le-Noble, France. *J Rheumatol* **29**:1308–20.

   This paper reviews the advantages and limitations of various radiologic/radiographic protocols that have been considered for use in clinical trials of DMOADs in patients with knee OA. It concludes that all such protocols have their problems.

60. Ledingham, J., Regan, M., Jones, A., and Doherty, M. (1995). Factors affecting radiographic progression of knee osteoarthritis. *Ann Rheum Dis* **54**:53–8.

61. Dougados, M., Gueguen, A., Nguyen, M., *et al.* (1991). Longitudinal radiologic evaluation of osteoarthritis in the knee. *J Rheum* **19**:378–84.

62. Massardo, L., Watt, I., Chushnaghan, J., and Dieppe, P. (1989). Osteoarthritis of the knee joint: an eight year prospective study. *Ann Rheum Dis* **48**:893–97.

63. *Dieppe, P.A., Cushnaghan, J., and Shepstone, L. (1997). The Bristol 'OA500' study: progression of osteoarthritis over three years and the relationship between clinical and radiographic changes at the knee joint. *Osteoarthritis Cart* **5**:87–97.

   This paper emphasizes the poor correlation between progression of clinical features of OA (e.g., pain, functional impairment) and the progression of radiographic features of OA.

64. Brandt, K.D., Smith, G., Kang, S.Y., Myers, S., O'Connor, B., and Albrecht, M. (1997). Effects of diacerhein in an accelerated canine model of osteoarthritis. *Osteoarthritis Cart* **5**:438–49.

11.3 Advantages and limitations of animal models in the discovery and evaluation of novel disease-modifying osteoarthritis drugs (DMOADs)

R.J. Griffiths and D.J. Schrier

Numerous animal models that mimic the pathological changes in OA have been described. They include spontaneous OA in several species; surgically induced models, generally produced by transection of the anterior cruciate ligament; OA induced by injection of either cytokines or the metabolic poison, monoiodoacetate; and, most recently, transgenic models. Although most studies have focused on the changes induced in the articular cartilage, in particular, each of these models reproduces some of the cardinal features of the disease in humans. These models are useful because they can be employed to probe the factors controlling the initiation and progression of the disease in a way that is not practical in human subjects. For example, knowledge of the time course of the disease in the model and access to joint tissues permits sequential biochemical characterization of the changes within the joint tissues. Effects of new drugs on these processes can be evaluated at a number of levels, for example, biochemical, histological, and imaging, permitting correlations between these techniques. The major drawback to the use of such models of OA is the lack of currently available disease-modifying OA drugs (DMOADs) needed to validate the predictive value of the models.

Spontaneous models of osteoarthritis

Spontaneous models of OA have been described in numerous species, including guinea pigs,[1,2] mice,[3–8] rats,[9] dogs[10] and primates[11] (Table 11.5). In general, these models evolve slowly and disease expression is somewhat variable. However, given their similarities to the human disease, the models have significant utility for study of the pathogenesis of OA. Such studies are beginning to yield valuable information that can be used to develop rational drug design strategies. Moreover, practical treatment paradigms have been developed that have encouraged the evaluation of novel compounds. Guinea pig and murine systems are particularly well suited for drug discovery.

Table 11.5 Animal models of OA

Method of induction	Species	Comments
Spontaneous	Guinea pig, mouse, rat, dog, primate	Variable onset and chronic time course (months); cause unknown; may be a surrogate for idiopathic human OA
Surgical. Usually induced by transection of the anterior cruciate ligament or meniscectomy	Dog, rabbit, guinea pig, rat, sheep	Chronic; more consistent than spontaneous models, but still require weeks to months
Intra-articular injection of cytokines, monoiodoacetate, papain	Mouse, rat, rabbit, guinea pig	Generally, acute cartilage damage; very consistent and rapid onset

The guinea pig model

The guinea pig model of spontaneous OA was first intensively studied during the 1980s.[1,2,12] In Dunkin-Hartley strain guinea pigs, degeneration of articular cartilage is preceded by changes in the underlying subchondral bone. Radiography and MRI indicate that the first changes occur as early as 4–8 weeks of age. Although significant bone remodelling is evident, the loss of trabecular bone initiates a sequence of events that leads to the destruction of the cartilage and, ultimately, of the joint architecture. By the age of 5 months, cartilage changes are evident in almost every animal. Loss of proteoglycan from the cartilage matrix and chondrocyte death are apparent first in the area of the medial tibial plateau that is not protected by the meniscus. Cartilage loss then progresses to cover a large area of the plateau. The femoral condyles are significantly involved by 9 months. By the time the guinea pigs reach 12 months of age, extensive full-thickness loss of cartilage is observed and the subchondral bone is exposed on both the medial femoral condyle and tibial plateau. Cathepsin B activity in the bone is elevated.[13] The ratio of 6-sulphated chondroitin to the 4-sulphated isomer on the glycosaminoglycan chains of articular cartilage proteoglycans is increasing dramatically by 8 weeks of age, but the 3-B-3 minus mimitope, typical of the OA proteoglycan phenotype, is not present before 9 weeks of age.[14]

A number of drug studies have been performed using this model. When diacerhein was administered daily for a year, with treatment beginning when the animals were 3 months old, the rate of progression of joint pathology was reduced by 50 per cent.[15] The magnitude of cartilage loss, osteophyte formation, and synovial hyperplasia were all reduced. The compound was shown to have protective effects on proteoglycan metabolism *in vivo*, increasing the half-life of the 4-sulphated isomer, with lesser effects on the 6-isomer of chondroitin sulphate. Doxycycline, and a chemically modified tetracycline (CMT), administered for 4–8 months, have also been shown to reduce cartilage fibrillation, thickening of the subchondral bone, and formation of subchondral cysts in this model.[16] In addition, the rate of collagen synthesis and the contents of hyaluronan and proteoglycan in the cartilage were greater after treatment with a CMT than in controls.

A major disadvantage of drug testing in the guinea pig model is the amount of compound required for long-term dosing. However, the similarity of the pathology to that of human OA and the availability of significant amounts of tissue make this model one of the most desirable for preclinical evaluation of DMOADs. Increasing evidence of the role that bone plays in the pathogenesis of OA adds to the attractiveness of this model (see Chapters 7.2.2.1 and 7.2.2.2).

Murine models

Nearly all strains of inbred mice will eventually develop some degree of OA, although the incidence and severity of articular lesions varies widely among strains.[5,17] Mice of the STR strain (STR/ORT and STR/IN) commonly develop a severe form of disease. Radiographic assessment of the knee suggests that the incidence and severity of OA are both more common in male STR/ORT mice than in females. A number of early pathologic changes are associated with the murine disease. Patellar displacement, chondro-osseous metaplasia in tendons and around the insertion sites of periarticular ligaments are observed in a large proportion of the animals. These changes are also associated with an up-regulation of cartilage collagen synthesis and decreased tensile strength in the anterior cruciate ligament.[18] Although these features are not universal, they are observed before any radiological evidence of disease is present, suggesting a strong relationship to subsequent cartilage degeneration. Cartilage lesions in this model appear first as superficial fibrillation on the medial tibial plateau, and progress to deep erosions that are accompanied by osteophyte formation. Sclerosis of the subchondral bone is observed only very late; in this respect, the pathophysiology of murine OA differs from that observed in guinea pigs (see above) and primates.

Murine models of OA hold certain advantages for the identification of potential molecular targets and drug discovery. The availability of genetically modified mice offers a precise way to evaluate disease pathogenesis. Genetic manipulations include the insertion of a human gene to cause overexpression of the protein of interest (transgenics) and the creation of knockout mice, in which the mouse gene of interest is deleted in embryonic stem cells and is therefore absent throughout the life of the animal.

The fact that OA lesions have been identified in a relatively broad range of murine strains permits flexibility in the selection of genetic backgrounds. However, the gradual and variable onset of disease makes the routine use of knockout and transgenic mice somewhat cumbersome. Also, the small amount of material that can be retrieved from individual joints may create difficulty in conducting routine biochemical analysis of joint tissues. Presumably, newer molecular technologies, requiring only very small tissue samples, will make the use of murine models more practical, and eliminate the need to pool large numbers of animals. A number of drug studies have been performed using the STR line of mice. Results of studies of nonsteroidal antiinflammatory drugs (NSAIDs) and steroids have been inconsistent. Pataki et al.[19] found that steroids and two NSAIDs (indomethacin and diclofenac) had no effect on OA pathology, while Maier and Wilhelmi[20] found that diclofenac inhibited, but indomethacin exacerbated, cartilage damage. Recent studies have also shown that Ro 32-3555, a broad-spectrum matrix metalloproteinase (MMP) inhibitor, inhibited radiographic joint-space narrowing (presumed to be a surrogate for articular cartilage loss) and osteophyte formation. The therapeutic benefit of the compound was confirmed by histological data that showed significant protection against cartilage destruction.[21]

Surgical models

Because spontaneous models generally evolve very slowly and vary in terms of the incidence and severity of OA, a number of surgical approaches have been used to induce consistent OA lesions that develop rapidly. Surgical approaches have most often been used in dogs[22,23] and rabbits,[24,25] although guinea pigs[26,27] and rats[28] have also been used. In the dog, transection of the anterior cruciate ligament causes a change in joint mechanics that leads initially to cartilage hypertrophy. Within a few weeks after ligament transection, the cartilage begins to thicken. The water content of the cartilage increases, presumably due to damage to the collagen network. The increase in tissue bulk is not due only to water, however, because both the content and concentration of proteoglycans are increased and there is evidence of increased synthesis of proteoglycans and also of collagen and non-collagenous proteins. Marked osteophyte formation is apparent by about three months. The time required for cartilage degeneration, with fibrillation, loss of surface tissue, and chondrocyte cloning, is variable, depending on the procedure and size of animal used. Dorsal root ganglionectomy dramatically accelerates the course of this process[29] (see Chapter 7.2.4.1).

In rabbits, a number of meniscal and ligament procedures have been developed, including combinations of cruciate ligament (medial and collateral) transection, total or partial meniscectomy, and meniscal tears. Generally, the goal is to induce a lesion with characteristics of OA that is not so aggressive as to induce necrotic cell death or to be resistant to pharmacological intervention.

Because the sequence of events that occurs in surgical models of OA is synchronized and somewhat accelerated by the surgical procedure, such

models are used frequently in pharmacological studies and studies of pathogenetic mechanisms. Recent reports that orally administered glucosamine is effective in both rabbits and dogs,[30,31] were encouraging because of the suggestive evidence that glucosamine exhibited DMOAD activity in human clinical trials[32] (please see cautionary note regarding these results, however, in Chapter 11.4.2). In the preclinical studies, glucosamine, an amino monosaccharide that is utilized in the synthesis of disaccharide units of glycosaminoglycan, was combined with manganese ascorbate and chondroitin sulfate. Presumably, the provision of these cartilage matrix precursors promoted matrix synthesis and repair of articular cartilage. In a rabbit model, treatment with glucosamine reduced the severity of histopathologic changes of OA. In a canine model, treatment reduced the synovial fluid concentration of chondroitin sulfates with an increased chain length, altered sulfation pattern and structure. These proteoglycan fragments, which are recognized by monoclonal antibodies such as 7D4 and 3-B-3, are considered to be early indicators of OA pathology.

In cruciate-deficient dogs, therapeutic doses of corticosteroid[33] and tiaprofenic acid[34] have been shown to reduce the severity of structural damage in the unstable joint. Steroid was effective both orally (prednisone, 0.25 mg/kg/day) and after intra-articular injection (triamcinolone hexacetonide, single dose of 5 mg). Steroid treatment also prevented osteophyte formation and reduced stromelysin levels. However, using a lower dose of steroid, that is, the equivalent of only 5 mg of prednisone per day for a 70 kg human, Myers et al.[35] found no effect of the steroid on joint pathology. The results with tiaprofenic acid and tenidap are somewhat controversial, given the lack of efficacy of NSAIDs as DMOADs in humans. In rabbits, NSAIDs showed no effect on OA pathology in a ligament transection model.[36]

Dog and rabbit surgical models have been used also to evaluate therapeutic agents with novel mechanisms of action or to test as a unique indication for an existing therapeutic agent. Both species have been used to evaluate the interleukin-1 receptor antagonist (IRAP), a protein that blocks the action of IL-1. In dogs, treatment with IRAP, given biweekly by intra-articular injection, resulted in a dose-dependent reduction in cartilage lesions and osteophytes.[37] Similar results were observed in rabbits that received IRAP by gene transfer.[38]

Studies with calcitonin in the canine cruciate-deficiency model have suggested that an agent used for treatment of osteoporosis may be effective also for OA.[39,40] Calcitonin administration reduced the severity of articular cartilage damage, urinary concentrations of pyridinium crosslinks, and serum concentrations of hyaluronan and keratan sulphate. On the other hand, bisphosphonates, anti-resorbtive agents that inhibit bone resorbtion by osteoclasts and have been shown to be effective in osteoporosis, may not be optimal therapy for OA. In the canine cruciate-deficiency model, administration of a bisphosphonate in a dose that was effective in inhibiting resorption and formation of subchondral cancellous bone (in which formation is coupled to resorption) did not ameliorate the severity of OA pathology in a relatively short-term study. Indeed, the treatment with the bisphosphonate resulted in a decrease in the uronic acid concentration of the articular cartilage, relative to that in OA cartilage from control dogs, suggesting that bisphosphonate treatment may inhibit the repair response in OA cartilage and could lead to softening of the cartilage as a result of a decrease in proteoglycan concentration.[40] Furthermore, concern has been raised that bisphosphonate treatment may have adverse effects on subchondral bone in the OA joint (see Chapter 7.2.2.1).

Dog and rabbit models have been used also to evaluate the efficacy of pentosan polysulphate (an agent that binds growth factors). When administered with IGF-1, this agent conferred protection against cartilage damage and resulted in reductions in levels of matrix metalloproteinases (MMPs) and increases in levels of tissue inhibitor of matrix metalloproteinases (TIMP) in the cartilage.[41] Paradoxically, intra-articular injection of IGF-1 in rats results in the production of osteophytes.[42]

Doxycycline was markedly effective in a canine cruciate-deficiency model in which the severity and rapid development of joint damage were accelerated by deafferentation of the ipsilateral hind limb, prior to transection of the ligament[63] (see Chapter 7.2.4.1). The agent reduced the loss of articular cartilage and dramatically reduced the levels of MMPs in the cartilage.[43]

Other agents that are shown to be effective in rabbit or dog models of OA include MMP inhibitors,[44] sodium hyaluronate,[45,46] 6,7-dihydroxycoumarin (esculetin),[47] diacerhein,[48] and L-NIL (a selective inhibitor of NO synthase)[49] (Table 11.5). Notably, diacerhein was not effective in an accelerated canine model of OA produced by deafferentation of the hind limb prior to cruciate ligament transection, but it significantly reduced the severity of cartilage damage in the neurologically intact cruciate deficient dog.[50] This suggests that the effects of DMOADs may depend upon the stage of OA at which the drug is administered, that is, drugs that may be effective in the initial stages of the disease may be ineffective in advanced or rapidly progressive disease, and vice versa.

Reagent-induced models

A large number of chemical reagents and biologic mediators have been used to develop models with macroscopic or histopathological lesions similar to those of OA. Intra-articular injection of MMPs;[51] papain;[52] cytokines, for example, IL-1;[53] growth factors, for example, transforming growth factor-β (TGFβ);[54] and monoiodoacetate,[55] has been shown to induce pathological changes in the joint that resemble OA. A major impetus for this approach is the desirability of having a practical and efficient time frame for *in vivo* studies of potential DMOADs in drug discovery programs. Also, it is often useful to compartmentalize the pathophysiology and study the effects of only a single cytokine. Such models are commonly used in intermediate proof of concept studies that if positive, may lead to studies in more complex models of OA (Table 11.5).

Models induced by genetic manipulation

An exciting recent development has been the description of OA models induced by gene transfer of MMP-13- and TGFβ.[56,57] Such models offer the opportunity to look at the effects of a single mechanism in the development of OA. For MMP-13, a transgenic model was made by utilizing a tetracycline-regulated cartilage-specific promoter to target a constitutively active human MMP-13 in the articular cartilage of mice. Normally, MMPs are synthesized as precursors that are activated after secretion by proteolytic removal of a pro-region. This requirement was circumvented by use of an enzymatically active variant of the enzyme. Because the MMP-13 plays an important role in matrix remodelling and development of the growth plate and other skeletal tissues, a tetracycline system was used to repress MMP-13 expression during embryogenesis. Subsequent expression of this transgene caused pathologic changes similar to those observed in OA, for example, articular cartilage ulceration, with loss of cartilage matrix proteoglycans, cleavage of type II collagen by collagenase, and synovial hyperplasia. These results indicate that excessive MMP-13 activity can result in articular cartilage degradation and joint pathology.

The TGFβ model was induced by adenoviral transfer and overexpression in knee joints of C57BL/6 mice. Expression of active TGFβ induced synovial hyperplasia and chondro-osteophyte formation at the chondrosynovial junctions. It appears that the effects of TGFβ were related to the incorporation and subsequent expression of the gene by the synovial lining layer, because depletion of the lining resulted in a dramatic decrease in the severity of the joint pathology, with reduction of chondro-osteophyte formation and decreased accumulation of extracellular matrix in synovium. These effects suggest that TGFβ may play a significant role in the pathophysiology of OA.

Advantages of animal models

Animal models have long played an important role in the search for new therapeutic agents and the models described earlier in the chapter are

Table 11.6 Advantages associated with the use of animal models

- ◆ Well-defined time course
- ◆ Easy access to joint tissue
- ◆ Amenable to quantitation using a variety of techniques
- ◆ Permit validation of biomarkers
- ◆ Permit measurement of function/pain

frequently used. These models have both advantages and limitations that need to be recognized so that interpretation of the data obtained from such studies can be placed in the proper context. OA may be caused by a number of factors and the variety of techniques used to induce OA in animals reflects this. It is, therefore, not realistic to expect that any one model can mimic all facets of the human condition (Table 11.6).

In humans, the time course of OA progression can be highly variable and the duration of pre-existing disease very difficult to determine. In contrast, in most animal models (with the exception of the spontaneous models), the onset of the disease can be controlled, permitting accurate assessment of the sequence of events that occur after the initial insult. In addition, it may be possible to introduce experimental manipulations that alter the rate at which gross changes are produced, for example, in the canine cruciate ligament transection model, dorsal root ganglionectomy exacerbates the disease and shortens the timeframe over which pathologic changes develop. This opportunity to control the experimental situation is useful in that it permits the study of drug effects at various times after disease onset, that is, the drug can be dosed either at a time when there is minimal damage or when significant damage has already occurred. This may afford insights into which patient population is most likely to derive benefit in clinical trials.

Easy access to joint tissues

Access to joint tissue is a key advantage of animal models. The ability to sample cartilage and other joint tissues permits measurement of key biochemical/biomechanical properties of these tissues in a way that is rarely possible in humans. Obviously, the larger the animal species the greater the amount of cartilage available for study. This is one of the reasons that the lapine and canine models have been used much more extensively in OA research than rodent models.

Quantitation by a variety of techniques

The ability to quantify the progression of disease with a variety of methods is something that is possible only in models. For example, it is possible to obtain images of the joint using radiographs or magnetic resonance imaging while the animal is alive and then to perform histological and biochemical analysis of the cartilage after sacrifice. This permits assessment of the sensitivity of various imaging techniques for the detection of changes in the articular cartilage and other joint tissues. Even though biochemical changes may precede any macroscopic or even microscopic changes, correlation between the earliest detectable changes at the biochemical level and alterations in a signal measured by an imaging technique can be examined.

Correlation of measurements of biomarkers with measurements on cartilage

Biochemical markers of cartilage damage are being studied increasingly as potential diagnostic/prognostic indicators of OA and tools for assessment of drug effects. It is hoped that identification of a marker of progressive cartilage destruction might provide more rapid feedback regarding the efficacy of a DMOAD than is possible with radiography or MRI. Many such markers are being examined (Chapter 11.4.7); the use of animal models can provide an early indication of whether they may be applicable to the human disease. For example, serum levels of a neoepitope detected in an assay that monitors the appearance of a collagenase cleavage product of type II collagen have been shown to be elevated in a rat model of arthritis.[58] By correlating the kinetics of the appearance of this marker in serum with histological and biochemical analyses of the cartilage itself, it should be possible to evaluate how faithfully the marker reflects pathologic processes in the tissue.

Evaluation of functional status/pain

Measurements of structural changes of OA in the joints of animal models can be correlated with measures of functional status and pain. In humans, the relationship between functional status, as measured by composite clinical endpoints such as the Western Ontario and McMaster Universities Osteoarthritis Index (WOMAC) scale, and structural changes within the joint is a matter of intense interest and research. Although it is hoped that a drug designed to slow the progression of structural changes would have a favorable impact on joint pain and functional impairment, there is no a priori reason to believe, however, that this will be the case and the correlation between progression of radiographic features of OA and progression of the severity of pain and functional impairment is poor. Furthermore, it is by no means clear how long treatment will be required before any change in structure is transmitted into a measurable clinical effect. One of the most elegant methods devised to study this question in animals was employed in studies in the hamster by Otterness and Bliven[59] in which induction of acute or chronic joint damage by intra-articular injection of varying amounts of lipopolysaccharide led to cartilage degeneration of varying severity. Function was measured by monitoring the distance each animal traveled on a running wheel within its cage.

In larger animals, such as the dog, force-plate analysis has been used to assess indirectly the loading of the arthritic joint,[60] an endpoint that the FDA accepts as a surrogate for pain. This type of analysis can be used to investigate the effects of NSAIDs and other drugs that may improve functional status but do not prevent cartilage damage. More importantly, it may be used to study the impact of DMOADs on functional status. A key issue in this area of research is the uncertainty that exists with respect to the time required for a drug that prevents cartilage degradation to result in improvement in the functional status of humans with OA (Table 11.6). Indeed, there is no clear evidence at present that an effective DMOAD will have beneficial effects on pain and function in patients with OA.

Limitations of animal models

Lack of drugs with DMOAD activity in humans to validate animal models

There are, of course, limits to what can be learned from animal models of OA (Table 11.7). Because the etiology of OA is poorly understood, it is not possible to measure how well any given model really mimics the human disease. Clearly, confidence can be gained in a model if evidence is obtained that a drug that produces a beneficial effect in the model produces an effect of similar magnitude in humans. For example, it would be virtually impossible today to conduct a trial of a novel immunosuppressive agent for prevention of kidney transplant rejection in humans without first conducting such a study in primates, because drug regimens currently used in humans are highly effective in preventing kidney rejection (at least over the first year after transplant), and this efficacy has been shown to be replicated in primates. Therefore, before embarking on human studies it is prudent to test the drug in a highly predictive pre-clinical model, if one exists.

In OA, however, the situation is different. Although models are available that detect symptom-modifying activity of drugs known to be efficacious in the clinic, for example, cyclooxygenase (COX) inhibitors, the lack of any known DMOAD precludes such an analysis of the predictive power of any animal model of OA. In a three-year study of the effects of diacerhein in

Table 11.7 Limitations associated with the use of animal models

- Lack of any DMOADs to validate models
- Physiological differences between animals and humans
- Large species/slow time course

humans with hip OA, a significant reduction in the rate of joint-space width narrowing was observed in the diacerhein-treatment group, relative to the placebo group, among those subjects who completed the trial.[61] In retrospect, the results of prior studies in guinea pig and canine models of OA (see above) may predict the results of this clinical trial in humans. However, given the virtual absence of positive DMOAD studies in humans, the predictive power of any animal model is not yet clear. Nonetheless, positive results in one or more animal models provide reassurance that there is some justification for conducting the expensive long-term trials necessary to detect a DMOAD effect in humans.

Physiologic differences between animals and humans

One species difference is particularly appropriate in a discussion of OA: considerable efforts have been made by the pharmaceutical industry to develop inhibitors of MMPs, particularly of those that degrade type II collagen. In humans, two forms of interstitial collagenase have been identified—MMP-1 and -13. However, it seems likely that no rodent homologue of MMP-1 exists. Furthermore, the tissue distribution of MMP-13 in rodents differs considerably from that in humans: human MMP-13 is largely restricted to OA cartilage, whereas in rodents, MMP-13 is widely expressed.[62] The broad tissue distribution of MMP-13 in rodents could be potentially misleading in studying drug effects. Higher species, such as the guinea pig, rabbit and dog, express both MMP-1 and -13 and, therefore, are more appropriate for the study of such inhibitors. This emphasizes how helpful a thorough understanding of the mechanism of action of a drug may be in selecting an appropriate species for testing.

Slow time course with large animals

As indicated above, although there are models in mice, rats, and guinea pigs, several OA models employ higher species, such as the rabbit and dog. In the early stages of drug evaluation, it is preferable to use a small animal species because of the relatively small amount of drug required and the ease of housing smaller animals. However, even with these species, the duration of each experiment is usually measured in months rather than weeks. This is in contrast to rodent models of rheumatoid arthritis, in which the time frame is much shorter. Furthermore, use of larger animals requires specialized husbandry, large amounts of drug, and carries higher costs.

Conclusion

Modern drug discovery focuses on a greater understanding of the molecular processes that cause pathology and employs *in vitro* systems using human reagents to optimize potency and selectivity of a drug for a particular molecular target. It differs from the way in which many older drugs were discovered. For example, the original COX inhibitors were discovered by testing compounds *in vivo*, in models such as carrageenan paw edema and adjuvant arthritis. The target enzyme for these drugs was identified only after they had been in clinical practice for many years. However, it was the discovery of the presence of two distinct isoforms of the target enzyme (COX-1 and -2) that allowed the discovery of a new generation of drugs (selective COX-2 inhibitors) with improved tolerability and safety. These drugs were first identified by screening compounds against the isolated enzymes *in vitro*. Once sufficient potency and selectivity was achieved, this was followed by testing in the animal models used to identify the first generation inhibitors (i.e., nonselective COX inhibitors). This change in the process means that animal models have a different role in drug discovery today than they did in the past. They are now used to probe the effects of a drug, targeting a specific mechanism rather than to help identify the mechanism. Animal models have, therefore, become a bridge between *in vitro* testing systems, using human reagents and clinical trials in humans. They play an important role in confirming, in a complex physiological system, that the targeted pathway is important and in identifying any additional biological effects that may result from administration of the drug.

Key points

1. OA occurs spontaneously in many species.

2. Pathological changes similar to those observed in humans with OA can be induced by a variety of experimental manipulations. However, transection of the anterior cruciate ligament and meniscectomy are the only models that have a direct counterpart in humans.

3. A drug-induced effect in animal models of OA provides encouragement that similar effects may be observed in humans. However, the predictive power of any given model is not yet understood.

4. Manipulations of the mouse genome will permit the development of new models that may address some of the current limitations of existing models.

References

(An asterisk denotes recommended reading.)

1. *Bendele, A.M., Hulman, J.F., and Bean, J.S. (1989). Spontaneous osteoarthritis in Hartley Albino guinea pigs: effects of dietary and surgical manipulations. *Arthritis Rheum* **32**:S106.

    This is a comprehensive description of one of the most widely used small animal models.

2. Bendele, A.M. and Hulman, J.F. (1988). Spontaneous cartilage degeneration in guinea pigs. *Arthritis Rheum* **31**:561–5.

3. Das-Gupta, E.P., Lyons, T.J., Hoyland, J.A., Lawton, D.M., and Freemont, A.J. (1993). New histological observations in spontaneously developing osteoarthritis in the STR/ORT mouse questioning its acceptability as a model of human osteoarthritis. *Int J Exp Pathol* **74**:627–34.

4. Okabe, T. (1989). Experimental studies on the spontaneous osteoarthritis in C57 black mice. *J Tokyo Med Coll* **47**:546–57.

5. Stanescu, R., Knyszynski, A., Muriel, M.P., and Stanescu, V. (1993). Early lesions of the articular surface in a strain of mice with very high incidence of spontaneous osteoarthritis-like lesions. *J Rheumatol* **20**:102–10.

6. Garofalo, S., Vuorio, E., Metsaranta, M., Rosati, R., Toman, D., Vaughan, J., *et al.* (1991). Reduced amounts of cartilage collagen fibrils and growth plate anomalies in transgenic mice harboring a glycine-to-cysteine mutation in the mouse type II procollagen a1-chain gene. *Proc Natl Acad Sci USA* **88**:9648–52.

7. Nakata, K., Ono, K., Miyazaki, J-I., Olsen, B., Muragaki, Y., Adachi, E., *et al.* (1993). Osteoarthritis associated with mild chondrodysplasia in transgenic mice expressing a1 (IX) collagen chains with a central deletion. *Proc Natl Acad Sci USA* **90**:2870–4.

8. Van der Kraan, P.M., Vitters, E.L., Van de Putte, L.B., and Van den Berg, W.B. (1989). Development of osteoarthritic lesions by 'metabolic' and 'mechanical' alterations in the knee joints. *Am J Pathol* **135**:1001–14.

9. Smale, G., Bendele, A.M., and Horton, W.E. (1995). Comparison of age-associated degeneration of articular cartilage in Wistar and Fischer 344 rats. *Lab An Sci* **45**:191–4.

10. Alexander, J.W. (1992). The pathogenesis of canine hip dysplasia. *Vet Clin NA: Small Animal Prac* **22**:503–11.

11. Carlson, C.S., Loeser, R.F., Jayo, M.J., Weaver, D.S., Adams, M.R., and Jerome, C.P. (1994). Osteoarthritis in cynomolgus macaques: a primate model of naturally occurring disease. *J Orthop Res* **12**:331–9.

12. Meacock, S.C.R., Bodmer, J.L., and Billingham, M.E.J. (1990). Experimental osteoarthritis in guinea pigs. *J Exp Path* **71**:279–93.

13. Meijers, M.H.M., Bunning, R.A.D., Russell, R.G.G., and Billingham, M.E.J. (1994). Evidence for cathepsin B involvement in subchondral bone changes during early natural osteoarthritis in the guinea pig. *Br J Rheum* **33** (Suppl. 1):90.

14. Osborne, D.J., Woodhouse, S., and Meacock, S.C.R. (1994). Early changes in the sulfation of chondroitin in guinea-pig articular cartilage, a possible predictor of osteoarthritis. *Osteoarthritis Cart* **2**:215–23.

15. Carney, S.L., Hicks, C.A., Tree, B., and Broadmore, R.J. (1995). An *in vivo* investigation of the effect of anthroquinones on the turnover of aggrecans in spontaneous osteoarthritis in the guinea pig. *Inflamm Res* **44**:182–6.

16. De Bri, E. and Lei, W. (2000). Biochemical and histological effects of tetracyclines on spontaneous osteoarthritis in guinea pigs. *Image Anal Stereol* **19**:125–31.

17. Yamamota, H. and Iwase, N. (1998). Spontaneous osteoarthritic lesions in a new mutant strain of the mouse. *Exp-Anim* **47**:131–5.

18. Anderson-MacKenzie, J.M., Billingham, M.E., and Bailey, A.J. (1999). Collagen Remodeling in the anterior cruiciate liament associated with developing spontaneous murine osteoarthritis. *Biochem Biophys Res Commun* **258**:763–7.

19. Pataki, A., Graf, H.P., and Witzemann, E. (1990). Spontaneous osteoarthritis of the knee joint in C57BL mice receiving chronic oral treatment with NSAIDs or prednisolone. *Agents Actions* **29**:210–17.

20. Maier, R. and Wilhelmi, G. (1987). Osteoarthrosis-like disease in mice: effects of anti-arthrotic and antirheumatic agents. In D.J. Lott, M.K. Jasani, and G.F.B. Birdwood (eds), *Studies in Osteoarthrosis, Pathogenesis, Intervention, Assessment*. Chichester: John Wiley, pp. 75–83.

21. Brewster, M., Lewis, E.J., Wilson, K.L., Greenham, A.K., and Bottomley, K.M. (1998). Ro 32-3555, an orally active collagenase selective inhibitor, prevents structural damage in the STR/ORT mouse model of osteoarthritis. *Arthritis Rheum* **41**:1639–44.

22. Pond, M.J. and Nuki, G. (1973). Experimentally-induced osteoarthritis in the dog. *Ann Rheum Dis* **32**:387–8.

23. *Brandt, K.D. (1994). Insights into the natural history of osteoarthritis provided by the cruciate-deficient dog: an animal model of osteoarthritis. *Ann NY Acad Sci* **732**:199–205.

    This is a comprehensive description of one of the most widely used large animal models.

24. Vasilev, V., Merker, H.J., and Vidinov, N. (1992). Ultrastructural changes in the synovial membrane in experimentally-induced osteoarthritis of rabbit knee joint. *Histol Histopathol* **7**:119–25.

25. Vignon, E., Mathieu, P., Bejui, J., Descotes, J., Hartmann, D., Patricot, L.M., *et al.* (1991). Study of an inhibitor of plasminogen activator (tranexamic acid) in the treatment of experimental osteoarthritis. *J Rheumatol* **27**(Suppl.):131–3.

26. Layton, M.W., Arsever, C., and Bole, G.G. (1987). Use of the guinea pig myectomy osteoarthritis model in the examination of cartilage-synovium interactions. *J Rheumatol* **125**:125–6.

27. Bendele, A.M. and White, S.L. (1987). Early histopathologic and ultrastructural alterations in femorotibial joints of partial medial meniscectomised guinea pigs. *Vet Pathol* **24**:436–43.

28. Stoop, R., Buma, P., van der Keraan, P.M., Hollander, A.P., Billinghurst, R.C., Meijers, T.H.M., Poole, A.R., and van den Berg, W.B. (2001). Type II collagen degradation in articular cartilage fibrillation after anterior cruciate ligament transection. *Osteoarthritis Cart* **9**:308–15.

29. Vilensky, J.A., O'Connor, B.L., Brandt, K.D., Dunn, E.A., and Rogers, P.I. (1994). Serial kinematic analysis of the canine knee after L4-S1 dorsal root ganglionectomy: implications for the cruciate deficiency model of osteoarthritis. *J Rheumatol* **21**:2113–17.

30. Lippiello, L., Woodward, J., Karpman, R., and Hammand, T.A. (2000). *In vivo* chondroprotection and metabolic synergy of glucosamine and chondroitin sulfate. *Clin Orthop* **381**:229–40.

31. Johnson, K.A., Hulse, D.A., Hart, R.C., Kochevar, D., and Chu, Q. (2001). Effects of an orally administered mixture of chondroitin sulfate, glucosamine hydrochloride and manganese ascorbate on synovial fluid chondroitin sulfate 3B3 and 7D4 epitopes in a canine cruciate ligament transection model of osteoarthritis. *Osteoarthritis Cart* **9**:14–21.

32. Reginster, J.Y., Deroisy, R., Rovati, L.C., *et al.* (2001). Long term effects of glucosamine sulphate on osteoarthritis progression: a randomised, placebo-controlled clinical trial. *Lancet* **357**:251–6.

33. Pelletier, J.P. and Martel-Pelletier, J. (1989). Protective effects of corticosteroids on cartilage lesions and osteophyte formation in the Pond-Nuki dog model of osteoarthritis. *Arthritis Rheum* **32**:181–93.

34. Pelletier, J.P. and Martel-Pelletier, J. (1991). *In vivo* protective effects of prophylactic treatment with tiaprofenic acid or intraarticular corticosteroids on osteoarthritic lesions in the experimental dog model. *J Rheumatol* **27**(Suppl.):127–30.

35. Myers, S.L., Brandt, K.D., and O'Connor, B.L. (1991). Low dose prednisone treatment does not reduce the severity of osteoarthritis in dogs after anterior cruciate ligament transection. *J Rheumatol* **18**:1856–62.

36. Kuo, S.Y., Chu, S.J., Hsu, C.M., Chen, C.M., Chang, M.L., and Chang, D.M. (1994). An experimental model of osteoarthritis in rabbit. *Chung Hua I Hsueh Tsa Chih* **54**:377–81.

37. Caron, J.P., Fernandes, J.C., Martel-Pelletier, J., Tardif, G., Mineau, F., Geng, C., and Pelletier, J.P. (1996). Chondroprotective effect of intraarticular injections of interleukin-1 receptor antagonist in experimental osteoarthritis. Suppression of collagenase-1 expression. *Arthritis Rheum* **39**:1535–44.

38. Fernandes, J., Tardif, G., Martel-Pelletier, J., Lascau-Coman, V., Dupuis, M., Moldovan, F., Sheppard, M., Krisnan, B.R., and Pelletier, J.P. (1999). *In vivo* transfer of interleukin-1 receptor antagonist gene in osteoarthritic rabbit knee joints: prevention of osteoarthritis progression. *Am J Pathol* **154**: 1159–69.

39. Manicourt, D.H., Altman, R.D., Williams, J.M., Devogelaer, J.P., Druetz-Van Egeren, A., Lenz, M.E., Pietryla, D., and Thonar, E.J. (1999). Treatment with calcitonin suppresses the responses of bone, cartilage and synovium in the early stages of canine experimental osteoarthritis and significantly reduces the severity of the cartilage lesions. *Arthritis Rheum* **42**:1159–67.

40. Myers, S.L., Brandt, K.D., Burr, D.B., O'Connor, B.L., and Albrecht, M. (1999). Effects of a bisphosphonate on bone histomorphometry and dynamics in the canine cruciate deficiency model of osteoarthritis. *J Rheumatol* **26**:2645–53.

41. Rogachevsky, R.A., Dean, D.D., Howell, D.S., and Altman, R.D. (1994). Treatment of canine osteoarthritis with insulin-like growth factor (IGF1) and sodium pentosan polysulfate. *Ann N Y Acad Sci* **732**:392–4.

42. Okazaki, K., Jingushi, S., Ikenoue, T., Urabe, K., Sakai, H., Ohtsuru, A., Akino, K., Yamashita, S., Nomura, S., and Iwamato, Y. (1999). Expression of insulin-like growth factor I messenger ribonucleic acid in developing osteophytes in murine experimental osteoarthritis and in rats inoculated with growth hormone secreting tumor. *Endocrinology* **140**:3821–30.

43. Yu, L.P., Jr., Smith, G.N., Jr., Brand, K.D., Myers, S.L., O'Connor, B.L., and Brandt, D.A. (1992). Reduction of the severity of canine osteoarthritis by prophylactic treatment with oral doxycycline. *Arthritis Rheum* **35**:1150–9.

44. MacPherson, L.J., Bayburt, E.K., Capparelli, M.P., Carroll, B.J., Goldstein, R., Justice, M.R., Zhu, L., Hu, S., Melton, R.A., Fryer, L., Goldberg, R.L., Doughty, J.R., Spirito, S., Blancuzzi, V., Wilson, D., Obyrne, E.M., Ganu, V., and Parker, D.T. (1997). Discovery of CGS 27023A, a non-peptidic, potent, and orally active stromelysin inhibitor that blocks cartilage degradation in rabbits. *J Med Chem* **40**:2525–32.

45. Kobayashi, K., Amiel, M., Harwood, F.L., Healy, R.M., Sonoda, M., Moriya, H., and Amiel, D. (2000). The long-term effects of hyaluronan during development of osteoarthritis following partial meniscectomy in a rabbit model. *Osteoarthritis Cart* **8**:359–65.

46. Smith, G.N., Myers, S.L., Brandt, K.D., and Mickler, E.A. (1998). Effect of intraarticular hyaluronan injection in experimental canine osteoarthritis. *Arthritis Rheum* **41**:976–85.

47. Yamada, H., Watanabe, K., Saito, T., Hayashi, H., Niitani, Y., Ito, A., Fujikawa, K., and Lohmander, L.S. (1999). Esculetin (dihydrocoumarin) inhibits the production of matrix metalloproteinases in cartilage explants, and oral administration of its prodrug, CPA-926, suppresses cartilage destruction in rabbit experimental osteoarthritis. *J Rheumatol* **26**:654–62.

48. *Smith, G.N., Myers, S.L., Brandt, K.D., Mickler, A., and Albrecht, M.E. (1999). Diacerhein treatment reduces the severity of osteoarthritis in the canine cruciate-deficiency model of osteoarthritis. *Arthritis Rheum* **42**:545–54.

Demonstration of the disease-modifying effects of a drug in an animal model. The effect was subsequently confirmed in a randomized controlled trial in humans with hip OA (see Ref. 61).

49. Pelletier, J.P., Jovanovic, D.V., Lascau-Coman, V., Fernandes, J.C., Manning, P.T., Connor, J.R., Currie, M.G., and Martel-Pelletier, J. (2000). Selective inhibition of inducible nitric oxide synthase reduces progression of experimental osteoarthritis *in vivo*—possible link with the reduction in chondrocyte apoptosis and caspase 3 level. *Arthritis Rheum* **43**:1290–99.

50. Brandt, K.D., Smith, G., Kang, S.Y., Myers, S., O'Connor, B., and Albrecht, M. (1997). Effects of diacerhein in an accelerated canine model of osteoarthritis. *Osteoarthritis Cart* **5**:438–49.

51. Kikuchi, T., Sakuta, T., and Yamaguchi, T. (1998). Intra-articular injection of collagenase induces experimental osteoarthritis in mature rabbits. *Osteoarthritis Cart* **6**:177–86.

52. Kopp, S., Mejersjo, C., and Clemensson, E. (1983). Induction of osteoarthrosis in the guinea pig knee by papain. *Oral Surg. Oral Med Oral Pathol* **55**:259–66.

53. Schrier, D.J., Flory, C.M., Finkel, M., Kuchera, S.L., Lesch, M.E., and Jacobson, P.B. (1996). The effects of the phospholipase A2 inhibitor, manoalide, on cartilage degradation, stromelysin expression and synovial fluid cell count induced by intraarticular injection of human recombinant interleukin-1 alpha in the rabbit. *Arthritis Rheum* **39**:1292.

54. Van-Beuningen, H.M., Glansbeek, H.L., Van der Kraan, P.M., and Van den Ber, W.B. (2000). Osteoarthritis-like changes in the murine knee joint resulting from intra-articular transforming growth factor-beta injections. *Osteoarthritis Cart* **8**:25–33.

55. Clark, K.A., Heitmeyer, S.A., Smith, A.G., and Taiwo, Y.O. (1997). Gait analysis in a rat model of osteoarthrosis. *Physiol Behav* **62**:951–4.

56. Neuhold, L.A., Killar, L., Weigusng, Z., Sung M-LA, Warner, L., Kulik, J., Turner, J., Wu, W., Billinghurst, C., Meijers, T., Poole, A.R., Babij, P., and Degennaro, L.J. (2001). Postnatal expression in hyaline cartilage of constitutively active human collagenase-3 (MMP-13) induces osteoarthritis in mice. *J Clin Invest* **107**:35–44.

57. Bakker, A.C., Van de loo, F.A.J., Van Beuningen, H.M., Sime, P., Van Lent, P.L.E.M., Van der Kraan, P.M., Richards, C.D., and Van den Berg, W.B. (2001). Overexpression of active TGF-beta-1 in the murine knee joint: evidence for synovial layer dependent chondro-ostephyte formation. *Osteoarthritis Cart* **9**:128–36.

58. Song, X., Zeng, L., Jin, W., *et al.* (1999). Secretory leukocyte protease inhibitor suppresses the inflammation and joint damage of bacterial cell wall induced arthritis. *J Exp Med* **190**:535–42.

59. *Otterness, I.G., Bliven, M.L., Milici, A.J., and Poole, A.R. (1994). Comparison of mobility changes with histological and biochemical changes during LPS-induced arthritis in the hamster. *Am J Pathol* **144**: 1098–108.

This study serves as one of the best examples of how a small animal model can be used to relate functional responses to biochemical and histological changes within the OA joint.

60. Toutain, P.L., Cester, C.C., Haak, T., and Laroute, V. (2001). A pharmacokinetic/pharmacodynamic approach vs. a dose titration for the determination of a dosage regimen: The case of nimesulide, a Cox-2 selective nonsteroidal antiinflammatory drug in the dog. *J Vet Pharmacol Ther* **24**:43–55.

61. Dougados, M., Nguyen, M., Berdah, L., Mazieres, B., Vignon, E., and Lesquesne, M. (2001). Evaluation of the structure-modifying effects of diacerein in hip osteoarthritis. *Arthritis Rheum* **44**:2539–47.

62. Mitchell, P.G., Magna, H.A., Reeves, L.M., Lopresti-Morrow, L.L., Yocum, S.A., Rosner, P.J., *et al.* (1996). Cloning of matrix metalloproteinase-13 (MMP-13, collagenase-3) from human chondrocytes, expression of MMP-13 by osteoarthritic cartilage and activity of the enzyme on type II collagen. *J Clin Invest* **97**:761–8.

11.4 Assessment of changes in joint tissues in patients treated with disease modifying osteoarthritis drugs (DMOADs): monitoring outcomes

11.4.1 Radiographic grading system

Geraldine Hassett, Deborah J. Hart, and Tim D. Spector

Radiographic assessment has been widely used as an outcome measure in OA. Kellgren and Lawrence proposed the first standardized system. This is a global grading system in which composite scores are derived. Joint-specific definitions with separate measurements of individual radiographic features are thought to better reflect OA that occurs in each joint. A number of validated atlases are now available that score individual features in each joint affected by OA. All grading systems rely on the reproducibility of the X-rays and grading systems. This is particularly true for the assessment of radiographic progression of OA. This chapter will cover the history of the development of radiographic systems, how they apply to individual joints, problems inherent with measurement at the hip, knees, hands, and lumbar spine and finally a section on OA progression.

History and problems of existing radiographic grading systems

In the past, attempts to classify OA have set out to identify similar features of the disease and to apply changes in these features globally in all joints. It has now been shown that classification criteria cannot be developed to cover changes in this way, as OA manifests differently in each joint group it affects. The time sequence of exactly when articular cartilage is lost, subchondral bone alters, and new bone is formed, remains unclear. Choosing one as a marker for OA may lead to problems of misclassification should a different feature commonly appear first in a particular joint. Indeed classification of OA at some sites may be easier than at others. For example in the knee, osteophytes may be more prevalent and more closely associated with knee pain,[1] whereas in the hip, joint-space narrowing more strongly associates with pain and may be of more use in the definition than osteophytes alone.[2] Altman *et al.*, in 1987, demonstrated that for progression of OA, the most useful radiographic variables differed according to the anatomic site (hand, hip, and knee), with results indicating that there should be different approaches toward the evaluation of OA progression at specific joint regions.[3]

Radiographs are the most common method of classifying OA and have been widely used as an outcome measure, particularly in epidemiological and clinical studies. Despite advantages of widespread availability, permanency of the record, reproducibility, and good standardization, there are limitations. Reproducibility of radiographic grading can be poor, and there are inconsistencies in interpreting existing criteria thus affecting prevalence estimates in populations. For nearly 40 years the radiological definitions of Kellgren and Lawrence,[4] have been accepted as a gold standard, but there are many problems associated with this system.

The method of grading radiographic OA was developed by Kellgren and Lawrence in 1957, and adopted by the World Health Organisation (WHO) in Rome in 1961 as the accepted gold standard for cross-sectional and longitudinal epidemiological studies. The original written definitions of the grading of radiographs were given in 1957 (Table 11.8), and it was intended that an atlas should accompany the definitions. However, the corresponding photographs used in a subsequent atlas[5] in some cases did not exactly match the written grades. For example, Grade 2 was described as 'presence of definite osteophyte with minimal joint space narrowing', and this was later described[6] as 'definite osteophyte but joint space unimpaired'. Definitions of the Kellgren and Lawrence grading system as presented in 1963 are given in Table 11.8. These inconsistencies in interpretations of the system have led to problems of different classification in epidemiological studies by groups who believe that they have all applied the standard criteria. The Kellgren and Lawrence grading system has subsequently been criticized for its reliance on the presence of the osteophyte for classification of disease.[7] The time sequence of when bony changes occur and articular cartilage is lost is still controversial. Thus, according to Kellgren and Lawrence, presence of a narrowed, sclerotic joint with deformity cannot be classified as osteoarthritic

Table 11.8 Description of the radiological features of the Kellgren and Lawrence grading system of osteoarthritis (Atlas 1963)

The following radiological features were considered evidence of osteoarthrosis:

(a) Formation of osteophytes on the joint margins or, in the case of the knee joint, on the tibial spines

(b) Periarticular ossicles; these are found chiefly in relation to the distal and proximal interphalangeal joints

(c) Narrowing of the joint cartilage associated with sclerosis of the subchondral bone

(d) Small pseudocystic areas with sclerotic walls usually situated in the subchondral bone

(e) Altered shape of bone ends, particularly in the head of the femur.

These changes have been graded numerically:

0	None	No features
1	Doubtful	Minute osteophyte, doubtful significance
2	Minimal	Definite osteophyte, unimpaired joint space
3	Moderate	Moderate diminution of joint space
4	Severe	Joint space greatly impaired with sclerosis of sub-chondral bone

unless an osteophyte is also present. There also remains a problem of how to classify those individuals with a Grade 1, doubtful osteophyte. Is it correct to classify these people with Grade 1 as a normal group, or treat them as an affected group with early changes of OA? It has been suggested that since no clear consensus exists as to whether Grade 1 subjects are cases or controls, they should be treated as a separate grade.[8] This could be achieved by either excluding Grade 1 from the analysis or treating them as a separate subgroup. The imperfections of the Kellgren and Lawrence criteria were discussed at the 3rd International Symposium on Rheumatic Disease in New York in 1966.[9] However, it was decided that in the absence of any improved, validated criteria the Rome criteria should stand. There is an increasing acceptance that OA may not represent one disorder but that it is a disease spectrum with a series of subsets that lead to similar clinical and pathological alterations. The prevalent view that OA should no longer be thought of as a single disease, but as a group of 'osteoarthritic diseases' has been emphasized.[10] The first step in classifying these diseases is to develop joint-specific definitions and criteria, and abandon trying to develop a single criterion that incorporates manifestations of the whole spectrum of the disease. A number of groups, aware of these existing problems, have developed new criteria for classifying OA radiographically, and have focused on improving radiographic criteria, particularly in solving the problems of emphasis on the osteophyte in the Kellgren and Lawrence atlas. These groups have selected particular joints and developed criteria relating to the differing pathological processes of OA that present as common individual features, which accompany OA in that joint site. However despite the major academic group's criticism of the Kellgren and Lawrence grade, the system refuses to die, and is still widely used in clinical trials for subject inclusion.

Features of osteoarthritis on radiographs and their utility

Radiographically OA is characterized by joint-space narrowing due to changes in articular cartilage, and by changes in the subchondral and marginal bone, which manifest as osteophyte, cysts, and eburnation. A number of methods of radiographic assessment have been proposed each taking into account some of these features. The following descriptions attempt to interpret these changes radiographically.

Osteophytes

An osteophyte is a fibrocartilage-capped bony growth. On a radiograph, marginal osteophytes appear as new spurs or lips of bone around the edges of a joint and are variable in size. They originate at tendon insertions and capsular attachments. They frequently predominate in one side of the joint and develop initially in areas of relatively normal joint space. They can also occur in central areas of the joint in which remnants of articular cartilage still exist. These central osteophytes frequently lead to a bumpy contour on a radiograph. Osteophytes can be very large and can increase the size of a joint. They are almost always seen in association with some degree of cartilage loss except in the interphalangeal joints of the hands. Some authors have proposed that the presence of osteophytes be attributed to age, rather than OA.[11] However, studies such as that by Brandt *et al.* examining pathological correlates of OA by arthroscopy and radiography, found that patients with osteophytes and normal articular cartilage on arthroscopy were younger than the patient group as a whole, suggesting that osteophytes cannot be explained on the basis of age alone.[12]

Joint-space narrowing

Cartilage in a degenerating joint initially becomes thinned and roughened—'fibrillation'. Later, larger areas of erosions begin and this progressive cartilage loss leads to a common radiographic sign of OA narrowing and loss of joint space. In general, cartilage loss is most pronounced in areas of maximum weight bearing, for example the medial tibio-femoral compartment of the knee. Guidelines recommend that the measure of joint-space width

(JSW) determined on radiography should be used as a proxy for joint-space narrowing. Currently articular cartilage preservation is considered the primary outcome measure in OA studies and thus JSW, an indirect measure of articular cartilage loss, is an important primary endpoint in both epidemiological studies and clinical trials.

Sclerosis

Generally after evidence of joint-space loss, eburnation becomes apparent followed by sclerosis—an increased localized area of density at the joint margin seen as a dense white line extending vertically into deeper regions of the subchondral bone. Initially the radiodense region may be uniform, leading to radiolucent lesions reflecting subchondral cyst formation. Reproducibility for grading sclerosis is often poor, as it is dependent on film penetration, and the assessment is subjective and difficult to quantify.

Tibial spiking

A major radiological text states that 'spiking' (i.e., an increase in height and reduction in angle) of the tubercles of the intercondylar eminence of the tibial plateau is an early sign of OA of the knee joint.[13] Most imaging centres uniformly report on spiking, without clear evidence of its significance. One study found spiking was more marked in OA patients, but did not look at other features of OA.[14] A recent much larger population study found a modest association with degree of spike angle and presence of osteophyte and joint-space narrowing. However, in subjects with otherwise normal radiographs for OA, there was no association of spiking and pain, and isolated spiking was not found to be a useful measure for the diagnosis of knee OA.[15]

Joint-specific radiographic features

The hand

Osteoarthritis of the distal and proximal interphalangeal joints (DIP/PIP) of the hand and the trapeziometacarpal joints of the thumb base (1st CMC) are extremely common, especially in middle-aged, post-menopausal women. Metocarpophalangeal joint involvement is rare, except in the elderly. Osteoarthritis of the hand is characterized by the presence of multiple affected joints and is usually symmetrical. Osteoarthritis of the DIP joints are more prevalent than OA of the PIPs, which may be absent in the presence of DIP OA. Interrelationships of joint involvement and symmetry in the hand have been studied. A study confirmed that clustering, commonly affecting the DIP and 1st CMC joints, was greater than expected with increasing age.[16] The most important determinants of pattern of involvement in the hand were in order of importance, symmetry, clustering by row (DIP), then by ray (DIP followed by PIP).

Clinically, OA of the DIP and PIP joints present as bony enlargements around the joint, clinically known as Heberden's and Bouchard's nodes, respectively. These nodes may not always be seen as a radiographic bony deformity, and may also be undetectable in the presence of X-ray changes.[17] Malalignments and flexion deformity may also occur in severe cases of OA. X-rays of the hands reveal prominent osteophyte and joint-space narrowing. In OA the wavy contour of the distal phalanx resembles the wings of a bird (Seagull sign).[13] There is sometimes mild to moderate subluxation at the distal or proximal joints producing a zig–zag contour. Occasionally, at the joint margin are what appear to be fractured osteophytes that have broken away from the articular surface.

OA of the wrist, in the absence of trauma, is rare except at the trapeziometacarpal joint. Subluxation of the metacarpal base with resultant joint-space loss is commonly seen, as well as osteophytosis and fragmentation of bone (Fig. 11.11).

The hip

In the hip joint the most common feature of OA is joint-space narrowing. This narrowing follows several patterns, with superolateral loss being the most common, whilst medial and concentric losses affect only a minority. In later stages of OA, the femoral head may also appear flattened with resulting proximal migration of the femur. Osteophytes appear most commonly on the superolateral acetabular surface, and less commonly on the femoral head and neck. Lateral acetabular osteophytes have the appearance of a lip extending from the articular surface (Fig. 11.12). If the normal acetabular surface extends, this can often be misclassified as a mild osteophyte. In population studies acetabular osteophytes are only weakly associated with hip pain and are not a useful indicator on their own of disease. Other features commonly seen at the hip are sclerosis and cysts.

Radiographs of hips are obtained with patients in supine or standing positions, and internal rotation of the feet. Weight bearing knee radiographs are considered necessary to assess accurately JSN in tibio-femoral OA.[18] Thus, a number of authors have examined the influence of the radiographic method on joint-space estimation of the hip.[19–21] Conrozier et al. demonstrated a significant decrease in JSW of the hip only in a subgroup of patients with JSW less than 2.5 mm, when comparing supine and weight bearing films.[19] The detected difference was larger in radiographs centred on the hip than those centred as a pelvic X-ray. In contrast, Auleley et al. found concordant measurements of JSW on standing and supine radiographs in the same patient.[22] The use of the *faux profil* (oblique view) has also been proposed in addition to the standard standing antero-posterior view.[23] In a recent study, a difference of 10° of internal rotation of the foot did not induce bias in the JSW measured on pelvic X-ray of hip OA.[24] Therefore it remains unclear as to whether hip X-rays should be taken supine or standing, as there has been conflicting results in the literature. Taken together nevertheless, these studies show that weight bearing affects

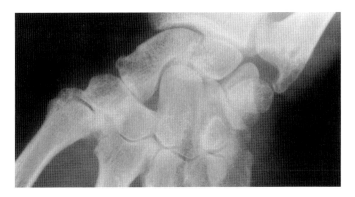

Fig. 11.11 Subluxation of the metacarpal base and osteophytosis.

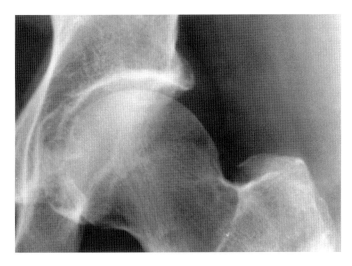

Fig. 11.12 Lateral acetabular margin showing mild osteophyte formation.

JSW in hip OA. Despite this, JSW on plain radiographs remains a reliable outcome measure for hip OA.

The knee

The knee is made up of three compartments: medial and lateral tibio-femoral joint (TFJ) and the patello-femoral joint (PFJ). Common features of knee OA on radiographs are osteophyte, narrowed joint space, sclerosis, and cysts. Three views of the knee have been proposed for the study of the tibio-femoral joint: (1) antero-posterior extended view,[25,26] (2) antero-posterior semi-flexed view,[26,27] and (3) postero-anterior flexed view.[28] TFJ space narrowing is traditionally best visualized on anterior-posterior extended view films that are useful for the assessment of the joint space in both the medial and lateral compartments. Problems in the reproducibility of the extended view may occur in two ways: positional problems (i.e., variable knee flexion), which may result in large changes in JSW, and precision of measurement. A coefficient of variation of 20–40 per cent has been estimated using conventional views and it is likely to be the major source of error.[29] One small study examined the reproducibility of extended and semi-flexed views of the medial compartment using computerized joint-space measurement in optimal conditions.[30] The coefficient of variation (CV) was 9 per cent for the traditional method and 5 per cent for a standing semi-flexed method, suggesting the latter may become more widely used. Buckland-Wright et al. propose the use of a semi-flexed view, however compared to the fully extended view it does not significantly improve the precision and accuracy of joint-space measurement in the medial compartment of patients with OA, but only those of the lateral compartment.[31] Using guidelines defining the radiographic procedure, both the conventional extended view and the semi-flexed view appear reproducible in the measurement of JSW.[31,32] For the flexed and semi-flexed views, the use of fluroscopy is necessary to capture the joint space well.[27] However, in numerous centres fluroscopy is not available and the real benefit from using fluroscopy remains to be evaluated.

OA of the patello-femoral compartment is often seen in conjunction with the TFJ, and to a lesser extent on its own. The patello-femoral view is useful for assessing joint-space narrowing and osteophyte on the patella side of the joint. Traditionally two views of the PFJ have been used; the lateral, in approximately 30° of flexion and the skyline (30–60° flexion) or sunrise view.[33] Studies have examined the relative merits of skyline versus lateral view for assessing the patello-femoral joint. In a small study of hospital cases Jones et al. found grading of the skyline view was more reproducible than the lateral view, and allowed more precise localization of change.[34] This has been confirmed in a larger population-based study that also suggested that different osteophytes are detected by the two views, and may be complimentary.[35]

Lumbar spine

Vertebral osteophytes are a characteristic feature of intervertebral disc degeneration. Early classification criteria for disc degeneration utilized a combination of radiographic features including the presence of osteophytes, disc-space narrowing, and vertebral endplate sclerosis.

In 1958, Kellgren and Lawrence reported that the prevalence of disc degeneration in the general population gradually increased with age, reaching 85 per cent in men and 71 per cent in women over the age of 65.[4] Relatively few studies concerning radiological disc degeneration have been performed, and therefore there remains uncertainty about the role of individual radiographic features in the definition and course of disease. Indeed a recent study showed that lumbar degenerative disease is more common in the United Kingdom than in a mountain village in Japan, and that differences exist in the prevalence of both osteophytosis and disc degeneration between the two countries.[36] The general mechanism for 'degeneration' of the spine is thought to be disc narrowing with subsequent osteophyte formation, these results therefore suggest that there may be alternative mechanisms in different ethnic groups. One study found that isolated osteophytes predict the subsequent development of disc-space narrowing.[37]

Longitudinal studies are needed to evaluate the radiographic features that best define lumbar disc degeneration and their association with clinical disease.

Methods of grading features of osteoarthritis

The hand

Kallman *et al.* were the first to produce an atlas of features of hand OA to include a graded scale of severity of osteophyte formation, narrowing of the joint space, subchondral sclerosis, subchondral cysts, lateral deformity, and cortical collapse.[38] Osteophyte and narrowing were to be graded using a 0–3 scale, and the other features scored present or absent (Table 11.9). In developing the atlas, Kallman also graded all films using Kellgren and Lawrence for comparison. Grade 1 Kallman was to correspond to Kellgren and Lawrence Grade 2 (definite osteophyte), and Grade 1 Kellgren and Lawrence (doubtful osteophyte) scored 0 on the Kallman scale. The grading scale appeared to be reliable when used cross-sectionally and in longitudinal data, and also compared well to the Kellgren and Lawrence scale. All features performed well for intra-observer reproducibility, but for interobserver reproducibility, osteophyte, and narrowing, Kellgren and Lawrence performed best, with cysts, deformity and collapse performing less well. The interobserver agreement was best for dichotomous variables (96–99 per cent) and for multiple categories readers agreed most for osteophyte (86 per cent) followed by narrowing (79 per cent) and Kellgren and Lawrence (78 per cent). Reliability was good overall for osteophyte (interclass correlation, ICC = 0.71), narrowing (ICC = 0.70), sclerosis (ICC = 0.60), and was best for Kellgren and Lawrence (ICC = 0.74). It was less good for cysts and deformity. Percentage agreement was higher within than between readers, and again highest for dichotomous variables (98–99 per cent). Osteophyte performed best (93 per cent) followed by narrowing (88 per cent) and Kellgren and Lawrence (85 per cent). Reliability within readers was better than between readers for all measures. For the longitudinal data, readers also studied films 20–25 years apart. The authors suggested that one reader may be appropriate for longitudinal film data, as the different readers all determined progression similarly and intra-reader reliability was almost perfect. Kallman *et al.* recommended different methods for reading X-rays for longitudinal studies. Firstly, paired films were read side by side and assigned a progression score for time sequence and magnitude of change, in the films this carried the advantage of an increase in sensitivity, although films were subject to 'time sequence' bias. Secondly, serial films were read one at a time in random order to eliminate 'time sequence' bias. The Kallman grading system is reproducible for both cross-sectional and longitudinal studies, and has been validated in other population studies,[39] the only problem being the quality of the reproduced standard films, which are difficult to read. The presence of the osteophyte remains the best way of defining OA of the hand.

Individual scoring of features as proposed by Kallman for hand OA can be time consuming, which may be disadvantageous for clinical and epidemiological studies dealing with large patient samples. Kessler *et al.*, demonstrated the reliability of a hand scale based on a simple dichotomy of whether or not OA is present by grouping several radiographic features, to assess the prevalence of hand OA and to measure the number of joints being included in the disease process.[40] They based their scale on JSN, on the assumption that it is the major radiological feature of OA, and therefore other radiological parameters were only used in conjunction with JSN. The average reading time required for one antero-posterior hand radiograph with the Kessler hand scale was five minutes, compared with 10–15 minutes per hand for the Kallman method. The scale had good inter and intra-reader reliability for all the individual joints, with the highest reliability being for PIP joints. This scale may prove useful in large epidemiological studies.

A recent overview on the methodology of clinical trials in hand OA, were unable to recommend a particular radiographic grading system as the most appropriate radiographic method to be used in studies assessing the

Table 11.9 Rating method used in scales for grading individual features of OA[*]

Feature	Grade
Osteophytes	0, None
	1, Small (definite) osteophyte(s)
	2, Moderate osteophyte(s)
	3, Large osteophyte(s)
Joint space narrowing[†]	0, None
	1, Definitely narrowed
	2, Severely narrowed
	3, Joint fusion at least one point
Subchondral sclerosis	0, Absent
	1, Present
Subchondral cysts	0, Absent
	1, Present
Lateral deformity[‡]	0, Absent
	1, Present
Collapse of central joint cortical bone	0, Absent
	1, Present

[*] Modified from Ref. 24.

[†] Narrowing between bone end plates, not osteophyte bridging.

[‡] Malalignment of at least 15 degrees.

structure-modifying effects of a drug in hand OA.[41] However, they suggested that five methods should be considered: (1) Kellgren and Lawrence score; (2) Kallman grading scale; (3) Verbruggen numerical scoring methods; (4) Buckland-Wright macroradiography; and (5) global assessment of the presence/absence of OA.

The hip

Similar radiographic features have been tested by Croft *et al.* to classify OA of the hip.[2] The features measured were (1) minimum joint space at 4 points around the joint arc read by transparent ruler; (2) size of largest osteophyte; and (3) subchondral sclerosis. A composite score was also used. Joint-space narrowing was more reproducible than osteophyte size; intra-observer kappas of 0.81 versus 0.44, and intra-observer 0.70 versus 0.33. Narrowing of the joint space was more strongly associated with pain than osteophyte presence (56 versus 34 per cent), suggesting that joint-space narrowing may be of more importance in defining hip OA than the presence of osteophyte. Scott *et al.* studied 1 363 women in the United States of America and found that of the individual variables joint-space narrowing correlated best with pain, although a combination of osteophyte and joint-space narrowing provided the best overall predictor of pain.[42]

The narrowest point of the hip for measurement of joint-space narrowing can be chosen manually by the reader of the film or automatically after digitization of the film.[43] Measurement of the joint-space area calculated after digitization of the films rather than the JSW has also been proposed, but this technique may be less sensitive to change.[44] Computer analyses of digitalized films and macroradiography have also been proposed for the measurement of JSW.[43,45]

Lane *et al.*, developed new indices for the presence and severity of radiographic features of OA in the hip and hand, and disc degeneration in the thoracic and lumbar spine.[46] Individual radiographic features are scored and then a summary grade is derived directly from the assessment of selected radiographic features. The interobserver agreement for the right hip (ICC 0.82 for narrowing, 0.74 for osteophytes, 0.85 for summary grade, and kappa 0.67 for sclerosis), and intra-observer (ICC 0.81 for narrowing, 0.82 for osteophytes, 0.82 for summary grade, kappa 0.61) was good.

The reproducibility of measurements of JSW is approximately ± 0.2 mm for the hip.[22] In a recent study the minimum clinically detectable decrease in width over 12 months was 0.6 mm.[44] Radiographic hip OA progression has been reported to vary from 0.1–0.6 mm/year.[24,44,47]

The knee

Ahlback performed one of the earliest investigations into features of knee OA in 1968.[48] This atlas made recommendations on views to be used as well as gradings for measuring articular space, although these were crudely described and based on a subjective assessment likely to lead to variable interpretation. Spector et al. developed an atlas for the knee using individual features[49] and subsequently updated it to include the skyline view.[50] Individual features of osteophyte and joint-space narrowing were graded on a 0–3 scale, and sclerosis graded present or absent. This atlas also included a patello-femoral view, which was previously ignored in the Kellgren and Lawrence system. Reproducibility of reading lateral patello-femoral radiographs has however not been as good as tibio-femoral views.[51,52] Data has shown the skyline view is more reproducible for defining patello-femoral OA than the lateral view.[34,35] The atlas and its criteria for knee OA has been validated for observer reproducibility, and also compared to the Kellgren and Lawrence scale.[49] Features performed well within observers for both tibio-femoral and patello-femoral narrowing and osteophyte, and less well between observers; patello-femoral measurements between observers were poor. The individual features measured compared well to Kellgren and Lawrence grades.

The criteria of the Spector atlas were compared to a number of other criteria for classifying knee OA in a general population sample of 1954 knees.[1] The individual features graded from the atlas performed similarly well compared to Kellgren and Lawrence grades, precision ruler measurements, and automated digital analysis of joint-space loss.[53] However, in analysis of predictors for knee pain in this group, using the Spector atlas Kellgren and Lawrence Grade 2 definite osteophytes (medial or lateral) were better predictors than narrowing. This suggests that, for reading conventional X-rays of the knee for epidemiological studies, the osteophyte may be the best predictor of clinical disease and that joint-space narrowing may be more useful for assessing disease severity or progression.

Another atlas for knee radiographs has been produced assessing eight features of OA; medial and lateral osteophytes, joint-space narrowing, sclerosis, osteophytes of the tibial spines, and chondrocalcinosis. It was designed by Scott et al. as a scheme for equal weight scoring of selected 'fields' of the joint. Four readers read these signs in 30 films for reliability as well as reading the films for a Kellgren and Lawrence grade. The results were good for all measures with ICC ranging from 0.63–0.83 for interreader and 0.82–0.95 for intra-reader. The poorest measures were sclerosis and tibial spiking. All measures were comparable to Kellgren and Lawrence grades, and narrowing performed as well as osteophyte grading.[54] Recently Cooke et al. have proposed a revised Scott scheme in an attempt to increase the sensitivity of the grading system to progressive deterioration and to specific biomechanical variables of deformity.[55] They included the new fields of tibial erosion and subluxation and removed tibial osteophytes and sclerosis. The worst affected compartment only was scored on frontal standardized knee images, which were used to define knee alignment variables. The interobserver reliability score was good at kappa 0.92.

However, photographic atlases in general and in particular of the knee have several potential problems. Altman et al. produced an atlas for the Osteoarthritis Research Society (OARS), which permits the scoring of individual features and includes the skyline view of the patello-femoral compartment and is considered by many as the current standard radiographic atlas for OA.[56] Potential limitations of this atlas have been suggested including: (1) ordinal grades for JSN and osteophyte size do not increase in a strictly geometric fashion, (2) variation in magnification and intensity of photographs, (3) uncommon shapes of osteophytes are presented on several knee radiographs, (4) no radiographs for the medial and lateral aspects of the femoral trochlea in the skyline view, (5) concurrence of several features within the same X-ray photograph may distract the observer and lead to bias when matching the study film and atlas image for more than just the individual item of interest, (6) cumbersome to use, and (7) due to high costs of photographic reproduction the atlas is not readily available to all investigators. Nagaosa et al. have therefore developed an atlas of line drawings for the assessment and grading of narrowing and osteophyte on knee radiographs, to try and overcome some of the above problems.[57] Joint-space narrowing and osteophytes were included in the line drawings as they are accepted as the cardinal features of radiographic structural OA. As with previous standard atlases each feature was scored 0–3 to allow direct comparison with the OARS atlas. Antero-posterior radiographs were taken with weight bearing in full extension and skyline views were taken according to the method of Laurin. Tracings of two representative radiographs from several hundred normal films, one male and one female, showing normal bone contours for each radiographic view and having normal JSWs in each compartment were made. These sets were designated 0 for JSN. Copies of these tracings were subsequently adjusted to show grades 1, 2, and 3 JSN in each compartment, calculated as 33, 66, or 99 per cent reductions of the interbone distance evident on the Grade 0 joint-space narrowing set. In addition to make the drawings as biological and representative as possible, the tibia was shifted more medially, the patella more laterally, with no reduction in the contralateral compartment with progressive joint-space narrowing. The maximum size of Grade 3 osteophyte was selected from a hospital-based sample of patients with knee OA. Selection of radiographs showing the biggest as well as the most typical shape and direction at each site were chosen. Hand tracings were made of Grade 3 osteophytes, and then Grades 1 and 2 osteophytes were drawn to be one-third and two-thirds, respectively, the length and width of the Grade 3 osteophyte. The shape and direction of the osteophyte showed some variation at each site, particularly at the lateral tibial plateau and medial femoral trochlea, where a standard set of line drawings and a secondary optional set were produced. Three observers (after training for a period) then scored 50 sets of bilateral knee films four times, the first and third reading using the OARS atlas, the second and fourth the line drawing atlas. Reproducibility for both features was generally good using either atlas, though JSN showed better reproducibility than osteophyte. Reproducibility between observers was lower than the within observer agreement, and did not improve with the second reading. Overall there was no clear difference between the two systems. Comparison of the two atlas systems was made for grades obtained for each feature. Grades for JSN of the lateral tibio-femoral compartment were significantly lower ($p < 0.001$), whereas those for the lateral and medial patello-femoral compartments were significantly higher ($p < 0.001$), in the line drawing atlas than in the OARS atlas. No differences were seen for grading of medial tibio-femoral joint-space narrowing. Grades for lateral tibial osteophyte were higher ($p = 0.029$), whereas grades for medial femoral osteophyte were lower ($p < 0.001$), in the line drawing atlas than in the OARS atlas. No differences were seen for other osteophyte grades. The discordance between the two atlases shows that they are not equivalent instruments. The authors felt that the line drawing atlas had more representative images of common osteophyte shape and direction at all sites, and because the grades of osteophyte and JSN are arithmetically calculated they are logically justified. Further studies are required to determine whether employment of such an interval rather than ordinal scale produces differences in population study findings or assessment of knee OA progression. Future developments of this atlas envisaged by the authors include: (1) an increase in the number of grades, (2) inclusion of a minus one grade for JSN so as to record joint spaces that are thicker than the mean for each sex, (3) development of similar atlases for other joint sites, and (4) production of transparencies that may be directly overlaid onto the X-ray film.

In a preliminary study of radiographic OA progression in 32 pairs of knees it was found that joint-space narrowing followed by osteophyte were the best variables in assessing progression.[3] We have assessed reproducibility of progression in 20 patients with knee OA 4 years apart and found changes in joint-space narrowing measured by atlas to be internally more reproducible (kappa = 0.71) than changes in osteophyte (kappa = 0.50). Changes in joint-space narrowing may be better for assessing progression, although these findings need to be confirmed. On current evidence we believe that the osteophyte grade is the best way of defining OA of the knee in population studies, and that changes in knee joint-space narrowing, with or without osteophyte, should be used for progression.

Lumbar spine

Quantitative measurement of disc height has been found to be unreliable, but semi-quantitative classification, Grades 0–3 demonstrate good inter-observer agreement.[58,59] The atlas of Lane *et al.* scores individual radiographic features and then generates a summary grade directly from the assessment of the selected radiographic features, that allows for the independent variation in these features, which are often noted in degenerative disc disease.[46] The interobserver agreement for the lumbar spine (ICC 0.95 for narrowing, 0.91 for osteophytes, 0.93 for summary grade, and kappa 0.55 for sclerosis), and intra-observer (ICC 0.92 for narrowing, 0.96 for osteophytes, 0.90 for summary grade, and kappa 0.59 for sclerosis) was good. They found that the assignment of these summary grades is as reliable as those demonstrated by studies of the Kellgren–Lawrence type of global grading system.

A summary of the reproducibility for within and between observers for all radiographic grading systems is presented in Table 11.10.

Grading progression of radiographic changes

Relatively little is known of the determinants of progression of OA. Several recommendations for assessing OA progression exist but there is still no consensus on the definition of radiological progression in OA and therefore the need for standardized methodology remains a challenge.[25,26,60,61] Obtaining reproducible radiographs on successive visits is a pre-requisite for reliable assessment of OA progression, particularly when using quantitative measures.[25] Development of standardized methodology will generate consistency in data and permit direct comparison of radiographs between different studies. Methods assessing the radiological progression of OA can be divided into categorical and continuous variables. Categorical variables such as the Kellgren and Lawrence grade permit definition of progression by a change of at least one grade during the study. However these grades may have a ceiling effect and are not linear over their range (i.e., change from Grades 1 to 2 may not be equivalent to the change from Grades 3 to 4). Current qualitative methods such as the atlases are best at detecting and grading new abnormalities, such as osteophytes, but not as good at quantifying changes in these abnormalities (e.g., increase in osteophyte size).[62] Ravaud *et al.* propose that for continuous variables, the results should be presented as a mean change over the study, for example, JSW as a mean change per unit of time or as a dichotomous variable (progression Yes/No).[62] As a dichotomous variable it is necessary to establish a cut-off point above which the value obtained for change in the continuous variable will define progression. These changes over time must exceed the variability inherent in repeat radiographs and in the measurement process.

JSW is considered the primary endpoint in the assessment of the radiological progression of OA. The concept of cut-offs for JSW measurement has been introduced.[63,64] Cut-offs on JSW measurements are necessary to decide whether the difference observed between two successive measures in the same subject constitutes a relevant change (organic), or a change related to the variability inherent in repeating radiographs and in the measurement process. That is, the cut-offs define statistically relevant changes (i.e., a change reflecting organic modification of JSW rather than measurement error) and not clinically relevant change (i.e., a change related to clinically relevant structural outcome measure in OA). Ravaud *et al.* examined the variability in knee radiography and its implications for radiological progression in medial compartment tibio-femoral OA.[48] Ten healthy volunteers had both knees X-rayed using three imaging modalities: (1) knee X-ray without specific guidelines, (2) knee X-ray using specific guidelines without fluoroscopy, and (3) knee X-ray using specific guidelines with fluroscopy at baseline and two weeks later. Twenty patients with symptomatic

OA underwent standard X-rays at baseline and two hours later. From Ravaud's study in healthy volunteers the cut-off point defining minimal relevant change in JSW of the medial compartment of the knee should be at least 1.29 mm for X-rays without guidelines, 0.73 mm for X-rays with guidelines but without fluoroscopy, and 0.59 mm for X-rays performed using guidelines and fluroscopy. The use of guidelines and fluroscopy will spare only 5 per cent of patients, compared with the use of guidelines alone, and there was no significant statistical difference between the two approaches. In contrast the use of guidelines even without fluroscopy was found to spare 32 per cent of patients compared with the absence of guidelines. These cut-offs may vary according to the radiological procedure, the measuring instrument, the reader, and the sample of studied patients. Therefore Ravaud *et al.* propose that each study should generate their own individual cut-off points. This could be achieved if each study repeated radiographs over a short interval (e.g., one or two days apart) in a representative sample of patients to determine the reproducibility of the radiographic procedure and to derive a specific cut-off for the study in question.[62]

Landmarks have been recommended for measuring JSW in OA clinical trials.[26] In addition, it has been suggested that for hip OA a paired reading procedure with landmarks for JSW should be recommended in longitudinal studies.[65] Auleley *et al.* examined 104 subjects with ACR clinical and radiological diagnosis for hip OA, at baseline and 3 years. In their study the paired X-rays were read in 4 procedures. Radiographs were read as single (with and without landmarks), paired, or chronologically ordered, depending on whether the patient's identity or time sequence or both were known or unknown. When assessed with the single reading procedure, the Kellgren and Lawrence grade changed in 44 (42 per cent) compared with change in 35 (34 per cent) and 33 (32 per cent) patients, when assessed with the chronologically ordered or paired reading procedures, respectively. When assessed with the single reading procedure, the joint-space narrowing grade changed in 38 (37 per cent) compared with change in 30 (29 per cent) and 24 (23 per cent) patients when assessed with the chronologically ordered or paired reading procedures, respectively. The JSW progression was less with the single reading procedure without landmarks (−0.47 mm) than with the other reading procedures (at least −0.58 mm for the single with landmarks). Therefore measurement of JSW progression on single radiographs without landmarks would require 10 per cent more patients than on single radiographs with landmarks in longitudinal studies. Thus, reading procedures for JSW of the hip with landmarks is clearly contrasted with the reading procedure without landmarks.

The recommended features to be recorded for the hip and knee are summarized in Table 11.11.

Conclusion

Current studies suggest that no single global system is suitable for the assessment of OA at all sites. Instead, individual radiographic features should be given different weight in each joint affected by OA. At the hip, measurement of JSW is simple, reproducible, and might be preferred for the assignment of OA in epidemiological studies. This may not be true at the knee, where precise location for joint-space measurement, and tricompartmental structure of the joint, make assessment of this feature more difficult, and assessment of the osteophyte potentially more useful. All methods of assessment such as composite indices (i.e., Kellgren and Lawrence, Kallman Grade), and individual radiographic features (JSN, osteophytes) or measurement of JSW, usually show acceptable cross-sectional and longitudinal reproducibility. Reproducibility of radiographs over time is a prerequisite for reliable assessment of OA progression, particularly when using quantitative measures and therefore a set of recommended guidelines should be followed in epidemiological studies and clinical trials.[25,26]

It can be seen that considerable advances have been made over the last thirty years in solving the problem of definition and criteria in OA, but we are still lacking a universal definition and classification of the disease. Radiological site, and perhaps compartment specific definition of the

Table 11.10 Summary of reproducibility of radiographic grading scales for interobserver and intra-observer

Joint	Feature	Kallman (1990) (P) Inter	Kallman (1990) (P) Intra	Hart (1993) (P) Inter	Hart (1993) (P) Intra	Lane (1993) (P) Inter	Lane (1993) (P) Intra	Croft (1990) (P) Inter	Croft (1990) (P) Intra	Spector (1992) (P) Inter	Spector (1992) (P) Intra	Cooper (1992) (H) Inter	Cooper (1992) (H) Intra	Scott (1993) (P) Inter	Scott (1993) (P) Intra
DIP	OP	+++	+++	++	+++	+++	+++								
	N	+++	+++	+++	++	+++	+++								
	S	++	+++			+	++								
PIP	OP	+++	++	+++	+++	+++	+++								
	N	+++	++	++	+++	+++	+++								
	S	++	+++			+	++								
CMC	OP	+++	+++	++	+++										
	N	++	+++	+++	+++										
	S	+++	++												
SPINE	OP					+++	+++								
	N					+++	+++								
	S					+	+								
KNEE TFJ	OP									++	+++	++	+++	++	+++
	N									+	+++	++	+++	+++	+++
	S									+	++	+	++	+	+++
KNEE PFJ	OP									++	+++	++	+++		
	N									+	+++	+	+++		
	S									+	++	+	++		
HIP	OP					+++	+++	+	+						
	N					+++	+++	+++	+++						
	S					+++	++	+	++						

+, poor; ++, good; +++, excellent.

OP, osteophyte; N, joint space narrowing; S, sclerosis.

TF, tibio-femoral; PF, patello-femoral.

H, hospital based; P, population based.

Table 11.11 Radiographic features to be recorded in cases of hip and knee OA*

Feature	Assessment of hip	Assessment of knee	
		TFJ	PFJ
Joint-space narrowing	Graded 0–3 Millimetre measurement, (calliper optional)	Graded 0–3 Graded in 10ths of millimetres, Perhaps with calliper	Graded 0–3
Osteophytes	Superior and inferior femoral Graded 0–3, acetabular is difficult to judge and should be noted	Graded 0–3	Grade 0–3
Subchondral bony sclerosis	Femoral/acetabular sclerosis graded present/absent	Graded present/absent	Graded present/absent
Attrition	Collapse of subchondral bony plate graded present/absent	Graded present/absent	
Subchondral bony cyst	Femoral/acetabular bony cyst graded 0–3		
Femoral migration	Superior and lateral migration should be noted present/absent		
Subluxation			Medial or lateral subluxation to be noted
Overall severity of OA	Kellgren and Lawrence or modified	Kellgren and Lawrence or modified	

TFJ, tibiofemoral joint; PFJ, patellofemoral joint.

*Modified from Ref. 52.

disease is now recognized as the major tool available in defining OA and the way forward. There is general consensus that the grading of osteophytes and joint-space narrowing at the major sites using validated atlases is an important advance, and a number of atlases with similar grading scales for most joints are available for general use.[46,51,56]

Key points 1

♦ Radiographs are the standard for classification of structural changes in OA

♦ Kellgren and Lawrence is a global grading system

♦ Structural changes and their significance are joint specific Joint-specific definitions and criteria now developed

Key points 2

♦ All grading methods show acceptable cross-sectional and longitudinal reproducibility

♦ Photographic atlases are the current standard method of grading

♦ Measurement variability can be due to radiographic procedure, patient positioning, site of measurement, measuring methods, or the reader

♦ Recommended guidelines should be followed in epidemiological studies and clinical trials

Key points 3

♦ No consensus on the definition of radiological progression in OA

♦ Methods for assessing progression can be divided into continuous and categorical variables

♦ JSW cut-offs to define relevant change over time should be derived

♦ Landmarks recommended for JSW measurement

♦ Reproducible radiographs are a prerequisite to reliable assessment

References

(An asterisk denotes recommended reading.)

1. Spector, T.D., Hart, D.J., Byrne, J., Harris, P.A., Darce, J.E., and Doyle, D.E. (1993). Definition of osteoarthritis of the knee for epidemiologic studies. *Ann Rheum Dis* **52**:790–4.

2. Croft, P., Cooper, C., Wickham, C., and Coggon, D. (1990). Defining osteoarthritis of the hip for epidemiological studies. *Am J Epidemiol* **132**:514–22.

3. Altman, R.D., Fries, J.F., Bloch, D., Carstens, J., Cooke, T.D., Genant, H., et al. (1987). Radiographic assessment of progression in osteoarthritis. *Arthritis Rheum* **30**:1214–25.

4. Kellgren, J.H. and Lawrence, J.S. (1957). Radiological assessment of osteoarthritis. *Ann Rheum Dis* **16**:494–501.

5. Kellgren, J.H., Jeffrey, M.R., and Ball, J. (1963). *The Epidemiology of Chronic Rheumatism: Atlas of Standard Radiographs* (Vol. 2). Oxford: Blackwell scientific.

6. Lawrence, J.S. (1977). *Rheumatism in Populations*. London: Heinemann.

7. Wood, P.H.N. (1976). Osteoarthritis in the community. *Clin Rheum Dis* **2**:495–507.

8. Spector, T.D. and Hochberg, M.C. (1994). Methodological problems in the epidemiological study of osteoarthritis. *Ann Rheum Dis* **53**:143–6.

9. Bellamy, N., Bennett, P.H., and Burch, T.A. (1967). New York Symposium on Population Studies in Rheumatic Diseases: New Diagnostic Criteria. *Bull Rheum Dis* **17**:453–58.

10. Dieppe, P. and Kirwan, J. (1994). The localisation of osteoarthritis. *Br J Rheumatol* **33**:201–4.

11. Hernborg, J. and Nilsson, B.E. (1973). The relationship between osteophytes in the knee joint, osteoarthritis and ageing. *Acta Orthop Scand* **44**:69–74.

12. Brandt, K.D., Fife, R.S., Braunstein, E.M., and Katz, B. (1991). Radiographic grading of the severity of knee osteoarthritis: Relation of the Kellgren and Lawrence grade to a grade based on joint space narrowing, and correlation with arthroscopic evidence of articular cartilage degeneration. *Arthritis Rheum* **34**:1381–6.

13. Resnick, D. and Niwayama, G. (1988). *Diagnosis of Bone and Joint Disorders* (2nd ed.). Philadelphia: WB Saunders.

14. Reiff, D.B., Heron, C.W., and Stoker, D.J. (1991). Spiking of the tubercles of the intercondylar eminence of the tibial plateau in osteoarthritis. *Br J Radiol* **64**:915–7.

15. Donelly, S., Jawad, S., Hart, D.J., Doyle, D.V., and Spector, T.D. (1995). Does spiking of the tubercles predict osteoarthritis of the knee? *Br J Rheumatol* (s1) **34**:36.

16. Egger, P., Cooper, C., Hart, D.J., Doyle, D.V., Coggon, D., and Spector, T.D. (1995). Patterns of joint involvement in osteoarthritis of the hand: The Chingford Study. *J Rheumatol* **22**:1509–13.

17. Hart, D.J., Spector, T.D., Egger, P., Coggon, D., and Cooper, C. (1994). Defining osteoarthritis of the hand for epidemiological studies: The Chingford Study. *Ann Rheum Dis* **53**:220–3.

18. Leach, R.E., Gregg, T., and Siber, F.J. (1970). Weight bearing radiography in osteoarthritis of the knee. *Radiology* **97**:265–6.

19. Conrozier, T., Lequesne, M.G., Tron, A.M., Mathieu, P., Berdah, L., and Vignon, E. (1997). The effects of position on the radiographic joint space in osteoarthritis of the hip. *Osteoarthritis Cart* **5**:17–22.

20. Evison, G., Reilly, P.A., Gray, J., and Calin, A. (1987). Comparison of erect and supine radiographs of the hip. *Br J Rheumatol* **26**:393–4.

21. Hansson, G., Jerre, R., Sanders, S.M., and Wallin, J. (1993). Radiographic assessment of coxarthrosis following slipped capital femoral epiphysis: A 32 year follow-up study of 151 hips. *Acta Radiol* **34**:117–23.

22. Auleley G.-R, Rousselin, B., Ayral, X., Edouard-Noel, R., Dougados, M., and Ravaud, P. (1998). Osteoarthritis of the hip: agreement between joint space width measurements on standing and supine conventional radiographs. *Ann Rheum Dis* **57**:519–23.

23. Lequesne, M.G. and Laredo J.-D. (1998). The faux profil (oblique view) of the hip in the standing position. Contribution to the evaluation of osteoarthritis of the hip. *Ann Rheum Dis* **57**:676–81.

24. *Auleley, G.-R., Duche, A., Drape, J.L., Dougados, M., and Ravaud, P. (2001). Measurement of joint space width in hip osteoarthritis: influence of joint positioning and radiographic procedure. *Rheumatology* **40**:414–9.

    Recent paper examining important issue of the influence of joint positioning and radiographic procedure on JSW in OA.

25. Dieppe, P.A. (1995). Recommended methodology for assessing the progression of osteoarthritis of the hip and knee joints. *Osteoarthritis Cart* **3**:73–7.

26. *Altman, R., Brandt, K., Hochberg, M., Moskovitzt, Bellamy, N., Bloch, D.A., et al. (1996). Design and conduct of clinical trials in patients with osteoarthritis: recommendations from a task force of the Osteoarthritis Research Society. *Osteoarthritis Cart* **4**:217–43.

    Core set of recommendations that all researchers and clinicians interested in OA should be familiar with.

27. Buckland-Wright, J.C. (1995). Protocols for precise radioanatomical positioning of the tibio femoral and patello femoral compartments of the knee. *Osteoarthritis Cart* **3**(Suppl. A):71–80.

28. Messieh, S.S., Fowler, P.J., and Munro, T. (1990). Anteroposterior radiographs of the osteoarthritic knee. *J Bone Joint Surg* **72B**:639–40.

29. Spector, T.D. (1995). Measuring joint space in knee osteoarthritis: Position or precision? *J Rheumatol* **22**:807–8.

30. Buckland-Wright, J.C., Macfarlane, D., Williams, S., and Ward, R. (1995). Joint space width measured more accurately and precisely in semi-flexed than extended view of OA Knees. *Br J Rheumatol* (s1) **34**:121.

31. Buckland-Wright, J.C., MacFarlane, D.G., Williams, S.A., and Ward, R.J. (1995). Accuracy and precision of joint space width measurement in standard and macro-radiographs of osteoarthritis knees. *Ann Rheum Dis* **54**:872–80.

32. Ravaud, P., Auleley, G.R., Chastang, C., Rousselin, B., Paolozzi, L., Amor, B., et al. (1996). Knee joint space width measurement: An experimental study of the influence of radiographic procedure and joint positioning. *Br J Rheumatol* **35**:761–6.

33. Rosenberg, T.D., Paulos, L.E., Parker, R.D., Coward, D.B., and Scott, S.M. (1988). The 45 degree posterior-anterior flexion weightbearing radiographs of the knee. *J Bone Joint Surg* **70A**:1479–83.

34. Jones, A.C., Ledingham, J., McAlindon, T., Regan, M., Hart, D., MacMillan, P.J., et al. (1993). Radiographic assessment of patello-femoral osteoarthritis. *Ann Rheum Dis* **52**:655–8.

35. Ciccuttini, F.M., Baker, J., Hart, D.J., and Spector, T.D. (1996). Choosing the best method of radiological assessment of patello-femoral arthritis. *Ann Rheum Dis* **55**:134–6.

36. Yoshimura, N., Dennison, E., Wilman, C., Hashimoto, T., and Cooper, C. (2000). Epidemiology of Chronic Disc Degeneration and Osteoarthritis of the lumbar spine in Britain and Japan: A Comparative Study. *J Rheumatol* **27**:429–33.

37. Symmons, D.P.M., van Hemert, A.M., Vandenbroucke, J.P., and Valkenburg, H.A. (1991). A longitudinal study of back pain and radiological changes in the lumbar spines of middle aged women. II. Radiographic Findings. *Ann Rheum Dis* **50**:162–6.

38. Kallman, D.A., Wigley, F.M., Scott, W.W., Jr., Hochberg, M.C., and Tobin, J.D. (1989). New radiographic grading scales of osteoarthritis of the hand. Reliability for determining prevalence and progression. *Arthritis Rheum* **32**:1584–91

39. Hart, D.J., Harris, P.A., and Chamberlain, A. (1993). Reliability and reproducibility of grading radiographs for osteoarthritis of the hand. *Br J Rheumatol* **32**:S1:137.

40. Kessler, S., Dieppe, P., Fuchs, J., Strumer, T., and Gunther, K.P. (2000). Assessing the prevalence of hand osteoarthritis in epidemiological studies. The reliability of a radiological hand scale. *Ann Rheum Dis* **59**:289–92.

41. *Lequesne, M.G. and Maheu, E. (2000). Methodology of clinical trials in hand osteoarthritis: conventional and proposed tools. *Osteoarthritis Cart* **8**:S64–S69.

    Excellent up to date review of methodology in hand OA.

42. Scott, J.C., Nevitt, M.C., Lane, H.K., et al. (1992). Association of individual radiographic features of hip osteoarthritis with pain. *Arthritis Rheum* **35**(Suppl.):s81

43. Buckland-Wright, J.C. (1994). Quantitative radiography of osteoarthritis. *Ann Rheum Dis* **63**:268–75.

44. Dougados, M., Gueguen, A., Nguyen, M., Berdah, L., Lequesne, M., and Mazieres, B., et al. (1996). Radiological progression of hip osteoarthritis: definition, risk factors and correlations with clinical status. *Ann Rheum Dis* **55**:356–62.

45. Conrozier, T.H., Tron, A.M., Mathieu, P., and Vignon, E. (1995). Quantitative assessment of radiographic normal and osteoarthritic hip joint space. *Osteoarthritis Cart* **3**(Suppl. A):81–7.

46. Lane, N.E., Nevitt, M.C., Genant, H.K., and Hochberg, M.C. (1993). Reliability of new indices of radiographic OA of the hand and hip and lumbar disc degeneration. *J Rheumatol* **20**:1911–8.

47. Goker, B., Doughan, A.M., Schnitzer, T.J., and Block, J.A. (2000). Quantification of progressive joint space narrowing in osteoarthritis of the hip. Longitudinal analysis of the contralateral hip after total hip arthroplasty. *Arthritis Rheum* **43**:988–94.

48. Ahlback, S. (1968). Osteoarthritis of the knee: A radiographic investigation. *Acta Radiol* **277**(Suppl.):7–72.

49. Spector, T.D., Cooper, C., Cushnaghan, J., et al. (1992). *A Radiographic Atlas of Knee Osteoarthritis.* London: Spinger.

50. Burnett, S.J., Hart, D.J., Cooper, C., and Spector, T.D. (1994). *A Radiographic Atlas of Osteoarthritis.* London: Springer.

51. Cooper, C., Cushnaghan, J., Kirwan, J., Dieppe, P.A., Rogers, J., McAlindon, T., et al. (1992). Radiological assessment of the knee joint in osteoarthritis. *Ann Rheum Dis* **51**:80–2.

52. Cooper, C., McAlindon, T., Snow, S., Vines, K., Young, P., Kirwan, J., et al. (1994). Mechanical and constitutional risk factors for symptomatic knee osteoarthritis: differences between medial, tibio-femoral and patellofemoral disease. *J Rheumatol* **21**:307–13.

53. Dacre, J.E. and Huskisson, E.C. (1989). The automatic assessment of knee radiographs in osteoarthritis using digital image analysis. *Br J Rheumatol* **28**:506–10.

54. Scott, W.W., Lethbridge-cejku, M., Reichle, R., Wigley, F.M., Tobin, J., and Hochberg, M.C. (1993). Reliability of grading scales for individual radiographic features of osteoarthritis of the knee. *Invest Radiol* **28**:497–501.

55. Derek, T., Cooke, V., Kelly, B.P., Harrison, L., Mohamed, G., and Khan, B. (1999). Radiographic grading for knee osteoarthritis. A revised scheme that relates to alignment and deformity. *J Rheumatol* **26**:64–4.

56. Altman, R.D., Hochberg, M., Murphy, W.A., Wolfe, F., Jr., and Lequesne, M. (1995). Atlas of Individual Radiographic Features in Osteoarthritis. *Osteoarthritis Cart* **3**(Suppl. A):3–70.

57. *Nagaosa, Y., Mateus, M., Hassan, B., Lanyon, P., and Doherty, M. (2000). Development of a logically devised line drawing atlas for grading of knee osteoarthritis. *Ann Rheum Dis* 59:587–95.

  First line drawing atlas produced, which now provides an alternative to the standard photographic atlas for radiographic grading of the knee.

58. Saraste, H., Brostrom, L.-Å., Aparisi, T., and Axdorph, G. (1985). Radiographic Measurement of the lumbar spine. A clinical and experimental study in man. *Spine* 10:236–41.

59. Andersson, G.B., Schultz, A., Nathan, A., and Irstam, L. (1981). Roentgenographic measurement of lumbar intervertebral disc height. *Spine* 6:154–8.

60. Dieppe, P., Brandt, K.D., Lohmander, S., and Felson, D.T. (1995). Detecting and Measuring Disease Modification in Osteoarthritis. The Need for Standardized Methodology. *J Rheumatol* 22:201–3.

61. Group for the respect of ethics and excellence in science for the registration of drugs used in the treatment of osteoarthritis. (1996). *Ann Rheum Dis* 55:552–7.

62. *Ravaud, P., Ayral, X., and Dougados, M. (1999). Radiographic progression of hip and knee osteoarthritis. *Osteoarthritis Cart* 7:222–9.

  Summary of difficulties in defining progression of OA and discussion of categorical versus continuous data when reporting results.

63. Ravaud, P., Giraudeau, B., Auleley, G.-R, Drape, J.-L, Rousselin, B., Paolozzi, L., *et al.* (1998). Variability in knee radiological progression in medial knee osteoarthritis. *Ann Rheum Dis* 57:624–9.

64. Ravaud, P., Giraudeau, B., Auleley, G.-R., Edouard-Noel, R., Dougados, M., and Chastang, Cl. (1999). Assessing smallest detectable change over time in continuous structural outcome measures: application to radiological change in knee osteoarthritis. *J Clin Epidemiol* 52:1225–30.

65. *Auleley, G.-R. (2000). Radiographic assessment of hip osteoarthritis progression: impact of reading procedures in longitudinal studies. *Ann Rheum Dis* 59:422–7.

  Emphasizes the importance of the reading procedure when assessing progression of OA and introduces the concept of landmarks.

11.4.2 Quantitation of radiographic changes

Steven A. Mazzuca

Accepted diagnostic criteria and semiquantitative scales for grading the severity of the radiographic features of OA are clinically useful despite the inherent limitations of conventional joint radiography. However, studies of purported biomarkers of cartilage deterioration and pharmacological modification of structural damage in OA require quantitative assessment of the thickness of articular cartilage. Much of what we know about quantitative changes in knee OA is based on data derived from the conventional standing AP radiograph, in which the knee is imaged in full extension. Conventional knee radiography suffers from several serious limitations in standardization of the radioanatomic position of the knee in serial examinations (i.e., knee flexion and rotation, parallel alignment of the medial tibial plateau, and X-ray beam). Poor standards for joint positioning in previous studies of the radiographic progression of knee OA are likely to have obscured our understanding of the rate, variability, and determinants of radiographic joint-space narrowing (JSN) (the surrogate for articular cartilage thickness) in patients with this disease. Recent advances in methods to standardize the positioning of the knee under fluoroscopy, or with empirically derived procedures for flexion/rotation of the knee and angulation of

the X-ray beam, afford more reproducible measurement of radiographic joint-space width (JSW) in repeated examinations than is possible with conventional examination procedures. It can be anticipated that the implementation of these protocols for standardizing the position of the joint in current and future studies of OA progression will facilitate the acquisition of important new information about risk factors for OA progression, biomarkers of articular cartilage degeneration, and the efficacy of putative structure-modifying drugs for OA.

The purposes of this chapter are to: (1) describe recent advances in the measurement of radiographic changes of OA; (2) illustrate how these advances have influenced our current understanding of the nature and rate of OA progression; and (3) discuss how future studies of OA progression, based on current quantitative approaches, may produce new knowledge that will be of high relevance to clinical practice. The issues pertinent to this area are largely distinct from those addressed by Drs. Flores and Hochberg in Chapter 1. The radiographic and clinical diagnostic criteria for OA described in that chapter are based on observations of the presence and apparent severity of radiographic abnormalities (e.g., osteophytes or sclerosis of subchondral bone) and clinical findings, such as joint pain and crepitus. These dichotomous and semi-quantitative approaches are highly robust for clinical purposes, not because conventional methods of joint radiography can be relied upon to afford an accurate representation of the state of articular cartilage, but because accepted diagnostic criteria and semiquantitative scales for grading the severity of the radiographic features of OA are clinically useful *despite* the inherent limitations of conventional joint radiography.

As detailed below, to measure progressive radiographic changes of OA accurately requires control of numerous technical factors affecting the radioanatomic position of the joint. In conventional radiography, failure to adequately standardize the position of the joint, relative to the central ray of the X-ray beam, in serial examinations may obscure progressive radiographic changes of OA and, in particular, changes in the radiographic JSW, the surrogate for thickness of articular cartilage. This chapter will concentrate on measurement of radiographic JSN in the OA knee. The knee is an appropriate focal point for this discussion because of the numerous advances in radiographic imaging of this joint that have occurred over the past five years. Moreover, because of the high prevalence of knee OA and the fact that it is a major cause of chronic disability in the elderly,[1,2] the knee is the common focus of studies of risk factors, biomarkers of progression, and modification of OA structural damage by disease-modifying OA drugs (DMOADs). Discussions of the measurement of radiographic changes in other joints in which OA is highly prevalent (e.g., the hip and joints of the hand) can be found elsewhere.[3,4]

Overview of measurement

The key features of good measurement are validity and reliability. Validity is defined as *accuracy* in measurement. This is to say that an instrument is considered to possess validity to the extent that a measured estimate of the parameter in question (and variation in estimates between subjects) correspond closely to the true values of the parameter, as determined by the accepted criterion measure or 'gold standard.' With respect to measurement of radiographic JSW in, for example, the tibiofemoral compartment, the criterion is the sum of the actual thicknesses of the articular cartilage on the tibial plateau and adjacent femoral condyle (Fig. 11.13).

The reliability of an instrument is defined as its *reproducibility* or *precision*. In studies of the reliability of measurements of JSW, reproducibility is typically demonstrated by determining the extent to which measured JSW in a sample of knees varies in repeated radiographic examinations, over an interval too brief to permit an actual change in the thickness of articular cartilage. The most straightforward expression of reproducibility is the standard error of measurement (SE_m). Conceptually, the SE_m is the mean of the within-subject standard deviations (SD) of repeated measurements in a sample.[5] The precision of a measure can be interpreted directly

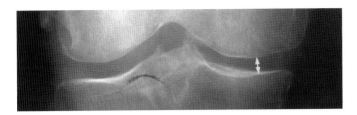

Fig. 11.13 Location of minimum joint-space width (arrows) in the medial tibiofemoral compartment of an OA knee.

from the SE_m. For example, in a set of JSW measurements with a demonstrated SE_m equal to 0.25 mm, the 95 per cent confidence interval ($\pm 2\,SE_m$) would be ± 0.50 mm for an individual estimate of JSW. Therefore, when evaluating JSN in a subsequent radiographic examination, a change in JSW in an individual knee would need to be >0.5 mm to be interpreted as being greater than the margin of error of the baseline estimate of JSW.

An alternative expression of reproducibility is the coefficient of variation (CV). The CV for a set of repeated JSW measurements is

$$CV = \frac{SE_m}{Mean\ JSW} \times 100\%$$

While expression of reproducibility as the CV affords a readily interpretable estimate of the magnitude of variation due to measurement error, relative to a typical value of JSW, it can also be the source of ambiguity. For example, if a measurement procedure were determined to have an SE_m equal to 0.28 mm in separate samples of normal and OA knees (in which the means of JSW were 5.1 and 3.2 mm, respectively), the resulting CVs (5.5 and 8.1 per cent, respectively) would obscure the fact that the absolute precision (SE_m) of JSW measurements was identical in the two samples. Therefore, when comparing the reproducibility of radiographic and mensural techniques on the basis of reported CVs, care should be taken to ascertain the extent to which any apparent discrepancy is due to a difference in measurement precision and/or a difference between reference groups with respect to mean JSW.

Elements of radioanatomic positioning of the joint

Since publication of the classic monograph by Ahlback[6] and the supporting paper by Leach *et al.*,[7] the conventional standard for plain knee radiography has been the bilateral weight-bearing anteroposterior (AP) view with both knees in full extension. This view has been the accepted radiographic technique for characterizing the bony changes of OA (e.g., osteophytosis, subchondral sclerosis), but is severely limited as a means by which to visualize accurately the thickness of the articular cartilage. This limitation stems from several shortcomings of the technique with respect to radioanatomic positioning of the knee (lack of knee flexion, misalignment of the X-ray beam, variable radiographic magnification) and has resulted in inconsistent descriptions of the rate of JSN in knee OA.[8]

Knee flexion

Imaging of the human knee in weight-bearing flexion more closely represents the normal anatomic position of the tibiofemoral joint during standing or walking than the fully extended view.[9,10] As shown below, numerous investigations confirm that extension of the joint exaggerates the impression of the thickness of the cartilage on the articular surface and does not reflect the region of the tibiofemoral compartment most likely to exhibit cartilage damage in OA.

Resnick and Vint[11] described 6 patients in whom the standing AP view significantly underestimated joint-space loss that was evident in a posteroanterior (PA) 'tunnel' view, in which the knee was flexed to 60–70°. When Messieh *et al.*[12] compared the standing AP view to an alternative tunnel view (with 30° of knee flexion) in 64 patients, they found 10 knees that exhibited normal joint space on the fully extended view, but marked narrowing on the flexion view. Arthroscopy confirmed that a radiographic image of an OA knee in 30° of flexion was more likely than a view of the knee in full extension to display the region of the tibiofemoral compartment in which cartilage damage was most prevalent (i.e., the posterior aspect of the femoral condyle).[12] However, other degrees of flexion were not examined. In radiographs of knees with advanced OA (i.e., medial JSW <2 mm), Buckland-Wright *et al.*[9,13] demonstrated that full knee extension exaggerated the apparent width of the joint space by an average of 1.5 mm (125 per cent), compared to 5–10° of knee flexion.

X-ray beam alignment

In many subjects, full extension of the knee tilts the medial tibial plateau at an angle, so that it is not parallel to a horizontally directed X-ray beam.[14] Skewed alignment of the central ray of the X-ray beam and the plane of the tibial plateau results in an incomplete or indistinct image of the floor of the joint space that hampers measurement of JSW. Using fluoroscopic imaging as the gold standard, Ravaud *et al.*[15] demonstrated the medial tibial plateau of the average radiographically normal knee in full extension, tilted downward at an angle of 3.4°. Accordingly, they determined that 5° downward angulation of the X-ray beam in the extended view radiograph of the normal knee yielded more accurate measurements of tibiofemoral JSW than did 10° angulation.[15]

The position of the central X-ray beam relative to the center of the joint space is also important. In a bilateral standing AP view, the central ray of the X-ray beam intersects the plane of the joint at a single point—between the two knees. All other points in the image are subject to some degree of parallax distortion because of the divergence of the beam in a cone-shaped manner around the central ray. The degree of distortion increases with increasing angulation (i.e., increasing distance from the central ray). Even in a unilateral examination, in which the beam is directed at the center of the joint space, the degree of misdirection of the beam necessary to alter the results is not large. Fife *et al.*,[16] found a 17 per cent decrease in JSW when the point of focus of the X-ray beam was displaced by only 1 cm from its original alignment centered at the mid-point of the patella.

Radiographic magnification

Although radiographic magnification is not generally taken into account in clinical knee radiography, the distance between the center of the joint and the X-ray film will affect the degree of magnification of the joint space in the radiograph. This distance can be large, and is influenced by factors such as obesity (common in subjects with knee OA) and restriction of joint movement because of pain or soft tissue contracture. In an assessment of radiographic magnification in conventional standing AP radiographs,[17] the difference in diameter between X-ray images of two identical spherical markers, one placed over the head of the fibula and the other taped to the film cassette, revealed as much as 35 per cent magnification of the image. The effects of radiographic magnification (and of changes in magnification in serial examinations) are minimized in PA examinations of the knee, in which the patella is in contact with the X-ray cassette (see below).

Protocols for standardized knee radiography

Several teams of investigators have developed and tested protocols for knee radiography which, in various ways, negate the shortcomings of the conventional standing AP view with respect to joint flexion, alignment with the X-ray beam, and/or radiographic magnification. The first generation of

Table 11.12 First-generation (fluoroscopically assisted) protocols for standardized knee radiography

| Investigator | View | Standards for fluoroscopically assisted positioning of the knee | | | Number of knees* | SE$_m$† (mm) |
		Flexion/extension of the knee	Angulation of the X-ray beam	Rotation of the knee		
Buckland-Wright et al.[17]	AP	5–10° flexion, as needed, to superimpose (±1 mm) the anterior and posterior Margins of the medial tibial plateau	Horizontal	Tibial spines centered below femoral notch	10 N 25 OA	0.11 0.19
Ravaud et al.[15]	AP	Full extension	As needed, to bring the medial tibial plateau into sharpest focus into sharpest focus	Tibial spines Centered below femoral notch	20 N	0.31
Piperno et al.[18]	PA	Schuss position: i.e., patellae in contact with film cassette and coplanar with the tips of the great toes (20–30° flexion)	As needed, to bring the medial tibial plateau into sharpest focus	Tibial spines centered below femoral notch	10 N 10 OA	0.35 0.24

* Results for normal (N) and OA knees are presented separately.

† Standard error of measurement.

(a)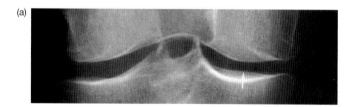

(b)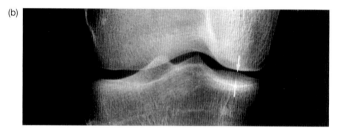

Fig. 11.14 Examples of satisfactory and unsatisfactory positioning of the knee: (a) illustrates alignment of the medial tibial plateau and central X-ray beam, as defined by superimposition ±1 mm of the anterior and posterior margins of the medial plateau (arrow), and proper rotation of the knee (i.e., centering of the tibial spines beneath the femoral notch). (b) represents unsatisfactory alignment, as reflected by displacement of the anterior and posterior margins of the medial tibial plateau (arrows), and poor knee rotation.

such protocols[15,17,18] used fluoroscopy to guide knee flexion and/or adjustment of the angle of the X-ray tube to align the medial tibial plateau with the central ray of the X-ray beam. A comparison of the key elements of radioanatomic positioning of the knee in these protocols is shown in Table 11.9. Each protocol described a unilateral examination that calls for rotation of the foot to center the tibial spines under the femoral notch (Fig. 11.14a). These protocols vary from one another, however, with respect to the orientation of the knee relative to the X-ray source (i.e., AP or PA) and the degree of flexion and/or angulation of the X-ray beam required, to align the medial tibial plateau parallel with the central ray of the X-ray beam.

A noteworthy feature of the protocol of Buckland-Wright[17] is the operational definition of parallel radioanatomic alignment as superimposition (±1 mm) of the anterior and posterior margins of the medial tibial plateau (Fig. 11.14). This criterion may not be more effective in achieving true alignment of the plateau with the X-ray beam than the subjective judgment required by the other two protocols, which call for angulation of the beam to bring the tibial plateau into sharpest focus during fluoroscopy. However, this definition of alignment lends itself better to objective confirmation by

a third party, as would be required in quality control procedures needed for use of these standardization techniques in multicenter studies of biomarkers of OA progression, or of the modification of structural damage by a DMOAD.

With respect to the reproducibility of JSW measurement, each of these protocols represents an advance over the measurement precision possible in conventional radiographic images.[19] As shown in Table 11.12, investigators have reported absolute precision (SE$_m$) of 0.11–0.35 mm in repeated measurements of medial tibiofemoral JSW in OA and/or normal knees. Corresponding CVs were all <10 per cent—notably smaller than the 15–20 per cent generally attributed to JSW measurements in conventional extended view images of the knee.[8]

In a recent field test we conducted of the fluoroscopically assisted semiflexed AP view,[20] technologists from 5 clinical radiology units were instructed in the performance of this examination and in the conduct of quality assurance checks of the resulting radiographs (including knee flexion and rotation) according to the semiflexed AP protocol.[17] After the technologists had demonstrated their proficiency with the technique, a sample of 44 subjects exhibiting a spectrum of radiographic severity of knee OA (Grade 0–III by the Kellgren–Lawrence criteria[21]) underwent semiflexed AP examinations in two randomly selected units, with repeat examinations 7–10 days later in the same units.

Independent evaluations of the technical quality of the radiographs indicated that the technologists had some difficulty achieving and self-correcting the superimposition of anterior and posterior margins of the tibial plateau. Thirty-six per cent of films in this field test were judged independently to be unsatisfactory in meeting the protocol standard for knee flexion (i.e., superimposition ±1 mm of the anterior and posterior margins of the medial tibial plateau). Within-unit percentages of substandard films ranged from 20–56 per cent.

When both images were technically satisfactory with respect to knee flexion and rotation, reproducibility of minimum JSW measurements in paired examinations performed in the same unit (SE$_m$ = 0.25 mm, CV = 7.1 per cent) was only slightly poorer than that demonstrated originally by Buckland-Wright et al.[17] in radiographs of similarly high quality performed in his laboratory (SE$_m$ = 0.19 mm, CV = 5.5 per cent). However, in paired examinations of the same knee in which one or both radiographs were technically flawed with respect to flexion or rotation, measurement precision suffered considerably (SE$_m$ = 0.31–0.40 mm, CV = 8.9–10.2 per cent). It remains to be seen whether large-scale implementation of fluoroscopically assisted protocols in a multicenter biomarker study or DMOAD trial (rather than only in the laboratories in which they were developed and validated) can be accomplished without serious reduction in the precision of measurement of JSW.

Fluoroscopically assisted protocols for knee radiography are not without practical limitations. For example, in the clinical radiology department

Table 11.13 Second generation (non-fluoroscopically assisted) protocols for standardized knee radiography

Investigator		Standards for non-fluoroscopically assisted positioning of the knee				
	View	Flexion/extension of the knee	Angulation of the X-ray beam	External foot rotation	Number of knees[*]	SE_m † (mm)
Ravaud et al.[25]	AP	Full extension	5° caudal angulation	15°	20 N	0.37
					36 OA	0.32
Buckland-Wright et al.[22]	PA	1st MTP joints beneath the front surface of the X-ray cassette; patellae in contact with the X-ray cassette and aligned vertically with 1st MTP joints	Horizontal	15°	74	0.11
Peterfy et al.[23]	PA	Schuss position: i.e., patellae in contact with film cassette and coplanar with the tips of the great toes (20–30° flexion)	10° caudal angulation	10°	18 N	0.1
					19 OA	0.1

[*] Results for normal (N) and OA knees are presented separately.

† Standard error of measurement.

MTP, metatarsophalangeal.

required for the fluoroscopic examination, competition for personnel and equipment is common: hence, the clinical research project finds itself in competition with the barium enema or the urgent imaging study, ordered for a patient with acute head trauma. Furthermore, the per-examination cost of fluoroscopically assisted knee radiographs is considerably greater than that for conventional radiography. Finally, although well within occupational safety limits, the radiation exposure resulting from 10–15 seconds of positioning (and repositioning) the knee under the fluoroscope (87–130 mR) can increase radiation exposure to the extremities several-fold beyond that entailed in a conventional radiographic examination of the knee (32 mR).

Concerns about these limitations have recently led investigators to pursue empirically derived standardization procedures that do not require fluoroscopy and minimize subjective judgments concerning knee flexion and alignment.[15,22,23] A comparison of the key elements of radioanatomic positioning of the knee in these second-generation protocols is presented in Table 11.13. Like the first-generation protocols described above, they differ from one another with respect to orientation (AP or PA), degree of knee flexion, beam angulation, and foot rotation. Nevertheless, each appears to yield measurements of JSW that are at least as reproducible as those in which alignment of the tibial plateau and the central ray of the X-ray beam is determined by fluoroscopy. Indeed, the semiflexed MTP protocol of Buckland-Wright[22] and the PA flexion view of Peterfy[23] appear to permit more precise measurement of JSW than the full-extension AP procedure recommended by Ravaud et al.[15] (Table 11.13) and, surprisingly, the fluoroscopically assisted protocols described in Table 11.12.

An unexpected finding in the original report of the semiflexed MTP view[22] that bears serious implications for the quality control of knee radiography in future studies is that this technique does not assure radioanatomic alignment of the tibial plateau and X-ray beam (Fig. 11.14). Only 25 of 78 semiflexed MTP radiographs (32 per cent) resulted in superimposition (±1 mm) of the anterior and posterior margins of the medial plateau. While this percentage is somewhat higher than that observed in an extended view of the same knee (13 per cent), this level of technical quality is far below the uniformly high level (100 per cent alignment) demonstrated by Buckland-Wright with the fluoroscopically assisted semiflexed AP view.[17] Our recent field test of the semiflexed MTP protocol[24] confirmed that only about 30 per cent of semiflexed MTP examinations result in an image of the knee in which the medial plateau and X-ray beam are aligned satisfactorily. However, we also found that alignment, or the degree of misalignment, of the medial plateau in the initial examination was reproduced ±1 mm in 89 per cent of repeat examinations. We estimated the SE_m of minimum medial JSW measurements in the semiflexed MTP view to be 0.30 mm,[24] that is, larger than reported originally by the author of the protocol (0.11 mm).[22] However, about 50 per cent of the discrepancy was attributable to the non-standard computational method for SE_m used by Buckland-Wright et al.[22] No published accounts of field tests of Peterfy's PA flexion view[23] are available.

Effects of radioanatomic positioning on JSN in knee OA

We recently examined the effect of chance alignment of the medial tibial plateau and X-ray beam in serial extended knee radiographs of cohorts from previous studies of the JSN in knee OA.[25] Subjects with definite OA at baseline and repeat extended knee radiographs taken at 2–3 year intervals were identified in a population-based research cohort in Indianapolis and two clinical OA cohorts drawn from Bristol and Nottingham, England, respectively. Alignment was determined by consensus of 2 readers and was considered satisfactory if anterior and posterior margins of the medial tibial plateau were superimposed ±1 mm (Fig. 11.14A). Readers were blinded to the identity of the subject and films were read in random order. Minimum medial JSW was measured manually with a calipers and a magnifying lens fitted with a 1-cm graticule (0.20 mm subdivisions).[26]

Satisfactory alignment of the medial tibial plateau and X-ray beam occurred fortuitously in only 21–41 per cent of the standing AP knee radiographs within the three cohorts (Table 11.14). In data from the combined cohorts, the proportion of baseline and follow-up radiographs deemed satisfactory with respect to tibial plateau alignment (34 and 29 per cent, respectively) was comparable to that reported by Buckland-Wright et al.[22] for the semiflexed MTP view (32 per cent). When paired standing AP images were examined, satisfactory alignment in *both* images of the pair was present for only 10–20 per cent of knees within each cohort.

Figure 11.15 illustrates JSN in subsets of knees from the Indianapolis cohort in which satisfactory alignment occurred fortuitously in both examinations and in neither examination. Most of the 21 knees with satisfactory alignment in both examinations exhibited a consistent degree of JSN over $2\frac{1}{2}$–3 years; in the remainder, JSW did not change beyond the margin of measurement error for our procedure (SE_m = 0.20 mm). In sharp contrast, the 46 knees with misalignment in one or both examinations exhibited a wide range of changes in JSW—including many with an apparent increase in JSW beyond the margin of error.

Table 11.14 contains quantitative summaries of absolute JSN (the difference between serial measures of JSW) and the annualized rate of JSN in OA knees in each cohort and in all cohorts combined. In the population-based Indianapolis cohort, the rate of JSN in knees with satisfactory alignment of the medial tibial plateau in both images was more than twice as rapid as that in the entire cohort and nearly threefold more rapid than that

Table 11.14 Frequency of occurrence of alignment of the medial tibial plateau and joint space narrowing (JSN) in serial standing AP radiographs of OA knees from three research cohorts

	Cohort			
	Indianapolis	Bristol	Nottingham	Combined
Source of cohort	Population	Clinic	Clinic	
Size of cohort (number of knees)	100	157	145	402
Mean interval between examinations (yrs)	2.6	3.0	2.3	2.7
Satisfactory alignment at 1st examination (%)	39	33	39	34
Satisfactory alignment at 2nd examination (%)	41	21	33	29
Satisfactory alignment at both examinations (%)	20	10	17	15
Absolute JSN, mm (mean ± SD)				
◆ All knees	0.29 ± 1.04	0.35 ± 1.52	0.49 ± 1.06	0.37 ± 1.25
◆ Knees with satisfactory alignment in both examinations	0.69 ± 0.69*	0.56 ± 0.72	0.73 ± 0.70	0.67 ± 0.70†
Annualized rate of JSN, mm/yr (mean ± SD)				
◆ All knees	0.11 ± 0.40	0.12 ± 0.51	0.21 ± 0.46	0.14 ± 0.46
◆ Knees with satisfactory alignment in both examinations	0.27 ± 0.27*	0.19 ± 0.24	0.32 ± 0.30	0.25 ± 0.26†

* Mean JSN in knees with satisfactory alignment in both images > that in knees with misalignment in one or both images, $P < 0.10$.

† Mean JSN in knees with satisfactory alignment in both images > that in knees with misalignment in one or both images, $P < 0.01$.

Compared to all knees in each cohort and in all cohorts combined, the subsets of knees with fortuitous alignment in the baseline and follow-up examinations exhibited significantly more rapid and less variable JSN.

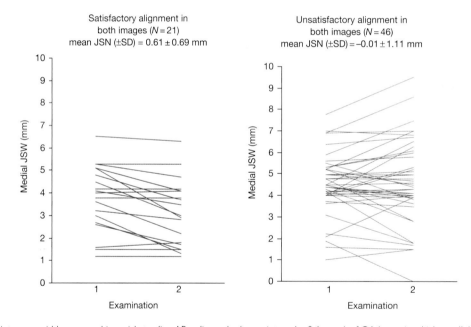

Satisfactory alignment in both images (N = 21)
mean JSN (±SD) = 0.61 ± 0.69 mm

Unsatisfactory alignment in both images (N = 46)
mean JSN (±SD) = −0.01 ± 1.11 mm

Fig. 11.15 Changes in joint-space width measured in serial standing AP radiographs (mean interval = 2.6 years) of OA knees in which parallel alignment of the medial tibial plateau and X-ray beam was observed in both radiographs (left) and misalignment was observed in one or both radiographs (right). JSW in knees exhibiting satisfactory radioanatomic alignment either narrowed to a consistent degree over 2–3 years or remained unchanged. In contrast, knees with unsatisfactory alignment exhibited a wide variety of changes in JSW (including numerous, improbable increases in JSW) that obscured any change in mean JSW.

previously reported for population-based samples (0.27 mm/yr vs 0.06–0.10 mm/yr[27,28]). In the 2 clinical cohorts, the subsets of knees with tibial plateau alignment in both images exhibited a mean rate of JSN about 50 per cent more rapid than that in the full cohorts.

Due to the small number of knees with satisfactory alignment in both images, the difference in mean JSN between knees with alignment in both images vs misalignment in one or both radiographs approached significance only in the Indianapolis cohort ($P = 0.06$). However, in combined data from all cohorts, JSN was significantly more rapid among knees with satisfactory alignment than in misaligned knees ($P < 0.004$).

Moreover, the SD of JSN in well-aligned pairs of images from each cohort was consistently smaller than that for the entire cohort. Between-subject variance in JSN among knees with satisfactory alignment in both images was significantly less than that in knees with misalignment ($0.001 < P < 0.05$ within individual cohorts, $P = 0.006$ in combined cohorts).

These data suggest that true JSN (i.e., JSN not confounded by changes in the alignment of the tibial plateau and X-ray beam in serial X-ray examinations) occurs more rapidly, and with less between-subject variability, than was previously thought to be characteristic of OA.

Implications for future studies

The findings in the above study bear important implications for the design of future studies to predict or modify progression of knee OA. Consider first a hypothetical randomized controlled trial of a purported DMOAD in which cumulative JSN in the placebo group (measured in serial conventional standing AP radiographs) is conservatively assumed to be 0.50 ± 1.00 mm over $2\frac{1}{2}$ years (i.e., 0.20 ± 0.40 mm/yr $\times$ 2.5 yrs, as suggested by the literature[8]).

If the drug slows the rate of JSN by 30 per cent in the treatment group and variances of JSN within the treatment and placebo groups remain equal, cumulative JSN over $2\frac{1}{2}$ years in the active treatment group would be 0.35 ± 1.00 mm. In this scenario, data from 1400 subjects (700/group) would be required to achieve 80 per cent power (2-tailed $\alpha = 0.05$) to detect a significant difference in JSN between the treatment groups. Alternatively, if alignment of the medial tibial plateau with the X-ray beam were achieved in all radiographs in this trial, the above data could lead one to anticipate that JSN over $2\frac{1}{2}$ years would be 0.50 ± 0.50 mm (0.20 ± 0.20 mm/yr $\times$ 2.5 yrs) in the placebo group and 0.35 ± 0.50 mm in the active treatment group (reflecting a 30 per cent reduction in the mean annual rate of JSN). Therefore, all other factors being equal, medial tibial plateau alignment in both the baseline and close-out radiograph would permit detection of a 30 per cent drug effect with only 352 subjects (176/group)—a 75 per cent reduction in sample size, in comparison with a similar trial using the conventional standing AP radiograph.

These data relate also to studies of modifiable and non-modifiable risk factors for knee OA. Numerous studies examining risk factors for incidence and progression of knee OA, as reflected in serial standing AP radiographs, have found that the variables associated with incident knee OA (e.g., age, female sex, previous knee injury, dietary intake and serum levels of vitamin D, quadriceps weakness) tend not to predict progression of structural damage.[29–34] This has led to conjecture that risk factors for incident OA differ from those for progressive OA.[34,35] However, incident OA is defined by the appearance of a definite osteophyte, while progression entails observable JSN.[21] We have shown that the apparent change in the size of osteophytes is unaffected by longitudinal changes in knee positioning, in sharp contrast to measurement of JSN.[25] Therefore, better-than-chance prediction of JSN is probably more difficult than prediction of the appearance, or growth, of osteophytes if radioanatomic positioning of the knee is not standardized.

Random measurement error, as illustrated in Fig. 11.15, can be expected to lead to underestimation of the significance of the predictive value of risk factors and biomarkers of OA progression. However, changes in the radioanatomic alignment of the medial tibial plateau in serial X-ray examinations may also introduce *systematic* error into JSN data. This may lead to overestimation of the strength of predictors of JSN or of the size of the effect of a purported DMOAD, if changes in the radioanatomic position of the knee reflect features of OA other than the loss of articular cartilage (e.g., joint pain, periarticular muscle spasm). Such features may restrict knee movement and alter the position of the joint—and, thereby, JSW—in follow-up X-ray examinations, while being unrelated to loss of articular cartilage. For example, we have found that mean JSW in the standing AP radiograph of OA knees of patients with severe standing knee pain (due to washout of their usual pain medications) was significantly *smaller* ($P = 0.005$) than when the examination was repeated 3–4 weeks later (Table 11.15), after resumption of the patient's analgesic or non-steroidal anti-inflammatory drug and a 50 per cent decrease in the severity of joint pain.[36] In contrast, mean JSW was unaffected by knee pain in fluoroscopically assisted semiflexed AP radiographs obtained concurrently. Changes in knee pain also had no effect on JSW in standing or semiflexed AP radiographs of knees of patients who reported nothing worse than moderate pain on standing after washout.[36]

The above data suggest that false JSN (change in radiographic JSW due to a change in joint pain or some feature of OA other than actual loss of articular cartilage) may confound the detection of true JSN in the conventional standing AP radiograph. An example of a study of OA risk factors that may have been susceptible to the confounding of false and true JSN is

Table 11.15 Change (mean $\pm$ SE) in WOMAC pain score and in joint space width (JSW) in knee radiographs obtained with extended and semiflexed views, after adjustment for the within-subject correlation between knees. Changes reflect the values observed after resumption of usual pain medications, relative to those obtained immediately after a washout of analgesics/NSAIDs

	Flaring knees[*] (N = 12)	Non-flaring knees (N = 15)	P-value
WOMAC pain score	-8.7 ± 1.1[†]	-3.5 ± 0.9[†]	0.0004
JSW in extended views, mm	0.20 ± 0.06[†]	-0.04 ± 0.04	0.0053
JSW in semiflexed views, mm	0.08 ± 0.05	0.02 ± 0.05	0.369

[*] Knees for which patients rated standing knee pain as 'severe' or 'extreme' after washout and in which pain decreased after resumption of treatment.

[†] $P \leq 0.005$ for paired t-tests of mean > 0.

an analysis of the Framingham cohort,[37] in which low dietary intake of vitamin C was considered to predict both incident knee pain *and* JSN in conventional knee radiographs. Based on the above, if incident pain had limited knee extension at follow-up, compared to that achieved in the absence of knee pain at baseline, the slight loss of extension could have disproportionately reduced JSW in the follow-up radiographs of knees that had become painful subsequent to the baseline examination. While, as indicated in Chapter 9.10, low vitamin C intake predicted OA progression also in asymptomatic knees, the *overall* predictive value of vitamin C intake in that study may have been exaggerated by the effects of incident knee pain during the follow-up exam.

The effect of longitudinal changes in knee pain on JSW in the standing AP radiograph is relevant also to two recent reports from randomized controlled trials of the purported disease-modifying properties of glucosamine sulfate.[38,39] Both studies reported concomitant pain relief and *widening* of mean JSW in the treatment group. However, if relief of knee pain by glucosamine enabled subjects to extend their knee to a greater degree during the follow-up examination than was possible at baseline, artifactual increases in JSW could have been seen disproportionately, if not selectively, in subjects in that treatment group. Conversely, frequent increases in knee pain among subjects in the placebo group may have resulted in artifactual JSN (as described above) in a disproportionate number of subjects in that group. It should be pointed out that even though mean pain scores of subjects in these two trials indicate that the typical subject had only mild-to-moderate knee pain at baseline,[38,39] the variability of pain scores suggest strongly that some patients in the active treatment groups had severe knee pain at baseline that was relieved to some degree at follow-up. To the extent that these subjects experienced relief of severe knee pain by glucosamine, and to the extent that subjects in the placebo group developed severe pain during follow-up, differences between treatment and placebo groups with respect to JSN may have been exaggerated.

Summary

Much of what we know about quantitative changes in knee OA, especially the thinning of articular cartilage as reflected by radiographic JSN, is based on data derived from the conventional standing AP radiograph. This technique suffers from several serious limitations, however, with respect to standardization of the radioanatomic position of the knee in serial examinations. Poor control of joint positioning (flexion and rotation, parallel alignment of the medial tibial plateau, and X-ray beam) in previous studies of the radiographic progression of knee OA using conventional knee radiography has likely obscured our understanding of the rate, variability, and determinants of radiographic JSN in patients with this disease. Recent advances in methods to standardize the radioanatomic positioning of the knee in repeated examinations afford significantly more reproducible measurement of radiographic JSW than is possible with conventional examination procedures. Implementation of these standardization protocols in future studies of OA progression can be anticipated to facilitate the acquisition of important new information about risk factors for OA progression, biomarkers of articular cartilage damage, and pharmacological modification of tissue damage in patients with OA.

Key points

1. Much of what we know about quantitative changes in knee OA, especially the thinning of articular cartilage as reflected in radiographic JSN, is based on data derived from the conventional standing AP radiograph, in which the knee is imaged in full extension.

2. Conventional knee radiography suffers from several serious limitations with regard to standardization of the radioanatomic position of the knee in serial examinations.

3. Poor control of joint positioning (knee flexion and rotation, parallel alignment of the medial tibial plateau, and X-ray beam) in previous studies of the radiographic progression of knee OA using conventional knee radiography, is likely to have obscured our understanding of the rate, variability, and determinants of radiographic JSN in patients with this disease.

4. Recent advances in methods to standardize the radioanatomic positioning of the knee under fluoroscopy, or with empirically derived procedures for flexion/rotation of the knee and angulation of the X-ray beam, afford more reproducible measurement of radiographic JSW in repeated examinations than is possible with conventional examination procedures.

5. The implementation of these standardization protocols in current and future studies of OA progression can be anticipated to facilitate the acquisition of important new information about risk factors for OA progression, biomarkers of articular cartilage deterioration, and pharmacological modification of structural damage in OA.

Acknowledgement

Supported in part by grants from the National Institutes of Health (AR20582, AR43348, AR43370).

References

(An asterisk denotes recommended reading.)

1. Yelin, E. and Callahan, L.F. (1995). The economic cost and social and psychosocial impact of musculoskeletal conditions. *Arthritis Rheum* **38**:1351–62.

2. Gabriel, S., Crowson, C., and O'Fallon, W. (1995). Costs of osteoarthritis: estimates from a geographically defined population. *J Rheumatol* **22** (Suppl. 4):23–5.

3. Buckland-Wright, C. (1998). Quantitation of radiographic changes. In K Brandt, M Doherty, and S Lohmander (eds), *Osteoarthritis*. Oxford: Oxford University Press, pp. 459–72.

4. Buckland-Wright, J.C. and Macfarlane, D.G. (1995). Radio-anatomic assessment of therapeutic outcome in osteoarthritis. In K Kuettner and V Goldberg (eds), *Osteoarthritic disorders*. Rosemont, IL: American Academy of Orthopaedic Surgeons, pp. 51–66.

5. *Bland, M.J. and Altman, D.G. (1996). Statistics notes: measurement error. *Brit Med J* **313**:744.

   This is a straightforward explanation of the concept of measurement error, with guidelines for estimating the magnitude of such error in repeated measurements.

6. Ahlback, S. (1968). Osteoarthritis of the knee: a radiographic investigation. *Acta Radiol* **277**(Suppl.):7–72.

7. Leach, R.E., Gregg, T., and Siber, F.J. (1970). Weight bearing radiography in osteoarthritis of the knee. *Radiology* **97**:265–68.

8. *Mazzuca, S.A., Brandt, K.D., and Katz, B.P. (1997). Is conventional radiography suitable for evaluation of a disease-modifying drug in patients with knee osteoarthritis? *Osteoarthritis Cart* **5**:217–26.

   This review of the literature summarizes what is known, based on conventional radiographic methods, about JSW and JSN in knee OA and offers estimates of the sample size and duration of treatment needed for DMOAD trials in which outcomes are derived from conventional and standardized radiographic protocols.

9. Buckland-Wright, C. (1997). Current status of imaging procedures in the diagnosis, prognosis and monitoring of osteoarthritis. *Baillieres Clin Rheumatol* **11**:727–48.

10. Maquet, P. (1976). *Biomechanics of the Knee*. Berlin: Springer.

11. Resnick, D. and Vint, V. (1980) The 'tunnel' view in assessment of cartilage loss in osteoarthritis of the knee. *Radiology* **137**:547–8.

12. Messieh, S.S., Fowler, P.J., and Munro, T. (1990). Anteroposterior radiographs of the osteoarthritic knee. *J Bone Joint Surg* **72B**:639–40.

13. Buckland-Wright, J.C., Edwards, M., Greaves, I.D., *et al.* (1998). Comparison of OA knee joint space width in standing extended and semiflexed views (abstract). *Trans Orthop Res Soc* **23**:711.

14. Mesquida, V., Mazzuca, S.A., Piperno, M., *et al.* (1998). Reproducibility of measurements of medial tibiofemoral joint space width in the schuss view and sensitivity to joint space narrowing over 1 year in osteoarthritic knees (abstract). *Trans Orthop Res Soc* **23**:879.

15. Ravaud, P., Auleley, G.R., Chastang, C., *et al.* (1996). Knee joint space width measurement: an experimental study of the influence of radiographic procedure and joint positioning. *Br J Rheumatol* **35**:761–6.

16. Fife, R.S., Brandt, K.D., Braunstein, E.M., *et al.* (1991). Relationship between arthroscopic evidence of cartilage damage and radiographic evidence of joint space narrowing in early osteoarthritis of the knee. *Arthritis Rheum*, **34**:377–82.

17. *Buckland-Wright, J.C., Macfarlane, D.G., Williams, S.A., *et al.* (1995). Accuracy and precision of joint space width measurements in standard and macroradiographs of osteoarthritic knees. *Ann Rheum Dis* **54**:872–80.

   This study demonstrates the separate contributions of alignment of the medial tibial plateau and correction for radiographic magnification to the reproducibility of JSW measurements in repeated plain standing AP and semiflexed AP knee radiographs and in standardized macroradiographs of normal and OA knees. Comparisons of techniques within this study with respect to the reproducibility of JSW measurements are highly instructive. However, because the computational methods for estimating SE$_m$ in this study are not based on parametric statistics (as recommended by Bland and Altman[5]), care should be taken when comparing the results of this study to those of other studies.

18. Piperno, M., Hellio Le Graverand, P., Conrozier, T., Bochu, M., Mathieu, P., and Vignon, E. (1998). Quantitative evaluation of joint space width in femorotibial osteoarthritis: comparison of three radiographic views. *Osteoarthritis Cart* **6**:252–9.

19. Mazzuca, S. and Brandt, K.D. (1999). Plain radiography as an outcome measure in clinical trials of OA. *Rheum Dis Clin NA* **25**:467–80.

20. *Mazzuca, S.A., Brandt, K.D., Buckland-Wright, J.C., *et al.* (1999). Field test of the reproducibility of automated measurements of medial tibiofemoral joint space width derived from standardized knee radiographs. *J Rheumatol* **26**:1359–65.

   This field test of the semiflexed AP view illustrates the extent to which the reproducibility of a protocol for standardizing the radioanatomic position of the knee, as originally determined under ideal conditions, may decrease somewhat when transported for use in clinical radiology departments, such as those that participate in multicenter studies of the radiographic progression of OA.

21. Kellgren, J.H. and Lawrence, J.S. (1957). Radiographic assessment of osteoarthritis. *Ann Rheum Dis* **16**:494–502.

22. Buckland-Wright, J.C., Wolfe, F., Ward, R.J., Flowers, N., and Hayne, C. (1999). Substantial superiority of semiflexed (MTP) views in knee osteoarthritis: a comparative radiographic study, without fluoroscopy, of

standing extended, semiflexed AP, and schuss views. *J Rheumatol* **26**:2664–74.

23. Peterfy, C.G., Li, J., Duryea, J., Lynch, J.A., Miaux, Y., and Genant, H.K. (1998). Nonfluoroscopic method for flexed radiography of the knee the allows reproducible joint space width measurement (abstract). *Arthritis Rheum* **41**(Suppl 9):S361.

24. Mazzuca, S.A., Brandt, K.D., Buckwalter, K.A., Lane, K.A., and Katz, B.P. (2002). Field test of the reproducibility of the semiflexed metatarsophalangeal (MTP) view in repeated radiographic examinations of subjects with osteoarthritis of the knee. *Arthritis Rheum* **46**:109–13.

25. *Mazzuca, S.A., Brandt, K.D., Dieppe, P.A., Doherty, M., Katz, B.P., and Lane, K.A. (2001). Effect of alignment of the medial tibial plateau and X-ray beam on apparent progression of osteoarthritis in the standing anteroposterior knee radiograph. *Arthritis Rheum* **44**:1786–94.

    This study of conventional standing AP radiographs in OA research cohorts from the United States of America and England, shows how the lack of standards for radioanatomic positioning of the knee in previous studies of the knee OA may obscure the true rate and variability of JSN. In contrast, detection of changes in the size of marginal osteophytes was not affected by uncontrolled changes in the position of the knee in serial standing AP radiographs.

26. Lequesne, M. (1995). Quantitative measurements of joint space during progression of osteoarthritis: chondrometry. In: K Kuettner and V Goldberg (eds), *Osteoarthritic disorders*. Rosemont, IL: American Academy of Orthopedic Surgeons, pp. 427–44.

27. Neuhauser, K.B., Anderson, J.J., and Felson, D.T., (1994). Rate of joint space narrowing in normal knees and knees with osteoarthritis. *Arthritis Rheum* **37**(Suppl. 9):S423.

28. Lethbridge-Çejku, M., Hochberg, M.C., Scott, W.W. Jr., Plato, C.C., and Tobin, J.D. (1995). Longitudinal change in joint space of the knee: data from the Baltimore Longitudinal Study of Aging. *Arthritis Rheum* **38** (Suppl. 9):S626.

29. Felson, D.T., Anderson, J.J., and Naimark, A. (1989). Obesity and knee OA. The Framingham study. *Ann Intern Med* **109**:18–24.

30. Davis, M.A., Ettinger, W.H., Neuhaus, J.M., Cho, S.A., and Hauck, W.W. (1989). The association of knee injury and obesity with unilateral and bilateral osteoarthritis of the knee. *Am J Epidemiol* **130**:278–88.

31. Schouten, J.S.A.G., Ouweland, F.A. van den, and Valkenburg, H.A. (1992). A 12-year follow up study in the general population on prognostic factors of cartilage loss in osteoarthritis of the knee. *Ann Rheum Dis* **51**:932–7.

32. McAlindon, T.E., Felson, D.T., Zhang, Y., *et al.* (1996). Relation of dietary intake and serum levels of Vitamin D to progression of osteoarthritis of the knee among participants in the Framingham study. *Ann Intern Med* **125**:353–9.

33. Slemenda, C.W., Heilman, D.K., Brandt, K.D., *et al.* (1998). Quadriceps muscle weakness. A risk factor for knee osteoarthritis in women? *Arthritis Rheum* **41**:1951–9.

34. Cooper, C., Snow, S., McAlindon, T.E., *et al.* (2000). Risk factors for the incidence and progression of radiographic knee osteoarthritis. *Arthritis Rheum* **43**:995–1000.

35. Felson, D.T. Epidemiology of osteoarthritis. (1998). In KD Brandt, M Doherty, and LS Lohmander (eds). *Osteoarthritis*. Oxford: Oxford University Press, pp. 13–22.

36. *Mazzuca, S.A., Brandt, K.D., Buckwalter, K.A., Lane, K.A., and Katz, B.P. (2002). Knee pain reduces joint space width in conventional standing anteroposterior radiographs of osteoarthritic knees. *Arthritis Rheum* **46**:1223–7.

    This small clinical study provides evidence that changes in joint pain can alter JSW in the standing AP radiograph of the OA knee. These data are relevant to clinical trials of the disease-modifying and symptomatic effects of purported DMOADs when radiographic outcomes are derived from the conventional standing AP view. Systematic reduction of symptoms in the active treatment group may permit subjects randomized to that group to extend the knee more fully than was possible in earlier examination(s), thereby increasing the radiographic joint space. This may exaggerate the difference between treatment groups with respect to JSN.

37. McAlindon, T.E., Jacques, P., Zhang, Y., *et al.* (1996). Do antioxidant micronutrients protect against the development and progression of knee osteoarthritis? *Arthritis Rheum* **39**:648–56.

38. Reginster, J.Y., Deroisy, R., Rovati, L.C., *et al.* (2001). Long-term effects of glucosamine sulphate on osteoarthritis progression: a randomized, placebo-controlled clinical trial. *Lancet* **357**(9252):251–6.

39. Pavelka, K., Gatterova, J., Olejarova, M., *et al.* A long-term, randomized, placebo-controlled, confirmatory trial on the effects of glucosamine sulfate on knee osteoarthritis progression (abstract). *Osteoarthritis Cart*, **8**(Suppl.):S6–7.

11.4.3 Magnetic resonance imaging
Charles G. Peterfy

Since its development more than two decades ago, magnetic resonance imaging (MRI) has become the imaging method of choice for evaluating internal derangement of the knee and other joints. Despite this, however, MRI has thus far played only a minor role in the study or management of OA. The principal reason for this has been the lack of effective therapies to combat this disease. In the absence of a therapy, clinical practice has no need for methods of identifying patients most appropriate for the therapy or for determining how well the therapy worked. However, new insights into the pathophysiology of OA coupled with advances in molecular engineering and drug discovery have spawned a host of new treatment strategies and rekindled the hope of achieving long-term control of this disorder.

This explosion in drug development has created a demand for better ways of monitoring disease progression and treatment response in patients with OA. Noninvasive imaging techniques, particularly MRI, have drawn considerable attention in this regard. This interest has been intensified by the growing acceptance of structure modification as an independent therapeutic objective in arthritis. Underlying this therapeutic strategy is the classic disease-illness debate: must therapies that effectively slow or prevent structural abnormalities in arthritis necessarily show an immediate parallel improvement in clinical symptoms and function, so long as they ultimately yield clinical benefits for the patient? Elucidating the structural determinants of the clinical features in arthritis has, accordingly, become a key objective for academia as well as the pharmaceutical industry.

MRI is particularly well suited for imaging arthritic joints. In addition to delineating the anatomy, MRI is capable of quantifying a variety of compositional and functional parameters of articular tissues relevant to the degenerative process and OA. Moreover, since MRI is a nondestructive technique, multiple parameters can be analyzed in the same region of tissue and frequent serial examinations can be performed on even asymptomatic patients. With more than 9000 MRI systems present worldwide, lack of availability is less of a limitation than in the past. Moreover, the cost of MRI is decreasing. This is because of both market forces and technical innovations, such as small extremity scanners. These small MRI systems, which allow only the extremity of interest to be placed within the magnet while the rest of the body remains outside (Fig. 11.16), offer a number of advantages over conventional whole-body MRI in certain settings. These include significantly lower cost (potentially less than one-quarter that of conventional MRI), improved patient comfort and safety, including fewer biohazards associated with aneurysm clips, pacemakers, etc.; and greater convenience and versatility.[1] In some cases, these systems are small enough to support office-based MRI of the extremities. The demand for such technology may increase as structure-modifying therapies enter the market.

Accordingly, the imaging tools that ultimately will be used to direct patients with OA to specific therapies and to monitor treatment effectiveness and safety are currently being refined and validated in rigorous multicenter and multinational clinical trials aimed at gaining regulatory approval of putative new therapies. As these trials approach completion,

(a)

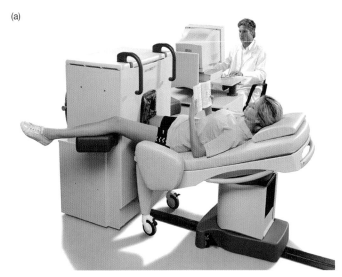

(b) 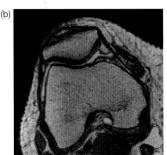   (c)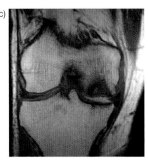

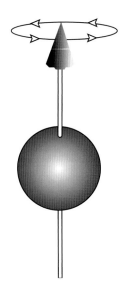

Fig. 11.17 The nuclear magnetic moment. Spinning (precessing) anatomic nuclei ('spins') generate small local magnetic fields analogous to the spinning planets. The magnitude of the magnetic moment depends on the rate of precession, or frequency, of the nucleus. The vector sum of individual magnetic moments for a pool of hydrogen nuclei ('protons') in fat or water is the essential parameter measured in clinical MRI.

Fig. 11.16 Dedicated extremity MRI. Recently introduced dedicated extremity MRI systems reduce imaging cost and improve patient comfort and safety. In contrast to conventional whole-body MRI, only the limb is inserted into the dedicated extremity scanner—the remainder of the patient remains outside (a). This obviates problems associated with claustrophobia. The low magnetic field strength virtually eliminates any hazards associated with metallic objects near the magnet or in the patient. Also, dedicated systems cost only a fraction of the cost of whole-body scanners, and because of their small size and light weight, offer convenient and inexpensive siting. In addition to these practical and economic advantages, dedicated extremity MRI provides high quality images of articular anatomy (b) and (c). (b) Transverse image through the patella acquired using a dedicated extremity system (Artoscan: Lunar, Madison, WI). (c) Coronal image of the knee acquired with the same system shows complete denuding of articular cartilage, bone attrition, and subarticular marrow changes in the femur in the medial femorotibial compartment.

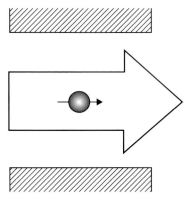

Fig. 11.18 Longitudinal magnetization. Protons placed within the strong magnetic field (large open arrow) in the bore of a MRI magnet tend to align their magnetic moments (small arrow) with this large magnetic field. The magnitude of this net longitudinal magnetic moment and therefore the maximal signal that could be generated during imaging varies directly with the field strength of the MRI magnet.

there will be an increased demand for expertise and experience in evaluating disease progression and treatment response with these techniques, and the emergence of MRI systems specifically designed for this market. This chapter reviews these innovations in MRI of OA and points to areas where further advances may be anticipated in the future.

MR imaging technique

The clarity and detail with which MRI depicts cross sectional anatomy makes interpretation of the images appear deceptively simple. In reality, MRI is a highly sophisticated technology, and while a detailed understanding of quantum physics may not be necessary to view the images, some background knowledge is essential to understand the findings as well as to critically assess conclusions drawn from investigations that employ this technology. The following brief review of basic principles and terminology used in MRI is provided, therefore, not only to serve as an aid to understanding the remainder of the chapter, but also to help investigators outside the discipline of Radiology take better advantage of the growing number of

studies in the literature that use MRI. For the interested reader, there are several excellent books and articles that delve deeper into MRI physics and its applications in medicine.[2–7]

Basic principles

MR imaging is based on the natural magnetic behavior of atomic nuclei as they spin about their axes (Fig. 11.17). Although a number of different nuclei (e.g., sodium, phosphorus, hydrogen) could theoretically be used to generate MR images, only hydrogen is present in sufficient quantities within biological tissues to be feasible for clinical imaging. When the nuclei within a tissue are placed within the very high magnetic field in the bore of an MR imaging magnet, they show a net tendency to align their nuclear magnetic moments along this static magnetic field (longitudinal magnetization) (Fig. 11.18). Exposure of these protons to a second field (radio frequency

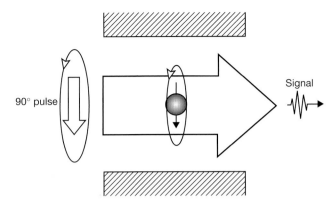

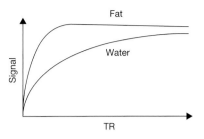

Fig. 11.21 Effect of TR on signal intensity. Repetition time (TR) is the time between successive rf pulses in an imaging sequence. Typically, 192–256 repetitions are necessary to generate an MR image. If the TR is less than five times the T1 of a substance, there is insufficient time for complete recovery of longitudinal magnetization and signal intensity is decreased. Therefore, as TR is shortened, substances with long T1 relaxation times (e.g., free water) begin to loose signal first, while substances with short T1 relaxation times (e.g., fat) retain signal until TR is very short. Short-TR sequences thus generate T1 contrast among tissues and are called T1-weighted.

Fig. 11.19 Transverse magnetization. Protons that are longitudinally aligned with the high magnetic field (large open arrow) in the MRI magnet bore will realign (resonate) with a second relatively smaller magnetic field (small open arrow) if this new field is tuned to the precessional frequency of these protons. Since this resonant frequency is in the same range as radio waves, this second field is called a radio-frequency (rf) pulse. If the rf pulse is oriented transverse to the static magnetic field of the MRI magnet, it is said to have a 90° flip angle. If the rf pulse is also made to rotate in the transverse plane, the realigned (flipped) magnetic moment (small solid arrow) will also rotate transversely and induce an alternating current (by Faraday's Law) in receiver wires in an imaging coil placed near the patient. This induced current is the basis for the MR image.

principal determinants of the imaging time; typically, a sequence of 192–512 rf pulses is used to generate an MR image), slow-T1 substances, such as water, are not given sufficient time to recover between the pulses, and therefore exhibit low signal intensity, while fast-T1 substances, such as fat, show high signal intensity (Fig. 11.21). Short-TR[1] sequences therefore generate contrast (relative signal intensity difference) among tissues on the basis of differences in T1 and are accordingly referred to as T1-weighted (Fig. 7).

Subtle T1 contrast (e.g., between articular cartilage and synovial fluid) is usually overshadowed on T1-weighted images by the far greater difference in signal intensity that exists between fat and most other tissues (Fig. 11.22). However, by selectively suppressing the signal intensity of fat, it is possible to expand the scale of image intensities across smaller differences in T1 and thus to augment residual T1 contrast (Fig. 11.23). Another application of fat suppression is to increase contrast between fat and other substances, such as methemoglobin and gadolinium (Gd)-containing contrast material, which also show rapid T1 relaxation. The most widely used technique for fat suppression is based on the chemical-shift phenomenon: since the frequency of protons in fat differ from that of protons in water the magnetization of fat (or water) can be selectively suppressed by a specifically tuned rf pulse at the beginning of the sequence (Fig. 11.24).

A similar technique can also be used to suppress the signal of water indirectly through a mechanism called magnetization transfer. In this case, direct suppression of tightly constrained protons in macromolecules like collagen, which are thermodynamically coupled to freely mobile protons in bulk water, evokes a transfer of magnetization from the water proton pool to the macromolecular pool to maintain equilibrium. This manifests as a loss of longitudinal magnetization, and therefore signal intensity, from water in proportion to the relative concentrations of the two proton pools in the tissue and the specific rate constant for the equilibrium reaction. Since collagen (unlike fat) is strongly coupled to water in this way, cartilage and muscle exhibit pronounced magnetization-transfer effects[8–11] (Fig. 11.25). Magnetization-transfer techniques are therefore useful for imaging the articular cartilage, and could potentially be used to quantify the collagen content of this tissue.

Image contrast is also influenced by T2 relaxation. This phenomenon manifests as a loss of transverse magnetization, and therefore signal, over time as neighboring protons exposed to the transverse rf pulse gradually fall out of phase with each other. As for T1 relaxation, the rate of T2 relaxation, or 'dephasing', of a group of protons depends on their local microenvironment and therefore varies among different tissues. Freely mobile water protons (e.g., in synovial fluid) show slow T2 relaxation, and therefore retain signal over time, while constrained or 'bound' water protons (e.g., by collagen or proteoglycan) show rapid T2 relaxation and signal decay (Figs 11.22 and 11.26).

In addition to the effects of neighboring protons on each other (T2 relaxation), fixed magnetic-field heterogeneities in a specimen also cause

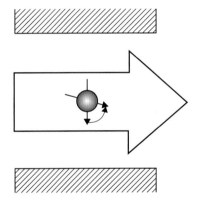

Fig. 11.20 T1 relaxation. When the rotating 90° rf pulse is turned off, the transversely oriented magnetic moment (small solid arrow) realigns with the static field of the magnet (large open arrow). This recovery of longitudinal magnetization is called T1 relaxation, and the parameter, T1, is a measure of the rate of this recovery. If the 90° rf pulse is repeated before longitudinal magnetization has fully recovered, only this smaller longitudinal component is flipped into the transverse plane and the image signal is correspondingly lower—these protons are said to be partially saturated.

pulse) that is rotating and perpendicular to the original static field of the magnet (90° radio frequency, rf, pulse) realigns the protons transversely (transverse magnetization) (Fig. 11.19). This rotation of one magnetic field against another induces an alternating electrical current in receiver coils near the patient in proportion to the magnitude of the net magnetic moment of these transversely aligned protons. This signal is then used to generate the MR images by computerized Fourier transformation.

Once the rf pulse is turned off, the protons relax to their original alignment with the static field of the magnet (Fig. 11.20). This process of recovering longitudinal magnetization is called T1 relaxation. T1 relaxation varies from tissue to tissue depending on the microenvironments of the different proton populations. In general, fat shows rapid T1 relaxation, while water shows slow T1 relaxation (Fig. 11.21). Under conditions of rapid rf pulsing (the time between repeated 90° rf pulses in an MRI pulse sequence is called the repetition time, TR; the number and duration of the TR are the

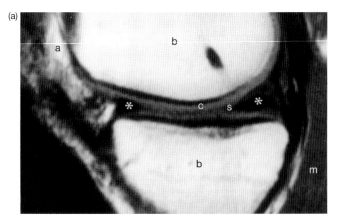

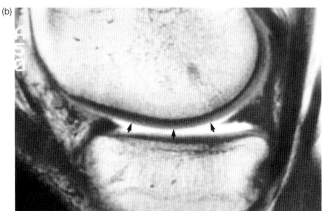

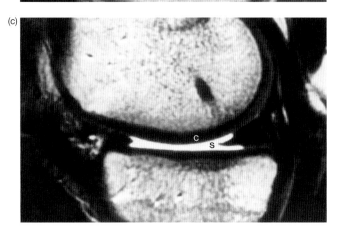

Fig. 11.22 T-weighted MRI. (a) Sagittal T1-weighted spin-echo image of a knee depicts structures that contain fat (*f*) (short T1) with high signal intensity, and structures that contain water (long T1) with low signal intensity. The small differences in T1 relaxation time among synovial fluid (*s*), articular cartilage (*c*) and muscle (*m*) are not sufficient to generate substantial contrast among these structures on this image. It is difficult, therefore, to delineate the articular cartilage surface. (b) Sagittal T1-weighted image of the same knee immediately following intra-articular injection of Gd-containing contrast material that shortens the T1 of water, depicts the synovial fluid with high signal intensity, and clearly delineates the cartilage-fluid interface (*arrows*). (c) T2-weighted spin-echo image of the same knee before Gd-containing contrast injection depicts fat (relatively short T2) with intermediate signal intensity and water in synovial fluid (long T2) with high signal intensity. Water in articular cartilage and muscle is relatively bound (short T2); these structures therefore show low signal intensity. High intrinsic contrast between cartilage and synovial fluid makes this technique useful for delineating the articular surface.

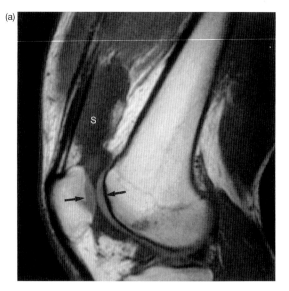

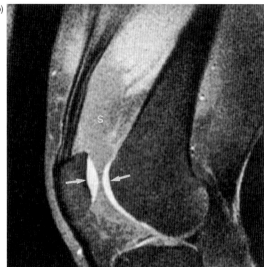

Fig. 11.23 Augmenting T1 contrast with fat suppression. (a) Sagittal, T1-weighted spin-echo image of a knee acquired with a somewhat shorter TR (300 msec) than usual (500–700 msec) depicts the articular cartilage (*arrows*) with a slightly higher signal intensity than the adjacent synovial fluid (*s*). Contrast between cartilage and water is greater on this shorter-TR image than on the conventional T1-weighted image shown in Fig. 11.22(a) (TR = 600 msec), but is still overshadowed by the greater T1 contrast between fat and other tissues in the image. (b) The same sequence repeated with fat suppression generates greater contrast between articular cartilage (*arrows*) and synovial fluid as their pixel intensities are rescaled across a broader range of grayscale values. The same effect can be achieved with water-selective excitation.

protons to dephase and loose transverse magnetization. The combined effects of these two causes of proton dephasing and signal loss is called T2* (this is the formal notation in MR physics for the sum of the two relaxation components defined above, i.e., T2 + T2′ = T2*) relaxation. Signal lost to fixed magnetic heterogeneity, but not that lost to T2 relaxation, can be recovered by rephasing the protons with a 180° rf pulse (spin-echo, SN) or to a lesser extent by rapidly reversing the magnetic gradient (gradient-echo, GRE). Long echo time (TE) sequences thus generate contrast among tissues on the basis of T2 (Figs 11.22 and 11.26), and when combined with a long TR to minimize the effects of T1 on contrast, are referred to as T2-weighted.

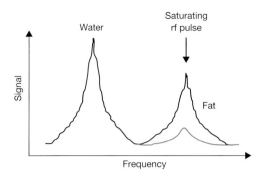

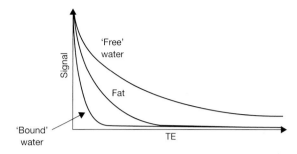

Fig. 11.24 Frequency-selective fat suppression. The chemical-shift phenomenon separates the resonant frequencies of water and fat (by 220 Hz at a magnetic field strength of 1.5 T). This allows the longitudinal magnetization of either of these proton pools to be selectively suppressed by a rf pulse tuned to the correct resonant frequency. Since the resonant frequency and the magnitude of the chemical shift both depend on magnetic field strength, this method of fat suppression is dependent on the homogeneity of the static magnetic field and is not feasible at very low field strengths.

Fig. 11.26 Effect on TE on signal intensity. Echo time (TE) is the time between the initiating rf pulse and a subsequent 180° rephasing rf pulse (spin-echo) or gradient reversal (gradient-echo). The longer the TE, the greater the decay of transverse magnetization (and therefore signal intensity) by T2 or T2* relaxation. Substances with long T2 relaxation times (e.g., free water) retain the most signal intensity on long-TE (T2-weighted) sequences. Structures, such as tendons and menisci, that contain highly immobile water protons (bound water), show such rapid T2 relaxation that no attainable TE is short enough to recover any signal. These structures therefore appear dark on even the shortest TE sequences.

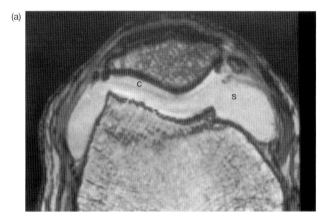

(a)

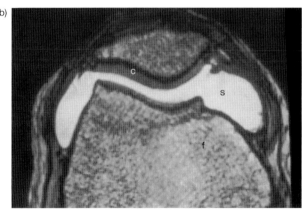

(b)

Fig. 11.25 Magnetization-transfer contrast. (a) Transverse (axial) T2*-weighted gradient-echo image of a knee shows poor contrast between articular cartilage (c) and adjacent synovial fluid (s). (b) Same image acquired with the addition of a magnetization-transfer pulse, which causes signal loss in collagen-containing tissues, such as articular cartilage (c) and muscle, but not synovial fluid (s) or fat (f).

Local perturbations of the magnetic field typically arise at interfaces between substances that differ considerably in magnetic susceptibility (the degree to which a substance magnetizes in the presence of a magnetic field), such as between soft tissue and gas, metal, or heavy calcification. Severe T2* at these sites is referred to as magnetic susceptibility effect. SN technique

corrects for fixed magnetic heterogeneities and therefore can provide images with true T2 contrast. GRE technique is faster than SN, but does not correct for these effects and therefore provides only T2*-weighted images, which are highly vulnerable to magnetic susceptibility effects, such as those caused by metallic prostheses. Magnetic susceptibility effects are more severe on high field strength magnets.

Finally, diffusion of protons (i.e., water) within a specimen during the acquisition of an MR image will result in loss of phase coherence among the protons and therefore a loss in signal. This effect is usually insignificant in conventional MRI but can be augmented with the use of strong magnetic field gradients such as those employed in MR microimaging. Water diffusivity is thus an additional tissue parameter measurable with MRI[12,13] (see below).

Both T1-weighting (short TR) and T2-weighting (long TE) involve discarding MR signal. If these effects are eliminated, signal intensity reflects only the proton density. Accordingly, long-TR/short-TE images are often referred to as proton-density-weighted. However, even the shortest finite TE attainable is too long to completely escape T2 relaxation, and extremely long TRs (>2500 msec) are not practical for imaging in vivo. Therefore, even so called proton-density-weighted images contain some T1 and T2 contrast. To generate true proton-density images (e.g., for purposes of quantifying water content) multiple scans must be acquired and TR and TE extrapolated to infinity and zero respectively (see below).

The dimensions of the individual volume elements, or voxels, comprising it, define the spatial resolution of an MR image. All signals within a single voxel are averaged. Therefore, if an interface with high signal intensity on one side and low signal intensity on the other side passes through the middle of a voxel, the interface is depicted as an intermediate signal intensity band the width of the voxel (Fig. 11.27). This effect is known as partial-volume averaging. Voxel size is determined by multiplying the slice thickness by the size of the in-plane subdivisions of the image, the pixels (picture elements). Pixel size, in turn, is determined by dividing the field of view by the image matrix, which most commonly ranges between 256×128 and 256×256. The smaller the voxel, the greater the spatial resolution. However, as voxel size decreases, so does signal-to-noise ratio (S/N). Accordingly, high-resolution imaging requires sufficient S/N to support the spatial resolution. S/N can be increased by shortening TE (less T2 decay), increasing TR (more T1 recovery), imaging at higher field strength (greater longitudinal magnetization) or utilizing specialized coils, which reduce noise (small surface coil, quadrature coil, phased array of small coils).[14,15] Specialized sequences, such as three-dimensional (3D) GRE also provide greater S/N.

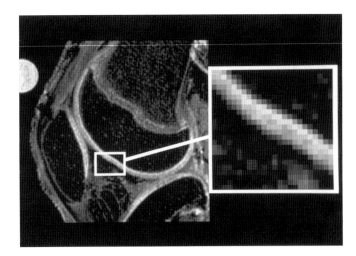

Fig. 11.27 Partial volume averaging. The smallest element of an MR image is the individual voxel (pixel size × slice thickness). Different signal intensities within a single voxel are averaged. This effect is most noticeable at high contrast interfaces as shown in the magnified view of the femoral cartilage on this sagittal, fat-suppressed, T1-weighted gradient-echo image of a knee.

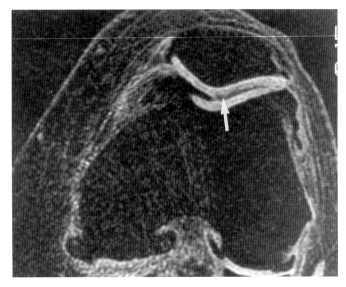

Fig. 11.28 Imaging cartilage with fat suppression. Transverse, thin-partitioned, fat-suppressed 3D gradient-echo image of a 62-year-old man with OA of the knee delineates cartilage with high resolution. Fibrillation of the surface of the patellar cartilage (*arrow*) is visible on this image.

Source: Peterfy, C., Majumdar, S., Lang, P., van Dijke, C.F., Sack, K., and Genant, H.K. 1994. MR imaging of the arthritic knee: improved discrimination of cartilage, synovium and effusion with pulsed saturation transfer and fat-suppressed, T1-weighted sequences. *Radiology* **191**:413–19; reproduced with permission.

Imaging articular cartilage

MRI appearance of articular cartilage

The signal behavior of articular cartilage on MRI reflects the complex biochemistry and histology of this tissue. It is the high water content (proton density) of articular cartilage that forms the basis for MR signal. Water content in this tissue depends on the delicate balance between the swelling pressure of the aggregated proteoglycans and the counter resistance provided by the fibrous collagen matrix, but in general terms, changes in cartilage proton density tend to be relatively small (typically less than 20 per cent). Since the water constitutes approximately 70 per cent of the weight of normal articular cartilage, proton density itself offers little scope for generating image contrast between cartilage and adjacent synovial fluid. However, this fundamental MRI signal in cartilage is modulated by a number of processes, including T1 relaxation, T2 relaxation, magnetization transfer, water diffusion, magnetic susceptibility, and interactions with contrast agents, and these provide a rich palette of mechanisms for delineating cartilage morphology and probing its composition.

The T1 of articular cartilage at 1.5 Tesla is approximately 700 ms. This is shorter than the T1 of both adjacent synovial fluid (1500 ms) and subarticular marrow fat (200 ms). However, the gray scale on a conventional T1-weighted SE image is so dominated by fat that the contrast between articular cartilage and adjacent synovial fluid is normally difficult to appreciate (Fig. 11.27). Intrinsic T1-contrast can be augmented slightly by shortening TR, but a more powerful approach is to suppress the fat signal or selectively excite protons in water, and rescale the smaller residual T1 contrast across the image. This generates images in which articular cartilage is depicted as an isolated high signal intensity band in sharp contrast with adjacent low signal intensity joint fluid, and nulled fat in adipose tissue (e.g., Hoffa's fat pad) and bone.[9,16] Fat suppression also eliminates chemical-shift artifacts that distort the cartilage–bone interface and complicate dimensional measurements. Augmentation of T1 contrast in this way can be combined with higher through-plain spatial resolution and greater S/N ratio by using a 3D GRE technique (3D spoiled-GRE) (Fig. 11.28). Fat-suppressed, T1-weighted 3D spoiled-GRE is easy to use and widely available, and has become a popular MRI technique for delineating articular cartilage morphology.[9,16–20]

More recently, projection-reconstruction spiral imaging (PRSI) techniques have been developed to image the articular cartilage with ultra-short TE (<0.2 ms) and even greater contrast, less chemical-shift effects, and lower vulnerability to magnetic susceptibility artifacts (Fig. 11.29).[21] Other advantages of this technique include the potential for spectroscopic determination of water content and T2. However, the technique is currently not widely available, and involves long image reconstruction times.

T2 relaxation is another tissue characteristic that can be harnessed to image the articular cartilage. Fibrillar collagen in the articular cartilage immobilizes tissue water protons and promotes dipole–dipole interactions among them. This increases T2 relaxation and, therefore, signal decay. The T2 of normal articular cartilage increases from approximately 30 ms in the deep radial zone to 70 ms in the transitional zone[22] (Fig. 11.30). Above the transitional zone, the superficial tangential zone shows extremely rapid T2 relaxation because of its densely matted collagen fibers. This radial heterogeneity of T2 gives articular cartilage a laminar appearance on all but extremely short-TE images.[23] The pattern of T2 variation can be explained to some extent by the heterogeneous distribution of collagen in this tissue, but is also affected by the orientation of collagen fibrils relative to the static magnetic field (B_0). T2 anisotropy in cartilage manifests as decreased signal decay in regions where the collagen fibrils are oriented at 55° to B_0.[23–26] This so-called 'magic-angle' phenomenon is responsible for areas of mildly elevated signal intensity in the radial zone of appropriately oriented cartilage segments on intermediate-TE images (Fig. 11.31). It is also one explanation for the slower T2 seen in the transitional zone. Collagen fibrils in this zone are slightly sparser than in the radial zone, but more importantly they are also highly disorganized. Accordingly, a significant proportion of the fibrils in the transitional zone will be angled at 55° to B_0, regardless of the orientation of the knee in the magnet. With sufficiently long TE (<80 ms) normal articular cartilage appears diffusely low in signal intensity even in regions normally affected by this magic-angle phenomenon.

Superimposed upon these histological and biochemical causes of laminar appearance in articular cartilage are patterns created by truncation artifact.[27,28] This manifests as one or several thin horizontal bands of low signal intensity midway through the cartilage on short-TE images. Truncation artifacts are less common on high-resolution images, but usually present on fat-suppressed 3D spoiled-GRE images generated with most clinical protocols (Fig. 11.32).

Long-TE images provide high contrast between articular cartilage and adjacent synovial fluid, but poor contrast between cartilage and bone.

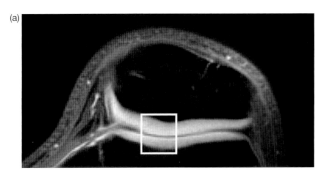

(a)

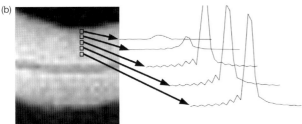

(b)

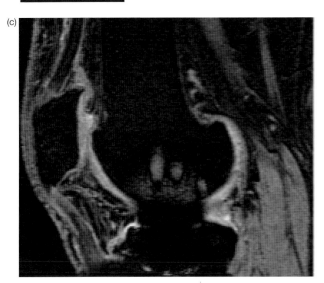

(c)

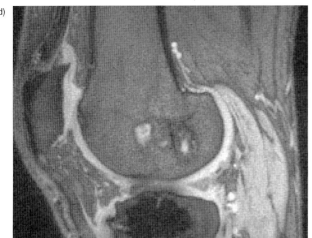

(d)

Fig. 11.29 Projection-reconstruction spiral imaging of cartilage. (a) Water frequency image (TE = 200 ms, 0.2-mm in-plane resolution, 8-min scan time). (b) Spectra from the voxels indicated in (a), showing increasing peak area and decreasing width towards articular surface. This indicates increasing water

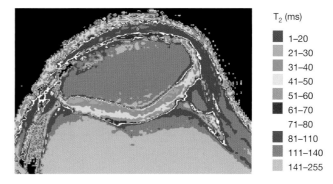

T₂ (ms)

- 1–20
- 21–30
- 31–40
- 41–50
- 51–60
- 61–70
- 71–80
- 81–110
- 111–140
- 141–255

Fig. 11.30 T2 relaxation of normal adult articular cartilage. T2 map generated from multi-slice, multi-echo (11 echoes: TE = 9,18,… 99 ms) spin-echo images acquired at 3 T shows increasing T2 towards the articular surface.

Source: Courtesy of Dardzinski, B.J. University of Cincinnati College of Medicine.

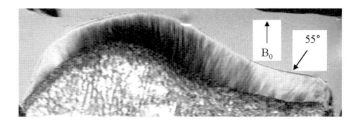

B_0

55°

Fig. 11.31 Magic-angle phenomenon in articular cartilage. High-resolution spin-echo image of the patellar cartilage shows low signal intensity due to T2 relaxation in the radial zone of the central portion of the cartilage, where collagen is aligned with the static magnetic field (B_0.) Increased signal intensity (arrow) indicative of prolonged T2 can be seen in areas where the collagen is oriented at approximately 55° relative to B_0.

Source: Courtesy of Goodwin, D., and Dunn, J., Dartmouth Medical School.

Shorter-TE images improve cartilage bone contrast, but are vulnerable to magic-angle effects. Fast SE (FSE) combines T2 effects with magnetization transfer to decrease signal intensity in articular cartilage.[29,30] Signal loss due to magnetization transfer results from equilibration of longitudinal magnetization between nonsaturated freely mobile protons in water and saturated restricted protons in macromolecules, such as collagen, that have been irradiated off the resonant frequency of free water during multi slice imaging.[8,9,11,29–31] The effect is exaggerated with FSE imaging because of the multiple 180° rf/pulses used with this technique. Accordingly, intermediate-TE (~40 ms) FSE images show relatively low signal intensity in articular cartilage while preserving high signal intensity in synovial fluid and subjacent bone marrow to delineate the articular cartilage with high contrast. Both intermediate- and long-TE FSE images offer relatively good morphological delineation of articular cartilage in less time than is required for high-resolution fat-suppressed 3D-GRE images. The choice of which TE to use depends on the objectives of the imaging, and how they relate to the range of normal and pathological T2 heterogeneity found in articular cartilage.

In addition to delineating cartilage morphology, T2 relaxation can be used to probe the status of the collagen matrix in this tissue. This is because

density and T2-relaxation times. (c) Gradient-recalled echo image from a patient with osteochondral allografts. Metal artifact obscures the articular cartilage. (d) Spectral maximum intensity image (SMIP) of projection-reconstruction spiral imaging of the same slice shows reduced artifacts.

Source: (b) Gold, G., Thedens, D., Pauly, J., Fechner, K., Bergman, G., Beaulieu, C., and Macovski, A. 1998. MR imaging of articular cartilage of the knee: new methods using ultrashort Tes. *AJR* **170**:1223; reproduced with permission. (d) Gold, G., *et al.* 1998. *Topics in MRI* **9**:377–92.

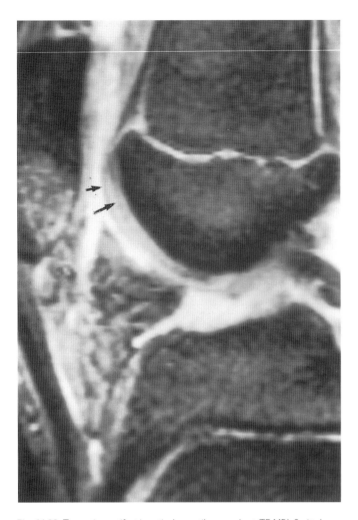

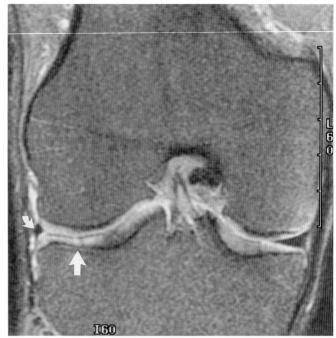

Fig. 11.32 Truncation artifact in articular cartilage on short-TE MRI. Sagittal short-TE gradient-echo image of the knee shows a thin, low signal intensity lamina (*long arrow*) midway between the cartilage surface (*short arrow*) and the subarticular bone. This central lamina is believed to represent an artifact related to the spatial resolution of the image.

Fig. 11.33 Abnormal MRI signal in osteoarthritic cartilage. Coronal, fat-suppressed, T2-weighted fast spin-echo image of the knee of a patient with remote lateral meniscectomy shows focal high signal intensity (*straight arrow*) in the cartilage over the lateral tibial plateau indicative of chondromalacia. Signal intensity in the cartilage elsewhere in the knee is also mildly elevated suggesting an element of diffuse chondromalacia in this patient. Note the small residual lateral meniscus (*curved arrow*).

as the collagen network breaks down, tissue water in articular cartilage becomes more fluid and correspondingly less affected by T2 relaxation (see below). Consistent with this, foci of high signal intensity are often seen within the cartilage of knees of patients with OA on T2-weighted images (Figs 11.33–11.35). These signal abnormalities have been reported to correspond to arthroscopically demonstrable abnormalities.[32,33] However, they have also been observed in cartilage that appeared normal by arthroscopy.[33–35] This raises questions about the sensitivity of arthroscopy for assessing articular cartilage integrity—at least in very early disease.

A careful assessment of the sensitivity and specificity of subjective evaluations of T2 abnormalities in articular cartilage, using images attainable with conventional MRI hardware and software and histological assessment as the gold standard has yet to be reported. Moreover, most studies that have looked at T2 abnormalities in cartilage have provided only cross sectional information. Longitudinal data describing the natural history of this potential marker of cartilage matrix integrity and its association with subsequent cartilage loss and joint failure are scant. In one study,[36] however, five (33 per cent) of 15 meniscal surgery patients followed over three years post surgery developed a total of six T2-lesions in otherwise normal appearing articular cartilage. Two of these lesions progressed to focal cartilage defects during the study (Fig. 11.36), while three persisted and one

regressed. Interestingly, the four lesions that did not progress were in patients who had undergone meniscal repair, while the lesions that progressed were in patients who had meniscal resection. Accordingly, abnormal T2 may identify cartilage at risk of future loss.

Water diffusion in cartilage also contributes to signal loss on T2-weighted MR images. This is because water molecules that have changed positions during a portion of the MRI acquisition can no longer be rephased properly and so do not contribute maximally to the net signal. This loss of phase coherence is proportional to the distance traveled by the diffusing water protons and is, therefore, worse on long-TE images. The presence of proteoglycans, particularly chondroitin sulfate, in normal cartilage inhibits water diffusion and keeps this effect relatively small; although with very strong gradients and specialized phase-sensitive pulse sequences, water diffusion can be demonstrated and even quantified in normal articular cartilage.[13] With cartilage degeneration and proteoglycan loss, however, water diffusion has been shown to increase considerably. Accordingly, diffusion may play a more significant role in cartilage signal modulation in osteoarthritic joints.

Burstein et al.[13] showed that treatment of a bovine cartilage sample with trypsin (for proteoglycan removal) resulted in a 20 per cent increase in the measured rate of diffusion. They also showed that a 35 per cent compression of a bovine cartilage sample corresponded with a 19 per cent reduction in the rate of diffusion. Diffusion-weighted imaging of cartilage has also recently been demonstrated *in vivo*. Gold *et al.*[37] were able to measure diffusion rates for water in cartilage using an in-plane resolution of 1.3×1.7 mm that were consistent with values determined *in vitro* at high resolution by Xia, *et al.*[12] Increases in the available gradient strength on clinical systems will be required to fully evaluate the clinical utility of diffusion-weighted imaging for OA. Using a local extremity gradient coil designed to improve the sensitivity and spatial resolution of imaging the

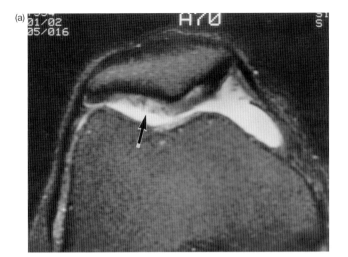

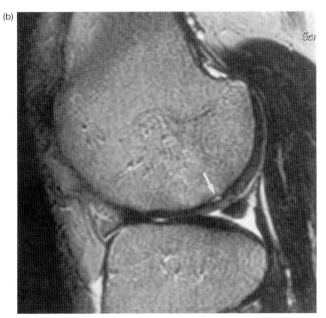

Fig. 11.34 Patterns of abnormal cartilage signal. (a) Transverse fat-suppressed, T2-weighted fast spin-echo image of a different patella shows transmural signal increase and surface fraying in the cartilage over the lateral facet (*arrow*). (b) Sagittal T2-weighted fast spin-echo image of an osteoarthritic knee shows an isolated focus of increased signal intensity (*arrow*) in the deep cartilage of the weight-bearing region of the medial femoral condyle. The overlying cartilage shows slightly increased signal intensity (compare with adjacent cartilage), but otherwise appears intact. This deep signal pattern may reflect early basal delamination of the cartilage resulting from mechanical failure and may not be apparent on arthroscopy.

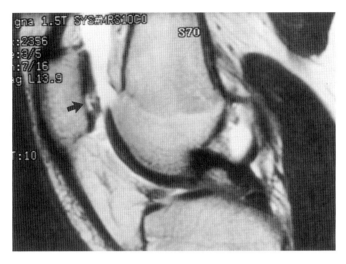

Fig. 11.35 Traumatic delamination of articular cartilage. Sagittal T2-weighted spin-echo image of a knee immediately following transient dislocation of the patella shows focal high signal intensity (*arrow*) in the patellar cartilage extending from the surface to the subchondral cortex. In the deep calcified zone, this signal abnormality takes on a linear configuration and parallels the subchondral cortex. This pattern is consistent with traumatic delamination of the articular cartilage at the tide mark.

knee with MRI, Frank *et al.*[38] were able to achieve a spatial resolution of the $350 \times 350 \mu m$ in-plane with a slice-thickness of 5 mm. Further advances in local gradient coils and improvements in system gradients will greatly aid the study of cartilage diffusion.

In addition to effects on water diffusion, there was loss of proteoglycan from cartilage matrix results in decreased ^{23}Na-ion concentration through the associated decrease in fixed negative charge density. Estimation of *in vivo* ^{23}Na concentration of cartilage by ^{23}Na NMR has been proposed as a means to provide an early marker for proteoglycan loss.[39–43]

Despite a high natural abundance in biological systems, the signal from ^{23}Na is approximately 10 per cent of the ^{1}H signal due to a lower NMR

sensitivity than protons. NMR sensitivity is defined as $\gamma^3 I(I+1)$, where γ is the gyromagnetic ratio and I is the spin.[44] The NMR signal is directly proportional to the sensitivity of the nuclei. ^{23}Na imaging is at an initial disadvantage because of these basic differences in the NMR properties of the two nuclei.

The transverse relaxation time (T2) of ^{23}Na for cartilage exhibits a bi-exponential behavior, with a fast T2 component between 0.7 and 2.3 ms and a slow T2 component between 8 and 12 ms.[45] The *in vivo* longitudinal relaxation time (T1) of ^{23}Na ranges between 14 and 20 ms.[45] Rapid transverse relaxation times make imaging more difficult due to the rapid loss of signal during the echo time. ^{23}Na imaging is aided by a relatively short T1, which allows rapid signal averaging to partially overcome the poor sensitivity and short transverse relaxation times. Spatial resolution is generally the major concern in ^{23}Na imaging due to the reduced signal strength. Clinical feasibility of ^{23}Na imaging was first demonstrated in 1988.[46,47] Granot[46] acquired *in vivo* sodium images from various tissue structures (including knees) by employing a 3D sequence with short repetition (45 ms) and GRE times (6 ms), concluding that sodium imaging of body organs is clinically feasible.

Several groups have shown for *in vitro* studies that enzymatic degradation of proteoglycans leads to changes in ^{23}Na relaxation rates.[39,40,42,48] Reddy *et al.*[45] demonstrated that ^{23}Na MRI can differentiate between regions of proteoglycan depletion from healthy cartilage when imaging *in vitro* bovine patella. In addition, they also obtained ^{23}Na images from a healthy volunteer with a 4 Tesla MRI scanner at an in-plane resolution of 1.25×2.5 mm and a slice thickness of 4 mm. ^{23}Na imaging was also shown to be sensitive to the mechanical deformation of cartilage. Shapiro *et al.*[49] found that during recovery after exercise (50 deep knee bends), a 15 per cent decrease in the thickness of the lateral facet of the subject's patella cartilage resulted in a 20 per cent reduction in ^{23}Na signal intensity. A possible cause for the loss in signal was attributed to the expulsion of saline from the cartilage during compression. An *in vitro* comparison of normal versus PG-depleted cartilage showed that both specimens exhibited a decrease in T1 and T2 during compression.[50]

^{23}Na imaging has been shown to have great potential in characterizing the physiological and mechanical state of cartilage. The major limiting factor to wide clinical usage of these techniques is the available signal

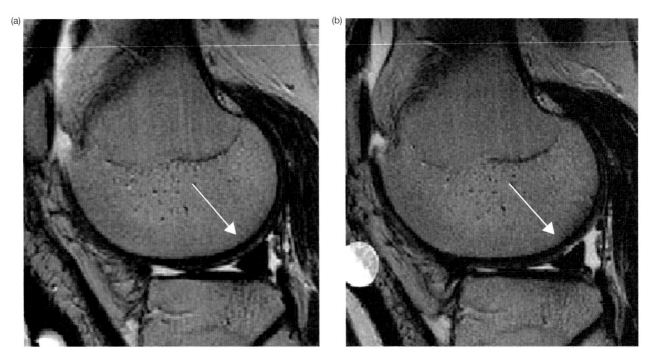

Fig. 11.36 Progression of T2 lesions in articular cartilage. Serial sagittal T2-weighted fast spin-echo images show a focal T2 lesion (*arrow*) in the femoral cartilage adjacent to the posterior horn of the lateral meniscus at baseline. (a) Follow-up imaging nine months later (b) shows a partial-thickness (Grade 2.0) defect at that exact location. *Source*: Peterfy, C.G. 2000. Scratching the surface: articular cartilage disorders in the knee. *MRI Clin NA* **8**(2):409–30.

strength on the standard 1.5 Tesla system. All of the studies described above were performed on systems ranging from 1.9–4 Tesla. Improvements in RF coil sensitivity,[51] stronger gradients for shorter echo times, and greater clinical access to high field systems are prerequisites for ^{23}Na imaging of cartilage to move from the research environment to the clinical setting.

Another interesting marker of cartilage matrix integrity is Gd-DTPA^{2-} uptake.[52–54] Under normal circumstances anionic Gd-DTPA^{2-} introduced into the synovial fluid (either by IV or direct intra-articular injection) is repelled by the negatively charged proteoglycans in normal cartilage. However, in areas of decreased glycosaminoglycan content where the fixed negative charge density of cartilage is reduced, Gd-DTPA^{2-} can diffuse into the cartilage and enhance T1 relaxation. These areas are depicted as conspicuous foci of high signal intensity in the otherwise low signal intensity cartilage on inversion recovery images. Cartilage T1 values correlate almost linearly with proteoglycan content in the range normally found in cartilage. However, quantifying T1 can be time consuming and impractical for most clinical studies. Further work is necessary to establish the optimal method for acquiring this imaging data. Additional studies are also needed to define the relationship between this marker of proteoglycan matrix damage and elevated T2 as a marker of collagen matrix damage (Fig. 11.37). Whether one precedes the other and exactly how predictive each of these are—alone or in combination—for subsequent cartilage loss, the development of other structural features of OA, and ultimately for clinical manifestations of OA, have yet to be established. In addition to the use of Gd-DTPA^{2-}, proteoglycan content of cartilage can be probed with cationic contrast agents, such as manganese,[55,56] or, as discussed above, by imaging sodium instead of hydrogen.[57]

Monitoring changes in articular cartilage with MRI

Morphological markers of articular cartilage include both quantitative measures, such as thickness and volume, and semiquantitative measures, that grade cartilage integrity by a variety of scoring methods. Intermediate-TE and long-TE FSE images are usually adequate for most current clinical applications and in circumstances when lengthier high-resolution techniques are

not justified (Figs 11.32 and 11.38). However, thin-partitioned, fat-suppressed 3D spoiled-GRE images are preferable for delineating cartilage morphology. Advantages of this latter technique include greater contrast, higher resolution, wide availability, ease of use, stable performance, no chemical-shift artifact, and reasonable acquisition time (7–10 min.). Disadvantages include longer acquisition times than those required for FSE imaging and vulnerability to magnetic susceptibility and metallic artifacts. These artifacts range from mild distortions arising near small postoperative metallic fragments, or gas bubbles introduced into the joint by vacuum phenomenon, to severe distortions caused by metallic implants or other orthopedic hardware following tibial plateau fracture or cruciate ligament repair. Failure of fat-suppression due to regional field heterogeneities is generally not a problem because of the cylindrical shape of the knee, but can arise if the knee is bent or if the patella protrudes excessively. Typically, however, failed fat-suppression in the region of the patella usually involves the marrow and superficial soft tissues, but does not reach the articular cartilage.

Several studies have evaluated the diagnostic accuracy of fat-suppressed 3D spoiled-GRE for identifying areas of cartilage loss in the knee. In a comparison of 3D spoiled-GRE with and without fat suppression, T2*-weighted GRE, and conventional T1-weighted, proton-density-weighted and T2-weighted SE sequences in 10 elderly cadaver knees, Recht *et al.*[17] found fat-suppressed, 3D spoiled-GRE (flip angle = 60°, TE = 10 msec, voxel size = 469 × 938 × 1500 μm) to have the greatest sensitivity (96 per cent) and specificity (95 per cent) for demonstrating patellofemoral cartilage lesions visible on pathological sections. Disler *et al.*[20] similarly showed the same technique *in vivo* to have 93 per cent sensitivity and 94 per cent specificity for arthroscopically visible cartilage lesions.

Most scoring methods reported thus far simply count articular cartilage defects and grade them according to the depth of the cartilage loss (e.g. 0, normal thickness; 1, superficial fraying or isolated signal abnormality; 2, partial-thickness loss; 3, full-thickness loss) (Fig. 11.36). Various more complex schemes, which take into account different patterns of cartilage involvement and the distribution of these changes in the knee, have been developed recently.[58] However, the surrogate validity of any of these schemes has not yet been thoroughly established. There is considerable face

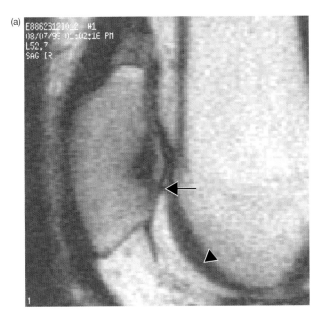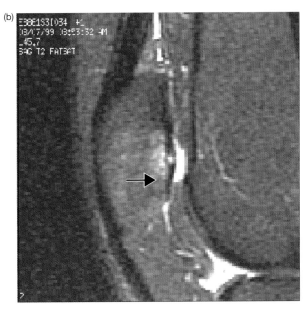

Fig. 11.37 Imaging cartilage matrix damage. (a) Sagittal inversion-recovery image of a knee following IV administration of Gd-DTPA shows a region of high signal intensity (*arrow*) in the patellar cartilage indicative of abnormal uptake of anionic Gd-DTPA^{2-}, and therefore, local proteoglycan depletion. Cartilage in the trochlear groove (*arrowhead*) shows low signal intensity indicative of repulsion of Gd-DTPA^{2-} by negatively charged proteoglycans. (b) Fat-suppressed, T2-weighted image of the same knee prior to Gd-DTPA^{2-} injection shows a smaller focus of increased signal intensity (*arrow*) in the same location indicative of local collagen matrix loss. This is associated with subarticular marrow edema in the patella.

Source: Courtesy of Synarc, Inc., with permission.

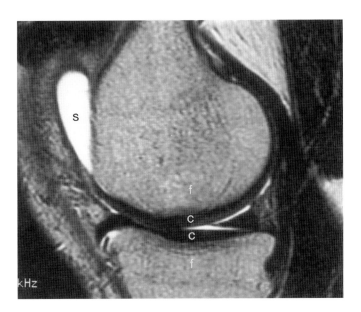

Fig. 11.38 Fast spin echo imaging of cartilage. Sagittal T2-weighted fast spin-echo image of the knee shows high contrast between the low signal intensity articular cartilage (c) and adjacent high signal intensity synovial fluid (s) and intermediate signal intensity subchondral marrow fat (f).

validity to the link between cartilage loss and clinical outcomes in OA, but the amount of cartilage loss that is clinically relevant has not yet been determined. The issue is complicated by the multi-factorial nature of joint failure and the oversimplification that mono-structural models suffer. Nevertheless, cartilage loss is currently the most broadly accepted metric of structural progression in OA. Unresolved issues of surrogate validity not withstanding, semiquantitative scoring of cartilage loss can be relatively

precise and resolve progression in one year. In a recent study of 29 patients with OA in whom the articular cartilage was scored in 15 locations in the knee using a seven-point scale, the intra-class correlation coefficient between two specially trained radiologists was 0.99.[58] A subsequent examination of 30 subjects from an ongoing cohort study of 3075 elderly men and women imaged with a 15-min MRI protocol (T2-weighted FSE) found similar inter-reader precision for femorotibial cartilage using the same scoring method (ICC = 0.91).[59]

Aside from semiquantitative scoring, a number of quantitative markers of cartilage morphology have been developed, including cartilage volume. This measurement can be derived from segmented images of the articular cartilage on fat-suppressed 3D spoiled-GRE images using any one of a variety of image analysis packages currently available (Fig. 11.39). A number of studies have validated the technical accuracy of these methods and established the precision error to range from 2–4 per cent coefficient of variation (SD/mean volume)[11,60,61] (Fig. 11.40). In a recent investigation, 16 elderly women with OA of the knee were imaged with MRI at yearly intervals for two years. The mean annual rate of cartilage loss was determined to be (-6.7^{+-} 5.2 per cent for the femur, -6.33^{+-} 4.3 per cent for the tibia and -3.4^{+-} 2.9 per cent for the patella) based on linear regression of the three time-points.[62]

Limitations of cartilage volume quantification include assumptions used to model cartilage volume change over time. For practical reasons, a linear model is usually the only feasible assumption for most clinical trials and epidemiological studies involving four or fewer time points. More complicated models (quadratic, etc.) may turn out to be more accurate, but until careful natural history studies have refined these models, curve-fitting challenges limit their use in most studies. Regardless, measurement precision for cartilage volume change combines errors related both to the measurement technique and the cartilage loss model used.

Other limitations of cartilage volume as a marker of disease severity and structural progression include insensitivity to small focal defects. These are more easily identified by semiquantitative scoring, or by regional cartilage volume mapping.[63] Measurement precision and therefore statistical power

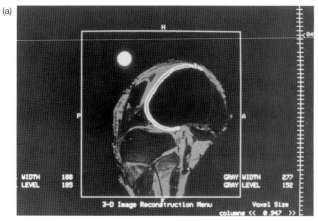

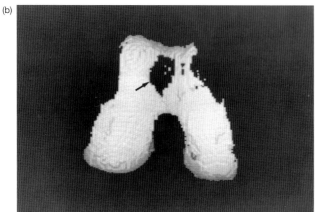

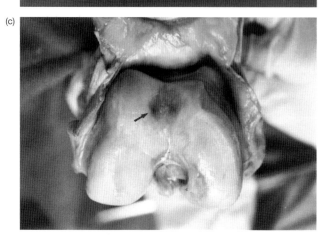

Fig. 11.39 Segmentation and 3D rendering of articular cartilage. (a) One slice of a T1-weighted, fat-suppressed 3D gradient-echo acquisition of the knee is shown with disarticulation boundaries traced around the articular cartilage of the femur during segmentation and 3D reconstruction of this cartilage. (b) 3D surface rendering (viewed from an anterior vantage point) of this femoral cartilage delineates a large focal defect in the trochlear groove (*arrow*). (c) Gross anatomical findings correlate well with the surface rendered 3D image.

Source: Peterfy, C., van Dijke, C.F., Janzen, D.L., Glüer, C., Namba, R., Majumdar, S., Lang, P., and Genant, H.K.1994. Quantification of articular cartilage in the knee with pulsed saturation transfer and fat-suppressed MR imaging. *Radiology* **192**:485–91; with permission.

decreases as the subdivisions get smaller. Accordingly, the trade off between sensitivity and measurement precision must be carefully balanced. One highly refined method of depicting regional variations in cartilage quantity is thickness-mapping[64,65] (Fig. 11.41). As intuitive as cartilage thickness

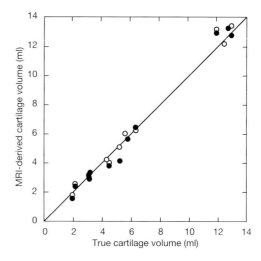

Fig. 11.40 Technical accuracy of volumetric quantification of cartilage with MRI. The graph depicts cartilage volumes determined from fat-suppressed, T1-weighted 3D gradient-echo images (*open circles*) and magnetization transfer subtraction images (*closed circles*) plotted against volumes measured directly by water displacement. A total of 12 cartilage plates (six patellar, three tibial, three femoral) from six knees were included. Line represents theoretical 100 per cent accuracy.

Source: Modified from Peterfy, C., van Dijke, C.F., Janzen, D.L., Glüer, C., Namba, R., Majumdar, S., Lang, P., and Genant H.K. 1994. Quantification of articular cartilage in the knee with pulsed saturation transfer and fat-suppressed MR imaging. *Radiology* **192**:485–91; with permission.

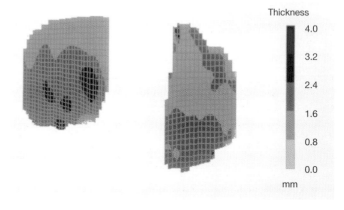

Fig. 11.41 Mapping cartilage thickness with MRI. Geometric model of the tibial cartilages was generated from contour curves using parametric bicubic B-spline representations of manually segmented MR images. Regional cartilage thicknesses (perpendicular to the cartilage–bone interface) are depicted at intervals of 0.8 mm and shown in shades of orange.

may seem, however, questions remain as to whether the minimum, maximum, or average thickness is the most relevant, how to deal with multiple lesions, and to what extent the location of a lesion (e.g., weight bearing, non weight-bearing) is important.

Perhaps the greatest limitation of all markers of cartilage morphology, however, is their fundamentally irreversible nature and relatively slow responsiveness. Regardless of how precisely change in cartilage morphology can be measured, its rate of change cannot be driven any faster than the disease process itself. For a solution to this problem, one must look upstream to earlier stages in the disease process of cartilage degeneration. Accordingly, there has been a great deal of interest in developing MRI markers of cartilage composition.

MRI in markers of cartilage composition relate principally to the collagen matrix or constituent proteoglycans. The most promising markers of collagen matrix integrity include T2 relaxation and magnetization transfer coefficient. Markers of proteoglycan integrity include water diffusion, Gd-DTPA^{2-} uptake, and ^{23}Na concentration.

As discussed above, disruption of the fibrillar organization of collagen or actual decrease in collagen content reduces T2 relaxation and increases signal intensity on T2-weighted images. Areas of elevated signal in otherwise low signal-intensity cartilage on long-TE MR images, therefore, represent foci of chondromalacia. While several studies have verified this relationship between T2 relaxation and fibrillar collagen in cartilage, none have meticulously established the diagnostic accuracy (e.g. area under ROC curve, with histological verification) of subjective readings using MRI acquisition techniques that are applicable to multi-center studies or generalizable to clinical use. More importantly, the validity of cartilage T2 as a surrogate marker of matrix integrity depends on its predictive power for subsequent cartilage loss. While there is considerable face validity to this model and some anecdotal longitudinal evidence to support it, further prospective validation is needed. If this hypothesis is indeed true, then abnormal cartilage T2 may identify cartilage at risk of future loss and thereby identify patients in need of aggressive therapy, hopefully before the point of no return. In addition to subjective evaluations of focal signal abnormalities in articular cartilage, regional changes in T2 relaxation can be quantified and monitored over time with multi-echo SE imaging.[15,22] Limitations of this approach include technical trade offs between image acquisition time and the number of echoes, spatial resolution and the attainable S/N ratio. Further surrogate validation and performance characterization of cartilage T2 are clearly needed.

Significantly less work has been done with magnetization transfer as a marker of collagen integrity in articular cartilage. Theoretically, this marker could be used almost exactly the same way that cartilage T2 is used. However, even less is known about its diagnostic accuracy, responsiveness to disease and therapy, dynamic range, and measurement precision. Accordingly, further characterization is needed.

As mentioned above, methods for evaluating the integrity of the proteoglycan matrix by probing regional variations in fixed negative charged density in articular cartilage have recently been developed. The histological and biochemical validity of this approach has been well demonstrated by a number of groups.[52–54] Using cartilage-nulling inversion recovery sequences at high spatial resolutions and high field strength, Bashir et al.[52] demonstrated high histological correlation of the distribution of anionic Gd-DTPA^{2-} with perichondrocytic glycosaminoglycan (GAG) depletion following incubation of cartilage explants with IL-1 (interleukin-1). Subsequent studies have shown a linear correlation between T1 associated with Gd-DTPA^{2-} and cartilage GAG ranging from 10–70 mg/ml as measured directly biochemically.[66] In a recent study by Trattnig et al.[54] areas of abnormal Gd-DTPA^{2-} uptake in cartilage specimens harvested at total knee replacement surgery corresponded to sites of collagen loss based on azan staining at histology. Unfortunately, this study did not report the correlation with areas of abnormal T2, if any were present. The study also reported marked inter-individual variation in the pattern of Gd-DTPA^{2-} uptake in eight normal volunteers that were examined, as well as marked differences in the diffusion times observed for cartilages of different thickness. Accordingly, while Gd-DTPA^{2-} uptake appears to be a valid method for quantifying GAG concentration and its distribution in articular cartilage, with good dynamic range properties relative to GAG concentration, the relationship of this marker to cartilage T2 has yet to be examined. Does abnormal Gd-DTPA^{2-} uptake precede abnormal T2 temporally? What is the relative performance of these two markers in terms of sensitivity, specificity, responsiveness to disease and therapy, dynamic range, predictive power for subsequent cartilage loss, other structural changes associated with OA, and clinical outcomes of OA? Finally, what is the optimal *in vivo* acquisition technique for cartilage Gd-DTPA^{2-} uptake as a marker? In this regard, cartilage T2 may be a simpler marker to use.

Imaging other articular components in OA

In addition to evaluating the articular cartilage, MRI is uniquely capable of imaging all of the other structures that make up the joint, including the synovium and joint fluid, articular bones, intra-articular menisci, labra and discs, cruciate ligaments, collateral and other capsular ligaments, and peri-articular tendons and muscles. Moreover, using the same voxel-counting technique employed for quantifying articular cartilage in 3D reconstructed images,[11,67] it is possible to determine the volume of each of these components within the same joint (Fig. 11.42).

Some degree of synovial thickening can be found in a majority of osteoarthritic joints.[68] Whether this synovitis contributes directly to articular cartilage loss in OA, or simply arises in reaction to the breakdown of cartilage by other causes remains a controversy.[69] However, synovitis may be important to the symptoms and disability of OA, and may pose different treatment requirements than those directed only towards 'chondroprotection'. MRI is capable of imaging thickened or inflamed synovium, but usually this requires the use of special techniques, such as magnetization-transfer subtraction,[9] fat-suppressed, T1-weighted imaging,[9] or intravenous injection of Gd-containing contrast material[9,70–72] (Fig. 11.43). By monitoring the rate of synovial enhancement with Gd-containing contrast over time using rapid, sequential MRI, it is, furthermore, possible to grade the severity of the synovitis in these patients. The majority of work in this area has, however, focused on rheumatoid arthritis.

Osseous changes in OA are superbly depicted by MRI. Both cortical and trabecular bone can be visualized with MRI, and because of the tomographic nature of this modality, MRI is better at delineating structures,

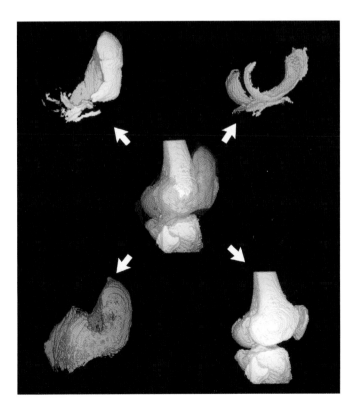

Fig. 11.42 'Exploded' 3D rendering of the knee imaged with MRI showing individual components (clockwise from the top left: synovial fluid, cartilage, bone marrow, thickened synovium) surrounding a composite image viewed from a posterolateral vantage point.

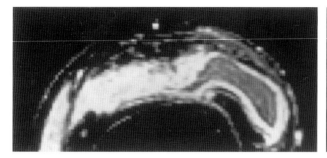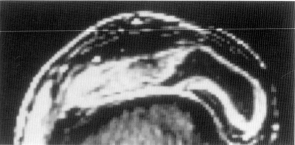

Fig. 11.43 Synovial imaging with MRI. Transverse images of the suprapatellar recess of the knee of a patient with rheumatoid arthritis using magnetization-transfer subtraction (*left panel*) and fat-suppressed T1-weighted gradient-echo (*right panel*) both delineate the thickened synovial tissue with high contrast.

Source: Peterfy, C., Majumdar, S., Lang, P., van Dijke, C.F., Sack, K., and Genant, H.K. 1994. MR imaging of the arthritic knee: improved discrimination of cartilage, synovium and effusion with pulsed saturation transfer and fat-suppressed, T1-weighted sequences. *Radiology* **191**:413–19.

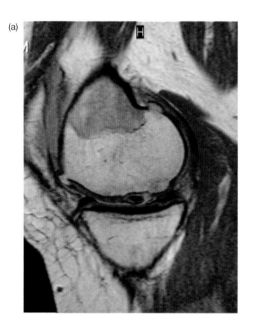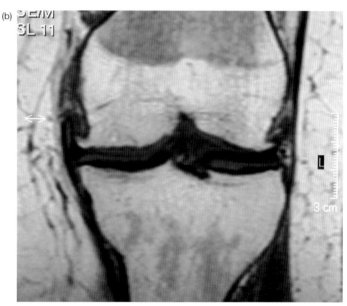

Fig. 11.44 Delineating osteophytes with MRI. Sagittal (a) and coronal (b) images of a knee of a patient with OA clearly delineate marginal and central osteophytes.

Source: Courtesy of Synarc, Inc., with permission.

such as osteophytes (Fig. 11.44) and subchondral cysts, that are often obscured by overlying structures on conventional radiographs. Using high-resolution MRI techniques[73,74] it may be possible to monitor trabecular changes in the subchondral bone (Fig. 11.45), in order to determine their importance in the development and progression of OA.

In addition to delineating the calcified components of a bone, MRI is uniquely capable of imaging the marrow. Subchondral marrow edema is occasionally associated with not only acute trauma but also progressive OA[75,76] (Fig. 11.46). Focal bone marrow edema in OA may be due to subchondral injuries caused by shifting articular contact points at sites of bio-mechanically failing cartilage, or pulsion of synovial fluid into uncovered subchondral bone. However, osteonecrosis, infection and infiltrating neoplasms could theoretically produce a similar MRI appearance. Conventional radiographs are usually unremarkable in areas of bone marrow edema; although, bone scintigraphy may show increased uptake in these areas.

The menisci in the knee (Fig. 11.47) and glenoid labrum in the shoulder are important to the stability and functional integrity of these joints. Equally important are the cruciate (Fig. 11.48) and collateral ligaments (Fig. 11.46) and the glenohumeral ligaments. The utility of MRI for evaluating these articular structures is already well established.[77]

Trade offs in imaging specific joints

The knee

Each joint poses different challenges to proper imaging with MRI. Most work thus far has focused on the knee, not only because the knee is frequently affected by OA and because loss of knee function can be severely disabling, but also because the knee is a comparatively easy joint to image. Reasons for this include the large size of this joint, which lowers demands on spatial resolution, and the relatively cylindrical shape of the knee, which minimizes perturbation of the static magnetic field—field homogeneity is critical to the performance of frequency-selective fat suppression or water excitation techniques, and important in quantitative studies based on signal intensity measurements. The cylindrical shape also allows the use of circumferential imaging coils, which show greater homogeneity than surface coils.[14] Additionally, since the knee is a relatively incongruent joint, contact areas between the hyaline cartilage plates in all but the most severely degenerated joints are small. Articular surfaces are therefore easy to separate from each other on MR images. Delineating the articular surfaces is facilitated by the relative abundance of synovial fluid in the knee, which provides high contrast at this interface on T2-weighted images and fat-suppressed,

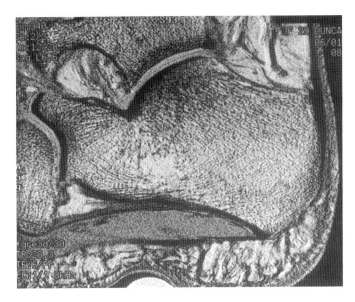

Fig. 11.45 High-resolution MRI of cortical and trabecular bone. Sagittal high-resolution gradient-echo image of the calcaneus delineates both cortical and trabecular bone with high detail.

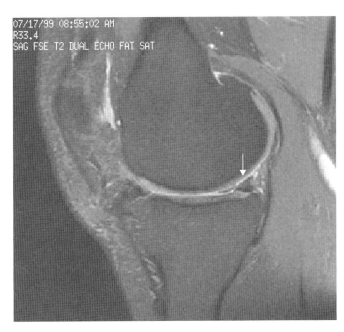

Fig. 11.47 MRI of the meniscus. Sagittal, fat-suppressed proton-density image shows a minimally displaced tear of the posterior horn of the medial meniscus. This is associated with partial-thickness thinning (*arrow*) of the femoral articular cartilage immediately adjacent to the torn meniscus.

Source: Courtesy Synarc, Inc., with permission.

These advantages, however, are offset to some extent by a number of disadvantages. Firstly, the knee is a highly complex joint composed of three articular compartments, one of which involves a sesamoid bone—the patella. The hyaline cartilage covering each of the articular surfaces accordingly shows somewhat different biomechanical properties and vulnerabilities. The joint contains two intra-articular ligaments, an intra-articular tendon, two menisci, intracapsular-extrasynovial fat pads, complex capsular ligaments (particularly laterally), and variable ontological remnants (plicas). Joint failure in the knee involves an equally complex interplay among these numerous articular constituents. Because the knee is a large joint, full coverage of the synovial cavity, including the suprapatellar recess, requires a relatively large field of view (12–18 cm). Since loose bodies tend to collect in the eddy pools within synovial recesses, incomplete coverage can result in important oversights. This can be particularly problematic in cases with large popliteal cysts dissecting down the calf. Larger fields of view, however, necessitate proportionately larger imaging matrices in order to maintain spatial resolution, and this increases the imaging time (imaging time = TR × number of phase encodings × number of acquisitions averaged).

The hip

Next to the knee, the hip is the most important joint affected by OA from a disability standpoint. Despite this, however, the hip has received only scant attention in terms of MRI evaluation for OA. This is at least in part because the hip poses significant challenges to proper imaging with MRI. It is a highly congruent joint, which makes separating the articular surfaces difficult. Delineation of the surfaces is further hampered by the relative lack of joint fluid in the tight synovial cavity of the hip. Moreover, the articular surfaces are highly curved, giving rise to severe partial-volume effects in all planes unless extremely high spatial resolution is employed. Accordingly, cartilage thickness measurements in the hip using MRI have been somewhat disappointing.[78] Achieving high spatial resolution in the hip is, itself, not an entirely straightforward matter. Since the hip is a relatively

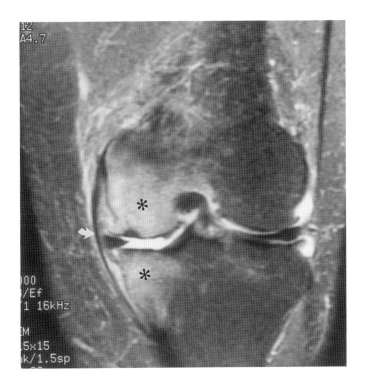

Fig. 11.46 Subchondral bone edema in OA. Coronal fat-suppressed T2-weighted fast spin-echo image of an osteoarthritic knee shows areas of full-thickness cartilage loss in the medial femorotibial joint associated with local bone marrow edema (*asterisks*). The intact medial collateral ligament is also delineated on this image (*arrow*).

T1-weighted images. Since the articular surfaces are only gently curved, partial-volume averaging is not a major problem. Because of these forgiving imaging features and the availability of surgical and arthroscopic therapies for many internal derangements of the knee, MRI experience with the knee is greater than for any other joint in the body.

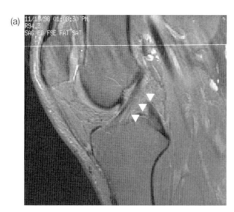
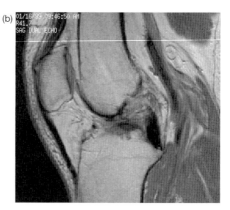

Fig. 11.48 MRI of the anterior cruciate ligament. (a) Sagittal, fat-suppressed proton-density weighted image shows an intact anterior cruciate ligament (*arrowheads*). (b) Similar image of a different knee shows a torn anterior cruciate ligament.

Source: Courtesy of Synarc, Inc., with permission.

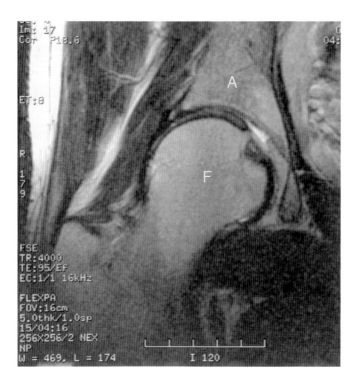

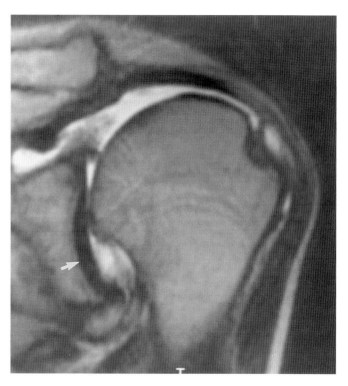

Fig. 11.49 MRI of the hip using phased array technique. Sagittal T2-weighted fast spin-echo image of a normal hip acquired using two imaging coils arranged in a flexible phased array shows high S/N despite the relatively high-resolution employed. The articular cartilage is well delineated with this technique. F, femoral head; A, superior acetabulum.

Fig. 11.50 MRI of OA shoulder. Oblique coronal (in plane with the long axis of the supraspinatus tendon), T2-weighted fast spin-echo image of an osteoarthritic shoulder with a chronically torn and retracted rotator cuff, shows superior subluxation of the humerus, and denuding of the cartilage over the humeral head. Relatively abundant articular cartilage is still present over the glenoid surface (*arrow*).

deep joint, signal drop off with small (< 5 cm) surface coils is usually prohibitive. Larger surface coils could be employed, but these offer lower resolution and do not provide homogeneous signal for quantitative measurements. The anatomy of the hip prevents the use of small circumferential coils, which could provide homogeneous images with high resolution. A large circumferential coil, such as the body coil, could be used in this way, but does not provide sufficient S/N to support the high spatial resolution needed. Multiple coils configured in a phased array about the hip offer high S/N along with high spatial resolution (Fig. 11.49) and are probably the best alternative for this purpose.

The shoulder

Like the hip, the shoulder is a congruent, ball-in-socket joint with closely opposing articular surfaces[79] (Fig. 11.50). Because of the angular shape of the shoulder, magnetic field heterogeneities tend to develop laterally near the greater tuberosity.[80] While the field appears relatively undisturbed at the glenohumeral joint, lateral heterogeneities can limit the performance of fat suppression and complicate evaluation of the rotator cuff. Accurate assessment of the tendons of the rotator cuff is important since the shoulder relies heavily on these structures for stability, and rotator cuff tear is an important risk factor for the development of OA in this joint.[81] Shoulder stability is also

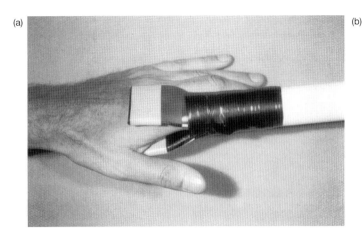
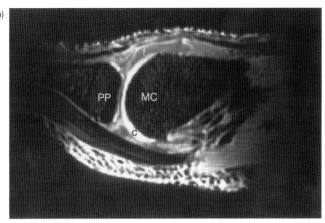

Fig. 11.51 MRI of the metacarpophalangeal joints. (a) Specialized imaging coil for finger joints is composed of two one-inch coils positioned on either side of the joint and housed in a plastic pipe. (b) Sagittal T1-weighted, fat-suppressed 3D gradient-echo image of a metacarpophalangeal joint acquired using the coil shown in (a) and conventional clinical MRI hardware and software shows high contrast between articular cartilage (c) and adjacent effusion (f) and subchondral bone. (PP, proximal phalanx; MC, metacarpal).

Source: Peterfy, C.G., van Dijke, C.F., Lu, Y, Nguyen, A., Connick, T., Kneeland, B., Tirman, P.F.J., Lang, P., Dent, S., and Genant, H.K. 1995. Quantification of articular cartilage in the metacarpophalangeal joints of the hand: accuracy and precision of 3D MR imaging. *AJR* **165**:371–5; with permission.

dependent on the integrity of the glenoid labrum and the glenohumeral ligaments. However, reliable imaging of these labrocapsular structures can be extremely difficult, particularly in the absence of joint distention by significant synovial effusion. This can be improved by intra-articular injection of saline[82] or Gd-containing MRI contrast material (MR arthrography).[83,84]

Hand and finger joints

The joint most commonly affected by OA is the distal interphalangeal joint of the finger. The major challenge to imaging this small joint is the demand on spatial resolution. For this reason, small-bore, high-field magnets, and small circumferential imaging coils are usually necessary.[10] The metacarpophalangeal joints are less frequently affected by OA, but are larger joints, and have been successfully imaged using conventional clinical MRI systems[67] (Fig. 11.51).

Conclusion

MRI is clearly a tool of unprecedented capabilities for evaluating joint disease and its potential treatments. MRI's unparalleled tissue contrast allow it to directly examine all components of a joint simultaneously and thus evaluate the joint as a whole organ and OA as a disorder of organ failure, in which dysfunction may result from anyone of a number of different causes. Especially intriguing is the unique potential of this technology for identifying very early changes associated with cartilage degeneration, and its ability to quantify subtle morphological and compositional variations in different articular tissues over time. Employing these techniques, MRI may provide more objective measures of disease progression and treatment response than are currently attainable by other methods. This will facilitate both the assessment of new therapies for OA and investigations of the pathophysiology in this disorder. Investigators dealing with OA and other articular disorders should become more sophisticated in MRI so that they can take full advantage of its unique capabilities and take a more active hand in directing its development.

Key points

The advantages of MRI for imaging arthritis include:

1. Multiplanar 2D and 3D image data
2. Unparalleled tissue contrast

    a. whole organ evaluation of joint

    b. potential for compositional analysis of tissues

3. Digital image format
4. Noninvasive/high patient tolerance
5. Widely available

References

(An asterisk denotes recommended reading.)

1. *Peterfy, C.G., Roberts, T., and Genant, H.K. (1996). Dedicated extremity MRI: an emerging technology. In J.B. Kneeland (ed.). *Radiol Clin NA*. Vol. 35. Philadelphia, PA: W.B. Saunders, pp. 1–20.
   This article reviews the pros and cons of small MRI systems for imaging the knee.
2. Abragam, A. (1983). *The Principles of Nuclear Magnetism*. London: Oxford University Press.
3. Budinger, T. and Lauterbur, P. (1984). Nuclear magnetic resonance technology for medical studies. *Science* **226**:288–98.
4. Haacke, E. and Tkach, J. (1990). Fast MR imaging: techniques and clinical applications. *Am J Roentgenol* **155**:951–64.
5. Pykett, I. (1982). NMR imaging in medicine. *Sci Am* **246**:78–88.
6. Young, S. (1988). *Magnetic Resonance Imaging: Basic Principles*. New York: Raven Press.
7. König, S. and Brown, R. (1984). Determinants of proton relaxation in tissue. *Magn Reson Imag* **1**:437–49.
8. Woolf, S.D., Chesnick, S., Frank, J.A., Lim, K.O., and Balaban, R.S. (1991). Magnetization transfer contrast: MR imaging of the knee. *Radiology* **179**:623–8.
9. Peterfy, C.G., Majumdar, S., Lang, P., van Dijke, C.F., Sack, K., and Genant, H. (1994). MR imaging of the arthritic knee: improved discrimination of cartilage, synovium and effusion with pulsed saturation transfer and fat-suppressed T1-weighted sequences. *Radiology* **191**:413–19.
10. Hall, L.D. and Tyler, J.A. (1995). Can quantitative magnetic resonance imaging detect and monitor the progression of early osteoarthritis? In K.E. Kuetner and V.M. Goldberg (eds), *Osteoarthritic Disorders*. Rosemont, IL: American Acadamy of Orthopaedic Surgeons, pp. 67–84.
11. *Peterfy, C.G., van Dijke, C.F., Janzen, D.L., *et al.* (1994). Quantification of articular cartilage in the knee by pulsed saturation transfer and fat-suppressed MRI: optimization and validation. *Radiology* **192**:485–91.

This article describes the basic technique of cartilage volume quantification using MRI.

12. Xia, Y., Farquhar, T., Burton-Wuster, N., Ray, E., and Jelinski, L.W. (1994). Diffusion and relaxation mapping of cartilage-bone plugs and excised disks using microscopic magnetic resonance imaging. *Magn Reson Med* **31**:273–82.

13. Burstein, D., Gray, M.L., Hartman, A.L., Gipe, R., and Foy, B.D. (1993). Diffusion of small solutes in cartilage as measured by nuclear magnetic resonance (NMR) spectroscopy and imaging. *J Orthop Res* **11**:465–78.

14. Kneeland, J.B. and Hyde, J.S. (1989). High-resolution MR imaging with local coils. *Radiology* **171**:1–7.

15. Mosher, T., Dardzinski, B., and Smith, M. (2000). Human articular cartilage: influence of aging and early symptomatic degeneration on the spatial variation of T2—preliminary findings at 3 T. *Radiology* **241**:259–66.

16. Chandnani, V.P., Ho, C., Chu, P., Trudell, P., and Resnick, D. (1991). Knee hyaline cartilage evaluated with MR imaging: a cadaveric study involving multiple imaging sequences and intraarticular injection of gadolinium and saline solution. *Radiology* **178**:557–61.

17. Recht, M.P., Kramer, J., Marcelis, S., *et al.* (1993). Abnormalities of articular cartilage in the knee: analysis of available MR techniques. *Radiology* **187**:473–8.

18. Recht, M.P., Pirraino, D.W., Paletta, G.A., Schils, J.P., and Belhobek, G.H. (1996). Accuracy of fat-suppressed three-dimensional spoiled gradient-echo FLASH MR imaging in the detection of patellofemoral articular cartilage abnormalities. *Radiology* **198**:209–12.

19. Disler, D.G., McCauley, T.R., Kelman, C.G., *et al.* (1996). Fat-suppressed three-dimensional spoiled gradient-echo MR imaging of hyaline cartilage defects in the knee: comparison with standard MR imaging and arthroscopy. *Am J Roentgenol* **167**:127–32.

20. Disler, D.G., McCauley, T.R., Wirth, C.R., and Fuchs, M.C. (1995). Detection of knee hyaline articular cartilage defects using fat-suppressed three-dimensional spoiled gradient-echo MR imaging: comparison with standard MR imaging and correlation with arthroscopy. *Am J Roentgenol* **165**:377–82.

21. Gold, G., Thedens, D., Pauly, J., *et al.* (1998). MR imaging of articular cartilage of the knee: new methods using ultrashort TEs. *Am J Roentgenol* **170**:1223–6.

22. *Dardizinski, B., Mosher, T., Li, S., Van Slyke, M., and Smith, M. (1997). Spatial variation of T2 in human articular cartilage. *Radiology* **205**:546–50.

This article discusses the basic technique of T2 mapping in articular cartilage with high-field strength MRI.

23. Tim, D.J., Suh, J.-S., Jeong, E.-K., Shin, K.-H., and Yang, W.I. (1999). Correlation of laminated MR appearance of articular cartilage with histology, ascertained by artifical landmarks on the cartilage. *J Magn Reson Imaging* **10**:57–64.

24. Xia, Y., Farquhar, T., Burton-Wurster, N., and Lust, G. (1997). Origin of cartilage laminae in MRI. *JMRI* **7**:887–94.

25. Rubenstein, J.D., Kim, J.K., Morava-Protzner, I., Stanchev, P.L., and Henkelamn, R.M. (1993). Effects of collagen Orientation on MR imaging characteristics of bovine cartilage. *Radiology* **188**:219–26.

26. Erickson, S.J., Prost, R.W., and Timins, M.E. (1993). The 'magic angle' effect: background physics and clinical relevance. *Radiology* **188**:23–5.

27. Erickson, S.J., Waldschmidt, J.G., Caervionke, L.F., and Prost, R.W. (1996). Hyaline cartilage: truncation artifact as a cause of trilaminar appearance with fat suppressed three dimensional spoiled gradient recalled sequences. *Radiology* **201**:260–4.

28. Frank, L.R., Brossman, J., Bucton, R.B., and Resnick, D. (1997). MR imaging truncation artifacts can create a false laminar appearance in cartilage. *Am J Roentgenol* **168**:547–54.

29. Yao, L., Gentili, A., and Thomas, A. (1996). Incidental magnetization transfer contrast in fast spin-echo imaging of cartilage. *JMRI* **6**:180–4.

30. Miyazaki, M., Takai, H., Kojima, F., and Kassai, Y. (1994). *Control of Magnetization Transfer Effects in Fast SE Imaging.* Chicago, IL: Radiological Society of North America, p. 306.

31. Santyr, G.E. (1993). Magnetization transfer effects in multislice MR imaging. *Magn Reson Imaging* **11**:521–2.

32. Broderick, L.S., Turner, D.A., Renfrew, D.L., Schnitzer, T.J., Huff, J.P., and Harris, C. (1994). Severity of articular cartilage abnormality in patients with osteoarthritis: evaluation with fast spin-echo MR vs arthroscopy. *Am J Roentgenol* **162**:99–103.

33. Rose, P.M., Demlow, T.A., Szumowski, J., and Quinn, S.F. (1994). Chondromalacia patellae: fat-suppressed MR imaging. *Radiology* **193**:437–40.

34. Yulish, B.S., Montanez, J., Goodfellow, D.B., Bryan, P.J., Mulopulos, G.P., and Modic, M.T. (1987). Chondromalacia patellae: assessment with MR imaging. *Radiology* **164**:763–6.

35. Quinn, S.F., Rose, P.M., Brown, T.R., and Demlow, T.A. (1994). MR imaging of the patellofemoral compartment. *MRI Clin NA* **2**:425–39.

36. Zaim, S., Lynch, J.A., Li, J., Genant, H.K., and Peterfy, C.G. (2001). *MRI of Early Cartilage Degeneration Following Meniscal Surgery: A Three-Year Longitudinal Study.* Glasgow, Scotland: International Society for Magnetic Resonance in Medicine, 2001.

37. Gold, G.E., Butts, K., Fechner, K.P., *et al.* (1998). *In Vivo Diffusion-Weighted Imaging of Cartilage.* 6th Annual Meeting of the International Society of Magnetic Resonance in Medicine, Sydney, Australia, p. 1066.

38. Frank, L.R., Wong, E.C., Luh, W., Ahn, J.M., and Resnick, D. (1999). Articular cartilage in the knee: mapping of the physiologic parameters at MR imaging with a local gradient coil—preliminary results. *Radiology* **210**:241–6.

39. Foy, B.D., Gray, M.L., and Burstein, D. (1989). NMR parameters of interstitial sodium in cartilage (abstract). Amsterdam: Society of Magnetic Resonance in Medicine, p. 1108.

40. Jelicks, L.A., Paul, P.K., O'Byrne, E.M., and Gupta, R.K. (1993). Hydrogen-1, sodium-23, and carbon-13 MR spectroscopy of cartilage degradation *in vitro. J Magn Reson Imag* **3**:565–8.

41. Paul, P.K., O'Byrne, E.M., Gupta, R.K., and Jelicks, L.A. (1991). Detection of cartilage degradation with sodium NMR (letter). *Br J Rheumatol* **30**:318.

42. Bashir, A., Gray, M., and Burnstein, D. (1995). Sodium T1 and T2 in control and defraded cartilage: implications for determination of tissue proteoglycan content. In *Proceedings of the 14th annual meeting of the Society of Magnetic Resonance in Medicine*, 1995. Nice: Society of Magnetic Resonance in Medicine, p. 1896.

43. Insko, E., Reddy, R., Kaufman, J., Kneeland, J., and Leigh, J. (1996). Sodium spectroscopic evaluation of early articular cartilage degradation. In *Proceedings of the 4th annual International Society of Magnetic Resonance in Medicine.* New York: International Society of Magnetic Resonance in Medicine, p. 1098.

44. Callaghan, P. (1991). *Principles of Nuclear Magnetic Resonance Microscopy.* New York, NY: Oxford University Press.

45. Reddy, R., Insko, E.K., Noyszewski, E.A., Dandora, R., Kneeland, J.B., and Leigh, J.S. (1998). Sodium MRI of human articular cartilage *in vivo. Magn Reson Med* **39**:697–701.

46. Granot, J. (1988). Sodium imaging of human body organs and extremities *in vivo. Radiology* **167**:547–50.

47. Ra, J.B., Hilal, S.K., Oh, C.H., and Mun, I.K. (1988). *In vivo* magnetic resonance imaging of sodium in the human body. *Magn Reson Med* **7**:11–22.

48. *Insko, E.K., Kaufman, J.H., Leigh, J.S., and Reddy, R. (1999). Sodium NMR evaluation of articular cartilage degradation. *Magn Reson Med* **41**:30–4.

This article describes an application of sodium imaging of articular cartilage in the knee.

49. Shapiro, E., Saha, P., Kaufman, J., *et al.* (1999). *In vivo* evaluation of human cartilage compression and recovery using 1H and 23Na MRI. In *Proceedings of the 7th annual meeting of the International Society of Magnetic Resonance in Medicine.* Philadelphia: International Society of Magnetic Resonance in Medicine, p. 548.

50. Regatte, R.R., Kaufman, J.H., Noyszewski, E.A., and Reddy, R. (1999). Sodium and proton MR properties of cartilage during compression. *J Magn Reson Imaging* **10**:961–7.

51. Wu, E., Gao, E., Cham, E., *et al.* (1999). Application of HTS RF Coil for sodium imaging on a high field system. In *Proceedings of the 7th Annual Meeting of the International Society of Magnetic Resonance in Medicine*, Philadelphia: International Society of Magnetic Resonance in Medicine, p. 2115.

52. Bashir, A., Gray, M.L., and Burstein, D. (1996). Gd-DTPA as a measure of cartilage degradation. *Magn Reson Med* **36**:665–73.

53. *Bashir, A., Gray, M.L., Hartke, J., and Burstein, D. (1999). Nondestructive imaging of human cartilage glycosaminoglycan concentration by MRI. *Magn Reson Med* **41**:857–65.

This article presents an MRI technique for quantifying proteoglycan concentration in articular cartilage.

54. Trattnig, S., Mlynarkck, V., Breilenseher, M., *et al.* (1999). MR visualization of proteoglycan depletion in articular cartilage via intravenous injection of Gd-DTPA. *Magn Reson Imaging* **17**:577–83.

55. Kusaka, Y., Grunder, W., Rumpel, H., Dannhauer, K-H., and Gersone, K. (1992). MR microimaging of articular cartilage and contrast enhancement by manganese ions. *Magn Reson Med* **24**:137–48.

56. Fujioka, M., Kusaka, Y., Morita, Y., Hirasawa, Y., and Gersonde, K. (1994). Contrast-enhanced MR imaging of articular cartilage: a new sensitive method for diagnosis of cartilage degeneration. 40th Annual Meeting, *Orthopaedic Research Society*, New Orleans, 1994.

57. Lesperance, L.M., Gray, M.L., and Burstein, D. (1992). Determination of fixed charge density in cartilage using nuclear magnetic resonance. *J Orthop Res* **10**:1–13.

58. Peterfy, C.G., White, D., Tirman, P., *et al.* (1999). Whole-organ evaluation of the knee in osteoarthritis using MRI. *European League Against Rheumatism*, Glasgow, Scotland, 1999.

59. Wildy, K., Zaim, S., Peterfy, C., Newman, B., Kritchevsky, S., and Nevitt, M. (2001). Reliability of the Whole-Organ review MRI scorring (WORMS) method for knee osteoarthritis (OA) in a multicenter study. *65th Annual Scientific Meeting of the American College of Rheumatology*, San Francisco, CA, Nov. 11–15, 2001.

60. Eckstein, F., Sitteck, H., Gavazzenia, A., Milz, S., Putz, R., and Reiser, M. (1995). Assessment of articular cartilage volume and thickness with magnetic resonance imaging (MRI). *Trans Orthop Res Soc* **20**:194.

61. Burgkart, R., Glaser, C., Hyhlik-Dürr, A., Englmeier, K-H., Reiser, M., and Eckstein, F. (2001). Magnetic resonance imaging-based assessment of cartilage loss in severe osteoarthritis: Accuracy, precision and diagnostic value. *Arthritis Rheum* **44**:2072–7.

62. Peterfy, C., White, D., Zhao, J., Van Dijke, C., and Genant, H. (1998). *Longitudinal Measurement of Knee Articular Cartilage Volume in Osteoarthritis.* San Diego: American College of Rheumatology.

63. Pilch, L., Stewart, C., Gordon, D., *et al.* (1994). Assessment of cartilage volume in the femorotibial joint with magnetic resonance imaging and 3D computer reconstruction. *J Rheumatol* **21**:2307–21.

64. Cohen, Z.A., McCarthy, D.M., Ateshian, G.A., *et al.* (1997). *In vivo* and *in vitro* knee joint cartilage topography, thickness, and contact areas from MRI. *Orthopaedic Research Society*, San Francisco, February 1997.

65. Eckstein, F., Gavazzeni, A., Sittek, H., *et al.* (1996). Determination of knee joint cartilage thickness using three-dimensional magnetic resonance chondro-Crassometry (3D MR-CCM). *Magn Reson Med* **36**:256–65.

66. Bashir, A., Gray, M.L., Hartke, J., and Burstein, D. (1998). *Validation of Gadolinium-Enhanced MRI for GAG Measurement in Human Cartilage.* Philadelphia, PA: International Society of Magnetic Resonance in Medicine.

67. Peterfy, C.G., van Dijke, C.F., Lu, Y., *et al.* (1995). Quantification of articular cartilage in the metacarpophalangeal joints of the hand: accuracy and precision of 3D MR imaging. *Am J Roentgenol* **165**:371–5.

68. Fernandez-Madrid, F., Karvonen, R.L., Teitge, R.A., Miller, P.R., An, T., and Negendank, W.G. (1995). Synovial thickening detected by MR imaging in osteoarthritis of the knee confirmed by biopsy as synovitis. *Magn Reson Imaging* **13**:177–83.

69. Brandt, K.D. (1995). Insights into the natural history of osteoarthritis and the potential for pharmacologic modification of the disease afforded by study of the cruciate-deficient dog. In K.E. Kuetner and V.M. Goldberg (eds), *Osteoarthritic Disorders.* Rosemont, IL: American Academy of Orthopaedic Surgeons, pp. 419–26.

70. Palmer, W.E., Rosenthal, D.I., Shoenberg, O.I., *et al.* (1995). Quantification of inflammation in the wrist with gadolinium-enhanced MR imaging and PET with 2-[F-18]-fluoro-2-deoxy-D-glucose. *Radiology* **196**:645–55.

71. König, H., Sieper, J., Sorensen, M., and K.-J., W. (1991). Contrast-enhanced dynamic MR imaging in rheumatoid arthritis of the knee joint: follow-up study after cortisol drug therapy. *77th Scientific Assembly and Annual Meeting of the Radiological Society of North America*, Chicago, IL, 1991.

72. Yamato, M., Tamai, K., Yamaguchi, T., and Ohno, W. (1993). MRI of the knee in rheumatoid arthritis: Gd-DTPA perfusion dynamics. *J Comput Assist Tomogr* **17**:781–5.

73. Weinstein, R.S. and Majumdar, S. (1994). Fractal geometry and vertebral compression fractures. *J Bone Min Res* **9**:1797–802.

74. Majumdar, S., Genant, H.K., Grampp, S., Jergas, M.D., and Gies, A.A. (1994). Analysis of trabecular structure in the distal radius using high-resolution magnetic resonance images. *Euro Radiol* **4**:517–24.

75. Vellet, A.D., Marks, P., Fowler, P., and Mururo, T. (1991). Occult posttraumatic lesions of the knee, prevalence, classification, and short-term sequelae evaluated with MR imaging. *Radiology* **178**:271–6.

76. Felson, D., Chaisson, C., Hill, C., *et al.* (2001). The association of bone marrow lesions with pain in knee osteoarthritis. *Ann Intern Med* **134**:541–9.

77. *Resnick, D. (1995). Internal derangements of joints. In D. Resnick (ed.). *Diagnosis of Bone and Joint Disorders* (Vol. 5) (3 ed.). Philadelphia, PA: W.B. Saunders, pp. 3063–9.
    Excellent discussion of clinical MRI of the knee.

78. Hodler, J., Trudell, D., Pathria, M.N., and Resnick, D. (1992). Width of the articular cartilage of the hip: quantification by using fat-suppression spin-echo MR imaging in cadavers. *Am J Roentgenol* **159**:351–5.

79. Hodler, J., Loredo, R., Longo, C., Trudell, D., Yu, J., and Resnick, D. (1995). Assessment of articular cartilage thickness of the humeral head: MR-anatomic correlation in cadavers. *Am J Roentgenol* **165**:615–20.

80. Peterfy, C. (1998). Technical considerations. In L. Steinbach, P. Tirman, C. Peterfy, J. Feller (eds), *Shoulder Magnetic Resonance Imaging.* Philadelphia, PA: Lippencott-Raven, pp. 37–63.

81. Peterfy, C., Genant, H., Mow, V., and Bigliani, L. (1998). Evaluating arthritic changes in the shoulder with MRI. In L. Steinbach, P. Tirman, C. Peterfy, and J. Feller (eds), *Shoulder Magnetic Resonance Imaging.* Philadelphia, PA: Lippencott-Raven, pp. 221–37.

82. Tirman, P.F.J., Stauffer, A.E., Crues, J.V., *et al.* (1993). Saline magnetic resonance arthrography in the evaluation of glenohumeral instability. *Arthroscopy* **9**:550–9.

83. Palmer, W.E., Brown, J.H., and Rosenthal, D.I. (1994). Labral-ligamentous complex of the shoulder: evaluation with MR arthrography. *Radiology* **190**:645–51.

84. Tirman, P.F.J., Bost, F.W., Garvin, G.J., *et al.* (1994). Posterosuperior glenoid impingement: MRI and MR arthrographic findings with arthroscopic correlation. *Radiology* **193**:431–6.

85. Ateshian, G.A., Kwak, S.D., Soslowsky, L.J., and Mow, V.C. (1994). A stereophotogrammetric method for determining in situ contact areas in diarthroidial joints, and a comparison with other methods. *J Biomech* **27**:111–24.

11.4.4 Arthroscopic evaluation of knee articular cartilage

Xavier Ayral

Research into potential disease-modifying drugs for OA (DMOADs) requires standardized and reproducible outcome measurements that evaluate changes in the joint. Since many of the potential DMOADS are directed at altering the breakdown of articular cartilage, measurement of the quantity, integrity, and/or quality of articular cartilage would prove of value.[1]

Arthroscopy provides a direct, inclusive, magnified view of the six articular surfaces of the knee. Over the last few decades, arthroscopy has been established to be of value for diagnosis and surgical intervention in numerous disorders of the knee. An evolving methodology uses knee arthroscopy in clinical research, utilizing baseline and follow-up arthroscopy to monitor the course of knee OA[2,3] and to compare the natural history in one cohort of patients to an intervention in another one.[4]

Factors that have interfered with the development of arthroscopy for clinical research include the following:

♦ the invasive nature of arthroscopy,

♦ the lack of a validated, standardized scoring system of chondropathy, and

♦ the lack of standardized guidelines for video recording the articular cartilage surfaces during arthroscopy.

Can arthroscopy be simplified?

Local anesthesia

Therapeutic arthroscopy is often performed under general or spinal anesthesia. The procedure requires a preoperative and operative anesthetist consultation, with as much as two days of hospitalization. Explorative arthroscopy conducted for research purposes can be simplified by the use of local anesthesia administered subcutaneously and intra-articularly. Lidocaine or marcaine can provide skin and synovial anesthesia. With the use of local anesthesia, arthroscopy is almost always performed on an outpatient basis or as a day-case procedure.

Explorative arthroscopy under local anesthesia is safe, reliable, accurate, well tolerated, relatively inexpensive, and is an alternative to arthroscopy under general or spinal anesthesia.[2,4–6] Nevertheless, performance of arthroscopy under local anesthesia requires specific training, even for experienced arthroscopists.

Small glass-lens arthroscope

Knee arthroscopy is often performed with a 4.0 mm glass lens arthroscope requiring a 5.5 mm trochar. In some patients with contracted ligaments or residual muscle tension (because of local anesthesia), the posterior part of femorotibial compartments may not be accessible with a standard 4.0 mm scope. The 2.7 mm arthroscope has a similar field of view as the 4.0 mm arthroscope and most often permits the inspection of all compartments. Continuous knee irrigation provided by the 2.7 mm arthroscope is adequate to clear the joint of blood and debris, allowing a clear field for visualization.[2] Technically, the 25 or 30-degree angle provides a wide field and a better view. The images obtained by smaller diameter (1.8 mm, about 16-gauge) fiberoptic arthroscopes (sometimes called 'needlescopes') appear to be insufficient for clinical research on cartilage, as they tend to underestimate cartilage lesions.[7]

Tourniquet

An inflated thigh tourniquet is routinely used under general or spinal anesthesia for therapeutic arthroscopy to minimize bleeding. Post-operative thigh rehabilitation is often necessary due to the potential deleterious effect of the tourniquet on nerve and muscle recovery.[8] A tourniquet cannot be tolerated under local anesthesia but bleeding during explorative arthroscopy is a potential problem for correct visualization. In association with joint irrigation, some arthroscopists include epinephrine in the local anesthesia to reduce bleeding.[2]

Joint lavage

Ayral et al. found that one month after explorative arthroscopy, 82 per cent of the patients felt improved.[2] It is believed that the lavage performed during the procedure (usually one liter of normal saline) prompted clinical improvement of joint symptoms. This beneficial effect of joint lavage has been reported in controlled studies[9–11] and might partially counterbalance the invasive nature of the technique. This beneficial effect of arthroscopy should be kept in mind when evaluating the benefits of any potential DMOAD.

How to score chondropathy?

Articular cartilage lesions can be defined by three baseline parameters: depth, size, and location. Over the years, several arthroscopic classification systems have been devised in an attempt to describe and categorize the articular cartilage damage.[12–17]

Previous classifications

Some systems take into account only the depth of the lesions[12,13] and give qualitative information on the surface appearance of articular cartilage. They do not provide a quantitative approach to cartilage lesions.

Some systems[14–17] combine the depth and the size of the most severe chondropathy of the articular surface under a single and inaccurate descriptive category.

Guidelines for a quantitative system providing accurate information on depth, size, and location of cartilaginous lesions could be the following:

1. All the different articular cartilage lesions of a given articular surface must be evaluated, and not only the most severe chondropathy, in order to score the overall articular cartilage breakdown.

2. Depth and size of each cartilage lesion must be rated separately.

3. The evaluation of depth must distinguish chondromalacia, superficial fissures, deep fissures, and exposure of subchondral bone.

4. The evaluation of size must be as accurate as possible to allow detection of change with time.

A system for scoring chondropathy can be applied globally to the joint or specifically to each of the three compartments of the knee. Nevertheless, without quantitative joint mapping, the description of the location of chondropathy on a given articular surface remains qualitative.

Newer classifications

Noyes and Stabler

In 1989, Noyes and Stabler proposed a system for grading articular cartilage lesions at arthroscopy.[18] They separate the description of the surface appearance, the depth of involvement, and the diameter and location of the lesions. The diameter of each lesion is estimated by the examiner in millimeters using a graduated probing hook, and the lesions are reported on a knee diagram. Depending on the diameter and depth of the lesion, a point scaling system is used to calculate the score of chondropathy for each compartment, and, finally, to calculate an overall joint score.

This system is the first attempt to score chondropathy; we offer this critique:

1. In this system, all the chondral lesions are represented on the knee diagram as a full circle with a single diameter defined by the graduated hook. This is a semiobjective estimate of size because most cartilage lesions are not circular, but rather oval or irregularly shaped. Moreover, degenerative cartilage lesions often have the appearance of escharotic skin lesions, with the deepest breakdown located at the central point, surrounded by more superficial cartilage lesions. A diameter cannot be attributed to this 'surrounding lesion,' which is crown-shaped.

2. In this system, any lesion less than 10 mm in diameter is not considered clinically significant and, therefore, no points are subtracted: this induces a lack of sensitivity. In monitoring the outcome of DMOAD, all lesions, even the smallest, must be described.

3. The point scaling system proposed to score, simultaneously, depth and diameter of chondral lesions, is arbitrary. It is not based on statistical methodology, or on clinical assessment of the severity of the lesions.

4. This system has not been validated.

Ayral et al.

In 1993, Ayral et al. proposed two methods for scoring chondropathy.[2,19,20] The first method is a subjective approach based on overall assessment of chondropathy by the investigator, reported on a set of 100 mm visual analog scales (VAS) in which '0' indicates the absence of chondropathy and '100' the most severe chondropathy.[2] One VAS is used for each articular surface of the knee: patella, trochlea, medial femoral condyle, lateral femoral condyle, medial tibial plateau, and lateral tibial plateau. A VAS score is calculated for each of the three compartments of the knee and is obtained by averaging the VAS scores from the two corresponding articular surfaces of the compartment.

The second method is a more objective and analytic approach that includes an articular diagram of the knee with grading for location, depth, and size of all the different cartilaginous lesions[19,20] (Fig. 11.52 and Table 11.16).

Location. Areas defined include the patella, trochlea, medial femoral condyle, medial tibial plateau, lateral femoral condyle, and the lateral tibial plateau.

Depth. The system is based on the classification of chondropathy proposed by the French arthroscopists Beguin and Locker[12] (Fig. 11.53):

1. Grade 0, normal cartilage.

2. Grade I, chondromalacia, including softening with or without swelling.

3. Grade II, superficial fissures, either single or multiple, giving a 'velvet-like' appearance to the surface; Grade II also includes superficial erosion. Fissures and erosions are less than one-half thickness and do not reach the subchondral bone.

4. Grade III, deep fissures of the cartilage surface, down to subchondral bone, which is not directly visualized but may be touched with an arthroscopy probe; Grade III lesions are more than one-half thickness and may take different aspects: a 'shark's mouth-like' aspect, or a

detached chondral flap, due to a single deep fissure; a 'crab meat-like' aspect due to multiple deep tears; Grade III also includes deep ulceration of the cartilage creating a crater which remains covered by a thin layer of cartilage.

5. Grade IV, exposure of subchondral bone with intact bone surface or with cavitation.

In knee OA, cartilage breakdown often shows a combination of different grades, the most severe grade being surrounded by milder lesions (Fig. 11.52).

Size. The size and shape of each grade of chondropathy is recorded on a knee diagram (Fig. 11.52) by the arthroscopist: this step is crucial for evaluation. Then, the size is evaluated as a percentage of the articular surface. The percentage can be calculated by computer using numerization of the drawing on the knee diagram, or calculated directly from the diagram by a trained investigator.

Location, depth, and size of the different chondropathies are reported on a special form (Table 11.16). This form lists ten different quantitative variables, that is, sizes of chondropathy from Grades 0–IV for each compartment. The comparison of chondropathy severity between patients and/or between arthroscopies performed at different times in the same patient, required the integration of these different quantitative variables into a single score of chondropathy. For this purpose, the French Society of Arthroscopy carried out a prospective multicenter study that resulted in the establishment of two systems of assessing chondropathy: the SFA scoring system[19,20] and the SFA grading system.[19]

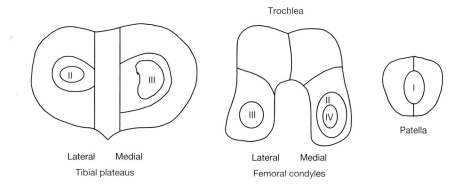

Fig. 11.52 An example of articular cartilage lesions visualized by arthroscopy and recorded on a knee diagram (right knee) with grades according to the Beguin and Locker classification.[12]

Table 11.16 Calculation of SFA score from one example of articular cartilage lesions visualized by arthroscopy and recorded on case record form (see Fig. 11.52)

Grade *	Location								
	Medial compartment			Lateral compartment			Femoropatellar compartment		
	Femur	Tibia	Mean value	Femur	Tibia	Mean value	Patella	Trochlea	Mean value
0	60†	65	62.5	80	75	77.5	80	100	90
I	0	0	0	0	0	0	20	0	10
II	30	0	15	0	25	12.5	0	0	0
III	0	35	17.5	20	0	10	0	0	0
IV	10	0	5	0	0	0	0	0	0

SFA score = size (%) of Grade I lesions × 0.14 + size (%) of Grade II lesions × 0.34 + size (%) of Grade III lesions × 0.65 + size (%) of Grade IV lesions × 1.00.

Medial score: (15 × 0.34) + (17.5 × 0.65) + (5 × 1.00) = 21.475.

Lateral score: (12.5 × 0.34) + (10 × 0.65) = 10.75.

Femoropatellar score: 10 × 0.14 = 1.4.

* 0, normal; I, softening-swelling; II, superficial fissures; III, deep fissures; IV, exposure of subchondral bone (Beguin and Locker classification[12]).

† Example: the number represents the size of the corresponding grade expressed in percentage of the corresponding whole articular surface. Each column totals 100%.

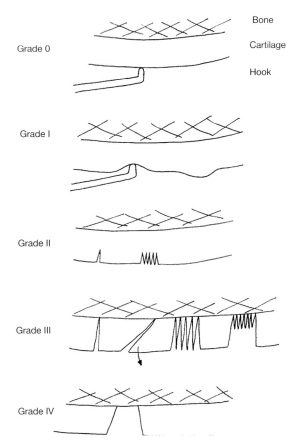

Fig. 11.53 Depth of articular cartilage lesions, according to the classification proposed by Beguin and Locker.[12] Grade 0, normal articular cartilage; Grade I, softening with or without swelling (chondromalacia); Grade II, superficial fissures; Grade III, deep fissures down to bone; Grade IV, exposure of subchondral bone.

The SFA score is a continuous variable graded between '0' and '100'. The score is obtained for each compartment as follows:

SFA score = A + B + C + D; where

♦ A = size (per cent) of Grade I lesions × 0.14
♦ B = size (per cent) of Grade II lesions × 0.34
♦ C = size (per cent) of Grade III lesions × 0.65
♦ D = size (per cent) of Grade IV lesions × 1.00

Size (per cent) = average per cent of surface for the medial femoral condyle and medial tibial plateau (medial tibiofemoral compartment), lateral femoral condyle and lateral tibial plateau (lateral tibiofemoral compartment), or trochlea and patella (patellofemoral compartment).

The coefficients of severity of chondropathy (0.14, 0.34, 0.65, 1.00) were obtained by parametric multivariate analysis.[20]

The SFA grade is a semiquantitative variable. The above numbers (size (per cent) of Grades 0–IV lesions) are placed in a formula to provide a summary grade (or category of chondropathy severity of the compartment) for each of the knee compartments. The formula for each compartment was obtained by non-parametric multivariate analysis, using a tree-structured regression.[19] There are six categories for the patellofemoral compartment and five categories for the medial and lateral tibiofemoral compartments.

The validation of arthroscopic quantification of chondropathy using the VAS score and SFA scoring and grading systems

Ayral *et al.* investigated their system for practicality of chondroscopy in terms of simplicity, reliability, validity, clinical relevance, sensitivity to change, and discriminant capacity.

Simplicity

Arthroscopy will always be an invasive procedure because of the stab incision required, but can be rendered less complex by the use of local anesthesia, performance on an outpatient basis, elimination of the tourniquet, and use of a small-bore glass lens arthroscope[2] (see Chapter 2).

Reliability

Intraobserver reliability of chondropathy measurement using either VAS score of chondropathy, or SFA score and SFA grade is good and better than interobserver reliability.[2,3] Thus, it appears that a single trained investigator should review arthroscopy videotapes from a clinical study. For multicenter studies, training sessions will be needed to improve interobserver evaluations of depth and size of the cartilage lesions.[21]

Validity

Intrinsic validity was evaluated by calculating the correlations between the different arthroscopy scales (VAS score and SFA systems). A strong correlation was found between these different systems,[3] which appear to be of complementary interest and are used together, at this time, in clinical trials in OA. The VAS and the SFA scores are more appropriate to detect minimal changes in severity of chondropathy over time, as they represent a continuous variable. The SFA grade permits classification of a population of OA patients into homogenous categories of chondropathy severity.

Extrinsic validity was evaluated by calculating the correlations between the arthroscopic quantification of chondropathy and radiological joint-space narrowing on weight-bearing X-rays with knees fully extended.[2,3] Arthroscopic and roentgenographic evaluations of chondropathy are closely correlated. Nevertheless, arthroscopy appears to be more sensitive than plain radiographs. Mild cartilage lesions, but also severe and deep cartilage erosions, may remain undetected, even on weight-bearing radiographs.[2,3]

Clinical relevance

Ayral *et al.* evaluated clinical relevance in two cross-sectional studies of the severity of chondropathy of medial tibiofemoral knee OA[3] and of post-traumatic patellofemoral chondropathy.[22] Correlations were investigated between cartilage damage and the clinical characteristics of the patients, including demographic data, baseline characteristics, and clinical activity of OA. There was a statistically significant correlation between medial and patellofemoral cartilage damage and patient age and the body mass index.[3,22] Pain was not correlated with cartilage damage,[3,22] and functional disability (Lequesne's index) was only correlated with patellofemoral cartilage breakdown.[22] Conversely, a longitudinal study performed with a one-year arthroscopy follow-up in 41 patients suffering from medial tibiofemoral knee OA, showed that changes in the severity of cartilage lesions correlated with changes in functional disability (Lequesne's index) and quality of life (AIMS2).[3]

Sensitivity to change

Arthroscopy demonstrated statistically significant worsening in cartilage lesions of medial tibiofemoral knee OA between two arthroscopic evaluations, performed one year apart in 41 patients.[3] Sensitivity to change after only one year might be explained by the precision of the technique and enrollment of patients with active OA of the knee. These patients had prior failure of analgesics, NSAIDs, physical exercises, and intra-articular gluco-corticoid injection leading to joint lavage. It should be noted that arthroscopy did not find significant worsening of chondropathy in a 6-month trial of 46 patients with post-traumatic patellofemoral chondro-pathy,[22] and that several longitudinal arthroscopic studies noted reversible changes in occasional patients.[3,23]

Discriminant capacity

A preliminary study of repeated hyaluronic acid injections suggested that arthroscopy might be capable of identifying chondromodulating agents.[4]

Guidelines for video recording articular cartilage surfaces at knee arthroscopy

Arthroscopies conducted for research purposes are recorded on videotape and reviewed by a single reader. Video recording must be of a good quality.

Clarity of the image

Clarity of the video recording can be improved by:

♦ using a local intra-articular anesthesia with epinephrine to reduce bleeding,

♦ performing abundant articular lavage before starting to record, in order to remove debris and cellular material,

♦ continuously focusing the camera,

♦ maximizing light intensity by providing enough light for visualization but avoiding overexposure ('flash') of the articular cartilage, and

♦ removing any condensation on the camera or scope.

Complete exploration

The aim of arthroscopy is to explore the entire six articular surfaces of the knee joint. Areas of normal cartilage should receive as much attention as areas of damage, so that the reader can assess what percentage of the total cartilage is damaged. The arthroscopist can briefly assess any cartilage lesion, but should not focus on specific lesions before making a general examination by sweeping along the whole articular surface from medial to lateral edge, and inversely, and from back to front, in order to allow the reader to assess the size of any lesion. The exploration of each articular sur-face should be performed twice, and slowly, to ensure that no area is missed. The femoral condyles should be explored from 20–90° of knee flexion, whilst maintaining valgus or varus pressure, to allow the inspection of their posterior surfaces.

Perspectives

Arthroscopic quantification of chondropathy remains an invasive and time-consuming technique. Therefore, the SFA scoring and grading systems have been applied to the evaluation of chondropathy with magnetic resonance imaging. Drape *et al.* found that quantification of chondropa-thy with MR imaging by using the SFA systems was feasible and well corre-lated with anatomic cartilage breakdown assessed and quantified at arthroscopy.[24]

Arthroscopy also provides a direct visualization of the synovium and permits the evaluation of interrelations between synovitis and chondro-pathy in OA.[22,25]

Conclusions

Arthroscopy, performed under local anesthesia, should be considered as a relevant outcome measure of OA in clinical research. Arthroscopy could potentially lead to reducing the duration and number of patients in clinical trials on DMOADs in OA. In the field of monitoring cartilage lesions, arthroscopy could be used to validate non-invasive imaging techniques, such as MRI and weight-bearing radiographs in flexed or semi-flexed position.

Key points

1. Simplification of arthroscopy for research purposes is based on:

   local anesthesia,

   absence of a tourniquet,

   small glass-lens arthroscope, and

   outpatient basis.

2. Arthroscopic quantification of the severity of chondropathy is needed to monitor the lesions over time.

3. Quantification of chondropathy can be either global, using a 100 mm visual analog scale (VAS) of severity, or more analytic, by using the scoring and grading systems proposed by the French Society of Arthroscopy.

4. Arthroscopic quantification of chondropathy, using VAS score and SFA system, has been validated.

5. Arthroscopic quantification of chondropathy requires high-quality video recording of articular cartilage surfaces.

References

(An asterisk denotes recommended reading.)

1. Lequesne, M., Brandt, K., Bellamy, N., *et al.* (1994). Guidelines for testing slow acting drugs in OA. *J Rheumatol* **41**(Suppl.):65–71.

2. Ayral, X., Dougados, M., Listrat, V., *et al.* (1993). Chondroscopy: A new method for scoring chondropathy. *Sem Arthritis Rheum* **22**:289–97.

3. *Ayral, X., Dougados, M., Listrat, V., *et al.* (1996). Arthroscopic evaluation of chondropathy in osteoarthritis of the knee. *J Rheumatol* **23**:698–706.

   Establishment of a cutoff for the SFA score, above which the changes observed in a single patient can be attributed to disease progression and not to the vari-ability of the technique.

4. Listrat, V., Ayral, X., Patarnello, F., *et al.* (1997). Arthroscopic evaluation of potential structure modifying activity of hyaluronan (Hyalgan®) in osteoarthritis of the knee. *Osteoarthritis Cart* **5**:153–60.

5. Eriksson, E., Haggmark, T., Saartok, T., Sebik, A., and Ortengren, B. (1986). Knee arthroscopy with local anesthesia in ambulatory patients. *Orthopedics* **9**:186–8.

6. McGinty, J.B. and Matza, R.A. (1978). Arthroscopy of the knee. *J Bone Joint Surg* **60A**:787–9.

7. Ike, R.W. and Rourke, K.S. (1993). Detection of intra-articular abnormal-ities in OA of the knee. A pilot study comparing needle arthroscopy with standard arthroscopy. *Arthritis Rheum* **36**:1353–63.

8. Dobner, J. and Nitz, A. (1982). Postmeniscectomy tourniquet palsy and functional sequelae. *Am J Sports Med* **10**:211–4.

9. Ike, R.W., Arnold, W.J., Rothschild, E., and Shaw, H.L. (1992). The Tidal Irrigation Cooperating Group. Tidal irrigation versus conservative medical management in patients with OA of the knee: a prospective randomized study. *J Rheumatol* **19**:772–9.

10. Chang, R.W., Falconer, J., Stulberg, S.D., Arnold, W.J., Manheim, L.M., and Dyer, A.R. (1993). A randomized, controlled trial of arthroscopic surgery versus closed-needle joint lavage for patients with OA of the knee. *Arthritis Rheum* **36**:289–96.

11. Ravaud, P., Moulinier, L., Giraudeau, B., *et al.* (1999). Effects of joint lavage and steroid injection in patients with osteoarthritis of the knee. Results of a multicenter, randomized, controlled trial. *Arthritis Rheum* **42**:475–82.

12. Beguin, J. and Locker, B. (1983). Chondropathie rotulienne. In: *2ème journée d'arthroscopie du genou*, No.1. Lyon, pp. 89–90.

13. Insall, J.N. (1984). Disorders of the patellae. In: *Surgery of the Knee*. New York: Churchill Livingston, pp. 191–260.

14. Outerbridge, R.E. (1961). The etiology of chondromalacia patellae. *J Bone Joint Surg* **43B**:752–7.

15. Ficat, R.P., Philippe, J., and Hungerford, D.S. (1979). Chondromalacia patellae: a system of classification. *Clin Orthop Rel Research* **144**:55–62.

16. Bentley, G. and Dowd, G. (1984). Current concepts of etiology and treatment of chondromalacia patellae. *Clin Orthop Rel Res* **189**:209–28.

17. Casscels, S.W. (1978). Gross pathological changes in the knee joint of the aged individual: a study of 300 cases. *Clin Orthop Rel Res* **132**:225–35.

18. Noyes, F.R. and Stabler, C.L. (1989). A system for grading articular cartilage lesions at arthroscopy. *Am J Sports Med* **17**:505–13.

19. Dougados, M., Ayral, X., Listrat, V., *et al.* (1994). The SFA system for assessing articular cartilage lesions at arthroscopy of the knee. *Arthroscopy* **10**:69–77.

20. Ayral, X., Listrat, V., Gueguen, *et al.* (1994). Simplified arthroscopy scoring system for chondropathy of the knee (revised SFA score). *Rev Rhum Engl Ed* **31**:89–90.

21. Ayral, X., Gueguen, A., Ike, R.W., *et al.* (1998). Interobserver reliability of the arthroscopic quantification of chondropathy of the knee. *Osteoarthritis Cart* **6**:160–6.

22. *Ayral, X., Ravaud, P., Bonvarlet, J.P., *et al.* (1999). Arthroscopic evaluation of post-traumatic patellofemoral chondropathy. *J Rheumatol* **26**:1140–7.

    Quantification of cartilage damage and synovitis in post-traumatic patellofemoral chondropathy; triangular relationship among severity of cartilage damage, synovitis, and progression of cartilage damage.

23. Raatikainen, T., Vaananen, K., and Tamelander, G. (1990). Effect of glycosaminoglycan polysulfate on chondromalacia patella. A placebo controlled 1 year study. *Acta Orthop Scand* **61**:443–8.

24. *Drape, J.L., Pessis, E., Auleley, G.R., Chevrot, A., Dougados, M., and Ayral, X. (1998). Quantitative MR imaging evaluation of chondropathy in osteoarthritis of the knee. *Radiology* **208**:49–55.

    Quantification of chondropathy of knee OA with MR imaging by using the SFA score and grade; correlations between MR and arthroscopic findings; intra- and interobserver reliability of quantitative MR imaging.

25. Ayral, X., Mayoux-Benhamou, A., and Dougados, M. (1996). Proposed scoring system for assessing synovial membrane abnormalities at arthroscopy in knee osteoarthritis. *Br J Rheumatol* **35**(3 Suppl.):14–17.

11.4.5 Bone scintigraphy

Donald S. Schauwecker

Radiographic techniques, such as microfocal spot radiography magnification and computed tomography, provide excellent anatomic details of the joint. In OA, the articular cartilage, subchondral cysts, subchondral sclerosis, size and number of osteophytes, and other structural changes can be evaluated. Unfortunately, these anatomic changes are a historic record of the response of the joint to past insults; they are of no use in assessing current physiologic changes or disease 'activity' at the time of the radiographic examination.

Overview of scintigraphy

Scintigraphy is the nuclear medicine imaging technique in which radioactive isotopes are bound to pharmaceutical agents to form radiopharmaceuticals that, after injection, localize physiologically in the tissues. As will be described later, radiopharmaceuticals have been developed that bind to articular cartilage, remodeling bone and at sites of inflammation, all of which may be relevant to OA. Although scintigraphy offers the advantage of providing information about alterations in physiology that exist at the time of the study, it has two drawbacks: first, image resolution is much poorer than with radiography, because the number of gamma rays produced by the injected radiopharmaceutical is far smaller than the number of X-rays produced by the cathode ray tube used in radiography. Second, because bone cells respond to a wide variety of insults, such as trauma, infection, and tumor invasion, by increasing bone turnover, scintigraphy has high sensitivity but poor specificity. The physiologic information from scintigraphy, therefore, complements the anatomic information of the radiologic examination and clinical information gained from the history, physical examination, and laboratory studies.

The scintigraphic examination

From the point of view of the patient, a nuclear medicine bone scan, the most common study done for OA, is a relatively innocuous procedure. The patient lies on a table and receives an intravenous injection of radiopharmaceutical, Tc^{99m} diphosphonate, through a small gauge needle while a nuclear angiogram, or perfusion study, is obtained for a duration of about one minute. Images are obtained with a gamma camera, an instrument which detects gamma rays and localizes the source of the rays in a two-dimensional plane. The patient is then free to spend about 3 hours up and about, during which time the radiopharmaceutical localizes to the bone. Delayed imaging of the bone is then performed, which takes 30–60 minutes. If the gamma camera is rotated around the patient, it is possible to produce cross-sectional images in any plane, as may be obtained with MRI. This technique is called single photon emission computed tomography (SPECT).

The level of radiation exposure from a bone scan is about comparable to that which we receive naturally from the environment and is about 5–10 per cent of the government regulated maximum limit that individuals with occupational exposure to radiation are permitted to receive each year. Tc^{99m} diphosphonate is injected in quantities so small that they are below the pharmacological range. Reported adverse reactions to Tc^{99m} diphosphonate include hypersensitivity reactions, such as itching and skin rashes, and rare cases of dizziness (Bracco Diagnostics, Inc., Princeton, NJ, package insert). The reported rate of adverse reactions in 1984 was 0.5 per 100 000 administrations.[1] Thus, very rarely does anyone experience an adverse reaction from the procedure.

Approaches to imaging

The diarthrodial joint is an organ composed of several distinct structures, including cartilage, bone, and synovium, each of which is affected to a greater or lesser degree during the development of OA. In this chapter the use of scintigraphy for evaluation of these changes, and the correlation of scintigraphic data with clinical symptoms and radiographic changes will be reviewed.

Scintigraphy of articular cartilage

Because many of the early changes of OA occur in the articular cartilage, a cartilage-imaging agent might theoretically provide the best approach to evaluation of the OA joint. Two preliminary attempts have been made to develop a cartilage-imaging agent. In the first $[^{75}Se]bis[\beta$-$(N,N,N$-trimethylamino)ethyl]selenide diiodide was studied in normal adult guinea pigs. Moderate lesion-to-background ratios of about 10–20 : 1 were achieved.[2] However, attempts to extend this work to humans were unsuccessful because the radiopharmaceutical did not localize as well in human cartilage as in guinea pig cartilage.

In another study, a monoclonal antibody specific to link protein of human articular cartilage produced lesion-to-background ratios of 20–100 : 1 in rats and rabbits.[3] The investigators pointed out the advisability of utilizing an antibody to a unique constituent of OA cartilage to increase the clinical usefulness of the approach; however, no further publications have appeared using this approach since 1993. Accordingly, other approaches are employed today for scintigraphic evaluation of OA.

The perfusion bone-scan

Two approaches have been used to study the increases in joint perfusion that occur when inflammation is present. The first is the injection into the joint of Xe-133, which is then cleared from the joint at a rate proportional to the level of perfusion. Phelps et al.[4] described a biexponential washout curve of the intra-articular injection of Xe-133 and hypothesized that the faster component related to perfusion of the synovial membrane, while the slower represented washout of the radionuclide from adipose tissues of the joint. When results in 6 rabbits with surgically induced OA of the knee were compared with those in normal controls, the OA knee showed significantly greater synovial perfusion than the control knee. Before the development of modern gamma cameras, quantitative isotope dilution studies, such as Xe-133 clearance studies, were performed frequently, but they are rarely employed today largely because referring physicians and nuclear medicine specialists prefer images to pages of data. No Xe-133 clearance studies in patients with OA appear to have been published since 1972.

A more readily available indication of perfusion is the nuclear angiogram performed in conjunction with the bone scan. After injection of a bone-scanning agent, serial 2–4-second images of the joint are obtained with a gamma camera. In comparison with a normal joint, the OA joint exhibits increased perfusion. Interpretation is only qualitative, however, and is based upon direct comparison of the OA joint to a normal control. In general, this approach has proved less accurate in evaluation of OA joints than the evaluation of increased bone turnover on delayed bone images[5,6] (see below).

The delayed bone-scan

The most common scintigraphic approach to the study of OA is the use of delayed bone-scan images obtained 3–4 hours after intravenous injection of the bone-seeking radiopharmaceutical. Over the years, many agents that are incorporated into calcium hydroxyapatite crystals as the bone remodels have been used for this purpose. The current agents of choice are diphosphonates (e.g., Tc^{99m} medronate or Tc^{99m} oxidronate), which are incorporated onto the surface of microcrystals of calcium hydroxyapatite in the bone.[7] Given an adequate blood supply, the more rapid the rate of bone turnover, the greater the localization of the radiopharmaceutical. Most of the data on bone scintigraphy discussed below were obtained with this approach.

It has been known for years that bone-seeking isotopes are rapidly taken up by OA joints. Christensen[8] found that the distribution of ^{99m}Tc-methylene diphosphonate uptake was similar to the histochemical localization of acid and alkaline phosphatase activity in bone within the OA joint. In 1963, Danielsson et al.[9] described a relationship between isotope uptake and the radiographic severity and rate of progression of OA of the hip. The most intense uptake was seen in subchondral bone, at the osteochondral junction of osteophytes, and in the walls of bone cysts. Although the technique is non-specific, bone scintigraphy may be highly sensitive and may reveal more extensive and severe changes of OA than other imaging modalities.[10]

Sharif et al.[11] compared the results of bone scans with the synovial fluid concentration of putative markers of bone and cartilage turnover in 35 patients with knee OA and found a statistically significant correlation between the intensity of uptake in the scan and the synovial fluid concentration of osteocalcin, a biochemical marker of bone turnover. A weaker association was present between uptake on bone scan and the synovial fluid concentration of keratan sulfate and chondroitin sulfate epitopes, suggesting that cartilage turnover correlated less well with bone scintigraphy than does bone turnover. These observations reinforced the suggestion that scintigraphy provided an index of bone remodeling in OA.

Petersson et al.[12] were interested in detecting OA in the earliest stages, that is, when intervention might possibly prevent irreversible joint damage. They studied knee radiographs, delayed bone scans, and serum concentrations of cartilage oligomeric matrix protein (COMP) and bone sialoprotein (BSP) in 38 patients with knee OA, and found that serum concentrations of both COMP and BSP were higher in patients with delayed bone scan abnormalities than in those with normal scintigrams. Serum levels of COMP correlated positively with the magnitude of the increased uptake of radionuclide in the bone scan, while the serum concentration of BSP did not.

The resolution of bone scintigraphy is approximately 1 cm only. Therefore, in the following discussion, scintigraphic evaluation of OA in large joints, such as the hip and knee, will be considered separately from that in smaller joints, such as those in the fingers and toes. In large joints, semiquantitative measurements can be made by comparing pixel counts at various sites within the joint. The limited resolution of the gamma camera precludes such topographic comparison in smaller joints.

The indium-111-labeled leukocyte scan

Indium-111-labeled leukocytes are routinely used to study infection and inflammation such as osteomyelitis and septic arthritis. Thomas and Mullan described a patient with severe knee OA without infection who had a striking accumulation of indium-111-labeled leukocytes in the knee joint,[13] which they considered to represent intense synovial uptake due to the synovitis of active OA. The authors reported this case as an example of a false-positive scan in the investigation of suspected septic arthritis. However, no systematic attempt has been made to use indium-111-labeled leukocytes to study OA. It should be noted that the intensity of synovitis in OA is typically not great (see Chapter 5); the synovial fluid leukocyte count is usually less than 2000 cells mm.[3]

Studies in animal models of OA

Using an experimental model of secondary OA in the rabbit, Christensen showed that uptake of ^{99m}Tc-methylene diphosphonate was increased in the unstable knee within one week after surgical destabilization. Uptake was confined to sites at which osteophytes were forming.[14] Later, however, the same sites did not exhibit increased localization of the radiopharmaceutical, which was then seen in the subchondral bone beneath areas of cartilage damage.

In studies of a canine cruciate-deficiency model of OA, Brandt et al.[15] performed bone scans 6 and 12 weeks after anterior cruciate ligament transection and found that by 12 weeks, uptake in the OA knee was nearly double that in the contralateral stable knee, in which uptake did not change, relative to the baseline value. At sacrifice, 12 weeks after surgery, articular cartilage in the OA knee was thicker and more opaque than normal, while cartilage in the contralateral knee was normal. Osteophytes developed in the unstable knee, but not in the contralateral knee. Such bony changes, which may be either primary or secondary to early changes in the biomechanical properties of the cartilage, may contribute to the pathogenesis of cartilage damage (see Chapters 7.2.2.1 and 7.2.2.2).

Scintigraphic studies of hand OA in humans

Hutton et al.[16] utilized scintigraphy to predict radiographic changes in hand joints of subjects with OA, taking advantage of the fact that many joints within the hand are susceptible to OA and that progression of changes in hand joints is often rapid. In a cross-sectional survey of 33 patients with hand OA, in whom bone scans and plain radiographs were performed, the bone scans showed abnormalities in a number of joints that were normal on the plain radiograph. In several other cases, the radiograph showed evidence of OA but the bone scan was normal (Table 11.17).

The disagreement between the radiographic and scintigraphic findings illustrated in Table 11.17 are easily explained if the pattern of disease progression in OA is similar to that in many diseases of bone, such as osteomyelitis,[17] stress fracture,[18] and Paget's disease.[19] Initially, the bone suffers some insult or injury and responds with accelerated bone remodeling or turnover. At that stage, the bone scan will be positive but the radiograph will still be normal. Subsequently, increased bone remodeling may result in anatomic changes and both the bone scan and the radiograph will be abnormal. Later, if the insult has stabilized or healed, bone turnover may return to normal. At this stage, the bone scan will be normal, although anatomic changes may be present on the radiograph. Notably, 14 of the subjects in the Hutton et al.[16] study were followed for 3–5 years to relate the initial scintigraphic findings to subsequent development of OA.[20] Results indicated that positive scans at baseline were associated with a greater likelihood of subsequent radiographic evidence of OA progression than negative scans (Table 11.18). In several instances, initial scan abnormalities preceded radiographic changes of OA in the same joint by months or years. In some cases, scan positivity subsided as abnormalities in the involved joint stabilized on plain radiography (Table 11.18).

In a study of 28 patients with erosive hand OA and 24 with non-erosive hand OA,[21] the scan findings correlated significantly with the radiographic findings both at baseline and two years later. Joints in which the baseline bone scan was positive were significantly more likely to show radiographic progression and increased joint tenderness, relative to the baseline examination, than those in which the baseline scan was negative. The authors concluded that bone scintigraphy is useful for predicting clinical and radiographic progression of hand OA, with and without erosions.

The above results were corroborated by Buckland-Wright et al. who studied 32 patients with OA of the hand and wrist with serial magnification radiographs and 4-hour bone-scan images[22,23] and found that the intensity of the bone scan correlated well with the size and number of osteophytes, but not with joint-space width, subchondral sclerosis, or juxta-articular radiolucencies. One-year later, joints that had shown increased activity on the bone scan, exhibited growth in the size of the osteophytes, but no significant change in the number of osteophytes. In contrast, in those joints in which the baseline bone scan was essentially normal, little change was detected in the size and number of osteophytes. These data suggest that the onset of disease activity in the OA joint is marked by increased localization of the radiopharmaceutical, or followed eventually by radiographic changes of OA. As disease activity stabilizes, the bone scan subsequently returns to

normal. In individual patients, different stages in the evolution of OA may exist concurrently within joints of the same hand.

Other studies, however, have not fully confirmed the results of Hutton et al.,[20] Olejarova et al.[21] and Buckland-Wright et al.[22,23] For example, in a study by Balblanc et al.[24] in which hand radiographs and bone scans of 15 patients with symptomatic hand OA were obtained at baseline and again 4 years later, significant correlations between the radiographic score and the scintigraphic score were noted at entry and at the time of the follow-up examination. When bone uptake in the scintigram was quantitated by expressing the data as a joint-to-bone reference area ratio, it was found that joints in which an initially normal bone-scan had become positive, or in which both bone scans were abnormal, were more likely to show worsening of the radiographic score than those in which both bone scans were normal. However, in contrast to the results of the studies noted above,[20–23] quantification of isotope retention at baseline and changes in the scintigraphy score had no predictive value for progression of radiographic severity.

When Macfarlane et al. related blood pool and delayed bone scans to symptoms of hands with OA in 35 patients[25] and repeated the studies one year later to evaluate changes with time, they found poor correlation between the blood pool and delayed images; many more joints were positive on delayed imaging than blood pool imaging. Symptoms of OA of the hands were evaluated by two different methods: the articular index was determined by pressing on the individual joint and grading the patient's pain response on a four-point scale and patients were asked to indicate their overall level of pain on a standard 10 cm visual analog scale. The articular index correlated highly with the delayed bone images but not with the blood pool images, whereas the visual analog pain score correlated significantly with the blood pool images but not with the delayed images. The authors concluded that a larger study of longer duration might be helpful in determining the significance of the different information provided by the blood pool and delayed components of the bone scan.

Jónsson et al. prospectively studied 414 patients with non-inflammatory arthritis who were referred for whole body delayed bone-scans in whom a static image of the hands was also obtained.[26] Only low uptake of the radionuclide by subchondral bone was seen in various joints of subjects younger than age 40, but uptake increased in subjects in their fifth and sixth decades and then reached a plateau in all joints except the knee, in which uptake in the oldest subjects was lower than that in younger individuals. Uptake in the first carpometacarpal joint and patella was greater in women than in men and strong bilateral concordance of uptake in hands was observed. The authors concluded that bone scintigraphy is valuable for epidemiological studies of OA and can provide new information about age-related patterns and joint subsets, possibly indicating a difference in pathogenetic mechanisms of OA of various joints.

Table 11.17 Cross-sectional data from scintigraphic studies of subjects with OA of the hand*

Site	X-ray+, scan−	X-ray+, scan+	X-ray−, scan−	X-ray−, scan+
DIP	37	32	25	6
PIP	57	24	11	9
MCP	91	2	1	7
TB	17	55	12	17

DIP, distal interphalangeal joints; PIP, proximal interphalangeal joints; MCP, metacarpophalangeal joints; TB, thumb base; +, positive; −, normal.

* Numbers indicate the percentage of joints with each feature, based on analysis of all joints in the hand in 33 patients with OA.

Source: Taken from Ref. 16.

Table 11.18 Longitudinal data from scintigraphic studies of subjects with OA of the hand*

	Total number of joints	No change	Progression	Regression	Ankylosis
Normal	288	262 (91)	26 (9)	0	0
X-ray+, scan−,	59	43 (73)	8 (14)	6 (10)	2 (3)
X-ray+, scan+	81	46 (57)	30 (37)	3 (4)	2 (2)
X-ray−, scan+,	20	6 (30)	14 (70)	0	0

+, positive; −, normal; X-ray +; scan −, etc.

* Numbers indicate the total number of hand, in parentheses, the percentage of joints showing change in 14 patients with OA of the hand.

Source: Taken from Ref. 20.

Scintigraphic studies of knee OA in humans

Joints of the hand are too small to permit ready analysis of uptake within different areas of the joint. Hutton *et al.*[16] dealt with the limited resolution of bone scintigraphy by combining uptake in the first carpometacarpal joint and scaphotrapezoid joint, and calling this area 'thumb base.' The images of the remainder of the carpal bones were combined and called 'the wrist.' However, the knee is a much larger structure than the hand or wrist, and analysis of uptake in different areas of that joint is possible. McCrae *et al.* found four different image patterns on the delayed (4-hour) bone scan of OA knees (Fig. 11.54).[5] Generalized retention of isotope around the joint,

in either the early (flow) or late (bone) phase of the bone scan was less common than focal areas of uptake around the margin of the patella or in the subchondral bone, which were observed only in the late phase scans. As noted in the above studies of hand OA, some knees with abnormal scans were radiographically normal, while others that exhibited evidence of OA on the radiograph were normal on the scintigraphic study. Retention of isotope along the joint line correlated with joint pain and with subchondral sclerosis on the radiograph, while a generalized pattern of uptake was associated with the presence of osteophytes.[5]

Planar scintigraphy of the knee often superimposes activity in the patellofemoral compartment upon that in the medial and lateral tibiofemoral compartments. The early studies of McCrae *et al.* (see above)

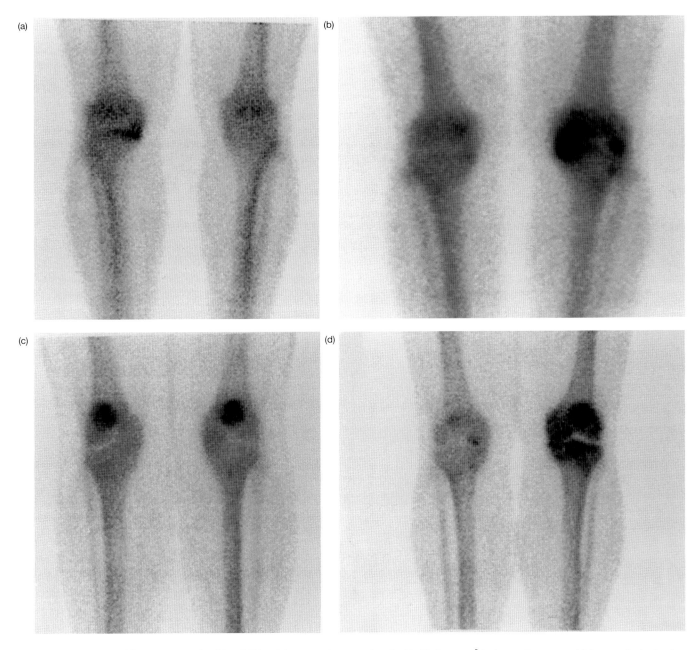

Fig. 11.54 Four patterns of OA are seen on the delayed (4-hour) bone-scan image, as described by McCrae *et al.*[5] In the tramline pattern (a), increased retention is seen along the joint line. This corresponded to the presence of joint pain and to subchondral sclerosis on the plain radiograph. In the extended pattern (b), uptake is seen in the subchondral bone. This was associated with more severely damaged knees, with joint-space narrowing, and subchondral sclerosis. The 'hot patella' sign (c), was associated with radiographic changes of patellofemoral OA. The generalized pattern (d), marked by a diffuse increase in uptake around the joint, was associated with joint pain and radiographic evidence of osteophytosis.

examined only the anterior view of the knee on bone scans.[5] However, a lateral view can separate activity in the patellofemoral compartment from that in the tibiofemoral compartment. Studying both anterior and lateral knee scans of 56 OA knees, Thomas *et al.* found that scintigraphy was no more sensitive than clinical evaluation or conventional radiography in identifying patellofemoral OA.[10]

Unfortunately, superimposition of structures can be a problem on the lateral as well as the anterior views. The best way to solve the problems associated with superimposition of activity is to use single photon emission computed tomography (SPECT). Collier *et al.* used arthroscopy as the 'gold standard' to determine the presence or absence of cartilage damage and synovitis in the patellofemoral, lateral, and medial compartments of the knee in 27 patients with OA[6] and found that SPECT was superior to either clinical evaluation or conventional radiography (Table 11.19). The authors proposed that non-invasive SPECT be used prior to arthroscopy and suggested that a negative SPECT could eliminate the need for arthroscopic evaluations for a torn meniscus, that while in knees with an increased SPECT uptake, the arthroscopist could concentrate on those areas of the joint that exhibited scan abnormalities.

Dieppe *et al.*[27] suggested that bone scintigraphy could predict progression of knee OA in patients who already exhibited clinical and radiographic evidence of the disease. In this study, patients who had knee radiographs and bone scans in 1986 underwent repeat radiography in 1991. Criteria for progression of knee OA were: (1) joint surgery; or (2) a decrease in the tibiofemoral joint space of more than 2 mm. Of the 94 patients enrolled in this study: 10 died, 9 were lost to follow-up over the 5-year interval, and 15 underwent knee surgery (22 knees). Bone scan abnormalities were noted in 87 knees at the initial evaluation, and 52 (60 per cent) exhibited progression of radiographic abnormalities or surgery during the 5-year period. Notably, of the 32 knees with severe scintigraphic abnormalities at the outset of the study, 28 (88 per cent) showed radiographic progression. On the other hand, *none* of the 55 knees in which knee scintigraphy was normal at entry into the study showed radiographic progression of OA.

Three caveats should be raised, however, with regard to this study. First, the criteria for joint surgery were not defined. This is important because the basis for the decision to proceed with arthroplasty varies markedly among clinicians. It is often related to joint pain and function, and may have had nothing to do with progression of joint pathology.[28] Second, the sequential knee films were plain radiographs, that is, an anteroposterior standing view in full extension and a lateral in 30° of flexion. Because no particular effort was made to standardize radioanatomic positioning for the serial radiographs, changes in joint-space width due to errors in beam alignment or increased knee flexion (e.g., as a result of joint pain; see Chapter 11.4.2) may have resulted in artifactual narrowing of the joint space in the standing anteroposterior view (see Chapter 11.5.1). Third, the bone scan results were interpreted only dichotomously, as 'normal' or 'abnormal;' criteria for grading were not defined nor was any attempt made to quantify radionuclide uptake.

Clarke *et al.*[29] studied 99 patients with knee OA clinically, radiographically, and with bone scintigraphy. Scintigraphic abnormalities correlated significantly with advancing Kellgren–Lawrence (K–L) radiographic grade and joint-space narrowing. Positive scintigraphic results correlated highly also with clinical evidence of bony swelling and greater levels of joint pain.

Mazzuca *et al.*[30] studied 182 overweight female patients who had radiographic evidence of unilateral knee OA on the conventional standing anteroposterior view. A region of interest was drawn around the medial tibia, lateral tibia, medial femur, lateral femur, and patella areas in the knee and compared to an internal control region of identical area in the distal tibia on the 3-hour delayed images. Results (Table 11.20) revealed that radionuclide uptake in the OA knee were significantly greater than that in the contralateral knee. Furthermore, uptake in the radiographically 'normal' contralateral knee was significantly greater than that in knees of normal non-arthritic subjects,[30] consistent with the observation that patients with unilateral idiopathic knee OA are at high risk for developing OA in the 'normal' knee. The authors also found that uptake in the medial femoral and medial tibial regions of interest was inversely related to joint-space width on the radiograph. The severity of knee pain was strongly related to the magnitude of radionuclide uptake (Table 11.20). The authors concluded that increased activity seen on the delayed bone scan is indicative of active OA. Continuing follow-up of subjects in this study will permit a determination of whether the increased activity in the 'normal' contralateral knee predicts development of radiographic changes of OA in that joint.

McAlindon *et al.*[31] recently studied 12 OA knees by MRI and compared the results with those seen on scintigraphy, using the classification developed by McCrae *et al.*[5] (Fig. 11.54). In that classification a 'tramline' scintigraphic pattern (Fig. 11.54(a)) correlated with the findings of hyperintense osteophytes in the proton density sequence for MRI imaging, indicating an increase in local fat content. The 'extended' scintigraphic pattern of knee

Table 11.19 Evaluation of knee compartments for cartilage damage and/or synovitis

Study	Sensitivity	Specificity	Accuracy (%)
Patellofemoral compartment			
Clinical evaluation	0.17	1.00	35
Conventional radiography	0.22	1.00	37
Radionuclide angiography	0.39	1.00	52
Planar bone scintigraphy	0.57	1.00	66
SPECT bone scintigraphy	0.91	1.00	93
Lateral tibiofemoral compartment			
Clinical evaluation	0.67	0.79	72
Conventional radiography	0.20	0.93	55
Radionuclide angiography	0.67	0.64	66
Planar bone scintigraphy	0.73	0.71	72
SPECT bone scintigraphy	0.93	0.50	72
Medial tibiofemoral compartment			
Clinical evaluation	0.86	0.50	76
Conventional radiography	0.71	1.00	79
Radionuclide angiography	0.76	0.88	79
Planar bone scintigraphy	0.86	0.88	86
SPECT bone scintigraphy	0.91	0.86	90

Source: Taken from Ref. 6.

Table 11.20 Tc^{99m} diphosphonate uptake in index, contralateral, and control knees. Ratio of counts/pixel in the region of interest to counts/pixel in an region of identical area in the distal tibia (mean ± SD)

Region of interest	Image	OA knee (N = 182)	Contralateral knees (N = 182)	Control knee (N = 20)
Medial tibia	AP	1.7 ± 0.6*	1.4 ± 0.4[†]	1.2 ± 0.3
Lateral tibia	AP	1.7 ± 0.5*	1.5 ± 0.4	1.4 ± 0.3
Medial femur	AP	1.7 ± 0.5*	1.5 ± 0.4	1.3 ± 0.4
Lateral femur	AP	2.1 ± 0.6*	1.8 ± 0.5[†]	1.4 ± 0.4
Patella	Lateral	2.4 ± 0.9*	2.2 ± 0.8[†]	1.6 ± 0.6

* Radionuclide uptake in the OA index knee was significantly greater than in the contralateral knee (adjusted $P < 0.05$).

[†] Radionuclide uptake in contralateral knees was significantly greater than that in control knees (adjusted $P < 0.01$) based on general estimating equation (GEE) models.

Source: Modified from Ref. 30.

OA (Fig. 11.54(b)) corresponded to an increased signal on STIR MRI images of the subchondral bone, which may represent inflammation, pseudocyst, or synovial leakage. Signal changes in MRI of the patellofemoral joint corresponded to radionuclide uptake in the patella.

Boegard et al.[32] studied 58 people with chronic knee pain with plain radiography, bone scintigraphy, and MRI. Good agreement was found between increased bone uptake and lesions in subchondral bone seen on the T2 STIR sequence of the MRI. However, agreement between increased bone uptake and osteophytes or cartilage defects, and between the intensity of bone uptake and MRI findings, was poor.

Clarke et al.[33] compared dual energy X-ray absorbtiometry at baseline and 18 months later with baseline bone scintigrams in patients with OA. Bone mineral density was lost more rapidly in patients whose baseline bone scans were positive than in those with a negative scan, suggesting that a positive bone scan reflects increased metabolic activity in subchondral bone that may predict the progression of OA.

Implications

Scintigraphy is not currently a component of the routine clinical evaluation of a patient with OA, although it can be helpful in research studies. The above data suggest that bone scintigraphy may prove useful in diagnosing *preclinical* OA, for example, in identifying involved joints before the appearance of clinical evidence of the disease. In addition, scintigraphy may predict future radiographic changes of OA. If the strong negative predictive value of bone scintigraphy reported by Dieppe et al.[27] is confirmed, the procedure would be useful in screening patients for enrollment in controlled clinical trials of disease-modifying drugs for OA. Indeed, use of a negative baseline bone scan as an exclusion criterion could sharply decrease the number of subjects required to demonstrate a statistically significant effect of the drug under study and, therefore, significantly reduce the cost of the study.

Second, the localization of disease activity seen on the bone scan could prove helpful in planning treatment. For example, relative disease activity in the knee can be determined separately for the patellofemoral and medial and lateral tibiofemoral compartments. If, as Dieppe et al.[27] have shown, a normal bone-scan tends to remain normal in patients with OA, it might be possible to use scintigraphy to help identify subjects who are candidates for an osteotomy or unicompartmental arthroplasty, rather than total joint replacement.

Conclusion

Correlation of scintigraphic findings with radiographic findings, while often good, is not always perfect. Scintigraphy reflects real-time physiology while the radiograph depicts anatomic changes that have occurred previously. Physiologic changes precede anatomic changes. As anatomic changes progress, scintigraphic and radiographic studies are both abnormal. Later, in the burned-out stage, the anatomy remains abnormal while scintigraphy returns to normal as the physiologic alterations subside.

The major limitations of bone scintigraphy are its poor spatial resolution, in comparison with plain radiography and computed tomography, and its poor specificity for OA.

The chief advantage of scintigraphy is its extreme sensitivity for activity of the disease at the time the scan is obtained: this may permit scintigraphy to predict future anatomic changes. Conversely, if, as suggested, scintigraphy proves to have a strong negative predictive value, it may be helpful in predicting joints that will not be affected by OA.

Summary

Radiographic studies such as plain films, computed tomography, and magnetic resonance imaging (MRI) can provide detailed anatomic information

about the OA joint, such as the number and size of osteophytes and thickness of the articular cartilage. However, although such anatomic information reveals a history of what has happened to the joint in the past, it may not tell what is happening currently and cannot predict what will happen in the future. Scintigraphic studies do not offer the fine anatomic detail of radiographic studies, but the radiopharmaceuticals employed provide an image of the joint, which is based upon the current local physiology and biochemistry. Therefore, they can be used to reveal what is going on in the joint at the time of the study. The routine bone scan appears to correlate well with findings of plain radiography, magnetic resonance imaging, and computed tomography, as well as with joint tenderness on the clinical examination. More important, it may be able to predict anatomic changes of OA that will be present in future radiographic studies.

Key points

1. Conventional radiography provides detailed anatomic information while scintigraphy provides poor anatomic information but excellent real-time physiological information.

2. Because bone cells respond to a wide variety of insults, such as trauma, infection, and tumor by increased bone turnover, scintigraphy has high sensitivity but poor specificity.

3. Because physiologic changes precede anatomic changes, scintigraphic and radiographic changes follow the following sequence:

   - Scintigraphy positive, radiography normal
   - Scintigraphy positive, radiography abnormal
   - Scintigraphy negative, radiography abnormal

4. Conventional radiology provides a history of what has happened in the past. Scintigraphy may predict changes that will be seen on future conventional radiographs.

5. Optimal scintigraphic visualization of the patellofemoral and medial and lateral tibiofemoral joints is obtained with single photon emission computed tomography (SPECT).

References

(An asterisk denotes recommended reading.)

1. **Atkins, H.L.** (1986). Reported adverse reactions to radiopharmaceuticals remain low in 1984. *J Nucl Med* **27**:327.

2. **Yu, W.K.S., Shaw, S.M., Bartlett, J.M., Van Sickle, D.C., and Mock, B.H.** (1989). The biodistribution of [^{75}Se]bis [β-(N,N,N-trimethylamino)ethyl] selenide diiodide in adult guinea pigs. *Nucl Med Biol* **16**:255–9.

3. **Cassiede, P., Amedee, J., Vuillemin, L., et al.** (1993). Radioimmunodetection of rat and rabbit cartilage using a monoclonal antibody specific to link proteins. *Nucl Med Biol* **20**:849–55.

4. **Phelps, P., Steele, A.D., and McCarty, D.J.** (1972). Significance of Xenon-133 clearance rate from canine and human joints. *Arthritis Rheum* **15**:360–70.

5. *****McCrae, F., Shouls, J., Dieppe, P., and Watt, I.** (1992). Scintigraphic assessment of osteoarthritis of the knee joint. *Ann Rheum Dis* **51**:938–42.

   This study of 100 subjects represents the first description of different patterns of uptake on bone scans of patients with knee OA and relates scan patterns to clinical and radiographic features.

6. *****Collier, B.D., Johnson, R.P., Carrera, G.F., et al.** (1985). Chronic knee pain assessed by SPECT: comparison with other modalities. *Radiology* **157**:795–802.

   Single photon emission computed tomography (SPECT) is more sensitive, and provides superior anatomic localization of increased activity than planar bone scintigraphy, conventional radiography or clinical examination.

7. **Francis, M.D.** (1969). The inhibition of calcium hydroxyapatite crystal growth by polyphosphonates and polyphosphates. *Calc Tiss Res* **3**:151–62.

8. Christensen, S.B. (1985). Osteoarthrosis: changes of bone, cartilage and synovial membrane in relation to bone scintigraphy. *Acta Orthop Scan* **56**(Suppl. 214):1–43.

9. Danielsson, L.G., Dymling, J.F., and Heripret, G. (1963). Coxarthrosis in man studied with external counting of ^{85}Sr and ^{47}Ca. *Clin Orthop* **31**:184–99.

10. Thomas, R.H., Resnick, D., Alazraki, N.P., Daniel, D., and Greenfield, R. (1975). Compartmental evaluation of osteoarthritis of the knee: a comparative study of available diagnostic modalities. *Radiology* **116**:585–94.

11. Sharif, M., George, E., and Dieppe, P.A. (1995). Correlation between synovial fluid markers of cartilage and bone turnover and scintigraphic scan abnormalities in osteoarthritis of the knee. *Arthritis Rheum* **38**:78–81.

12. Petersson, I.F., Boegård, T., Dahlström, J., Svensson, B., Heinegård, D., and Saxne, T. (1998). Bone scan and serum markers of bone and cartilage in patients with knee pain and osteoarthritis. *Osteoarthritis Cart* **6**:33–9.

13. Thomas, P.A. and Mullan, B. (1995). Avid In-111 labeled WBC accumulation in a patient with active osteoarthritis of both knees. *Clin Nucl Med* **20**(11):973–5.

14. Christensen, S.B. (1983). Localization of bone-seeking agents in developing experimentally induced osteoarthritis in the knee joint of the rabbit. *Scand J Rheumatol* **12**:343–9.

15. Brandt, K.D., Schauwecker, D.S., Dansereau, S., Meyer, J., O'Connor, B., and Myers, S.L. (1997). Bone scintigraphy in the canine cruciate deficiency model of osteoarthritis. Comparison of the unstable and contralateral knee. *J Rheumatol* **24**:140–5.

16. Hutton, C.W., Higgs, E.R., Jackson, P.C., Watt, I., and Dieppe, P.A. (1986). ^{99m}TcHMDP bone scanning in generalized nodal osteoarthritis. I. Comparison of the standard radiograph and four-hour bone scan image of the hand. *Ann Rheum Dis* **45**:617–21.

17. Howie, D.W., Savage, J.P., Wilson, T.G., and Paterson, D. (1983) The technetium phosphate bone scan in the diagnosis of osteomyelitis in childhood. *J Bone Joint Surg* **65A**:431–7.

18. Zwas, S.T., Elkanovitch, R., and Frank, G. (1987). Interpretation and classification of bone scintigraphic findings in stress fractures. *J Nucl Med* **28**:452–7.

19. Wellman, H.N., Schauwecker, D.S., Robb, J.A., Khairi, M.R., and Johnston, C.C. (1977). Skeletal scintimaging and radiography in the diagnosis and management of Paget's disease. *Clin Orthop* **127**:55–62.

20. Hutton, C.W., Higgs, E.R., Jackson, P.C., Watt, I., and Dieppe, P.A. (1986). ^{99m}TcHMDP bone scanning in generalized nodal osteoarthritis. II. The four hour bone scan image predicts radiographic change. *Ann Rheum Dis* **45**:622–6.

21. Olejarova, M., Kupka, K., Pavelka, K., Gatterova, J., and Stolfa, J. (2000). Comparison of clinical, laboratory, radiographic, and scintigraphic findings in erosive and nonerosive hand osteoarthritis. Results of a two-year study. *Joint Bone Spine* **67**(2):107–12.

22. Buckland-Wright, J.C., Macfarlane, D.G., and Lynch, J.A. (1995). Sensitivity of radiographic features and specificity of scintigraphic imaging in hand osteoarthritis. *Rev Rheum Engl Ed* **62**:14S–26S.

23. Buckland-Wright, J.C., Macfarlane, D.G., Fogelman, I., Emery, P., and Lynch, J.A. (1991). Technetium 99m methylene diphosphonate bone scanning in osteoarthritic hands. *Eur J Nucl Med* **18**:12–16.

24. Balblanc, J.C., Mathieu, P., Mathieu, L., *et al.* (1995). Progression of digital osteoarthritis: a sequential scintigraphic and radiographic study. *Osteoarthritis Cart* **3**:181–6.

25. *Macfarlane, D.G., Buckland-Wright, J.C., Lynch, J., and Fogelman, I. (1993). A study of the early and late ^{99}technetium scintigraphic images and their relationship to symptoms in osteoarthritis of the hands. *Br J Rheumatol* **32**:977–81.

    In this study, the blood pool scan correlated with the joint pain score but not with the tender joint index, while uptake on the delayed bone scan correlated with the tender joints but not the joint pain score. This may imply that the blood pool and delayed portions of the bone scan reflect different pathogenetic aspects of OA, which relate to different clinical features.

26. *Jónsson, H., Elíasson, G.J., and Pétursson, E. (1999). Scintigraphic hand osteoarthritis (OA)—prevalence, joint distribution, and association with OA at other sites. *J Rheumatol* **26**:1550–6.

    In a study of 414 patients without inflammatory arthritis, they found that bone scintigraphy provided epidemiological information, such as the age and sequence in which the joints showed increased activity as OA developed. This might lead to new ideas about age-related patterns and joint subsets, possibly indicating a difference in pathogenetic mechanism among joints in OA.

27. *Dieppe, P., Cushnaghan, J., Young, P., and Kirwan, J. (1993). Prediction of the progression of joint space narrowing in osteoarthritis of the knee by bone scintigraphy. *Ann Rheum Dis* **52**:557–63.

    This was the first major long-term study of bone scintigraphy. The authors concluded that a positive bone scan was a poor predictor of subsequent joint-space loss, but a negative bone scan strongly predicted lack of subsequent progression of knee OA. Limitations of this study, however, include the absence of standardized positioning of the knee in the serial radiographs, undefined criteria for grading bone scan uptake, and the absence of criteria for knee surgery, which was used as a surrogate for OA progression.

28. Wright, J.G., Coyte, P., Hawker, G., *et al.* (1995). Variation in orthopedic surgeons' perceptions of the indications for and outcomes of knee replacement. *Can Med Assoc J* **152**:687–97.

29. Clarke, S., Duddy, J., Wakeley, C., *et al.* (2000). Bony swelling predicts positive bone scintigraphy in mild to moderate knee osteoarthritis. *Arthritis Rheum* **43**:S337.

30. Mazzuca, S.A., Brandt, K.D., Schauwecker, D.S., *et al.* (2000). The utility of scintigraphy in explaining x-ray changes and symptoms of knee osteoarthritis. *Trans Orthop Res Soc* **25**:234.

31. McAlindon, T.E.M., Watt, I., McCrae, F., Goddard, P., and Dieppe, P.A. (1991). Magnetic resonance imaging in osteoarthritis of the knee: correlation with radiographic and scintigraphic findings. *Ann Rheum Dis* **50**:14–19.

32. *Boegard, T., Rudling, O., Dahlstrom, J., Dirksen, H., Petersson, I.F., and Jonsson, K. (1999). Bone scintigraphy in chronic knee pain: comparison with magnetic resonance imaging. *Ann Rheum Dis* **58**(1):20–6.

    This study of 58 middle-aged people with chronic knee pain showed a correlation between an increase in uptake on the bone scan and an increase in signal from subchondral bone during the T2 STIR sequence of the MRI.

33. Clarke, S., Duddy, J., Shepstone, L., *et al.* (1998). Loss of subchondral bone mineral density in knees at risk of progressive osteoarthritis (OA). *Arthritis Rheum* **41**:S86.

11.4.6 Ultrasonography
Stephen L. Myers

Glossary

Attenuation: a characteristic reduction in acoustic energy transmitted within a fluid or tissue medium.

Echogenicity: the echo-generating ability/capacity of a medium, described as strong (hyperechoic), weak (hypoechoic) or absent (anechoic).

Speckle: in ultrasound images, the granular appearance that is derived from the internal backscatter of incident ultrasound.

Transducer: electromechanical device that sends and receives ultrasound energy.

Ultrasound: inaudible high-frequency (>1 MHz) vibration in an elastic medium.

Ultrasonography/Sonography: acquisition of images produced by reflected (backscattered) ultrasound signals.

Pharmacological agents are now available that favorably influence disease progression in experimental models of OA.[1] This raises the possibility that such agents, which can alter pathogenetic mechanisms within the joint and are termed 'disease-modifying OA drugs' (DMOADs),[2] may have utility in the prevention or treatment of OA in humans. The exciting prospect of evaluating these drugs has prompted considerable interest in the identi-fication of sensitive and reliable methods to measure the progression of this disease.[3] As discussed in other chapters, modifications of standard radio-graphic and magnetic resonance imaging techniques have been proposed to improve the performance of these measures of OA severity and progression, but none of these methods have proved to be entirely satisfactory and bet-ter ways to evaluate the OA joint are needed.[4] External ultrasonography (i.e., diagnostic sonography), is a safe, non-invasive, and relatively inex-pensive technique that can readily distinguish synovial fluid from tendon, cartilage, and bone, and provide a real-time visual display of the anatomic relationships of articular and periarticular tissue in a two-dimensional imaging plane. It represents a powerful technology and, if appropriate instrumentation is developed, could prove useful for serial measurements of the thickness and surface characteristics of articular cartilage in clinical trials of DMOADs.

Production of the sonographic image

The objective of diagnostic sonography is to obtain and interpret images of living tissue by probing it with very high frequency (ultrasonic) sound waves. The equipment used to image the extremities typically employs pulse–echo ultrasound technology to produce a gray-scale image.[5–8] A basic understanding of this technology can help us interpret the images produced and some of their limitations.

An electrical ultrasound generator, or transducer, that emits acoustic energy at a characteristic acoustic frequency, is the primary element in any sonographic imaging system.[7] The transducer usually consists of multiple piezo-electric elements that are electronically coupled to operate in a phased mode. An alternating voltage applied to these elements results in their rapid expansion and contraction, producing a mechanical wave (or ultrasound wave) in the adjacent soft tissue. A coupling gel is applied between the transducer and skin surface to permit maximum acoustic energy transfer. Transducers are generally pulsed at a rate known as the pulse repetition frequency. As the signal pulse encounters each successive layer of tissue or body fluid, part of its energy is reflected, part transmitted, and a small fraction absorbed. Between pulses, the transducer acts as a receiver (or hydrophone) of backscattered echoes that produce small volt-age changes across the elements that, after extensive signal processing, are used to produce a gray-scale image.

The acoustic energy reflected from the tissues under the transducer-receiver is detected as a spectrum of ultrasonic echoes. This 'A-mode' signal is amplified, processed, and then temporarily stored as an acoustic charac-terization of that site. To obtain a two-dimensional 'B-mode' image that can be more readily interpreted, multiple A-mode signals are displayed in a lin-ear array. These signals can be obtained, one at a time, by moving the trans-ducer laterally to a series of adjacent locations, or from an aligned array of multiple transducers that work in concert. In either case, the lateral distance between the location of the first and last signal corresponds to the x-axis of the B-mode sonographic image (Fig. 11.55). The y-axis of this image repres-ents the time-of-flight/2, that is, one-half the time required for the ultra-sound pulse to travel from the transducer to a tissue interface, such as a tendon, and to be reflected from this point back to the surface as an echo. Thus, the position of the echo on the y-axis indicates its distance from the transducer. In 'gray-scale' sonography, the acoustic intensity of the echo cor-responds to the echogenicity of the target tissue, and, therefore, to the bright-ness of the displayed image. Tissues that reflect very little acoustic energy, such as synovial fluid, appear hypoechoic or anechoic. In contrast, tendon and bone are highly reflective and, therefore, highly echogenic (Fig. 11.56). The high-speed image acquisition and display capabilities of the sonography equipment that are available today yield a real-time image and, when neces-sary, the operator can redirect the transducer to optimize the quality of the image. Observations made during voluntary movements, such as contrac-tion of the quadriceps muscle, can help identify anatomical landmarks and improve the visualization of structures, such as tendons and bursae.[8]

Acoustic properties of connective tissue

The usefulness of diagnostic sonography, and how far it can 'see' into the body, depend upon the characteristics of the transducer, its placement, and the acoustic properties of the target tissue. The absorption, reflection, and transmission of incident sound energy by tissue are related to the frequency of the ultrasound waves emitted by the transducer, and these parameters determine the sonographic appearance of each tissue or organ, and the res-olution and accuracy of the imaging system.[7–12]

Body fluids, including blood and hyaluronan-rich fluids, such as synovial fluid, transmit sound efficiently. This can be expressed in terms of tissue acoustic impedance, which relates the pressure in a sound wave to the size and velocity of the wave in the tissue; the impedance of blood (1.5×10^6 kg per m^2) is similar to that of skeletal muscle and fat.[7,9,13] The speed-of-sound in blood (1540 m per sec, Table 11.21) is nearly five times faster than that of sound traveling through air. Although sound travels at approxi-mately the same velocity (1430–1630 m per sec, Table 11.21) through blood, fat, and muscle, more acoustic energy is absorbed and scattered by muscu-loskeletal tissue than by body fluids. This difference in acoustic impedance, or attenuation, among tissues is frequency-dependent, and is expressed as an attenuation coefficient that ranges from 9 dB per m in blood to 1900 dB per m in bone (Table 11.21). The speed-of-sound in cortical bone is much faster (2888–3406 m per sec) than that in blood or other tissues.

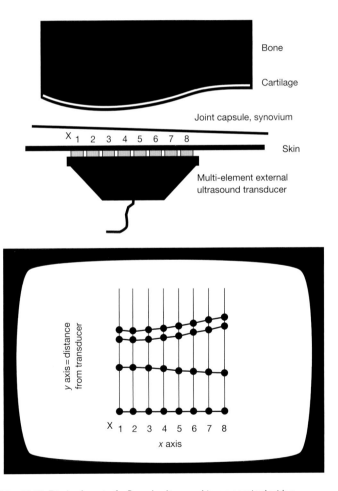

Fig. 11.55 Display format of a B-mode ultrasound image acquired with a multi-element external transducer. Pulse–echo data representing the tissues under each element of the transducer are displayed along the x-axis of the video screen to create a two-dimensional image. The position of each echo signal on the y-axis of the image corresponds to the distance between the transducer and the tissue that produced the echo.

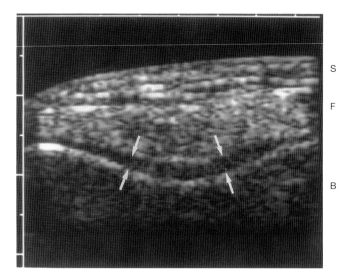

Fig. 11.56 External sonographic image of the femoral trochlea in a patient with OA. Transverse view, B-mode scan obtained with a diagnostic (7.5 MHz) transducer positioned above the superior pole of the patella, with the knee in 90° of flexion. Note skin (S); suprapatellar fat pad (F); nearly anechoic band of articular cartilage (between arrows); and subchondral bone (B). The cartilage on the lateral portion of the trochlea (on left) is 30–40% thinner than that in the midline, or on the medial portion.

Table 11.21 Velocity and attenuation of ultrasound in connective tissues

Tissue	Speed of sound (meters/second)	Sonic attenuation coefficient at 1 MHz (decibels/meter)
Blood	1540	9
Aqueous humor	1500	7
Muscle	1630	350
Fat	1430	60
Tibial bone	2888	1900*
Skull bone	3050	870
Articular cartilage (human)	1658	na
Articular cartilage (bovine)	1700	na

na, not available.

* Measured at 5 MHz.

However, because bone has a very high acoustic impedance (5×10^6 kg per m^2) and reflects and absorbs incident acoustic energy, rather than transmitting it,[6,11,12] external sonography reveals only the cortical surface of the bone. Like bone, calcifications in tendon or other soft tissue, and most foreign bodies, are highly echogenic.[6]

The speed-of-sound in non-calcified articular and periarticular tissues, including cartilage, tendon, muscle, and fat, and their acoustic attenuation coefficients, resemble those of blood more than that of bone[9,12,13] (Table 11.21). It is important to point out that adjacent tissues cannot be distinguished with sonography unless their acoustic impedance differs, because this difference determines how much incident acoustic energy each will reflect.[7] When the speed-of-sound in adjacent tissues differs, the direction of travel of an ultrasound wave passing from one to the other is altered, or refracted, at the interface. The complex interactions of the ultrasound signal and target tissues yield backscattered echo patterns that produce a granular appearance, or speckle, in the image. This appearance is related to the system resolution (transducer point response), and permits differentiation of the tissues.[10]

The effective imaging range of external ultrasound is inversely proportional to the operating frequency. Precise measurements of skin thickness have been obtained with a 20 MHz transducer array designed specifically for this application,[14] but tissue penetration at this frequency is insufficient to permit study of even superficial joints or tendons. Most diagnostic sonography systems used clinically to evaluate the musculoskeletal system have a center frequency of 3–10 MHz.[6] The spatial resolving power of the system is proportional to its center frequency, and the theoretical maximum resolving power that can be achieved at an imaging frequency of 7.5 MHz is approximately 0.2 mm.[10] Soft tissue structures several inches below the skin can be imaged with such equipment, and diagnostic sonography is often used to localize structures such as tumors or foreign bodies, no more than a few millimeters in diameter.

Inflammatory pannus, tenosynovitis, tendon rupture, and joint effusions in the hands and wrists of patients with rheumatoid arthritis have been identified using high-resolution 13 MHz clinical ultrasound imaging systems.[15–17] Images have been obtained of osteophytes and mucous cysts in the distal interphalangeal joints of patients with OA. Joint-space widening is considered sonographic evidence of synovitis in such images.[16] Published, peer-reviewed data are inadequate to assess the role of ultrasound for assessment of subchondral cysts or synovitis in OA,[17] but the clinical use of such scanners by rheumatologists is increasing, particularly in Europe.[18]

External sonography of the knee and hip

External sonography readily detects synovial effusions in the knee and other joints because the synovial fluid is readily distinguished as a black, anechoic area in the image.[19] Because of its higher fat content, synovium is less echogenic than the fibrous joint capsule and it can be identified as a distinct echo band between the capsule and the anechoic synovial fluid.[20–23] Synovitis and hypertrophic synovial villi are often present in OA, and 73 per cent of patients with symptomatic knee OA had sonographic evidence of synovitis,[17] almost always in the suprapatellar pouch. There is limited evidence, even in rheumatoid arthritis, that sonography provides a reliable estimate of the severity of synovial proliferation,[21] but advances in three-dimensional ultrasonic imaging may eventually make this possible.[24] Power Doppler sonography provides information on tissue fractional blood volume and flow, and a measure of local perfusion.[25] It can, therefore, detect soft-tissue hyperemia in inflammatory musculoskeletal diseases and shows promise in the evaluation of synovitis. In small studies, a qualitative decrease in synovial perfusion has been observed in patients with inflammatory knee synovitis after intra-articular injection of corticosteroid,[25] and synovial hyperemia was correlated with some laboratory indices of inflammation.[26]

Images of the articular surface of portions of the femoral condyles of humans can be obtained with external sonography.[6,20–30] Optimal, full-thickness images of the cartilage are obtained, however, only when the transducer-receiver can be positioned perpendicular to the articular surface. The patient must be able to maintain the knee in a flexed position for several minutes, and careful positioning of the joint and transducer are required because of the contours of the femoral condyles and the acoustic barrier created by the patella.[27] Extraneous echoes from the intervening skin and subcutaneous fat, muscle, tendon, joint capsule, and synovium tend to reduce the quality of the cartilage image.

Normal articular cartilage has a characteristic appearance in images obtained with sonography. The cartilage image is a uniformly hypoechoic band with a smooth surface that typically follows the contour of the subchondral bone (Fig. 11.56). The interface between the synovial fluid and the articular surface produces a thin line of echoes,[23,28–30] while the lower limit of the articular cartilage is defined by echoes from the highly echogenic interface between the hyaline cartilage and the calcified cartilage and subchondral bone.[31] In such images, the width of the hypoechoic band provides an estimate of cartilage thickness.[20] The fibrocartilaginous menisci yield a more intense, relatively homogeneous, pattern of echoes, which distinguish them from articular cartilage. Although defects in the menisci have been detected with external sonography[32,33] the technique is considered unreliable.[8]

The anatomy of the knee imposes strict limits on the chondral surfaces that can be evaluated with external ultrasound. A transverse view of the trochlea (Fig. 11.56) can be obtained when the joint is positioned in 80–120° of flexion.[20,30] Even though this degree of flexion cannot always be achieved in patients with knee OA, the possibility that this view might be used to evaluate the severity of OA has been explored because it depicts the thickness and contour of that portion of the trochlear cartilage that is loaded by contact with the patella.[30] Longitudinal views, obtained 1–2 cm medial or lateral to the midline of this portion of the trochlea and aligned with the femoral shaft, have been used to complement these transverse images.[29] Notably, neither patellar nor tibial cartilage nor the central, habitually loaded regions of the femoral condyles that are typically the site of fibrillation in early OA, can be adequately evaluated with external sonography.

In sonograms of the OA knee, the normal, well-defined boundary between articular cartilage and soft tissue often appears blurred.[23,28] A non-homogeneous appearance, or lack of clarity of the normally hypo-echoic cartilage matrix is considered a sonographic feature of OA cartilage,[23] although an age-related increase in the internal echogenicity of human cartilage has also been suggested.[17] Some investigators have concluded that subjective estimates of the severity of OA, based on the degree of blurring and thinning of the cartilage, may be more useful than efforts to measure cartilage thickness from these images.[27] In one series, measurements of cartilage thickness were least reliable when areas of eburnated bone were present, but good correlation was reported between the severity of chondral ulceration in gross specimens obtained at the time of knee arthroplasty and the grade of OA severity in preoperative sonograms.[27]

The average thickness of the cartilage on the normal human femoral trochlea, as determined by external sonography, is 2.1–2.3 mm.[20,27–29] A strong correlation ($r = 0.86$) has been shown between such measurements and measurements of cartilage thickness obtained with contrast-enhanced magnetic resonance imaging.[20] Notably, the precision of values obtained with ultrasound cannot exceed the 0.2 mm limit imposed by the operating frequency of the transducer. In cartilage obtained from patients at the time of knee arthroplasty, histologic measurements of the thickness of trochlear cartilage did not differ significantly from the values obtained by preoperative sonography.[29] In another study, sonograms from both knees of 60 patients with symptomatic and radiographic evidence of OA showed the articular cartilage on the trochlea was significantly thinner than that in age-matched controls.[28] Although most of the subjects with OA in these series[27–29] had advanced disease, the mean thickness of the trochlear cartilage (1.4 mm) was only 36 per cent less than that in normal knees. Measurement of cartilage thickness at the trochlea by any method is unlikely to be a sensitive indicator of disease progression. In general, external sonography of the OA knee does not appear well suited to studies of disease progression.

At the hip, external sonograms obtained with a hand-held 5 MHz linear array transducer have been used to determine the apparent thickness of the articular cartilage of the femoral head in adults with no radiographic evidence of OA.[33] These images showed the cartilage as a relatively sonolucent band, immediately adjacent to an echogenic, curvilinear band (Fig. 11.57) that represented the subchondral bone of the anterior femoral head. Measurements of joint space obtained from these sonograms had a coefficient of variation of 19 per cent and were less reproducible than those obtained in plain radiographs or magnetic resonance imaging of the same joint. The detection of joint effusion with hip sonography, or of effusion and synovitis with Doppler sonography, can be helpful in the clinical assessment of the painful hip.[19] For example, Foldes et al.,[34] in a study of 50 patients with various diseases of the hip, found sonographic evidence of joint effusion in 35, which was confirmed by arthocentesis in 30. Thirty-two of the 35 had nocturnal pain. Sonographic evidence of hip effusion and nocturnal pain both diminished after aspiration of the joint, which, in

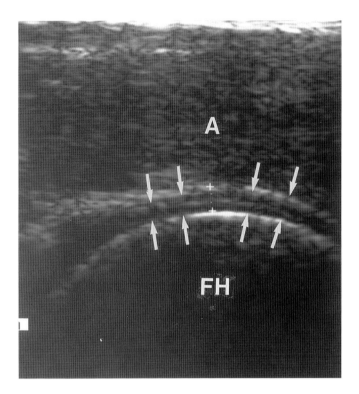

Fig. 11.57 External sonographic image of the normal hip. Longitudinal scan obtained with a 5 MHz transducer. Note the acetabulum (A) and the nearly anechoic band (between the arrows) representing the articular cartilage. The echogenic band under the cartilage indicates the subchondral bone of the femoral head (FH). A measurement of cartilage thickness (2.5 mm) was obtained with the cursors (+) superimposed on the image.

some cases, was followed by intra-articular injection of corticosteroid. The authors reported that the sensitivity of sonography in detecting hip joint effusion was 92 per cent and the specificity 70 per cent. In comparison, the sensitivity of nocturnal pain for detection of a hip effusion was somewhat lower (85 per cent), although the specificity was higher (94 per cent).

In a study by Bierma-Zeinstra et al.,[35] among 224 subjects with hip pain who were referred for imaging studies by a general practitioner, ultrasonography revealed the presence of an effusion in 38 per cent.[35] After adjustment for age and radiographic severity of OA, a significant relationship was noted between pain and ultrasonic evidence of effusion. Although, in contrast to the study by Foldes et al.,[34] a relationship between nocturnal pain and joint effusion was not apparent, this could have been due to the fact that patients in the study by Foldes et al. had more advanced disease than those in the study by Bierma-Zeinstra et al.

Investigational sonography of OA cartilage

Of the methods now available for evaluation of articular cartilage in OA, only direct, arthroscopic inspection of the joint can quantitate roughening of the articular surface, detect swelling or changes in turgor of the cartilage, or map the extent of chondral ulceration.[36] Arthroscopy, however, reveals little about the thickness of the cartilage, which varies with location on the femoral condyle. Cartilage thickness may be increased in early OA,[37] but diminishes with progression of the disease. Interest has arisen, therefore, in the possibility that intra-articular sonography could be used to complement and enhance radiographic and arthroscopic assessment of the knee.

The feasibility of mapping the thickness of the articular cartilage with high frequency, 20 MHz ultrasound, was established in *ex vivo* studies of the human acetabulum.[38] These pioneering studies showed that echoes from the smooth articular surface of normal cartilage could be distinguished from the hypoechoic cartilage matrix and from deeper echoes produced by the osteochondral junction. The accuracy of thickness measurements in this series was approximately 0.08 mm, or about the same as that reported for 20 MHz measurements of skin thickness.[14] Sonographic analysis of the acetabulum revealed that while this surface was nearly spherical, the contour of the calcified osteochondral interface was far more variable.

Recently, a pulse–echo technique, similar to that used to evaluate the acetabulum, was employed with a focused 25 MHz transducer to determine *in vitro* the velocity of sound in normal and OA human articular cartilage, and the thickness of the cartilage on canine and human femoral condyles.[39,40] The speed of sound in normal human articular cartilage averaged 1658 ± 185 m per s, and a slightly lower value, 1581 ± 148 m per s, was obtained for OA cartilage. Although the water, proteoglycan, and collagen content of OA cartilage differ from those of normal cartilage, no significant correlation was found between the speed of sound in OA cartilage and any of these variables. These data allay concern[38] that changes in the biochemical composition of the cartilage matrix in OA could affect the precision of sonographic measurements of cartilage thickness.

Investigators in several laboratories have used ultrasound to obtain B-mode cross-sectional images of canine,[39] porcine,[41] human,[30,40,42,43] rodent,[31,44,45] and bovine[46,47] articular cartilage specimens immersed in degassed saline. Typically, after the specimen has been excised, a high-frequency transducer (18–50 MHz) has been moved over the articular surface to image the cartilage and, in some cases, the attached subchondral bone. In images of normal cartilage, the interface between the saline bath and articular surface is seen as a smooth, echogenic band (Fig. 11.58), while the cartilage matrix is hypoechoic. The interface between the cartilage and calcified cartilage/subchondral bone produces a second, distinct band of strong echoes. Important species-specific differences in the sonographic appearance of normal cartilage have not been described. However, the internal echogenicity of the cartilage matrix varies from laboratory to laboratory because the image depends on transducer frequency and the other design characteristics of the imaging system, as well as on the composition and geometry of the target tissue.

B-mode images of OA cartilage reflect the severity of fibrillation and ulceration of the articular surface. The surface of severely fibrillated cartilage completely disrupts the saline-cartilage interface, so that the fibrillated matrix is seen as a band of chaotic internal echoes that extends from the cartilage surface into the matrix (Fig. 11.59). In contrast, mechanical abrasion of the surface of normal cartilage with fine sandpaper, producing a minor degree of fibrillation, significantly increased the number and intensity of the surface echoes representing the saline–cartilage interface, but left the deeper matrix echo free.[39]

In specimens of OA cartilage in which fibrillation extended only 0.1–1.2 mm beneath the articular surface, the width of the surface echo band in B-mode scans obtained with a 25 MHz transducer was proportional to the depth of fibrillation ($r = 0.78$).[40] Other work suggests that alternative ultrasonic techniques, measuring either the scattering by the cartilage surface of 10–30 MHz ultrasonic waves[41] or the frequency-dependent intensity of this acoustic backscatter,[43,45,46] could also provide a quantitative measure of the degree of cartilage fibrillation. These methods might eliminate the requirement for controlled scanning across and perpendicular to the joint surface needed to acquire an optimal B-mode image. In a pilot study of the ultrasonic backscatter method, confocal microscopic imaging was used to measure surface roughness (5–100 μm) in unfixed specimens of human OA cartilage. The data suggested a good correlation between the reflected (backscattered) acoustic power and the roughness of the surface, arguing that this parameter might be useful for intra-articular sonographic evaluation of the joint surface.[46]

Several laboratories have evaluated the thickness of articular cartilage with B-mode ultrasound. The distance between the echo bands produced

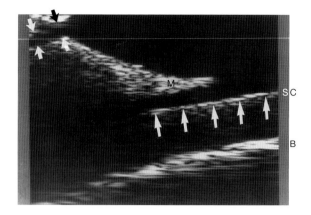

Fig. 11.58 Sonographic image of human tibial plateau obtained *ex vivo* with a high frequency (25 MHz) B-mode scanner. Note the wedge-shaped medial meniscus (M) and the echogenic band representing the subchondral bone (B). Echoes from the saline–cartilage interface (SC) delineate the smooth surface of the hypoechoic articular cartilage (arrows), except where the cartilage is eclipsed by the overlying meniscus. A defect produced by cutting the relatively echogenic meniscus with a scalpel is seen as an area of diminished echogenicity (short arrows) in the upper left corner of the figure.

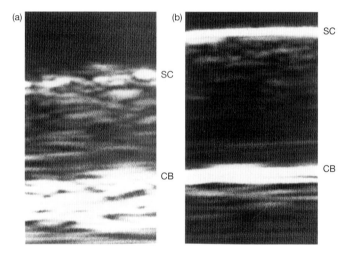

Fig. 11.59 High frequency (25 MHz) B-mode sonographic images, obtained *ex vivo*, of a specimen of cartilage and subchondral bone from a patient with OA (a) and from an individual with normal cartilage (b). Note the saline–cartilage (SC) and cartilage–bone (CB) echo bands. In the specimen from the patient with OA, the normally smooth SC interface is disrupted by superficial fibrillation of the articular surface and the cartilage is thinned.

by the saline–cartilage and cartilage–bone interfaces in images of a full-thickness specimen of normal articular cartilage has been shown to be proportional to the thickness of the tissue.[38,40] Measurements of this distance in scans obtained *in vitro* with a 25 MHz transducer permitted estimations of human cartilage thickness with a precision of approximately 0.1 mm and a mean coefficient of variation less than 2 per cent.[40] The thickness of OA cartilage determined from such scans showed a high degree of correlation ($r = 0.87$) with measurements of the distance between the surface and the zone of calcified cartilage in histological sections of the cartilage cut in the plane of the scan. Similar measurements of patellar cartilage thickness have been made with a 50 MHz scanning ultrasound microscope in a rat model of experimental OA,[44] and in normal rats of different ages.[31] The precision of the measurements was approximately 4 μm, and in the OA specimens, fibrillation between 40 and 50 μm deep was readily detected. For the relatively thin rat cartilage (160–400 μm), excellent correlation was seen between ultrasonic and histological measurements of cartilage thickness ($r = 0.89$). Additional work from the same laboratory has demonstrated the feasibility of computer-generated, three-dimensional reconstruction of rat patellar cartilage, and a high degree of correlation between manual and automated measurements of cartilage thickness.[48] Ultimately, the thickness and fibrillation of the articular cartilage may not be the optimal parameters for the ultrasonic assessment of osteoarthritic changes. For example, increases in internal echogenicity were seen in 50 MHz scans of rat patellar cartilage, which had been damaged and moderately thinned by intra-articular injection of iodoacetate.[42] Similarly, the internal echogenicity, or acoustic scatter, in images of bovine articular cartilage obtained with a 22 MHz scanner[47] increased by approximately 18 per cent, relative to the control, after depletion of the cartilage matrix proteoglycans by digestion of tissue samples with chondroitinase ABC. In contrast, collagenase digestion of the cartilage had no significant effect on internal echogenicity, although it markedly reduced the intensity of acoustic reflection at the articular surface. Digestion with either enzyme induced a significant decrease in cartilage stiffness in these experiments. Notably, the changes in the mechanical and acoustic properties of the cartilage described above occurred in the presence of a smooth, visually intact articular surface that would have appeared normal at the time of arthroscopy or by magnetic resonance imaging.

Summary and Conclusion

Diagnostic ultrasonic imaging, or ultrasonography, is a rapidly evolving imaging technique whose clinical value in the evaluation of some musculoskeletal problems has been established. Conventional external ultrasonography is useful for non-invasive examination of the articular and periarticular soft tissues but provides only limited information about the articular cartilage. Technological advances will be required if ultrasonography is to become a practical tool for the assessment of cartilage changes in patients with OA.

Recent studies support the view that high-frequency (e.g., 20–30 MHz) sonography may be useful in the evaluation of articular cartilage changes in OA. Considering the acoustic characteristics of connective tissue, this technique may be practical only when the transducer can be placed within the joint, that is, through an invasive procedure, probably coupled with arthroscopy.[49] Using such a device, the arthroscopist could supplement visual inspection of the joint with measurements of cartilage thickness, surface fibrillation, and other acoustic and/or biomechanical properties, and thereby substantially increase the information obtained by diagnostic arthroscopy of the OA knee.

Key points

1. Ultrasound can be used to produce full-thickness images of the articular cartilage and soft tissues, but is blocked by cortical bone.

2. Ultrasound images of normal articular cartilage show definite surface and cartilage–bone margins within which the non-calcified hyaline cartilage, like synovial fluid, appears hypoechoic or anechoic.

3. Ultrasound images of OA cartilage show loss of the normal sharpness of the synovial space–cartilage interface, diminished clarity of the band representing the hyaline articular cartilage, and thinning of the cartilage.

4. Additional technological development is needed before high-resolution ultrasound can be used *in vivo* to evaluate structural and compositional changes in articular cartilage in OA.

References

(An asterisk denotes recommended reading.)

1. Brandt, K.D. (1995). Toward pharmacologic modification of joint damage in osteoarthritis. *Ann Intern Med* **122**:874–5.

2. Lequesne, M., Brandt, K., Bellamy, N., Moskowitz, R., Menkes, C.J., Pelletier, J.P., *et al.* (1994). Guidelines for testing slow-acting and disease-modifying drugs in osteoarthritis. *J Rheumatol* **41**(Suppl.):65–71.

3. Adams, M.E. and Wallace, C.J. (1991). Quantitative imaging of osteoarthritis. *Sem Arthritis Rheum* **20**:26–39.

4. Gold, G.E., Beaulieu, C.F. (2001). Future of magnetic resonance imaging of articular cartilage. *Sem Musculoskeletal Radiol* **5**(4):313–27.

5. *Hashimoto, B.E., Kramer, D.J., and Wiitlal, L. (1999). Applications of musculoskeletal sonography. *J Clin Ultrasound* **27**:293–318.
   This is a good review of diagnostic ultrasonography.

6. Kaplan, P.A., Matamoros, A., Jr., and Anderson, J.C. (1990). Sonography of the musculoskeletal system. *Am J Roent* **155**:237–45.

7. Hussey, M. (1985). *Basic Physics and Technology of Medical Diagnostic Ultrasound*. New York: Elsevier, pp. 12–119.

8. Fornage, B.D. (1992). Musculoskeletal and soft tissue. In: C. A. Mittelstaedt (ed.), *General Ultrasound*. New York: Churchhill Livingstone, pp. 1–58.

9. Wells, P.N. (1993). Physics of ultrasound. In: P.A. Lewin and M.C. Ziskin (eds.), *Ultrasonic Exposimetry*. Boca Raton: CRC Press, pp. 9–45.

10. Harris, R.A., Follett, D.H., Halliwell, M., and Wells, P.N.T. (1991). Ultimate limits in ultrasonic imaging resolution. *Ultrasound Med Biol* **17**:547–58.

11. Newman, J.S., Adler, R.S., Bude, R.O., and Rubin, J. (1991). Detection of soft-tissue hyperemia: value of power Doppler sonography. *Am J Roent* **163**:385–9.

12. Kratochwil, A. (1978). Ultrasonic diagnosis in orthopaedic surgery. In: M. de Vlieger, J.H. Holmes, A. Kratochvil, *et al.* (eds), *Handbook of Clinical Ultrasound*. New York: J Wiley and Sons, pp. 945–53.

13. Sanders, R.C. (1984). Sonography of fat. In: R.C. Vaunder and M. Hill (eds.), *Ultrasound Annual 1984*. New York: Raven Press, pp. 71–94.

14. Turnbull, D.H., Starkoski, B.G., Harasiewicz, K.A., and Semple, J.L. (1995). A 40–100 MHZ B-scan ultrasound backscatter microscope for skin imaging. *Ultrasound Med Biol* **21**:79–88.

15. Grassi, W., Tittarelli, E., Blasetti, P., Pirani, O., and Cervini, C. (1995). Finger tendon involvement in rheumatoid arthritis. Evaluation with high-frequency sonography. *Arthritis Rheum* **38**:786–94.

16. Grassi, W., Filippucci, E., Farina, A., and Cervini, C. (2000). Sonographic imaging of the distal phalanx. *Sem Arthritis Rheum* **29**:379–84.

17. *Gibbon, W.W. and Wakefield, R.J. (1999). Ultrasound in inflammatory disease. *Radiol Clin NA* **37**:633–51.
   This paper provides a good review of the sonographic evaluation of synovitis and erosive arthropathy.

18. Koski, J.M. (2000). Ultrasound guided injections in rheumatology. *J Rheumatol* **7**:2131–8.

19. Fessell, D.P., Jacobson, J.A., Craig, J., Habra, G., Prasad, A., Radliff, A., and van Holsbeeck, M.T. (2000). Using sonography to reveal and aspirate joint effusions. *Am J Roent* **174**:1353–62.

20. Ostergaard, M., Court-Payen, M., Gideon, P., Wieslander, S., Cortsen, M., Lorenzen, I., *et al.* (1995). Ultrasonography in arthritis of the knee. A comparison with MR imaging. *Acta Radiol* **36**:19–26.

21. *Fiocco, U., Cozzi, L., Rubaltelli, L., Rigon, C., De Candia, A., Tregnaghi, A., Gallo, C., Favaro, M.A., Chieco-Bianchi, F., Baldovin, M., and Todesco, S. (1996). Long-term sonographic follow-up of rheumatoid and psoriatic proliferative knee joint synovitis. *Br J Rheumatol* **35**:155–63.
   This paper correlates ultrasonic and clinical findings in patients before and after synovectomy.

22. Derks, W.H.J., De Hooge, P., and Van Linge, B. (1986). Ultrasonographic detection of the patellar plica in the knee. *J Clin Ultrasound* **14**:355–62.

23. *Grassi, W., Lamanna, G., Farina, A., and Cervini, C. (1999). Sonographic imaging of normal and osteoarthritic cartilage. *Sem Arthritis Rheum* **28**:398–403.
   This paper includes state-of-the-art images of articular cartilage obtained with external ultrasonography in a clinical setting.

24. Adler, R.S. (1999). Future and new developments in musculoskeletal ultrasound. *Radiol Clin NA* **37**:623–31.

25. Newman, J.S., Laing, T.J., McCarthy, C.J., and Adler, R.S. (1996). Power Doppler sonography in synovitis: Assessment of therapeutic response-preliminary observations. *Radiology* **198**:582–4.

26. Giovagnorio, F., Martinoli, C., and Coari, G. (2001). Power Doppler sonography in knee arthritis—a pilot study. *Rheumatol Int* **20**:101–4.

27. McCune, W.J., Dedrick, D.K., Aisen, A.M., and MacGuire, A. (1990). Sonographic evaluation of osteoarthritic femoral condylar cartilage. Correlation with operative findings. *Clin Orthop* **254**:230–5.

28. Iagnocco, A., Coari, G., and Zappini, A. (1992). Sonographic evaluation of femoral condylar cartilage in osteoarthritis and rheumatoid arthritis. *Scand J Rheumatol* **21**:201–3.

29. Martino, F., Ettorre, G.C., Angelelli, G., *et al.* (1993). Validity of echographic evaluation of cartilage in gonarthrosis. *Clin Rheumatol* **12**:178–83.

30. Aisen, A., McCune, W.J., MacGuire, A., *et al.* (1984). Sonographic evaluation of the cartilage of the knee. *Radiology* **153**:781–4.

31. Cherin, E., Saied, A., Pellaumail, B., Loeuille, D., Laugier, P., Gillet, P., Netter, P., and Berger, G. (2001). Assessment of rat articular cartilage maturation using 50-MHz quantitative ultrasonography. *Osteoarthritis Cart* **9**:178–86.

32. Gerngross, H. and Sohn, C. (1992). Ultrasound scanning for the diagnosis of meniscal lesions of the knee joint. *Arthroscopy* **8**:105–10.

33. Jonsson, K., Buckwalter, K., Helvie, M., Niklason, L., and Martel, W. (1992). Precision of hyaline cartilage thickness measurements. *Acta Radiol* **33**:234–9.

34. Foldes, K., Balint, P., Gaal, M., Buchanan, W.W., and Balint, G.P. (1992). Nocturnal pain correlates with effusions in diseased hips. *J Rheumatol* **19**:1756–8.

35. Bierma-Zeinstra, S.M.A., Bohnen, A.M., Verhaar, J.A.N., Prins, A., Ginai-Karamat, A.Z., and Lameris, J.S. (2000). Sonography for hip joint effusion in adults with hip pain. *Ann Rheum Dis* **59**:178–82.

36. Ike, R.W. (1993). The role of arthroscopy in the differential diagnosis of osteoarthritis of the knee. *Rheum Dis Clin NA* **19**:673–96.

37. Adams, M.E. and Brandt, K.D. (1991). Hypertrophic repair of canine articular cartilage in osteoarthritis after anterior cruciate ligament transection. *J Rheumatol* **18**:428–35.

38. Rushfeldt, P.D. and Mann, R.W. (1981). Improved techniques for measuring *in vitro* the geometry and pressure distribution in the human acetabulum—Ultrasonic measurement of acetabular surfaces, sphericity and cartilage thickness. *J Biomech* **14**:253–60.

39. Sanghvi, N.T., Snoddy, A.M., Myers, S.L., Brandt, K.D., Reilly, C.R., and Franklin, T.D. Jr. (1990). Characterization of normal and osteoarthritic cartilage using 25 MHZ ultrasound. Ultrasonics, Ferroelectrics and Frequency Control Society 1990 Ultrasonics Symposium Proceedings, *Institute of Electronic and Electromechanical Engineering* **3**:1413–6.

40. Myers, S.L., Dines, K., Brandt, K.D., and Albrecht, M.E. (1993). Experimental assessment by high frequency ultrasound of articular cartilage thickness and osteoarthritic changes. *J Rheumatol* **22**:109–16.

41. Kim, H.K.W., Babyn, P.S., Harasiewicz, L., Pritzker, F.P.H., and Foster, F.S. (1995). Imaging of immature articular cartilage using ultrasound backscatter microsocopy at 50 MHz. *J Orthop Res* **13**:963–70.

42. Senzig, D.A. and Forster, F.K. (1992). Ultrasonic attenuation in articular cartilage. *J Acoust Soc Am* **92**:676–80.

43. Adler, R.S., Dedrick, D.K., Laing, T.J., Chiang, E.H., Meyer, C.R., Bland, P.H., *et al.* (1992). Quantitive assessment of cartilage surface roughness in osteoarthritis using high frequency ultrasound. *Ultrasound Med Biol* **18**:51–8.

44. Saied, A., Cherin, E., Gaucher, H., Laugier, P., Gillet, P., Floquet, J., Netter, P., and Berger, G. (1997). Assessment of articular cartilage and subchondral bone: Subtle and progressive changes in experimental osteoarthritis using 50 MHz echography in vitro. *J Bone Mineral Res* **12**:1378–86.

45. Chiang, E.H., Adler, R.S., Meyer, C.R., Rubin, J.M., Dedrick, D.K., and Laing, T.J. (1994). Quantitative assessment of surface roughness using backscattered ultrasound: the effects of finite surface curvature. *Ultrasound Med Biol* **20**:123–35.

46. Chiang, E.H., Liang, T.J., Meyer, C.R., Boes, J.L., Rubin, J.M., and Adler, R.S. (1997). Ultrasonic characterization of in vitro osteoarthritic articular cartilage with validation by confocal microscopy. *Ultrasound Med Biol* **23**:203–13.

47. Toyras, J., Rieppo, J., Nieminen, M.T., Helminen, H.J., and Jurvelin, J.S. (1999). Characterization of enzymatically induced degradation of articular cartilage using high frequency ultrasound. *Phys Med Biol* **44**:2723–33.

48. Lefebvre, F., Graillat, N., Cherin, E., Berger, G., and Saied, A. (1998). Automatic three-dimensional reconstruction and characterization of articular cartilage from high-resolution ultrasound acquisitions. *Ultrasound Med Biol* **9**:1369–81.

49. Disler, D.G., Raymond, E., May, D.A., Wayne, J.S., and McCauley, T.R. (2000). Articular cartilage defects: in vitro evaluation of accuracy and inter-observer reliability for detection and grading with US. *Radiology* **215**:846–51.

11.4.7 Defining and validating the clinical role of molecular markers in osteoarthritis

L. Stefan Lohmander and A. Robin Poole

Osteoarthritis is associated with a loss of the normal balance between synthesis and degradation of the structural components of the extracellular matrix that are necessary to provide articular cartilage and bone with their normal biomechanical and functional properties. Concomitantly, synovitis also develops which is usually much less pronounced than in rheumatoid arthritis (RA). These processes result in the destruction of joint cartilage, extensive remodeling of subchondral bone, and changes in the form and function of the affected joints, which cause pain and physical disability.

Current therapy of OA is largely symptom-based, and is focused on decreasing pain and improving function with analgesics, non-steroidal anti-inflammatory drugs, or arthroplasty. It is not disease modifying. However, new disease-modifying treatments have been introduced for the management of joint disease in RA[1,2] by blocking the action of the cytokines TNF-α or interleukin-1.[1,2] It is possible that the same type of treatment may decrease the rate of joint destruction in OA.

The ability to reproducibly and sensitively monitor disease activity, its progression, and outcome such as in interventional trials is critical to the development of new disease-modifying treatment strategies in OA. There are three general means by which OA can be assessed:

1. patient-related measures of joint pain, impairment and disability (algofunctional scores such as WOMAC[3] or KOOS,[4] and others);

2. measurements of the structural (anatomical) changes in the affected joints (plain radiographs,[5] magnetic resonance imaging,[6] arthroscopy,[7] high frequency ultrasound[8]); and

3. measurements of the disease process exemplified by changes in metabolism or functional properties of the articular cartilage, subchondral bone or other joint tissues (body fluid markers of cartilage and bone metabolism,[9] bone scintigraphy,[10] measurement of cartilage compression resistance by indentation or streaming potentials[11]).

These different dimensions of outcome are, in turn, related to the concept of defining an endpoint for use in measuring OA disease development or for use in a clinical trial when comparing two different treatments. What is the gold standard endpoint, what is the core measure? In the context of the clinical trial, the clinical endpoint(s) that measures how a patient feels, functions, or survives would appear to be most relevant. Other measures and endpoints may be relevant as well, but need to be validated against this gold standard for their value to be established, and be classified as surrogate outcome measures.

- ◆ Clinical endpoint—a characteristic or variable that measures how a patient feels, functions, or survives

- ◆ Biomarker—evaluated as an indicator of a biological, pathological, or other process, or response to a therapeutic intervention

- ◆ Surrogate endpoint—a measure or marker intended to substitute for a clinical endpoint

All existing measures of structural change and of the disease process in OA (see above) may be defined as biomarkers, representing potential surrogate endpoints for clinical outcome. However, not even plain radiography, used for many years to monitor development of OA,[12,13] fulfils the criteria of a validated surrogate measure for clinical outcome in OA. Even with improved techniques for patient positioning and imaging, plain X-ray examination remains at best an indirect measure of the consequences of articular cartilage destruction. It is not a measure of the disease process or of the product of the process. Magnetic resonance imaging will no doubt find increasing use as a measure of joint changes in OA. Until methods are clearly established to monitor joint cartilage quality or composition by MRI, the technique suffers from the same weakness as X-ray examination: it provides only an indirect measure of the current disease process, in that it documents outcome, not process.

The validation of a biomarker as a surrogate endpoint/measure is a complex process. If one critical question is how well a putative surrogate endpoint reflects patient preference and quality of life, an equally critical question is how well it accounts for adverse effects that may cancel out all or part of the apparent treatment benefit. Further, even if a surrogate endpoint/measure is identified and validated, beneficial effects may occur via pathways that do not include the surrogate.

- ◆ How well do surrogate endpoints and measures reflect patient preference and quality of life?

- ◆ Beneficial effects may occur through a pathway that does not include surrogate endpoint

- ◆ Surrogates do not always account for adverse effects that may cancel out all or part of treatment benefit

Methods that could provide rapid information about the metabolic processes in arthritic joint cartilage, which would predispose or lead to change, would thus be of considerable value to evaluate the role of new and existing interventions in OA.[13]

The destruction of joint cartilage and associated remodeling of bone in OA involves changes in the degradation, synthesis, and the altered release of matrix molecules, which are reflected by their presence, usually intact or fragmented, in joint fluid, blood, and urine. Such molecular biomarkers of cartilage and bone matrix turnover, and the proteases, growth factors, and cytokines involved in these events, could be used in diagnosis, prognosis, and to monitor joint disease activity and treatment in conditions such as RA and OA, and to identify disease mechanisms at the molecular level. A number of reviews and examples (Table 11.22) are available.[9,14–22]

Although many publications have described the altered content of molecular markers of cartilage, bone, or synovial metabolism in joint fluid, serum, and urine in OA, their validation as surrogate measures in OA is still awaited.

The word 'biomarker' has been used in many different contexts in OA. Cytokines, growth factors, acute phase proteins, enzymes and their inhibitors, cartilage and bone matrix components and their fragments, antibodies to cartilage collagen, and membrane proteins of chondrocytes have been proposed as biomarkers for OA. We will, in this chapter, focus on biomarkers that are directly associated with the turnover of joint tissue, such as matrix molecules and proteases that may be involved in their generation. We will review aspects of current research on these 'molecular markers of OA,' and discuss the requirements for a marker to fulfil its promise as a surrogate of a clinical outcome/endpoint.

The relationship between marker concentration and joint pathology

Our understanding of the relationship between changes in marker concentrations in a body fluid compartment and changes in skeletal matrix metabolism is limited. For example, the concentration of a marker of cartilage matrix degradation in joint fluid may depend not only on the rate of degradation of cartilage matrix, but also on other factors such as the rate of elimination and clearance of the molecule or fragment in question from the joint fluid compartment,[23] the amount of cartilage matrix remaining in the joint[24] and whether it is a product of the degradation of a newly synthesized molecule, the rate of its synthesis, and the balance between these two events (Figs 11.60 and 11.61). Since the clearance of macromolecules from the joint fluid compartment to the lymphatics or directly to capillaries may be increased by inflammation,[23,25–27] differences in the rates of release of markers from joint cartilage into joint fluid between control joints and diseased joints with inflammation may actually be underestimated. An estimate of the degradation rate of a cartilage matrix molecule in arthritis, based on the joint fluid concentration of its fragments, is therefore very difficult to achieve and the changes must be seen as relative at best.

1. Is the relationship known between the marker concentration and the metabolic turnover in joint cartilage or bone or synovium of the molecule in question?

2. Concentrations of a marker in different body fluid compartments such as joint fluid, blood, or urine is influenced by rate of clearance from one compartment and delivery into another. Synovial inflammation, liver, and kidney functions may determine this.

3. The specificity of the marker molecule for a specific tissue such as bone or joint cartilage or synovium. Can diseased cartilage or bone be distinguished?

4. Metabolism and partial degradation of markers and their fragments en route may change concentrations and the structure of fragments from one compartment to another. This may influence detection.

In spite of these confounding factors, marker concentrations in joint fluid, in general, do indeed reflect changes in the turnover of cartilage and bone matrix molecules in OA.[9] For example, the temporal changes in joint fluid concentrations of fragments of aggrecan, cartilage oligomeric matrix protein (COMP), type II collagen, collagen II C-propeptide, and bone sialoprotein after joint injury and in developing OA, are consistent with the changes in metabolic rate observed for these molecules in animal models in vivo and in human osteoarthritic cartilage in vitro[9,14–22,24,28–39] and with increased human subchondral bone turnover in vivo.[39] Loss of proteoglycan into synovial fluid in an experimental model of OA may not, however, always reflect cartilage change.[37]

The identification of the specific source of the molecule/fragment can be a problem with regard to both process and tissue. An increased rate of release of a marker may occur as a result of a net increase in degradation (resulting in net loss), or as a result of an increased rate of degradation in the presence of an increased rate of synthesis. We therefore need markers that are specific for both degradative and synthetic events. An example of the former is the cleavage of type II collagen,[33,36,40–43] and of the latter the

Table 11.22 Molecular markers in synovial fluid, serum, or urine in human osteoarthritis

Marker[*]	Process[**]	OA markers in synovial fluid[†‡] (references)	OA markers in serum or urine[†‡] (references)
Cartilage			
Aggrecan			
Core protein epitopes	Degradation	⇑ (24, 28, 32, 80, 104)	
Core protein cleavage site specific neoepitopes	Degradation	⇑ (89–92)	
Keratan sulfate epitopes	Degradation	⇑ (45, 106, 123)	⇑ ⇔ ⇓ (45, 71, 73–75 105, 106)
Chondroitin sulfate epitopes (846, 3B3, 7D4, etc.)	Synthesis/degradation	⇑ or ⇓ (32, 45, 115–117, 123)	⇑ ⇔ (45)
Chondroitin sulfate ratio 6S/4S	Synthesis/degradation	⇓ (107, 123)	
Small proteoglycans	Synthesis/degradation	⇑ (108)	
Cartilage collagens			
Type II collagen C-propeptide	Synthesis	⇑ (30, 34, 41, 44)	⇓ (34)
Type II collagen α chain fragments and neoepitopes	Synthesis/degradation	⇑ (40)	⇑ (19, 42, 43, 93)
Synovium			
Hyaluronan	Synthesis/release		⇑ ⇔ (58–60)
Matrix metalloproteinases and inhibitors			
Stromelysin (MMP-3)	Synthesis/secretion	⇑ (28, 72, 110, 123)	⇑ ⇔ (109, 110)
Interstitial collagenase (MMP-1)	Synthesis/secretion	⇑ (28, 110)	
Tissue inhibitors of metalloproteinases	Synthesis/secretion	⇑ (28, 110)	⇑ (111)
Type III collagen N-propeptide	Synthesis/degradation	⇑ (112, 114)	⇑ (112–114)
Cartilage/Synovium			
Cartilage oligomeric matrix protein (COMP)	Synthesis/degradation	⇑ (29, 102, 115)	⇑ ⇔ (81–85, 102, 115)
YKL-40 or gp-39	Synthesis/degradation	⇑ (116–118)	⇑ (116–118)
Cytokine/growth factor/acute phase protein			
Tumor necrosis factor p75 receptor	Regulation of TNFα activity		⇑ (77)
C-Reactive protein	Systemic inflammation		⇑ (77, 102, 119, 120)
Transforming growth factor β_1	Can induce inflammation and/or skeletal turnover		⇑ (77, 102)
Bone			
Bone sialoprotein	Synthesis/degradation	⇑ ⇔ (31)	⇑ ⇔ (83, 84)
Osteocalcin	Synthesis	⇑ (112, 121, 122)	⇑ ⇓ (112, 121, 122)
3-hydroxypyridinium crosslinks	Degradation of type I collagen in bone		⇑ (15, 18, 19, 20, 97, 98, 99, 113)

⇑ ⇔ ⇓, increased, unchanged, or decreased concentrations, respectively, compared with healthy controls.

[*] Markers have been assigned a predominant tissue source with regard to marker occurrence in joint fluid, serum, and urine.

[**] As discussed in this chapter (see e.g. Figs 11.60–11.62) some individual marker levels may change both as a result of changes in synthesis and in degradation.

[†] A predominant increase or decrease, respectively, is assigned on the basis of representative publications on 'active', not end-stage OA.

[‡] Some representative literature references are given, but this is not intended to be a comprehensive review of the literature.

synthesis of type II procollagen where the release of the C-propeptide reflects its synthesis.[30,34,44]

Even with a molecular marker being unequivocally identified as a consequence of specific proteolytic events, the specific process or source needs to be carefully considered. For example, fragments could result from the degradation of a newly synthesized matrix molecule that has not yet been incorporated into a functional matrix, a molecule recently incorporated into cell-associated matrix, or be derived from a resident matrix molecule that is a critical functional part of the mature matrix (Fig. 11.62). The ensuing consequences for cartilage function may well be different. In general, markers are not specific to these processes, perhaps with the exception of collagen II and aggrecan cleavage markers. Specific neoepitope containing degradation fragments containing crosslinks may be specific for the degradation and loss of 'mature', functional type II collagen from the tissue

matrix.[37,38,40,42–44] In contrast, other type II collagen fragments not containing crosslinks may result from degradation of both newly synthesized and mature collagen, particularly in OA where this has been observed.[38,39]

A largely unresolved question is the specific cartilage matrix compartment (pericellular, territorial, or interterritorial matrix), from which a molecular marker present in joint fluid, blood, or urine may originate. Newly synthesized molecules are mainly seen in pericellular sites. Metabolic rates of these cartilage matrix compartments may differ significantly. Assay of some low-abundance epitopes associated with altered sulfation of chondroitin sulfate on the proteoglycan aggrecan in OA may help identify populations of newly synthesized aggrecan molecules.[14,45–47]

That molecules or their fragments, which are present in joint fluid and which we know are normally resident in cartilage, may primarily be generated locally from joint cartilage, may or may not be true. It relies, in turn, on the assumption that the molecule in question is significantly more abundant in healthy or arthritic cartilage than in any other joint tissue, or that its metabolic rate in cartilage is higher than in other joint tissues. Careful comparisons within patients of joint fluid versus serum concentrations of a marker may help in determining its source.[45] While it may be true that cartilage contains a far greater total mass of joint aggrecan compared to, for example, the meniscus,[24] the total mass of COMP in the menisci of the knee may approach that in the joint cartilage of the knee.[48] COMP is produced in increased amounts in OA[49] but it is also synthesized by synovial cells exposed to cytokines such as interleukin-1.[50,51] Synovitis in OA has a significant effect on serum COMP.[52] Therefore, its significance as a marker of a specific event in a joint tissue remains unclear. However, this

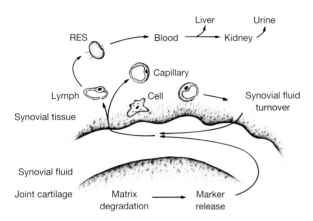

Fig. 11.60 Molecular fragments generated by degradation of cartilage matrix, or released from synovial tissue or bone into the joint fluid compartment are cleared by bulk flow through the synovial tissue matrix into the lymphatic vessels or directly into blood vessels.[23] Some fragments are eliminated or further degraded in the regional lymph nodes. Many, and possibly most products of cartilage matrix metabolism are taken up and degraded in the liver, some in the kidney (e.g. osteocalcin). Some specific types of fragments, such as collagen cross-links, are not further metabolized, and are found in urine.

Source: Taken from Ref. 14 with permission.

does not detract from the overall value of COMP in identifying pathological changes in joint disease, which may be associated with inflammation. The same applies to YKL-40 or gp-39, a glycoprotein produced by chondrocytes and synovial cells in OA.[53–55] Since its content in serum is closely correlated with C-reactive protein[55] it may be a measure of synovitis, as in the case of COMP. Hyaluronan concentrations in serum, which are correlated with synovitis in RA,[56] is also correlated with joint-space width and disease progression in OA,[57,58] where it is frequently increased.[59,60] Both chondrocytes and synovial cells produce MMP-3 (stromelysin-1),[61,62] but the cell number and rates of synthesis in synovial tissue may be higher in the inflamed synovium than in cartilage, so that a significant proportion of the MMP-3 detected in joint fluid originates in the synovium. The specific source of the molecule or molecular fragment identified in joint fluid may, thus, not always be entirely evident, and is likely often more complex than originally proposed.

The question of the tissue source(s) of markers of cartilage metabolism is even more relevant for markers assayed in serum or urine samples (Fig. 11.61). Canine joint cartilage represents less than 10 per cent of all the hyaline cartilages,[63] so what is measured in a body fluid may originate from many sites in the body. Sources of the marker other than cartilage must also be considered. In monoarticular disease, any markers released from the affected joint are mixed with markers released from normal cartilages. Hence, determinations of cartilage markers in serum or urine may be of more use in polyarticular or systemic disease, and may be less likely to be useful in monoarticular disease where measurement of joint fluid may provide a more accurate insight into the local pathology. However, experimental studies in the rabbit have revealed that surgical induction of monoarticular experimental OA is indeed reflected by elevations in serum of the collagenase generated cleavage epitope in type II collagen (S Laverty, AR Poole, et al., unpublished). This holds some promise for serum analyses of biomarkers also in localized joint disease.

As discussed above, factors that affect the generation and clearance of the marker from the joint fluid, serum, or urine compartment must be carefully considered in interpreting marker data. Physical activity can change the concentrations of some markers in both synovial fluid and serum.[64–66] Circadian variations in metabolism lead to alterations in the generation of bone derived urinary collagen crosslinks and osteocalcin.[67,68] The lymph nodes and the liver are responsible for the elimination of a great part of the molecular fragments released from cartilage and other connective tissues. Again, any change in the function of these organ systems will affect the

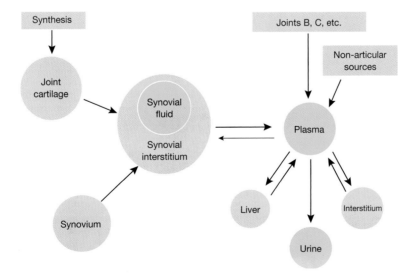

Fig. 11.61 Biomarker concentrations in body fluid compartments are influenced by many processes.

Source: Modified from Ref. 23.

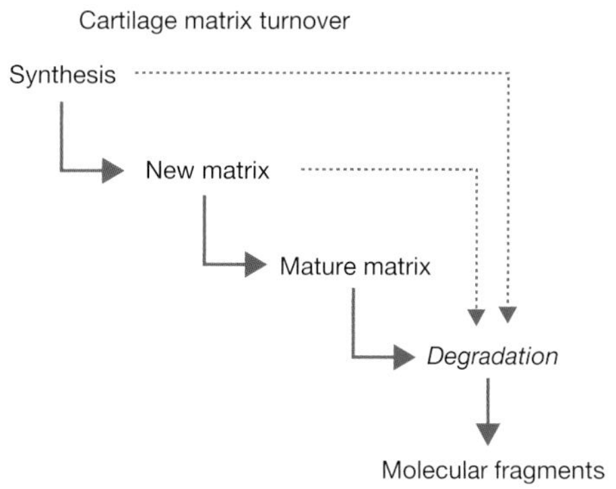

Fig. 11.62 Fragments of cartilage matrix molecules may be generated by degradation of: newly synthesized molecules that are never incorporated into the functional matrix, molecules that have recently been incorporated into a functional matrix, and molecules that have been long-time members of the 'resident' functional matrix. At the current time, it is not always possible to distinguish these different sources of fragments. Another source of heterogeneity is the origin of fragments from pericellular, territorial, and interterritorial matrix, as well as from superficial and deep layers of the joint cartilage.

clearance of cartilage markers from serum[17,18] (Figs 11.60 and 11.61). For example, the serum concentration of hyaluronan is greatly affected by liver function since this is its principal organ for clearance. But its serum concentration is also influenced by peristalsis since it is most concentrated in the lymphatics draining the intestine.[69] It should also be remembered that biomarkers might vary in content with age, with respect to menopause, and between the sexes.[17,18,70,71] Carefully matched populations are thus required to control for such differences. It is therefore important to characterize variations in marker levels dependent upon factors other than disease.

Potential uses of markers

The demands on a marker may differ, depending on its usage—whether it is to be used as a research tool, a diagnostic, prognostic, or an evaluative test. For example, research opportunities are offered by the use of markers to investigate interrelationships between proteases, inhibitors, proteolysis, and inflammation and between the synthesis and degradation of a molecule, as in the case of type II collagen. Analyses of joint fluids in OA have provided hypothesis-generating insights into the dynamic interactions between matrix molecules and events in which they are involved, and have provided valuable insights into the pathobiology and dynamics of disease development.

The *diagnostic test* focuses on the ability to detect differences between affected and non-affected individuals, often expressed in terms of sensitivity and specificity of the test. Markers could serve as diagnostic tests in helping to distinguish joints with OA from unaffected joints or other joint diseases. The concentration of keratan sulfate in serum was originally suggested to serve as a diagnostic test for generalized OA.[73] Subsequent experience has not fulfilled this promise,[45,74] although this marker reflects altered cartilage proteoglycan degradation in specific situations including familial OA.[22,75,76] A considerable overlap exists between affected and non-affected individuals for most markers. Recent results suggest good discrimination between OA patients and controls by analysis of a group of serum markers that include the 846 epitope of aggrecan, the tumor necrosis factor p75 receptor, transforming growth factor receptor, and C-reactive protein, pointing to the differences in skeletal and systemic cytokine activity in these patient groups.[77] Other studies have shown differences in knee joint fluid concentrations of aggrecan fragments, COMP fragments, and matrix metalloproteinases and their inhibitors between healthy reference groups, RA, reactive arthritis, and OA.[21,28,29,32,78,79] While these investigations show

significant differences of mean values between the study groups with only moderate overlap, interpretation is confounded by the fact that comparisons between groups are cross-sectional and retrospective.[17,18] These studies should therefore be regarded only as hypothesis-generating, and will require confirmation in prospective studies.

A marker might also be used for a test evaluating *disease severity* rather than its presence or absence. In OA, disease severity (or stage) is measured, for example, by the Kellgren-Lawrence grade of radiological changes (which measures joint remodeling as well as destruction); by the amount of cartilage loss measured at arthroscopy, or by the patient's degree of functional impairment. Several reports have suggested that assay of molecular markers of cartilage metabolism may provide complementary information on joint disease stage.[24,80,81] While further experience in this area is needed, molecular markers clearly have the potential to provide unique information on joint cartilage quality not currently available by other modalities of staging.

Assays of molecular markers developed for patients with arthritis have also been promoted as *prognostic markers* and tested to see whether they predict the onset or progression of OA. For example, it was shown that levels of serum hyaluronan (but not keratan sulfate) in patients with clinically diagnosed knee OA at study entry, predicted subsequent progression of knee OA at the 5-year follow-up.[58] An increase in serum COMP during the first year after study entry was associated with radiographic progression of OA.[82–84] Similar data for disease progression were shown for bone sialoprotein, which was inversely correlated with bone changes in OA, including osteophytes.[84]

Studies on patients with early RA have revealed that elevated serum levels of COMP and reduced levels of the chondroitin sulfate epitope 846 can distinguish the rate of progression of skeletal damage.[85] Such reports describe results obtained on well-defined patient groups but these are of limited size, and often do not specify the strength of the relationship between marker levels and disease progression. However, they indicate that opportunities exist for the use of prognostic markers in longitudinal studies of larger patient cohorts.

Measures of disease dynamics that evaluate the ongoing repair and degradative processes occurring within a joint might prove to be of value as prognostic measures. Thus, the measurement in OA knee joint fluids of the marker of type II collagen synthesis has been shown to correlate with mechanical risk factors for knee OA such as obesity and varus alignment.[86]

Markers offer the opportunity to predict responses to therapy. For example, the collagenase generated cleavage neoepitope of cartilage type II collagen that is released into serum has been shown to correlate with experimental chondroprotection in a polyarthritis model in rats.[41] Similarly, longitudinal changes in cartilage turnover caused by intra-articular treatment with steroids can be determined.[87] In patients with RA, therapy with methotrexate has been shown to reduce a marker of bone resorption, suggesting suppression of bone erosions.[88] Studies of this kind are of importance in drug development in the preclinical as well as in the clinical trial setting and in examining responses to future treatment in individual patients. If such studies can be accelerated by use of prognostic surrogate markers for clinical endpoints, the benefits are considerable.

Structural analysis of molecules and their fragments released from or remaining in the cartilage matrix can yield important information on matrix turnover and the protease(s) responsible. Results obtained on aggrecan fragments may serve as an example. The cleavages of core protein that generate the fragments released into joint fluid, and of those remaining in the matrix, are consistent with two different types of proteolytic activity in cartilage matrix in OA.[89–91] One of these activities generates fragments consistent with the action of a 'classic' matrix metalloprotease such as MMP-3, while the cleavages that generate other fragments are consistent with the action of other proteases called aggrecanases.[91,92] Similar and ongoing structure analyses of cleavage products of cartilage collagens, proteoglycans, and matrix proteins have yielded additional information on the role of different proteases in disease development, critical for our understanding of cartilage degradation in OA.[33,40,49,91–93] This information may in turn be used to predict responsiveness to treatment specific for a prote-olytic activity such as that of a collagenase or an aggrecanase. The useful-ness of this concept relies on the clear demonstration and knowledge of disease mechanisms, and on the availability of agents specific for these processes.

The *evaluative test*, on the other hand, focuses on the ability of the marker to monitor change over time in the individual patient, often expressed as sensitivity to change or effect size. The effect size is dependent on the amount of change for the test, divided by the baseline variation in the test. Knowledge of longitudinal within-patient variability and correla-tions with other measures of disease activity is thus important, although there are only few published studies.[72] Molecular markers that can monitor a response to therapy in OA, may be valuable as sensitive surrogate meas-ures of outcome in therapeutic trials, in the ideal case providing 'early warning' and indications of clinical outcome. Here, advances in our under-standing of disease mechanisms assisted by molecular analysis of cleavage products released in and from human cartilage and bone, as outlined in the preceding paragraph, will be critical. Obviously, with the current lack of known disease-modifying treatments in OA, the validation of this particu-lar role of molecular markers still remains. Experience from the treatment of rheumatoid patients is also limited, but suggests that cartilage and bone molecular markers are responsive to treatment.[79,88,94] Randomized, con-trolled clinical trials of new disease-modifying treatments of OA and RA will represent important opportunities to validate OA markers as surrogate outcome measures. Such studies are underway with the collagenase-generated cleavage neoepitope of type II collagen in patients with RA treated with a disease-modifying antibody to TNF-α. Responses following initiation of treatment have been identified and are being related to clinical responses (Poole, A.R., Ionescu, M., and Keystone E., unpublished). Similar investigations with bone markers in the treatment of patients with osteo-porosis (OP) have demonstrated their prognostic value in determining therapeutic responses.[95]

Given that markers reflect the dynamic state of cartilage or bone metabolism, it is likely that markers will be used clinically to evaluate the dynamic changes in disease as in OP,[95,96] as prognostic tools to identify those at high risk of rapid progression, or as measures of response to treat-ment, to identify the responders and assess the degree of response. Other potential uses of markers (e.g. as diagnostic tests) will possibly be less attractive.

Markers in osteoporosis—a paradigm for osteoarthritis?

Biochemical markers of bone formation and bone resorption that utilize commercially available assays based on serum and urine, have a proven value in assessing disease activity and responses to therapy in OP. They are primarily indices of bone turnover, the dynamic balance between resorp-tion and formation of bone matrix, something that is also fundamentally altered in OA, particularly in subchondral bone. As will likely be the case for OA, comparisons of different assays that presumably measure the same type of bone activity such as resorption, are not necessarily consistent in their sensitivity to change or discriminant validity. Some markers are measured with more precision than others; others may be more specific for certain bone locations, and still others may have variable rates of metabolism by liver and other organs and may therefore not always accurately reflect bone turnover. Despite these limitations, bone marker studies have been used to identify women with and at risk for OP, high bone turnover states, and to follow treatment, especially with therapy aimed at diminishing bone turnover.[95,96]

In transferring the concepts of OP to OA, several caveats are in order: (1) Alterations in subchondral bone turnover in OA, while not necessarily systemic as in OP, can be measured in serum and urine.[97–100] Cartilage turnover in a single joint may not be so easily detected in serum and may

require synovial fluid sampling. (2) Variations in clearance from synovial fluid caused by varying degrees of inflammation, is a concern unique to arthritis. (3) As discussed in a previous section of this chapter, a number of practical barriers will make it harder to validate the clinical usefulness of markers in OA compared to OP. Obtaining synovial fluid is more difficult, and having access to persons to determine expected levels of markers in synovial fluid in non-diseased joints is extremely difficult. Serum levels would be much easier to determine in normals, but may not be as relevant unless they reflect more fundamental differences in skeletal turnover, which may in fact predispose towards the development of OA rather than being a consequence of the disease. Such an example is the reduction in the serum content of the C-propeptide of type II collagen seen in patients with OA, which is in contrast to the elevations seen in OA cartilage.[34] (4) Precise and accurate bone mineral density assessments in OP to provide a very well-defined endpoint have provided a consensus 'gold standard' that has enabled drug development and simplified prognostic studies of bone markers. Similar quantitative measures of disease status in an OA joint are not yet possible, since such a 'gold standard' endpoint does not as yet exist for this disease.

Markers may therefore be more difficult to validate and use clinically in OA than they have been in OP. (5) A further obvious hindrance in OA is the lack of agents that can predictably and reproducibly alter the metabolism of joint cartilage, whereas PTH and other hormones, steroids, and bisphos-phonates can produce clear changes in bone turnover.

Validating markers

Different aspects of validity are discussed in more detail in a previous review.[101] As an example, we suggest criteria to validate a prognostic marker (Table 11.23). Each of the criteria is necessary but not sufficient on its own, for validation. First, a prognostic marker should have a strong biological rationale. The marker should be identifiable in and specific for cartilage or bone or be a protease, cytokine, or growth factor, or some other such molecule. A prognostic marker should correlate strongly with subse-quent clinical, patient relevant change of OA in an individual (see above). If the level of a marker is abnormal at baseline, then the risk of subsequent joint deterioration may be magnified. The evaluation of the course of OA should be made by measures that are accepted and independent of the marker. The marker should be detectable in all OA patients or their joints and should correlate with other appropriate measures of disease dynamics, if these are available. Importantly, some markers may identify skeletal changes or molecular processes that are not measurable by other means at this time, so a lack of clinical correlations is not necessarily a negative. If joint biology suggests that a marker is relevant at all disease stages, the marker should be

Table 11.23 Suggested criteria for validating a marker of OA prognosis—all are necessary

1. Clear biological rationale (face validity). Marker identifiable in cartilage, synovium, or bone. The marker's role in pathogenesis of OA is at least partly understood.

2. Marker measured at baseline in a body fluid predicts the course of OA (predictive validity). The course of OA at baseline and follow-up is determined independently of marker measurement using conventional clinical means.

3. Marker present in sufficient concentrations in appropriate tissue or fluid from patients with OA. Correlates with other measures of disease dynamics (construct validity).

4. Marker validated in patients with spectrum of mild/severe disease and OA of different etiologies (e.g. post-traumatic vs primary) (content validity).

5. Marker measurement is reliable (reproducible) and described in sufficient detail so as to be replicable by others.

found in identifiable concentrations in those with different stages of disease and disease of different etiologies.

It is possible that measurement of a combination of markers, or ratios between markers, will prove to be more useful than one single marker.[12,13,18,20,77,102] Further, while 'snap-shot' measurement values of biomarkers are often used to compare with other outcomes, such as loss of joint cartilage mass by radiography, it is possible that measuring the 'area under the curve' generated by several timed measurements may compare better to cumulative cartilage loss.

Markers might also serve as valuable predictors of responsiveness to treatment. Such a putative marker should be assayed first at baseline (more than one measurement may be necessary to identify this) and then in a longitudinal manner following treatment. Those who 'respond' to treatment, defined by the marker or independently of the marker, may have a different marker level at baseline than those who did not respond to treatment. For a marker of treatment response, measures at baseline and after treatment must be obtained. Normalization or change in the level of marker may occur in those who respond to treatment. Thus, markers should be capable of indicating an effect of the treatment such as decreased degradation or enhanced matrix synthesis.

For all suggested uses of markers, but perhaps in particular for markers used to monitor treatment response, and to help identify adverse side effects, we shall require knowledge of the variability both over time in the individual and between individuals in representative and stable cohorts of appropriate size. Such data can be used in power analyses to calculate the required number of patients and the required response to treatment in a clinical trial setting. Only few such data have yet been presented.[72,103] Similarly, we will need marker data for age- and gender-matched groups of joint-healthy and arthritic individuals at different stages of disease development. On the basis of such data, sensitivity and specificity for diagnostic tests may be calculated. Again, only few such calculations have been presented.[21] The future use of markers for any of the uses proposed here will, finally, require the general availability of both reproducible assays (and standards) that measure known molecules or fragments thereof in a reproducible and accurate manner. A detailed knowledge of the molecular events they measure and how these are related to the pathology of OA is essential.

Conclusion

In conclusion, molecular markers for OA could serve different purposes. Since markers reflect ongoing dynamic changes associated with the skeleton as a whole as well as with joint disease, they are likely to serve as measures of prognosis and responses to treatment, as well as a means of gaining valuable insights into the pathobiology of this joint disease and identifying disease subsets. Obviously, some markers may serve multiple functions. To function adequately in the study and treatment of OA, they should meet a clearly defined and generally accepted set of standards. It is only when these markers have met such criteria that they will be acceptable to the research and clinical community and will become more widely used.

Acknowledgements

The Swedish Medical Research Council, Lund University Medical Faculty and Hospital, the King Gustaf V 80-year Fund, Kock Foundation (to LSL), and Shriners Hospitals for Children, Canadian Institutes of Health Research, Canadian Arthritis Network and National Institute of Ageing (NIH) (to ARP).

References

1. Jiang, Y., Genant, H.K., Watt, I., *et al.* (2000). A multicenter, double-blind, dose-ranging, randomized, placebo-controlled study of recombinant human interleukin-1 receptor antagonist in patients with rheumatoid arthritis. Radiologic progression and correlation of Genant and Larsen scores. *Arthritis Rheum* **43**:1001–9.

2. Lipsky, P., van der Heijde, D., St. Clair, E.W., *et al.* (2000). Infliximab and methotrexate in the treatment of rheumatoid arthritis. *N Engl J Med* **343**:1594–602.

3. Bellamy, N., Buchanan, W.W., Goldsmith, C.H., Campbell, J., and Stitt, L.W. (1988). Validation study of WOMAC: A health status instrument for measuring clinically important patient relevant outcomes to antirheumatic drug therapy in patients with osteoarthritis of the hip or knee. *J Rheumatol* **15**:1833–40.

4. Roos, E.M., Roos, H.P., and Lohmander, L.S. (1999). WOMAC osteoarthritis index—additional dimensions for use in subjects with post-traumatic osteoarthritis of the knee. *Osteoarthritis Cart* **7**:216–21 www.koos.nu.

5. Spector, T.D. and Cooper, C. (1993). Radiographic assessment of osteoarthritis in population studies: whither Kellgren and Lawrence? *Osteoarth Cart* **1**:203–6.

6. Peterfy, C.G. (2001). Role of MR imaging in clinical research studies. *Sem Musculoskelet Radiol* **5**(4):365–78.

7. Dougados, M., Ayral, X., Listrat, V., *et al.* (1994). The SFA system for assessing articular cartilage lesions at arthroscopy of the knee. *Arthroscopy* **10**:69–77.

8. Myers, S., Dine, K., Albrecht, M., Brandt, D., Wu, D., and Brandt, K. (1995). Experimental assessment by high frequency ultrasound of articular cartilage thickness and osteoarthritic changes. *J Rheumatol* **22**:109–16.

9. Lohmander, L.S. (1994). Articular cartilage and osteoarthrosis—The role of molecular markers to monitor breakdown, repair and disease. *J Anatomy* **184**:477–92.

10. Dieppe, P., Cushnagan, J., Young, P., and Kirwan, J. (1993). Prediction of the progression of joint space narrowing in osteoarthritis of the knee by bone scintigraphy. *Ann Rheum Dis* **52**:557–63.

11. Bonassar, L.J., Frank, E.H., Murray, J.C., *et al.* (1995). Changes in cartilage composition and physical properties due to stromelysin degradation. *Arthritis Rheum* **38**:173–83.

12. Dieppe, P. (1995). Recommended methodology for assessing the progression of osteoarthritis of the hip and the knee. *Osteoarthritis Cart* **3**:73–7.

13. Dieppe, P., Brandt, K.D., Lohmander, L.S., and Felson, D. (1995). Detecting and measuring disease modification in osteoarthritis—The need for standardised methodology. *J Rheumatol* **22**:201–3.

14. Lohmander, L.S. (1991). Markers of cartilage metabolism in arthrosis. A review. *Acta Orthop Scand* **62**:623–32.

15. Poole, A.R. (1994). Skeletal and inflammation markers in aging and osteoarthritis. Implications for early diagnosis and monitoring of the effects of therapy. In: D Hammerman (ed.), *Osteoarthritis: Public Health Implications for an Aging Population*. Baltimore: Johns Hopkins University Press, pp. 187–214.

16. Saxne, T. and Heinegård, D. (1995). Matrix proteins: potentials as body fluid markers of changes in the metabolism of cartilage and bone in arthritis. *J Rheumatol* **22**(Suppl. 43):71–4.

17. Lohmander, L.S., Saxne, T., and Heinegård, D (eds). (1995). Molecular markers of joint and skeletal diseases. *Acta Orthop Scand* **66**(suppl. 266):1–212.

18. Poole, A.R. (1999). NIH White Paper: Biomarkers, The Osteoarthritis Initiative. A basis for discussion. www.nih.gov/niams/news/oisg

19. Garnero, P., Rousseau, J.C., and Delmas, P.D. (2000). Molecular basis and clinical use of biochemical markers of bone, cartilage, and synovium in joint diseases. *Arthritis Rheum* **43**:953–68.

20. Otterness, I.G. and Saltarelli, M.J. (2000). Using molecular markers to monitor osteoarthritis. In: G.C. Tsokos *et al.* (eds), *Modern Therapeutics in Rheumatic Diseases*. Totowa, New Jersey: Humana Press pp. 215–36.

21. Lohmander, L.S., Roos, H., Dahlberg, L., and Lark, M.W. (1995). The role of molecular markers to monitor disease, intervention and cartilage breakdown in osteoarthritis. *Acta Orthop Scand* **66**(Suppl. 266):84–7.

22. Thonar, E.J-M.A., Shinmei, M., and Lohmander, L.S. (1993). Body fluid markers of cartilage changes in osteoarthritis. *Rheum Dis Clin NA* **19**:635–57.

23. Simkin, P.A. and Bassett, J.E. (1995). Cartilage matrix molecules in serum and synovial fluid. *Curr Opin Rheumatol* **7**:346–51.

24. Dahlberg, L., Ryd, L., Heinegård, D., and Lohmander, L.S. (1992). Proteoglycan fragments in joint fluid—influence of arthrosis and inflammation. *Acta Orthop Scand* **63**:417–23.

25. Pejovic, M., Stankovic, A., and Mitrovic, D.R. (1995). Determination of the apparent synovial permeability in the knee joints of patients suffering from osteoarthritis and rheumatoid arthritis. *Br J Rheumatol* **34**:520–4.

26. Myers, S.L., Brandt, K.D., and Eilam, O. (1995). Even low grade synovitis accelerates the clearance of protein from the canine knee. Implications for measurement of synovial fluid 'markers' of osteoarthritis. *Arthritis Rheum* **38**:1085–91.

27. Page-Thomas, D.P., Band, D., King, B., and Dingle, J.T. (1987). Clearance of proteoglycan from joint cavities. *Ann Rheum Dis* **46**:934–7.

28. Lohmander, L.S., Hoerrner, L.A., and Lark, M.W. (1993). Metalloproteinases, tissue inhibitor and proteoglycan fragments in knee synovial fluid in human osteoarthritis. *Arthritis Rheum* **36**:181–9.

29. Lohmander, L.S., Saxne, T., and Heinegård, D. (1994). Release of cartilage oligomeric matrix protein (COMP) into joint fluid after injury and in osteoarthrosis. *Ann Rheum Dis* **53**:8–13.

30. Lohmander, L.S., Yoshihara, Y., Roos, H., Kobayashi, T., Yamada, H., and Shinmei, M. (1996). Procollagen II C-propeptide in joint fluid. Changes in concentrations with age, time after joint injury and osteoarthritis. *J Rheumatol* **23**:1765–9.

31. Lohmander, L.S., Saxne, T., and Heinegård, D. (1996). Increased concentrations of bone sialoprotein in joint fluid after knee injury. *Ann Rheum Dis* **55**:622–6.

32. Lohmander, L.S., Ionescu, M., Jugessur, H., and Poole, A.R. (1999). Changes in joint cartilage aggrecan metabolism after knee injury and in osteoarthritis. *Arthritis Rheum* **42**;534–44.

33. Billinghurst, R.C., Dahlberg, L., Ionescu, M., *et al.* (1997). Enhanced cleavage of type II collagen by collagenases in osteoarthritic articular cartilage. *J Clin Invest* **99**:1534–45.

34. Nelson, F., Dahlberg, L., Reiner, A., *et al.* (1998). Evidence for altered synthesis of type II collagen in patients with osteoarthritis. *J Clin Invest* **102**:2115–25.

35. Rizkalla, G., Reiner, A., Bogoch, E., and Poole, A.R. (1992). Studies of the articular cartilage proteoglycan aggrecan in health and osteoarthritis: evidence for molecular heterogeneity and extensive molecular changes in disease. *J Clin Invest* **90**:2268–77.

36. Kojima, T., Mwale, F., Yasuda, T., Girard, C., Poole, A.R., and Laverty, S. (2001). The comparative degradation of type IX and type II collagens and proteoglycan in articular cartilage in early experimental inflammatory arthritis. *Arthritis Rheum* **44**:120–7.

37. Myers, S.L., Brandt, K.D., and Albrecht, M.E. (2000). Synovial fluid glycosaminoglycan concentration does not correlate with severity of chondropathy or predict progression of osteoarthritis in a canine cruciate deficiency model. *J Rheumatol* **27**:753–63.

38. Poole, A.R. (2000). Cartilage in health and disease. In: W. Koopman (ed.), *Arthritis and Allied Conditions. A Textbook of Rheumatology* (14th ed.). Philadelphia: Lippincott, Williams and Wilkins, pp. 226–84.

39. Poole, A.R. and Howell, D.S. (2001). Etiopathogenesis of osteoarthritis. In: R.W. Moskowitz, D.S. Howell, V.M. Goldberg, and H.J. Mankin (eds), *Osteoarthritis: Diagnosis, and Management* (3rd ed.) London: W.B. Saunders pp. 29–47.

40. Lohmander, L.S., Atley, L.M., Pietka, T.A., and Eyre, D.R. (2000). The release of cross-linked peptides from type II collagen into joint fluid and serum is increased in osteoarthritis and after joint injury. *Trans Orthop Res Soc* **25**:236.

41. Song, X-Y., Zeng, L., Jin, W., *et al.* (1999). Secretory leukocyte-protease inhibitor suppresses the inflammation and joint damage of bacterial cell wall-induced arthritis. *J Exp Med* **190**:535–42.

42. Downs, J.T., Lane, C.L., Nestor, N.B., *et al.* (2001). Analysis of collagenase-cleavage of type II collagen using a neoepitope ELISA. *J Immunol Methods* **247**:25–34.

43. Christgau, S., Garnero, P., Fledelius, C., *et al.* (2001). Collagen type II c-telopeptide fragments as an index of cartilage degradation. *Bone* **29**:209–15.

44. Shinmei, M., Ito, K., Matsuyama, S., Yoshihara, Y., and Matsuzawa, K. (1993). Joint fluid carboxy-terminal type II procollagen peptide as a marker of cartilage collagen. *Osteoarthritis Cart* **1**:121–8.

45. Poole, A.R., Ionescu, M., Swan, A., and Dieppe, P.A. (1994). Changes in cartilage metabolism in arthritis are reflected by altered serum and synovial fluid levels of the cartilage proteoglycan aggrecan—implications for pathogenesis. *J Clin Invest* **94**:25–33.

46. Visco, D.M., Johnstone, B., Hill, M.A., Jolly, G.A., and Caterson, B. (1993). Immunohistochemical analysis of 3-B-3(-) and 7-D-4 epitope expression in canine osteoarthritis. *Arthritis Rheum* **36**:1718–25.

47. Slater, R.R., Jr, Bayliss, M.T., Lachiewicz, P.F., Visco, D.M., and Caterson, B. (1995). Monoclonal antibodies that detect biochemical markers of arthritis in humans. *Arthritis Rheum* **38**:655–9.

48. Hauser, N., Geiss, J., Neidhart, M., Paulsson, M., and Häuselmann, H.J. (1995). Distribution of CMP and COMP in human cartilage. *Acta Orthop Scand* **66**(Suppl. 266):72–3.

49. DiCesare, P.E., Carlson, C.S., Stolerman, E.S., Hauser, N., Tulli, H., and Paulsson, M. (1996). Increased degradation and altered tissue distribution of cartilage oligomeric protein in human rheumatoid and osteoarthritic cartilage. *J Orthop Res* **14**:946–55.

50. Recklies, A.D., Baillargeon, L., and White, C. (1998). Regulation of cartilage oligomeric matrix protein synthesis in human synovial cells and articular chondrocytes. *Arthritis Rheum* **41**:997–1006.

51. Dodge, G.R., Hawkins, D., Boesler, E., Sakai, L., and Jimenez, S.A. (1998). Production of cartilage oligomeric matrix protein (COMP) by cultured human dermal and synovial fibroblasts. *Osteoarthritis Cart* **6**:435–40.

52. Vilim, V., Vytasek, R., Olejarova, M., *et al.* (2001). Serum cartilage oligomeric matrix protein reflects the presence of clinically diagnosed synovitis in patients with knee osteoarthritis. *Osteoarthritis Cart* **9**:612–8.

53. Volck, B., Ostergaard, K., Johansen, J.S., Garbarsch, C., and Price, P.A. (1999). The distribution of YKL-40 in osteoarthritic and normal human articular cartilage. *Scand J Rheumatol* **28**:171–9.

54. Hakala, B.E., White, C., and Recklies, A.D. (1993). Human cartilage gp-39, a major secretory product of articular chondrocytes and synovial cells is a mammalian member of a chitinase protein family. *J Biol Chem* **268**:25803–10.

55. Conrozier, T.H., Cartier M-C, Mathieu, P., *et al.* (2000). Serum levels of YKL-40 and C-reactive protein in patients with hip osteoarthritis and healthy subjects: a cross-sectional study. *Ann Rheum Dis* **59**:828–31.

56. Poole, A.R. and Dieppe P.A. (1994). Biological markers in rheumatoid arthritis. *Sem Arthritis Rheum* **23**(Suppl. 2):17–31.

57. Sharma, L., Hurwitz, D.E., Thonar E-JMA, *et al.* (1998). Knee adduction moment, serum hyaluronan level, and disease severity in medial tibiofemoral osteoarthritis. *Arthritis Rheum* **41**:1233–40.

58. Sharif, M., George, E., Shepstone, L., *et al.* (1995). Serum hyaluronic acid level as a predictor of disease progression in osteoarthritis of the knee. *Arthritis Rheum* **38**:760–7.

59. Goldberg, R.L., Lenz, M.E., Huff, J., Glickman, P., Katz, R., and Thonar, EJ-MA. (1991). Elevated plasma levels of hyaluronate in patients with osteoarthritis and rheumatoid arthritis. *Arthritis Rheum* **34**:799–807.

60. Hedin, P-J., Weitoft, T., Hedin, H., Engström-Laurent, A., and Saxne, T. (1991). Serum concentrations of hyaluronan and proteoglycan in joint disease. Lack of association. *J Rheumatol* **18**:1601–5.

61. Hutchinson, N.I., Lark, M.W., MacNaul, K.L., *et al.* (1992). *In vivo* expression of stromelysin in synovium and cartilage of rabbits injected intraarticularly with interleukin-1 beta. *Arthritis Rheum* **35**:1227–33.

62. Wolfe, G.C., MacNaul, K.L., Buechel, F.F., *et al.* (1993). Differential *in vivo* expression of collagenase messenger RNA in synovium and cartilage. Quantitative comparison with stromelysin messenger RNA levels in human rheumatoid arthritis and osteoarthritis patients and in two animal models of acute inflammatory arthritis. *Arthritis Rheum* **36**:1540–7.

63. Atencia, L.J., McDevitt, C.A., Nile, W.B., and Sokoloff, L. (1989). Cartilage content of an immature dog. *Connective Tiss Res* **18**:235–42.

64. Roos, H., Dahlberg, L., and Hoerrner, L.A., (1995). Markers of cartilage matrix metabolism in human joint fluid and serum—The effect of exercise. *Osteoarthritis Cart* **3**:7–14.

65. Neidhart, M., Müller-Ladner, U., Frey, W., *et al.* (2000). Increased serum levels of non-collagenous matrix proteins (cartilage oligomeric matrix protein and melanoma inhibitory activity) in marathon runners. *Osteoarthritis Cart* **8**:222–9.

66. Manicourt, D-H., Poilvache, P., Nzeusseu, A., *et al.* (1999) Serum levels of hyaluronan, antigenic keratan sulfate, matrix metalloproteinase 3, and tissue inhibitor of metalloproteinases 1 change predictably in rheumatoid arthritis patients who have begun activity after a night of bed rest. *Arthritis Rheum* **42**:1861–9.

67. Bollen, A.M., Martin, M.D., Leroux, B.G., and Eyre, D.R. (1995). Circadian variation in urinary excretion of bone collagen cross-links. *J Bone Min Res* **10**:1885–90.

68. Gundberg, C.M., Markowitz, M.E., Mizruchi, M., and Rosen, J.F. (1985). Osteocalcin in human serum: a circadian rhythm. *J Clin Endocrinol Met* **60**:736–9.

69. Laurent, T.C. and Fraser, R.E. (1992). Hyaluronan. *FASEB J* **6**:2397–404.

70. Poole, A.R., Witter, J., Roberts, N., *et al.* (1990). Inflammation and cartilage metabolism in rheumatoid arthritis. Studies of the blood markers hyaluronic acid, orosomucoid and keratan sulfate. *Arthritis Rheum* **33**:790–9.

71. Lohmander, L.S. and Thonar, EJ-MA. (1994). Serum keratan sulfate concentrations are different in primary and posttraumatic osteoarthritis of the knee. *Trans Orthop Res Soc* **19**:459.

72. Lohmander, L.S., Dahlberg, L., Eyre, D., Lark, M., Thonar EJ-MA., and Ryd, L. (1998). Longitudinal and cross-sectional variability in markers of joint metabolism in patients with knee pain and articular cartilage abnormalities. *Osteoarthritis Cart* **6**:351–61.

73. Sweet, M.B., Coelho, A., Schnitzler, C.M., *et al.* (1988). Serum keratan sulfate levels in osteoarthritis patients. *Arthritis Rheum* **31**:648–52.

74. Spector, T.D., Woodward, L., Hall, G.M., *et al.* (1992). Keratan sulphate in rheumatoid arthritis, osteoarthritis, and inflammatory diseases. *Ann Rheum Dis* **51**:1134–7.

75. Thonar, EJ-MA., Masuda, K., Häuselmann, H.J., Uebelhart, D., Lenz, M.E., and Manicourt, D.H. (1995). Keratan Sulfate in body fluids in joint disease. *Acta Orthop Scand* **66**(Suppl. 266):103–6.

76. Bleasel, J.F., Poole, A.R., Heinegård, D., *et al.* (1999). Changes in serum cartilage marker levels indicate altered cartilage metabolism in families with the osteoarthritis-related type II collagen gene COL2A1 mutation. *Arthritis Rheum* **42**:39–45.

77. Otterness, I.G., Zimmerer, R.O., Swindell, A.C., Poole, A.R., Ionescu, M., and Weiner, E. (2001). Analysis of 14 molecular markers for monitoring osteoarthritis. Segregation of the markers into clusters and distinguishing osteoarthritis at baseline. *Osteoarthritis Cart* **8**:180–5.

78. Saxne, T., Heinegård, D., Wollheim, F.A., and Pettersson, H. (1985). Difference in cartilage proteoglycan level in synovial fluid in early rheumatoid arthritis and reactive arthritis. *Lancet*, **8447**:127–8.

79. Saxne, T., Heinegård, D., and Wollheim, F.A. (1987). Cartilage proteoglycans in synovial fluid and serum in patients with inflammatory joint disease. *Arthritis Rheum* **30**:972–9.

80. Saxne, T. and Heinegård, D. (1992). Synovial fluid analysis of two groups of proteoglycan epitopes distinguishes early and late cartilage lesions. *Arthritis Rheum* **35**:385–90.

81. Clark, A.G., Jordan, J.M., Vilim, V., *et al.* (1999). Serum cartilage oligomeric matrix protein reflects osteoarthritis presence and severity. *Arthritis Rheum* **42**:2356–64.

82. Sharif, M., Saxne, T., Shepstone, L., *et al.* (1995). Relationship between serum cartilage oligomeric matrix protein levels and disease progression in osteoarthritis of the knee joint. *Br J Rheumatol* **34**:306–10.

83. Petersson, I.F., Boegård, T., Svensson, B., Heinegård, D., and Saxne, T. (1998). Changes in cartilage and bone metabolism identified by serum markers in early osteoarthritis of the knee joint. *Br J Rheumatol* **37**:46–50.

84. Conrozier, T., Saxne, T., Fan, C.S.S., *et al.* (1998). Serum concentrations of cartilage oligomeric matrix protein and bone sialoprotein in hip osteoarthritis: a one year prospective study. *Ann Rheum Dis* **57**:527–32.

85. Månsson, B., Carey, D., Alini, M., *et al.* (1995). Cartilage and bone metabolism in rheumatoid arthritis. Differences between rapid and slow progression of disease identified by serum markers of cartilage metabolism. *J Clin Invest* **95**:1071–7.

86. Kobayashi, T., Yoshihara, Y., Yamada, H., and Fujikawa, K. (2000). Procollagen II C-propeptide as a marker for assessing mechanical risk factors of knee osteoarthritis: efffects of obesity and varus alignment. *Ann Rheum Dis* **59**:982–4.

87. Robion, F., Doizé, B., Bouré, L., *et al.* (2001). Use of synovial fluid markers of cartilage synthesis and turnover to study effects of repeated intra-articular administration of methylprednisolone acetate on articular cartilage *in vivo*. *J Orthop Res* **19**:250–8.

88. Yasser, M., Miedaney, E., Abubakr, I.H., and Baddini, M.E. (1998). Effect of low dose methotrexate on markers of bone metabolism in patients with rheumatoid arthritis. *J Rheumatol* **25**:2083–7.

89. Sandy, J.D., Flannery, C.R., Neame, P.J., and Lohmander, L.S. (1992). The structure of aggrecan fragments in human synovial fluid: Evidence for the involvement in osteoarthritis of a novel proteinase which cleaves the glu 373–ala 374 bond of the interglobular domain. *J Clin Invest* **89**:1512–6.

90. Lohmander, L.S., Neame, P., and Sandy, J.D. (1993). The structure of aggrecan fragments in human synovial fluid: Evidence that aggrecanase mediates cartilage degradation in inflammatory joint disease, joint injury and osteoarthritis. *Arthritis Rheum* **36**:1214–22.

91. Lark, M.W., Bayne, E.K., Flanagan, J., *et al.* (1997). Aggrecan degradation in human cartilage. Evidence for both aggrecanase and matrix metalloproteinase activity in normal, osteoarthritic and rheumatoid joints. *J Clin Invest* **100**:93–106.

92. Mort, J.S. and Poole, A.R. (2001). Mediators of inflammation, tissue destruction and repair. D. Proteases and their inhibitors. In: J.H. Klippel, L.J. Crofford, J.H. Stone, and C.M. Weyand (eds), *Primer on the Rheumatic Diseases*, (12th ed) Atlanta: Arthritis Foundation, pp. 72–81.

93. Hollander, A.P., Heathfield, T.F., Webber, C., *et al.* (1994). Increased damage to type II collagen in osteoarthritic cartilage detected by a new immunoassay. *J Clin Invest* **93**:1722–32.

94. Saxne, T., Heinegård, D., and Wollheim, F.A. (1986). Therapeutic effects on cartilage metabolism in arthritis as measured by release of proteoglycan structures into the synovial fluid. *Ann Rheum Dis* **45**:491–7.

95. Delmas, P., Hardy, P., Garnero, P., and Dain, M-P. (2000). Monitoring individual responses to hormone replacement therapy with bone markers. *Bone* **26**:553–60.

96. Hanson, D.A., Weis, M.A.E., Bollen, A-M., Maslan, S.L., Singer, F.R., and Eyre, D.R. (1992). A specific immunoassay for monitoring human bone resorption: Quantitation of type I collagen cross-linked N-telopeptides in urine. *J Bone Min Res* **7**:1251–8.

97. Astbury, C., Bird, H.A., McLaren, A.M., and Robins, S.P. (1994). Urinary excretion of pyridinium crosslinks of collagen correlated with joint damage in arthritis. *Br J Rheumatol* **33**:11–5.

98. Thompson, P.W., Spector, T.D., James, I.T., Henderson, E., and Hart, D.J. (1992). Urinary collagen crosslinks reflect the radiographic severity of knee osteoarthritis. *Br J Rheumatol* **31**:759–61.

99. Seibel, M.J., Duncan, A., and Robins, S.P. (1989). Urinary hydroxypyridinium crosslinks provide indices of cartilage and bone involvement in arthritic diseases. *J Rheumatol* **16**:964–70.

100. Sowers, M., Lachance, L., Jamadar, D., *et al.* (1999). The associations of bone mineral density and bone turnover markers with osteoarthritis of the hand and knee in pre- and perimenopausal women. *Arthritis Rheum* **42**: 483–9.

101. Lohmander, L.S. and Felson, D. (1998). Defining and validating the clinical role of molecular markers in osteoarthritis. In: K. Brandt, M. Doherty, and S. Lohmander (eds), *Osteoarthritis*. Oxford: Oxford University Press, pp. 519–30.

102. Otterness, I.G., Weiner, E., Swindell, A.C., Zimmerer, R.O., Ionescu, M., and Poole, A.R. (2001). An analysis of 14 molecular markers for monitoring osteoarthritis. Relationship of the markers to clinical end-points. *Osteoarthritis Cart* **9**:224–31.

103. Lohmander, L.S. (1995). Molecular markers to monitor outcome and intervention in osteoarthritis (promises, promises …). *Br J Rheumatol* **34**: 599–601.

104. Lohmander, L.S., Dahlberg, L., Ryd, L., and Heinegård, D. (1989). Increased levels of proteoglycan fragments in knee joint fluid after injury. *Arthritis Rheum* **32**:1434–42.

105. Mehraban, F., Finegan, C.K., and Moskowitz, R.W. (1991). Serum keratan sulfate—quantitative and qualitative comparisons in inflammatory versus noninflammatory arthritides. *Arthritis Rheum* **34**:383–92.

106. Manicourt, D.H., Fujimoto, N., Obata, K., and Thonar, E.J. (1994). Serum levels of collagenase, stromelysin-1, and TIMP-1. Age- and sex-related differences in normal subjects and relationship to the extent of joint involvement and serum levels of antigenic keratan sulfate in patients with osteoarthritis. *Arthritis Rheum* **37**:1774–83.

107. Shinmei, M., Miyauchi, S., Machida, A., and Miyazaki, K. (1992). Quantitation of chondroitin 4-sulfate and chondroitin 6-sulfate in pathologic joint fluid. *Arthritis Rheum* **35**:1304–8.

108. Witsch-Prehm, P., Miehlke, R., and Kresse, H. (1992). Presence of small proteoglycan fragments in normal and arthritic human cartilage. *Arthritis Rheum* **35**:1042–52.

109. Zucker, S., Lysik, R.M., Zarrabi, M.H., *et al.* (1994). Elevated plasma stromelysin levels in arthritis. *J Rheumatol* **21**:2329–33.

110. Clark, I.M., Powell, L.K., Ramsey, S., Hazleman, B.L., and Cawston, T.E. (1993). The measurement of collagenase, tissue inhibitor of metalloproteinases (TIMP), and collagenase-TIMP complex in synovial fluids from patients with osteoarthritis and rheumatoid arthritis. *Arthritis Rheum* **36**:372–9.

111. Chevalier, X., Conrozier, T., Gehrmann, M., *et al.* (2001). Tissue inhibitor of metalloprotease-1 (TIMP-1) serum level may predict progression of hip osteoarthritis. *Osteoarthritis Cart* **9**:300–7.

112. Sharif, M., George, E., and Dieppe, P.A. (1995). Correlation between synovial fluid markers of cartilage and bone turnover and scintigraphic scan abnormalities in osteoarthritis of the knee. *Arthritis Rheum* **38**:78–81.

113. Garnero, P., Piperno, M., Gineyts, E., Christgau, S., Delmas, P.D., and Vignon, E. (2001). Cross sectional evaluation of biochemical markers of bone, cartilage, and synovial tissue metabolism in patients with knee osteoarthritis. Relations with disease activity and joint damage. *Ann Rheum Dis* **60**:619–26.

114. Sharif, M., George, E., and Dieppe, P.A. (1996). Synovial fluid and serum concentrations of aminoterminal propeptide of type III procollagen in healthy volunteers and patients with joint disease. *Ann Rheum Dis* **55**:47–51.

115. Saxne, T. and Heinegård, D. (1992). Cartilage oligomeric matrix protein: a novel marker of cartilage turnover detectable in synovial fluid and blood. *Br J Rheumatol* **31**:583–91.

116. Johansen, J.S., Jensen, H.S., and Price, P.A. (1993). A new biochemical marker for joint injury. Analysis of YKL-40 in serum and synovial fluid. *Br J Rheumatol* **32**:949–55.

117. Harvey, S., Weisman, M., O'Dell, J., *et al.* (1998). Chondrex: a new marker of joint disease. *Clin Chem* **44**:509–16.

118. Johansen, J.S., Hvolris, J., Hansen, M., Backer, V., Lorenzen, C., and Price, P.A. (1996). Serum YKL-40 levels in healthy children and adults. Comparison with serum and synovial fluid levels of YKL-40 in patients with osteoarthritis or trauma of the knee joint. *Br J Rheumatol* **35**:533–9.

119. Sharif, M., Elson, C.J., Dieppe, P.A., and Kirwan, J.R. (1997). Elevated C-reactive protein levels in osteoarthritis. *Br J Rheumatol* **36**:140–1.

120. Spector, J.D., Hart, D.J., Nandra, D., *et al.* (1997). Low level increases in serum C-reactive protein are present in early osteoarthritis of the knee and predict progressive disease. *Arthritis Rheum* **40**:723–7.

121. Campion, G.V., Delmas, P.D., and Dieppe, P.A. (1989). Serum and synovial osteocalcin (bone Gla protein) levels in joint disease. *Br J Rheumatol* **28**:393–8.

122. Sowers, M., Lachance, L., Jamadar, D., *et al.* (1999). The associations of bone mineral density and bone turnover markers with osteoarthritis of the hand and knee in pre- and perimenopausal women. *Arthritis Rheum* **42**:483–9.

123. Sharif, M., Osborne, D.J., Meadows, K., Woodhouse, S.M., Colvin, E.M., Shepstone, L., and Dieppe, P.A. (1996). The relevance of chondroitin and keratan sulphate markers in normal and arthritic synovial fluid. *Br J Rheumatol* **35**:951–7.

12 Design of clinical trials for evaluation of structure modifying drugs and new agents for symptomatic treatment of osteoarthritis

Nicholas Bellamy

In recent years, there has been increasing attention on standardizing several aspects of OA clinical trials methodology. Issues relating to the conduct of OA studies have been captured in the Osteoarthritis Research Society International (OARSI) Task Force Guidelines,[2] the Society's attention focusing more recently on developing an international consensus on the conduct of future hand OA studies.[4] Issues in OA outcome measurement have been discussed at several Outcome Measures in Rheumatology Clinical Trials (OMERACT) Conferences, with OMERACT 3[5] and OMERACT 5[6] meetings being of particular relevance. Recognition of the importance of OA in the World Health Organization's Bone and Joint Decade Initiative is especially encouraging.[7] Subsequent meetings in various regions and the emergence of the National Institutes of Health—OA Initiative, and draft US Federal Drugs and Administration (FDA) OA Guidelines all highlight the growing importance of OA research. These initiatives have been facilitated by several years of productive international basic and applied research in OA. Given the emergence of Guidelines documents, this chapter will address conceptual challenges, implementation issues, and provide a future perspective.

Research architecture alternatives

In the hierarchy of research designs, the double-blind randomized controlled trial remains pre-eminent. It is the most appropriate design for large-scale comparative studies of StMOADs and SyMOADs. Although sample size requirements may be greater than for a comparable crossover study, the design offers simplicity without any danger of carryover effects.[8] Furthermore, crossover designs are not suitable where the intervention has a relatively slow onset and offset of action. There have been relatively few studies reported in recent years using crossover designs, most investigators and agencies prefer data analysis and interpretation based on parallel designs. Although there has been much interest in the N-of-1 trial design,[9] which is a multiple crossover design, it has been rarely used in comparative studies in OA, and used relatively infrequently even in clinical practice for the evaluation of SyMOADs.[10] The necessity for multiple crossovers, blinding procedures, and Baysean mathematics, reduces the viability of this design for widespread use in clinical practice applications, while its operational complexity, reductionist philosophy, and inferior statistical performance limit its value in new drug development.

In general, non-randomized comparative group designs and one-group non-comparative open designs lack the necessary rigor essential for assessing the relative and absolute, efficacy and tolerability, of anti-rheumatic compounds. They are, however, the standard design options for cohort or longitudinal observation studies (LOS).

Trial duration

Trial duration is contentious, and depends on goals and objectives. Pain relief from fast-acting SyMOADs can be detected in a matter of days. However, longer-term studies over 6–12 weeks are required to demonstrate persistence of that effect. The duration of follow-up in studies of slow-acting SyMOADs may be 4–6 months, in pharmacoeconomic studies of SyMOADs 1–2 years, and in studies of StMOADs it may be 2–3 years. The duration of follow-up for StMOAD studies will depend on the mechanism of action, the pharmacodynamics, and the level of commitment to evaluating the clinical consequences of structural conservation.

Comparator groups

Placebo control groups involving fully informed volunteer patients should be used, where ethically acceptable, in situations where efficacy has not yet been established. Once efficacy has been established, the use of a placebo group is generally unnecessary, and usually inappropriate. At that point active comparator groups are appropriate in order to assess the differential response to competing alternatives. Studies of slow-acting SyMOADs and StMOADs are complicated by the clinical necessity and ethical obligation to provide opportunity for relief of symptoms and/or premature withdrawal. In the case of slow-acting SyMOADs the potential effect of co-therapy on the primary clinical outcome becomes an issue. In the case of StMOAD studies, it is important to control and limit the implications of access to co-therapies that may have purported positive (Glucosamine sulphate),[11] or negative (Indomethacin)[12] effects on joint structure, through patient selection criteria, randomization, and trial management procedures. In early proof of concept studies of StMOADs, the patient's capacity and willingness to continue on protocol is paramount in determining success in measuring structure modifying effects. It is likely, therefore, in such studies, that all normal reasonable and appropriate symptomatic measures would be offered to maintain patients on protocol for as long as possible. While the dual classification SyMOAD and StMOAD has been employed it is reasonable to speculate that there will in the future exist a spectrum of agents that might be subclassified as follows:

- Exclusively SyMOAD
- Predominantly SyMOAD
- Predominantly StMOAD
- Exclusively StMOAD

Indeed, the current debate as to whether an agent should be classified as a drug or a device is likely to continue, and further expand the list of acronyms.

Patient selection

Patient selection brings together a group of patients who fulfill specified inclusion and exclusion criteria, and serves several purposes.

Patient selection increases the homogeneity of the sample, by including patients who are potential responders to active treatment, and at the same time reducing the probability of adverse events by excluding higher risk patients; however, it may reduce generalizability of the study results. Increased homogeneity may have a positive impact on sample size requirements, and therefore on study costs, accrual, and timelines. It should be noted that study results are generalizable to similar patients, managed in the same way, under similar conditions. For aforementioned reasons, the statistical efficiency of studying a relatively homogeneous group of compliant patients with potentially responsive disease needs to be weighed against the more limited generalizability of the study result.

Confirmation of the diagnosis of OA is essential, otherwise the study can only address the issue of joint pain, rather than a specific pathologic entity. Furthermore, patient self report of OA may be unreliable, necessitating diagnosis by criteria,[13] supported by appropriate imaging confirming current, not historic, structural status.[14–16] The OARSI Guidelines describe suitable patient groups, and propose specific selection criteria.[2]

In SyMOAD studies, patients are often selected on the basis of having demonstrated their potential responsiveness to an anti-inflammatory drug, by meeting flare criteria during a washout period. Flare criteria are usually phrased in terms of a minimum percentage increase in pain. It should be noted that for studies using analytic methods based on OARSI responder criteria,[17] patients whose baseline pain, function, and patient global assessment values are below the threshold for minimum improvement, will lack the necessary response potential and should not be included. Current OARSI responder criteria do not attempt to address response definition in patients with very low symptom severity at baseline.

In StMOAD studies, a number of patient groups might be selected.

1. Subjects at risk of developing OA (e.g., prior injury known to be associated with the development of OA) in studies assessing the ability of a drug or device to prevent OA.

2. Patients with established OA (with or without symptoms) in studies assessing the ability of a drug or device to retard or stop further disease progression.

3. Patients with established OA (with or without symptoms) in studies assessing the ability of a drug or device to repair damaged joint tissue.

Randomization and stratification

In a comparative trial, the relative effectiveness of two anti-rheumatic drugs can be demonstrated only if the two treatment groups are known to be prognostically similar. However, there is considerable variability in the response to anti-inflammatory drugs, and the key determinants of this variability have proven extremely difficult to define. As a result, randomization has generally been used to increase the probability that treatment groups are comparable. It should be noted, that randomization does not guarantee group comparability, it only increases the probability that prognostically important factors have been evenly distributed.[8]

In contrast, stratification is a process in which patients are categorized into two or more groups with respect to certain defined variables of potential prognostic importance, so that their distribution is guaranteed.[8] Identification of stratification variables has proven difficult. The initial pain level might be used as a stratification variable in SyMOAD studies, since there is a positive relationship between initial pain rating and subsequent pain relief[18] (Table 12.1). Despite this observation stratification is rarely performed, any resulting baseline differences being dealt with by using adjustment procedures for baseline imbalance. Given the potential association between obesity and disease progression, the body mass index (BMI) might be used as a stratification variable in StMOAD studies. It should be noted, that while there may be current enthusiasm for targeting patients at increased risk of rapidly progressive OA, there is no evidence whether the disease process in this group is more or less amenable to disease modification than that in other OA subgroups. Stratification would not ordinarily be employed alone, and when used, it is a prelude to randomization: so-called stratified randomization.

Blinding

Studies may be single-, double-, triple-, or unblinded.[8] Usually, the test treatments are given in an identical format, either as indistinguishable compounds or using the 'double-dummy' technique, so as to create a double-blind. When only a single-blinded technique is used, either the patient, or, more usually, the assessor, can be compromised by an expectation bias that may either enhance or abrogate the clinical result. In a triple-blinded format, not only the patient and assessor are blind, but also a third party, who has responsibility for administering certain aspects of the trial—for example, termination of the study on ethical grounds if adverse reactions or response failure are unexpectedly frequent or severe in one or other treatment group. In a triple-blinded scheme, such decisions can be made without prejudice.

The importance of double-blinding in SyMOAD trials is unchallenged. Its value in StMOAD trials, where the principal outcome is based on a structural image, is equally important, but for less obvious reasons. In such studies, radiographic or magnetic resonance (MR) images may be read blind by a third party. However, StMOAD trials are usually of several years' duration, and the lack of blinding of patients and assessors may cause an expectation bias, one result of which may be that patients on traditional therapy will terminate prematurely because of therapeutic nihilism on the part of the patient, or the assessor, or both. Furthermore, since studies usually assess clinical as well as imaging outcomes, it is important to use blinding procedures in StMOAD trials.

Intervention

The term, intervention, is applied to the use of a specific treatment in a study.[8] The agent tested may be given a fixed dose, or may be titrated according to a predetermined schedule or to the requirements of the patient. Although clinical practice is best simulated by the titration strategy—because it commits patients neither to excessive nor inadequate therapy, and thereby minimizes response failures because of either inefficacy or adverse reactions—it renders dose-based comparative analyses difficult, because of the small residual sample size at each dose level. In contrast, a fixed-dose strategy permits conclusions to be drawn about the efficacy and tolerability of a single specified dose, but fails to address the issue of optimal therapy in routine clinical practice.

For SyMOAD studies, drug administration may be preceded, punctuated, or followed by a 'washout' period—such periods may be NSAID-free or totally drug free.[19] For practical and ethical reasons, 'rescue' analgesia with acetaminophen is usually allowed during the washout period. Because withdrawal may be poorly tolerated by some patients, premature advancement ('trap door' provision) to the active treatment phase may be required. In spite of these problems, washout periods are advantageous in that they allow assessment of the baseline status of study patients, and amplify any subsequent response to active SyMOAD therapy, thereby minimizing sample size requirements for detecting statistically significant within-group improvements. Also, they facilitate assessment of patient responsiveness and absolute

Table 12.1 Standardised Response Mean (SRM) and correlation between initial pain rating and pain relief scores in OA

Pain scale	SRM	Correlation
VA	0.97	0.49
Numerical	0.91	0.48
CCAS	0.94	0.43
Likert	0.84	0.50
Pain faces 1	0.78	0.55
MPQ (total)	0.74	0.50
Pain faces 2	0.70	0.34
Reversed ladder	0.50	0.48

Source: Adapted from Bellamy et al. 1999. *Curr Med Res Opin* **15**(2) 113–19.[18]

magnitude of the change, minimize carryover effects from prior treatments, and allow clinical baselines to be re-established in crossover studies. Finally, when performed at the end of a trial, washout periods serve to redefine group comparability and the persistence of patient responsiveness.

Cointervention

Cointervention refers to the administration of another potentially efficacious treatment at the same time as the intervention.[20] It can take many forms, including concomitant use of analgesic drugs, hospitalization, physiotherapy, and surgery. Because these activities often have a major biasing effect, and confound interpretation of trial results, cointervention should be minimized, monitored, and taken into account in interpreting trial data. Because pain relief is the principal outcome measure in most SyMOAD trials, such caution is particularly relevant for concomitant analgesics, given their ubiquitous use, whether they are officially permitted or not. Unrecognized differential analgesic consumption rates can minimize between-group differences in pain control, and lead incorrectly to the assumption that no difference exists. Analgesic consumption is a surrogate measure of pain control and, therefore, is itself an important end-point.

Contamination

Contamination is rarely a problem in well-managed clinical trials of antirheumatic drugs. It occurs when an individual, instead of receiving the intended medication, receives a drug specifically designated for individuals in one of the other treatment groups.[20] Its biasing effects are obvious, and if the effects are unrecognized, patients will be analyzed according to the drug that they were scheduled to receive, rather than that which they truly received.

Compliance

Compliance is a measure of the extent to which a patient adheres to the protocol, in general, and to drug ingestion, in particular.[20] It can be measured in four ways: by direct observation, patient report (verbal or diary), pill counting, and plasma drug-level monitoring. Each method has its limitations, so that non-compliant patients can appear compliant, and vice versa. Even when the monitoring procedure is satisfactory, there is no standard definition for any level of compliance below which the therapeutic response is significantly compromised. In clinical trials, a level of compliance greater than 80 per cent is often considered acceptable. Furthermore, because enrolment is entirely voluntary, and because patients are in pain and under close supervision, compliance levels are generally high, and patient report (by diary) and pill counting are probably adequate in short-term studies. However, in studies of StMOADs, in which the treatment period must be several years in length, compliance may be a problem. The so-called faintness-of-heart test may be useful in trying to estimate whether the patient is a suitable candidate for long-term study.

Outcome assessment

The timing and nature of outcome assessments should respect both the potential adverse and beneficial effects of test compounds.[3] Although adverse reactions to SyMOADs and purported StMOADs can occur at any time after administration, the induction-response (efficacy) interval for fast-acting SMOADs will be shorter than for slow-acting SMOADs and both, in turn, will be shorter than that for StMOADs. The experience with disease-modifying antirheumatic drug therapy in rheumatoid arthritis is that certain toxic effects (e.g., thrombocytopenia) occur more rapidly than others (e.g., anemia) because of physiological variability in the half-life of the target cells. For both safety and scientific rigor, patients should be appropriately monitored for both clinical and laboratory tolerance to drugs

and devices, in accordance with their known pharmacokinetic and pharmacodynamic profiles. It may not be necessary to measure all variables at every time point, some may be required to assess toxicity, others efficacy, and still others, both.

Adverse events

Clinical tolerance can be monitored by spontaneous patient report, or open-ended or close-ended questioning. In general, the more rigorous the probe, the greater the incidence of 'intolerance' and the more difficult the task of attributing it to the studied drug. Even in a healthy population there is a background level of transient symptoms, such as headache, diarrhoea, and dyspepsia. For this reason, the term 'adverse event' is often used in preference to the term 'drug side-effect'. In general adverse events are characterized according to nature, timing, severity, and consequence. They can be formerly classified according to the COSTART[21] and WHO-ARD[22] systems.

Health status measurement

Health Status Measures (HSMs) used to assess drug efficacy outcomes, should be able to detect the smallest clinically important change, be reliable and responsive, and also be valid with respect to capturing the dimensionality of the clinical response profile.[3]

Irrespective of the specific protocol, five major and five minor criteria are important in selecting evaluative indices for clinical trials[3] (Table 12.2). The five major criteria are as follows.

Criterion 1

The measurement process must be ethical. Measurement procedures that are painful, embarrassing, or hazardous to study subjects raise ethical issues. Such issues must be fully disclosed to participants and, if possible, less invasive procedures sought. The necessity for data collection must be carefully weighed against the risks, and the final procedures reviewed by an independent committee versed in judging ethical issues in biomedical research.

Criterion 2

Validity should be adequate for achieving measurement objectives.[3] There are four types of validity: face, content, criterion, and construct.

1. *Face validity*. A measure has face validity if informed individuals (investigators and clinicians) judge that it measures at least part of the defined phenomenon.

2. *Content validity*. An instrument can have face validity but fail to capture the dimension of interest in its entirety. A measure, therefore, has content validity if it is comprehensive; that is, it encompasses all relevant aspects of the defined attributes. Like face validity, content validity is subjective, but can be conferred either by a single individual or by a group of individuals using one of several consensus-development techniques. In general, evaluative instruments for clinical trials should include measures that comprehensively probe symptoms that occur frequently and are clinically important to patients. The definition of importance is best decided by groups of patients, polled to assess the dimensionality of their symptoms, or by clinical investigators whose decision is based on their perception of the symptoms of the patient. If not supplemented by patient-based assessments, the latter approach may be considered paternalistic.

3. *Criterion validity*. Criterion validity is assessed statistically by comparing the new HSM against a concurrent independent criterion or standard (concurrent criterion validity), or against a future standard (predictive criterion validity). It is, therefore, an estimate of the extent to which a measure (e.g., the perceived difficulty of the patient in walking) agrees with the true value of an independent measure of health

Table 12.2

Major criteria

- ◆ The measurement process must be ethical
- ◆ Reliability should be adequate for achieving measurement objectives
- ◆ Validity (face, content, criterion, and construct) should be adequate for achieving measurement objectives
- ◆ Responsiveness must be adequate, that is, the technique must be able to detect a clinically important statistically significant change in the underlying variable
- ◆ The feasibility of data collection and instrument application should not be constrained unduly by time or cost

Minor criteria

- ◆ The technique should have been designed for a specific purpose
- ◆ The technique should have been validated in individuals or populations of patients having similar characteristics to future study populations
- ◆ Utilization of the technique should have been adopted by other clinical investigators
- ◆ Performance should have been maintained in subsequent applications under similar study conditions
- ◆ The method of deriving scores, particularly in composite indices, should be both credible and comprehensive

status (e.g., the actual observed performance of the patient in walking a set distance or for a defined period of time), either present or future. The attainment of concurrent criterion validity is usually frustrated by the lack of any available standard, whereas predictive criterion validity is not immediately relevant to many evaluative objectives.

4. *Construct validity.* Construct validity is of two types: convergent and discriminant. Both represent statistical attempts to demonstrate adherence between instrument values and a theoretical manifestation (construct) or consequence of the attribute. Convergent construct validity testing assesses the correlation between scores on a single health component, as measured by two different instruments. If the coefficient is positive and appreciably above zero, the new measure is said to have convergent construct validity. In contrast, discriminant construct validity testing compares the correlation between scores on the same health component, as measured by two different instruments (e.g., two different measures of physical function), and between scores on that health component and each of several other health components (e.g., separate measures of social and emotional function). A measure has discriminant construct validity if the proposed measure correlates better with a second measure, accepted as more closely related to the construct, than it does with a third, more distantly related measure. Validity, like reliability, has no absolute level, and its adequacy depends on the measurement objective.

Criterion 3

Reliability should be adequate for achieving measurement objectives.[3] Reliability is a synonym for consistency, or agreement, and is the extent to which a measurement procedure yields the same result on repeated applications, when the underlying phenomenon has not changed. Because repeated measures rarely equal one another exactly, some degree of inconsistency is common. This form of measurement error is referred to as noise or random error. Low levels of reliability are reflected in the magnitude of the standard deviation and result in increased sample size requirements for clinical trials using such instruments. In contrast to systematic error, that is,

bias, random error can be minimized by increasing sample size. Although there is no absolute level of acceptable reliability, and depending on the method used, reliability coefficients should, in general, exceed 0.80.

Criterion 4

An evaluative index must be responsive to change, that is, be capable of detecting differential change in health status occurring in two or more groups of individuals exposed to competing interventions. This is an absolute prerequisite for an evaluative instrument and requires careful documentation. Not only should the instrument be responsive in general, but it should also be specifically responsive in the clinical setting in which it is to be applied.[23] In the older literature statistical *p*-values were often used to compare the relative responsiveness of different measures. More recently, effect sizes, standardized response means, and on occasion the relative efficiency statistic have been employed for that purpose.

Criterion 5

The feasibility of data collection should not be constrained by time, cost, complexity, or burden. Feasibility is one of the three components of the OMERACT Filter, which has been promoted as a basis for instrument selection.[24] Measurement procedures that are complex and excessively lengthy run the risk of patient and assessor fatigue, with a resultant decline in data quality. Similarly, measurement methods that are excessively expensive may lack general applicability.

Structuring efficacy outcome assessment

There are two constructs and two recent consensus developments that have shaped outcome assessment procedures in OA clinical trials. The original 5Ds paradigm, proposed by Fries, remains popular and relevant.[25] In that schema, health outcomes are classified according to Death, Disability, Discomfort, Drug(Iatrogenic), and Dollar (Costs). The paradigm is useful for considering the major dimensions of health. The World Health Organization (WHO) has revised its original classification system based on impairment, disability, and handicap,[26] to accommodate more of the positive and personal aspects of health, and is based on impairment, abilities and participation, also encompassing personal and environmental factors.[27] Both the Fries paradigm and the WHO classification could be thought of as generic and applicable to a variety of disease states.

From an OA-specific standpoint, the OMERACT 3 Conference marked the achievement of an international multi-stakeholder consensus on core set measures for future OA clinical trials.[5] The core set measures are as follows:

- ◆ Pain
- ◆ Function
- ◆ Patient Global Assessment
- ◆ Imaging for studies of ≥ 1 year

These decisions were subsequently ratified by the OARSI Clinical Trials Guidelines Task Force,[2] which in addition set down recommendations for measurement techniques, instruments, and basic research methodology. A more recent OARSI Task Force has developed an extension of that proposal, specifically directed at future hand OA studies.[4] The measurement section of the draft document mirrors the earlier document in many respects, and emphasizes the same domains for core set measurement. One of the added complexities in OA, compared to RA, is that measurement may be confined to one anatomic area or indeed a single joint, which is used to represent the disease as a whole. The key joint areas are the hips, knees, and hands.

Instrument developers have used very different strategies to arrive at the item content, subscale composition, and scaling, which are peculiar to the different measures. There is no doubt that instrument responsiveness is extremely important. However, it is also important to recognize the extreme conceptual differences that underpin different instruments. In brief, the differences relate to the following issues:

- Level of OA patient involvement in developing the item inventory
- Procedures used to reduce ambiguity, gender-specificity, and redundancy
- Methods used to assess reliability, validity, and responsiveness
- Recall timeframe over which questions are posed
- Scaling format
- Interviewer vs patient self-administration
- Weighting and aggregation procedures used to derive subscale and total index scores
- Rigor and standardization of the procedures used in the development of alternate-language translations

Review of selected outcome measures

In recent years a number of disease-specific OA outcome measures have developed. They differ conceptually from one another, but share a common focus on the symptoms of patients with OA. Some are unidimensional, others are either aggregated or segregated multidimensional indices.

Disease-specific OA measures

Australian/Canadian (AUSCAN) Hand Osteoarthritis Index

Developed in 1995, the AUSCAN Index is a valid, reliable, and responsive tri-dimensional patient self-reported questionnaire, containing 15 questions, within three dimensions (Pain, 5 questions; Stiffness, 1 question; and Physical function, 9 questions), and employed in the evaluation of hand OA.[28] Today the AUSCAN Index is used in clinical research and clinical practice applications, and is available in ten different alternate-language forms, which have been developed using a rigorous standardized translation/validation process. Different versions of the AUSCAN Index have specific applications. It is important therefore that users contact the originator at the AUSCAN website at www.auscan.org, to obtain the AUSCAN questionnaire best suited to their needs, and for the latest version of the AUSCAN User Guide. The AUSCAN Index is suited to flexible delivery in paper format for office, institutional, or home completion, and for interviewer administration by telephone. A weighting system termed the Patient Assessment of the Relative Importance of Symptoms (PARIS) sectogram has been developed as a basis for calculating priority-weighted total AUSCAN scores.[29]

Cochin Hand OA Index

The Cochin Hand OA Index was developed in Paris.[30] Originally developed for use in rheumatoid arthritis patients, the index has recently been validated in OA patients. The Index is valid, reliable, and responsive to change. The Index contains 18 questions, responses to which are scaled on 6-point Likert scales. The Index divides the 18 responses into five areas: in the kitchen, dressing, hygiene, at the office, and other.

Functional Index for Hand Osteoarthritis (FIHOA) (Dreiser Index)

The FIHOA is a unidimensional function index for hand OA.[31] The Index contains 10 questions, and offers alternative question stems. Data on reliability, validity, and responsiveness that have been published, and a limited number of alternate-language translations created. In the validation study of the Cochin Index, the FIHOA was less responsive than the Cochin Index, and in a comparative study, the FIHOA was also less responsive than the

AUSCAN. Therefore, based on these two early experiences, it appears that the FIHOA is less sensitive, and requires larger sample sizes than either the AUSCAN or Cochin Indices.

Indices of Clinical Severity (Algofunctional Indices, Lequesne Indices)

The separate Indices of Clinical Severity for knee and hip OA, developed by Lequesne and colleagues were early entrants into the field.[32] The indices contain elements that tap into pain, stiffness, maximum distance walked and activities of daily living, and assume a total score in the range 0–24. Originally developed as interviewer-administered indices, based on composite scores generated from the simple summation of component items, the Indices of Clinical Severity have been translated into various languages, have proven popular, mainly in some European studies, have been recently self-administered and the data disaggregated into component subscale scores.

Western Ontario and McMaster Universities (WOMAC) Osteoarthritis Index

Developed in 1982, the WOMAC Index is a valid, reliable, and highly responsive tri-dimensional patient self-reported questionnaire, containing 24 questions, within three dimensions (Pain, 5 questions; Stiffness, 2 questions; and Physical function, 17 questions), and employed widely in the evaluation of knee and hip OA.[33,34] Over the last 20 years there has been extensive experience with variations in phraseology, time frame, scaling format, and presentation of the WOMAC Index. Today the WOMAC Index is used extensively in clinical research and practice, and is available in over 60 different alternate-language forms, which have been developed using a rigorous standardized translation/validation process. Several of the different versions of the WOMAC Index have very specific applications. It is important therefore that users contact the originator at the WOMAC website at www.womac.org, to obtain the WOMAC questionnaire best suited to their needs, and for the latest version of the WOMAC User Guide. The WOMAC Index is suited to flexible delivery in paper format for office, institutional, or home completion, for interviewer-administration by telephone, and for touch screen computer-based administration using the Quali-Touch™ system. A weighting system termed the Patient Assessment of the Relative Importance of Symptoms (PARIS) sectogram has been developed as a basis for calculating priority-weighted total WOMAC scores.[35]

It is of note that in recent years different research groups have recommended both the shortening,[36] and lengthening[37,38] of the original WOMAC Index. At the present time, the unmodified 3.1 series Index remains the standard, and most widely used form of the index.

General arthritis measures

In contrast to the disease-specific OA outcome measures, there are two important general arthritis measures that can be used in OA, and are particularly useful in situations where a measure of the combined, rather than separate, effects of upper and lower extremity joint involvement are required. They do not provide joint-specific information, but have been widely used and have been validated in several alternate languages.

Arthritis Impact Measurement Scales (AIMS[39] and AIMS2[40])

The Arthritis Impact Measurement Scales (AIMS)[39] has been extensively validated in different clinical settings, and in several alternate-language forms. AIMS is a multidimensional self-administered index using 45 items to probe nine separate dimensions of mobility, physical activity, dexterity, social role, social activity, activities of daily living, pain, depression, and anxiety. Using a Guttman scaling technique, each response carries a specific value and a standardization procedure is applied to bring each dimension to a common scale (0–10). The AIMS2 is a modification of the original instrument in which some items have been modified, deleted, or added, but the majority of the items left unchanged. Three new subscales (arm function, ability to work, support from family and friends) and three new assessments (satisfaction with current level of function, prioritization of three areas for improvement, and specific impact of arthritis on health status) have been added.

Health Assessment Questionnaire (HAQ)[41]

The Health Assessment Questionnaire (HAQ)[41] developed by Fries and colleagues has been extensively validated and is available in a large number of alternate-language forms. Pain is measured using a single 15-cm horizontal visual analog scale, whilst disability is divided into eight categories (dressing and grooming, arising, eating, walking, hygiene, reach, grip, and activities), responses being scored on a 4-point ordinal scale. A recent publication has suggested that the original version of the HAQ may be preferable to at least some of the available alternatives.

Generic health status measures

Finally, there are a number of generic health status measures which are neither disease-specific, nor joint-specific, but which offer opportunity to compare health outcomes across different disease states, and which in the case of the Health Utilities Index™ (HUI™), generate a utility-based measure suitable for a type of health economic analysis termed cost-utility analysis.

EuroQoL[42]

The EuroQoL is a standardized generic instrument capable of providing a utility value. The five-part questionnaire captures elements of mobility, self-care, main working activity, pain and mood, and social relationships. It takes only a few minutes to complete and is suitable for use as a postal questionnaire. The instrument generates a single numeric index of health status, and therefore can be used as a measure of health outcome in both clinical and economic evaluation.

Health Utilities Index™[43]

The Health Utilities Index (HUI™) is based on a multi-attribute health status classification system. The system measures eight attributes: vision, hearing, speech, physical mobility, dexterity, cognition, pain and discomfort, and emotion. This self-administered questionnaire takes less than 10 minutes to complete, measures health-related quality of life and produces a utility score. The HUI™ is available in several alternate-language forms and has been used in over 300 clinical applications. Information on the HUI™ can be obtained at www.healthutilities.com.

Short-Form 36 (SF-36)[44]

The SF-36 and its shorter variants are widely used for the assessment of generic health status. The SF-36 questionnaire has been translated and validated in multiple alternate-language forms, normative values being available in several jurisdictions and for several health states. The SF-36 measures three major health attributes (functional status, well-being, and overall evaluation of health) and eight health concepts:

- limitations in physical activities because of health problems (10 items);
- limitations in social activities because of physical or emotional problems (two items);
- limitations in usual role activities because of physical health problems (four items);
- bodily pain (two items);
- general mental health (psychological distress and well-being) (five items);
- limitations in usual role activities because of emotional problems (three items);
- vitality (energy and fatigue) (four items); and
- general health perceptions (five items).

Miscellaneous measures

The aforementioned indices represent the state-of-the-art in OA outcomes assessment in rheumatology. Measures of joint geometry (goniometry, plurimetry, intercondylar distance, intermalleolar straddle), performance (walk time, ascent time), inflammation (tenderness,[45] swelling, erythema, flares), and time to surgery remain relevant but are not part of the OMERACT or OARSI core set measures, either because of concerns regarding their clinimetric properties, or because they represent surrogates for more immediate measures of disease consequence.[3]

Statistical issues

Statistical issues can be subdivided into those relating to sample size calculation and those relevant to statistical analysis of the resulting data. Both are quite complex, and those readers less experienced in this area of clinical research may find it advantageous to recruit a biostatistician to the research team.

Sample size estimation

Sample size requirements may be calculated from several standard formulae that differ, depending on the trial design and whether the analysis compares means or proportions.[3] In addition to setting the Type I (α) and Type II (β) error rates, the calculation requires definition of the minimum clinically important difference (Δ) to be detected and the variance (SD) or, in the case of proportions, the differential event rates of interest. (The Type I error is the risk that the investigator takes the risk of erroneously concluding that a difference between treatments exists, and the Type II error is the risk of erroneously concluding that no difference exists, when the converse is true.) The key difficulty, currently, is in obtaining estimates of the Δ and SD for comparisons of mean values. Some 10 years after our own publication of parameters for sample size calculation in OA clinical trials, the OA parameter tables remain the only published proposal in the rheumatology literature.[46] This is disappointing and suggests that the issue has not received the attention it deserves. There were, however, discussions at the OMERACT 5 conference on the definition of difference in the context of OA. There is not a single definition. Acronyms for at least four aspects of 'difference' were discussed and defined. They were as follows: Minimum Change Potentially Detectable (MCPD),[6] Minimum Percentage Change Potentially Detectable (MPCPD),[6] Minimum Perceptible Clinical Improvement (MPCI),[5,47] and Minimum Clinically Important Difference (MCID).[6] Estimates for some but not all outcome measures are available. We have been particularly interested in developing estimates for the WOMAC Index and have illustrated known values in Table 12.3.

Statistical analysis

The study results should be analyzed and presented in a way that demonstrates both their clinical importance and their statistical significance. Two types of analytic philosophy are commonly used: explicative or per protocol; and management or intention to treat.[48] In the explicative approach, all patients failing to complete the study exactly according to protocol are excluded from analysis. In contrast, in a management trial, all patients entered into the trial are included in the analysis. Although the former strategy is operationally simple, it runs the risk of producing a biased result, usually by eroding any true differences in drug efficacy or tolerability. In the management strategy, patient dropouts, that often represent important drug-dependent events, are included in the analysis. For this reason, the management approach is currently the preferred method for analysis in most studies. We recommend that if an explicative strategy is used, the analysis be duplicated using a management approach, to establish the stability of the result and the integrity of the conclusions. One of the contentious issues in intention-to-treat analyses relates to the method of handling dropouts, or withdrawals from therapy. The longer the duration of follow-up, the greater the potential problem. Withdrawals due to side effects are dealt with reasonably simply, since their endpoint is discrete, that is, unable to continue by reason of intolerance. In contrast, withdrawals due to inefficacy are more problematic. In either event, the options available for the efficacy analysis are to impute post-discontinuation health status data, using one of several techniques, which include Last Observation Carried Forward (LOCF), Best Observation Carried Forward (BOCF), Worst Observation Carried Forward (WOCF), and various imputation techniques, including Hot-Deck imputation. In Hot-Deck imputation, patients continuing the study are matched with patients discontinuing the study, according to specified criteria. Then one patient is selected at random, and that patient's data used to impute missing data for the discontinued patient.

In addition to these basic approaches, which often employ statistical methods appropriate to the analysis of repeated measurements of continuous variables, it may be important to examine the time-dependent rate at which patients withdraw from treatment due to inefficacy, intolerance, or both. Methods applicable to the comparison of multiple proportions, such as Log Rank Chi-square may be required for these analyses, as well as for other efficacy comparisons and some tolerability comparisons.

Finally, OARSI have recently published responder criteria for OA hip and knee studies.[17] The criteria are in the form of two propositions, differing in the emphasis placed on pain reduction. The criteria are joint- and intervention-class specific. In contrast to the American College of Rheumatology Responder Criteria for Rheumatoid Arthritis (ACR 20),[49] the OARSI responder criteria are based on a required absolute as well as a required percentage change in one or more variables. A preliminary evaluation of these criteria suggests that they agree well with patient-based and key informant-based estimates of response.

Table 12.3 Definitions of difference for the WOMAC Index for individual OA patients[6]

		Pain	Stiffness function	Physical
MCPD	LK	1 unit	1 unit	1 unit
	VA	1 mm	1 mm	1 mm
MPCPD	LK	5%	12.5%	1.5%
	VA	0.2%	0.5%	0.06%
MPCI	VA	9.7%	10	9.3

MCPD, minimum change potentially detectable; MPCPD, minimum percentage change potentially detectable; MPCI, minimum perceptible clinical improvement.

Interpretation and application

Caution is necessary in extrapolating results of a study and in generalizing them to other patient groups (e.g., the elderly) that may differ in their response, be they beneficial or adverse. The results of a trial should be reviewed, therefore, in the appropriate clinical context. Furthermore, they should be interpreted with respect to other relevant data from trials of similar or different design, and knowledge gained from case reports and case series. It should be recognized that different variables have different sample size requirements, and that where several variables have been measured there are issues of multiple statistical comparisons to be considered. Finally, it is important to be aware of the possible existence of unpublished studies, some of which may contain negative results. With respect to published trials, the Cochrane Collaborative Project has greatly facilitated the identification, evaluation, and meta-analysis of data from randomized clinical trials. This tremendously important initiative has attracted considerable interest and international collaboration. This endeavor should contribute significantly to the practice of evidence-based medicine, and thereby directly benefit patients with OA.

Future perspective

While the basic architecture of clinical trials is unlikely to radically change, further development of some components can be anticipated. Outcome measurement in particular continues to evolve. One of the most difficult challenges in measurement is in combining measures on different dimensions into a summated or total score. Andersson et al.[50] have studied the consequences of using different indices to categorize the outcome of orthopedic surgery (Table 12.4). Using the Judet and Judet scale,[50] it would be concluded that 97.5 per cent of outcomes were good. However, a completely different conclusion would be reached using the Harris scale.[50] A study by Langan and Weiss made similar observations.[3] Both studies illustrate the complexities of placing more importance on some aspects of the disease than on others (weighting), and the consequence of combining information (aggregation) and then categorizing the final score (transformation). It also indicates that data from composite indices require cautious interpretation. This issue dates back to the early rheumatology and orthopaedic literature, and was well recognized by the clinimetric pioneer John Lansbury.[3]

Conclusion

The basic building blocks of clinical trial design are well described, and often used. The most important developments of recent years have been the development of the OMERACT 3 Consensus on Core Set Measures, the OARSI Task Force Guidelines on Clinical Trials, the OARSI Hand OA Guidelines, the OARSI Responder Criteria, attempts to define MCPD, MPCPD, MPCI, and MCID values and the globalization of HSMs. At this point, the major challenge is often in operational aspects of an endeavor, rather than the conceptual. Designing clinical trials often requires making trade offs between the ideal and the practical, between the 'real-world' and

Table 12.4 Comparative results (as %) of categorizing the outcomes of orthopaedic surgery using seven different rating scales on the same group of 27 patients

	Judet and Judet	Stinchfield et al.	Merle d'Aubigne	Shepherd	Larson	Harris	Andersson and Möller-Nielsen
Good	97.5	62.5	35	49	49	36	36
Fair	2.5	28.5	17	33	13	24	38
Bad	0.0	9.0	48	18	38	40	26

Source: Courtesy of the Editor of the *Journal of Bone and Joint Surgery.* Adapted from Ref. 50 and published.

the experimental situation. The conduct of short-term and longer-term trials of SyMOADs is complicated by the requirement to provide rescue analgesia, the influence of which is not readily discernible. In contrast, the conduct of long-term clinical trials of StMOADs, is challenging with respect to compliance and retention. Some such studies require demonstration that structural conservation, where achieved, has clinical meaningful consequence within a reasonable time frame. Given the relatively low correlation between clinical and imaging scores (especially in mild to moderate OA), the potential for progressive involvement of multiple joints in different anatomic configurations and the relatively slow rate of clinical deterioration, demonstrating the clinical consequence of structural conservation represents a significant clinimetric challenge.

Summary

The terminology and acronyms used to classify agents has evolved as a function of time and understanding. An earlier classification based on Fast Acting Symptom Modifying OA Drugs (FASMOADs), Slow Acting Symptom Modifying OA Drugs (SASMOADs), and Disease Modifying OA Drugs (DMOADs),[1] has been replaced by one based on purported structure modifying OA drugs (StMOADs), and symptom modifying OA drugs (SyMOADs).[2] Regardless of taxonomy the scientific evaluation of new agents requires the application of rigorous methodologies. The key elements are a clearly specified hypothesis, an appropriate research architecture, appropriately selected patients, outcome measures that are valid reliable and responsive, sufficient statistical power, trial management and data management procedures that meet quality control and ethical standards, and appropriate statistical methodologies. Given that efficacy, tolerability, and safety are each determined by formal measurement procedures, the validity, reliability, and particularly the responsiveness of the measurement procedures employed are quintessential to the enterprise, and, as a consequence, decisions regarding what to measure and how to conduct measurement are fundamental methodological questions.[3] It should not be assumed, because OA is generally a more indolent, slowly progressive disorder than the inflammatory arthropathies, that outcome assessment is simpler. On the contrary, measurement options are more complex because of a tendency for the condition to either be confined to a single joint, or to show different patterns of multi-joint involvement in different patients.

References

(An asterisk denotes recommended reading.)

1. Lequesne, M., Brandt, K., Bellamy, N., et al. (1994). Guidelines for testing slow acting drugs in osteoarthritis. J Rheumatol 21(Suppl. 41):65–73.

2. *Osteoarthritis Research Society (OARS) Task Force Report. (1996). Design and conduct of clinical trials in patients with osteoarthritis: Recommendations from a task force of the Osteoarthritis Research Society. Osteoarthritis Cart 4:217–43.
   The OARSI Task Force Guidelines are a landmark paper in OA. The Guidelines are recommendations, not regulations, and remain amenable to modification. The Guidelines represent an international consensus at a high level between key stakeholders and, as such, provide a firm basis for designing and conducting future clinical trials in OA.

3. *Bellamy, N. (1993). Musculoskeletal Clinical Metrology. Dordrecht: Kluwer Academic Publishers, pp. 1–365.
   This reference work overviews many of the principles that underpin outcome assessment in musculoskeletal clinical trials and reviews many of the instruments used currently.

4. *Maheu, E. and Altman, R.D. (2001). Osteoarthritis Research Society International Hand OA Task Force: design and conduct of clinical trials on osteoarthritis (OA) of the hand. Osteoarthritis Cart 9(Suppl. B):S1.
   The new OARSI Hand OA Guidelines provide specific instructions with respect to the future conduct of OA hand studies. Like the OARSI Task Force Guidelines, they are recommendations not regulations, and are amenable to

modification. They represent an international consensus on fundamental elements in the design of future clinical trials in hand osteoarthritis.

5. *Bellamy, N., Kirwan, J., Boers, M., et al. (1997). Recommendations for a core set of outcome measures for future phase III clinical trials in knee, hip and hand osteoarthritis—consensus development at OMERACT III. J Rheumatol 24(4):799–802.
   OMERACT 3. This publication describes the process by which an international consensus was reached on core set measures for future clinical trials in OA.

6. *Bellamy, N., Carr, A., Dougados, M., et al. (2001). Towards a definition of difference in OA. J Rheumatol 28:427–30.
   OMERACT 5. This paper provides an insight into the complexities of defining difference in OA. There are several different definitions of difference. Considerable further elucidation of this issue remains to be undertaken.

7. Brooks, P.M. (2001). Reporting of the Sixth Joint WHO/ILAR/Task Force Meeting on Rheumatic Diseases, January 16th, 2000, Geneva, Switzerland. J Rheumatol 28(11):2540–3.

8. Friedman, L.M., Furberg, C.D., and De Mets, D.L. (1998). Fundamentals of clinical trials. New York: Springer, pp. 1–361.

9. Guyatt, G.H., Heyting, A., Haeschke, et al. (1991). N of 1 randomized trials for investigating new drugs. Control Clin Trials 11:88–100.

10. March, L., Irwig, L., Schwarz, J., et al. (1994). N of 1 trials comparing a non-steroid antiinflammatory drug with paracetamol in osteoarthritis. Br Med J 3089:1041–5.

11. Reginster, J.Y., Deroisy, R., Rovati, L.C., et al. (2001). Long-term effects of glucosamine sulphate on osteoarthritis progression: a randomised, placebo-controlled clinical trial. Lancet 357:251–6.

12. Walker, F.S., Revell, P., Hemmingway, A., Low, F., Rainsford, K.D., and Rashad, S. (1989). Comparative effects of azaproprazone on the progression of joint pathology in osteoarthritis. In: K.D. Reinsford (ed.), Azaproprazone: 20 Years of Clinical Use. Kluwer Academic Publishers, pp. 239–53.

13. Altman, R. (1991). Criteria for classification of clinical osteoarthritis. J Rheumatol 22(Suppl. 27):10–12.

14. Altman, R.D., Hockberg, M., Murphy, W.A., et al. (1995). Atlas of individual radiographic features in osteoarthritis. Osteoarthritis Cart 3:3–70.

15. Burnett, S., Hart, D.J., Cooper, C., and Spector, T.D. (1994). A Radiographic Atlas of Osteoarthritis. London: Springer.

16. Kellgren, J.H. and Lawrence, J.S. (1957). Radiological assessment of osteoarthritis. Ann Rheum Dis 16:494–501.

17. *Dougados, M., Le Claire, P., van der Heijde, D., et al. (2000). Response criteria for clinical trials on osteoarthritis of the knee and hip: A report of the Osteoarthritis Research Society International Standing Committee for Clinical Trials Response Criteria Initiative. Osteoarthritis Cart 8(6):395–403.
   OARSI Responder Criteria. This publication reports a key development in the elucidation of responder criteria. The criteria are joint- and intervention-specific and take the form of two propositions that vary principally in the emphasis placed on pain relief. Response is defined by a combination of absolute as well as percentage improvements on one or more clinical core set variables.

18. Bellamy, N., Campbell, J., and Syrotuik, J. (1999). Comparative study of self-rating pain scales in osteoarthritis patients. Curr Med Res Opin 15(2):113–19.

19. Rosenbloom, D., Brooks, P., Bellamy, N., and Buchanan, W.W. (1985). Clinical Trials in Rheumatic Diseases. New York: Praeger Scientific Publishers, pp. 19–69.

20. Sackett, D.L., Haynes, R.B., Guyatt, G.H., and Tugwell, P. (1991). Clinical Epidemiology a Basic Science for Clinical Medicine. Toronto: Little, Brown and Company, pp. 1–440.

21. US Department of Commerce. (1989). National Technical Information Service. COSTART: Coding Symbols for Thesaurus of Adverse Reaction Terms, 3E. Springfield: US Department of Commerce, National Technical Information Service.

22. World Health Organization. (1990). The WHO Adverse Reaction Dictionary. Uppsala: WHO Collaborating Centre for International Drug Monitoring.

23. Norman, G.R. and Streiner, D.L. (2000). Biostatistics: the Bare Essentials. Hamilton: BC Decker, pp. 1–321.

24. Boers, M., Brooks, P., Strand, V., and Tugwell, P. (1998). The OMERACT Filter for outcome measures in rheumatology. J Rheumatol 25:198–9.

25. **Fries, J.F. and Bellamy N.** Introduction. (1991). In N. Bellamy (ed.), *Prognosis in the Rheumatic Diseases*. Dordrecht: Kluwer Academic Publishers, pp. 1–10.

26. World Health Organisation. (1980). *Classification of Impairments, Disabilities and Handicaps*. Geneva: WHO.

27. World Health Organisation. ICIDH-2. (1997). *An International Classification of Impairments, Activities and Participation*. Geneva: World Health Organisation.

28. **Bellamy, N., Campbell, J., Haraoui, B.,** *et al.* (2002). Clinimetric properties of the AUSCAN Osteoarthritis Hand Index: an evaluation of reliability, validity and responsiveness. *Osteoarthritis Cart* **10**:863–9.

29. **Bellamy, N., Buchbinder, R., Hall, S.,** *et al.* (1998). PARIS Sectogram: a novel method for weighting and aggregating the AUSCAN Osteoarthritis Hand Index. *Arthritis Rheum* **41**(Suppl. 9): S145.

30. **Poiraudeau, S., Chevalier, X., and Conrozier, T.** (2001). Reliability, validity and sensitivity to change of the Cochin Hand Functional Disability Scale in hand osteoarthritis. *Arthritis Cart* **9**(6):570–77.

31. **Drieser, R.L., Maheu, E., Guillou, G.B.,** *et al.* (1995). Validation of an algofunctional index for osteoarthritis of the hand. *Rev Rhum* **62**(Suppl. 6):43S–53S.

32. **Lequesne, M.G., Mery C. Samson, M., and Gerard, P.** (1987). Indexes of severity for osteoarthritis of the hip and knee: Validation-value in comparison with other assessment tests. *Scand J Rheum* **65**(Suppl.):85–9.

33. **Bellamy, N., Buchanan, W.W., Goldsmith, C.H., Campbell, J., and Stitt, L.W.** (1988). Validation study of WOMAC: a health status instrument for measuring clinically important patient relevant outcomes to antirheumatic drug therapy in patients with osteoarthritis of the hip or knee. *J Rheumatol* **15**:1833–40.

34. **Bellamy, N., Buchanan, W.W., Goldsmith, C.H., Campbell, J., and Stitt, L.** (1988). A validation study of WOMAC: a health status instrument for measuring clinically important patient relevant outcomes following total hip or knee arthroplasty in osteoarthritis. *J Orthop Rheum* **1**:95–108.

35. **Bellamy, N., Wells, G.A., and Campbell, J.** (1994). PARIS Sectogram: a method for weighting and aggregating the WOMAC Osteoarthritis Index. *Osteoarthritis Cart* **2**(Suppl. 1):37.

36. **Whitehouse, S.I., Lingard, E.A., and Learmonth, I.D.** (Kinemax Outcomes Group Boston, M.A. and Bristol, United Kingdom). (2000). A reduced WOMAC function scale—derivation and validation. *Arthritis Rheum* **43**(Suppl. 9):S393.

37. **Klassbo, M., Larsson, E., Mannevik, E., and Roos, E.** (2000). Hip dysfunction and osteoarthritis outcomes score (HOOS). An extension of the Western Ontario and McMaster Universities Osteoarthritis Index (WOMAC). 5th World Congress of the OARSI, Barcelona. *Osteoarthritis Cart* **8**(Suppl. B):S76.

38. **Roos, E.M., Roos, H.P., Ekdahl, C., and Lohmander, S.** (1998). Knee injury and osteoarthritis outcomes score (KOOS)—validation of a Swedish version. *Scand J Med Sci Sports* **8**(6):439–48.

39. **Meenan, R.F., Gertman, P.M., and Mason, J.H.** (1980). Measuring health status in arthritis: The Arthritis Impact Measurement Scales. *Arthritis Rheum* **23**:146–52.

40. **Meenan, R.F., Mason, J.H., Anderson, J.J., Guccione, A.A., and Kazis, L.E.** (1992). AIMS2—the content and properties of a revised and expanded Arthritis Impact Measurement Scales health status questionnaire. *Arthritis Rheum* **35**:1–10.

41. **Fries, J.F., Spitz, P., Kraines, R.G., and Holman, H.R.** (1980). Measurement of patient outcome in arthritis. *Arthritis Rheum* **23**:137–45.

42. **Hurst, N.P., Jobanputra, P., Hunter, M., Lambert, M., Lochhead, A., and Brown, H.** (Economic and Health Outcomes Research Group). (1994). Validity of Euroqol—a generic health status instrument—in patients with rheumatoid arthritis. *Br J Rheumatol* **33**:655–62.

43. **Feeny, D., Furlong, W., Barr, R.D., Torrance, G.W., Rosenbaum, P., and Weitzman, S.** (1992). A comprehensive multiattribute system for classifying the health status of survivors of childhood cancer. *J Clin Oncol* **10**:923–8.

44. **Ware J.E. Jr. and Sherbourne, C.D.** (1992). The MOS 36-item Short-Form Health Status survey (SF-36): 1. Conceptual framework and item selection. *Med Care* **30**:473–83.

45. **Doyle, D.V., Dieppe, P.A., Scott, J.** *et al.* (1981). An articular index for the assessment of osteoarthritis. *Ann Rheum Dis* **40**:75–8.

46. **Bellamy, N., Carette, S., Ford, P.M.,** *et al.* (1992). Osteoarthritis antirheumatic drug trials. III. Setting the delta for clinical trials—results of a consensus development (Delphi) exercise. *J Rheumatol* **19**:451–7.

47. **Ehrich, E.W., Davies, G.M., Watson, D.J.,** *et al.* (2000). Minimal Perceptible Clinical Improvement with the Western Ontario and McMaster Universities Osteoarthritis Index Questionnaire and global assessments in patients with osteoarthritis. *J Rheumatol* **27**:2635–41.

48. **Sackett, D.L. and Gent, M.** (1979). Controversy in counting and attributing events in clinical trials. *N Engl J Med* **301**:1410–12.

49. **Felson, D.T., Anderson, J.J., Boers, M.,** *et al.* (1993). The American College of Rheumatology preliminary core set of disease activity markers for rheumatoid arthritis clinical trials. *Arthritis Rheum* **36**:729–40.

50. **Anderson, G.** (1972). Hip assessment: a comparison of nine different methods. *J Bone Joint Surg Br* **54B**:621–5.

Appendices

A1 The American College of Rheumatology (ACR) criteria for the classification and reporting of osteoarthritis

Table A1.1 ACR criteria for the classification and reporting of OA of the hip*

Hip pain and at least 2 of the following 3 features:

ESR <20 mm/hour

Radiographic femoral or acetabular osteophytes

Radiographic joint-space narrowing (superior, axial, and/or medial)

* This classification method yields a sensitivity of 89% and a specificity of 91%.

ESR, erythrocyte sedimentation rate (Westergren).

Source: From Altman, R., Alarcón, G., Appelrouth, D., *et al.* (1991). The American College of Rheumatology criteria for the classification and reporting of osteoarthritis of the hip. *Arthritis Rheum* **34**:505–14.

Table A1.2 ACR criteria for the classification and reporting of OA of the knee

Clinical and laboratory	Clinical and radiographic	Clinical*
Knee pain + at least 5 of 9:	Knee pain + at least 1 of 3:	Knee pain + at least 3 of 6:
Age >50 years	Age >50 years	Age >50 years
Stiffness <30 minutes	Stiffness <30 minutes	Stiffness <30 minutes
Crepitus	Crepitus + osteophytes	Crepitus
Bony tenderness		Bony tenderness
Bony enlargement		Bony enlargement
No palpable warmth		No palpable warmth
ESR <40 mm/hour		
RF <1:40		
SF OA		
92% sensitive	91% sensitive	95% sensitive
75% specific	86% specific	69% specific

ESR, erythrocyte sedimentation rate (Westergren); RF, rheumatoid factor; SF OA, synovial fluid signs of OA (clear, viscous, or white blood cell count <2000/mm^3).

* Alternative for the Clinical category would be 4 of 6, which is 84% sensitive and 89% specific.

Source: From Altman, R., Asch, E., Bloch, G., *et al.* (1986). Development of criteria for the classification and reporting of osteoarthritis: classification of osteoarthritis of the knee. *Arthritis Rheum* **29**:1039–49.

Table A1.3 ACR criteria for the classification and reporting of OA of the hand

Hand pain, aching, or stiffness, and 3 or 4 of the following features:

  Hard tissue enlargement of 2 or more of 10 selected joints[*]

  Hard tissue enlargement of 2 or more DIP joints

  Fewer than 3 swollen MCP joints

  Deformity of at least 1 of 10 selected joints

MCP, metacarpophalangeal.

[*] The 10 selected joints are the second and third distal interphalangeal (DIP), the second and third proximal interphalangeal, and the first carpometacarpal joints of both hands. This classification method yields a sensitivity of 94% and a specificity of 87%.

Source: From Altman, R., Alarcón, G., Appelrouth, D., *et al.* (1990). The American College of Rheumatology criteria for the classification and reporting of osteoarthritis of the hand. *Arthritis Rheum* **33**:1601–10.

A2 Lequesne's algofunctional lower limb indices

Table A2.1 Algofunctional Index for hip OA

Pain or discomfort	
During nocturnal bedrest	
None or insignificant	0
Only on movement or in certain positions	1
With no movement	2
Morning stiffness or regressive pain after rising	
1 minute or less	0
More than 1 but less than 15 minutes	1
15 minutes or more	2
After standing for 30 minutes	0–1
While ambulating	
None	0
Only after ambulating some distance	1
After initial ambulation and increasingly with continued ambulation	2
After initial ambulation, not increasingly	1
With prolonged sitting (2 hours)	0–1
Maximum distance walked (may walk with pain)	
Unlimited	0
More than 1 km, but limited	1
About 1 km (0.6 min), (in about 15 min)	2
From 500 to 900 m (1.640–2.952 ft or 0.31–0.56 min) (in about 8–15 min)	3
From 300–500 m (984–1.640 ft)	4
From 100–300 m (328–984 ft)	5
Less than 100 m (328 ft)	6
With one walking stick or crutch	1
With two walking sticks or crutches	2
*Activities of daily living**	
Put on socks by bending forward	0–2
Pick up an object from the floor	0–2
Climb up and down a standard flight of stairs	0–2
Can get into and out of a car	0–2

* Without difficulty, 0; with small difficulty, 0.5; moderate, 1; important difficulty, 1.5; unable, 2.

Source: Reproduced with the kind permission of the author, Dr Michel Lequesne.

Table A2.2 Algofunctional Index for knee OA

Pain or discomfort	
During nocturnal bedrest	
None or insignificant	0
Only on movement or in certain positions	1
With no movement	2
Morning stiffness or regressive pain after rising	
1 minute or less	0
More than 1 but less than 15 minutes	1
15 minutes or more	2
After standing for 30 minutes	0–1
While ambulating	
None	0
Only after ambulating some distance	1
After initial ambulation and increasingly with continued ambulation	2
After initial ambulation, not increasingly	1
While getting up from sitting without the help of arms	0–1
Maximum distance walked (may walk with pain)	
Unlimited	0
More than 1 km, but limited	1
About a km (0.6 min), (in about 15 min)	2
From 500–900 m (1.640–2.952 ft or 0.31–0.56 min) (in about 8–15 min)	3
From 300–500 m (984–1.640 ft)	4
From 100–300 m (328–984 ft)	5
Less than 100 m (328 ft)	6
With one walking stick or crutch	1
With two walking sticks or crutches	2
Activities of daily living*	
Able to climb up a standard flight of stairs	0–2
Able to climb down a standard flight of stairs	0–2
Able to squat or bend on the knees	0–2
Able to walk on uneven ground	0–2

* Without difficulty, 0; with small difficulty, 0.5; moderate, 1; important difficulty, 1.5; unable, 2.

Source: Reproduced with the kind permission of the author, Dr Michel Lequesne.

A3 WOMAC osteoarthritis Index

The WOMAC Index is a disease-specific, tri-dimensional self-administered questionnaire, for assessing health status and health outcomes in osteoarthritis of the knee and/or hip. The questionnaire contains 24 questions, targeting areas of pain, stiffness and physical function, and can be completed in less than 5 minutes. Usually patient self-administered, the Index is amenable to electronic data capture (EDC) formats using mouse-driven curser, touch screen, and to interview administration by telephone. Available in over 60 alternative language forms, there are several different forms of the WOMAC Index suitable for different clinical practical and clinical research applications. The most recent version of the Index is WOMAC 3.1, which is a joint targeted version of the Index, which for most purposes has superseded earlier versions of the Index.

Questionnaire Content

Pain Subscale:
  1. Walking on flat surface
  2. Going up/down stairs
  3. At night
  4. Sitting/lying
  5. Standing upright

Stiffness Subscale:
  6. After first awakening
  7. After periods of inactivity

Physical Function Subscale:
  8. Descending stairs
  9. Ascending stairs
10. Getting out of chair
11. Remaining in standing position
12. Bending
13. Walking on flat surface
14. In/out of car
15. Shopping
16. Socks/stockings on
17. Getting out of bed
18. Socks/stockings off
19. Lying in bed
20. In/out bath
21. Sitting
22. Toileting
23. Heavy domestic duties
24. Light domestic duties

Alternate language translations (as of September 2002):

ARGENTINA	JAPAN
AUSTRALIA	LATVIA
AUSTRIA	LITHUANIA
BELGIUM (FRENCH, FLEMISH)	MALAYASIA (CANTONESE, ENGLISH, MALAY)
BRAZIL (JAPANESE)	MEXICO
BULGARIA	NETHERLANDS
CANADA (ENGLISH, FRENCH)	NEW ZEALAND
CHILE	NORWAY
CHINA (MANDARIN)	PERU (JAPANESE)
COLUMBIA	PHILIPPINES (TAGALOG)
COSTA RICA	POLAND
CROATIA	PORTUGAL
CZECH REPUBLIC	ROMANIA
DENMARK	RUSSIA
ECUADOR	SINGAPORE (MANDARIN, ENGLISH)
EGYPT	SLOVAKIA
ESTONIA	SLOVENIA
FINLAND	SOUTH AFRICA (ENGLISH, AFRIKAANS)
FRANCE	SPAIN
GERMANY	SWEDEN
GREECE	SWITZERLAND (GERMAN, FRENCH, ITALIAN)
GUATEMALA	TAIWAN (MANDARIN)
HONG KONG (CANTONESE)	THAILAND
HUNGARY	TURKEY
ICELAND	UK
ISRAEL	USA (ENGLISH, SPANISH, FLORIDA)
ITALY	VENEZUELA

The WOMAC Index has been subject to a multiple validation studies, and is reliable, valid and responsive. The VA (100 mm) form of the Index may be slightly more responsive than the LK (5-point) form of the Index, but both have proven very responsive in various research environments. The Index may be presented with or without access to prior scores, our preference being for the latter. The time-frame may be varied from last 24 hours to last one month, depending on the trial design and research question. The object of measurement may be tailored to individual patients using the signal version of the instrument, although overall we have favoured using the entire instrument. The WOMAC Index is relevant to both clinical research and clinical practice applications.

Use of the WOMAC Index is supported by a User Guide. Information about the WOMAC Osteoarthritis Index and the User Guide can be obtained direct from the constructor (Professor Nicholas Bellamy) at www.womac.org.

A4 Protocols for radiography

J. Christopher Buckland-Wright

Procedures for standardizing the position of joints during radiography are essential if assessment for diagnosis and disease progression is to be made reliable. Indeed the use of validated published procedures or protocols are essential to maintain quality control in a technique involving several steps with respect to both the numbers of personnel and technical procedures.[1–3] The radiographic protocols are based upon the principal of minimizing any distortion in the radiographic image of the joint.[3,4] This is achieved by positioning the joint such that the central ray of the X-ray beam passes between the margins of the joint space, so that the margins and the space are optimally defined when the joint is in a position of functional loading, that is weight bearing as during normal activity.

Protocol for dorsipalmar radiography of the hand and wrist

The optimal position for joint assessment is obtained with the fingers held together and in line with the wrist and forearm when laid flat on the X-ray film holder. In this position the joints will be under muscular load along its own axis, providing a reproducible method for evaluating joint space. Radiography of both hands in ulnar deviation and with the fingers spread is inadvisable as the degree of joint-space narrowing cannot be assessed reliably in this view.

Preparation for radiography

1. The X-ray tube is positioned so that the central ray of the X-ray beam is vertical and perpendicular to the film, with a film-to-focus distance (FFD) of 1 m.
2. A sheet of paper the size of the X-ray film is placed over the film holder.

Radiography

1. Each hand is X-rayed separately.
2. The hand is laid flat on the X-ray film holder with the thumb slightly extended. The fingers are held together and in line with the axis of the wrist and forearm.
3. The centre of the wrist and hand is aligned with the centre of the X-ray beam, by placing the positioning light of the tube directly over the head of the third metacarpal bone.
4. The radiograph is taken immediately after this position is obtained.
5. Following the exposure, the outline of the wrist and hand is drawn on the paper, to facilitate joint repositioning at subsequent visits.
6. The other extremity is X-rayed, following the procedure described above.

No correction for radiographic magnification is required since the extremities are in almost direct contact with the film.

Protocol for posteroanterior radiography of the tibiofemoral compartment of the knee in the standing semi-flexed position (MTP view) without fluoroscopy

Although, the anteroposterior standing extended view of the knee has been widely used to assess the tibiofemoral compartment, recent studies[5–7] have demonstrated that this view does not reliably assess the thickness of the articular cartilage detected radiographically as the joint-space width. A most reliable and reproducible method for assessing this compartment is the non-fluoroscopic radiographic procedures for the semiflexed view[7] of the knee. This technique has been found to accurately position the joint and is a reproducible method for repositioning the joint at successive examinations and for measuring cartilage loss from joint-space width measurement. This simple technique, which does not require fluoroscopy, allows this method to be used in a wide variety of conditions without the need for specialist equipment.

Preparation for radiography

1. The X-ray tube is positioned so that the central ray of the X-ray beam is horizontal, parallel to the floor, and perpendicular to the X-ray film held within an erect film holder, and with a film-to-focus distance (FFD) set at 1 m.
2. A large sheet of paper or the back of the patient's envelope is used to help position the patient at repeat visits. A black-line is drawn 3 inches from the long-edge of the sheet of paper or envelope. The paper, or envelope, is then placed immediately in front and under the film holder so that the black-line drawn on the paper is positioned directly below and in line with the front of the film cassette. The paper is then fixed to the floor with adhesive tape.
3. Pen or tape marks the floor or platform to which the sheet of paper is taped so that the sheet of paper can be repositioned in the same place with respect to the film holder and X-ray tube at each subsequent examination. The patient's name must be written on the sheet of paper.
4. The patients must be barefoot.
5. Identify the position of the tibiofemoral joint-space by locating the inferior border of the patella and the superior margin of the tibial tuberosity, trace this line around to the side of the knee and mark the skin with a felt tip pen. This mark will be used to help align the centre of the X-ray beam with the joint space (see 7 below).

Radiography

1. The patient stands with both knees facing the film cassette in an erect film holder.

2. Both knees are radiographed together in the Postero-Anterior view. The patient is asked to stand with their feet slightly externally rotated (so that the angle between the feet is approximately 15°) and not close together.

3. The joint of the first metatarso-phalangeal (MTP) joint of each foot is positioned directly below and in line with the front of the film cassette (Fig. A5.1). The position of the MTP joint, with respect to the film, is also defined by the black line already drawn on the sheet of paper.

4. The patient is asked to bend the knees until the anterior surface of each knee touches the middle and front of the film cassette. (In this position the tibial plateau should be at right angles to the film.) The patient may need to be provided with hand support.

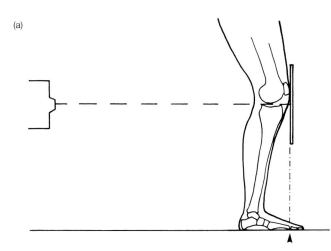

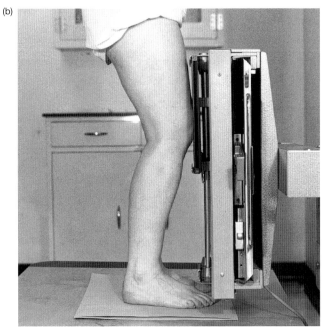

Fig. A5.1 (a) Alignment of the leg relative to the X-ray tube, right, and the film cassette in the vertical holder, left, in the anteroposterior view of the knee in the semiflexed or MTP position. The arrow marks the position of the MTP joint, which is in line with the front of the film cassette. (b) General view of the X-ray equipment for the posteroanterior view of the knee in the MTP position. The first metatarsophalangeal (MTP) joint is placed in line with the front of the film cassette and the knees are flexed until they touch the cassette. A map of the feet is drawn on the patient's envelope or card to help reposition the patient at repeat visits.

5. The outline of the feet is drawn on the paper, to help reposition the joint at repeat visits.

6. The tube is positioned so that the X-ray beam is directed at the back of the knees.

7. The tubes positioning light is used to align the centre of the X-ray beam midway between the knees and in the same horizontal plane as the centre of the joints, defined by the joint space (see 5 above), and which lies above the horizontal skin crease of the popliteal fossa.

8. The radiograph is taken immediately after this position is obtained.

Protocol for anterioposterior radiography of the tibiofemoral compartment of the knee in the standing semi-flexed position with fluoroscopy

The radiographic protocols that were first developed for the knee, employed fluoroscopic screening in order to optimally position the joint for radiography.[3,6] Fluoroscopic guidance in the positioning of the joint ensures that radioanatomically the compartment is in the same position within and between patient examinations. This method is used in therapeutic trials.[8]

Preparation for radiography

1. The X-ray tube is positioned so that the central ray of the X-ray beam is horizontal and parallel to the floor, and with a film-to-focus (FFD) distance set to 1 m.

2. A large sheet of paper, or the back of the patient's X-ray envelope, is placed immediately in front of the film holder and fixed to the floor with adhesive tape.

3. The floor is marked so that the sheet of paper can be repositioned in exactly the same place, relative to the film holder and X-ray tube, for each patient and at each subsequent visit.

4. A metal sphere (5 mm), mounted in semi-radiolucent material (to improve the definition of the margin of the ball), is placed on the head of the fibula of each knee.

Radiography

1. Each knee is X-rayed separately in the anteroposterior view.

2. The centre of the joint, defined by the joint space, is aligned with the center of the X-ray beam with the aid of the positioning light of the tube (Fig. A5.2).

3. With the patient standing straight, the back of the heel is placed on the back edge of the sheet of paper, which is in line with the front edge of the film cassette.

4. With the heel fixed, the foot is internally or externally rotated until the tibial spines appear centrally placed relative to the femoral notch.

5. The knee is flexed until the tibial plateau is horizontal and perpendicular to the X-ray film. The precise position of the knee is confirmed visually with the aid of fluoroscopy. The tibial plateau is horizontal when the anterior and posterior margins of the medial compartment are superimposed.

6. The radiograph is taken immediately after this position is obtained.

7. Following the exposure, the outline of the foot is drawn on the paper, to facilitate joint repositioning at subsequent visits.

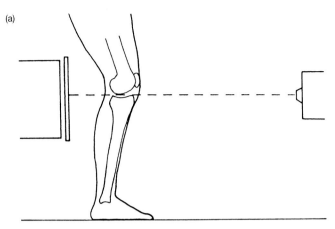

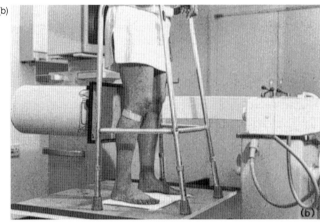

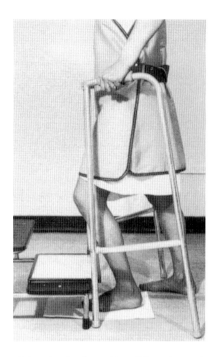

Fig. A5.3 General view showing the position of the patient and associated equipment for a skyline view of the patellofemoral compartment.

Fig. A5.2 (a) Diagram of the leg in the standing semi-flexed position and its position relative to the X-ray tube on the right and the film cassette placed in front of the image intensifier tube to the left. In this position the tibial plateau is horizontal, parallel to the central X-ray beam (broken line) and perpendicular to the X-ray film. (b) General view of the X-ray equipment for this view of the knee. The metal sphere is taped to the side of the knee. With this equipment, a table was used to raise the subject so that the knees were level with the horizontal X-ray beam.

3. For computing radiographic magnification, a metal sphere (5 mm), as described above, is placed on the anterior surface of the knee.

Radiography

1. Each knee is radiographed separately.

2. With the patient standing, the foot of the knee under examination is placed on the sheet of paper, with the front part of the foot under the step. The knee is flexed to 30° from the vertical. In this position, the anterior surface of the patella is positioned above and, a little in front of, the toes. The patient's stability is maintained by a support frame (Zimmer or 'walker' frame) and, in this instance, by resting the front edge of the tibia against the crossbar of the frame (Fig. A5.3).

3. The radiographic plate is placed on the step positioned below the knee.

4. The tube is positioned vertically above the patellofemoral joint. This may require the tube to be moved to a position above the head of the patient.

5. With the aid of the positioning light of the tube the central ray of the X-ray beam is directed so as to project through the patellofemoral joint space.

6. The radiograph is taken immediately after this position is obtained.

7. The outline of the foot is drawn on the paper, to facilitate joint repositioning at subsequent visits.

Protocols for axial radiography of the patellofemoral compartment

The axial or skyline view is more precise than the lateral view of the joint at localizing changes in the medial and lateral facets of the patello-femoral joint.[9] Examination of this compartment in the skyline view is obtained with the patient standing and the knee flexed to 30° from the vertical[3] (Fig. A5.3). In this position the joint is under load, ensuring the articular surfaces are in apposition, providing a more reliable assessment of cartilage thickness than when the patient is radiographed in the supine position.[3,4,10]

Preparation for radiography

1. The X-ray tube is positioned so that the X-ray beam is directed vertically downwards and the film-to-focus distance (FFD) is set to 1.5 m.

2. A large sheet of paper is placed partly under the step and at the front of the patient's support (Fig. A5.3), and fixed to the floor with adhesive tape using pre-existing marks. Marks on the floor are used to reposition the sheet of paper, the step, and patient support in exactly the same place, for each patient and at each subsequent visit.

Protocol for anteroposterior radiography of the hip

Radiographic studies of hip OA have shown that a more reliable assessment of articular cartilage thickness is obtained with the patients standing rather than when lying down[11] and with the feet internally rotated[10] (with an angle subtended between the feet of 15–20°. It is beneficial when assessing JSW to centre the X-ray beam on the hip joint, since displacement of the

X-ray tube away from the centre of the joint can significantly alter the JSW measurement.[10]

Preparation for radiography

1. The X-ray tube is positioned so that the central ray of the X-ray beam is horizontal and parallel to the floor, and with the film-to-focus distance (FFD) set to 1 m.

2. A large sheet of paper, or the back of the patient's X-ray envelope, is placed immediately in front of the film holder and fixed to the floor with adhesive tape using pre-existing marks, for the reasons given above.

3. To identify the position of the femoral head, the skin overlying the femoral pulse (or at a point 2.5 cm distally along the perpendicular bisector of the line joining the pubic symphesis and the anterior superior iliac spine) should be marked. Should this surface mark be located with the patient supine, it will need to be reconfirmed when the patient stands, since the skin often moves between the two positions.

4. A metal sphere (10 mm), as described above, is placed on the skin overlying the greater trochanter.

Radiography

1. Each hip is X-rayed separately.

2. With the patient standing straight, the backs of the heels are placed on the back edges of the sheet of paper. The center of the joint under examination, defined by the skin mark over the femoral head, is aligned with the center of the X-ray beam.

3. Each foot is internally rotated to be in the range 5–10°, so that the inside edge of the big toes touch. The angle subtended between the long axes of the feet should be approximately 15–20°.

4. Care should be taken to ensure that the pelvis is neither rotated nor tilted, and that the anterior superior iliac spines are equidistant from the plane of the film placed behind the patient.

5. The radiograph is taken immediately after this position is obtained.

6. Following the exposure, the outline of the feet is drawn on the paper, to facilitate joint repositioning at subsequent visits.

References

1. Buckland-Wright, J.C. (1994). Quantitative radiography of osteoarthritis. *Ann Rheum Dis* **53**:268–75.

2. Altman, R., Brandt, K., Hochberg, M., and Moskowitz, R. (1996). Design and conduct of clinical trials in patients with osteoarthritis. *Osteoarthritis Cart* **4**:217–43.

3. Buckland-Wright, C. (1995). Protocols for precise radio-anatomical positioning of the tibio-femoral and patello-femoral compartments of the knee. *Osteoarthritis Cart* **3**(Suppl. A):71–80.

4. Buckland-Wright, J.C. (1999). Radiographic assessment of osteoarthritis: comparison between existing methodologies. *Osteoarthritis Cart* **7**:430–3.

5. Buckland-Wright, J.C. (1997). Current status of imaging procedures in the diagnosis, prognosis and monitoring of OA. In N. Bellamy (ed.), *Osteoarthritis*. *Bailliére's Clin Rheumatol* **11**(4):727–48.

6. Buckland-Wright, J.C., Macfarlane, D.G., Williams, S.A., and Ward, R.J. (1995). Accuracy and precision of joint space width measurements in standard and macro-radiographs of osteoarthritic knees. *Ann Rheum Dis* **54**:872–80.

7. Buckland-Wright, J.C., Wolfe, F., Ward, R.J., Flowers, N., and Hayne, C. (1999). Substantial superiority of semiflexed (MTP) views in knee osteoarthritis: a comparative radiographic study, without fluoroscopy, of standing extended, semiflexed (MTP), and schuss views. *J Rheumatol* **26**:2664–74.

8. Buckland-Wright, J.C., Macfarlane, D.G., Lynch, J.A., and Jasani, M.K. (1995). Quantitative microfocal radiography detects changes in OA knee joint space width in patients in placebo-controlled trial of NSAID therapy. *J Rheumatol* **22**:937–43.

9. Cicuttini, F.M., Baker, J., Hart, D.J., and Spector, T.D. (1996). Choosing the best method for radiological assessment of patellofemoral osteoarthritis. *Ann Rheum Dis* **55**:134–6.

10. Buckland-Wright, J.C. (1998). Quantitation of radiographic changes. In: K.D. Brandt, S. Lohmander, and M. Doherty (eds), *Osteoarthritis* (1st ed.). Oxford: University Press, pp. 459–72.

11. Conrozier, T., Lequesne, M., Tron, A.M., *et al.* (1997). The effects of position on the radiographic joint space in osteoarthritis of the hip. *Osteoarthritis Cart* **5**:17–22.

Index